Fundamentals of Anaesthesia

Third Edition

Edited by
Tim Smith
Colin Pinnock
Ted Lin

Associate Editor
Robert Jones

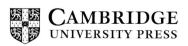

CAMBRIDGE
UNIVERSITY PRESS

CAMBRIDGE
UNIVERSITY PRESS

University Printing House, Cambridge CB2 8BS, United Kingdom

Cambridge University Press is part of the University of Cambridge.

It furthers the University's mission by determining knowledge in the pursuit of education, leaning and research at the highest international levels of excellence.

www.cambridge.org
Information on this title: www.cambridge.org/9780521692496

First published by Greenwich Medical Media 1999
Second edition published 2003
Third edition published by Cambridge University Press 2009
4th printing 2013

Printed by Grafos SA, Arte sobre papel, Barcelona, Spain

A catalogue record for this publication is available from the British Library

Library of Congress Cataloguing in Publication data
Fundamentals of anaesthesia / edited by Tim Smith, Colin Pinnock,
Ted Lin ; associate editor, Robert Jones. – 3rd ed.
    p.   ;   cm.
Includes bibliographical references and index.
ISBN 978-0-521-69249-6 (hardback)
1. Anesthesia.   I. Smith, Tim, 1960–   II. Title.
[DNLM: 1. Anesthesia.   2. Analgesia.   WO   200   F9813   2008]
RD81.F78   2008
617.9′6 – dc22   2008028629

ISBN 978-0-521-69249-6 Paperback

Additional resources for this publication at www.cambridge.org/smith

Fundamentals of Anaesthesia

Third Edition

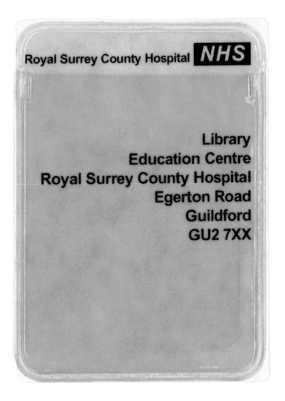

to Beccy, Jane, Linda and Marlene

Contents

Contributors

Dr B. L. Appadu
Consultant Anaesthetist
Peterborough General Hospital
Peterborough

Dr I. T. Campbell
Reader in Anaesthesia
University of Manchester

Dr G. Cavill
Consultant Anaesthetist
Wansbeck General Hospital
Northumberland

Dr H. B. J. Fischer
Consultant Anaesthetist
Alexandra Hospital
Redditch

Dr S. Graham
Consultant Anaesthetist
The James Cook University Hospital
Middlesbrough

Dr A. K. Gupta
Director of Neurocritical Care and Consultant
    Anaesthetist
Addenbrooke's Hospital
Cambridge

Dr R. M. Haden
Consultant Anaesthetist
Alexandra Hospital
Redditch

Dr C. D. Hanning
Consultant Anaesthetist
Leicester Royal Infirmary
Leicester

Dr S. A. Hill
Consultant Anaesthetist
Southampton General Hospital
Southampton

Dr J. M. James
Consultant Anaesthetist
Birmingham Heartlands Hospital
Birmingham

Dr R. P. Jones
Associate Specialist in Anaesthesia
Withybush Hospital
Haverfordwest

Dr K. M. Kerr
Consultant Anaesthetist
Alexandra Hospital
Redditch

Dr E. S. Lin
Consultant Anaesthetist
Glenfield Hospital
Leicester

Dr D. Liu
Consultant Anaesthetist
Bedford Hospital
Bedford

Professor C. J. Lote
Professor of Experimental Nephrology
University of Birmingham
Birmingham

Dr T. J. McLeod
Consultant Anaesthetist
Birmingham Heartlands Hospital
Birmingham

Dr M. C. Mushambi
Consultant Anaesthetist
Leicester Royal Infirmary
Leicester

Dr J. R. Neilson
Consultant in Haematology
Russells Hall Hospital
Dudley

Dr J. P. Nolan
Consultant Anaesthetist
Royal United Hospital
Bath

Dr A. Ogilvy
Consultant Anaesthetist
Leicester General Hospital
Leicester

Dr M. Paleologos
Royal North Shore Hospital
Sydney
Australia

Dr S. M. Parr
Consultant Anaesthetist
Solihull Hospital
Solihull

Dr C. A. Pinnock
Consultant Anaesthetist
Alexandra Hospital
Redditch

Professor I. Power
Professor of Anaesthesia, Critical
   Care and Pain Medicine
Royal Infirmary Hospital
Edinburgh

Dr A. M. Sardesai
Consultant Anaesthetist
Addenbrooke's Hospital
Cambridge

Dr J. Skoyles
Consultant Anaesthetist
Nottingham City Hospital
Nottingham

Dr T. C. Smith
Consultant Anaesthetist
Alexandra Hospital
Redditch

Dr J. Stone
Consultant Microbiologist
Gloucester Royal Hospital
Gloucester

Dr J. L. C. Swanevelder
Consultant Anaesthetist
Glenfield Hospital
Leicester

Dr A. J. Stronach
Consultant Anaesthetist
Alexandra Hospital
Redditch

Dr M. Tidmarsh
Consultant Anaesthetist
City General & Maternity Hospitals
Carlisle

Dr L. A. G. Vries
Consultant Anaesthetist
Alexandra Hospital
Redditch

Professor A. R. Wolf
Professor of Anaesthesia
Bristol Children's Hospital
Bristol

Dr J. K. Wood
Consultant Haematologist
Leicester Royal Infirmary
Leicester

Preface to the first edition

The advent of a syllabus for the FRCA examination, itself a requirement of the STA, seemed to me to provide an ideal opportunity for a dedicated revision textbook. It will therefore be of no surprise to readers that this volume mirrors closely the syllabus for the primary FRCA in both structure and content.

Having enlisted the willing help of my two co-editors, Tim Smith and Ted Lin, we set about recruiting authors to contribute. Chapter authors have been chosen for their ability and known prowess as teachers and a deliberate policy of not inviting 'usual' contributions from frequently seen names was taken. Having said that, several primary examiners appear as contributors and within each chapter coverage of revision topics has been kept as appropriate to the examination as possible.

To reduce the variability that is the bane of multi-author texts I have personally edited every chapter to ensure consistency of style and it is a reflection of the workload involved that it has taken three years to complete this project. I am grateful to all contributing authors for their tolerance and good humour during alteration of their golden prose.

Whilst no single book can cover the entire syllabus as a 'one stop' aid, the majority of material covered in the examination is detailed within these pages. Some items lately included in the syllabus, after completion of the manuscript, will be added in future editions (such as the anatomy pertaining to ankle block). Candidates will, however, be well served if this book is used as a general basis for revision.

I am extremely grateful to Rob Jones, who has been responsible for generating virtually all the artwork within this text, the few other diagrams being credited to their sources.

Thanks are also due to both my co-editors for their extensive work and dedication. If this volume enables any candidate to pass the primary examination, who would not have done so otherwise, then our job will have been well done.

C. A. Pinnock
July 1999

Preface to the second edition

I am delighted that the success of *Fundamentals* has enabled us to proceed to an early second edition. It will be apparent to the familiar reader that this edition has undergone rather more than a simple facelift. A great deal of feedback from both examiners and candidates has been used to modify and shape this current volume. New authors have been brought in to Section 1 to revise and modify the clinical chapters where necessary (incorporating several important and new areas of emerging knowledge), whilst resuscitation and trauma chapters have been updated by their original writers. Anatomy has been extended in scope to reflect subjects that are currently popular in the Primary FRCA.

In Section 2, there are new chapters on neurology and endocrinology, and an extra chapter on neonatal physiology has been incorporated to satisfy the demands of the examination syllabus.

Section 3 has been updated comprehensively with the removal of some drugs now lapsed and the incorporation of newer agents that have become available. By popular demand a new chapter on clinical trial design rounds off the pharmacology section.

It is, however, Section 4 that has undergone the most radical changes. I am very grateful to Ted Lin for the completely new physics and equipment chapters, which provide excellent core revision in these important areas. A greater number of diagrams (and many revised graphics) throughout the book and a completely new index complete the modifications over the first edition.

I thus believe that the second edition of *Fundamentals* is an even better revision aid to the Primary FRCA examination and will build on the reputation of its forerunner. Once again my thanks go to my three co-editors for their hard work and determination.

Colin Pinnock
October 2002

Preface to the third edition

I am privileged to have led the creation of the third edition of this popular Primary FRCA text, ably helped by my three co-editors. Once again, feedback from users of the book has helped enormously in developing *FoA3*. The Royal College of Anaesthetists' publication of the Primary syllabus within the Competency-based Training Framework has led us to include that knowledge base, uniquely referenced to *Fundamentals*, in a new Appendix. A number of new contributors have enhanced the proportion of current and past examiners amongst our writers. The greater use of colour allows the reader to navigate more easily, and changes to technique boxes make that information easier to assimilate. This edition contains a number of new chapters in addition to widespread updates, and has been thoroughly copy-edited by Hugh Brazier to an unrivalled standard of consistency over the previous editions.

Whilst all chapters have been reviewed, there are a number of significant changes.

- Section 1 contains a significantly updated chapter in the growing field of preoperative assessment, and a brand new chapter on resuscitation. The inclusion of the DAS algorithms for airway management is a particular bonus.
- In Section 2 Ted Lin has written an additional chapter specifically covering the physiology of pain, and Colin Pinnock has edited haematology to bring it more in line with the current syllabus.
- Section 3 has a new chapter on analgesic drugs, taking account of the substantial developments in this area. The new chapter on mechanisms of drug action puts clear emphasis on the current thinking on the mechanism of anaesthesia.
- In Section 4, Ted Lin has put together a clear and concise statistics chapter, which will make preparation for this part of the exam straightforward. The inclusion of aspects of ultrasound and MRI scanning here and in the clinical section follows its incorporation into the syllabus.

Despite suggestions to expand *Fundamentals* to cover anaesthesia to higher levels and in greater depth, we have adhered to our original aim of providing a textbook specifically designed around the RCA Primary Fellowship. In so doing, we have been better able to adapt to changes in that exam as well as in anaesthetic core knowledge. The result is a much more effective exam preparation tool, which in turn is frequently used as a starting point for anaesthetists (and indeed others) of all grades including consultants, some of whom achieved exam success helped by the first edition. Finally, I am particularly grateful to Colin for his help and advice during my turn at leading the editorial process.

We were saddened to hear of the death of Dr Andy Ogilvy, author of Section 2, Chapter 11, as this edition was in preparation.

Tim Smith
March 2008

How to use this book

FoA3 is not just a book. It is a tool to enable the reader to develop both their anaesthetic practice and an understanding of the scientific principles of anaesthesia.

The book has been structured to correlate closely with the syllabus of the Primary FRCA. The knowledge sections of the syllabus are listed in the Appendix, and each section of the syllabus is cross-referenced to the relevant page(s) of the text to facilitate revision.

Acknowledgements

A number of organisations have kindly allowed us to use illustrations, tables and other material in these pages. We gratefully acknowledge the help given by the parties listed below in granting permission to use the material cited.

Association of Anaesthetists of Great Britain and Ireland
Section 1, Chapter 2
  Figure IA5: Clinical features of anaphylaxis
  Figure IA6: First clinical features of anaphylaxis
  Figure IA7: Management of a patient with suspected anaphylaxis
Section 1, Chapter 3
  Figure IN6: Recommendations for standards of monitoring during anaesthesia and recovery
Section 1, Chapter 4
  Figure PO1: Criteria to be met before transfer from recovery room to general ward
Section 1, Chapter 5
  Figure SC9: Indications for intubation and ventilation for transfer after brain injury
  Figure SC10: Transfer checklist for neurosurgical patients
Section 4, Chapter 3
  Figure EQ41: AAGBI checklist for anaesthetic equipment

British Journal of Anaesthesia (BMJ Publishing Group / Oxford University Press)
Section 1, Chapter 4
  Figure PO11: DVT risk group classification
Section 4, Chapter 3
  Figure EQ20: Mapleson classification system for breathing systems

Difficult Airway Society (UK)
Section 1, Chapter 2

Figure IA11: Unanticipated difficult intubation during routine induction of anaesthesia
Figure IA12: Unanticipated difficult intubation during rapid sequence induction
Figure IA13: Failed intubation: rescue techniques for the 'can't intubate, can't ventilate' situation

European Resuscitation Council and **Resuscitation Council** (UK)
Section 1, Chapter 8
  Figure RS1: Causes of airway obstruction
  Figure RS2: Algorithm for in-hospital resuscitation
  Figure RS3: Adult basic life support algorithm
  Figure RS4: Adult choking algorithm
  Figure RS5: Adult advanced life support algorithm
  Figure RS7: Bradycardia algorithm
  Figure RS8: Tachycardia algorithm
  Figure RS9: Paediatric BLS algorithm
  Figure RS10: Paediatric foreign-body airway obstruction algorithm
  Figure RS11: Paediatric ALS algorithm

European Society of Regional Anaesthesia
Section 1, Chapter 7
  Figure RA19: ESRA good practice guidelines for thromboprophylaxis and CNB

Pharmacokinetics of Anaesthesia, ed. C. Prys-Roberts and C. C. Hug. Oxford: Blackwell, 1984
Section 3, Chapter 4
  Figure PK9: Mapleson's water analogue models

Royal College of Anaesthetists
Appendix: Primary FRCA syllabus

The Sourcebook of Medical Illustration, ed. P. Cull. Carnforth: Parthenon Publishing Group, 1989
Section 1, Chapter 7
  Figure RA7: Patient positions for spinal anaesthesia

Abbreviations

2,3-DPG	2,3-diphosphoglycerate	AP	anaesthetic proof
5-HT	5-hydroxytryptamine	APC	activated protein C
A	adenine	APC	antigen-presenting cell
A	ampere	APCR	activated protein C resistance
A&E	accident and emergency	APG	anaesthetic proof category G
ABC	airway, breathing, circulation	APL	adjustable pressure-limiting
ABV	arterial blood volume	APTT	activated partial thromboplastin time
AC	alternating current	AQP	aquaporin
ACC	anterior cingulate cortex	ARDS	acute respiratory distress syndrome
ACE	angiotensin-converting enzyme	ARR	absolute risk reduction
ACh	acetylcholine	ASA	American Society of Anesthesiologists
ACT	activated clotting time	ASIC	acid-sensing ion channel
ACTH	adrenocorticotropic hormone	ASIS	anterior superior iliac spine
ACTH-RH	adrenocorticotropic hormone-releasing hormone	ATLS	advanced trauma life support
		ATP	adenosine triphosphate
ADCC	antibody-dependent cell-mediated cytotoxicity	ATPS	ambient temperature and pressure saturated
		AUC	area under curve
ADH	antidiuretic hormone	AV	atrioventricular
ADP	adenosine diphosphate	AVNRT	AV nodal re-entry tachycardia
ADR	adverse drug reaction	AVRT	AV re-entry tachycardia
ADROIT	Adverse Drug Reactions Online Information Tracking	bd	twice a day
		BDNF	brain-derived neurotrophic factor
AED	automated external defibrillator	BLS	basic life support
AER	audio evoked response	B_M	B memory cell
AF	atrial fibrillation	BMI	body mass index
AIDS	acquired immune deficiency syndrome	BMR	basal metabolic rate
ALS	advanced life support	$BMRO_2$	basal metabolic rate of oxygen consumption
AMD	airway management device	BNP	brain natriuretic peptide
AMP	adenosine monophosphate	BP	blood pressure
AMPA	α-amino 3-hydroxy 5-methyl 4-isoxazolepropionic acid	BP	boiling point
		bpm	beats per minute
Ang I	angiotensin I	BSA	body surface area
Ang II	angiotensin II	BSER	brain-stem evoked responses
ANOVA	analysis of variance	BTPS	body temperature and pressure saturated
ANP	atrial natriuretic peptide	c	centi
ANS	autonomic nervous system	C	cytosine
ANSI	American National Standards Institute	Ca	arterial compliance
AP	action potential (in cardiac physiology)	CAM	cell adhesion molecules
AP	anteroposterior	cAMP	cyclic adenosine monophosphate

C_AO_2	alveolar oxygen content
CaO_2	arterial oxygen content
CAPD	continuous ambulatory peritoneal dialysis
CBF	cerebral blood flow
CBG	corticosteroid-binding globulin
CBV	cerebral blood volume
CCK	cholecystokinin
CcO_2	capillary oxygen content
cd	candela
CFAM	cerebral function analysing monitor
CGRP	calcitonin gene-related peptide
CI	cardiac index
CI	confidence interval
CK	creatinine kinase
CL	confidence limit
Cl	clearance
C_L	lung compliance
$CMRO_2$	cerebral metabolic rate of oxygen consumption
CNB	central nerve block
CNS	central nervous system
CO	cardiac output
CO_2	carbon dioxide
CoA	co-enzyme A
COAD	chronic obstructive airways disease
COMT	catechol-O-methyl transferase
COP	colloid osmotic pressure
COPA	cuffed oropharyngeal airway
cos	cosine
COSHH	control of substances hazardous to health
COX	cyclo-oxygenase
CP	creatine phosphate
CPAP	continuous positive airway pressure
CPD-A	citrate phosphate dextrose adenine
CPK MB	creatinine phosphokinase (cardiac isoenzyme)
CPP	cerebral perfusion pressure
CPP	coronary perfusion pressure
CPR	cardiopulmonary resuscitation
C_R	respiratory system compliance
CRPS	complex regional pain syndrome
CSE	combined spinal–epidural
CSF	cerebrospinal fluid
CSM	Committee on Safety of Medicines
CT	computerised tomography
CTZ	chemoreceptor trigger zone
CV	controlled ventilation
CvO_2	mixed venous oxygen content
CVP	central venous pressure
CVS	cardiovascular system
Cw	chest wall compliance
d	deci
D	dopaminergic
da	deca
DAG	diacylglycerol
D&C	dilatation and curettage
DC	direct current
DCR	dacryocystorhinostomy
DDAVP	1-deamino-8-arginine vasopressin
DHEA	dehydroepiandrosterone
DIC	disseminated intravascular coagulation
DIT	di-iodothyronine
DLCO	diffusing capacity of the lungs for carbon monoxide
DNA	deoxyribonucleic acid
DNAR	do not attempt resuscitation
DNR	do not resuscitate
$\dot{D}O_2$	oxygen delivery
DRG	dorsal root ganglion
DVT	deep venous thrombosis
Ea	arterial elastance
EAR	expired air respiration
EBC	effective blood concentration
EC	effective concentration
ECA	electrical control activity
ECF	extracellular fluid
ECF-A	eosinophil chemotactic factor of anaphylaxis
ECFV	extracellular fluid volume
ECG	electrocardiogram
ECMO	extracorporeal membrane oxygenation
ECV	effective circulating volume
ED_{50}	effective dose in 50% of population
ED_{95}	effective dose in 95% of population
EDP	end-diastolic point
EDPVR	end-diastolic pressure–volume relationship
EDRF	endothelium-derived relaxing factor
EDTA	ethylenediaminetetra-acetate
EDV	end-diastolic volume
EEG	electroencephalogram
Ees	ventricular systolic elastance
EF	ejection fraction
EM	electromagnetic
EMD	electromechanical dissociation
EMF	electromotive force
EMG	electromyogram
EMLA	eutectic mixture of local anaesthetic
EMS	emergency medical service
ENT	ear nose and throat

EPO	erythropoietin	G	guanine
EPSP	excitatory postsynaptic potential	GABA	gamma-aminobutyric acid
ER	endoplasmic reticulum	GCS	Glasgow coma scale
ER	extraction ratio	GDNF	glial cell line-derived neurotrophic factor
ERC	European Resuscitation Council	GDP	guanine diphosphate
ERK	extracellular signal-regulated kinase	GFR	glomerular filtration rate
ERPC	evacuation of retained products of conception	GH	growth hormone
		GI	gastrointestinal
ERV	expiratory reserve volume	GIT	gastrointestinal tract
ESP	end-systolic point	GlyR	glycine receptor
ESPVR	end-systolic pressure–volume relationship	GMP	guanosine monophosphate
ESR	erythrocyte sedimentation rate	GP	glycolytic phosphorylation
ESRA	European Society of Regional Anaesthesia	GPCR	G-protein-coupled receptor
ESV	end-systolic volume	GTN	glyceryl trinitrate
ET	endothelium	GTP	guanosine triphosphate
ETC	oesophageal–tracheal combitube	h	hecto
$ETCO_2$	end-tidal carbon dioxide	h	hour
ETT	endotracheal tube	H_2	histamine receptor 2
f	femto	HAFOE	high airflow oxygen enrichment
f	frequency of breaths	HAS	human albumin solution
F	gas flow	Hb	haemoglobin
F/M	feto maternal ratio	HbA	adult haemoglobin
FA	fatty acid	HbCO	carboxyhaemoglobin
FAC	fractional area change	HbF	fetal haemoglobin
F_ACO_2	fractional alveolar carbon dioxide concentration	HBF	hepatic blood flow
		Hbmet	methaemoglobin
$FADH_2$	flavine adenine dinucleotide	HbS	sickle haemoglobin
FBC	full blood count	Hbsulph	sulphaemoglobin
FDC	F-decalin	HCG	human chorionic gonadotrophin
FDP	fibrin degradation product	HCO_3^-	bicarbonate
Fe^{2+}	ferrous iron state	Hct	haematocrit
$F_{\bar{E}}CO_2$	fractional mixed expired carbon dioxide concentration	HD	haemodialysis
		HDL	high density lipoprotein
FEMG	frontalis electromyogram	HDN	haemolytic disease of the newborn
FEV%	ratio of FEV_1 to FVC	HDU	high dependency unit
FEV_1	forced expiratory volume in one second	HELLP	haemolytic anaemia elevated liver enzymes low platelets
FFA	free fatty acids		
FFP	fresh frozen plasma	HER	hepatic extraction ratio
FFT	fast Fourier transform	HFJV	high-frequency jet ventilation
FG	fat group	HIV	human immunodeficiency virus
FGF	fresh gas flow	HME	heat and moisturiser exchanger
F_IO_2	fractional inspired oxygen concentration	HMWK	high molecular weight kininogen
FNHTR	febrile non-haemolytic transfusion reactions	HPL	human placental lactogen
		HPV	hypoxic pulmonary vasoconstriction
FRC	functional residual capacity	HR	heart rate
FSH	follicle-stimulating hormone	Hz	hertz
FTPA	F-tripropylamine	I	current
FVC	forced vital capacity	I : E	inspiratory : expiratory ratio
G	giga	IABP	intra-aortic balloon pump

IC	insular cortex
ICAM	intercellular adhesion molecule
ICF	intracellular fluid
ICP	intracranial pressure
ICU	intensive care unit
IDDM	insulin dependent diabetes mellitus
IgA	immunoglobulin A
IgE	immunoglobulin E
IGF	insulin-like growth factor
IgG	immunoglobulin G
iGluR	ionotropic glutamine receptor
IgM	immunoglobulin M
IHD	ischaemic heart disease
IL	interleukin
ILCOR	International Liaison Committee on Resuscitation
IM	intramuscular
IML	intermediolateral
INR	international normalised ratio
IO	intraosseous
IOP	intra-ocular pressure
IP$_3$	inositol triphosphate
IPSP	inhibitory postsynaptic potential
IR	infrared
IRV	inspiratory reserve volume
ISI	international sensitivity index
ISPTA	spatial-peak temporal-average intensity
IT	implant tested
ITP	idiopathic thrombocytopaenia purpura
IU	International units
IV	intravenous
IVC	inferior vena cava
IVIg	intravenous immunoglobulin
IVRA	intravenous regional anaesthesia
J	joule
JVP	jugular venous pressure
k	kilo
K	kelvin
KCCT	kaolin clotting time
KE	kinetic energy
LAK	lymphokine-activated killer
LAP	left atrial pressure
Laser	light amplification by stimulated emission of radiation
LBP	lipopolysaccharide binding protein
LC	locus coeruleus
LCNT	lateral cutaneous nerve of the thigh
LD$_{50}$	lethal dose 50%

LDL	low density lipoprotein
LED	light-emitting diode
LH	luteinising hormone
LIS	lateral intracellular space
LMA	laryngeal mask airway
LMW	low molecular weight
LMWH	low molecular weight heparin
LOH	loop of Henle
LOR	loss of resistance
LOS	lower oesophageal sphincter
LT	leukotriene
LV	left ventricle
LVEDP	left ventricular end-diastolic pressure
LVEDV	left ventricular end-diastolic volume
LVF	left ventricular failure
LVH	left ventricular hypertrophy
LVSW	left ventricular stroke work
LVSWI	left ventricular stroke work index
μ	micro
m	metre
m	milli
M	mega
M	muscarinic
MAC	minimum alveolar concentration
MAO	monoamine oxidase
MAOI	monoamine oxidase inhibitor
MAP	mean arterial pressure
MCH	mean cell haemoglobin
MCV	mean cell volume
MDP	maximum diastolic potential
MEA	microwave endometrial ablation
MEFR	mid-expiratory flow rate
MEPP	miniature endplate potential
MEWS	modified early warning system
MFR	mannosyl–fucosyl receptor
MG	muscle group
MH	malignant hyperthermia
MHC	major histocompatability
MI	myocardial infarction
MIA	mechanically insensitive afferent
MIC	minimum inhibitory concentration
MILS	manual in line stabilisation
MIR	minimum infusion rate
MIRL	membrane inhibitor of reactive lysis
MIT	mono-iodothyronine
MMC	migratory motor complex
mmHg	millimetres of mercury (pressure)
MODS	multiple organ dysfunction syndrome

mol	mole	PABA	para-aminobenzoic acid
MONA	morphine, oxygen, nitrates, aspirin	PAC	pulmonary artery catheter
MPAP	mean pulmonary arterial pressure	P_ACO_2	partial pressure of carbon dioxide – alveolar
mRNA	messenger RNA	$PaCO_2$	partial pressure of carbon dioxide – arterial
MSA	mechanically sensitive afferent	PACWP	pulmonary artery capillary wedge pressure
MRSA	methicillin-resistant *Staphyloccocus aureus*	PADP	pulmonary artery diastolic pressure
MUGA	multigated scan	PAF	platelet activating factor
MV	minute volume	PAG	periaqueductal grey
MW	molecular weight	PAH	para-aminohippuric acid
n	nano	P_AO_2	partial pressure of oxygen – alveolar
N	newton	PaO_2	partial pressure of oxygen – arterial
nAChR	nicotinic acetylcholine receptor	PARS	patient at risk score
NADH	nicotinamide adenine dinucleotide	PART	patient at risk team
NADPH	nicotinamide adenine dinucleotide phosphate	Paw	airway pressure
NaHCO₃	sodium bicarbonate	PBP	penicillin-binding protein
NANC	non-adrenergic non-cholinergic	PCA	patient controlled analgesia
Nd-YAG	neodymium yttrium aluminium garnet	PCC	prothrombinase complex concentrates
NGF	nerve growth factor	PCEA	patient-controlled epidural analgesia
NIBP	non-invasive blood pressure	PCO_2	partial pressure of carbon dioxide
NIST	non-interchangeable screw thread		
NK	natural killer	PCWP	pulmonary capillary wedge pressure
NK	neurokinin receptor	PD	photodiode
NMDA	N-methyl-D-aspartate	PDE	phosphodiesterase enzyme
NMJ	neuromuscular junction	PDGF	platelet-derived growth factor
NNH	number needed to harm	PDPH	post-dural puncture headache
NNT	number needed to treat	PE	potential energy
NO	nitric oxide	PE	pulmonary embolus
NREM	non-rapid eye movement	$P_{\bar{E}}CO_2$	partial pressure end-tidal carbon dioxide
NRM	nucleus raphe magnus	PEA	pulseless electrical activity
NSAID	non-steroidal anti-inflammatory drug	PEEP	positive end-expiratory pressure
NTP	normal temperature and pressure	PEFR	peak expiratory flow rate
NTS	nucleus tractus solitarius	PFC	perfluorocarbon
NV	nausea and vomiting	PGE	prostaglandin E
NWC	number of words chosen	PGG	prostaglandin G
Ω	ohm	PGH	prostaglandin H
O/G	oil/gas	PGI	prostaglandin I
O/W	oil/water	Pi	inorganic phosphate
OCI	oesophageal contractility index	PIH	prolactin inhibiting hormone
ODC	oxyhaemoglobin dissociation curve	PIP_2	phosphatidylinositol bisphosphate
OP	oxidative phosphorylation	PK	prekallikrein
OPAC	oximetric pulmonary artery catheter	PLOC	provoked lower oesophageal contractions
OR	odds ratio	PMN	polymorphonuclear neutrophils
Osm	osmole	PNMT	phenylethanolamine N-methyl transferase
π	osmotic pressure	PO_2	partial pressure of oxygen
p	pico	PONV	postoperative nausea and vomiting
P	probability	PPAR	peroxisome proliferator-activated receptor
Pa	pascal	PPF	plasma protein fraction
PA	pulmonary artery	PPHN	persistent pulmonary hypertension of the newborn

ppm	parts per million		Σ	sum of
PPP	pentose phosphate pathway		s	second
PRI	pain rating index		S/N	signal to noise ratio
PRST	pressure, rate, sweating, tears		SA	sinoatrial
PSI	pounds per square inch		SAGM	saline adenine glucose mannitol
PSVT	paroxysmal supraventricular tachycardia		SaO_2	arterial oxygen saturation
PT	prothrombin time		SARS	severe acute respiratory syndrome
PTC	post tetanic count		SD	standard deviation
PTH	parathyroid hormone		SEM	standard error of the mean
PTT	partial thromboplastin time		SFH	stroma-free haemoglobin
PTTK	partial thromboplastin time with kaolin		SI	stroke index
PV	pressure volume		SI	Système International d'Unités (International System of Units)
PVC	poly vinyl chloride			
PVD	peripheral vascular disease		SIADH	syndrome of inappropriate ADH secretion
PVG	periventricular grey		SIMV	synchronised intermittent mandatory ventilation
PVR	pulmonary vascular resistance			
Q	flow		sin	sine
Q	charge		SIRS	systemic inflammatory response syndrome
$\dot{Q}$	cardiac output		SL	semilunar
Qs	shunt flow		SLE	systemic lupus erythematosus
R	resistance (electrical)		SLOC	spontaneous lower oesophageal contractions
R	universal gas constant		SMP	sympathetically maintained pain
RAP	right atrial pressure		SNGFR	single-nephron glomerular filtration rate
RAS	reticular activating system			
RAST	radioallergosorbent test		SNP	sodium nitroprusside
RBC	red blood cell		SO_2	oxygen saturation
RBF	renal blood flow		SpO_2	pulse oximeter oxygen saturation
RDS	respiratory distress syndrome		SR	sarcoplasmic reticulum
Re	Reynolds number		SRS-A	slow reacting substance of anaphylaxis
REM	rapid eye movement		SSRI	selective serotonin reuptake inhibitor
RH	relative humidity			
RIMA	reversible inhibitor of monoamine oxidase A		STOP	suction termination of pregnancy
			STT	spinothalamic tract
RMP	resting membrane potential		SV	stroke volume
RNA	ribonucleic acid		SVC	superior vena cava
RNU	regional neurosurgical unit		SVI	systemic vascular index
ROC	receptor-operated ion channel		SvO_2	mixed venous oxygen saturation
RPF	renal plasma flow		SVP	saturated vapour pressure
RQ	respiratory quotient		SVR	systemic vascular resistance
rRNA	ribosomal RNA		SVWI	stroke volume work index
RR	relative risk		SW	stroke work
RRR	relative risk reduction		T	absolute temperature
RS	respiratory system		T	tera
RSI	rapid sequence induction		T	thymine
RT_3	reverse tri-iodothyronine		$t_{1/2}$	half-life
RV	residual volume		T_3	tri-iodothyronine
RV	right ventricle		T_4	thyroxine
RVM	rostral ventromedial medulla		tan	tangent
RVSWI	right ventricular stroke work index		TBPA	thyroxine-binding prealbumin
			TBG	thyroxine-binding globulin
			TBV	total blood volume

TBW	total body water
Tc	cytotoxic T cell
TCA	tricyclic antidepressant
TCR	T-cell receptor
TCRE	transcervical resection of endometrium
TENS	transcutaneous electrical nerve stimulation
T_H	T helper cell
THC	terahydro-cannabinol
THR	total hip replacement
TIVA	total intravenous anaesthesia
TKR	total knee replacement
TLC	total lung capacity
TLV	total lung volume
T_m	tubular maximum
TNF	tumour necrosis factor
TOE	transoesophageal echocardiography
TOF	train of four
TP	threshold potential
t-PA	tissue-type plasminogen activator
TPP	thiamine pyrophosphate
TRALI	transfusion-related acute lung injury
TRH	thyrotropin-releasing hormone
tRNA	transfer RNA
TRP	transient receptor potential
TRPV1	transient receptor potential vanilloid 1
TSH	thyroid-stimulating hormone
TT	thrombin time
TTN	transient tachypnoea of the newborn
TUR	transurethral resection
TURBT	transurethral resection of bladder tumour
TURP	transurethral resection of the prostate
TXA_2	thromboxane A_2
U&E	urea and electrolytes
UBF	uterine blood flow
UFH	unfractionated heparin
UK	United Kingdom
UOS	upper oesophageal sphincter
URT	upper respiratory tract
URTI	upper respiratory tract infection
UTP	uridine triphosphate
UV	ultra violet
v	velocity
V	volt
$\dot{V}/\dot{Q}$	ventilation/perfusion
VA	alveolar volume
V_{BL}	blood volume
VC	vital capacity
VCO_2	carbon dioxide flux
VD	anatomical dead space
Vd	volume of distribution
VER	visual evoked response
VF	ventricular fibrillation
VIC	vaporiser inside circle
VIE	vacuum-insulated evaporator
V_{INT}	interstitial fluid volume
VIP	vasoactive intestinal peptide
VLDL	very low density lipoprotein
VMA	vannilyl mandelic acid
VO_2	oxygen uptake in the lungs
VOC	vaporiser outside circle
VPC	ventricular premature contractions
V_{PL}	plasma volume
VPN	ventral posterior nucleus of the thalamus
V_{RBC}	red blood cell volume
VRE	vancomycin-resistant enterococci
VRG	vessel-rich group
V_T	tidal volume
VT	ventricular tachycardia
V_TCO_2	volume of carbon dioxide per breath
vWF	von Willebrand's factor
W	watt
WBC	white blood cell
WCC	white cell count
WHO	World Health Organization
WPW	Wolff–Parkinson–White

CHAPTER **1**

Preoperative management

G. Cavill and K. Kerr

PREOPERATIVE ASSESSMENT
Screening
Preoperative assessment clinic
Preoperative assessment of functional capacity
Preoperative visit
The airway
American Society of Anesthesiologists (ASA)
  scoring system

PREPARATION FOR ANAESTHESIA
Premedication
Preoperative factors

CONCURRENT MEDICAL DISEASE
Respiratory disease
Cardiovascular disease
Haematological disease
Musculoskeletal disease
Renal disease
Endocrine disease

CONCURRENT MEDICATION

CONCURRENT SURGICAL DISEASE
Intestinal obstruction
Acute abdominal emergencies

The safe conduct of anaesthesia requires meticulous preoperative assessment, preparation and planning. In the case of elective procedures this should occur well in advance of surgery, allowing a comprehensive review of concurrent disease, medication and social issues. This is often carried out in a dedicated preoperative assessment clinic by a multidisciplinary team comprising nursing and medical staff as well as pharmacists and specialist technicians.

Whilst patients undergoing emergency surgery may not benefit from such a structured approach to their preoperative management, they must nevertheless undergo rigorous systematic review and preparation to ensure optimum care.

Preoperative assessment

Screening

When elective surgery is first planned, a screening questionnaire may be used to provide information regarding comorbidity that may require early preoperative review or intervention. A need for additional specialist input can be identified and acted upon at this stage.

Preoperative assessment clinic

During subsequent preoperative assessment a general medical history is taken, detailing concurrent disease and its management.

- Correspondence in the clinical notes may provide a useful outline of a disease process, giving some indication of its stability, as well as information on previous hospital admissions, current medication and recent investigation results.
- A history should be taken of previous anaesthetic experience. A family history of problems associated with anaesthesia must be noted and may require further investigation.
- The patient's general health should be assessed. In particular a history of reflux should be noted, along with smoking and alcohol habits.
- A history of recreational drug use may be appropriate.
- A list of current medication, including dosage and recent changes, is essential, along with a history of any allergic or other adverse drug reactions. The nature of the allergy or reaction should be recorded.
- Particular attention must be paid to drugs requiring specific perioperative management, such as anticoagulants or insulin.

A general physical examination must be carried out prior to anaesthesia and surgery.
- Of particular importance is a focused examination of the cardiorespiratory system. This aims to ensure control of conditions such as hypertension, but also to

Fundamentals of Anaesthesia, 3rd edition, ed. Tim Smith, Colin Pinnock and Ted Lin. Published by Cambridge University Press. © Cambridge University Press 2008.

detect features such as new cardiac murmurs. The latter may require further investigation.

- A functional assessment is particularly important in patients with cardiorespiratory disease. This will be considered in more detail below.
- An assessment of the cervical spine should be made in patients with conditions likely to limit neck movement. Radiological examination is seldom necessary, but limitation of movement should be defined and recorded. The presence of neurological symptoms or signs will require further evaluation.
- The presence and location of any loose or damaged teeth should be noted, as well as dentures, crowns and orthodontic appliances.
- Airway assessment is of fundamental importance, and is generally carried out at the time of the anaesthetist's preoperative visit.

Preoperative assessment of functional capacity

Functional capacity (what a patient can physically do) not only describes exercise tolerance but gives an indication of functional reserve (the extent to which that patient can be physically challenged). This is particularly important in the preoperative assessment of surgical patients with cardiac disease.

Gross limitation or deterioration of functional capacity is of particular significance, and indicates the need for further assessment, including investigation and specialist opinion. When considered along with clinical (mainly cardiac) factors and the planned surgical procedure, an estimate of functional capacity helps us to make an assessment of perioperative risk.

We can express functional capacity in so-called *metabolic equivalent* (MET) units (Figure PR1). A MET is expressed in terms of oxygen utilisation, and quantifies the estimated amount of energy expended at different levels of physical activity.

---

1 MET equates to 3.5 millilitres of oxygen per kilogram body weight per minute

Metabolic equivalents of common daily activities

1 MET	walk 100 metres on level ground
4 MET	climb a flight of stairs or walk up a hill
>10 MET	strenuous exercise

Figure PR1 MET units

A functional capacity corresponding to <4 MET (unable to climb a flight of stairs) is associated with increased perioperative risk. A more detailed assessment can be made by referring to an activity scale such as the Duke Activity Status Index. The answers to series of questions related to daily activities provide a score related to functional capacity. Great care is needed in making such assessments, as function may be limited by factors such as arthritis or neurological disease. In such cases more specific symptoms such as orthopnoea or paroxysmal nocturnal dyspnoea are helpful in identifying cardiac disease as the factor limiting functional capacity.

A number of baseline investigations may be carried out at the time of preoperative assessment. These typically include a full blood count, electrolytes and a 12-lead electrocardiogram (ECG). Pulmonary function tests may prove helpful in some patients with respiratory disease. There are, however, comprehensive guidelines available to minimise unnecessary investigations in fit young patients. Further investigation must be guided by underlying disease and functional status. Additional blood tests, for example, might be required to assess thyroid or liver function.

In some cases there may be a need for radiological investigation, echocardiography and, occasionally, cardiopulmonary exercise testing. Such investigations should only be sought following discussion with experienced clinicians. These investigations place a heavy demand on technicians and may themselves carry risks for the patient. The likely benefits must therefore be carefully weighed up.

Some patients with serious comorbidity may be referred by the preoperative assessment clinic at this stage for further assessment by a senior anaesthetist.

Written information regarding anaesthesia and specific surgical procedures is often provided to patients at this time.

Preoperative visit

A preoperative visit by an anaesthetist is essential, and increasingly occurs on the day of surgery. Such a visit provides an opportunity for the anaesthetist to introduce himself and give a brief explanation of his role.

A general medical and surgical history is often already available, and can be discussed in further detail. Specific issues regarding previous anaesthesia and associated problems are discussed. Earlier examination findings should be available following preoperative assessment. Examination of dentition and neck movement, along with an assessment of the airway, must be made at this stage. A plan of care, including proposed anaesthetic technique, postoperative analgesia and fluid management, can be outlined to the patient.

A discussion regarding the risks and benefits of proposed procedures is usually much appreciated. This also provides an opportunity to discuss any concerns the patient may have regarding specific issues such as postoperative nausea and vomiting, and duration of immobility following regional anaesthesia.

An effective preoperative visit should do much to allay anxiety, leaving the patient well-informed and confident in those caring for him or her. It may well preclude the need for premedication.

The airway

Failure to achieve adequate oxygenation and ventilation is responsible for a significant proportion of anaesthesia-related morbidity and mortality. Inadequate ventilation and difficult intubation are everyday hazards in anaesthesia and can prove catastrophic. Given the fundamental importance of adequate oxygenation, recognition of the 'difficult to ventilate' patient is essential. A number of factors are associated with difficulty in mask ventilation:

- Obesity (BMI > 26)
- Beard
- Edentulous
- Snoring
- Age > 55

Ease of intubation has been graded according to the best possible view obtained on laryngoscopy (Cormack & Lehane 1984). Grades 3 and 4 are difficult intubations:

- Grade 1: Whole of glottis visible
- Grade 2: Glottis incompletely visible
- Grade 3: Epiglottis but not glottis visible
- Grade 4: Epiglottis not visible

The reported incidence of difficult intubation varies, but is around 1 in 65 intubations. Despite careful history and examination, 20% of difficult intubations are not predicted. The consequences may be disastrous. A history of previous difficult intubation is important but a history of straightforward intubation several years earlier may be falsely reassuring as the patient's weight, cervical spine movement and disease process may all have changed. Some congenital conditions may predict a difficult intubation, e.g. Pierre Robin syndrome, Marfan's syndrome or cystic hygroma. Pathological conditions can make intubation difficult, e.g. tumour, infection or scarring of the upper airway tissues.

Airway assessment

As airway assessment, investigation and management becomes increasingly refined, the search for a single, reliable predictor of the difficult airway continues. A number of bedside tests are available to the anaesthetist wishing to make an assessment for features which might predict potential airway difficulties. However, unexpected airway problems can and do arise despite the ever-increasing array of assessment tools available to us. This should be borne in mind at all times.

In the modified Mallampati scoring system the patient sits opposite the anaesthetist with mouth open and tongue protruded. The structures visible at the back of the mouth are noted (Mallampati *et al.* 1985, Samsoon & Young 1987), as follows:

- Class 1: Faucial pillars, soft palate and uvula visible
- Class 2: Faucial pillars and soft palate visible, uvula masked by base of tongue
- Class 3: Only soft palate visible
- Class 4: Soft palate not visible

The Wilson risk factors may provide additional predictive information on the airway. The Wilson risk factors each score 0–2 points, to give a maximum of 10 points. A score >2 predicts 75% of difficult intubations, although as with the Mallampati system there is a high incidence of false positives. The Wilson risk factors (Wilson *et al.* 1988) are:

- Obesity
- Restricted head and neck movements
- Restricted jaw movement
- Receding mandible
- Buck teeth

A number of tests of neck and jaw movement may be used to evaluate these further:

- Inability to flex the chin onto the chest indicates poor neck movement. Once the neck is fully flexed, a patient should be able to move his or her head more than 15° to demonstrate normal occipitoaxial movement.
- Limitation of neck (atlanto-occipital joint) extension may be predictive of difficult intubation. The normal angle of extension is >35°.
- Reduced jaw movements are demonstrated by poor mouth opening (particularly if of less than two fingers' width) and by inability to protrude the lower teeth beyond the upper.
- Limited mouth opening clearly creates potential airway difficulties, and may reflect limitation of temperomandibular joint movement. This may be

evident as a reduced inter-incisor distance (the distance between the lower and upper incisors). A distance of <3.5 cm is predictive of a difficult airway.

The mandibular space length and its measurement have received much attention in the quest to accurately predict airway difficulties:

- The thyromental distance, described by Patil in 1983, is the distance between the chin and the thyroid notch with the neck fully extended. A distance of less than 6.5 cm (about 3 finger breadths) predicts difficulty.
- The sternomental distance was described by Savva in 1994; it is the distance from the suprasternal notch to the chin with the neck fully extended. A distance of less than 12 cm predicts difficulty.
- The hyomental distance is that from the chin to the hyoid bone. A distance of less than 4 cm (about 2 finger breadths) predicts difficulty.

No one test can predict airway difficulties with a high degree of sensitivity or specificity, but a combination of tests may be helpful. Careful assessment of the airway and consideration of more than one factor is therefore recommended. The modified Mallampati classification produces a high incidence of false positives. A thyromental distance of less than 6.5 cm and Mallampati class 3 or 4, however, predicts 80% of difficult intubations.

Radiological features may aid prediction of a difficult intubation, but they are not routinely performed. These include:

- Reduced distance between occiput and spine of C1 and between spines of C1 and C2
- Ratio of mandibular length to posterior mandibular depth >3.6
- Increased depth of mandible

Other rarely used investigations include indirect laryngoscopy, ultrasonography, CT and MRI imaging.

American Society of Anesthesiologists (ASA) scoring system

The ASA scoring system describes the preoperative physical state of a patient (Saklad 1941) and is used routinely for every patient in the UK. It makes no allowances for age, smoking history, obesity or pregnancy. Anticipated difficulties in intubation are not relevant. Addition of the postscript E indicates emergency surgery. There is some correlation between ASA score and perioperative mortality, although it was never intended for use in perioperative risk prediction. Definitions applied in the ASA system are given in Figure PR2.

Code	Description	Perioperative mortality
P1	A normal healthy patient	0.1%
P2	A patient with mild systemic disease	0.2%
P3	A patient with severe systemic disease	1.8%
P4	A patient with severe systemic disease that is a constant threat to life	7.8%
P5	A moribund patient who is not expected to survive without the operation	9.4%
P6	A declared brain-dead patient whose organs are being removed for donor purposes	

Figure PR2 ASA classification

Preparation for anaesthesia

Premedication

As more day surgery is performed and more patients are admitted to hospital close to the scheduled time of surgery, premedication has become less common. The main indication for premedication remains anxiety, for which a benzodiazepine is usually prescribed, sometimes with metoclopramide to promote absorption. Premedication serves several purposes: anxiolysis, smoother induction of anaesthesia, reduced requirement for intravenous induction agents, and possibly reduced likelihood of awareness. Intramuscular opioids are now rarely prescribed as premedication. The prevention of aspiration pneumonitis in patients with reflux requires premedication with an H_2 antagonist, the evening before and morning of surgery, and sodium citrate administration immediately prior to induction of anaesthesia. Topical local anaesthetic cream over two potential sites for venous cannulation is usually prescribed for children. Anticholinergic agents may be prescribed to dry secretions or to prevent bradycardia, e.g. during squint surgery. Usual medication should be continued up to the time of anaesthesia.

Preoperative factors

Starvation

It is routine practice to starve patients prior to surgery in an attempt to minimise the volume of stomach contents

Adults
- Clear fluids and water up to 2 hours preoperatively
- Food, sweets and milky drinks up to 6 hours preoperatively
- No chewing gum on day of surgery

Children
- Clear fluids and water up to 2 hours preoperatively
- Breast milk up to 4 hours preoperatively
- Formula/cow's milk up to 6 hours preoperatively
- Food and sweets up to 6 hours preoperatively

Figure PR3 Starvation guidelines

and hence decrease the incidence of their aspiration. Aspiration of solid food particles may cause asphyxiation, and aspiration of gastric acid may cause pneumonitis (Mendelson's syndrome). Guidelines for preoperative starvation are becoming less restrictive as more information becomes available. Milky drinks are not allowed because their high fat content increases gastric transit time.

There is evidence that chewing gum before surgery significantly increases gastric fluid volume, particularly in children.

Recently published national guidelines give recommendations for patients undergoing elective surgery as shown in Figure PR3.

Patients undergoing emergency surgery should be treated as if they have a full stomach. Normal fasting guidance should be followed where possible.

Prolonged periods of starvation give rise to problems. Dehydration may occur, particularly in children and in patients who are pyrexial or who have received bowel preparation. Infants may become hypoglycaemic. In patients with cyanotic heart disease, sickle cell disease or polycythaemia dehydration may precipitate thrombosis. In jaundiced patients the hepatorenal syndrome may be precipitated. It is thus essential that these patients receive intravenous therapy while they are being starved.

Fluid status
Healthy patients can balance daily fluid intake and output. Adults exchange approximately 5% of body water each day, while infants exchange about 15% and so are at greater risk of dehydration. A patient's fluid status may be affected by the underlying disease process or by its treatment (Figure PR4), and there may be associated electrolyte disturbances. In certain conditions such as trauma, infection

	Increased	Decreased
Input	Excessive IV fluids	Nausea
		Dysphagia
		Nil by mouth orders
		Coma
		Severe respiratory disease
Output	Sweating	Syndrome of inappropriate ADH secretion (SIADH)
	Diarrhoea (including bowel preparation)	Renal impairment
	Vomiting	
	Polyuria	
	Haemorrhage	
	Burns	

Figure PR4 Disturbances of fluid balance

or ileus, fluid is redistributed rather than lost from the body, but will nonetheless still require replacing to maintain fluid balance. If patients have been ill for longer periods, malnutrition may also be a problem.

Fluid balance should be assessed preoperatively in all patients who are at risk of disturbances, which is most likely in emergencies. A history of any of the above will direct clinical examination. Postural hypotension, tachycardia and hypotension may be found in volume depletion, while a raised jugular venous pressure (JVP) and peripheral oedema may be found in volume overload. Skin turgor, or fontanelle tension in infants, is a useful guide, and assessment of urine output is very important. Oliguria is defined as a urine output of less than $0.5 \, \text{ml kg}^{-1}$ per hour. Relevant investigations include serum electrolytes, urea and creatinine. Urea raised proportionally more than the creatinine value indicates dehydration.

Correction of fluid balance
Therapy should be guided by central venous pressure (CVP), urine output, blood pressure, heart rate and electrolyte balance. Where fluid overload is diagnosed, fluid restriction and possibly diuretic therapy are required. If fluid depletion is diagnosed, replacement of the lost fluid, plus maintenance fluids, is required. Hypovolaemia resulting from blood loss necessitates red cell transfusion. If

plasma has been lost, as in burns patients, plasma protein fraction (PPF) will be required. Maintenance fluid requirements are 40 ml kg^{-1} per day in adults (greater for children). Excessive administration of 5% dextrose to correct dehydration may lead to hyperglycaemia and hyponatraemia, while excessive administration of 0.9% saline may cause hypernatraemia and peripheral and pulmonary oedema.

Electrolyte disturbances

Disturbances of electroytes may be due to the underlying disease process, to drugs, particularly diuretics, or to iatrogenic causes. It is rare for a patient to exhibit overt clinical signs, but electrolyte disturbances present several potential problems for the anaesthetist (Figure PR5). It is particularly important to assess the volume status of the patient who has an electrolyte disturbance. Electrolyte disturbances are more likely to be acute and hence more serious in patients presenting for emergency surgery.

Preoperatively, hyponatraemia may be longstanding, commonly due to diuretics, and this situation rarely requires treatment. More acutely, preoperative hyponatraemia is often due to inappropriate intravenous therapy on the ward. Treatment should comprise the administration of intravenous normal saline and, if there are signs of fluid overload, diuretics. Severe symptomatic hyponatraemia has a high mortality, and is seen most commonly as part of the TUR (transurethral resection) syndrome (see Section 1, Chapter 6, page 107). Hyponatraemia should be treated promptly with diuretics and only rarely with hypertonic saline. Too rapid correction of severe acute hyponatraemia may result in subdural haemorrhage, pontine lesions and cardiac failure. Hypernatraemia is mainly a problem when associated with volume depletion, and it should be corrected by administration of 5% dextrose intravenously, taking care not to fluid-overload the patient.

Chronic changes in plasma potassium are well tolerated, but acute changes are associated with ECG changes and cardiac dysrhythmias (Figure PR6). It is the ratio of intracellular to extracellular potassium that is relevant to myocardial excitability. Where the disturbance is chronic, this ratio will be nearly normal. Hypokalaemia may be treated by giving potassium either orally or intravenously. Care must be taken in the presence of renal insufficiency or low cardiac output states, as hyperkalaemia may result. A flow-controlled pump should be used to control the intravenous infusion rate if the concentration of potassium exceeds 40 mmol l^{-1}, and ECG monitoring will be required

as ventricular fibrillation may occur if hypokalaemia is corrected too quickly. Hyperkalaemia should be treated over several days by the administration of calcium resonium. If ECG changes are noted, or if more rapid correction of acute changes is required preoperatively, insulin (20 units in 100 ml 20% dextrose over 30–60 minutes) may be given. This may be repeated, depending on the next serum potassium. Intravenous calcium (10 ml 10% calcium gluconate) immediately (but temporarily) improves automaticity, conduction and contractility.

Smoking

A heavy smoker is anyone who smokes 20 or more cigarettes per day. Smoking causes several perioperative problems: increased airway reactivity; increased sputum production and retention; bronchospasm; coughing and atelectasis associated with an increased risk of postoperative chest infection. Associated diseases include ischaemic heart disease and chronic obstructive pulmonary disease. Up to 15% of the haemoglobin in smokers combines with carbon monoxide to form carboxyhaemoglobin, reducing the oxygen-carrying capacity of blood. After 12–24 hours of stopping smoking the effects of carbon monoxide and nicotine are significantly reduced, and after 6–8 weeks ciliary and immunological activity are restored. All smokers should be encouraged to abstain prior to theatre. Nicotine replacement therapy may prove helpful.

Concurrent medical disease

It is important to be aware of any medical condition affecting a patient and to ensure that its management prior to surgery is optimal. Emergency cases present particular problems, as nausea or vomiting may have caused the patient to omit usual medication. An understanding of the pharmacology and possible interactions of concurrent medication with anaesthetic drugs is also essential.

Respiratory disease
Viral infection

The commonest respiratory problem of relevance to anaesthesia is viral upper respiratory tract infection (URTI), which causes increased bronchial reactivity, particularly in asthmatics, persisting for 3–4 weeks following resolution of the URTI. Current or recent URTI is also associated with an increased incidence of postoperative chest infection. Hence, unless surgery is urgent, such patients should be postponed for 4 weeks.

Problems	Causes
Hyponatraemia	
Confusion, fits and coma possible	Excess water intake (particularly intravenously)
If water excess: hypertension, cardiac failure, anorexia and nausea	Diuretics
	TUR syndrome
	Impaired water excretion (SIADH, hypothyroidism, cardiac failure, nephrotic syndrome)
Hypernatraemia	
Rarely symptoms if simple water loss	Reduced intake (impaired consciousness, unable to swallow, no water)
If severe, there may be muscle weakness, signs of volume depletion and coma	Increased insensible loss (fever, hot environment, hyperventilation)
	Impairment of urinary concentrating mechanism (diabetes insipidus, hyperosmolar non-ketotic coma or diabetic ketoacidosis)
Hypokalaemia	
Muscular weakness	Diuretics
Potentiates non-depolarising muscle relaxants	Gastrointestinal loss (diarrhoea, vomiting, fistula, ileus, villous adenoma of large bowel)
Cardiac arrhythmias	Recovery phase of diabetic ketoacidosis and acute tubular necrosis
Rhythm problems if on digoxin	Post relief of urinary tract obstruction
	Reduced intake
	Cushing's syndrome
	Hyperaldosteronism
Hyperkalaemia	
Spurious if blood sample haemolysed	Acute or chronic renal disease
Cardiac arrest may occur if plasma $K^+ > 7$ mmol l^{-1}	Shift of K^+ out of cells (tissue damage)
	Acidosis (particularly diabetic ketoacidosis)
	Increased intake
	Drugs impairing secretion (K^+ retaining diuretics)
	Addison's disease
	Tissue breakdown (rhabdomyolysis)

Figure PR5 Problems and causes of electrolyte disturbances

Asthma

Asthma is common, affecting 10–20% of the population. In many patients the condition is mild and requires only occasional treatment, but in others there may be frequent and severe attacks requiring hospital admission and, in a few patients, ventilation on the intensive care unit. There are two main groups, although there is some overlap: **early-onset** asthma (atopic or extrinsic) and **late-onset** asthma (non-atopic or intrinsic). The symptoms of asthma are wheeze, cough, chest tightness and dyspnoea. They are

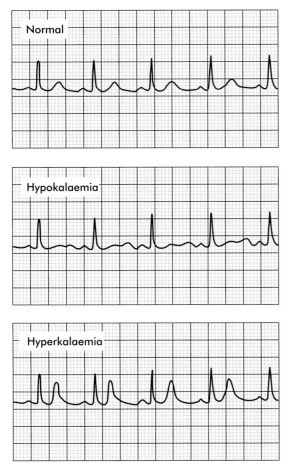

Figure PR6 ECG changes associated with hypo- and hyperkalaemia

suppression and prevent the normal stress response to surgery, and thus perioperative hydrocortisone cover may be required. Usual bronchodilator therapy should be continued preoperatively. It is common practice to prescribe a preoperative dose of inhaled β_2 adrenoreceptor agonist immediately prior to the patient going to theatre, and to ensure that the patient brings his or her inhaler to theatre in case it is required postoperatively. As bronchospasm may be precipitated by anxiety, benzodiazepine premedication is often prescribed. Sedative drugs are contraindicated in anyone experiencing an acute exacerbation of asthma.

Assessment of the severity of asthma may be made from the history: frequency of attacks, whether the patient has ever been admitted to hospital with an attack or has ever required ventilation, whether oral steroids are ever necessary and if so how frequently. Nocturnal cough and frequent waking with symptoms indicate poor control of asthma. A chest radiograph in an asthmatic patient who is currently well is often normal, and is not necessary preoperatively. In longstanding cases there may be hyperinflation of the lungs. Pulmonary function tests provide a useful indication of the degree of airflow obstruction: in particular, the forced expiratory volume in 1 second (FEV_1) and the peak expiratory flow rate (PEFR) are used. If a patient's normal PEFR is known, the current state of the asthma may be ascertained from preoperative measurement of PEFR. If the patient has experienced a recent exacerbation, with an increase in symptoms, reduced PEFR and increased requirement for medication, it is appropriate to postpone elective surgery until the condition has returned to normal, which may take several weeks. Where surgery is urgent, steps should be taken to optimise the patient's condition in the time available by the use of a nebulised β_2 adrenoreceptor agonist and, if it is severe, the commencement of enteral or parenteral steroids.

Chronic obstructive pulmonary disease

Chronic bronchitis and emphysema are different pathologically but frequently co-exist as chronic obstructive pulmonary disease. A patient's condition may fall anywhere in a spectrum from solely chronic bronchitis to solely emphysema, with the majority of patients possessing symptoms and signs of both. The main feature of both diseases is generalised airflow obstruction.

Chronic bronchitis is defined as daily cough with sputum production for at least three consecutive months a year for at least two consecutive years. It develops as a result of longstanding irritation of the bronchial mucosa,

caused by an inflammatory reaction within the bronchial wall which results in bronchospasm, mucosal swelling and viscid secretions. In atopic asthma exposure to allergens results in the formation of immunoglobulin E (IgE), which causes a type 1 or anaphylactic antigen–antibody hypersensitivity reaction.

The treatment of mild asthma is the occasional or regular use of inhaled selective β_2 adrenoreceptor agonists such as salbutamol or terbutaline. Some patients may be using prophylactic inhaled sodium chromoglycate. In moderate cases regular inhaled corticosteroids are required. More severely affected patients may also be taking oral theophylline or regular oral steroids. Acute exacerbations of asthma may be treated with short courses of high-dose oral steroids. Regular steroids may cause adrenocortical

nearly always by tobacco smoke. The disease is more common in middle and later life, in smokers than in non-smokers, and in urban than in rural dwellers. Pathologically there is hypertrophy of mucus-secreting glands and mucosal oedema, leading to irreversible airflow obstruction. Air becomes 'trapped' in the alveoli on expiration causing alveolar distension, which may result in associated emphysema. Chronic bronchitis is a progressive disease, worsening with each acute exacerbation. Eventually respiratory failure develops, characterised by hypoxia, polycythaemia, pulmonary hypertension and cor pulmonale. Rarely, chronic hypercapnia may lead to loss of the central response to carbon dioxide, resulting in a 'blue bloater' whose hypoxia is the only stimulus to ventilation. If these patients undergo general anaesthesia they are extremely difficult to wean and to extubate. Symptoms of chronic bronchitis are cough with sputum, dyspnoea and wheeze. Clinical signs include hyperinflation of the chest, variable inspiratory and expiratory wheeze and often basal crackles, which may disappear after coughing. Peripheral oedema and raised jugular venous pressure are found with cor pulmonale, and there may be cyanosis.

Emphysema is defined as enlargement of the air spaces distal to the terminal bronchioles with destructive changes in the alveolar wall. The main cause of emphysema is smoking, although the rare genetic deficiency of α_1 antitrypsin may cause severe emphysema in young adults. The complications of emphysema include rupture of a pulmonary bulla leading to pneumothorax, and later respiratory failure and cor pulmonale may occur. Classically emphysematous patients are described as 'pink puffers'. The only symptom of emphysema is exertional dyspnoea, or dyspnoea at rest as the condition worsens. The main clinical sign of emphysema is a hyperinflated chest.

The treatment of chronic obstructive pulmonary disease is mostly symptomatic, once the patient has stopped smoking. Bronchodilators are useful if there is an element of reversible airways obstruction. Patients may be prescribed inhaled β_2 agonists, ipratropium bromide and theophylline. Diuretic therapy may be used to control right-sided heart failure. Patients who are hypoxic with pulmonary hypertension may be on domiciliary oxygen therapy, a bad prognostic indicator.

There are no characteristic radiological abnormalities due to chronic bronchitis, but coexisting emphysema may result in the appearance of hyperinflation with low flat diaphragms, loss of peripheral vascular markings and prominent hilar vessels (bat winging) and bullae. The heart is narrow until cor pulmonale develops. The presence of bullae supports the diagnosis of emphysema, and occasionally a giant emphysematous bulla will be seen, in which case surgical ablation may improve symptoms and lung function. Preoperative pulmonary function tests may help determine which of the two pathological conditions predominates. Arterial blood gas analysis is indicated to assess gas exchange if a patient has severe dyspnoea on mild or moderate exertion.

If there is a history of recent onset of green sputum production rather than white, and clinical signs support a diagnosis of chest infection, surgery should if possible be postponed and a course of antibiotics and physiotherapy commenced.

Pulmonary function tests

Peak expiratory flow rate (PEFR) is the rate of flow of exhaled air at the start of a forced expiration, and is measured using a simple flowmeter. Reduced values compared to predicted values for age, height and sex indicate airflow obstruction. Serial measurements are useful for monitoring disease progress and for demonstrating a response to bronchodilator therapy.

Spirometric tests of lung function are easy to perform. If a subject exhales as hard and as long as possible from a maximal inspiration, the volume expired in the first second is the forced expiratory volume in 1 second (FEV_1) and the total volume expired is the forced vital capacity (FVC). The measured values are compared to predicted values for age, height and sex. The ratio of FEV_1 to FVC (FEV%) is most useful (normal range 65–80%). Obstructive airways disease, e.g. asthma, reduces the FEV_1 more than the FVC, so the FEV% is low. Restrictive airways disease, e.g. pulmonary fibrosis, reduces the FVC and, to a lesser degree, the FEV_1, so the FEV% is normal or high (Figure PR7).

Arterial blood gas analysis may be useful, and interpretation should be systematic. Look first at the pH value (acidosis or alkalosis) to determine the direction of the primary change. Although there may be partial compensation for the underlying abnormality, there is never full or over-compensation. Then look at the PCO_2, which is determined by alveolar ventilation. A low PCO_2 (hyperventilation) indicates a respiratory alkalosis or respiratory compensation for a metabolic acidosis. Conversely a raised PCO_2 (hypoventilation) indicates a respiratory acidosis. The PCO_2 does not increase above normal to compensate for a metabolic alkalosis. Next, consider the standard bicarbonate value (HCO_3^-). This is defined as the extracellular fluid (ECF) bicarbonate concentration the patient would have if the PCO_2 were normal. If standard

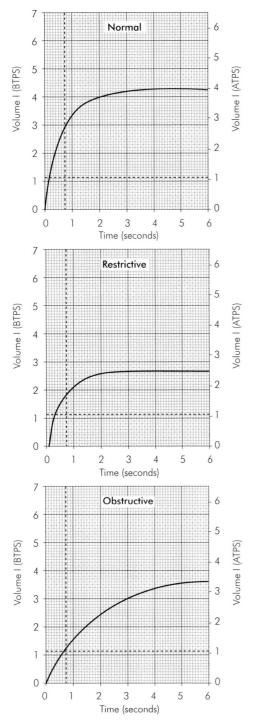

Figure PR7 Spirometric tests in obstructive and restrictive pulmonary disease

bicarbonate is raised, there is either a metabolic alkalosis or metabolic compensation for a respiratory acidosis. If the standard bicarbonate is low, there is a metabolic acidosis or metabolic compensation for a respiratory alkalosis. The base excess is defined as the number of mmol of HCO_3^- which must be added to (or removed from) each litre of ECF to return the ECF pH to 7.4, if the PCO_2 were normal. A negative base excess (a base deficit) indicates metabolic acidosis, so is found with a low standard bicarbonate, and a positive base excess, which is found with a raised standard bicarbonate, indicates metabolic alkalosis. Finally, the PO_2 should be examined. A low PO_2 indicates hypoxaemia and a raised PO_2 indicates that the patient is receiving additional oxygen.

Cardiovascular disease
Hypertension

Hypertension occurs in 15% of the UK population. Although mean systemic diastolic and systolic arterial pressure rise with increasing age, hypertension is defined by arbitrarily set levels (Figure PR8). In 97% of these patients the cause is unknown, and they are said to have 'essential' or primary hypertension. In the remaining 3% hypertension is secondary to renal or endocrine disease, coarctation of the aorta, drugs or pregnancy. It is important that hypertension is adequately controlled preoperatively.

Whilst degree of hypertension is traditionally defined in terms of diastolic blood pressure, the problem of isolated systolic hypertension is a topic currently receiving much

Degree of hypertension	Diastolic pressure (mmHg)	Prognosis with anaesthesia
Mild	90–104	No evidence that treatment makes any difference to outcome
Moderate	105–114	Not really looked at but presumably increased risk, particularly if evidence of end organ damage
Severe	>114	Probably increased risk of ischaemia, arrhythmia and poor outcome: therefore cancel and treat

Figure PR8 Degrees of hypertension and relevance to anaesthesia

interest. Isolated systolic hypertension is most prevalent in the elderly population and is a significant risk factor for stroke as well as cardiovascular morbidity in this group.

The pathogenesis of primary hypertension is not understood, but it is known that systemic vascular resistance is increased, leading to a possible decrease in cardiac output by 15–20%. Additionally, the level of sympathetic nervous system activity is high, resulting in a greater than normal response to any stimulus. In a hypertensive patient there is a much greater fall than normal in systemic arterial pressure on induction of anaesthesia due to a fall in cardiac output resulting from decreases in both heart rate and stroke volume. This exaggerated fall is lessened in controlled hypertension. Importantly, there is an increased risk of postoperative myocardial infarction in hypertensive patients. Hypertension is associated with other diseases of relevance to the anaesthetist such as ischaemic heart disease, peripheral vascular disease (PVD), renal disease, cerebrovascular disease and diabetes mellitus. At preoperative assessment the anaesthetist should look for evidence of any of these conditions and for end organ damage due to hypertension. An ECG may reveal left ventricular hypertrophy (LVH) or ischaemic heart disease. Serum urea, electrolytes and creatinine may reveal renal impairment, and serum glucose may show diabetes. Chest x ray may reveal left ventricular enlargement, and distended upper pulmonary lobe veins indicate left ventricular failure. In advanced failure there is generalised hazy opacification spreading out from the hilum and possibly Kerley 'B' lines or pleural effusions.

Drug treatment

Usual antihypertensive therapy should be continued on the day of surgery. Antihypertensive agents tend to potentiate the hypotensive effects of general anaesthesia. Thiazide diuretics are a common first-line treatment for hypertension, particularly in the elderly. Thiazide treatment can often result in hypokalaemia or hyponatraemia. Beta-adrenergic antagonists are frequently employed in conjunction with a thiazide. Despite their advantages during anaesthesia (depression of the cardiovascular response to laryngoscopy and to surgical stimulation), beta-blockers may cause problems: bradycardia, atrioventricular block, decreased myocardial contractility, bronchoconstriction and altered response to inotropes. If beta-blockers are stopped preoperatively, hypertension, arrhythmias and myocardial ischaemia are increased intraoperatively, as is postoperative myocardial ischaemia. Calcium channel antagonists are also prescribed for hypertension. Diltiazem and verapamil may cause bradycardia.

Angiotensin-converting enzyme (ACE) inhibitors are also used for the treatment of cardiac failure, and these agents are associated with hypotension and hyperkalaemia. Drugs more recently introduced for the treatment of hypertension include angiotensin II type 1 receptor antagonists and imidazoline receptor antagonists.

Sedative premedication is often prescribed for hypertensive patients to reduce endogenous catecholamine levels that may exacerbate the hypertension.

Ischaemic heart disease (IHD)

In the UK 12–20% of patients undergoing surgery have preoperative evidence of myocardial disease. This is almost always due to atheroma, although rarely other disease processes may be responsible. With increasing age atheromatous plaques form in the intima of arteries. These plaques grow and evolve with time, decreasing blood flow through a vessel and possibly occluding it. The rate of progression of individual plaques within any patient is variable, and this explains why, although peripheral vascular and cerebrovascular disease will often coexist with coronary artery disease, the patient may be asymptomatic of these other conditions.

IHD may be diagnosed from a history of angina or myocardial infarction (MI). It may also be the underlying cause of a conduction defect or arrhythmia. A guide to the severity of angina is the exertion necessary to precipitate an attack. The distance that is regularly walked on the flat before an attack occurs should be elicited in the history. It may be that angina is only occasional, such as when climbing more than one flight of stairs or in very cold weather. If angina is precipitated by minimal exertion or is even occurring at rest (unstable angina), the patient has severe myocardial insufficiency and anaesthesia may present problems. If elective surgery is proposed, this should be cancelled and the patient investigated further with a view to cardiac intervention. It is important to establish the timing of any previous MI. Perioperative MI has a mortality of up to 70%. The risk of perioperative MI is 0.1–0.2% when there is no history of previous MI. The overall risk of reinfarction with a history of previous MI is 6–7%, this varying in relation to the time elapsed since that MI. The introduction of thrombolysis has reduced the reinfarction rate.

The progressive, episodic nature of IHD has led many workers to attempt to make predictions about the postoperative risk of cardiac complications following major non-cardiac surgery.

Perioperative assessment of cardiac risk

The Goldman cardiac risk index was one of the earlier multifactorial scoring systems designed to predict clinical risk. There have been a number of modifications, notably by Detsky *et al.* (1986), but despite such modifications and the introduction of alternative scoring systems, overall predictive accuracy has remained disappointingly limited.

However, much of the work supports the likelihood that certain factors consistently reduce perioperative cardiac morbidity and mortality. These include preoperative optimisation of cardiac status, aggressive invasive monitoring and prompt treatment of intraoperative haemodynamic disturbance.

The modified cardiac risk index has proved useful in the development of guidelines for the preoperative assessment of patients with ischaemic heart disease. In 1996 the American College of Cardiology (ACC) and the American Heart Association (AHA) introduced guidelines for the evaluation of perioperative cardiac risk in patients undergoing non-cardiac surgery. These guidelines were updated in 2002 and consider clinical factors, functional capacity and the nature of the proposed surgery when evaluating patients preoperatively. Clinical predictors of perioperative cardiac risk include cardiac and non-cardiac factors, stratified as major, intermediate and minor (Figure PR9). A functional capacity of less than 4 MET (unable to climb a flight of stairs) is associated with increased cardiac risk. Surgery-specific risk is considered in terms of type of non-cardiac surgery and the anticipated degree of haemodynamic stress associated with the planned procedure (Figure PR10). Cardiovascular risk is defined in terms of myocardial infarction, heart failure and death. An algorithmic process is used to identify patients who might benefit from further investigation (such as echocardiography and radionuclide scanning) or therapeutic intervention.

These guidelines have enabled us to move away from the previously quoted intervals of 3 and 6 months' delay when considering perioperative risk following MI. Indeed, some patients would now be considered for elective surgery within 1 month of an MI. In other words, patients with cardiac disease awaiting elective surgery can be considered on a more individual basis with respect to their perioperative risk.

The electrocardiogram

A 12-lead ECG is essential in males aged >45 years, females aged >55 years, diabetics aged >40 years and in all patients

Major
- Unstable coronary syndromes
  - Acute or recent myocardial infarction with evidence of important ischaemic risk by clinical symptoms or non-invasive study
  - Unstable or severe angina (Canadian class III or IV)
- Decompensated heart failure
- Significant arrhythmias
  - High grade atrioventricular block
  - Symptomatic ventricular arrhythmias in the presence of underlying heart disease
  - Supraventricular arrhythmias with uncontrolled ventricular rate
- Severe valvular disease

Intermediate
- Mild angina pectoris (Canadian class I or II)
- Previous myocardial infarction by history or pathological Q waves
- Compensated or prior heart failure
- Diabetes mellitus (particularly insulin-dependent)
- Renal insufficiency

Minor
- Advanced age
- Abnormal ECG (left ventricular hypertrophy, left bundle branch block, ST–T abnormalities)
- Rhythm other than sinus (e.g. atrial fibrillation)
- Low functional capacity (inability to climb one flight of stairs)
- History of stroke
- Uncontrolled systemic hypertension

ACC/AHA Guideline Update for Perioperative Cardiovascular Evaluation for Noncardiac Surgery: executive summary. *Anesth Analg* 2002; **94**: 1052–64.

Figure PR9 Clinical predictors of increased perioperative cardiovascular risk

with a history suggestive of IHD (Figure PR11). Left axis deviation indicates IHD, while right axis deviation may be normal. Only 50% of old MIs will be seen. An exercise ECG may be indicated in patients in at-risk groups, e.g. those undergoing peripheral vascular surgery, if the resting ECG is normal, there is no LVH and no previous MI. Continuous ambulatory ECG may be useful if the patient's ability to exercise is limited. Although abnormal rhythms may be detected clinically, an ECG is needed to confirm diagnosis. Rate and rhythm should be noted (Figure PR12), and a 24-hour ECG may be useful.

High (cardiac risk often >5%)
- Emergent major operations, particularly in the elderly
- Aortic and other major vascular surgery
- Peripheral vascular surgery
- Anticipated prolonged surgical procedures associated with large fluid shifts and/or blood loss

Intermediate (cardiac risk generally <5%)
- Carotid endarterectomy
- Head and neck surgery
- Intraperitoneal and intrathoracic surgery
- Orthopaedic surgery
- Prostate surgery

Low (cardiac risk generally <1%)
- Endoscopic procedures
- Superficial procedure
- Cataract surgery
- Breast surgery

ACC/AHA Guideline Update for Perioperative Cardiovascular Evaluation for Noncardiac Surgery: executive summary. *Anesth Analg* 2002; **94**: 1052–64.

Figure PR10 Surgery-specific cardiac risk for non-cardiac surgery (combined incidence of cardiac death and nonfatal myocardial infarction)

Conduction abnormalities	Degrees of heart block
	Bundle branch block
Arrhythmias	Multifocal ventricular
	Ectopics
	Episodes of VT or VF
QRS	Presences of Q waves
	Poor R wave progression
ST segment	>1 mm depression
	>2 mm depression
T wave	Isoelectric
	Inverted
	Reverted

Figure PR11 ECG abnormalities associated with myocardial ischaemia

Sinus tachycardia has several common causes such as anxiety, pyrexia, cardiac failure and anaemia. Supraventricular tachycardia may be due to a congenital conduction

Rate	Rhythm	Diagnosis
Normal	Irregular	Multiple ectopics
Fast	Regular	Sinus tachycardia
		Atrial flutter
		Supraventricular tachycardia
Fast	Irregular	Atrial fibrillation
		Atrial flutter with variable block
Slow	Regular	Complete heart block
Fast and slow	Irregular	Sick sinus syndrome

Figure PR12 Diagnosis of arrhythmias

abnormality. IHD is the main cause of the other arrhythmias, although thyroid disease should not be forgotten. Atrial tachyarrhythmias should be controlled preoperatively with digoxin or amiodarone therapy. Complete heart block, any form of bifascicular block and sick sinus syndrome require preoperative pacing. Multifocal ventricular ectopics are more significant than unifocal ectopics, indicating IHD. Atrial ectopics are not usually significant.

Other cardiac investigations

Echocardiography uses ultrasound to study blood flow, the structure of the heart and the movement of valves and cardiac muscle. Ventricular volumes, ejection fraction and gradients across valves can be estimated. The ejection fraction is particularly useful: it is normally over 60%; if it is less than 40% serious problems associated with anaesthesia should be anticipated.

Chest x ray may show cardiomegaly, with a cardiothoracic ratio of >0.5. Seventy per cent of patients with cardiomegaly have an ejection fraction of less than 50%.

Radionucleotide scanning provides a relatively non-invasive means of accurately assessing myocardial function. In blood pool scanning [99]technetium-labelled red blood cells are injected intravenously and then both the amount of blood in the heart at each stage of the cardiac cycle and the shape of the cardiac chambers can be determined. The scanning camera may be linked to ECG and pictures collected over multiple cardiac cycles (multigated or MUGA scans). In perfusion scintigraphy, acute MI may be detected by 'hot spot' scanning. This technique also uses [99]technetium, which is taken up into the acutely infarcted myocardial tissue thus revealing the position and

1st code letter	2nd code letter	3rd code letter	4th code letter	5th code letter
Paced chamber	Sensed chamber	Response to endogenous depolarisation	Programmable functions	Antiarrhythmic function
I	II	III	IV	V
V (ventricle)	V (ventricle)	T (trigger)	P (rate)	S (scanning)
A (atrium)	A (atrium)	I (inhibited)	M (multiprogrammable)	E (externally activated)
D (double)	D (double)	D (double)	C (communicating)	
	O (none)	O (none)	R (rate responsive)	
			B (impulse burst)	
			N (normal rate competition)	
			O (none)	

Figure PR13 Generic pacemaker code

extent of the damage. Conversely, 'cold spot' scanning uses [201]thallium to demonstrate areas of myocardial ischaemia and scarring. [201]Thallium behaves like a potassium ion and is distributed throughout the heart muscle depending on coronary blood flow. It is taken up by normal myocardium, so areas that are not being perfused show on the scan as perfusion defects. A coronary vasodilator, such as dipyridamole, may then be given. A fixed perfusion defect indicates scar tissue while a reperfusion defect indicates ischaemia. Reperfusion defects are more significant because ischaemia may develop perioperatively whereas a fixed perfusion defect cannot deteriorate.

Pacemakers

The need for cardiac pacing results from disease of the conducting system of the heart, which may or may not be associated with general ischaemic heart disease. The most common scenario is that of an elderly patient without associated cardiac conditions.

A variety of pacemakers may be encountered, depending on the age of the unit. Modern pacemakers operate through a lead in the atrium, ventricle or both. Depolarisation arising endogenously may either inhibit or trigger a paced beat. Pacemakers are classified using a five-letter code as in Figure PR13.

As an illustration, an AAI unit paces atrially and will be inhibited by sensing an endogenous depolarisation in the atrium. In contrast a VVT unit paces ventricularly and is triggered if an endogenous depolarisation is sensed in the ventricle.

Most modern units are dual units which work in DDD mode, providing atrial pacing in the presence of atrial bradycardia and ventricular pacing after an atrial depolarisation (endogenous or paced) if a spontaneous ventricular beat is absent.

The characteristics of an implanted pacemaker can sometimes be changed externally, either by application of magnets or by radiofrequency generators. The most usual indication for this is a change of demand to fixed rate. The most modern units require a cautious approach to the use of magnets, which may expose a programmable unit to the risk of being re-set in a variable fashion. All patients who have an implanted pacemaker have a registration card with details of the device (see Figure PR14)

Preoperative assessment should be directed to determining the type of unit and its characteristics. Examination of the cardiovascular system should be undertaken in detail. Chest x ray will help identify the pulse generator siting and lead placement and number. The use of surgical diathermy is associated with various hazards, as detailed below.

Surgical diathermy and pacemakers

Use of surgical diathermy in the presence of an indwelling pacemaker may produce the following problems:
- Ventricular fibrillation: most common when the pacemaker unit is an older type
- Inhibition of demand function
- Unpredictable setting of programmable types
- Asystole
- Unit failure

Coded information recorded at implantation on European Pacemaker Registration Card	Symptom	01–02	unspecified
		03–04	dizziness or syncope
		05	bradycardia
		06	tachycardia
		07–09	miscellaneous conditions
	ECG	01–04	sinus or unspecified
	Rhythm	05–07	second degree AV block
		08–10	complete heart block
		11–21	bundle branch or bifascicular block
	Aetiology	01–03	unspecified
		04–05	idiopathic or ischaemic
		06	post infarction
		07–11	miscellaneous conditions
ECG rhythm	(1) All beats preceded by a pacemaker spike: assume patient is pacemaker-dependent		
	(2) If native rhythm predominates: patient is unlikely to be pacemaker-dependent		
	(3) No evidence of pacemaker activity: magnet may be applied over pulse generator to switch to fixed-rate pacing		
	(4) If pacemaker spike is not followed by P or QRS wave suspect pacemaker malfunction (note: if pacemaker is activated by a magnet to pace at a fixed rate, the spike may fall in the refractory period and fail to stimulate the ventricle)		
Chest x ray	(1) Location of pulse generator		
	(2) Location of leads in atrium, ventricle or both		
	(3) If necessary, pulse generator model can be identified		

Bloomfield and Bowler (1989)

Figure PR14 Preoperative assessment of the pacemaker patient

Recommendations for the use of surgical diathermy in the presence of an indwelling pacemaker unit are as follows:
- Place the indifferent electrode on the same side as the operation and as far from the pacemaker unit as possible.
- Limit the use of diathermy as much as possible.
- Use the lowest current setting possible.
- Use bipolar diathermy (but power of coagulation is less).
- Monitor patient ECG constantly.
- Keep the pacemaker programmer available, where appropriate.

Valvular heart disease
The availability of echocardiography today means that any patient with suspected valve disease should be properly investigated and a diagnosis made prior to anaesthesia.

Valve angioplasty or replacement is sometimes indicated before elective surgery. Unfortunately, patients with significant valve disease may still present for emergency surgery. Any patient with a heart valve lesion, including replacement valves, requires prophylactic antibiotics for dental, genitourinary, obstetric, gynaecological and gastrointestinal procedures. The current recommended regimes are found in the British National Formulary. The main causes of valvular heart disease are shown in Figure PR15. Note that multiple valve lesions may coexist.

Aortic stenosis
The symptoms of aortic stenosis occur late and include angina, syncope, dyspnoea and sudden death. Clinical signs are difficult to assess but generally include plateau pulse, LVH and an aortic ejection systolic murmur which is similar in character to that of aortic sclerosis. The ECG

Valve regurgitation
- Congenital
- Rheumatic fever
- Infective endocarditis
- Syphilitic aortitis
- Valve ring dilatation, e.g. dilated cardiomyopathy
- Traumatic valve rupture
- Senile degeneration
- Damage to chordae and papillary muscles, e.g. MI

Valve stenosis
- Congenital
- Rheumatic fever
- Senile degeneration

Figure PR15 Causes of valvular disease

may show LVH with strain. On chest x ray, left ventricular enlargement may not be evident and the aortic valve may be calcified. Echocardiography determines the gradient across the valve and will provide information on ventricular function. If the valve gradient is greater than 50 mmHg, angioplasty or valve replacement should be considered. The main anaesthesia-related problems are fixed cardiac output, ventricular arrhythmias and incipient cardiac failure.

Aortic regurgitation

Aortic regurgitation gives rise to few symptoms until the left ventricle fails, when dyspnoea occurs. Clinical signs include a collapsing pulse, left ventricular enlargement and an early diastolic murmur. The ECG shows changes of LVH, and on chest x ray the heart will be enlarged. Echocardiography shows a dilated left ventricle and aortic root. Problems with respect to anaesthesia are poor myocardial reserve and cardiac failure.

Mitral stenosis

Symptoms of mitral stenosis are dyspnoea, tiredness and haemoptysis. Clinical signs include malar flush and a mid-diastolic murmur. Mitral stenosis may be complicated by systemic embolism or pulmonary hypertension. The ECG will often demonstrate atrial fibrillation (AF), P mitrale and right ventricular hypertrophy. On chest x ray there may be left atrial enlargement and pulmonary venous congestion. Patients with a small valve area on echocardiography or moderate symptoms need surgery. Specific problems with respect to anaesthesia include fixed cardiac output, pulmonary oedema, AF and anticoagulant therapy.

Mitral regurgitation

Progressive dyspnoea and tiredness are common symptoms of mitral regurgitation. Left ventricular enlargement and a pansystolic murmur are the predominant clinical signs. The ECG shows LVH, P mitrale and atrial fibrillation. Chest x ray demonstrates left-sided enlargement of the heart, particularly atrial enlargement, and indications of pulmonary oedema may be seen. Echocardiography is useful to assess left ventricular function. Specific problems with respect to anaesthesia include pulmonary oedema, AF and anticoagulant therapy.

Tricuspid valve lesions

Tricuspid stenosis is usually associated with mitral and aortic valve disease. Tricuspid regurgitation is usually due to right ventricular enlargement. Anaesthesia-related problems are usually due to the accompanying other valve disease rather than to the tricuspid lesion itself.

Pulmonary valve lesions

Pulmonary stenosis is usually congenital, and may be part of Fallot's tetralogy. Pulmonary regurgitation is rare, and most often secondary to pulmonary hypertension.

Haematological disease
Anaemia

A patient is considered anaemic if the haemoglobin is below the normal range and polycythaemic if it is above the normal range. For adult females this is $12–16$ g dl^{-1} and for adult males $13–17$ g dl^{-1}. In children the range varies: a child is considered to be anaemic if the haemoglobin value is less than 18 g dl^{-1} at birth, less than 9 g dl^{-1} at 3 months, less than 11 g dl^{-1} from 6 months to 6 years and less than 12 g dl^{-1} from 6 to 12 years.

The causes of anaemia are blood loss, inadequate production of erythrocytes and excessive destruction of erythrocytes. Anaemia may be classified by the mean cell volume of the erythrocyte (MCV) (Figure PR16). The mean cell haemoglobin (MCH) is also useful, and defines hypo- and normochromic types of anaemia.

Iron deficiency is the most common cause of anaemia, but the cause is often multifactorial. Those patients in whom anaemia should be suspected include all females of child-bearing age (due to menstrual loss), the elderly (due to poor diet and other diseases) and all patients who are undergoing gastrointestinal or gynaecological surgery (due to blood loss). Most patients suffering from anaemia are completely asymptomatic. If severely anaemic,

MCV	Cause
Microcytic	Iron deficiency (hypochromic)
	Thalassaemia (hypochromic)
	Chronic disease
Normocytic	Chronic disease (normochromic or hypochromic)
	Mixed deficiency
	Acute blood loss (normochromic)
Macrocytic	Alcohol (normochromic)
	B_{12} or folate deficiency (normochromic)
	Pregnancy
	Hypothyroidism (normochromic)
	Low-grade haemolytic anaemia with high reticulocyte count

Figure PR16 A classification of anaemia

symptoms may include tiredness and dyspnoea on exertion, and in the elderly angina, heart failure and confusion may be precipitated.

A full blood count also provides the platelet count (raised in acute blood loss and acute inflammation) and the white cell count (raised in infection). A differential white cell count distinguishes between neutrophilia (bacterial infection, inflammation) and lymphocytosis (viral infection). If the platelet count, white cell count and haemoglobin are all low, this indicates marrow aplasia or infiltration. Abnormalities which may be detected on examination of the blood film include a raised reticulocyte count (haemolytic anaemia, continued bleeding), sickle cells or malarial parasites. Further investigation may be indicated prior to blood transfusion, e.g. additional blood tests (ferritin, vitamin B_{12}, folate, reticulocyte count, direct Coombs test) or bone marrow aspiration.

Of most relevance to anaesthesia is a decrease in the oxygen-carrying capacity of the blood. Although anaemia decreases blood viscosity and hence improves blood flow, with a consequent increase in oxygen delivery to the tissues, once the haemoglobin is less than 10 g dl^{-1} the increase in blood flow no longer compensates for the decreased oxygen-carrying capacity. Some authorities consider a haemoglobin value of greater than 8 g dl^{-1}, rather than 10 g dl^{-1}, acceptable for anaesthesia.

A secondary anaemia-related problem is the fact that cardiac output increases in order to maintain oxygen flux.

In some patients this leads to cardiac failure and in all cardiac reserve is decreased, reducing the ability to compensate for the myocardial depressant effects of anaesthesia. It is important to remember that cyanosis is only evident clinically when the level of deoxyhaemoglobin equals or exceeds 5 g dl^{-1}. Hence in severely anaemic patients cyanosis is rarely seen.

In patients with chronic anaemia, there is an increase in 2,3-diphosphoglycerate (2,3-DPG) concentration in the reticulocytes which causes the oxygen dissociation curve to shift to the right, improving the offloading of oxygen in the tissues. Stored blood contains decreased levels of 2,3-DPG, which take 24 hours to reach normal levels following transfusion. Hence blood transfusion in an anaemic patient immediately prior to anaesthesia confers minimal advantage and may lead to fluid overload. For elective surgery, transfusion should be completed at least 24 hours earlier.

In patients who are acutely anaemic (for example due to recent blood loss), heart rate, arterial pressure, CVP and urine output should be closely monitored during fluid replacement to ensure normovolaemia is restored prior to anaesthesia. Blood should be transfused to achieve a haemoglobin of greater than 10 g dl^{-1} and a haematocrit of greater than 0.3. Administration of oxygen therapy will increase oxygen delivery by ensuring maximal saturation of the available haemoglobin and an increase in the dissolved oxygen in blood. Urgent surgery may be indicated to stop the bleeding, so resuscitation may need to be continued during anaesthesia and surgery.

Sickle cell disease
Sickle cell disease is due to a haemoglobinopathy which is inherited autosomally, resulting in the formation of haemoglobin S (HbS) instead of haemoglobin A (HbA). The S variant consists of two normal α chains and two abnormal β chains in which glutamic acid has been substituted by valine in the sixth amino acid from the N-terminal. Small decreases in oxygen tension cause HbS to polymerise and form pseudo-crystalline structures which distort the red blood cell membrane to produce the characteristic sickle-shaped cells. Sickled cells increase blood viscosity and obstruct blood flow in the microvasculature, leading to thrombosis and infarction. These sickled cells are also subject to abnormal sequestration. Patients homozygous for another haemoglobinopathy, HbC, suffer minimal morbidity, but patients heterozygous for HbS and HbC (haemoglobin SC disease) suffer from a mild form of sickle cell anaemia as the presence of HbC causes the HbS to sickle more easily.

Sickle cell anaemia results from a patient being homozygous for haemoglobin S. Sickle cell trait results from a patient being heterozygous for haemoglobin S. Patients with sickle cell trait are resistant to falciparum malaria, and it is in those areas of the world where falciparum malaria is endemic that the gene is particularly common: tropical Africa, north-east Saudi Arabia, east central India and around the Mediterranean. The prevalence of HbSS in the UK black population is around 0.25%, and the prevalence of HbAS in the same population is around 10%.

The main clinical problems for patients suffering from sickle cell anaemia are chronic haemolytic anaemia and infarction crises. Infarction crises may be precipitated by dehydration, infection, hypoxia, acidosis or cold, although they may also occur spontaneously. Crises are very painful, often involving bones or the spleen, and may also cause cerebrovascular accidents, haematuria due to renal papillary necrosis and chest pain due to pulmonary infarction. Patients with sickle cell trait have a normal haemoglobin and are clinically well. Most of their red blood cells contain less than 50% HbS, and sickling occurs only when the oxygen tension is very low.

Preoperatively all patients in the at-risk population for HbS should be screened. A Sickledex test detects the presence of HbS by precipitating sickling of the red blood cells on exposure to sodium metabisulphite. If this test is positive then electrophoresis is necessary to distinguish between the heterozygote and the homozygote. In an emergency situation, if the Sickledex test is positive but there is no history to suggest sickle cell anaemia and the haemoglobin, the reticulocyte count and the blood film are normal, then it is safe to assume that the patient has the trait only. Haematological advice should always be sought for patients with sickle cell anaemia. Evidence of renal, pulmonary or cerebrovascular complications should be assessed preoperatively. Blood transfusion prior to elective surgery may be indicated if the anaemia is particularly severe, and exchange transfusion will be necessary prior to major surgery to reduce the concentration of HbS to around 40%. An intravenous infusion should always be set up preoperatively to avoid dehydration, and heavy premedication should be avoided. Depending on the type of surgery planned, the surgeon should be sufficiently experienced to proceed without the use of a tourniquet, as its use is contraindicated in both the homozygote and the heterozygote.

Clotting abnormalities

If a patient has a history of liver disease or bleeding problems, or is taking anticoagulants, a clotting screen is indicated. Clotting may also be abnormal after massive blood transfusion or in pregnancy-induced hypertension. The activated partial thromboplastin time (APTT) measures factors VIII, IX, XI and XII in the intrinsic system. It is prolonged by warfarin therapy and liver disease. In contrast the prothrombin time (PT) measures factors I, II, VII and X in the extrinsic system and is prolonged by heparin therapy and in dilutional coagulopathy. The international normalised ratio (INR) is the ratio of the PT sample time to control time, a widely used indicator of clotting function. An INR of <2.0 is considered safe for most surgery.

Coagulation abnormalities due to liver disease should be corrected by vitamin K administration. The effects of warfarin should be temporarily reversed by fresh frozen plasma (FFP), not by vitamin K, which will prevent the recommencement of warfarin therapy. Heparin coagulopathy is corrected by stopping the heparin or, more urgently, by protamine. FFP is required to correct a dilutional coagulopathy, as may occur with massive blood transfusion.

Disseminated intravascular coagulation (DIC) is indicated by decreased platelets, increased fibrin degradation products, decreased fibrinogen and prolonged APTT and PT. The underlying cause should be identified and treated, and clotting corrected with FFP (or cryoprecipitate) and platelet transfusion.

Thrombocytopenia may be asymptomatic, but haematological advice should be sought and platelets are usually given to ensure a platelet count above 50×10^9. For specific factor deficiencies, such as haemophilia, the purified factor or FFP should be given immediately preoperatively.

Musculoskeletal disease

Although many musculoskeletal conditions may be encountered prior to anaesthesia and surgery, by far the most common of these is rheumatoid arthritis.

Rheumatoid arthritis

Rheumatoid arthritis is an autoimmune connective tissue disease. The dominant pathological feature is a chronic, destructive synovitis, which causes an inflammatory, typically symmetrical, deforming polyarthritis. Rheumatoid arthritis has many extra-articular features, which greatly influence the morbidity and mortality of the disease (Figure PR17). Approximately 70% of patients are positive for rheumatoid factor, which is a circulating IgM antibody to the patient's own IgG. The overall prevalence is approximately 1%, with a male to female ratio of 1 : 3. Over the age of 55 years 5% of women and 2% of men are affected.

Respiratory	Fibrosing alveolitis, pleural effusion, rheumatoid nodules, bronchiolitis, Caplan's syndrome
Cardiovascular	Pericarditis, pericardial effusion, vasculitis, heart block, cardiomyopathy, aortic regurgitation
Renal	Amyloidosis (may affect other systems), drug-induced
Neurological	Cervical cord compression, peripheral neuropathy, entrapment neuropathy, mononeuritis multiplex
Haematological	Anaemia of chronic disease, iron-deficiency anaemia (NSAIDs), marrow suppression (gold), thrombocytosis, Felty's syndrome
Ocular	Keratoconjunctivitis sicca, scleritis, episcleritis, scleromalacia perforans

Figure PR17 Extra-articular features of rheumatoid arthritis

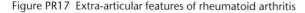

Rheumatoid arthritis is necessarily associated with a large number of drug-induced complications. Non-steroidal anti-inflammatory drugs (NSAIDs) are commonly used to treat pain and stiffness and may cause gastric erosions. The disease-modifying drugs used in the management of rheumatoid arthritis can similarly be associated with serious side effects. **Chloroquine** may cause haemolytic anaemia and ocular problems. **Sulphasalazine** rarely causes megaloblastic anaemia or hepatitis. **Oral gold** is less likely to cause marrow suppression or proteinuria than intramuscular gold. **Methotrexate** may cause marrow suppression or abnormal liver function. Although **penicillamine** may cause the nephrotic syndrome, it is also associated (rarely) with generalised marrow suppression and conditions which mimic myasthenia gravis or systemic lupus erythematosus. Some patients will be receiving systemic steroids for their disease and others may be taking immunosuppressant drugs.

Rheumatoid arthritis most commonly affects the joints of the hands and feet, but the larger joints of the hips, knees and elbows may also be involved. Twenty-five per cent of patients with rheumatoid arthritis have cervical instability. Not all will have longstanding disease and a quarter will have no clinical signs of cervical cord compression. The most common cervical problem is atlantoaxial subluxation, although subaxial subluxation may also occur. The atlantoaxial ligaments become lax and the odontoid peg is eroded, making neck flexion dangerous by risking cord

compression. Also of interest to the anaesthetist are limited mouth opening due to temporomandibular joint involvement and, rarely, airway obstruction due to dislocation of the cricoarytenoid joints. A hoarse voice suggests cricoarytenoid arthritis. Respiratory function may be additionally impaired by costochondrial joint disease, which can add to any restrictive defect.

It is therefore important to carefully assess the rheumatoid patient preoperatively for evidence of extra-articular involvement. A full blood count is essential and, if the patient is taking any disease-modifying drugs, serum electrolytes, urea and creatinine and liver function tests will also be necessary. Chest x ray and pulmonary function tests may be indicated. Neck mobility and mouth opening should be assessed clinically. A lateral x ray of the cervical spine in flexion and extension must be performed. If the gap between the odontoid peg and the posterior border of the anterior arch of the atlas is >3 mm (or >4 mm in those aged over 40 years), subluxation is present. Care should be taken when asking the patient to attempt maximal flexion of the cervical spine. Awake intubation may be indicated if a difficult intubation is anticipated, and if there is cervical spine involvement it will be necessary for the patient to wear a semi-rigid collar during anaesthesia to ensure perioperative cervical stability. If there is evidence of severe cervical spine instability, it is appropriate to refer the patient for surgical stabilisation.

Renal disease
Renal failure
Renal disease covers a wide spectrum of clinical pictures from decreased renal reserve, through varying degrees of renal impairment to end-stage renal failure. Up to 80% of excretory function may be lost before a rise in serum urea or creatinine is seen. The creatinine value gives a useful indication of the degree of renal failure. The corresponding urea value is more readily affected by dietary protein, tissue breakdown and hydration and is therefore less useful. The cause of renal impairment or failure is very relevant to anaesthesia because the underlying disease process may have other manifestations. Renal failure may be acute or chronic (Figure PR18).

The majority of renal patients presenting for anaesthesia will have chronic renal failure and most will be on a dialysis programme, involving either intermittent haemodialysis (HD) or continuous ambulatory peritoneal dialysis (CAPD). At preoperative assessment, the anaesthetist should establish the cause of renal failure and look for evidence of other systems affected by the same

Chronic renal failure
- Diabetic nephropathy
- Hypertensive nephropathy
- Chronic urinary tract obstruction
- Chronic glomerulonephritis
- Polycystic kidney disease
- Chronic bilateral pyelonephritis
- Collagen diseases
- Persisting acute renal failure

Acute renal failure
- Pre-renal
  - Severe hypotension (hypovolaemia, cardiac failure, septic shock, drug overdose)
  - Major vessel disease (thrombosis, aortic aneurysm)
  - Intravascular haemolysis
  - Rhabdomyolysis
- Renal
  - Acute tubular necrosis (acute ischaemia, drugs, bacterial endotoxins)
  - Vasculitis
  - Acute glomerulonephritis
  - Acute interstitial nephritis
  - Coagulopathies
  - Eclampsia
- Post-renal
  - Urinary tract obstruction (prostatic hypertrophy, renal or ureteric stones, surgical mishap)

Figure PR18 Causes of chronic and acute renal failure

Cardiovascular
- Premature atheroma
- Hypertension
- Left ventricular failure
- Pericardial effusions

Respiratory
- Pulmonary venous congestion or oedema
- Pneumonia

Haematological
- Normochromic normocytic anaemia
- Prolonged bleeding time due to platelet dysfunction
- Increased incidence of hepatitis B carriage

Gastrointestinal
- Delayed gastric emptying
- Increased gastric acidity
- Peptic ulceration
- Impaired liver function

Neurological
- Peripheral and autonomic neuropathies
- Encephalopathy

Biochemical
- Metabolic acidosis with compensatory respiratory alkalosis
- Hyperkalaemia
- Hypocalcaemia
- Hypoalbuminaemia

Figure PR19 Systemic effects of renal failure

disease process. Renal failure affects all systems of the body (Figure PR19).

Necessary investigations include urea and electrolytes, creatinine, full blood count, clotting screen, liver function tests and hepatitis B surface antigen. Chest x ray and ECG are also required. In evaluating the renal failure patient for anaesthesia, particular reference should be made to the fluid status. Twenty-four hours post-haemodialysis is the optimal time for elective surgery. Immediately following HD a patient may be volume-depleted. CAPD has far less effect on circulating volume and may be continued until surgery. Most patients will be chronically anaemic, but if asymptomatic and with no evidence of cardiovascular disease blood transfusion will probably not be necessary. Transfusion may precipitate fluid overload, and should be undertaken prior to or during the last HD before anaesthesia. Hypertension should be controlled and fluid balance

optimised. Acidosis and hyperkalaemia must be corrected by dialysis. The site of any arteriovenous fistula should be noted and arrangements made for it to be protected perioperatively by wrapping in gamgee. The limb with the fistula should **never** be used for intravenous access.

Endocrine disease

Patients suffering from endocrine disease should have their condition stabilised by consultation (where time allows) with the responsible physician. The most frequently encountered endocrine disease in surgical practice is diabetes mellitus, which is considered in more detail below and in Section 1, Chapter 5.

Diabetes mellitus

Diabetes mellitus is characterised by a persisting state of hyperglycaemia due to lack or diminished effectiveness of

	Primary	Secondary
Type I	Insulin-dependent diabetes mellitus	Pancreatic disease, e.g. pancreatitis, pancreatectomy, neoplastic disease, cystic fibrosis
Type II	Non-insulin-dependent diabetes mellitus	Excess production of insulin antagonists, e.g. growth hormone (acromegaly), glucocorticoids (Cushing's syndrome), thyroid hormones, catecholamines (phaeochromocytoma)
		Drugs, e.g. corticosteroids, thiazides
		Liver disease

Figure PR20 Classification of diabetes mellitus

endogenous insulin. It presents problems to the anaesthetist both in respect of the need to ensure adequate perioperative control of blood glucose and in respect of the known long-term complications of the condition. Diabetes mellitus may be classified as primary or secondary (Figure PR20). There are two types of primary diabetes mellitus: insulin-dependent diabetes mellitus (IDDM or type I) and non-insulin-dependent diabetes mellitus (NIDDM or type II). The prevalence in the UK is 2%, with a ratio of NIDDM : IDDM of 7 : 3. The aetiology of diabetes mellitus remains unclear, but it is known to be the result of environmental factors interacting with genetic factors. IDDM usually presents before the age of 40 years and NIDDM usually presents after the age of 50 years.

Glycosuria which has been detected on routine urine testing performed preoperatively may often be the first indication that a patient has diabetes. As there is individual variation in the renal threshold for glucose, diagnosis should be confirmed by examining blood glucose. The diagnosis of diabetes mellitus may be made from a random blood glucose of >11.1 mmol l^{-1} or a fasting blood glucose of >7.8 mmol l^{-1}. If the patient is a known diabetic, control may be assessed from the patient's diary of the results of home testing of blood glucose. Single random blood glucose estimations are of little value, although measurement of glycosylated haemoglobin is more useful,

reflecting blood glucose control over the previous 6–8 weeks.

The long-term complications of diabetes are equally likely in both IDDM and NIDDM, and are related to the duration of the disease and the effectiveness of blood sugar control. Complications are due to disease of both large blood vessels (atheroma) and small blood vessels (microangiopathy). Atheroma causes the same pathological changes as in non-diabetic patients, but the disease occurs earlier and is both more extensive and more severe. Atheroma is the cause of the increased incidence of IHD and PVD in diabetics. Diabetic microangiopathy is the cause of diabetic nephropathy, retinopathy and neuropathy. Diabetes is a common cause of autonomic neuropathy, which can be detected at the bedside by demonstrating postural hypotension. Diabetic patients frequently present for surgery for the complications of their disease, and preoperative assessment must include screening for evidence of other complications. An ECG and other cardiac investigations may be indicated. Serum urea, electrolytes and creatinine should be performed to assess renal function.

The management of approximately 50% of diabetics is by diet alone, while 20–30% require diet and an oral hypoglycaemic drug and 20–30% require diet and insulin. Oral hypoglycaemic agents fall into two groups, both of which depend on the presence of some endogenous insulin. **Sulphonylureas** act by augmenting insulin secretion and may also alter peripheral insulin receptor number and sensitivity. The commonly used sulphonylureas include glibenclamide, gliclazide and tolazamide. These drugs should be omitted on the day of surgery because of the risk of perioperative hypoglycaemia. Glibenclamide should be stopped 24 hours prior to surgery, and chlorpropamide 48 hours prior to surgery, because of their prolonged durations of action. In all cases blood sugar should be carefully monitored perioperatively.

The second group of oral hypoglycaemic agents are the **biguanides**. Metformin is the only available biguanide, and is often used in conjunction with a sulphonylurea. It enhances the peripheral action of insulin. Hypoglycaemia is very unusual with metformin, although it may cause lactic acidosis. Biguanide therapy should be stopped on the morning of surgery and blood glucose concentration monitored. Surgery itself is a cause of stress resulting in increased secretion of the catabolic hormones (cortisol, growth hormone and glucagon), which results in increased catabolism and may lead to diabetic ketoacidosis in both NIDDM and IDDM. Thus, NIDDM patients who are undergoing major surgery will require insulin in the perioperative period, and IDDM patients will experience an increase in their insulin requirements.

The two main types of insulin preparation are unmodified, rapid-onset, short-acting (soluble) insulin and modified, delayed-onset, intermediate- or long-acting insulin. The insulin regime used varies from patient to patient but involves a combination of short- and longer-acting insulins injected before meals and at bedtime. It is important to remember that IDDM patients need insulin even when they are being starved. Soluble insulin is the only form which can be given intravenously as well as subcutaneously, and it is used for perioperative control of blood glucose. The management of diabetic patients presenting for surgery is covered in Section 1, Chapter 5.

Concurrent medication

Concurrent medication may interact with drugs administered during anaesthesia. Furthermore, the surgical procedure itself may be affected by, or indeed affect, such medication. For this reason it is important that careful consideration is given to preoperative drug management. Medication may have to be continued, stopped or modified. Alternatively, anaesthetic technique may have to be modified to minimise the risk of adverse interaction. A change in mode of administration or formulation is sometimes required.

Examples of drugs that should be continued are anticonvulsants, most cardiovascular drugs (antihypertensives, antianginals, antiarrhythmics), bronchodilators, corticosteroids and antiparkinsonian drugs. All are important in terms of providing optimal control of underlying conditions.

It is seldom necessary to stop drugs preoperatively, but a number of possible exceptions are worthy of discussion. **Warfarin** should be stopped several days preoperatively and the patient heparinised. To minimise the risk of thromboembolism **oral contraceptives** and **hormone replacement therapy** are often stopped several weeks before surgery. **Lithium therapy** should be stopped 24 hours before surgery. Most drugs that have been stopped preoperatively can be restarted when oral intake resumes. Should this be delayed, alternative routes of administration may have to be sought.

Corticosteroids. It is occasionally necessary to modify dose and formulation of a drug perioperatively, as is the case with corticosteroid therapy. Adrenal suppression has not been reported with prednisolone doses below 5 mg daily. Patients on higher doses undergoing major surgery will require additional corticosteroid support administered as intravenous hydrocortisone.

Monoamine oxidase inhibitors (MAOI) irreversibly inhibit monoamine oxidase. Stopping these drugs 3 weeks prior to anaesthesia, to allow resynthesis of the enzyme, is no longer considered necessary, but anaesthetic technique may need to be modified. MAOIs interact with opioids, particularly pethidine, to cause cardiovascular and cerebrovascular excitation (hypertension, tachycardia, convulsions) or depression (hypotension, hypoventilation, coma). Hypertensive crises may be precipitated by sympathomimetic agents.

Tricyclic antidepressants competitively block norepinephrine reuptake by postganglionic sympathetic nerve endings. Patients taking these drugs are hence more sensitive to catecholamines, so sympathomimetics may cause hypertension and arrhythmias. Under the influence of anaesthesia arrhythmias and hypotension may be seen.

Low molecular weight heparins (LMWH) used in thromboprophylaxis must be considered when central nerve blockade is planned during anaesthesia. To minimise the risk of vertebral canal haematoma a period of at least 12 hours should elapse between administration of an LMWH and epidural or spinal anaesthesia. Similarly, heparin administration should be delayed for a period of 6 hours following central nerve blockade.

Platelet antagonists such as NSAIDs and aspirin may be stopped in certain circumstances, usually when there is a risk of excessive bleeding. Increasingly, patients with cardiac and peripheral or cerebral vascular disease present for surgery whilst taking clopidogrel, a potent platelet antagonist. This must be noted at preoperative assessment, as withdrawal is frequently required prior to anaesthesia and surgery. Anaesthetic risk relates mainly to regional anaesthetic techniques and the possibility of vertebral canal haematoma following epidural or spinal anaesthesia.

Whilst platelet antagonists should generally be stopped at least seven days before elective surgery, the underlying reason for their use must be considered. This is particularly the case for patients taking clopidogrel following percutaneous coronary artery stenting within the last 12 months. In such a case elective surgery should ideally be postponed. When this is not possible, advice should be sought from a cardiologist.

Herbal medicines have enjoyed an enormous increase in popularity recently. These drugs may not be declared by patients and should be actively sought at preoperative assessment. A number of such drugs are associated with complications such as bleeding, stroke and myocardial infarction, as well as interaction with more conventional drugs.

Garlic is a platelet inhibitor with potentially beneficial effects on blood pressure as well as serum lipid and cholesterol levels. There may be increased bleeding risk particularly if taken along with more conventional platelet antagonists. Patients should be advised to discontinue garlic for 7 days preoperatively.

Ginseng may be taken to counteract stress. The active components appear to have some effects similar to steroid hormones. The drug's ability to lower blood sugar makes hypoglycaemia a potential problem perioperatively. Ginseng may also have an anticoagulant effect. It should be discontinued for 7 days preoperatively.

St John's wort may be used in the treatment of mild to moderate depression. Effects are believed to be mediated by hypericin and hyperforin and result in the inhibition of serotonin, norepinephrine and dopamine reuptake. A central serotonin syndrome can be precipitated, characterised by autonomic, neuromuscular and cognitive effects. Enzyme induction is an important feature of this drug and may affect many of the drugs used during anaesthesia. It should be discontinued for 7 days preoperatively.

Valerian is readily available as a sedative drug and is commonly found in 'herbal sleep remedies'. This drug may potentiate the sedative effects of anaesthetic drugs. This effect is believed to be GABA-mediated. Physical dependence can occur, and so abrupt discontinuation is not recommended. Postoperative withdrawal symptoms can be treated with benzodiazepines.

Concurrent surgical disease
Intestinal obstruction

Patients with intestinal obstruction often have electrolyte disturbances due to vomiting or, if incomplete obstruction, diarrhoea. They may have been ill at home for several days and unable to take their usual medication for any concurrent medical condition. These patients may be dehydrated and possibly hypovolaemic due to gastrointestinal losses or to third space losses into the gut. Inappropriate intravenous fluid therapy on a surgical ward may have exacerbated the problems. Abdominal distension splints the diaphragm and decreases respiratory reserves. If longstanding, a chest infection may have developed. Fluid and electrolyte disturbances should be corrected prior to theatre, and preoperative chest physiotherapy may be useful. A nasogastric tube should be inserted before induction of anaesthesia in an attempt to empty the stomach and decrease the risk of perioperative regurgitation and aspiration.

Acute abdominal emergencies

All patients with an acute abdomen from whatever cause are at increased risk of regurgitation of stomach contents, and so a nasogastric tube should be inserted prior to theatre. Patients with testicular problems, e.g. torsion, should be included in this category because of the abdominal origin of the nerve supply of the testis.

References and further reading

ACC/AHA Guideline Update for Perioperative Cardiovascular Evaluation for Noncardiac Surgery: executive summary. *Anesth Analg* 2002; **94**: 1052–64.

American College of Physicians. Guidelines for assessing and managing the perioperative risk from coronary artery disease associated with major noncardiac surgery. *Ann Intern Med* 1997; **127**: 309–28.

Ang-Lee MK, Moss J, Yuan C. Herbal medicines and perioperative care. *JAMA* 2001; **286**: 208–16.

Bloomfield P, Bowler GMR. Anaesthetic management of the patient with a permanent pacemaker. *Anaesthesia* 1989; **44**: 42–6.

Cormack RS, Lehane J. Difficult tracheal intubation in obstetrics. *Anaesthesia* 1984; **39**: 1105–11.

Detsky AS, Abrams HB, Forbath N, Scott JG, Hilliard JR. Cardiac assessment for patients undergoing noncardiac surgery: a multifactorial clinical risk index. *Arch Intern Med* 1986; **146**: 2131–4.

Goldman L, Caldera DL, Nussbaum SR, *et al.* Multifactorial index of cardiac risk in noncardiac surgical procedures. *N Engl J Med* 1977; **297**: 845–50.

Gupta S, Sharma R, Jain D. Airway assessment: predictors of difficult airway. *Indian J Anaesth* 2005; **49**: 257–62.

Hlatky MA, Boineau RE, Higginbotham MB, *et al.* A brief-self administered questionnaire to determine functional capacity (the Duke Activity Status Index). *Am J Cardiol* 1989; **64**: 651–4.

Hopkins PM, Hunter JM (eds.). [*Endocrine and metabolic disorders in anaesthesia and intensive care.*] *Br J Anaesth* 2000; **85** (1): 1–153.

Mallampati SR, Gatt SP, Gugino LD, *et al.* A clinical sign to predict difficult tracheal intubation: a prospective study. *Can Anaesth Soc J* 1985; **32**: 429–34.

Mason R. Anaesthesia Databook: a Perioperative and Peripartum Manual, 3rd edn. London: Greenwich Medical Media, 2001.

National Institute for Health and Clinical Excellence (NICE). *Preoperative Tests: the Use of Routine Preoperative Tests for Elective Surgery.* Clinical Guideline 3. www.nice.org.uk.

Patil VU, Stehling LC, Zauder HL. Predicting the difficulty of intubation utilizing an intubation guide. *Anesthesiol Rev* 1983; **10**: 32–3.

Prys-Roberts C. Isolated systolic hypertension: pressure on the anaesthetist? *Anaesthesia* 2001; **56**: 505–10.

Royal College of Nursing (RCN). Perioperative Fasting in Adults and Children: an RCN guideline for the multidisciplinary team. London: RCN, 2005. www.rcn.org.uk.

Saklad M. Grading of patients for surgical procedures. *Anesthesiology* 1941; **2**: 281–4.

Samsoon GLT, Young JRB. Difficult tracheal intubation: a retrospective study. *Anaesthesia* 1987; **42**: 487–90.

Savva D. Prediction of difficult tracheal intubation. *Br J Anaesth* 1994; **73**: 149–53.

Sweitzer BJ. *Handbook of Preoperative Assessment and Management*. Philadelphia, PA: Lippincott Williams & Wilkins, 2000.

Wilson ME, Spiegelhalter D, Robertson JA, Lesser P. Predicting difficult intubation. *Br J Anaesth* 1988; **61**: 211–16.

Drug and Therapeutics Bulletin. Drugs in the peri-operative period.

(1) Stopping or continuing drugs around surgery, 1999; **37** (8).

(2) Corticosteroids and therapy for diabetes mellitus, 1999; **37** (9).

(4) Cardiovascular drugs, 1999; **37** (12).

CHAPTER 2

Induction of anaesthesia

S. M. Parr

Methods of induction

The objective of modern anaesthesia is to rapidly obtain a state of unconsciousness, to maintain this state, and then to achieve a rapid recovery. For any anaesthetic agent to be effective, whether administered intravenously or by inhalation, it must achieve a sufficient concentration within the central nervous system. Inhalational anaesthetic agents are administered by concentration rather than dose, and as the concentration delivered rapidly equilibrates between alveoli, blood and brain, this allows a way of quantifying the anaesthetic effect for each agent. The minimum alveolar concentration (MAC) is defined as that concentration of anaesthetic agent that will prevent reflex response to a skin incision in 50% of a population. MAC is, therefore, an easily defined measure of depth of anaesthesia. Intravenous induction agents are, in contrast, administered by dose rather than concentration. To administer a 'sleep dose' of an induction agent requires an assessment of the likely response from an individual and knowledge of the pharmacokinetics and pharmacodynamics of the particular agent used. Figures IA1 and IA2 summarise the main advantages and disadvantages of each route of administration. Regardless of the technique used, mini-mal standards of monitoring must be commenced prior to induction and maintained throughout anaesthesia (see Section 1, Chapter 3 for more details).

Intravenous induction

The intravenous route is the most common method of induction, allowing delivery of a bolus of drug to the brain, which results in rapid loss of consciousness. This is generally more acceptable to the patient than inhalational induction, and has the advantage of minimising any excitement phase. The rapid intravenous administration of a drug sufficient to achieve a plasma concentration which results in central nervous system depression will necessarily be associated with effects on other organ systems, in particular the cardiovascular system. The rapid smooth induction of anaesthesia by the intravenous route, therefore, coexists with an equally rapid onset of side effects. Hypotension, respiratory depression and rapid loss of airway control may provide cause for concern. Some of these potential problems can be minimised. Choosing an induction agent that demonstrates cardiovascular stability (such as etomidate) may be beneficial. The required dose may be reduced by premedication with benzodiazepines

Advantages
- Rapid onset
- Dose titratable
- Depression of pharyngeal reflexes allows early insertion of LMA
- Anti-emetic and anti-convulsive properties

Disadvantages
- Venous access required
- Risk of hypotension
- Apnoea common
- Loss of airway control
- Anaphylaxis

Figure IA1 Intravenous induction of anaesthesia

Advantages
- Avoids venepuncture
- Respiration is maintained
- Slow loss of protective reflexes
- End-tidal concentration can be measured
- Rapid recovery if induction is abandoned
- Upper oesophageal sphincter tone maintained

Disadvantages
- Slow process
- Potential excitement phase
- Irritant and unpleasant, may induce coughing
- Pollution
- May cause a rise in ICP/IOP

Figure IA2 Inhalation induction of anaesthesia

or pretreatment with intravenous opioids. Most importantly, whatever induction agent is chosen it should be administered at an appropriate dosage and suitable rate for the individual patient. This will depend on consideration of all relevant factors, taking special account of pre-existing morbidity. An additional potential problem of thiopental administration is that of inadvertent intra-arterial injection. The management of this is described in Figure IA3.

Inhalational induction

Venepuncture, especially for children, still remains a great fear, and many would see the avoidance of needles as the major advantage of inhalational induction. The slow speed of induction remains the major problem with this route. To achieve a sufficient concentration of inhalational agent in the central nervous system to produce unconsciousness requires adequate uptake by the lungs and sufficient distribution to the brain. The uptake of an inhaled agent is dependent on a number of factors: the inspired

Stop the injection
Leave the needle or cannula in place
Dilute immediately by injecting normal saline into the artery
Administer local anaesthetic and/or vasodilator directly into the artery
- Lidocaine 50 mg (5 ml 1% solution)
- Procaine hydrochloride 50–100 mg (10–20 ml 0.5% solution)
- Phenoxybenzamine (α adrenergic antagonist) 0.5 mg or infuse 50–200 μg per minute

Administer papaverine systemically 40–80 mg (10–20 ml 0.4% solution)
Consider sympathetic neural blockade
- Stellate ganglion or brachial plexus block (this produces prolonged vasodilatation to improve circulation and tissue oxygenation while improving clearance of the crystals)

Start IV heparin
Consider intra-arterial injection of hydrocortisone
Postpone non-urgent surgery

Figure IA3 Management of intra-arterial injection of thiopental

concentration, the alveolar ventilation, the blood/gas partition coefficient and the rate at which the agent is removed by the pulmonary circulation. Agents that are pleasant and non-irritant (regardless of concentration), and which have a low blood/gas partition coefficient (allowing rapid equilibration between inspired and alveolar concentrations), allow rapid induction and recovery.

An important advantage of the inhalational route over the intravenous route is the maintenance of airway control. If ventilation ceases, either because of profound respiratory depression or because of airway obstruction, the induction process will be reversed. This may be particularly important in patients with a compromised airway, where a gradual loss of consciousness with the preservation of ventilation maintains a degree of safety. The technique of an inhalational induction requires practice. Cooperative patients can sometimes be persuaded to take a vital capacity breath of isoflurane or sevoflurane in an attempt to speed up induction, but for the majority of cases volatile agents need to be introduced gradually. This is especially true with young children, who may be disturbed by anaesthetic masks and pungent volatile agents. In this situation the gradual introduction of the volatile agent and use of a cupped hand rather than a face mask is likely to meet with greater approval.

Anaphylaxis

Modern anaesthesia requires the use of several drugs to provide hypnosis, analgesia and muscular relaxation. In view of the large number of patients receiving anaesthesia annually, it is therefore not surprising that untoward reactions occasionally occur. An adverse reaction is likely to be more severe when drugs are administered by the intravenous route. In inhalational induction the relatively slow absorption of drugs across mucous membranes may offer a degree of immunological protection.

Anaphylactic reactions are immediate-type hypersensitivity reactions resulting from the interaction of antigens with specific IgE antibodies bound to mast cells and basophils. The mast cells and basophils respond by releasing vasoactive and bronchoconstrictive substances, which include histamine, leukotrienes (see Section 3, Chapter 13) and eosinophil chemotactic factor of anaphylaxis (ECF-A). Anaphylactic reactions occur in individuals who have become sensitised to an allergen. Anaphylactoid reactions are clinically indistinguishable from anaphylaxis but do not result from prior exposure to a triggering agent. They are often mediated via IgG causing activation of complement and the liberation of anaphylatoxins C3a, C4a and C5a. The frequency of allergic reactions to individual drugs is difficult to quantify. Approximate figures for the incidence of IgE-dependent anaphylaxis under anaesthesia are given in Figure IA4. Rocuronium appears to be developing a prevalence of IgE-dependent anaphylaxis similar to other

Muscle relaxants

comprising 70% of total, of which

- suxamethonium   43%
- vecuronium   37%
- pancuronium   13%
- atracurium   7%

Others

comprising 30% of total, of which

- latex   15%
- colloids   5%
- hypnotics   4%
- antibiotics   2%
- benzodiazepines   2%
- opioids   2%

Figure IA4 Substances identified in IgE-dependent anaphylaxis (incidence in %)

Cardiovascular collapse	88%
Bronchospasm	36%
Swelling of the face	24%
Generalised swelling	7%
Cutaneous signs rash	3%
erythema	45%
urticaria	9%

Association of Anaesthetists of Great Britain and Ireland.

Figure IA5 Clinical features of anaphylaxis

No pulse	26%
Difficult to inflate lungs	24%
Flush	18%
Desaturation	11%
Cough	7%
Rash	4%
ECG abnormality	2%
Urticaria	2%
Subjective	2%
Swelling	1%
No bleeding	0.5%

Adapted from Association of Anaesthetists of Great Britain and Ireland 2003.

Figure IA6 First clinical feature of anaphylaxis

steroid neuromuscular blocking agents. For details on latex allergy see Section 1, Chapter 5.

Recognition

Irrespective of the mode of triggering, all the clinical manifestations of an allergic reaction occur as a result of the liberation of vasoactive substances. The typical clinical features of anaphylaxis are hypotension, bronchospasm, oedema and the development of a rash (Figures IA5, IA6). Cardiovascular collapse is one of the most common early signs. This is usually the result of vasodilatation, and may be compounded by arrhythmias (usually supraventricular tachycardia), hypovolaemia and a reduction in venous return, which will be exacerbated if high inflation pressures are necessary to facilitate ventilation of the lungs. Bronchospasm is variable in its severity, from a transient degree of difficulty with ventilation to the situation where gas exchange is impossible despite the use of high airway pressures and slow inspiratory and expiratory times. The presence of weals and erythema near the point of venous access is usually a sign of localised histamine release, which usually does not require any treatment and resolves spontaneously within an hour. Generalised erythema, weals and oedema are signs of systemic histamine release, which may herald the onset of a major reaction.

Treatment

The prompt and aggressive treatment of a patient with a severe anaphylactic reaction is life-saving. 100% oxygen should be administered and consideration given to early intubation before the onset of angio-oedema. The administration of epinephrine is a priority, and if there is circulatory collapse 1 ml of 1 in 10 000 epinephrine should be administered IV at 1 minute intervals. Intravenous colloids are the most effective treatment to restore intravascular volume, and up to 2 litres may be infused rapidly (note that allergic reaction to colloids administered at this time is virtually unknown). Arrhythmias should be treated symptomatically. Bronchospasm can be difficult to overcome: although epinephrine is often effective, aminophylline and nebulised salbutamol may be useful for persistent bronchospasm. Intratracheal injections of local anaesthetic agents (such as lidocaine 100 mg) have also been advocated. Although such reactions are rare, all anaesthetists should rehearse a simulated 'anaphylaxis drill' at regular intervals (Figure IA7).

Follow-up

After a suspected drug reaction associated with anaesthesia the patient should be counselled and investigated. This is the responsibility of the anaesthetist who administered the drug, and should be conducted in consultation with a clinical immunologist. No tests or investigations of any kind should be performed until the resuscitation period is completed. Immediately after resuscitation (and at 1 hour and 6–24 hours after the reaction occurred) 10 ml venous blood should be taken into a plain glass tube, the serum separated and stored at −20 °C for estimation of serum tryptase concentration. Elevation of this enzyme indicates that the reaction was associated with mast cell degranulation. Blood samples in EDTA-containing tubes are useful for complement assays and haematology, the disappearance of basophils being indicative of a type I anaphylactic reaction. When more than one drug has been administered, skin-prick tests are useful to establish the

Initial therapy
(1) Stop administration of all agents likely to have caused the anaphylaxis
(2) Call for help
(3) Maintain airway, give 100% oxygen and lie patient flat with legs elevated
(4) Give epinephrine (adrenaline)
    IM 0.5–1 mg and repeated every 10 minutes as required according to the arterial pressure and pulse until improvement occurs
    IV 50–100 μg intravenously over 1 minute and repeated as required

Never give undiluted epinephrine 1 : 1000 intravenously
For cardiovascular collapse, 0.5–1 mg (5–10 ml of 1 : 10 000) may be required intravenously in divided doses by titration. This should be given at a rate of 0.1 mg per minute, stopping when a response has been obtained.
Paediatric doses of epinephrine depend on the age of the child.
Intramuscular epinephrine 1 : 1000 should be administered as follows:

>12 years	500 μg IM (0.5 ml)
6–12 years	250 μg IM (0.25 ml)
>6 months to 6 years	120 μg IM (0.12 ml)
<6 months	50 μg IM (0.05 ml)

(5) Start rapid intravenous infusion with colloids or crystalloids. Adult patients may require 2 to 4 litres of crystalloid.

Secondary therapy
(1) Give antihistamines (chlorpheniramine 10–20 mg by slow intravenous infusion)
(2) Give corticosteroids (100–500 mg hydrocortisone slowly IV)
(3) Bronchodilators may be required for persistent bronchospasm

(Adapted from Association of Anaesthetists of Great Britain and Ireland 2003.)

Figure IA7 Management of a patient with suspected anaphylaxis during anaesthesia

agent involved. These should be carried out by specialised departments with full resuscitation facilities.

RAST testing

The radioallergosorbent test (RAST) is an in vitro method of measuring circulating allergen-specific IgE antibodies. The allergen is first attached to a paper disc and is then incubated with serum from the patient. Circulating antibody will become bound and a second incubation is carried out with radiolabelled allergen-specific anti-IgE. The amount of bound radioactivity is related to the amount of specific IgE in the original serum. RAST capable of measuring IgE antibodies to thiopental, muscle relaxants and latex are available, among others.

Detailed written records should be kept of all events, especially the timing of administration of all drugs. The anaesthetist is responsible for submitting a 'yellow card' report to the Commission on Human Medicines (formerly the Committee on Safety of Medicines) and advising the patient about future anaesthesia. The Yellow Card database (Adverse Drug Reactions Online Information Tracking: ADROIT) collates reports of adverse drug reactions (ADRs) experienced by patients. The report must include an explanation to the patient and a full and detailed record in the case notes, with a copy to the general practitioner. The patient should also be given a written record of the reaction and be advised to wear a 'MedicAlert' bracelet. The patient should be referred to an allergist for further investigation, including skin-prick testing.

Management of the airway

A number of options exist for maintaining the patient's airway during anaesthesia:
- Face mask with a 'sniffing the morning air' position
- Face mask with Guedel airway
- Laryngeal mask airway (LMA)
- Tracheal intubation
  - oral
  - nasal

Face mask

The use of a face mask is the first step prior to using any intraoral methods. It is an essential skill for any anaesthetist but perhaps the most challenging airway skill. It has the advantage that it requires no further equipment or measures, but it uses at least one hand, is prone to leakage, and can be tiring. The anaesthetist is unable to attend to other relevant matters as freely. It is therefore only used during induction and for very short procedures. The Guedel airway is particularly useful to help maintain the patency of the airway, especially if nasal patency is a problem.

Laryngeal mask

The laryngeal mask comes in various forms (reuseable, disposable, standard and reinforced, and one with a gel-filled cuff) and sizes 1, 1 1/2, 2, 2 1/2, 3, 4 and 5, with guide patient weights to assist in selecting the size. The laryngeal mask provides a more reliable maintenance of the airway than the face mask, and is suitable for prolonged procedures.

Laryngeal masks are simple to introduce, allow spontaneous or controlled ventilation, and leave the anaesthetist's hands free to manage other aspects of the anaesthetic. They are not as stimulating as endotracheal tubes and will not traumatise the larynx. However, they do not protect the airway from aspiration reliably, may become dislodged intraoperatively, and may cause as much sore throat as an endotracheal tube. Although they do not damage the larynx, the distension of the pharynx can (rarely) lead to temporary vocal cord palsy.

Tracheal intubation

Indications

There are two major indications for tracheal intubation in the anaesthetised patient: first, to ensure airway patency and, second, to protect the airway from aspiration.

Airway patency

Assuming that the tracheal tube is kept clear of obstructions and free of kinks, tracheal intubation affords the anaesthetist the guarantee of a patent airway. This is particularly useful in the following situations:
- Prolonged operations such as neurosurgical, cardiac and extensive abdominal surgery
- Operations where access to the airway is difficult, such as head and neck surgery and patients in the prone position
- Operations involving excessive movement of the head and neck, where other forms of airway control may become dislodged
- Situations where it is difficult to achieve a clear airway with a laryngeal mask airway or face mask
- Situations where a major intraoperative complication develops (severe haemorrhage, anaphylaxis or malignant hyperpyrexia)

Protection from aspiration

A cuffed endotracheal tube forms an airtight seal at the level of the cuff and greatly reduces the risk of contamination of the lower respiratory tract. This is particularly useful in patients with an increased risk of regurgitation and during surgery when there may be extensive bleeding from the mouth, nose or oropharynx. Other indications for tracheal intubation include thoracic operations that require isolation of one lung and those patients in whom the aspiration of secretions from the lower respiratory tract is necessary.

Management of a difficult intubation

Clinical examination of the patient and bedside assessments of the airway are useful in identifying those patients posing the risk of a potentially difficult intubation, but it is not unusual to be confronted with a patient of normal appearance in whom the glottis cannot be visualised on direct laryngoscopy. The latest Triennial report into maternal mortality in the UK (CEMACH 2007) describes six cases of death directly attributable to anaesthesia. Whilst none of these were the result of unrecognised oesophageal intubation the lessons from previous reports should not be forgotten.

When faced with a potentially difficult airway it is important to remain calm. The degree of difficulty should be assessed and senior assistance sought if available. It is essential to ensure that the patient is adequately ventilated, oxygenated and anaesthetised at all times, but it may also be necessary to wake the patient up rapidly if a safe airway cannot be established. The drama of a difficult intubation can easily be turned into a crisis when there are multiple attempts at laryngoscopy in a hypoxic patient with a mouth full of blood and secretions. The use of rapidly redistributed intravenous induction agents such as propofol will allow rapid return of consciousness unless the patient has received significant amounts of volatile agent or further incremental doses of induction agent.

If ventilation by mask is easy and gas exchange can be maintained, there are a number of manoeuvres and aids available to improve the chances of correct endotracheal tube placement. These are detailed below.

(1) Positioning

The 'sniffing the morning air' position is the most important manoeuvre that can improve intubating conditions. The neck is flexed on the chest to about 35 degrees, which can usually be achieved with one pillow under the head. The head is then extended on the neck so that the face is tilted back 15 degrees from the horizontal plane. In this position the oral, pharyngeal and tracheal axes are aligned. The practice of placing one hand on the chin and the other on the back of the head to force the head into severe extension will not only push the larynx into an anterior position and make intubation more difficult, but also in patients with osteoporosis or rheumatoid arthritis it runs the risk of fracturing the odontoid peg against the body of C1. In very obese patients it may be necessary to place pillows under the shoulders and neck as well as the head to allow the head to be extended on the neck.

(2) Laryngoscopy technique

The Macintosh laryngoscope blade has a flange on its left side to keep the tongue out of the line of sight. The blade should be inserted into the right side of the mouth and advanced centrally towards the base of the tongue. The blade is then lifted to expose the epiglottis and advanced into the vallecula with continued lifting to expose the laryngeal opening. There is a natural tendency amongst inexperienced anaesthetists to advance the blade insufficiently and then lever the laryngoscope to try and achieve visualisation of the glottis, which will cause the proximal end of the blade to act as a lever on the upper incisors or gums, resulting in dental damage or bleeding. Other causes of difficulty include inserting the blade past the epiglottis and elevating the entire larynx, so that the oesophagus is visualised, or allowing the tongue to slip over the right side of the laryngoscope blade, impairing the view. Difficulty may be encountered in inserting the laryngoscope correctly in obese patients and large-breasted women, and it may occasionally be necessary to insert an unattached blade into the mouth and then reattach the handle. The use of external laryngeal pressure applied to the thyroid cartilage in a posterior direction can improve the view obtained at laryngoscopy. With respect to the grading of the view at laryngoscopy described by Cormack and Lehane (1984), a grade 3 may be changed into a grade 2 (Figure IA8).

(3) Gum elastic bougie

This simple device is a 60 cm long introducer, 5 mm in diameter, with a smooth angled tip at the end. The bougie is made from braided polyester with a resin coat, which provides both the necessary stiffness and flexibility to enable it to be passed into the larynx. It may be bent before insertion to aid placement, and is especially useful in cases where the glottic opening cannot be visualised. In this situation correct placement may be confirmed by the detection of clicks as the introducer is gently passed down into the trachea. The tracheal tube is then slid over the bougie into the trachea with a 90-degree anticlockwise rotation to facilitate passage through the larynx.

(4) Stylet

A pre-curved malleable stylet is placed within an endotracheal tube to enable the tube to be curved and to aid placement, especially when the larynx is more anterior. To

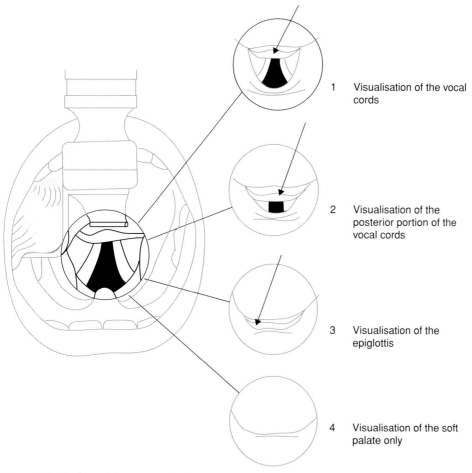

1   Visualisation of the vocal cords

2   Visualisation of the posterior portion of the vocal cords

3   Visualisation of the epiglottis

4   Visualisation of the soft palate only

Figure IA8 Grading of laryngoscopic views

avoid trauma to the larynx the stylet should not be allowed to protrude beyond the tip of the endotracheal tube.

(5) Lightwand

A lightwand (Trachlight) uses the principle of transillumination of the neck when a light is passed into the trachea. In this situation a distinct glow can be seen below the thyroid cartilage which is not apparent when the light is placed in the oesophagus. The light emitted by the wand should project laterally as well as forward, and there should be little associated heat production. The lightwand is usually advanced without the aid of a laryngoscope, and once in the trachea the internal stylet that gives the wand its stiffness can be retracted to allow the pliable wand to be advanced into the trachea and used as a guide for the placement of the endotracheal tube.

(6) Alternative laryngoscope blades

The standard Macintosh laryngoscope was introduced in 1943. It has a relatively short curved blade designed to rest in the vallecula and lift the epiglottis. Several alternative laryngoscope blades are available, some of which are described below.

Miller. A straight-bladed laryngoscope with a slight curve at the tip. The blade is longer, narrower and smaller at the tip, and is designed to trap and lift the epiglottis

McCoy. The McCoy levering laryngoscope (McCoy & Mirakhur 1993) has a 25 mm hinged blade tip controlled by a spring-loaded lever on the handle of the laryngoscope which allows elevation of the epiglottis without the use of excessive forces on the pharyngeal tissues.

Bullard. The Bullard laryngoscope is a rigid-bladed indirect fibreoptic laryngoscope with a shape designed to match the airway. The fibreoptic bundle passes along the posterior aspect of the blade and ends 26 mm from the distal tip of the blade, allowing excellent visualisation of the larynx. Intubation can be achieved using an attached intubating stylet with a preloaded endotracheal tube. This device requires a considerable amount of practice but is particularly useful in patients with upper airway pathology, limited mouth opening or an immobile or unstable cervical spine.

Prism. The Huffman prism is an example of a laryngoscope using refraction to aid visualisation of the larynx. It employs a modification of the Macintosh blade whereby a block of transparent plastic in a prism shape is attached to the proximal end of the blade. The ends of the prism are polished to provide optically flat surfaces, the nearest to the eye being cut at 90 degrees to the line of vision and the distal surface at 30 degrees. The net result to the view obtained is a refraction of approximately 30 degrees.

Polio. The Polio blade was originally designed to enable patients in an iron lung to be intubated. In the UK the 'polio blade' is actually a wedge adaptor located between the handle and blade of a standard Macintosh laryngoscope to give a 120-degree angle between the two. It allows the easier introduction of the blade in situations where the chest gets in the way of the handle.

Flexiblade. A flexible-bladed laryngoscope based on the Macintosh shape is now available. This takes the principle of the McCoy one step further in that the blade is multi-segmented and able to change its radius of curvature. This device may be manipulated to optimise the view of the cords during laryngoscopy.

(7) Laryngeal mask airway (LMA)

The laryngeal mask is a useful means of airway control in difficult and failed intubations. Note that the LMA has been shown to be life-saving in cases of failed intubation in obstetric anaesthesia (Gataure & Hughes 1995). A number of insertion methods have been advocated, and in the case of difficulty it seems wise to use a familiar technique. Anterior displacement of the mandible often prevents down-folding of the epiglottis, and is recommended in cases of difficulty. If intubation is difficult and the airway can be secured with a laryngeal mask there are then several choices available to the anaesthetist.

- Use the LMA to oxygenate the patient whilst allowing to wake up. Consider regional anaesthesia or securing the airway by alternative means.

- Use the LMA to maintain anaesthesia. The laryngeal mask can be used for both spontaneous and controlled ventilation. The laryngeal mask is in popular use for gynaecological surgery (such as laparoscopy) and there have been reports of its use in patients normally requiring intubation (such as coronary artery bypass grafting).

- Use the LMA to intubate the trachea. In adults a well-lubricated uncut cuffed 6 mm internal diameter endotracheal tube can be passed through the lumen of a size 3 or 4 laryngeal mask. The patient needs to be correctly positioned 'sniffing the morning air', and the laryngeal mask needs to be correctly sited with no downfolding of the epiglottis. The patient should be deeply anaesthetised with or without muscle relaxation to prevent coughing or laryngospasm. Rotation of the tube through 90 degrees will prevent the bevel of the tube catching on the bars of the laryngeal mask aperture, and the tube can then be passed into the trachea. If cricoid pressure has been applied this tends not to be compromised by the presence of a laryngeal mask, and it should be continued at least until the moment of intubation, when it may need to be momentarily released. If difficulty is encountered the position of the head and neck can be altered, firstly by extension at the atlanto-occipital joint and then with varying degrees of flexion of the neck. If an endotracheal tube larger than a size 6.0 is required a gum elastic bougie can be passed through the laryngeal mask into the trachea and an endotracheal tube railroaded over the bougie into place.

- A development of the LMA specifically designed for secondary intubation is now available. The intubating laryngeal mask is a shortened version of the usual device with a forwardly directed metal handle. The aperture has a single wider bar which is designed to elevate the epiglottis as a narrow endotracheal tube is advanced through the laryngeal mask lumen. The intubating laryngeal mask therefore has a role in the temporary establishment of the airway prior to securing it with a cuffed ET tube. The usual risks of aspiration during the process are, however, present.

(8) Other airway management devices

Several other devices are available for the management of the airway. These include:

- The combitube airway. This is a double-lumen device designed for blind placement in the pharynx. Its role is to allow ventilation of the lungs whether the tube enters the trachea or the oesophagus. There are eight supraglottic apertures and a single distal lumen. Two cuffs, a large-volume pharyngeal one and a small-volume distal one, create a seal, and both are fitted with pilot tubes. In practice it is most common that the combitube enters the oesophagus. Ventilation may not always be possible, and there have been instances of trauma and oesophageal damage.

- The cuffed oropharyngeal airway. This device is a modification of the standard Guedel airway, mainly differing in having a distal inflatable cuff.
- The airway management device (AMD). The AMD is a single-lumen device designed for blind placement. It has a double cuff, with each part having its own pilot balloon. There is limited experience with the AMD in practice.
- The laryngeal tube. This device is similar to the AMD but has two cuffs (small distal and large proximal) and a single pilot balloon. Early experience suggests that this device has a limited role in airway management. It has, however, been successfully used to aid nasotracheal intubation in difficult circumstances.

(9) Blind nasal intubation

In blind nasal intubation a nasotracheal tube is passed through the nose with the head extended at the atlantoaxial joint. The tip of the tube, if kept in the midline, will usually impact anteriorly, and flexion of the head will allow advancement of the tube into the larynx. If the tube is not in the midline it will tend to lodge in the pyriform fossa, and this usually shows as a bulge on the anterior aspect of the neck. If the tube enters the oesophagus it can often be relocated in the trachea by first withdrawing and then advancing again. This technique requires a great deal of practice and is not recommended for the novice. A topical vasoconstrictor solution (such as xylometazoline spray) should be used to minimise the risk of bleeding from the nasal mucosa.

(10) Retrograde intubation

Retrogade intubation involves the passage of a catheter through a cricothyroid incision upwards so as to protrude at the mouth. It is then possible to use the catheter to railroad an endotracheal tube into the larynx. For details of the practical method see Figure IA9. The technique may be carried out under local or general anaesthesia but it has complications (Figure IA10), and is not recommended for inexperienced hands.

- Pass a Tuohy needle attached to a saline-filled syringe through a cricothyrotomy puncture
- Verify penetration of the larynx by aspiration of air
- Angulate the needle 45 degrees cephalad with the bevel pointing anteriorly
- Push an epidural catheter through the needle until it appears at the mouth
- Anchor the catheter at its entry point in the neck
- Keeping the catheter tensioned, pass a lubricated endotracheal tube over the catheter, advancing until passage through the vocal cords is indicated by a 'click'
- If there is any obstruction to passage at this point, rotate the tube through 90 degrees, and if this fails try a smaller tube size

Figure IA9 Technique of retrograde intubation

- Bleeding
- Perforation of posterior wall of trachea with needle
- Subcutaneous emphysema of neck
- Pneumothorax
- Infection at puncture site

Figure IA10 Complications of retrograde intubation

Management of failed intubation

Failed intubation may be the result of an anticipated degree of difficulty with the airway or a totally unexpected event.

Unexpected

Figures IA11, IA12 and IA13, from the Difficult Airway Society, provide examples of drills to be followed. Figure IA11 is to be used when encountering an unanticipated difficult intubation during routine induction, Figure IA12 during a rapid sequence induction and Figure IA13 for when either of these sets of responses has failed to provide ventilation. The learning of such drills is mandatory. Generally patients do not come to harm because they cannot be intubated: they come to harm because of inadequate oxygenation, inadequate anaesthesia, trauma to the airway and aspiration. Persistent and prolonged attempts at intubation using conventional laryngoscopy cause oedema and bleeding in the airway with progressive difficulty in ventilation. Over-vigorous mask ventilation fills the stomach with gas, leading to an increasing likelihood of regurgitation.

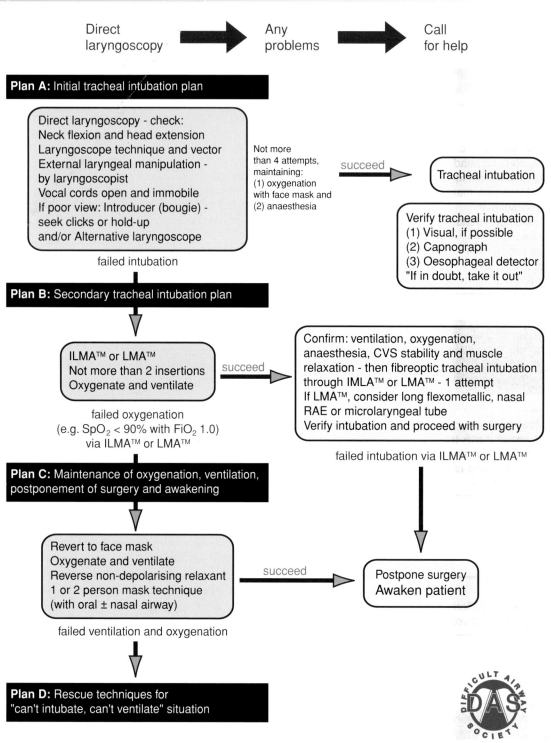

Figure IA11 Unanticipated difficult intubation during routine induction of anaesthesia.
Reproduced with permission from the Difficult Airway Society.

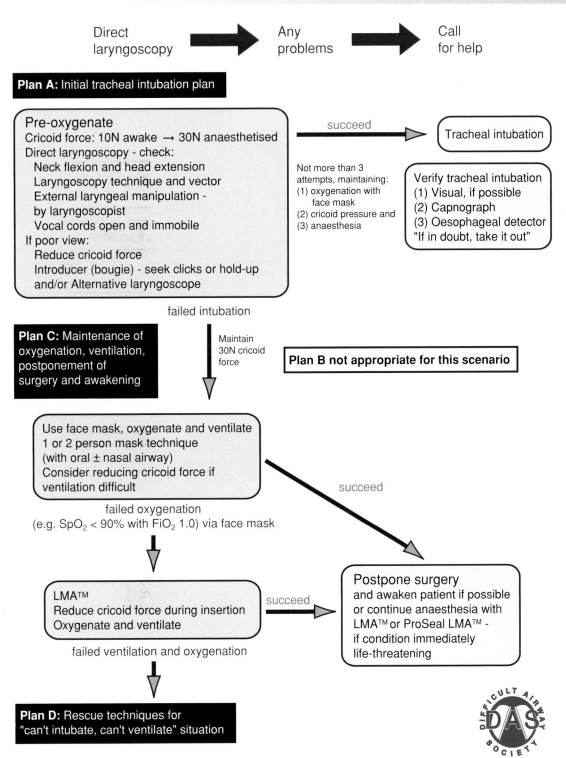

Figure IA12 Unanticipated difficult intubation during rapid sequence induction.
Reproduced with permission from the Difficult Airway Society.

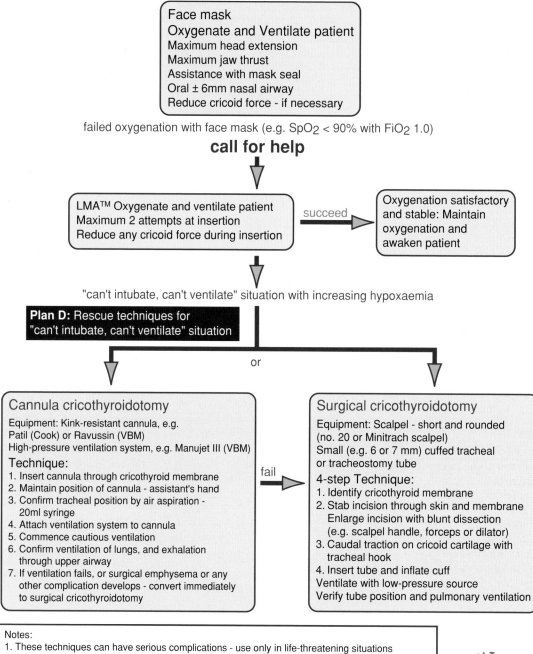

failed intubation and difficult ventilation (other than laryngospasm)

> **Face mask**
> **Oxygenate and Ventilate patient**
> Maximum head extension
> Maximum jaw thrust
> Assistance with mask seal
> Oral ± 6mm nasal airway
> Reduce cricoid force - if necessary

failed oxygenation with face mask (e.g. SpO_2 < 90% with FiO_2 1.0)

call for help

> LMA™ Oxygenate and ventilate patient
> Maximum 2 attempts at insertion
> Reduce any cricoid force during insertion

succeed →

> Oxygenation satisfactory and stable: Maintain oxygenation and awaken patient

"can't intubate, can't ventilate" situation with increasing hypoxaemia

Plan D: Rescue techniques for "can't intubate, can't ventilate" situation

or

Cannula cricothyroidotomy
Equipment: Kink-resistant cannula, e.g.
Patil (Cook) or Ravussin (VBM)
High-pressure ventilation system, e.g. Manujet III (VBM)
Technique:
1. Insert cannula through cricothyroid membrane
2. Maintain position of cannula - assistant's hand
3. Confirm tracheal position by air aspiration - 20ml syringe
4. Attach ventilation system to cannula
5. Commence cautious ventilation
6. Confirm ventilation of lungs, and exhalation through upper airway
7. If ventilation fails, or surgical emphysema or any other complication develops - convert immediately to surgical cricothyroidotomy

fail →

Surgical cricothyroidotomy
Equipment: Scalpel - short and rounded (no. 20 or Minitrach scalpel)
Small (e.g. 6 or 7 mm) cuffed tracheal or tracheostomy tube
4-step Technique:
1. Identify cricothyroid membrane
2. Stab incision through skin and membrane Enlarge incision with blunt dissection (e.g. scalpel handle, forceps or dilator)
3. Caudal traction on cricoid cartilage with tracheal hook
4. Insert tube and inflate cuff
Ventilate with low-pressure source
Verify tube position and pulmonary ventilation

Notes:
1. These techniques can have serious complications - use only in life-threatening situations
2. Convert to definitive airway as soon as possible
3. Postoperative management - see other difficult airway guidelines and flow-charts
4. 4mm cannula with low-pressure ventilation may be successful in patient breathing spontaneously

Figure IA13 Failed intubation: rescue techniques for the 'can't intubate, can't ventilate' situation. Reproduced with permission from the Difficult Airway Society.

A major problem relating to the use of a failed intubation drill is the timing of the decision as to when it should be implemented. Although there must be an early acceptance of failure it is probably reasonable to have three or four attempts at endotracheal intubation using some of the manoeuvres designed to aid success such as proper positioning of the patient, anterior laryngeal pressure and use of the gum elastic bougie. The use of totally unfamiliar equipment such as alternative laryngoscope blades is unlikely to be of help.

Anticipated

When a potentially difficult airway is recognised careful steps should be taken to assess the patient preoperatively. The previous medical history should be sought and past anaesthetic records scrutinised. The presence of respiratory or cardiac disease may require special attention during intubation or induction. The assessment of the airway should be particularly thorough and include mouth opening, neck extension, thyromental distance, nostril patency, Mallampati score and state of dentition.

Possible options in anticipated difficult intubation are:
- Awake intubation
- Intubation attempts after induction of anaesthesia
- Elective surgical tracheostomy under local anaesthesia
- Cricothyroid puncture and HFJV

Awake intubation is indicated in patients with congenital airway anomalies, in those with trauma to the face, airway

- Use sedative premedication cautiously, and not at all in the presence of severe airway compromise
- Anticholinergic premedication may be given to reduce secretions
- Prescribe aspiration prophylaxis (such as ranitidine and sodium citrate) preoperatively
- Check all equipment in the anaesthetic room, attach monitoring and secure intravenous access
- Prepare the airway by achieving local anaesthesia as described in Figure RA38 (Section 1, Chapter 7)
- Spray the nasal mucosa with a vasoconstrictor if this is the chosen route
- Having loaded the chosen endotracheal tube onto the fibreoptic scope proceed via mouth or nose until the larynx is visualised
- Pass the tube off the scope into the trachea and check for correct placement

Figure IA14 The technique of awake intubation

or cervical spine and in those with a history of previous difficult intubation. The practical technique of awake intubation is described in Figure IA14. Although awake intubation is an unpleasant experience for the patient it provides a number of advantages:
- The airway is preserved
- There is no loss of muscle tone (facilitating fibreoptic visualisation)
- Consciousness and respiration are unaffected

Confirmation of correct placement of endotracheal tube

After intubation of the trachea the tip of the endotracheal tube will ideally lie above the carina but below the vocal cords. The two major malplacements are accidental endobronchial intubation and accidental oesophageal intubation. Endobronchial intubation is generally the result of an endotracheal tube being cut to a length greater than necessary. It is more usual for the right main bronchus to become intubated, because of its more vertical alignment. The signs of accidental endobronchial intubation are an unexplained drop in oxygen saturation, higher than expected airway pressure (and a feel of poor compliance in the reservoir bag) and asymmetrical chest movement. If auscultation confirms endobronchial intubation, deflate the cuff, withdraw the tube until bilateral ventilation returns, then re-inflate the cuff.

Unrecognised oesophageal intubation is still a major cause of anaesthetic morbidity and mortality. Fortunately most oesophageal intubations are easily recognised, but there are still occasions where failure to recognise misplacement of the tube has serious, often fatal consequences. The oft-quoted maxim 'When in doubt take it out' is still valid. The methods used to verify the position of the endotracheal tube can be divided into clinical indications of correct tube placement and objective signs such

Clinical signs
- Direct visualisation of the tube through the cords
- Auscultation for breath sounds
- Chest movement with positive pressure ventilation
- 'Feel' of the reservoir bag
- (Absence of cyanosis)

Objective signs
- Carbon dioxide detectors
- Oesophageal detectors

Figure IA15 Confirmation of correct endotracheal tube placement

as tests based on the detection of CO_2 from expired gas (Figure IA15).

Clinical signs
Direct visualisation of the tracheal tube passing between the vocal cords
This simple method is one of the most reliable means of confirming correct intubation. Unfortunately, in grade 3 intubations and patients with an anterior larynx a satisfactory view may be impossible to obtain. Excessive movement of the head and neck, alterations in patient position, traction on the trachea or oesophagus and poor fixing of the tracheal tube are all potential causes of tube displacement.

Auscultation of breath sounds
This can and should be done repeatedly to ensure that the tube is still within the trachea whenever there has been movement of the tube or movement of the patient. Auscultation in both axillae to confirm symmetrical breath sounds will usually verify correct tube placement, although there have been occasions where transmitted sounds from oesophageal intubations have caused confusion. This is often the case in infants, where the presence of bilateral abnormal breath sounds should alert the anaesthetist to the possibility of oesophageal intubation. For this reason, in both adults and children, it is wise to auscultate in both axillae and in the epigastrium, as the gurgling sound of air entering the stomach is quite characteristic.

Observation of chest movement
This cannot be relied upon to distinguish oesophageal from tracheal intubation.

The 'feel' of the reservoir bag
The characteristic feel of the reservoir bag on manual ventilation is a good guide to the location of the tracheal tube. In particular, the rapid refilling of the bag during expiration is unlikely to occur in cases of oesophageal intubation. Unfortunately, there have been occasions where confusion has arisen, particularly in patients with poor compliance or high airway resistance. Oesophageal pressures tend to reflect intrapleural pressures, and the movement of the reservoir bag with spontaneous respiration cannot be regarded as an indication of tracheal intubation.

The appearance of cyanosis
Although oesophageal intubation will eventually cause severe decreases in oxygen saturation, there may be a delay of some minutes before cyanosis occurs. Cyanosis usually becomes apparent when there is 5 g of reduced haemoglobin per 100 ml blood (in cases of severe anaemia this may reflect oxygen saturations of 60%). Pre-oxygenation followed by a period of apnoea may delay the fall in oxygen saturation for up to 3 minutes, and normal oxygen saturations detected by a pulse oximeter should not be regarded as a sign of successful tracheal intubation. If a patient is making respiratory efforts through an unintubated trachea, recovery of consciousness may well occur before a significant reduction in oxygen saturation.

Objective signs
Identification of carbon dioxide in expired gas
Alveolar gas normally contains about 5% carbon dioxide. If the lungs are being perfused and effective alveolar ventilation is occurring then identification of carbon dioxide in exhaled gas by capnography should confirm correct tube placement. There are, however, a number of causes of false-negative results, where the tube is correctly placed but the capnograph waveform is absent (Figure IA16). There is also potential for false-positive results, where there is carbon dioxide passing out of a misplaced tube. This can occur after a period of vigorous mask ventilation with inflation of the stomach with gas containing carbon dioxide. The CO_2 waveform in this situation may initially appear normal but it rapidly diminishes to zero after a few breaths. Carbon dioxide in expired gas can also be detected chemically. pH-sensitive chemical indicator devices that reversibly change colour on exposure to CO_2 are available. These are often disposable devices that do not require a power source and are simple and safe in operation with a quick response time – but they may be relatively costly. In areas where sophisticated equipment is not available, bubbling expired gases through a diluted solution of bromothymol blue will cause a rapid colour change from a reddish blue to a greenish yellow on exposure to CO_2.

Oesophageal detector devices
The oesphageal detector device consists of a 60 ml syringe that can be attached to an endotracheal tube connector. A negative pressure applied to the lumen of the oesophagus will cause it to collapse, whereas the adult trachea contains cartilaginous rings and will not collapse under the same conditions. Aspiration of the plunger will therefore freely withdraw gas if the tube is in the trachea but will encounter resistance if the tube is located in the oesophagus. If the syringe is replaced by a self-inflating bulb then the

False-negative results
- Equipment failure
- Disconnection or apnoea
- Kinked or obstructed gas sampling tube
- Kinked or obstructed tracheal tube
- Dilution of expired gas by high fresh gas flow with sidestream sampling
- Severe airway obstruction
- Poor pulmonary perfusion (severe hypotension, pulmonary/air embolism)

False-positive results
- Tube in oesophagus after exhaled gases have been forced into stomach
- Tube in oesophagus after drinking carbonated beverages
- Distal end of endotracheal tube in pharynx

Figure IA16 Errors in confirmation of correct intubation

principle of use remains the same: compression of the bulb is followed by immediate refill if the tracheal tube is correctly placed, but if the tube is in the oesophagus the bulb will remain collapsed. Although these devices are simple and sensitive they may fail to confirm tracheal tube placement if the tube is partially obstructed or if the patient has bronchospasm or is morbidly obese.

Regurgitation and vomiting during induction

Regurgitation of gastric contents during induction risks pulmonary aspiration through the unprotected glottic opening.

Causes

There are multiple factors which may predispose to regurgitation and vomiting. The major causes are detailed in Figure IA17.

Prevention of pulmonary aspiration

It is important to prevent gastric contents from reaching the pharynx and then contaminating the lower respiratory tract. If there is a high risk of this then rendering the gastric contents as innocuous as possible should be considered (Figure IA18).

Gastric volume

The concept that a critical volume of 25 ml and pH of 2.5 is necessary to produce aspiration pneumonitis has been around since the time of Mendelson's original study (1946), and although these values may be somewhat arbitrary it

Factors that increase gastric volume	Full stomach
	Intestinal or pyloric obstruction
	Air inflation during mask ventilation
Factors that delay gastric emptying	Pregnancy
	Head injury
	Diabetic autonomic neuropathy
	Opioids
	Sympathetic stimulation: pain or anxiety
Incompetence of the gastro-oesophageal junction	Hiatus hernia
	Nasogastric tube in situ
	Scleroderma
Raised intra-abdominal pressure	Obesity
	Steep head-down position
	Pregnancy
Other causes	Peritonitis
	Pancreatitis
	Hypotension in the awake patient
	Drugs: opioids, ergometrine, magnesium, volatile agents
	Vagal stimulation (for example pressure on the epiglottis from a polio blade)

Figure IA17 Causes of regurgitation and vomiting

- Avoid oversedation
- Starve patient (elective procedure)
- Aspirate nasogastric tube
- Reduce gastric acidity
- Employ rapid sequence induction

Figure IA18 Guidelines for preventing pulmonary aspiration

is true that any mechanism that reduces gastric volume or acidity will tend to minimise the severity of aspiration pneumonitis. Ensure that the patient is starved. In recent years the value of conventional fasting regimes (6 hours for solids and 4 hours for liquids) has been challenged, and from these studies a few general conclusions can be drawn. Clear fluids are rapidly removed from the stomach, and in healthy adults and children clear fluid intake within 2–3 hours of induction does not affect gastric contents. Solid and semisolid food and milk products are not cleared from the stomach as rapidly. The application of suction to an orogastric or nasogastric tube allows liquid gastric contents to be removed from the stomach before the induction of anaesthesia. It cannot be relied upon, however, to completely empty the stomach. It has been argued that the presence of a gastric tube will interfere with the mechanics of the lower oesophageal sphincter and allow reflux of gastric contents, and that it should therefore be removed before a rapid sequence induction. In the authors' opinion the tube should be aspirated immediately before induction and left in situ open to allow the free passage of fluid and gas out of the stomach. Vomiting can be induced by the slow intravenous injection of up to 5 mg apomorphine. Not surprisingly this is rather unpleasant for the patient and cannot ever be recommended.

Gastric acidity

Gastric acidity may be reduced by the administration of an alkali or by deliberate inhibition of gastric acid production. Sodium citrate, magnesium trisilicate, H_2 blocking agents and proton pump inhibitors are the most commonly used agents.

- Sodium citrate is a clear, soluble, non-particulate alkali. 30 ml of 0.3 M sodium citrate is particularly effective at raising gastric pH, but may cause an increase in gastric volume. Failure to neutralise gastric acidity in some patients may be related to inadequate mixing with stomach contents. Unfortunately, the duration of action of sodium citrate is dependent on the rate of gastric emptying and may be as short as 20 minutes, thereby not providing adequate prophylaxis at the time of recovery. In some patients it is emetogenic.
- Magnesium trisilicate mixture contains magnesium trisilicate, magnesium carbonate and sodium carbonate made up with peppermint emulsion and chloroform water. Although an effective antacid, the solution is particulate in nature, and studies have suggested a link between the aspiration of gastric fluid containing particulate antacids and severe pulmonary reactions.
- H_2 receptor blockade by cimetidine or ranitidine will suppress acid secretion by gastric parietal cells.

Cimetidine 400 mg administered orally or intravenously will reduce gastric volume and raise pH in most patients after 1–2 hours. Unfortunately, cimetidine has a range of side effects when used long-term including mental confusion, dizziness and headaches as well as hypotension and arrhythmias following bolus administration. Cimetidine reduces hepatic blood flow and inhibits cytochrome P450 and will prolong the duration of action of drugs cleared by the liver such as warfarin, propanolol, phenytoin, diazepam and bupivacaine. Rantidine 150 mg orally is more rapid in onset, more effective and has a longer duration of action than cimetidine. Furthermore it is relatively free of side effects. For these reasons it is generally preferred to cimetidine for preoperative use.

- Omeprazole is a non-competitive proton pump inhibitor effectively suppressing the final step of gastric acid secretion. A single dose of omeprazole 40 mg will reduce gastric acidity for up to 48 hours. It has been used as a prophylactic agent for acid aspiration, and although a single dose will reduce gastric volume and acidity, better results have been obtained with two doses, the first given the evening before surgery.

Gastric emptying

Gastric emptying may be encouraged pharmacologically by drugs such as metoclopramide. Metoclopramide possesses central and peripheral antidopaminergic activity and will raise the lower oesophageal barrier pressure and accelerate gastric emptying within 10–20 minutes of an intravenous dose. Metoclopramide exhibits an inconsistent anti-emetic action secondary to inhibition of the chemoreceptor trigger zone. Extrapyramidal reactions are the commonest serious side effect, and can occur following a single dose of 10 mg.

Lower oesophageal sphincter tone

The lower oesophageal sphincter maintains closure of the distal oesophagus through tonic contraction of smooth muscle. The resulting pressure gradient between the distal oesophagus and the stomach is known as the lower oesophageal barrier pressure, and in healthy adults it is normally 30 mmHg. The sphincter cannot be relied upon to prevent reflux in a patient with gastric distension, obesity and pregnancy, and it is affected by various drugs. Dopaminergic and adrenergic stimulation decrease the lower oesophageal barrier pressure, whereas cholinergic stimulation increases it. Anticholinergic drugs such as atropine and glycopyrrolate will therefore decrease the contractility of the lower oesophageal sphincter, and may encourage reflux.

Cricoid pressure

The application of cricoid pressure to prevent passive regurgitation at induction of anaesthesia was proposed by Sellick (1961). The cricoid cartilage is a ring-shaped cartilage which when pressed backwards onto the vertebral column will occlude the upper end of the oesophagus. Sellick described having the head and neck extended, stabilising the cricoid cartilage between the thumb and second finger and applying pressure on the cricoid cartilage with the index finger. Firm pressure should be applied, sufficient to cause mild discomfort but not so severe as to cause breathing difficulties. The usual method of applying cricoid pressure is a modification of the original technique, with the patient in the 'sniffing the morning air' position and pressure applied with the thumb and index finger. If flexion of the neck occurs, hindering insertion of the laryngoscope, this can be prevented by the assistant placing the other hand behind the neck and applying gentle support. Lower oesophageal sphincter pressure decreases as anaesthesia is induced and cricoid pressure should, therefore, be applied whilst the patient is still awake and increased immediately consciousness is lost. Cricoid pressure should be maintained until the trachea has been intubated, the cuff inflated and the correct position of the tube confirmed. It should then be the responsibility of the anaesthetist to determine the moment at which cricoid pressure is released. Cricoid pressure should still be maintained if active vomiting occurs, as the risk of aspiration outweighs the potential risk of oesophageal rupture from high intra-oesophageal pressures. The application of cricoid pressure may prove difficult in patients with short, thick necks, and if pressure has been applied incorrectly the larynx may be pushed away from the midline, making the process of intubation more difficult.

Treatment of pulmonary aspiration

If regurgitation or vomiting occurs during induction, the upper airway should be cleared by immediately sucking out the pharynx and turning the patient head-down. If the patient is paralysed, tracheal intubation should be performed and the airway protected. If gastric contents are thought to have entered the trachea these should be aspirated before ventilation is commenced, as positive pressure will force the acidic contents further into the lungs. Attempted neutralisation of acid at this stage is ineffective, but the injection of 10 ml boluses of saline into the trachea followed by immediate suction is a useful form of bronchial lavage. Large volumes of saline will be absorbed and should, therefore, be avoided.

Early clinical signs of acid aspiration in the anaesthetised patient include a fall in arterial oxygen saturation and the presence of wheezing and ronchi, which may be localised to one lung. Aspiration of solid material causes plugging of the large airways and is often fatal. Bronchospasm, pulmonary oedema and ventilation perfusion mismatch all contribute to worsening arterial hypoxaemia, and often the only way to maintain adequate oxygenation is to institute a period of mechanical ventilation with 100% oxygen and the addition of positive end-expiratory pressure (PEEP). Bronchodilators and physiotherapy are often helpful, and prophylactic antibiotics should be administered, particularly in the case of gross soiling of the airways. Systemic steroids are of no benefit and may increase the risk of secondary bacterial infection.

Special circumstances

The full stomach

A patient with a full stomach requires a rapid sequence induction (RSI) to minimise the time from loss of consciousness to intubation with a cuffed endotracheal tube. Before beginning the induction it is necessary to minimise the pH and volume of gastric contents. This can be achieved by pharmacological methods if time allows, or by physical methods such as aspiration via a nasogastric tube (see above).

The term 'rapid sequence induction' is preferable to 'crash induction', which implies an element of panic that is clearly undesirable! Skilled assistance is mandatory, and the procedure should be explained to the patient in advance. Practical details of RSI are given in Figure IA19. Rocuronium is an alternative to suxamethonium for RSI when the latter is contraindicated, but the intubating conditions produced by rocuronium, although acceptable, are not yet considered comparable with those of suxamethonium.

The shocked patient

The patient with hypovolaemic shock poses a particular problem during the induction of anaesthesia. Conventional anaesthetic techniques reduce cardiac

- Place patient on tilting table
- Check all equipment
- Keep active suction readily to hand
- Attach monitoring and secure intravenous access
- Pre-oxygenate with 100% oxygen administered from a close-fitting face mask for 2 minutes
- Apply cricoid pressure (the role of a trained assistant)
- Administer a sleep dose of an appropriate induction agent intravenously
- Once consciousness has been lost administer suxamethonium 1 mg kg^{-1} intravenously
- When the patient is relaxed perform laryngoscopy and intubate the trachea
- Inflate the cuff and check position of the tube before releasing cricoid pressure
- Secure the tube

Figure IA19 Rapid sequence induction

contractility, cardiac output and systemic vascular resistance, and also attenuate the normal homeostatic responses to hypovolaemia. The potential end result of an induction in a hypovolaemic patient is cardiovascular collapse, with the 'unmasking' of the true extent of the hyovolaemia resulting from the removal and overburdening of the compensatory mechanisms.

The importance of adequate preoperative assessment of cardiovascular and intravascular volume cannot be over-stressed. Intravascular volume should be restored. In the case of active and continuing blood and fluid loss this may only be a temporary measure until surgical intervention stops the ongoing losses.

Adequate intravenous access is essential before induction. The dose of any induction agent should be considerably reduced, as not only is the conventional dose likely to cause too significant cardiovascular depression but also the preferential blood flow to essential organs exacerbates the effect of the given dose. Ketamine may be considered as an alternative induction agent owing to its sympatho-mimetic action. For further discussion of the management of trauma see Section 1, Chapter 9.

Head injury

A patient with a head injury may require intubation and ventilation for a number of reasons: to protect the airway from aspiration, to maintain adequate oxygenation, to allow controlled hyperventilation as a means of reducing intracranial pressure and to facilitate the management of convulsions. Intubation is often performed in emergency departments before transfer for CT scanning or neuro-surgery, and it is important that anaesthetists are aware that a protected airway and adequate oxygenation take priority over the wishes of neurosurgeons to be able to make a clinical examination of an unconscious patient. Great care should be taken to minimise rises in intracranial pressure in patients with a head injury. A slight (15 degree) head-up tilt is, therefore, beneficial. Patients with a head injury should be assumed to have a full stomach, and therefore require a rapid sequence induction. Head-injured patients must also be assumed to have suffered a cervical spine injury, and if this cannot be excluded the neck should be immobilised in the neutral position. The use of an induction agent such as thiopental or propofol will attenuate the rise in intracranial pressure associated with laryngoscopy and should be used even in unconscious patients. Coughing on the tracheal tube and turning of the head cause an increase in intracranial pressure, and should therefore be avoided.

Upper airway obstruction

Upper airway obstruction is always a matter of concern to the anaesthetist. Patients often require anaesthesia in order to assess the cause of the obstruction, and may require a period of endotracheal intubation or a formal tracheostomy. Inhalational induction is the preferred route in a patient with respiratory obstruction. This should be performed under controlled conditions by a senior anaes-thetist in an operating theatre environment using full monitoring. Equipment for a difficult intubation must be available, and if necessary a surgeon should be standing by to perform an emergency tracheostomy. The conduct of the induction will depend on the age and fitness of the patient and the severity of the obstruction. Venous access should be secured before induction unless the patient is a child, when crying can precipitate complete obstruction. Patients often prefer to sit up, and should be induced in this position. Halothane in 100% oxygen is a suitable agent, being potent and relatively non-irritant, and it should be introduced gradually and built up to an inspired concentration of 4–5%. Helium–oxygen mixtures have been advocated in airway obstruction due to the low density of helium, which results in greater flow under conditions of turbulence, but it is doubtful that any significant advantage results over the use of 100% oxygen as carrier for the volatile agent.

Sevoflurane is increasingly being used as an alternative to halothane in this situation. This is due in part to the declining availability of halothane but also to the lack of familiarity with the older drug among newer anaesthetists. Sevoflurane is reasonably effective, but whilst achieving more rapid onset of action it is difficult to achieve sufficient depth of anaesthesia without intravenous adjuncts.

With any form of airway obstruction the uptake of a volatile agent will be reduced, and it may take up to 15 minutes to achieve a sufficient depth of anaesthesia. Once the patient is deeply anaesthetised and breathing spontaneously then laryngoscopy may be performed. Alternatively, if the degree of obstruction is not too severe it may be possible to gently assist ventilation by hand, and if this is easy a dose of suxamethonium can be given and direct laryngoscopy performed. It is essential that the ability to ventilate the patient be confirmed before muscle relaxant drugs are given.

References and further reading

Association of Anaesthetists of Great Britain and Ireland. *Suspected Anaphylactic Reactions Associated with Anaesthesia, revised edn.* London: AAGBI, 2003. www.aagbi.org.

Cormack RS, Lehane J. Difficult tracheal intubation in obstetrics. *Anaesthesia* 1984; **39**: 1105–11.

Gataure PS, Hughes JA. The laryngeal mask airway in obstetrical anaesthesia. *Can J Anaesth* 1995; **42**: 130–3.

McCoy EP, Mirakhur RK. The levering laryngoscope. *Anaesthesia* 1993; **48**: 516–19.

Mendelson CL. Aspiration of stomach contents into lungs during obstetric anaesthesia. *Am J Obstet Gynecol* 1946: **52**: 191–205.

Confidential Enquiry into Maternal and Child Health. *Saving Mothers' Lives: Reviewing Maternal Deaths to Make Motherhood Safer, 2003–2005.* London: CEMACH, 2007. www.cemach.org.uk.

Sellick BA. Cricoid pressure to control regurgitation of gastric contents during induction of anaesthesia. *Lancet* 1961; **2**: 404–5.

CHAPTER 3
Intraoperative management

C. A. Pinnock

POSITIONING THE SURGICAL PATIENT

MAINTENANCE OF ANAESTHESIA
Techniques for maintenance of anaesthesia
  and analgesia
Prevention of awareness during surgery
Analgesia
Airway control
Controlled ventilation
Monitoring during anaesthesia
Management of intraoperative fluid therapy

CRITICAL INCIDENTS DURING ANAESTHESIA
Cyanosis
Hypertension
Hypotension
Cardiac arrhythmias
Bronchospasm
Respiratory obstruction (increased peak inspiratory
  pressure)
Hypercarbia and hypocarbia
Massive haemorrhage
Emboli
Malignant hyperthermia (hyperpyrexia) (MH)
Accidental pneumothorax

FAILURE TO BREATHE

The intraoperative period follows induction of anaesthesia and is terminated by discharge of the patient from the operating theatre into the recovery area. After leaving the confines of the anaesthetic room the first task is the safe positioning of the patient for surgery and the re-establishment of monitoring and the anaesthesia delivery system as soon as possible.

Positioning the surgical patient
Manipulation of a patient into the desired position for surgery carries its own problems. The main hazards are related to the effects of pressure and the physiological changes associated with a change in posture.

The anaesthetised patient is at risk of developing pressure sores in those areas where perfusion may be compromised. Likely sites are the occiput, the sacrum and the heel, all of which must be padded. External pneumatic compression devices applied to the lower limbs both confer a degree of protection from pressure effects and also improve circulation, which helps to prevent deep vein thrombosis. No patient should ever be allowed to lie with the legs crossed, and where possible an evacuable mattress should be used. Compartment syndrome, usually related to trauma or arterial surgery, and for which immediate fasciotomy is essential to save life or limb, can be a rare complication of prolonged lower limb compression in the lithotomy position.

The physiological effects which result from positioning are posture-related. In the respiratory system a reduction in functional residual capacity (FRC) and total lung volume (TLV) is usually seen, accompanied by ventilation and perfusion imbalance and a degree of mechanical embarrassment to the respiratory process.

Cardiovascular effects are generally the result of gravitationally dictated venous pooling which leads to a fall in preload and reduced cardiac output. Embarrassment of venous return due to abdominal compression is a specific complication of the prone position, but one that may be overcome by correct support so that the abdomen is unrestricted.

Steep head-down (Trendelenburg) positioning may increase intraocular pressure. Air embolism is a risk if the operative site lies above the right atrium.

It is particularly important to protect the patient in positions other than supine. Gel pads, tape and supports form part of this. The aim is always to provide a cushioning to pressure-sensitive areas, a position that avoids pressure on such areas and the avoidance of positions that cause excessive traction on ligaments. The eyes in the prone position must be taped closed and gel pads applied. A head ring is useful to avoid movement of the head so that the

Fundamentals of Anaesthesia, 3rd edition, ed. Tim Smith, Colin Pinnock and Ted Lin. Published by Cambridge University Press. © Cambridge University Press 2008.

eyes become under pressure. The neck requires careful attention during turning into the prone position, when the weight of the head could lead to excessive extension or rotation. In the final prone position the head should not be overextended.

The potential damage to nerves from the common positions is detailed in Figure IN1.

Maintenance of anaesthesia

Techniques for maintenance of anaesthesia and analgesia

The maintenance of anaesthesia may be conveniently divided into those techniques applied to patients who are self-ventilating and those techniques applied to patients who are receiving artificial ventilation of their lungs. Techniques suitable for self-ventilating patients are summarised in Figure IN2.

Local anaesthesia

Maintenance of anaesthesia by local anaesthetic techniques is covered in Section 1, Chapter 7.

General anaesthesia by inhalation of volatile agents

The ideal is to keep the patient safely asleep, pain free, and appropriately relaxed. This ideal cannot always be met. Unawareness (sometimes referred to as hypnosis) is an absolute priority. To an extent, hypnosis is related to the minimum alveolar concentration (MAC) of any specified volatile agent.

In unpremedicated subjects MAC (sometimes referred to as 1 MAC) is the alveolar concentration of a volatile anaesthetic (in oxygen) which will prevent movement in response to a standard surgical stimulus in one-half of the population. MAC is thus the ED_{50} (the effective dose in 50% of patients). MAC may be higher or lower in the other 50% of the population. MAC may, therefore, be considered to equal the median of a normal distribution of alveolar concentrations. It is important to consider where in the distribution an individual patient lies. The issue can only be resolved by clinical observation and monitoring. During anaesthesia (assuming normal respiratory function) the alveolar concentration of a volatile agent, or its MAC, is close to the concentration of the agent measured at the end of exhalation, the end-tidal concentration.

MAC is the standard way to compare the potencies of volatile agents, and is also useful because it is additive. Thus, if the patient inhales 0.5 MAC of one agent and 0.5 MAC of another agent, the MAC value is $0.5 + 0.5 = 1.0$.

MAC does not always relate to the 'depth' of anaesthesia. Various reasons apply, and these are listed in Figure IN3.

General anaesthesia by using IV agents via bolus or infusion

Various agents have been employed for intravenous techniques. **Thiopental** was widely used in the 1950s and 1960s for continuous IV anaesthesia but its accumulation in the tissues and hence prolonged recovery phase proved disadvantageous. **Ketamine** has proved useful in the Developing World. **Propofol** is currently popular in the UK and is in common use for total intravenous anaesthesia (TIVA). There are three popular techniques:

(1) An induction dose of propofol is followed by smaller bolus doses on an empirical basis. This technique is adequate for short procedures (<15 minutes).

(2) Manually controlled infusion. In this system blood concentrations of propofol are achieved by the use of a syringe pump which delivers the induction dose at a fixed rate (about 600 ml per hour) until verbal contact with the patient is lost. Maintenance of anaesthesia is continued at 6 mg kg^{-1} h^{-1} and the rate adjusted manually if the patient moves. The patient is allowed to breathe spontaneously a mixture of nitrous oxide in oxygen or oxygen in air. A 'stepdown' regimen is described, based on pharmacokinetic principles (e.g. after induction 10 mg kg^{-1} h^{-1} for 10 minutes, 8 mg kg^{-1} h^{-1} for 10 min and 6 mg kg^{-1} h^{-1} thereafter). Supplementary boluses of propofol may be needed to ensure adequate depth of anaesthesia.

(3) Target-controlled infusion. In this computer-controlled system the aim is to reach the effective blood concentration (EC) of propofol in μg ml^{-1} needed to prevent response to a surgical incision, and to keep it there. Minimum infusion rate (MIR), the infusion rate necessary to maintain EC, is the intravenous equivalent of MAC. The syringe pump, controlled by computer, is the equivalent of a vaporiser. If the target EC (say, 6 μg ml^{-1}) is set too low or too high the 'vaporiser concentration' can be adjusted as for an inhalational anaesthetic technique. Systems usually require programming for individual patient characteristics (age, weight, ASA status, concomitant opioid administration). Success depends on the software (a three-compartment pharmacokinetic model, a set of specific pharmacokinetic variables for propofol, and special instructions, or algorithms, to vary the rate of infusion).

Position	Nerve injury	Cause
Supine	supraorbital nerve	pressure from an endotracheal tube connector
	nerves innervating the eyeball	pressure by a face mask
	cranial nerve VII	pressure by a tight face-mask harness
	brachial plexus	traction injury due to incorrect positioning or from shoulder retainers in the Trendelenberg position
	radial nerve	pressure by screen supports
	ulnar nerve	pressure by the edge of the operating-table mattress

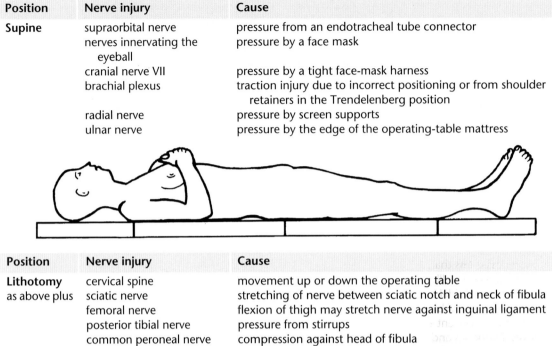

Position	Nerve injury	Cause
Lithotomy as above plus	cervical spine	movement up or down the operating table
	sciatic nerve	stretching of nerve between sciatic notch and neck of fibula
	femoral nerve	flexion of thigh may stretch nerve against inguinal ligament
	posterior tibial nerve	pressure from stirrups
	common peroneal nerve	compression against head of fibula
	saphenous nerve	compression against the medial tibial condyle
	obturator nerve	flexion at the obturator foramen

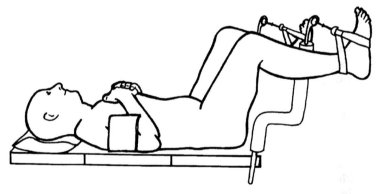

Position	Nerve injury	Cause
Prone	cervical spinal cord	overextension of the cervical spine
	brachial plexus	overdistension
	radial nerve	direct compression
	ulnar nerve	compression at the elbow against a mattress
	LCNT	pressure on the anterior superior iliac spine

Figure IN1 Nerve damage related to positioning

- Local anaesthesia by tissue infiltration, central or peripheral neural blockade
- General anaesthesia by inhalation of anaesthetic vapours with or without nitrous oxide
- General anaesthesia by intermittent manual or by target-controlled intravenous administration of anaesthetic agents, with or without inhalation of nitrous oxide
- General anaesthesia by intramuscular injection (ketamine)
- Hypnosis
- Acupuncture

Figure IN2 Anaesthetic techniques for self-ventilating patients

- Normally distributed
- Relate to movement and not to awareness (MAC for awareness is less than MAC for movement)
- Vary with age and wellbeing
- Inferred from end-tidal concentration (may not correlate with arterial blood concentration)
- Reduced by concurrent administration of sedatives, hypnotics and analgesics
- Increased by fear and by drug abuse (including alcohol)

Figure IN3 Characteristics of MAC values

Prevention of awareness during surgery

The primary purpose of maintenance of anaesthesia is to ensure the adequacy of anaesthesia so as to prevent awareness during surgery. Awareness may be defined as follows:

Awareness (explicit memory)

- Conscious awareness with recall but without pain. The patient recalls conversations in the operating theatre. The incidence is thought to be about 4/1000 in obstetrics and 2/1000 in non-obstetric surgery.
- Conscious awareness with recall and pain. The incidence is thought to be about 1/10 000 in elective surgery and 2/1000 in the 'shocked' patient.

Awareness (implicit memory)

- Perception without conscious awareness or recall. The patient denies recall, but may remember 'something' under hypnosis. Psychologists are sceptical about the existence of this phenomenon.

Awareness (deliberate)

- Surgery conducted under local anaesthesia is discussed in Section 1, Chapter 7.

- Surgery for spinal deformities under general anaesthesia. The 'wake-up' test to see whether surgery has affected the integrity of the spinal cord has been replaced by observing motor-evoked and/or somatosensory evoked potentials.

Recall after surgery under general anaesthesia can be a psychological disaster from which the victim may take months to recover (post-traumatic stress disorder). There remains no reliable means of measuring depth of anaesthesia or level of consciousness despite a large amount of research into automated real-time analysis of the EEG.

Recall is almost always linked to a general anaesthetic technique which has employed muscle relaxation and artificial ventilation (controlled ventilation). It may occur at any time: during induction (intubation of the trachea), during maintenance, and during emergence. Awareness may arise from several causes:
- Clinical fault (misjudged requirement)
- Technical fault (the anaesthesia system does not deliver the required mixture)
- Mixture of the above

Clinical observation remains the mainstay of the diagnosis of impending or actual awareness. This may be heralded by an increase in autonomic (sympathetic) activity, reflected by the following signs:
- Increase in pulse rate
- Increase in systemic arterial blood pressure
- Dilatation of the pupils
- Sweating
- Lacrimation
- Increase in metabolic rate
- Changes in the EEG (bispectral analysis, auditory evoked potentials)

It is important to note that there need not necessarily be an obvious sympathetic response. A significant change may not signify awareness (a 'false positive') but merely imply an increase in ascending spinal cord traffic as reflected in the EEG. Effective maintenance of anaesthesia as described in Figure IN4 minimises the risk of awareness.

Analgesia

With the exception of nitrous oxide (whose effect is limited) volatile anaesthetics are not analgesic agents but rather hypnotics and, to an extent, muscle relaxants. Thus a specific form of analgesia needs to be provided. This

- Constantly observe the patient
- Administer a muscle relaxant only when necessary
- Deliver 1 MAC of volatile agent, monitor and record MAC with an anaesthetic vapour analyser
- Provide good analgesia, for example by combining a general anaesthetic technique with a local anaesthetic block
- Monitor and record pulse rate, arterial blood pressure, pupil size, sweating, lacrimation, end-tidal carbon dioxide, core and skin temperature and the neuromuscular junction

Figure IN4 Recommendations for avoidance of awareness

might take the form of local or regional anaesthesia, augmented by opioids, with or without non-steroidal anti-inflammatory drugs (NSAIDs) orally, parenterally or rectally. For cultural and medico-legal reasons it is best to seek a patient's consent for rectal administration of any drug and to write that consent on the anaesthetic record.

Airway control

Airway control is a vital component of anaesthesia. Despite the best preoperative assessment it is not always possible to foresee problems. Control of the airway is to some extent dictated by the technique used for the maintenance of anaesthesia.

Spontaneous breathing

While oropharyngeal (Guedel) or nasopharyngeal airways are satisfactory (and sometimes essential), the laryngeal mask airway (LMA) has virtually replaced them. One reason is the ease with which it is possible to maintain the airway with no hands, freeing the anaesthetist to deal with other tasks. The LMA also provides, in most patients, a better and more secure airway. Provided the depth of anaesthesia and muscular relaxation is appropriate for the surgery, regurgitation of gastric contents and their aspiration into the trachea should be no more common, and perhaps even less common, than with other airways. Should artificial ventilation become necessary it can be readily commenced and maintained.

Artificial ventilation

Endotracheal anaesthesia was developed by Magill and Rowbotham in 1920, and early tracheal tubes were not cuffed. Today, endotracheal intubation with a cuffed tube is generally thought of as the 'gold standard' for controlled ventilation. However, in experienced hands it is feasible and usually safe to ventilate the lungs artificially with an LMA. Although there are fears about the risk of tracheal aspiration, there have been no reported deaths or serious morbidity even when the LMA has been used for emergency obstetric surgery or for resuscitation from cardiac arrest. The LMA has retrieved the situation when tracheal intubation was impossible. Recovery from anaesthesia and the establishment of spontaneous breathing have proved to be very smooth, and in contrast with intubation postoperative sore throats and transient cranial nerve palsies are uncommon.

At present the cuffed endotracheal tube is recommended in patients who are thought to have a full stomach, those with a radiologically proven hiatus hernia, severe oesophagitis or gross obesity, when airway access is difficult (prone position, intracranial surgery), and in prolonged surgery.

Controlled ventilation
Indications for controlled ventilation

The decision to use controlled ventilation, with or without a muscle relaxant, is often a personal one and depends upon the site, nature, extent and (to a degree) the likely duration of the operation. Posture and access to a secure airway are also important. Advice must be coloured by the gradual development of 'minimally invasive surgery' and by the increasing use of the laryngeal mask. Operations may be divided into 'surface' and 'non-surface'. Surface procedures should not need muscle relaxation and controlled ventilation. Consideration should be given to whether controlled ventilation is more or less likely than spontaneous breathing to affect functional residual capacity (FRC) and, hence, oxygenation. If the surgical technique is likely to impair the mechanics of breathing or there is a need to secure the airway with a cuffed tracheal tube, controlled ventilation should be employed. A patient who is already apnoeic from whatever cause (e.g. from drug overdose or head injury) will obviously require ventilation of the lungs.

The pattern of controlled ventilation

Controlled ventilation may be considered by evaluating its respective components as detailed in Figure IN5.

The aim is to choose a pattern of controlled ventilation which combines effective anaesthesia delivery with the best oxygen flux or 'oxygen availability' (oxygen delivery to the cell depends upon regional blood flow). The following factors are of importance: oxygen flux, cardiac output and saturation of haemoglobin with oxygen.

- Minute volume ventilation (MV)
- Tidal volume (VT) and hence the respiratory frequency (f)
- Ratio of inspiratory time to expiratory time (I : E ratio)
- Fresh gas inflow (FGF) from the anaesthetic apparatus
- Fractional inspired oxygen concentration (FiO_2)
- End-tidal carbon dioxide tension ($PETCO_2$)
- Airway pressure (consequent on the above)

Figure IN5 Components of controlled ventilation

Oxygen flux

The concept of oxygen flux relates to the delivery of oxygen to the tissues, and it is encapsulated in the following equation:

$$\text{Oxygen flux} = (\text{cardiac output} \times Hb\% \times Sat\% \times k) + Z$$

where k = Hüfner constant (1.39) and Z = the amount of oxygen dissolved in plasma.

Cardiac output

One of the main determinants of cardiac output is preload. Venous return to the heart depends not only upon posture and on the blood volume but on mean intrathoracic pressure. Increasing the mean intrathoracic pressure decreases venous return. During controlled ventilation mean intrathoracic pressure relates to the pattern of ventilation. Any positive pressure (that is, any pressure above atmospheric) will reduce venous return; thus, lowest positive pressure compatible with an adequate oxygen saturation (>96%) should be chosen.

Saturation of haemoglobin with oxygen

Saturation may be measured invasively by an arterial blood sample (SaO_2) or, more commonly, by non-invasive pulse oximetry (SpO_2). If the oxyhaemoglobin dissociation curve is shifted to the left (for example by hyperventilation or by hypothermia) the haemoglobin molecule will have a greater affinity for oxygen and will be less able to release oxygen to the tissues. In which case, no matter what the oxygen flux or availability, oxygen delivery to the tissues may be reduced. If, on the other hand, the curve is shifted to the right (for example by hypoventilation) the haemoglobin molecule will have a lesser affinity for oxygen and oxygen delivery to the tissues may be increased. Note that the shape and position of the curve is affected by body temperature, pH, and to some

degree by the concentration of 2,3-DPG in the red cells, but these are far less easy to manipulate than end-tidal carbon dioxide concentration. The choice of pattern of controlled ventilation is, therefore, always a compromise. Normocapnia is desirable.

Choosing a pattern of controlled ventilation: practical guidelines
Minute volume ventilation (MV)
The simplest method is to use a calculation based on body weight (for example 70 ml kg^{-1} per minute) which is unlikely to lead to underventilation of the lungs. The exhaled minute volume should be measured because, for various reasons (respiratory compliance, compliance of the anaesthesia system, leaks in the system, compression of the inspired gases), it may be less than both the inhaled and the prescribed volume.

Tidal volume (VT) and frequency of breathing (f)
The minute volume is divided into tidal volumes. A tidal volume of 10 ml kg^{-1} is reasonable for an adult. On this choice will depend the respiratory frequency (f) and, in combination with the minute volume and I : E ratio, the mean intrathoracic pressure. In the adult a respiratory frequency of 12–14 breaths per minute is usually suitable.

Ratio of inspiratory time to expiratory time (I : E ratio)
In adult patients with healthy lungs, choice is generally empirical. When the frequency of respiration is 10 breaths per minute, then inspiration of 2 seconds and expiration of 4 seconds, giving an I : E ratio of 1 : 2, is suitable. In obstructive airways disease, a longer time may be needed to allow full expiration.

Fresh gas inflow (FGF)
Choice of FGF will depend on the selected breathing system and, if an automatic ventilator is used, upon its design.

Fractional inspired oxygen concentration (FiO_2)
The value depends on the measured SpO_2, which should be kept above 93% (a value at which oxyhaemoglobin is very close to the steep part of the dissociation curve) and preferably at 96–100%.

End-tidal CO_2 concentration ($PETCO_2$)
The desired $PETCO_2$ (as a reflection of the $PaCO_2$) may be achieved by manipulation of alveolar ventilation using the above characteristics.

Airway pressure (Paw)

Airway pressure will be consequent on the decisions made on the above characteristics. It is a measure of the energy needed to deliver a given tidal volume and minute volume ventilation at a prescribed I : E ratio.

Monitoring during anaesthesia

In the UK the standards of monitoring are set out by the Association of Anaesthetists of Great Britain and Ireland (2007), and they are summarised in Figure IN6.

The devices necessary for minimal non-invasive monitoring are listed in Figure IN7.

Management of intraoperative fluid therapy

Intraoperative fluid therapy is required for several reasons. Preoperative starvation leaves a residual deficit that should be made up, direct loss of blood requires replacement, and the so-called third space creates an additional need for extracellular fluid replenishment.

Third space is a concept that was developed to explain the phenomenon of patients having undergone surgery whose fluid requirements were not explained by measurable loss. Experimentally, in such patients, the extracellular fluid volume had become depleted to a degree related to the extent of surgery, but the patient's body weight had not reduced. The fluid depletion of the extracellular space was said to have occurred due to the movement of fluid into a 'third space'. This concept is widely applied today. A useful formula for intraoperative fluid replacement is therefore:

$$\text{Input} = \text{basal requirements} + \text{deficit} \\ + \text{losses} + \text{third space}$$

Basal requirement of crystalloid for an adult is $2\,\text{ml}\,\text{kg}^{-1}$ per hour. Hartmann's is the usual solution of choice, because its ionic composition is close to that of plasma. Existing deficits from starvation are usually replaced in an empirical manner although CVP, if available, will give a useful guide. Direct loss of blood may be replaced by crystalloid at twice the estimated loss (up to 15% blood volume) or volume-for-volume with a colloid solution (gelatin or similar). Losses of greater than 15% blood volume should be replaced on a volume-for-volume basis with blood. If packed cells are used, additional plasma or colloid will be necessary. Whole blood is rarely supplied today. For the management of massive transfusion see later in this chapter.

The Association of Anaesthetists of Great Britain and Ireland regards it as essential that certain core standards of monitoring must be used whenever a patient is anaesthetised. These minimum standards should be uniform irrespective of duration, location or mode of anaesthesia.

(1) The anaesthetist must be present and care for the patient throughout the conduct of an anaesthetic.

(2) Monitoring devices must be attached before induction of anaesthesia and their use continued until the patient has recovered from the effects of anaesthesia.

(3) The same standards of monitoring apply when the anaesthetist is responsible for a local/regional anaesthetic or sedative technique for an operative procedure.

(4) A summary of information provided by monitoring devices should be recorded on the anaesthetic record. Electronic record keeping systems are now recommended.

(5) The anaesthetist must ensure that all equipment has been checked before use. Alarm limits for all equipment must be set appropriately before use. Audible alarms must be enabled during anaesthesia.

(6) These recommendations state the monitoring devices which are essential and those which must be immediately available during anaesthesia. If it is necessary to continue anaesthesia without a device categorised 'essential', the anaesthetist must clearly note the reasons for this in the anaesthetic record.

(7) Additional monitoring may be necessary as deemed appropriate by the anaesthetist.

(8) A brief interruption of monitoring is only acceptable if the recovery area is immediately adjacent to the operating theatre. Otherwise monitoring should be continued during transfer to the same degree as any other intra- or inter-hospital transfer.

(9) Provision, maintenance, calibration and renewal of equipment is an institutional responsibility.

Figure IN6 Recommendations for standards of monitoring during anaesthesia and recovery (Association of Anaesthetists of Great Britain and Ireland 2007)

Spontaneous breathing
- ECG
- Pulse oximeter
- Indirect BP
- Capnograph
- Inspired gas O_2 analyser
- Fresh gas O_2 analyser
- Anaesthetic vapour analyser

Artificial ventilation – all the above plus
- Airway pressure gauge
- Ventilation disconnect device
- Ventilation volume
- Peripheral nerve stimulator
- Temperature

Seriously ill – additional monitoring
- Central venous pressure
- Intra-arterial blood pressure measurement
- Transoesophageal echocardiographic devices
- Volumetric urine output

Figure IN7 Minimal monitoring

Critical incidents during anaesthesia

Cyanosis
Central cyanosis can usually be detected at an arterial oxygen saturation of about 80–85%, depending on whether the patient is anaemic. Note that absence of cyanosis does not necessarily mean normal arterial oxygen levels (Lumb 2005). Even at an oxyhaemoglobin saturation of 93% the patient is very close to the steep part of the saturation curve. At 89% saturation the PaO_2 is only 7.5 kPa, so that by the time central cyanosis is detectable the patient can be severely compromised. Cyanosis may be the result of failure to pre-oxygenate, airway obstruction, tracheal aspiration, drug overdose, a fall in cardiac output (haemorrhage, septicaemia, other surgical causes), inadequate ventilation and oxygenation (intubation of the right main bronchus, bronchospasm, laryngospasm), gross dehydration, and cardiac arrhythmias. Treatment depends upon the diagnosis, but the first act must be to cut off all volatile and intravenous anaesthetics and administer 100% oxygen.

Hypertension
Hypertension under anaesthesia may be defined as systolic arterial blood pressure >20% above the preoperative value. This usually happens because the depth of anaesthesia is inappropriate to the intensity of the stimulus. Hypercarbia during the surgery is another possibility; and, in the supposedly paralysed patient, when the neuromuscular junction has not been continually monitored, there may be a need for another dose of a muscle relaxant. Techniques to complement general anaesthesia (such as central and peripheral neural blockade) are not always successful, and inadequate depth may become revealed by a rise in arterial pressure.

Hypotension
Hypotension under anaesthesia may be defined as a systolic arterial blood pressure <20% below preoperative value. The most common causes of unwanted hypotension, apart from surgical consequences (of which haemorrhage is the most frequent) and central neural blockade, are bradycardias, hypovolaemia and drug overdose (which may be relative or absolute).

Cardiac arrhythmias
Cardiac arrhythmias are relatively common during general anaesthesia. Strangely, some preoperative arrhythmias (e.g. ventricular ectopics) may disappear during or after induction of anaesthesia, only to reappear on recovery. Others, particularly atrial fibrillation, or temperature-dependent sinus tachycardias, do not show this pattern.

Sinus bradycardia
This is a matter of definition, but an adult patient who arrives in the anaesthetic room with a heart rate of less than 60 beats per minute may, after induction and especially when an opioid is used, drop the heart rate to less than 40 beats per minute. The systemic arterial blood pressure may be adversely affected. In such patients, it may be wise to increase the heart rate before induction to 70 beats per minute or more by the judicious use of vagolytic agents. During maintenance of anaesthesia glycopyrrolate (0.2–0.6 mg) can be used.

Bradycardia
Bradycardia, proceeding to nodal rhythm, is typical of halothane anaesthesia. Other causes of bradycardia are consequent on vagal stimulation (traction on mesentery or extraocular muscles, for example).

Sinus tachycardia
The definition of sinus tachycardia is a matter of opinion. Adult heart rates above 100 beats per minute in the anaesthetic room usually mean inadequate preoperative medication, and during surgery (unless secondary to haemorrhage) inadequate anaesthesia or muscle relaxation.

Ventricular bigeminy

Ventricular bigeminy is associated with endotracheal intubation (a sympathoadrenal response). Given time the bigeminy will disappear, but if it does not intravenous lidocaine (50–100 mg) may be helpful.

The management of arrhythmias is shown in Figure IN8.

Bronchospasm

Bronchospasm during surgery may be detected clinically by listening to breath sounds in the anaesthesia system's expiratory limb or, in the presence of controlled ventilation, by observing an increase in ventilatory pressure or a decrease in tidal volume or both. Auscultation will confirm the finding. Capnography will show a rising end-tidal CO_2 concentration and a typical trace showing a prolonged and flattened expiratory curve (and occasionally a slightly lengthened inspiratory time).

The smoker, the asthmatic, the patient with chronic obstructive airways disease and the inadequately anaesthetised patient are all susceptible to bronchospasm. Preoperative physiotherapy and appropriate drug therapy should be arranged. Unexpected bronchospasm during anaesthesia in a patient with normal lungs is a matter for concern and may reflect tracheal aspiration, abutment of a tracheal tube on the carina, or an intraoperative drug hypersensitivity (e.g. hypersensitivity to an antibiotic). Bronchospasm may also be the first physical sign of impending pulmonary oedema.

Treatment of intraoperative bronchospasm should be instituted as follows. Stop the surgery and increase the inspired concentration of volatile agent. The vagus nerve should be blocked (with atropine or glycopyrrolate). Check the position of a tracheal tube. Give sympathomimetic agents (ephedrine, aminophylline). Aspirate the tracheobronchial tree. Stop the administration of any antibiotic. With drug hypersensitivity in mind, re-evaluate the patient's history. Continue to monitor end-tidal carbon dioxide and observe the ECG for evidence of a change in the ST segment. Analysis of an arterial blood sample may be helpful.

Respiratory obstruction (increased peak inspiratory pressure)

Respiratory obstruction should be very rare during maintenance of anaesthesia, but it demands instant relief. Inattention to detail (e.g. incorrect placement of Guedel or laryngeal mask airways or tracheal tubes, or their

Atrial fibrillation (AF)

Digoxin will reduce the ventricular response rate to atrial activity but takes too long to be effective in acute situations. Both amiodarone and verapamil can be employed to reduce ventricular rate. DC cardioversion is indicated for the acute onset of AF.

Atrial flutter

Drug control of the ventricular rate is not often successful. DC cardioversion or atrial pacing may restore sinus rhythm.

Atrial tachycardia with AV block

After halting glycoside therapy (and ensuring normokalaemia), lidocaine 1 mg kg^{-1} IV is the drug of choice. Alternatively DC cardioversion or atrial pacing may be effective.

Paroxysmal supraventricular tachycardia

Vagal tone should be increased by applying carotid sinus massage (or a Valsalva manoeuvre). Second-line treatment is verapamil 5–10 mg IV (contraindicated contemporaneously with beta-blockers). Alternatively, give adenosine by rapid IV injection of 3 mg over 2 seconds, if necessary followed by 6 mg after 2 minutes, then by 12 mg after a further 2 minutes. Other potential pharmacological agents include propranolol, quinidine, procainamide, disopyramide and digoxin. DC cardioversion can also be used.

Atrial ectopic beats

Treatment is not usually necessary.

Ventricular ectopic beats

Treatment is unnecessary, unless the ectopic beats are frequent (one in four), or 'R on T' type, in which situation an infusion of lidocaine or beta-blocker therapy is indicated.

Ventricular fibrillation

A single precordial thump should be administered, followed by immediate DC defibrillation if unsuccessful. If the rhythm does not respond to defibrillation, prior treatment with IV bretylium tosylate may help.

Ventricular tachycardia

In the acute situation when there is haemodynamic embarrassment DC cardioversion should be immediate. For brief episodes of VT, suitable pharmacological agents include lidocaine (drug of choice), flecainide, disopyramide, amiodarone and mexiletine.

Figure IN8 Management of intraoperative arrhythmias

dislodgement) may be one cause, and laryngeal spasm under too light anaesthesia another. The siting and patency of endotracheal tubes cannot always be relied upon: for example, the cuff may have been overinflated, causing herniation over the tracheal end. An increase in peak inspiratory pressure (during controlled ventilation) will be inevitable if there is respiratory obstruction or bronchospasm. Other causes of raised airway pressure include the insufflation of carbon dioxide into the peritoneal cavity (minimally invasive surgery), strong surgical retraction (intra-abdominal, intrathoracic), and inadequate anaesthesia.

Hypercarbia and hypocarbia

Hyper- and hypocarbia refer to high or low carbon dioxide tensions in arterial blood. The reference range for the homeostatically 'normal' tension in a patient with normal lungs remains constant throughout life (unlike the arterial oxygen tension, which tends to decrease) and varies from 4.8 to 5.3 kPa. Hyper- and hypocapnia refer to carbon dioxide tensions in end-expired, or end-tidal, gas, which is taken to represent fairly closely the concentration of carbon dioxide in most, but not all, alveoli and to reflect arterial carbon dioxide. Simultaneous sampling of arterial blood and end-tidal gas in the same patient should provide similar results, although arterial carbon dioxide is usually higher (by about 0.2–1.0 kPa), than end-tidal carbon dioxide. Since arterial sampling is uncommon in everyday anaesthesia but end-tidal sampling extremely common, the latter is usually equated with the former.

In spontaneously breathing patients end-tidal carbon dioxide concentration is determined by the response of the patient to a surgical stimulus, by the respiratory depressant effects of the anaesthetic agents, and by cardiac output. In artificially ventilated patients end-tidal carbon dioxide concentration is open to manipulation. As a general consensus, the value should be kept within the reference range (normocapnia).

Massive haemorrhage

Massive haemorrhage may be self-evident (a traumatised patient in an accident and emergency department), anticipated (elective cardiac, vascular, neurosurgical and obstetrical operations), or unexpected.

A sudden reduction in end-tidal carbon dioxide concentration may be a useful sign if the situation is not self-evident, but once the diagnosis is made, the steps detailed in Figure IN9 should be taken.

- Alert the surgeon to the problem
- Summon help (pairs of hands)
- Alert the consultant haematologist and the blood bank
- Request blood coagulation studies
- Maintain systemic arterial blood pressure by warmed intravenous infusions of blood, if available, and colloid or crystalloid
- Improve intravenous access
- Begin invasive monitoring (CVP, intra-arterial line)

Figure IN9 Management of massive haemorrhage

If more than 50% of the patient's blood volume requires replacement the situation becomes one of massive transfusion. Transfusion of large amounts of stored blood results in several unphysiological effects, mainly due to its composition. Stored blood has a potassium concentration of 5–20 mmol l^{-1}, a pH of 6.5–7.2 and a temperature of 4–6 °C. The initial acidosis that may be seen after transfusion is rapidly replaced by alkalosis as the citrate in the blood becomes metabolised. Transfused red cells rapidly take up the potassium, and thus transient hyperkalaemia will become normokalaemia, or hypokalaemia. Fluid warming is essential, and the device used should be able to cope with rapid rates of infusion. Because of dilutional effects a paucity of clotting factors and platelets will be seen. Treatment should be directed at the replacement of the relevant factors (using fresh frozen plasma or cryoprecipitates) and transfusion of platelet concentrates. Haematological advice as to how much of what is required is invaluable and will usually be based on the results of extensive testing of clotting function.

Mortality is related to the degree of embarrassment of organ oxygenation. High inspired oxygen concentrations are desirable, and the maintenance of adequate circulating volume and cardiac output should be high priorities.

Choice of blood products

Haematological advice may recommend, on a descending scale, red cells, fresh frozen plasma and possibly, when the situation is desperate, cryoprecipitate and platelets. It is best to assume that all these blood products will be needed.

Incompatibility reactions

Incompatibility reactions are extraordinarily rare, but in the very often crucial situations described above the overextended anaesthetist may be tempted to transfuse blood products without rigorous checking – which should never occur. A stock of uncrossmatched blood is usually available for use in the direst emergencies. This 'universal donor' blood is of blood group O negative. The risk of incompatibility reactions with transfusion of this is relatively minor.

Emboli

Intraoperative embolism most commonly results from thrombus, although other situations include gas, fat and rarely tumour or amniotic fluid.

Thrombus

The risk of developing intraoperative thrombosis is increased by various factors. These include:
* Smoking
* Immobility
* Malignancy
* Contraceptive pill
* Previous surgery
* Pelvic or lower limb surgery

Thrombus usually develops in the deep veins of the lower limb and pelvis and detachment of formed thrombus into the circulation results in venous thromboembolism, which may result in the clinical condition of pulmonary embolism. Measures to reduce the risk of thrombus formation should be taken in all patients. These include:
* Good hydration
* Preoperative low molecular weight heparin therapy
* Pneumatic leg compression
* Elastic stockings
* Spinal or epidural techniques (if appropriate)

Although rare, pulmonary embolism may occur during the intraoperative period. Diagnosis is usually made by a combination of signs such as unexplained tachyarrhythmias, hypoxia and an acute fall in end-tidal carbon dioxide concentration. Management consists of increasing FiO_2, haemodynamic support and thrombolytic therapy. Transfer to ICU is usually needed. Embolisation of fat or tumour results in a similar, though generally more severe, picture. Fat globules may be detectable in pulmonary secretions. Fat embolism is more common after long bone fractures and orthopaedic procedures where profound reaming of the intramedullary cavity is undertaken (such as femoral nailing). Amniotic fluid embolism is uncommon, and results in a profound derangement of clotting function which leads to severe disseminated intravascular coagulation (DIC).

Gas

Embolisation of gas results from the ingress of gas into the circulation via the venous route. The usual cause of room air embolism is the site of surgery being above the level of the right atrium, when air may enter an open vein. Air embolism via venous catheters may also occur. Laparoscopic procedures may result in embolisation of the insufflating gas (which is usually carbon dioxide).

The resulting clinical picture after gas embolism is dictated by the amount of gas which has entered the circulation (although in the case of carbon dioxide, little change will be seen). Embolisation of air at a rate exceeding $0.5 \, \text{ml kg}^{-1} \, \text{min}^{-1}$ will result in clinical signs, usually resulting from the air reaching the cardiac chambers. Features include:
* Millwheel murmur over the chest
* Fall in end-tidal CO_2
* Hypoxia
* Tachyarrhythmias
* Raised pulmonary artery pressure

After diagnosing air embolism further entry of gas should be prevented by flooding the operative site with saline and a wet pack. Venous pressure at the operative site should be increased and ventilation of the lungs with 100% oxygen applied (nitrous oxide should be stopped immediately). Occasionally gas can be aspirated through an existing central line, especially if the patient is turned laterally with the right side uppermost. Postoperative circulatory support and general supportive therapy on ICU may be required.

Malignant hyperthermia (hyperpyrexia) (MH)

MH is exceedingly rare but of great importance. The mortality rate in the 1970s was >70%, and although today it is closer to 25% even that is a high price to pay for what is often minor surgery. The reduction in mortality probably reflects an increased awareness of the condition, more intensive patient monitoring for sensitive indicators, such as end-tidal carbon dioxide tension, which assist early diagnosis, and the availability of an intravenous form of dantrolene sodium, a drug which has played an important role in the treatment of MH.

Pathophysiology

MH may represent a spectrum of conditions rather than a specific pharmacogenetic entity, as the inheritance is complex. Presentation under anaesthesia is usually that of a marked increase in metabolic rate arising from accelerated muscle metabolism. At cellular level the exact defect remains unclear, but dysfunction of the sarcoplasmic reticulum and abnormalities of intracellular ionic calcium transport occur, with a secondary effect of increased sympathetic nervous system activity. Agents known to

Cardinal physical signs
- Hyperthermia (core temperature rising by a minimum of 1–2 °C per hour)
- Respiratory acidosis (hypercarbia)
- Metabolic acidosis (with or without muscle rigidity)
- Cardiac arrhythmias
- Hypoxaemia
- Cyanosis (from a large rise in oxygen consumption plus ventilation perfusion defects)

Signs of abnormal muscle activity
- Failure of the jaw to relax after suxamethonium
- Rigidity of certain groups of muscles, but not necessarily all
- Hyperkalaemia
- Myoglobinuria and renal failure
- Rise in creatinine kinase (CK)

Other signs
- Disseminated intravascular coagulation (DIC)
- Cerebral and pulmonary oedema

Triggering agents
- ALL the inhalational agents including desflurane and sevoflurane
- Suxamethonium
- (Avoid if possible: phenothiazines, atropine)

Agents thought to be safe
- Thiopental
- Propofol
- Nitrous oxide
- Opioids
- Pancuronium
- Vecuronium
- Benzodiazepines
- Amide local anaesthetics

Figure IN10 Features of malignant hyperthermia (MH)

induce MH cause an enhanced release of calcium from the sarcoplasmic reticulum, and a generalised membrane permeability defect develops. Genetic studies indicate that the MH gene is on chromosome 19, in a position close to the ryanodine receptor gene. Features of MH are given in Figure IN10.

Clinical management of a suspected fulminant case
CALL FOR HELP. Then treat as in Figure IN11.

- Stop the use of all MH trigger agents
- Change the anaesthesia machine; and change from the circle system, if it is being used, to a non-rebreathing system
- Terminate surgery if possible
- Monitor the ECG and capnograph
- Alert the intensive care unit. Commence invasive monitoring
- Delegate one person to prepare dantrolene sodium 1 mg kg^{-1}
- Record core temperature, pulse rate and blood pressure every 5 minutes
- Estimate arterial pH and blood gases
- Treat hypercarbia with vigorous hyperventilation, acidosis with sodium bicarbonate 2–4 mmol kg^{-1}
- Maintain oxygenation
- Save one venous sample for serum CK and send one for electrolytes and serum calcium estimations
- Give IV dantrolene sodium 1 mg kg^{-1}. Repeat at 10-minute intervals if necessary, up to a maximum of 10 mg kg^{-1}

Figure IN11 Treatment of MH

Secondary management
Cool the patient and keep the first urine sample for myoglobin estimation. Measure urine output. If obvious myoglobinuria occurs, give intravenous fluids, and mannitol or frusemide to promote urine flow. The use of steroids is controversial, but may be indicated for cerebral oedema in severe cases. Repeat the serum CK estimation at 24 hours. Treat DIC if necessary. Dantrolene may need to be repeated for up to 24 hours, as re-triggering may occur.

Accidental pneumothorax
Accidental pneumothorax, uncommon in urgent, scheduled or elective surgery but to be expected during emergency surgery on patients admitted with trauma, may become more frequent with the use of interpleural anaesthesia and with today's emphasis on minimally invasive surgery, when it should more properly be renamed 'carbondioxidethorax'.

A patient with a pneumothorax should not be anaesthetised unless a chest drain with an underwater seal is in place. If, during anaesthesia, a pneumothorax is suspected, either unilateral or bilateral (e.g. by clinical observation, by percussion, by auscultation of the lungs, by hypoxia and hypercarbia, and by changes in the required ventilatory pressure accompanied by hypotension), surgery should be stopped and a chest drain with underwater seal promptly inserted. A tension pneumothorax is rapidly lethal and requires insertion of a large-bore cannula into the affected side. A formal chest drain can be subsequently sited.

Failure to breathe

Failure to breathe at the end of the procedure is commonly due to delayed recovery from the use of muscle relaxants. A full differential diagnosis is given in Section 1, Chapter 4 (pages 58–64).

At the end of the surgical procedure the aim is to have the patient pain-free, breathing spontaneously, cardiovascularly stable with reactive pupils, opening the eyes and mouth to command, and remembering nothing of the surgery. Delayed recovery from the use or abuse of muscle relaxants is less common than it used to be, although there may be occasional problems secondary to the use of suxamethonium and mivacurium (see Section 1, Chapter 4, Figure PO8). Monitoring of the neuromuscular junction throughout anaesthesia with a peripheral nerve stimulator has become much more widespread, reducing the empirical nature of relaxant dosage.

The reasons for greater than expected duration of muscle relaxant drugs include:

- Relative or absolute overdose of drug
- Impaired relaxant metabolism (suxamethonium or mivacurium apnoea)
- Electrolyte or acid–base imbalance
- Incorrect prescription of reversal agent
- Relative or absolute overdose of a volatile anaesthetic

References and further reading

Anderton JM, Keen RI, Neave R. *Positioning the Surgical Patient*. London: Butterworths, 1988.

Association of Anaesthetists of Great Britain and Ireland. *Recommendations for Standards of Monitoring During Anaesthesia and Recovery*, 4th edn. London: AAGBI, 2007.

Buck N, Devlin HB, Lunn JN. *The Report of a Confidential Enquiry into Perioperative Deaths*. London: Nuffield Provincial Hospitals Trust & The King's Fund, 1987.

Callum KG, Gray AJG, Hoile RW, *et al*. *Then and Now: the 2000 Report of the National Confidential Enquiry into Perioperative Deaths*. London: NCEPOD, 2000.

Lumb AB. *Nunn's Applied Respiratory Physiology*, 6th ed. London: Butterworth-Heinemann, 2005.

Lunn JN, Mushin WW. *Mortality Associated with Anaesthesia*. London: Nuffield Provincial Hospitals Trust, 1982.

Mushin WW, Rendell-Baker L, Thompson PW, Mapleson WW. *Automatic Ventilation of the Lungs*, 2nd edn. Oxford: Blackwell, 1969.

Rosen M, Lunn JN (eds). *Consciousness, Awareness and Pain in General Anaesthesia*. London: Butterworth, 1987.

Servant C, Purkiss S. *Positioning Patients for Surgery*. London: Greenwich Medical Media, 2002.

CHAPTER 4

Postoperative management

T. McLeod

Care of the unconscious patient

Emergence from anaesthesia, although usually uneventful, can be associated with major morbidity. In the immediate postoperative period, patients are at risk from respiratory and cardiovascular complications, which comprise approximately 70% and 20% of critical recovery room incidents respectively. The unconscious patient may develop upper airway obstruction or inadequate ventilation with subsequent hypoxaemia and hypercapnia, and is at increased risk of aspiration due to the absence of the protective airway reflexes. Ongoing blood loss and residual drug effects may compound cardiovascular compromise. The importance of observation and early intervention during this period has been recognised for many years. Hazards may be reduced by the provision of adequate postoperative recovery facilities along with fully trained staff, who should ideally be available at all times.

The recovery room

Recommendations for the situation and design of the recovery room and equipment required have been made by a working party of the Association of Anaesthetists of Great Britain and Ireland (2002).

Patient transfer from operating theatre

The design of trolleys should comply with the Association of Anaesthetists recommendations in that there is a need for oxygen cylinders, masks and tubing, airway support equipment, protective sides and a tilting mechanism. Portable monitoring equipment may be required. Care should be taken to avoid injury to eyes, dentition and peripheral nerves. Transfer to the recovery room should be undertaken by suitably trained staff under the supervision of the anaesthetist, who is additionally responsible for handing over information about relevant medical conditions, the anaesthetic technique, intraoperative problems and postoperative management to the recovery staff.

Management

Continuous observation must be made on a one-to-one basis by a nurse trained in recovery procedures until the patient is conscious and able to maintain his or her own

Fundamentals of Anaesthesia, 3rd edition, ed. Tim Smith, Colin Pinnock and Ted Lin. Published by Cambridge University Press. © Cambridge University Press 2008.

Level of consciousness

Fully conscious without excessive stimulation

Respiratory system

Upper airway	Able to maintain a clear airway
	Protective reflexes are present
Respiration	Satisfactory respiratory rate
	Satisfactory oxygenation

Cardiovascular system

Haemodynamically stable

No unexplained cardiac irregularity

Pulse rate acceptable

Blood pressure acceptable

No persistent bleeding

Peripheral perfusion adequate

Pain and nausea control

Effective pain control

Free of nausea

Adequate analgesic and anti-emetic provisions made

Temperature

Normothermic

No evidence of developing malignant hyperthermia

(Modified from Association of Anaesthetists of Great Britain and Ireland, 2002)

Figure PO1 Criteria to be met before transfer from recovery room to general ward

airway. Respiratory and cardiovascular parameters, pain severity, conscious level, drugs and IV fluids administered should be documented at appropriate intervals.

Clinical observations should be supplemented by pulse oximetry and blood pressure measurement, with an ECG, peripheral nerve stimulator, temperature monitor and capnography immediately available.

Patient discharge

Set criteria must be met before a patient is discharged to the ward (Figure PO1). The patient being transferred to the high dependency or intensive care unit is an obvious exception to this.

Postoperative complications

Postoperative complications may be from respiratory, cardiovascular or neurological causes, and include:

- Upper airway obstruction
- Postoperative hypoxaemia
- Inadequate pulmonary ventilation
- Hypertension
- Hypotension
- Cardiac arrhythmias
- Thromboembolism
- Shivering
- Failure to regain consciousness

Upper airway obstruction

The causes of oropharyngeal and laryngeal obstruction are shown in Figure PO2.

In the unconscious patient, the tongue may fall backwards and occlude the airway at the level of the oropharynx. This occurs because of a decrease in oropharyngeal muscle tone, which is related to the residual effects of general anaesthesia and inadequate recovery from muscle relaxants. Rarely, oropharyngeal obstruction results from a foreign body, e.g. failure to remove throat pack or post-traumatic airway oedema. Wound haematoma can occur after neck surgery (e.g. carotid endarterectomy, thyroidectomy, radical neck dissection) and can rapidly produce upper airway obstruction. Oedema formation resulting from external compression of the venous and lymphatic drainage of the head and neck will make matters worse.

	Oropharyngeal obstruction	Laryngeal obstruction
Common	Decreased muscle tone	Laryngospasm
	Secretions	Secretions
	Sleep apnoea	
Rare	Foreign body	Oedema
	Oedema	Bilateral recurrent laryngeal nerve palsy
	Wound haematoma	Tracheal collapse
	Neuromuscular disease	

Figure PO2 Causes of upper airway obstruction in the postoperative period

Laryngospasm is the commonest cause of laryngeal obstruction and is often associated with airway manipulation during emergence from anaesthesia, e.g. airway insertion at light levels of anaesthesia, or the presence of secretions or blood. After thyroidectomy, bilateral recurrent laryngeal nerve palsies and tracheal collapse can occur, although this is very rare. Laryngeal oedema secondary to prolonged or traumatic intubation can occasionally cause obstruction, although this is more likely in the paediatric than in the adult patient because of the smaller size of the airway.

Clinical features

The clinical signs of upper airway obstruction include absence of air movement, 'see-saw' motion of the chest and abdomen, and suprasternal and intercostal recession. Oxygen desaturation is a late sign. Incomplete laryngospasm typically produces stridor, an inspiratory 'crowing' noise, although this is absent if the laryngospasm is complete.

Management

Initial measures are directed at preventing the tongue from falling backwards and obstructing the airway. The unconscious patient should be recovered in the lateral position with the jaw supported. Blood and secretions should be cleared by suction and supplemental oxygen given via a face mask. If upper airway obstruction develops, the head should be tilted backwards and the jaw pushed forward by applying pressure behind the angle of the jaw. If this measure does not rapidly clear the airway then an oropharyngeal or nasopharyngeal airway should be inserted. Care should be taken on insertion of an oral airway as this may cause laryngospasm, coughing or vomiting in the waking patient and, if in doubt, a nasal airway should be passed. If this does not immediately rectify the situation then senior help should be sought and 100% oxygen administered via a tight-fitting mask. Continuous positive airway pressure (CPAP) at this stage may help to open the airway or 'break' the laryngospasm. However, in the presence of continued airway obstruction and falling oxygen saturation intravenous suxamethonium ($1-2$ mg kg^{-1}) should be given followed by manual ventilation with 100% oxygen and subsequent orotracheal intubation. In the rare event when this is not possible the failed intubation drill should be followed. Extubation of the trachea should occur when the patient has regained full muscle power and is awake. An algorithm for airway management is shown in Figure PO3.

Upper airway obstruction secondary to wound haematoma must be immediately treated. The surgeon and an experienced anaesthetist should be called, the airway supported, 100% oxygen administered and the trachea intubated. The wound stitches should be removed and the haematoma evacuated. It is important to remember that the airway anatomy may be grossly distorted, and it may be impossible to intubate the trachea. In this situation, a surgical airway will be required.

Postoperative hypoxaemia

Hypoxaemia is defined as an oxygen saturation of less than 90%. In the postoperative period it occurs due to a combination of factors, as listed in Figure PO4 (Mangat & Jones 1993). Prevention, early recognition and treatment are important because of the increased morbidity and mortality associated with this condition.

Clinical features

Clinical signs associated with hypoxaemia are non-specific and include central cyanosis, dyspnoea, tachycardia, arrhythmias, hyper- or hypotension and agitation. Cyanosis is a dusky, blue discoloration of the mucous membranes and skin. It is usually clinically detectable when the concentration of deoxygenated haemoglobin is greater than 5 g dl^{-1}. However, it may be absent in the hypoxaemic anaemic patient and present in the polycythaemic patient with a normal PaO_2 and is therefore an unreliable indicator of hypoxaemia.

Upper airway obstruction and alveolar hypoventilation are important causes of hypoxaemia in the postoperative period.

Ventilation–perfusion ($\dot{V}/\dot{Q}$) mismatch

There is about a 20% reduction in functional residual capacity (FRC) after induction of anaesthesia. This may lead to airway closure in dependent parts of the lung, resulting in ventilation–perfusion ($\dot{V}/\dot{Q}$) mismatch with subsequent hypoxaemia. The very young, elderly, obese and smokers are particularly at risk, as in these groups closing capacity may equal or exceed FRC, with resultant airway closure during tidal breathing. The reduction in FRC is greatest in the supine position, and oxygen saturation may be improved by sitting the patient up, provided he or she is awake enough.

Causes of $\dot{V}/\dot{Q}$ mismatch include atelectasis, bronchopneumonia, aspiration, pulmonary oedema and pneumothorax.

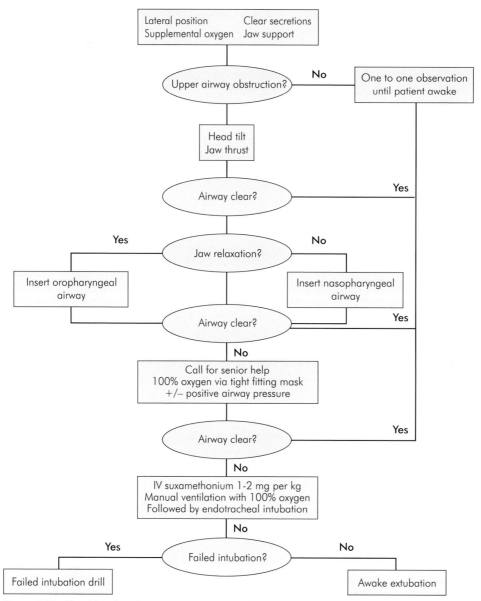

Figure PO3 Algorithm for airway management in the unconscious patient

Atelectasis

Postoperative pulmonary collapse or atelectasis is a common cause of hypoxaemia, particularly after upper abdominal and thoracic surgery. Onset is usually within 15 minutes of induction of anaesthesia, in both spontaneously breathing and mechanically ventilated patients, and lasts up to four days into the postoperative period. Absorption atelectasis has been implicated in the develo-

pment of postoperative pulmonary collapse. It develops when the rate of gas leaving the alveolus due to uptake into the blood exceeds the rate of inspired gas entering it. This occurs when the airway to an area of lung is closed or obstructed, usually with secretions or blood. It is also found in areas of lung with a marked reduction in $\dot{V}/\dot{Q}$ ratios. The rate of gas uptake is increased when insoluble gases such as nitrogen are replaced by soluble gases such as oxygen and

- Upper airway obstruction
- Alveolar hypoventilation
- Ventilation–perfusion mismatch
- Diffusion hypoxia
- Increased oxygen utilisation
- Low cardiac output states

Figure PO4 Causes of postoperative hypoxaemia

nitrous oxide in an anaesthetic mixture (Joyce & Baker 1995). Effective treatment includes adequate pain control, supplemental oxygen, chest physiotherapy and promotion of deep breathing exercises and coughing.

Bronchopneumonia

Bronchopneumonia may occur after major surgery, particularly if the patient is unable to clear respiratory tract secretions because of poor cough or inability to deep breathe. Treatment follows the same pattern as for atelectasis, with the addition of appropriate antibiotic therapy.

Aspiration

There is a significant risk of aspirating gastric contents in the postoperative period, as protective airway reflexes may be absent or impaired. Patients with delayed gastric emptying (e.g. bowel obstruction, obesity, pregnancy or an incompetent gastro-oesophageal sphincter) are at increased risk. Aspiration of liquid material results in a pneumonitis of varying severity dependent on the volume and acidity of the fluid. Severe pneumonitis is associated with aspiration of greater than 25 ml of fluid with a pH of less than 2.5. Aspiration of solid material results in bronchial or laryngeal obstruction, and, if not immediately relieved, can be fatal. In the supine position, due to the anatomy of the bronchial tree, aspiration is most likely to occur into the right lung, although, after a large aspiration, both lungs are often involved. The chance of aspiration may be reduced by recovering patients in the lateral position, and those at high risk should be extubated after full recovery of protective reflexes. The treatment of aspiration is detailed in Section 1, Chapter 2.

Pulmonary oedema

This is a relatively rare cause of $\dot{V}/\dot{Q}$ mismatch in the recovery room which usually occurs within an hour of the end of surgery. Causes include fluid overload or cardiac failure, and it may occur after relief of prolonged airway obstruction.

Pneumothorax

Pneumothorax may result from direct lung or airway trauma, rib fractures, central venous cannulation, brachial plexus block, intercostal nerve and interpleural blocks and after thoracic, neck or renal surgery. A pneumothorax due to barotrauma associated with mechanical ventilation is unusual unless ventilation pressures are high. Patients with emphysematous bullae are particularly at risk.

The characteristic features are pleuritic chest pain or breathlessness, but these may not be detected if the pneumothorax is small, or may be masked by the residual effects of anaesthesia. Spontaneously breathing patients with a pneumothorax of less than 20% of the lung field may be observed and the chest x ray repeated. Any patient with a larger pneumothorax or who is mechanically ventilated should be treated with an intercostal drain. A tension pneumothorax is associated with marked shift of the trachea and mediastinum away from the affected side, hypoxaemia, hyper-resonance to percussion and hypotension. It is a clinical diagnosis and a true medical emergency requiring immediate decompression by insertion of a chest drain at the fifth intercostal space in the anterior axillary line. A 14 gauge cannula should be inserted in the second intercostal space in the mid-clavicular line if a chest drain is not immediately available.

Diffusion hypoxia

At the end of anaesthesia nitrous oxide leaves the blood and enters the alveoli, diluting the gases already present. If the patient is breathing air, nitrogen will be absorbed into the blood at a slower rate than nitrous oxide enters the alveoli, resulting in a decrease in alveolar oxygen concentration and a potentially hypoxic gas mixture. In practice, the effect of diffusional hypoxia is transient and is simply overcome by administering supplemental oxygen for approximately 10 minutes in the immediate postoperative period.

Other causes of hypoxaemia

Hypoxaemia may also occur as a result of increased oxygen consumption (e.g. shivering, pyrexia) or increased tissue oxygen extraction. These both result in a reduction in mixed venous oxygen concentration. A variable amount of mixed venous blood is shunted from the right to the left side of the heart and mixes with oxygenated blood, producing a fall in PaO_2. The extent of this fall is dependent on the mixed venous oxygen concentration and the degree of right-to-left shunt.

Upper airway obstruction

Decreased ventilatory drive
• Inhalational anaesthetics
• Opioids
• Benzodiazepines
• Central nervous system trauma

Inadequate respiratory muscle function
• Incomplete reversal of neuromuscular blockade
• Neuromuscular disease
• Diaphragmatic splinting (obesity, abdominal distension)
• Thoracic or upper abdominal surgery
• Acute or chronic lung disease

Figure PO5 Causes of alveolar hypoventilation in the postoperative period

Inadequate pulmonary ventilation

Reduced alveolar ventilation has many causes in the postoperative period (Figure PO5). It results from a reduction in tidal volume or respiratory rate, or a combination of both, and by definition it produces a raised arterial carbon dioxide tension ($PaCO_2$). Hypoxaemia and respiratory acidosis may be associated features.

Decreased ventilatory drive

The commonest cause of central respiratory depression is the residual effect of inhalational anaesthetic agents or perioperative opioid administration. The effect of volatile anaesthetic agents is compounded, as they are predominantly excreted via the lungs.

An unconscious patient with low respiratory rate and pinpoint pupils is typical of opioid overdosage. Supportive treatment includes the administration of oxygen, maintenance of the airway and manual ventilation by mask or tracheal tube if required. Opioid-induced respiratory depression can be reversed by administration of naloxone, a competitive opioid antagonist. This agent should be given in small incremental doses of 50–100 µg intravenously in order to prevent reversal of analgesia. Tachycardia and hypertension associated with sudden development of pain increases myocardial oxygen consumption and may lead to ischaemia in susceptible patients. The onset of action of naloxone is within 1–2 minutes but the duration of action is only 20 minutes, which is shorter than that of many opioids, so a repeat dose may be required. The patient must not return to the ward until full recovery from the respiratory depressant effects of the opioid has occurred.

Benzodiazepines are often used as adjuncts to general anaesthesia. The elderly, sick and patients with liver disease are at risk of prolonged effects from these agents. Oversedation can be treated with flumazenil, a competitive benzodiazepine receptor antagonist. It is administered intravenously in 100 µg increments titrated against clinical response. Onset of action is within 30–60 seconds and duration of effect varies from 15 to 120 minutes.

Decreased ventilatory drive may be related to a period of intraoperative hyperventilation with a resultant marked decrease in $PaCO_2$ which may continue into the immediate postoperative phase. Neurosurgical and head-injury patients may also develop hypoventilation in the postoperative period as a direct result of central nervous system trauma.

Inadequate mechanical function of the respiratory muscles
Incomplete reversal of non-depolarising muscle blockade

This is distressing and potentially dangerous to the patient. It is an important cause of both hypoventilation and upper airway obstruction. There are many factors that contribute to incomplete reversal (Figure PO6). The use of short-acting non-depolarising muscle relaxants and neuromuscular monitoring to assess the degree of muscle blockade should help to avoid this complication.

Typically the inadequately reversed patient can initiate movements but cannot complete them, as a result of which they appear twitchy with uncoordinated actions. Patients

Hypothermia	
Respiratory acidosis	
Electrolyte abnormalities	Hypokalaemia
	Hypocalcaemia
	Hyponatraemia
	Hypermagnesaemia
Drug interactions	Volatile agents
	Calcium channel blockers
	Aminoglycosides
	Diuretics
Decreased excretion	Renal failure
	Liver failure

Figure PO6 Factors associated with prolonged neuromuscular blockade

may exhibit extreme distress and in addition complain of visual disturbance. Adequate muscle function may be confirmed clinically if the patient can lift his or her head off the pillow for 5 seconds; strength of hand grip is also assessed, but this is more subjective. A peripheral nerve stimulator may also be used, with a train-of-four ratio of greater than 70% and absence of fade after double burst stimulation indicating adequate recovery.

Treatment of inadequate reversal includes reassurance, along with sedation and ventilatory support if it is severe. All patients should receive supplemental oxygen, and a further dose of neostigmine 1.25–2.5 mg intravenously (maximum total dose 5 mg) may be given.

Suxamethonium apnoea

Recovery from the effect of suxamethonium is dependent on the enzyme plasma cholinesterase, which hydrolyses suxamethonium to succinyl monocholine and choline. Succinyl monocholine is further hydrolysed to succinic acid and choline. A prolonged neuromuscular block after suxamethonium administration is described as suxamethonium apnoea and can be due to both acquired (Figure PO7) and genetic factors (Davis *et al.* 1997).

Acquired: The majority of acquired causes produce a minor prolongation of apnoea of only a few minutes. Decreased cholinesterase synthesis occurs in liver disease and to a lesser extent in pregnancy and hypothyroidism. Drugs decrease the activity of the enzyme either by competing with suxamethonium at the binding site (either reversibly or irreversibly) or by inactivating it.

In cases of suxamethonium apnoea the type 1 block normally seen on using a nerve stimulator (absence of fade on train of four, no post-tetanic facilitation) progresses

Decreased plasma cholinesterase **concentration**
- Pregnancy
- Liver disease
- Chronic renal failure
- Haemodialysis
- Hypothyroidism

Decreased plasma cholinesterase **activity**
- Induction agents (etomidate and ketamine)
- Ester local anaesthetics
- Anticholinesterases

Figure PO7 Acquired causes of suxamethonium apnoea

through a transitional phase (development of tetanic fade and, later on, fade on train of four) or dual block and finally develops into a type 2 block (fade on train of four, post-tetanic facilitation).

Treatment of suxamethonium apnoea includes ongoing sedation and ventilation until there is spontaneous recovery of muscle function. Active measures such as administration of fresh frozen plasma have been used although risk of infection and cost have limited this practice. The patient may have to be managed in the intensive care unit if recovery is prolonged.

Inherited: The inheritance of abnormal cholinesterase is linked to several autosomal recessive genes, which are classified by their percentage inhibition of action when exposed to different substances (for example dibucaine or fluoride). Figure PO8 describes the different situations.

The degree of prolongation of action is related to the genetic inheritance of the enzymes. Heterozygotes for the normal enzyme will obviously have a normal response. Two to four hours of paralysis after a 1 mg kg^{-1} dose of suxamethonium will be seen in homozygotes for the silent

Type	Genotype		Dibucaine number	Fluoride number	Typical apnoea	Incidence
Normal	$E_1^u E_1^u$	homozygous	80	60	1–5 min	94%
Atypical	$E_1^u E_1^a$	heterozygous	60	50	10 min	1 : 25
Atypical	$E_1^a E_1^a$	homozygous	20	20	2 hours	1 : 3000
Silent	$E_1^u E_1^s$	heterozygous	80	60	10 min	1 : 25
Silent	$E_1^s E_1^s$	homozygous	minimal activity		2 hours	1 : 100 000
Fluoride-resistant	$E_1^u E_1^f$	heterozygous	75	50	10 min	1 : 300 000
Fluoride-resistant	$E_1^f E_1^f$	homozygous	65	40	2 hours	1 : 150 000

Note: u, a, s and f are the four commonest of 25 possible gene variants for plasma cholinesterase

Figure PO8 Inheritance of abnormal plasma cholinesterase

or atypical genes. Homozygotes for the fluoride-resistant gene will show a prolongation of effect of 1–2 hours. Most heterozygotes who have one normal and one abnormal gene will have a minor increase in duration of effect of about 20 minutes. Combinations of abnormal genes are rare, with an unpredictable result. For further details on inheritance see Section 3, Chapter 8.

Mivacurium apnoea

The action of mivacurium is mainly terminated by plasma cholinesterase, and thus the defective forms of this enzyme will result in prolonged action of the drug. This is usually in the region of 2–4 hours from a typical dose. Other elimination pathways include liver esterase metabolism and biliary and renal excretion.

Neuromuscular disease

Patients with neuromuscular disease may be particularly sensitive to the residual effects of general anaesthesia and to neuromuscular blocking agents which, if possible, should be avoided or used at a reduced dose with monitoring of neuromuscular function.

Diaphragmatic splinting

Obese patients, those with gastric distension, and post-thoracotomy or upper abdominal surgical patients can develop diaphragmatic splinting. Good pain relief with thoracic epidural or patient-controlled analgesia, chest physiotherapy, and nasogastric tube insertion where indicated can help prevent hypoventilation in these cases.

Pre-existing lung disease

Patients with chronic obstructive airways disease (COAD) are at increased risk of hypoventilation in the postoperative period. They may not be able to further increase their work of breathing to maintain an adequate $PaCO_2$, particularly if bronchospasm or excessive airway secretions are present.

Bronchospasm may occur in asthma, COAD, smokers and in patients with acute respiratory infection. It is commonly precipitated by upper airway irritation, either during airway manipulation or if secretions are present. Other causes of wheeze include aspiration, pulmonary oedema, and bronchospasm associated with anaphylaxis. Treatment of bronchospasm will depend on the underlying cause and the severity but should include supplemental oxygen and inhaled bronchodilator therapy.

Patient factors	Agitation Preoperative hypertension Pain
Inadequate ventilation	Hypoxaemia Hypercapnia
Drug interaction	Monoamine oxidase inhibitors
Bladder distension	
Malignant hyperpyrexia	
Endocrine (phaeochromocytoma)	

Figure PO9 Factors associated with hypertension in the immediate postoperative period

Hypertension

This is defined as a 20% or greater increase in preoperative systolic blood pressure and is often short-lived. It usually develops within 30 minutes of the end of surgery and may be precipitated by acute withdrawal of antihypertensive medication. There are multiple causes (Figure PO9) of which pain, preoperative hypertension and blood gas abnormalities are the commonest.

Management of high blood pressure is directed at establishing and treating the underlying cause, of which pain is the most common. Other causes include hypoxia, hypercapnia and intravascular fluid overload. Further measures at this stage are determined by the degree of hypertension and associated medical or surgical factors. In general, a moderate elevation in blood pressure of 30% of the preoperative value is well tolerated.

Postoperative hypertension is usually short-lived. Agents used to treat it should therefore be short-acting, and may include the following:

- Labetalol is a β_1 adrenoceptor antagonist with some α_1 adrenoceptor antagonist activity. 5 mg bolus doses administered intravenously act within 5 minutes and last for up to an hour.
- Esmolol is a very short-acting β adrenoceptor antagonist with a rapid onset of action. It is given as a bolus of 500 μg kg^{-1} over 60 seconds followed by an infusion at a rate of 50–300 μg kg^{-1} per minute dependent on clinical effect. Both labetalol and esmolol are contraindicated in asthmatics.
- Nifedepine, a calcium antagonist, given sublingually at a dose of 5–20 mg, is an effective means of reducing postoperative hypertension.
- Hydralazine, a direct-acting peripheral vasodilator, administered intravenously in 5 mg boluses has an

Frequent causes

Hypovolaemia	Blood loss or third space losses
Vasodilatation	Subarachnoid and extradural block
	Residual effects of anaesthetic and analgesic agents
	Rewarming
	Sepsis
	Anaphylaxis

Infrequent causes

	Arrhythmias
	Myocardial ischaemia/ infarction
	Heart failure
	Tension pneumothorax
	Pulmonary embolism
	Pericardial tamponade
	Hypothyroidism

Figure PO10 Causes of postoperative hypotension

- onset of action within 10–20 minutes but may cause tachycardia.
- Glyceryl trinitrate, a direct-acting arterial and venous dilator, is usually used intraoperatively to control blood pressure but can be administered at a rate of $0.2–8\ \mu g\ kg^{-1}$ per minute intravenously to rapidly reduce blood pressure in the postoperative period.

Hypotension

Hypotension occurs frequently in the recovery room and, in the majority of cases, is transient and benign. It is usually related to the residual effects of anaesthetic and analgesic drugs (Figure PO10).

Whilst the causes of hypotension are manifold, hypovolaemia due to inadequate perioperative fluid replacement or ongoing fluid loss is the most common. Sympathetic blockade associated with spinal anaesthesia or analgesia, with a resultant fall in systemic vascular resistance (SVR), is also an important cause of hypotension in the postoperative period. The reduction in SVR related to rewarming of a hypothermic patient may also cause a decrease in blood pressure, as may rarer causes such as anaphylaxis, cardiac arrhythmias, tension pneumothorax and pulmonary embolus.

Once hypotension is evident the cause must be sought and treatment initiated to prevent ischaemia to vital organs. The patient should be laid flat or slightly head-down and given supplemental oxygen whilst further assessment takes place.

The hypovolaemic patient has a tachycardia, with a low JVP, decreased urine output and poor peripheral perfusion, and there may be obvious blood loss, e.g. into drains. A rapid intravenous bolus of 250–500 ml of crystalloid or colloid should be given and the haemodynamic response assessed. Patients assumed to have normal left ventricular function who fail to respond to fluid therapy require central venous pressure monitoring. A pulmonary artery catheter may be required if left ventricular function is impaired. Ongoing blood loss may require further surgical intervention.

Patients with marked peripheral vasodilatation can be hypotensive despite adequate volume replacement. This is commonly seen after subarachnoid or extradural anaesthesia, where administration of vasoconstricting drugs with or without further intravenous fluid should be given. Marked vasodilatation also occurs in sepsis and anaphylaxis, where management is both supportive and guided at treating the specific underlying abnormality.

Eighty per cent of hypotensive patients in recovery will respond to intravenous fluid therapy alone. It is potentially dangerous to use vasopressor drugs in the face of inadequate fluid replacement, as they may cause ischaemia of the visceral organs such as the liver and kidneys, but they may be useful in severe hypotension whilst a diagnosis is being sought, and in the presence of vasodilatation. Vasopressor agents used include the following:

- Ephedrine, a sympathomimetic agent with α and β adrenoceptor agonist activity, produces peripheral vasoconstriction, and an increase in heart rate and myocardial contractility. It has a rapid onset of action when given intravenously in 3 mg boluses.
- Metaraminol, an α adrenoceptor agonist with some β adrenoceptor agonist activity, can also be used in the postoperative period. It has a rapid onset of action and is given in incremental doses of 0.5 mg titrated against effect.

Cardiac arrhythmias

The majority of arrhythmias in the postoperative period are benign. They may be related to hypercapnia, hypoxaemia, electrolyte and acid–base disturbance, pain, pre-existing cardiac disease, and myocardial ischaemia or infarction.

- Sinus bradycardia (pulse < 60 beats per minute) – this may be normal in the young, healthy patient, or may result from vagal stimulation, hypoxaemia and drug effects, e.g. β adrenoceptor antagonists, neostigmine. Treatment with intravenous glycopyrrolate 0.2–0.4 mg or atropine 0.2–0.6 mg will usually increase the heart rate.
- Sinus tachycardia (pulse > 100 beats per minute) – pain, hypovolaemia, anaemia, pyrexia and an increased metabolic rate can all produce a tachycardia. Tachycardia is usually harmless, and treatment of the underlying cause is all that is warranted in the majority of cases. If it is associated with myocardial ischaemia, treatment with a β-blocker may be required.
- Atrial or ventricular premature contractions – no specific treatment other than correction of hypercapnia and electrolyte abnormalities is usually required.
- Supraventricular tachycardia – management of this arrhythmia depends on the degree of haemodynamic instability. Hypoxaemia, hypercapnia and electrolyte imbalance should be corrected. Carotid sinus massage may result in the return of sinus rhythm. Intravenous adenosine 6 mg over 5 seconds followed by a further dose, 2 minutes later, of 12 mg if required is often effective, although it should not be used in the asthmatic patient. Esmolol or verapamil can also be used. Synchronised direct current (DC) cardioversion is indicated if the patient is haemodynamically compromised.
- Ventricular tachycardia – this is rare in the postoperative period but can progress to ventricular fibrillation and must be treated immediately. If the blood pressure and cardiac output are not compromised, an intravenous bolus of lidocaine 50–100 mg should be given over a few minutes followed by a lidocaine infusion of 1–4 mg per minute. DC cardioversion is indicated if hypotension is present.

Thromboembolism

Deep venous thrombosis (DVT) and pulmonary embolus (PE) are significant causes of morbidity and mortality in the postoperative period. The incidence of DVT is difficult to assess accurately, as many cases are not clinically detected. In the postoperative period 10–80% of patients may, depending on patient risk factors and type of surgery, develop DVT (Wheatley & Veitch 1997). The risk of subsequent PE in this group of patients is unknown, although up to 0.9% of all hospital admissions suffer fatal PE after DVT.

Deep venous thrombosis

The commonest sites for venous thrombosis are in the leg and pelvis, although any vein may be affected. The classic presentation of a painful calf which is red, swollen and warmer than the unaffected side is often not present, and many cases are asymptomatic. The investigation of choice for below-knee thrombosis is venography, although iliofemoral thrombosis can usually be detected with Doppler ultrasound.

The main aim of treatment in established venous thrombosis is to minimise the risk of subsequent PE. All patients with above-knee thrombosis must be formally anticoagulated for a period of 3 months. Treatment of below-knee thrombosis is controversial because, although a PE can occur with any DVT, it is rare in cases confined to veins situated below the knee. For this reason, formal anticoagulation is not always carried out in this group.

Prophylaxis

Effective prevention of DVT is an important aspect of perioperative care and requires accurate identification of the at-risk patient (Figure PO11). All moderate- and high-risk patients should be given prophylaxis. Prophylactic measures often vary from hospital to hospital, and local guidelines should be followed.

Physical methods available include the application of graduated compression or thromboembolic deterrent

Low-risk patients
- <40 yr old without additional risk factors
- Minor surgery (<30 min)

Moderate-risk patients
- >40 yr old
- Oral contraceptive medication
- Major surgery (>30 min)

High-risk patients
- Previous DVT/PE
- Major surgery for malignant disease
- Orthopaedic surgery to lower limbs

(Adapted from Wheatley & Veitch 1997, with permission.)

Figure PO11 DVT risk group classification

stockings and intermittent compression devices that work by preventing venous stasis. Early ambulation and leg exercises should be encouraged in the postoperative period.

Pharmacological methods include the subcutaneous administration of unfractionated and low molecular weight heparin. The main advantage of low molecular weight heparin is that it can be given as a once-daily dose, with a resultant improvement in patient acceptability.

Due to the increased risk of bleeding associated with pharmacological prophylaxis the mechanical methods are preferred in certain situations where the consequences of bleeding are severe, as in major head and neck surgery or neurosurgery.

Pulmonary embolus

This usually results from dislodgement of thrombus in the systemic veins or, rarely, from the right atrium (atrial fibrillation may promote thrombus formation) or right ventricle (postseptal/right ventricular infarction). It has a mortality of approximately 10%.

Clinical features depend on the size of the PE. A small embolus may present with exertional dyspnoea and lassitude, a moderate-sized embolus with pleuritic chest pain of sudden onset, haemoptysis and dyspnoea, and a massive embolus with severe chest pain, tachycardia, tachypnoea and syncope. Physical signs may be absent after a small PE. Larger infarcts may produce a tachycardia, gallop rhythm, right ventricular heave and a prominent 'a' wave in the jugular venous wave form. A pleural rub may be present, and signs and symptoms of DVT must be sought.

The investigation of choice is a ventilation–perfusion scan, looking for ventilated but non-perfused areas of lung. The ECG usually only shows a sinus tachycardia, although right ventricular hypertrophy, right axis deviation and right bundle branch block may be present after large emboli. The classical S wave in lead I, Q wave and inverted T wave in lead III is usually absent. The chest x ray is also often normal. Arterial blood gas sampling usually shows hypoxaemia and hypocapnia.

Anticoagulant therapy should be initiated, after confirmation of the diagnosis, to prevent further embolisation. In cases where a delay in ventilation–perfusion scan is expected, anticoagulation should be started on clinical suspicion alone. The duration of anticoagulation depends on the risk of further venous emboli, with treatment continuing for up to 6 months. Thrombolysis with streptokinase is occasionally used after large emboli.

Shivering

Post-anaesthetic shivering occurs in up to 65% of cases (Crossley 1993) and is related to age, gender, duration of anaesthesia and anaesthetic technique. The consequences of shivering include marked increases in minute ventilation and cardiac output secondary to greater oxygen demand and carbon dioxide production. This may have a detrimental effect particularly in the patient with cardiorespiratory disease. Shivering can also interfere with postoperative haemodynamic and oxygen saturation monitoring.

The incidence of post-anaesthetic shivering is increased in hypothermic patients, but not all patients who shiver are hypothermic. Prolonged anaesthesia is associated with postoperative shivering. Methods to prevent a fall in core temperature, such as raising ambient temperature in the operating theatre, warming intravenous fluids and using forced warm air blankets in the intra- and postoperative period, should be used in the at-risk patient. Premedication with anticholinergic agents is associated with an increased incidence of shivering. The use of propofol as opposed to thiopental as an induction agent, or clonidine, an α_2 adrenergic agonist, given at induction reduces the incidence of shivering in the postoperative period.

Treatment includes oxygen administration to prevent hypoxia, active warming and the use of specific drugs. Pethidine at a minimum dose of 0.35 mg per kilogram is the most effective opioid in the treatment of post-anaesthetic shivering, with a 95% success rate. Fentanyl and alfentanil have some effect although this is less marked and shorter in duration than with pethidine. Doxapram, an agent usually used as a respiratory stimulant, is also effective at a dose of 0.2 mg kg^{-1}.

Failure to regain consciousness

In most instances, failure to regain consciousness or postoperative confusion may be attributed to residual drug effects. Other causes include endocrine abnormalities such as hypoglycaemia or hypothyroidism, cerebral events including cerebrovascular accident or cerebral hypoxia, or existing physiological derangements such as hypothermia, hypoxia, hypercapnia or hypotension.

Residual drug effects may be reversed with specific antagonists if unconsciousness is particularly prolonged. These may include naloxone for opioids and flumazenil, up to 1 mg intravenously, for benzodiazepines.

Diabetic patients should have their blood sugar levels checked both intra- and postoperatively. Hypoglycaemia should be treated with 50 ml of 50% dextrose intravenously.

Patient factors
- Cardiorespiratory disease
- Obesity
- Elderly
- Shivering

Surgical factors
- Upper abdominal procedures
- Thoracic surgery

Physiological factors
- Hypovolaemia
- Hypotension
- Anaemia

Postoperative analgesic technique
- Patient-controlled analgesia
- IV opioid infusion
- Epidural infusion (both local anaesthetic agents and opioids)

Figure PO12 Indications for oxygen therapy in the postoperative period

Oxygen therapy

Indications

Supplemental oxygen should be administered for at least 10 minutes to all patients during emergence from anaesthesia to prevent the development of tissue hypoxia.

The indications for oxygen therapy to continue after emergence from anaesthesia are listed in Figure PO12 (Leach & Bateman 1993). Any patient who is at risk of developing tissue hypoxia or is already hypoxaemic should be given supplemental oxygen.

Techniques of administration

Delivery systems used in the postoperative period are listed in Figure PO13, and some are illustrated in Figure PO14. They may be subdivided into variable or fixed performance devices.

Variable-performance devices are so called because the inspired oxygen concentration (FIO_2) and degree of rebreathing vary from patient to patient and at different times in the same patient. This is dependent on the respiratory rate, inspiratory flow rate and length of expiratory pause. This type of device is most commonly used, as an accurate FIO_2 is not required in the majority of patients. The Hudson mask is a clear plastic facemask that is placed over the nose and mouth and, at a flow rate of 4 litres per minute, provides an FIO_2 of approximately 0.4. Addition of a reservoir bag to these masks increases the maximum

Variable performance
- Hudson mask
- MC mask
- Nasal cannulae
- Nasal catheter (nasopharyngeal catheter)

Fixed performance
- Venturi masks
- Anaesthetic breathing circuits

Figure PO13 Oxygen delivery systems in the postoperative period

obtainable FIO_2 to approximately 98%. Patient compliance is poor due to a claustrophobic feeling and the need to remove it during eating and drinking and for routine mouth care. Nasal cannulae provide a more comfortable and continuous method of oxygen delivery. At a flow rate of 2–4 litres per minute, these devices provide an FIO_2 comparable with the face mask.

The fixed-performance devices provide an accurate FIO_2 and avoid rebreathing. They may be further subdivided into high airflow oxygen enrichment (HAFOE) devices, e.g. Venturi masks, or lower flow devices such as anaesthetic breathing systems. Venturi masks use injectors of different sizes to deliver set oxygen concentrations varying from 24% to 60% by entraining air in oxygen using the Venturi principle. The appropriate oxygen flow rate for each mask is printed on the injector, which is also colour-coded. For example, a 24% oxygen valve requires an oxygen flow of 2 litres per minute and entrains 38 litres of air per minute. Patients who require these masks include those at risk of respiratory failure if given high oxygen concentrations, i.e. those who are reliant on a hypoxic drive for ventilation.

In patients who are taken to recovery with a laryngeal mask in situ, supplemental oxygen may be provided by a T-piece connected to it as an alternative to a Mapleson C. This may be run as simply an open-ended tube or as a fixed-performance device.

The use of anaesthetic breathing systems is reserved for the immediate postoperative period, when 100% oxygen may need to be delivered via a tight-fitting mask, for example when there is airway obstruction or laryngeal spasm.

Humidification

Humidification is only required when oxygen is delivered at high flow rates or when the upper airway humidification processes are bypassed, as occurs after tracheostomy or

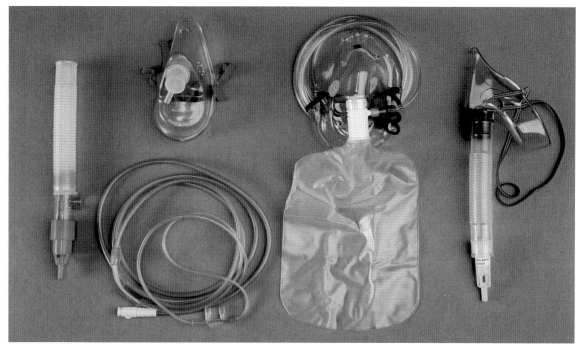

Figure PO14 Left to right: Venturi T-piece, Hudson facemask with nasal cannulae below, mask with oxygen reservoir bag, Ventimask

during prolonged tracheal intubation. It is therefore rarely required during the postoperative period.

Duration

There is no consensus on how long supplemental oxygen therapy should be given. However, the incidence of hypoxaemia is greatest on the second or third postoperative night after major surgery and the PaO_2 may not return to preoperative levels until the fifth night. Supplemental oxygen should therefore be given, where indicated, for at least three days postoperatively.

Complications

Supplemental oxygen administration is a safe technique. However, problems may occur when inappropriate methods are used. Two common problems are the occurrence of barotrauma and the risk of interference with hypoxic drive in certain patients.

Barotrauma

Barotauma occurs when oxygen is directly delivered to the lower airway without free outflow of any excess gas. The practice of placing a variable-performance face mask over the open end of a tracheal tube or laryngeal mask should be avoided as there have been reports of the oxygen inlet part of the face mask impacting on the male connector of the tracheal tube. This resulted in delivery of oxygen at a flow rate of 4 litres per minute and a pressure of 400 kPa, with fatal consequences. The use of a T-piece system, where excess gas is vented to the atmosphere, is a much safer alternative.

Loss of hypoxic ventilatory drive

Approximately 10% of patients with chronic respiratory failure depend on hypoxic ventilatory drive to maintain an adequate $PaCO_2$. In this group of patients administration of a high FiO_2 will cause hypoventilation, with subsequent CO_2 retention and respiratory acidosis. However, the fear of causing CO_2 retention must not prevent the provision of appropriate oxygen therapy. A PaO_2 of 7–8 kPa must be attained. At this level of PaO_2 a slight increase will have a marked effect on oxygen content as this equates to the steepest part of the oxygen–haemoglobin dissociation curve. In practice, 24–28% oxygen should be given in the first instance followed by blood gas analysis to assess clinical response. A higher FiO_2 should be administered if the PaO_2

Cardiovascular
- Tachycardia
- Hypertension
- Increased myocardial oxygen demand

Respiratory
- Decreased vital capacity
- Decreased functional residual capacity
- Decreased tidal volume
- Chest infections
- Basal atelectasis

Gastrointestinal
- Nausea and vomiting
- Ileus

Other effects
- Urinary retention
- Deep venous thrombosis
- Pulmonary embolus

Figure PO15 Adverse effects of postoperative pain

is too low and, if required, ventilatory support should be instituted to control the $PaCO_2$.

Postoperative analgesia

The provision of effective pain relief during the post-operative period is dependent on anaesthetic technique, type and extent of surgery and patient factors such as age and personality. In practice, a combination of opioid, non-steroidal anti-inflammatory drugs (NSAIDs) and local anaesthetic techniques is often used.

Good pain control not only alleviates patient distress but also prevents or modifies many adverse effects (Figure PO15). The increase in sympathetic activity associated with pain results in tachycardia, hypertension, and increased myocardial oxygen demand, which, in patients with cardiac disease, may produce myocardial ischaemia. Postoperative chest infection and basal atelectasis are more frequent in the patient who is unable to deep breathe or cough, such as after upper abdominal or thoracic surgery. Patient immobility associated with poor pain control increases the risk of thromboembolic disease.

Treatment of pain
Opioids

Opioids may be given via the following routes: intra-muscular, subcutaneous, intravenous, oral, intrathecal or extradural.

The dose of opioid required in the postoperative period shows marked interpatient variability. This is due to both pharmacokinetic and pharmacodynamic factors with up to a fivefold difference in plasma concentrations after identical doses of intramuscular opioid. There are also differences in opioid receptor sensitivity between patients.

The conventional regime of on-demand intramuscular opioid often fails to provide adequate pain relief as delays in administration, lack of patient awareness of availability and time taken for onset of action result in plasma levels falling below that required to produce analgesia. Usual dosage is 10–15 mg every 2–4 hours. There may be slow absorption in patients with poor peripheral perfusion. Subcutaneous opioid administration via indwelling cannulae is associated with similar limitations but avoids repeated needle insertion.

Intravenous opioids

Intravenous administration of opioid is generally more effective. A bolus dose can be followed by increments every few minutes until acceptable pain control is reached. This technique minimises the risk of serious side effects but is labour-intensive and is only suitable in the recovery room or high dependency unit.

Continuous intravenous administration via an infusion will ensure maintenance of adequate plasma levels but may be associated with over-sedation and respiratory depression mandating observation of the patient in a high dependency unit.

Patient-controlled analgesia (PCA) was developed to further improve opioid analgesia by accounting for the variation in opioid requirement from patient to patient and the reduction in opioid required with time. The theoretical advantage of this technique is that the patient should maintain a plasma concentration at around the minimum effective analgesic plasma concentration, with resultant good pain control and reduced side effects. It is safer than intravenous infusion techniques as the associated sedation when the patients are pain-free results in reduced usage. In practice, patients may not alleviate their pain completely with this technique because of their worries about addiction and side effects. The success of PCA is dependent on patient education during the preoperative visit, adequate pain control in the recovery room and regular review by nursing and anaesthetic staff. Morphine is the most commonly used opioid, although other drugs such as alfentanil and pethidine have been used with good effect. A demand dose of morphine 1 mg is used with a lock-out period of 5 minutes. The demand dose should be large enough to provide an analgesic effect but small enough to prevent unwanted side effects, and may have to be altered depending on the clinical effect. The lock-out period must be long enough to prevent repeat administration before the initial bolus has had a maximal effect. A maximum dose per hour can also be set to prevent inadvertent overdose although, due to the large variation in opioid requirements between patients, this may prevent some patients from attaining adequate pain relief. A background infusion can also be used with a PCA device, although there is no evidence to suggest that this is of benefit.

The main side effects associated with parenteral opioid administration are nausea and vomiting, and cardiorespiratory depression. The incidence of severe respiratory depression during PCA is approximately 0.5%, which compares favourably with the intramuscular route. The risk of this is increased in patients receiving background opioid infusions or other sedative drugs. The elderly and patients with pre-existing sleep apnoea also have an increased risk of respiratory depression.

Oral opioids

Patients who are able to tolerate oral intake may benefit from opioids given by this route. It is a particularly useful technique in children as it avoids needle or cannula insertion. A dose of morphine 0.2 mg kg^{-1} is adequate in most instances. First-pass metabolism results in lower plasma concentrations after oral than after parenteral administration of the same dose.

Spinal opioids

Opioid administration via the intrathecal or extradural route can provide excellent postoperative pain control. The commonest side effects associated with this technique are nausea, pruritus, sedation and urinary retention. Respiratory depression is an infrequent complication, but it can occur up to 24 hours after administration of intrathecal opioids, and therefore patients must be observed in the high dependency unit for a 24-hour period to monitor their respiratory status. Patients receiving extradural opioids are at a lower risk of developing respiratory depression but they must also be managed on a ward where this potentially fatal complication can be recognised and treated.

The conscious level of the patient is as important as the respiratory rate, if not more so. A patient with a decreased conscious level, with or without a low respiratory rate, requires immediate treatment. Intravenous naloxone given in titrated doses is effective at reversing the opioid-induced respiratory depression without reducing the analgesic effect.

Non-steroidal anti-inflammatory drugs

This group of drugs have both analgesic and anti-inflammatory properties. They are effective for treatment of mild to moderate postoperative pain and, after the first 24–36 hours, may be used as the sole analgesic in major surgical patients. NSAIDs also have an opioid-sparing effect with a reduction of opioid requirement after major surgery of greater than 20% when given regularly.

NSAIDs have several advantages over opioid analgesics. Their use is not associated with respiratory depression or gastric stasis and, as they are not controlled drugs, they are readily available. However, their use is associated with potentially serious side effects, which include gastrointestinal haemorrhage, gastric ulceration, renal impairment and an increased risk of postoperative bleeding due to impairment of platelet function. NSAIDs are contraindicated in patients with a history of peptic ulcer disease, gastrointestinal bleeding, renal impairment, previous hypersensitivity reactions to aspirin or NSAIDs, asthma, and bleeding diathesis. They should be avoided in the dehydrated or hypovolaemic patient and care should be taken when using NSAIDs in the elderly.

The salicylates are absolutely contraindicated in children less than 12 years of age. Reye's syndrome, an acute encephalopathy with fatty infiltration of the liver, is associated with administration of these drugs in this age group.

Local anaesthetics

Local infiltration, peripheral nerve blocks and epidural analgesia are often used to produce postoperative pain relief, both alone and in conjunction with other analgesic methods.

The advantage of local anaesthetic techniques is that profound analgesia can be produced without respiratory depression or nausea and vomiting. However, local anaesthetic toxicity may occur as a result of inadvertent intravenous administration or after large doses. In addition, although rare, peripheral nerve damage, haemorrhage, infection, accidental arterial or subarachnoid injection and pneumothorax can all occur, depending on the site of the block.

Pain assessment

Pain, by definition, is a subjective sensation and is difficult for an observer to accurately assess. The provision of a reliable and valid means of assessing pain is important because it allows the degree of improvement, after an analgesic intervention, to be documented in a reproducible way.

There are a number of specific pain assessment scales that are used in the postoperative setting to ensure that a history of the patient's pain is recorded in a useful form so as to inform treatment decisions. These include:

- Verbal rating scale (VRS)
- Numerical rating scale (NRS)
- Visual analogue scale (VAS)

In very young children, physiological and behavioural indicators are used. Older children may choose from ranked facial expressions on a chart.

The verbal rating scale is simple and easy to use. The patient is asked to rate the pain as 'none', 'mild', 'moderate', or 'severe' when at rest and on movement.

The numerical rating scale consists of a numerical scale representing the pain from 0 = 'no pain' to 10 (or 5) = 'the worst imaginable pain'.

The visual analogue scale consists of a 10 cm long line which represents a spectrum of pain intensity from 'no pain at all' on the extreme left through to 'the worst pain imaginable' on the extreme right. The patient is asked to mark the point on this line that corresponds to the severity of the pain. The VAS is primarily a research tool and, performed correctly, is arguably too complex for routine postoperative use. There is no obvious advantage of the more detailed methods in terms of practical patient management.

Acute pain service

The importance of effective postoperative pain relief, and the increased complexity of analgesic techniques such as PCA and continuous epidural infusions, has resulted in the formation of acute pain services in many hospitals. They provide a multidisciplinary approach to postoperative pain control with the involvement of anaesthetists, specialist nurses and clinical pharmacists. An acute pain service carries out regular patient assessment and provides backup for ward staff. It is also involved in 'in-house' training of medical and nursing staff to improve understanding of analgesic methods and pain assessment.

Postoperative nausea and vomiting

Postoperative nausea and vomiting (PONV) is one of the commonest complications in the postoperative period despite the use of modern-day anaesthetic techniques. It occurs in 20–40% of cases, resulting in patient discomfort and anxiety, and can produce significant morbidity in

Patient factors

Gender

Age

Anxiety

History of motion sickness

Previous PONV

Delayed gastric emptying

Obesity

Anaesthetic factors

Drugs	Opioids
	Intravenous induction agents
	Nitrous oxide
	Neostigmine
Technique	Gastric insufflation
	Subarachnoid block

Surgical factors

Emergency procedure

Day-case surgery

ENT surgery

Strabismus correction

Gynaecological procedures

Gastrointestinal surgery

Postoperative pain

Ileus, gastric distension

Figure PO16 Risk factors associated with PONV

some cases. Sudden increases in intraocular and intracranial pressure associated with vomiting may be detrimental in the ophthalmic and neurosurgical patient. Fluid and electrolyte disturbances can occur if the period of vomiting is prolonged.

PONV exhibits a multifactorial aetiology and is influenced by patient, anaesthetic and surgical factors (Figure PO16).

Females are 2.5 times more likely to develop PONV than males. The incidence also varies with age, with the lowest incidence found in infants aged less than 12 months and a peak in the 6- to 16-year-old age group, followed by a slight decrease during adult life. Inadequate starvation or delayed gastric emptying, from whatever cause, is associated with an increase in PONV, and anxiety may have its effect via this mechanism. The increased incidence in obesity may be related to anaesthetic problems associated with these patients, such as stomach insufflation and the development of hypoxaemia or hypercapnia, rather than with obesity itself.

Intravenous induction agents are incriminated to varying degrees. Propofol is associated with less PONV than thiopental and may have specific anti-emetic properties. Thiopental is less emetogenic than etomidate. Nitrous oxide is thought to be associated with PONV, possibly as a result of gut distension and raised pressure in the middle ear. Neuromuscular blocking agents are not implicated, but reversal with neostigmine has been shown to increase emesis. This is despite concurrent administration of atropine, which has anti-emetic properties. The development of hypotension after spinal anaesthesia is associated with almost twice the incidence of PONV when compared with those patients where hypotension did not occur.

Prevention

Prevention of PONV is difficult due to its multifactorial aetiology. The mainstay of management is the avoidance of emetogenic drugs and the use of anti-emetic agents.

A patient presenting for surgery at risk of PONV should receive anxiolytic and anti-emetic premedication. Anaesthesia should be induced using intravenous propofol in a controlled manner, taking care to avoid gastric insufflation with anaesthetic gases. Opioid drugs should be used sparingly and, where appropriate, NSAIDs and local anaesthetic techniques used instead. An oxygen/air/volatile mix or total intravenous anaesthesia should be used for maintenance of anaesthesia. Further anti-emetic therapy should be given intraoperatively and continued, on a regular basis, into the postoperative period.

Treatment

Vomiting in a semiconscious patient requires immediate action. The patient should be placed in the lateral position, the pharynx cleared of any secretions and supplemental oxygen administered.

The conscious patient should be reassured and supplemental oxygen administered, although this will only have a placebo effect unless hypoxaemia is the cause. Other underlying causes such as hypercapnia, hypotension or pain should be treated. The majority of patients, however, will require an anti-emetic (Rowbotham 1992).

There are several classes of drugs used for the treatment of PONV:

- D_2 – dopaminergic antagonists
- $5\text{-}HT_3$ – serotonergic antagonists
- H_1 – histaminergic antagonists
- M_3 – muscarinic antagonists

Prochlorperazine, a phenothiazine, is a dopamine antagonist acting on the chemoreceptor trigger zone whose use is limited by low efficacy, lack of an intravenous preparation and central nervous system side effects. Metoclopramide has antidopaminergic activity and a peripheral action on the gut, which increases gastric emptying and small intestine transit time. The incidence of side effects is less than 10% but there is little evidence supporting its efficacy in the doses routinely used. $5\text{-}HT_3$ antagonists such as ondansetron have been used much more frequently over the last few years with good effect, but they are often used as second-line treatment due to their high cost. Cyclizine, a histamine receptor antagonist with mild anticholinergic activity, is increasing in popularity as it is inexpensive and can be given orally, intramuscularly or intravenously.

Postoperative fluid therapy

The aims of postoperative fluid therapy are to maintain adequate hydration, blood volume, renal function and electrolyte balance. It is indicated in patients with preoperative fluid abnormalities or ongoing fluid losses, and also in any patient undergoing a major surgical procedure.

Physiology

Total body water (TBW) accounts for 50–70% of body weight dependent on age, sex, body habitus and fat content. TBW is distributed between three fluid compartments: the intravascular space (8% TBW), the interstitial space (32% TBW) and the intracellular space (60% TBW). The intravascular and interstitial space together form the extracellular fluid (ECF) compartment and are separated by the endothelial cells of the capillary wall, which are freely permeable to water and small ions, but not to proteins. The intracellular fluid (ICF) compartment is separated from the ECF by the cell membrane, which is selectively permeable to ions.

Surgical incision produces a neurohumoral or 'stress' response, with increasing levels of circulating catecholamines, vasopressin, aldosterone and cortisol and resultant sodium and water retention.

Postoperative fluid loss

There are many causes of fluid loss in the surgical patient (Figure PO17). Insensible losses from the skin and lungs

Insensible losses
- Sweating
- Respiration
- Faeces
- Urine output

'Third space' losses
- Haemorrhage
- Drains
- Nasogastric
- Vomiting
- Diarrhoea

Figure PO17 Causes of postoperative fluid loss in the surgical patient

are approximately $0.5\ ml\ kg^{-1}$ per hour. This figure increases by 12% for each degree rise in body temperature above 37 °C. 'Third space' loss is due to tissue oedema and is directly related to the extent of the surgical incision, varying from 1 to $15\ ml\ kg^{-1}$ per hour. The amount of ongoing loss is often difficult to quantify, and it may be difficult to accurately measure blood loss.

Clinical assessment
Regular clinical evaluation to detect any fluid deficit should be carried out in the postoperative period. Adequacy of volume status is associated with normal pulse, blood pressure, and jugular venous pressure, a urine output of at least $0.5\ ml\ kg^{-1}$ per hour, moist mucous membranes and warm extremities and good peripheral perfusion. Trends in haemodynamic parameters can guide further fluid management, and central venous or pulmonary artery occlusion pressure monitoring may be indicated in some cases. Assessment can be difficult in patients with residual effects of general or regional anaesthesia or on beta-blocker therapy, where normal responses (peripheral vasoconstriction, tachycardia) may be masked. Laboratory investigations including haemoglobin concentration, haematocrit and urea may be abnormal in moderate to severe fluid deficit.

Fluid replacement
It is difficult to predict fluid requirements in the postoperative period, particularly after major surgery. The fluid regime in Figure PO18 acts only as a guide to fluid therapy during this period, and emphasis must be placed on repeated clinical assessment. Patients undergoing minor surgery who will start drinking within a few hours of the procedure do not usually require additional intravenous fluids.

The choice of fluid replacement depends on which fluid compartment is depleted. Crystalloids, which are solutions of electrolytes and sugars in water, are distributed throughout the three fluid compartments depending on

Cause	Replacement fluid	Volume ($ml\ kg^{-1}\ h^{-1}$)	Comment
Insensible loss	5% dextrose or 4% dextrose/0.18% saline	1	
'Third' space loss	0.9% saline or	1–3	Minor surgery, e.g. hernia repair
	Hartmann's solution	3–5	Intermediate surgery, e.g. mastectomy
		5–10	Major surgery, e.g. THR
		10–15	Major plus surgery, e.g. aortic aneurysm repair
Blood loss	0.9% saline (3 × blood loss) or Colloid (1 × blood loss) or Packed red blood cells (1 × blood loss)		Aim for Hb of $10\ g\ dl^{-1}$

Figure PO18 Postoperative intravenous fluid regime

their sodium concentration. Isotonic fluids such as 0.9% saline remain predominantly within the ECF compartment, whereas hypotonic solutions such as 5% dextrose are distributed throughout the ECF and ICF. Colloids, which are solutions of high molecular weight proteins (blood and blood products), gelatins, starches or dextrans, are mainly confined to the intravascular compartment.

Insensible losses are replaced with 5% dextrose if there is no ECF loss. However, the majority of postoperative patients have a degree of ECF loss and require additional sodium. 4% dextrose/0.18% saline is then the fluid of choice. Potassium should be added to maintenance fluids after the first postoperative day at 1 mmol kg^{-1} per day. Estimated 'third space' loss is replaced with normal (0.9%) saline or a balanced salt solution such as Hartmann's solution. Blood loss is replaced with colloid on a one-to-one basis and, if the loss exceeds approximately 15% of the patient's blood volume, packed red blood cells to maintain the haemoglobin concentration at about 10 g dl^{-1}. Normal saline or Hartmann's solution can also be used to maintain intravascular volume, although a volume three times the estimated blood loss has to be infused.

Postoperative fluid therapy should continue until there is adequate oral intake, fluid deficits have been corrected and there are no major ongoing fluid losses.

Sequelae of anaesthesia

Complications occurring after surgery result from a combination of patient, surgical and anaesthetic factors. Morbidity directly attributable to anaesthetic practice is often relatively minor, e.g. postoperative sore throat, but can result in permanent disability, e.g. hypoxic brain damage. An increasing number of medico-legal claims are made against anaesthetists each year, which highlights the virtues of diligence, accurate record keeping, attention to detail and continued observation throughout the administration of anaesthesia and into the postoperative period.

The sequelae of anaesthesia are related to anaesthetic technique and patient positioning.

Eye trauma

Corneal abrasions can occur if the eyelids remain open during anaesthesia and the cornea is allowed to dry out. This is easily preventable by applying adhesive tape, which should be removed with care, to ensure that the eyelids remain closed. Corneal abrasion may also occur if the eye comes into direct contact with equipment such as laryngoscope blades or anaesthetic masks. Retinal ischaemia has been reported after prolonged eyeball compression, with resultant transient blindness. Eye pads should be used if the prone or lateral position is adopted.

Airway trauma

Instrumentation of the oropharynx with a laryngoscope blade, a laryngeal mask or oral airway can result in lip, tongue and gum abrasions. Care should be taken to prevent the lips or tongue from being caught on the teeth.

Broken teeth and damaged dental work not only put the patient at risk of aspiration but are also a cause of significant inconvenience after recovery. For this reason, dental damage is a major cause of litigation. Poor dentition, loose teeth and the presence of caps, crowns and bridges should be documented at the preoperative visit. Methods employed to decrease the risk of dental trauma include the use of nasal airways, mouth guards and fibre-optic intubation.

Up to 50% of patients complain of postoperative sore throat. This may be related to tracheal intubation, although it is often associated with airway or laryngeal mask insertion, nasogastric tube placement and administration of dry gases.

Musculoskeletal trauma

Muscle pains can occur in the postoperative period and are usually related to suxamethonium administration. Suxamethonium pains are more common in the young ambulant patient with large muscle bulk. During pregnancy and childhood the muscle pains are less intense. The onset is typically delayed by 24 hours and may mimic influenza-like symptoms. Administration of low-dose non-depolarising muscle relaxants, benzodiazepines or lidocaine before anaesthetic induction has been used in an attempt to reduce the muscle pains, with variable effect. Patients should be informed of the possibility of this complication.

Backache and neck pain can occur from poor patient positioning and as a result of stretched ligaments and relaxed skeletal muscle. Arms and legs can slip off operating tables or trolleys, if inadequately secured, with the potential for ligament and bony injuries.

Nerve injuries have been extensively reported, and are a result of direct compression or stretching of the nerve. Correct patient positioning and extensive padding of exposed sites are mandatory. The brachial plexus can be damaged if there is excessive abduction of the arm (>90 degrees) with the humeral head impinging on the axillary neurovascular bundle. The radial nerve, as it runs down the lateral border of the arm 3–5 cm above the lateral epicondyle, is at risk of being damaged by a blood pressure cuff. The ulnar nerve is exposed at the elbow and can be damaged by direct trauma or the blood pressure cuff. The common peroneal nerve can be damaged, when the patient is placed in the lithotomy position, as it passes laterally around the neck of the fibula, resulting in foot drop and loss of sensation on the dorsum of the foot. The saphenous nerve is also at risk in the lithotomy position when there is compression of the medial aspect of the leg against the leg support, and this results in loss of sensation along the medial aspect of the calf. Facial and supraorbital nerve palsies due to direct nerve compression have also been reported.

Skin damage

Bruising and skin breakdown over pressure areas can occur after prolonged procedures and in the elderly. The occiput, elbows and heels should be padded and the undersheet smoothed out. Skin contact with metal must be prevented because of the risk of electrical burns if diathermy is used. Excessively frequent blood pressure cuff inflation is associated with localised bruising and should be avoided. In the postoperative period, patients with residual local anaesthetic blocks or epidural analgesia are at increased risk of skin breakdown due to immobility and loss of sensation.

Medico-legal issues

After receiving a verbal or written complaint from a patient a copy of all the relevant clinical information should be made. A senior member of the anaesthetic department should be informed and, if in any doubt, advice should be sought from the relevant medical defence institution. Under no account must any documented information be altered. The importance of completing an accurate and legible anaesthetic form for every patient undergoing anaesthesia cannot be stressed enough.

References and further reading

Association of Anaesthetists of Great Britain and Ireland. *Immediate Postanaesthetic Recovery*. London: AAGBI, 2002.

Australian and New Zealand College of Anaesthetists and Faculty of Pain Medicine. *Acute Pain Management: Scientific Evidence*, 2nd edn. Melbourne: ANZCA, 2005.

Crossley AW. Postoperative shivering. *Br J Hosp Med* 1993; **49**: 204–8.

Davis L, Britten JJ, Morgan M. Cholinesterase: its significance in anaesthetic practice. *Anaesthesia* 1997; **52**: 244–60.

Joyce CJ, Baker AB. What is the role of absorption atelectasis in the genesis of peri-operative pulmonary collapse? *Anaesth Intensive Care* 1995; **23**; 691–6.

Leach RM, Bateman NT. Acute oxygen therapy. *Br J Hosp Med* 1993; **49**: 637–44.

Mangat PS, Jones JG. Perioperative hypoxaemia. In: Kaufman L (ed.) *Anaesthesia Review* **10**. Edinburgh: Churchill Livingstone, 1993: 83–106.

Moore A, Edwards J, Barden J, McQuay H. *Bandolier's Little Book of Pain*. Oxford: Oxford University Press, 2003.

Rowbotham DJ. Current management of postoperative nausea and vomiting. *Br J Anaesth* 1992; **69** (7 Suppl. 1): 46S–59S.

The Royal College of Surgeons of England and the College of Anaesthetists. *Pain after Surgery*. Report of a Working Party of the Commission on the Provision of Surgical Services (Chairman AA Spence), 1990.

Wheatley T, Veitch PS. Recent advances in prophylaxis against deep vein thrombosis. *Br J Anaesth* 1997; **78**: 118–20.

CHAPTER 5

Special patient circumstances

C. A. Pinnock and R. M. Haden

The pregnant patient

Obstetric anaesthesia requires detailed knowledge of the physiological changes associated with pregnancy. Whilst these are covered thoroughly in Section 2, Chapter 14, the salient points are outlined below to aid the reader.

As pregnancy progresses, the maternal blood volume increases and, although total haemoglobin increases, the haemoglobin concentration falls by dilution. The concentration of clotting factors increases, causing a tendency to deep vein thrombosis exacerbated by pressure on the pelvic veins from the increasingly bulky uterus. Cardiac output increases throughout pregnancy due to increases in stroke volume and heart rate. Thoracic volume rises so that although tidal volume remains comparable to pre-pregnancy values, there becomes an impression of hyperinflation. At the end of pregnancy $PaCO_2$ is reduced to 4 kPa. The hormonal changes of pregnancy cause relaxation of smooth muscle and ligaments, resulting in a reduction in lower oesophageal sphincter tone which, combined with increasing intra-abdominal pressure, leads both to functional hiatus herniae and oesophageal reflux. Gastric contents are more voluminous than usual and gastric emptying is slowed. In labour, gastric emptying virtually ceases.

Patients in the third trimester of pregnancy should not be allowed to lie in the supine position for any reason without left lateral tilt to displace the uterus, because the weight of the uterus compresses the inferior vena cava. The substantial reduction in venous return to the heart that follows may produce fainting. If compensatory vasoconstriction is abolished by epidural blockade, serious falls in cardiac output may result.

Analgesia in labour

Pain in labour is the result of a hollow organ, the uterus, contracting against an obstruction, the fetus, in an attempt to expel it. The pain is the result of tension in the uterine

Fundamentals of Anaesthesia, 3rd edition, ed. Tim Smith, Colin Pinnock and Ted Lin. Published by Cambridge University Press. © Cambridge University Press 2008.

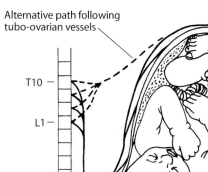

Alternative path following tubo-ovarian vessels

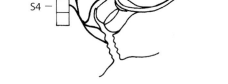

T10 —

L1 —

S2 —

S4 —

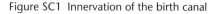

Figure SC1 Innervation of the birth canal

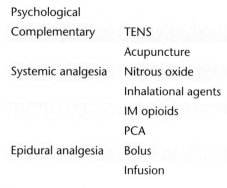

Psychological

Complementary	TENS
	Acupuncture
Systemic analgesia	Nitrous oxide
	Inhalational agents
	IM opioids
	PCA
Epidural analgesia	Bolus
	Infusion

Figure SC2 Methods of pain relief in labour

wall. The patient's response to the pain of contractions is a psychological response that depends on culture, history and preparation; therefore each patient must be taken on her own merits. The pain of labour is transmitted to the spinal cord via two routes, depending on the stage of labour. The impulses from the body and fundus of the uterus pass via the lower thoracic spinal roots, T10 to L1, while those from the cervix and birth canal pass via the sacral roots. The net result is that pain in the first stage of labour is perceived to be lower abdominal while in the second stage it changes focus to pelvis and perineum (see Figure SC1). Nociceptive impulses pass up the spinal cord and are interpreted in the brain. The various methods of providing analgesia in labour are detailed in Figure SC2.

Psychological methods
There is no doubt that adequate psychological preparation for labour significantly reduces pain. Breathing and relaxation techniques are taught routinely in antenatal classes. Self-hypnosis can also be successful in the suitably motivated patient.

Complementary methods
Transcutaneous electrical nerve stimulation (TENS) can work well if introduced early enough in labour. The technique depends on the gate theory of pain transmission (as described by Melzack & Wall 1965). Stimulation must be applied to the dorsal columns of the spinal cord in the mid-thoracic region, above the level of the affected nerve roots, i.e. T10. TENS is effective early in labour but begins to lose its effect after 5 cm cervical dilatation is reached. Acupuncture has been advocated for use in labour but it is not in common use in the UK.

Systemic analgesia
Systemic administration of analgesic drugs remains the mainstay of labour analgesia. Administration is usually by inhalation of nitrous oxide or anaesthetic vapours, or alternatively by intravenous or intramuscular administration of opioids.

Nitrous oxide is usually administered as a 50% mixture with oxygen (Entonox®). Effective use of nitrous oxide depends on beginning the inhalation before the painful part of the contraction so that an analgesic concentration is reached by the time a contraction becomes painful, which is difficult to achieve. Anaesthetic vapours have been advocated in sub-anaesthetic concentrations (such as isoflurane 0.2%) but have not achieved large-scale use.

Opioid analgesia may be given by either the intramuscular or the intravenous route. Local rules and preferences dictate the choice of opioid. Midwives may administer intramuscular opioids on their own responsibility, subject to local protocols relating to which drug, number of doses and accountability. Agents in widespread use include the agonists pethidine and diamorphine, while some units favour partial agonists such as meptazinol. All opioids have a reputation for causing fetal respiratory depression.

The intravenous route via a patient-controlled analgesia (PCA) device has not yet become popular, despite the

- Maternal refusal
- Bleeding diathesis
- Anatomical abnormalities
- Hypovolaemia
- Cardiac disease
- Neurological disease
- Sepsis

Figure SC3 Contraindications to epidural anaesthesia

advantages of patient control and lower total dose. PCA devices may be simple 'elastic recoil' systems with a reservoir refilled at a fixed rate or complex computer-controlled devices with adjustable background infusions and lock-out times. Pethidine remains the most popular drug for obstetric PCA.

Epidural analgesia

Epidural analgesia is the most effective form of labour analgesia, but has disadvantages in that it requires the availability of a trained anaesthetist and is accompanied by rare but potentially major complications. Epidural analgesia comes into its own in long or complicated labours, malpresentations (such as occipitoposterior position or breech) and pre-eclampsia, where control of the blood pressure and improvements in placental blood flow are vital to the well-being of both mother and fetus. Indications for epidural analgesia are numerous, and contraindications are listed in Figure SC3.

Contraindications to epidural analgesia

(1) **Maternal refusal** is the only absolute contraindication to the technique. If, after reasonable explanation of the risks and benefits, the patient refuses, then to continue constitutes assault. On this basis there is no need for written consent to epidurals in labour: first, a woman in labour is in pain and distressed and cannot, under those circumstances, be expected to make a balanced judgement and, second, if the basis of the service is request, then the fact that the patient, via her midwife, asks for this method of analgesia can be taken as verbal consent. This has not been tested in court. The available methods of analgesia should have been explained in antenatal classes and the patient should, therefore, be able to make an informed choice without lengthy explanation during labour.

(2) **Bleeding diathesis.** There is controversy about the provision of epidural and spinal blockade in patients with a bleeding tendency, whether this is congenital, such as haemophilia, or acquired, such as warfarinisation. It is generally accepted that any patient whose clotting times are more than 50% extended should probably not have an epidural (in practice this means an INR > 1.5). The potential problem is the vulnerability of the epidural venous plexus and concern that if an epidural vein is punctured there will be an uncontrolled bleed from it, causing a haematoma, which could compress the spinal cord. While this sequence of events is certainly possible, it is also exceptionally rare, occurring with the same incidence as spontaneous epidural haematoma.

The suitability of epidural analgesia for patients taking low-dose heparin or aspirin is also controversial. Aspirin causes a permanent block of platelet thromboxane A2, which affects any platelets in the circulation at the time the aspirin is administered. This continues for the life of any individual platelet, roughly 10 days from new. While this may appear to be a contraindication to epidural puncture, with its attendant risk of haemorrhage, the effect is quite limited because new, unaffected platelets are continually being produced. The best indicator of platelet function is the bleeding time, which suffers from poor reproducibility and a wide normal range. The ESRA guidelines on epidural use and anticoagulation are given in Section 1, Chapter 7 (Figure RA19).

In obstetric anaesthesia there are a number of other causes of acquired clotting failure which may contraindicate epidural puncture. Pre-eclampsia is associated with deranged clotting function, particularly if severe or late in pregnancy. The platelet count will give an indication of the severity of the problem before it becomes clinically important. The **HELLP** syndrome is a variant of pre-eclampsia (**H**aemolytic anaemia, **E**levated **L**iver enzymes and **L**ow **P**latelets). This condition is highly dangerous and causes extreme physiological upsets which can only be restored using the full facilities of an intensive care unit and haematological support. The pronounced coagulopathy that occurs in HELLP syndrome is a contraindication to epidural analgesia.

Intrauterine fetal death causes a failure of clotting as the fetus begins to macerate and breakdown products enter the maternal circulation. The process does not become significant until the fetus has been dead for more than about 5 days, but it is usual to measure clotting in this situation before an epidural is sited.

Placental abruption and other significant intrauterine bleeds may cause clotting failure secondary to the consumption of clotting factors in a vain attempt to stop bleeding from the spiral arteries. The spiral arteries pass through the myometrium to the placental bed and are usually closed off by uterine contraction after delivery. If the uterus is kept open by the presence of a fetus, blood clots or placental remnants the bleeding will continue until the uterus is emptied or the patient exsanguinates. The blood loss may not be seen as vaginal bleeding because it can remain concealed entirely within the uterus.

Amniotic fluid embolus causes a syndrome similar to major fat embolism, with clouding of consciousness, petechial haemorrhages, respiratory distress, hypotension and severe disseminated intravascular coagulation (DIC). This condition is rare but often fatal. Management consists of general supportive therapy and replacement of clotting factors and blood.

(3) **Anatomical abnormalities.** Previous back surgery or spina bifida are relative contraindications to epidural analgesia because of difficulty in identifying bony landmarks. If the patient has had a lumbar laminectomy or spinal fusion then it is wise to check the level of surgery from previous notes or x rays so that a level can be chosen for the puncture which has bony landmarks and avoids scar tissue or implanted metal. In spina bifida occulta, the landmarks are missing congenitally but the epidural space is relatively normal. The ligamentum flavum may, however, be absent. In the more severe forms of neural tube defect the epidural space and dural tube may be abnormal and so the situation is more complicated. None of the above situations is an absolute contraindication to epidural analgesia but the technique may be difficult or impossible, the spread of local anaesthetic in the epidural space may not be normal, and the resulting pattern of block may be patchy or deficient.

(4) **Hypovolaemia** must be corrected before any form of anaesthesia or analgesia, unless the situation is so dire that immediate surgery is the only way to reduce massive blood loss, in which case general anaesthesia will be indicated. In this situation, as with any hypovolaemic patient, induction must be carried out with extreme care. Sympathetic blockade caused by epidural or spinal anaesthesia in a hypovolaemic patient can have catastrophic consequences.

(5) **Cardiac disease** is often taken as a contraindication to central neural blockade. In general, the effects of epidural anaesthesia are falls in both cardiac preload and afterload, which can be controlled by the gentle administration of local anaesthetic agents and by judicious use of fluids and vasoconstrictors. Pregnancy itself carries such major vascular and cardiac changes that it is difficult to reach term unless there are reasonable cardiac reserves. Unfortunately, more and more patients with congenital cardiac disease, whether corrected or not, are being brought to term. In addition, the age of onset of major coronary artery disease is now falling within the childbearing years. These patients may be on the verge of major cardiac decompensation by the time they reach term. Each woman must be considered on her merits.

(6) **Neurological disease.** Chronic neurological disease is often quoted as a contraindication to local or regional anaesthesia, without evidence to confirm this view. Most of the chronic neurological disorders, such as multiple sclerosis, follow a relapsing and remitting course, usually deteriorating at times of physical or mental stress and following a slow progression downward. If at the time of childbirth (one of the stressful times likely to cause relapse) central nerve block is provided for analgesia or anaesthesia then it is likely that the relapse will be blamed on the technique, regardless of whether it is in fact to blame. Provided that this is explained and accepted by the patient there is no reason why this form of analgesia should be withheld.

(7) **Sepsis** at the proposed site of puncture is a contraindication to epidural anaesthesia, but there is usually a non-infected space available close by which can be used. Maternal pyrexia, however, should be taken as a contraindication because of the risk of blood-borne infection with a foreign body, the epidural catheter, in situ or a potential haematoma from epidural vein puncture providing an infective focus. Epidural analgesia limits maternal thermoregulation, and fetal death rate increases dramatically in maternal pyrexia, so it may be preferable to avoid the use of epidural anaesthesia in this situation.

Epidural technique

Detailed knowledge of the relevant anatomy is essential (Figure SC4). For further details of epidural technique, see Section 1, Chapter 7.

The epidural space is a potential space within the spinal canal. It is broadly triangular in shape with the apex posteriorly. The shape varies considerably from level to level, being more oval in the neck. Superiorly it is closed at the foramen magnum, where the spinal dura mater and the periosteum of the spinal canal fuse to form the intracranial dura mater. It is, therefore, impossible for a true epidural injection to extend intracranially. Inferiorly, the epidural space is closed at the sacrococcygeal ligament. The anterior boundary lies within the spinal canal, being formed by the posterior longitudinal ligaments of the spinal column, the vertebral bodies and the intervertebral discs. Posteriorly the space is bounded by the ligamenta flava (these may be

Boundaries	Superior	Closed at foramen magnum
	Inferior	Closed at sacrococcygeal membrane
	Anterior	Posterior longitudinal ligaments, vertebral bodies
	Posterior	Vertebral laminae, ligamenta flava
	Lateral	Open, pedicles and intervertebral foramina
Shape		Broadly triangular, apex posteriorly
Contents		Veins, arteries, fat, lymphatics, nerve roots and dural cuffs

Figure SC4 Anatomy of the epidural space

paired at each level or one pair of continuous ligaments – opinion varies) and the vertebral laminae. There may be a plane of cleavage between the ligamenta flava that can give an impression that there is no ligament when a needle passes through it. Laterally the epidural space is bounded by the pedicles and laminae of the vertebrae and by the intervertebral foramina, and thus it is not a closed space laterally. Interiorly the space contains the spinal dural sac and its contents: the spinal cord and nerve roots. The epidural space itself contains fat, arterioles, a complex of thin-walled valveless veins which drain into the azygos system, lymphatics and the spinal nerve roots after they cross the dura and before they exit through the intervertebral foramina. The nerve roots carry with them a cuff of dura that may extend out into the paravertebral space.

To reach the epidural space from the skin of the back, the tip of the needle must pass through successive layers of tissue. The bones over the lumbar area are palpated and the spaces between spinous processes identified. Once a suitable space has been identified (L2/3 is usually the easiest and most consistent to use) the needle is inserted through the skin, staying strictly on the midline, although a deliberate paramedian approach is acceptable. The first ligament encountered is the supraspinous ligament. This has a 'crunchy' consistency and is up to 1 cm thick. The interspinous ligament feels 'spongy' and can be up to 6 cm thick. The ligamentum flavum is very variable in thickness, up to 2 cm, but is usually tough and difficult to penetrate. The essence of the technique is that with the needle tip in the ligamentum flavum, nothing can be injected through the needle whereas after careful advancement, the tip will emerge into the epidural space and there will be a sudden total loss of resistance to injection.

Combined spinal–epidural in labour

Combined spinal–epidural (CSE) techniques may be used for analgesia in labour. An epidural needle is sited in the epidural space and a longer small-gauge spinal needle is then passed through it. A small dose of a mixture of bupivacaine and fentanyl is injected through the spinal needle, which is then withdrawn and an epidural catheter passed through the epidural needle. The spinal solution establishes analgesia for the early part of the first stage of labour and, when this analgesia becomes inadequate, the epidural catheter is used for further doses. The patient is allowed some mobility while the spinal solution is effective but this may be limited by the need for continuous monitoring of the fetus. Each unit must have written policies to establish the limits to mobility in labour.

Test doses

It is impossible to be absolutely sure of the correct placement of an epidural catheter until a dose of local anaesthetic agent has been injected. A test dose serves two purposes, first to identify vascular placement and second to identify intrathecal placement. To achieve this, a test dose must be small enough to do no harm if in the wrong place but large enough to show an effect. Most practitioners use a 3 ml dose of either 0.5% or 0.25% plain bupivacaine. There are advocates for both epinephrine-containing and dextrose-containing test doses but neither is in popular use.

In practice, 3 ml plain isobaric bupivacaine, placed directly into the CSF, will produce total spinal anaesthesia within 5 minutes. Hyperbaric bupivacaine (Heavy Marcain®) will have a less extensive result, and if it is placed intravenously there will be no noticeable effect. Larger volumes of local anaesthetic agent injected into the lumbar epidural venous plexus tend to pass backwards up the basilar vessels and cause a short-lived loss of consciousness or at least a period of light-headedness with lingual and circumoral paraesthesia. The rationale behind using an epinephrine-containing solution is that, on intravenous injection, there will be a measurable increase in heart rate. While this may be so, the increase so caused will be within the pulse rate variation of any woman in labour and so may not be distinguished from normal.

Having given the test dose and waited an appropriate time for an effect to appear, usually 5 minutes, the main dose may be given. Traditionally the choice is 0.25% or 0.5% plain bupivacaine by bolus top-ups of between 6 and

10 ml as necessary to relieve the pain. The top-ups may be given all in one position, usually semi-reclining, or half the dose may be given in each lateral position with 5 minutes between. This method, while still in widespread use, is being superseded by a variety of low-dose infusion techniques that have the advantage of reducing both the drug load and the unwanted effects of the traditional epidural, such as high-density motor block and an increased incidence of instrumental delivery.

The majority of infusion epidurals begin with a single top-up to rapidly establish the analgesia before commencing the infusion. Increasingly, the local anaesthetic agent in the top-up is supplemented by small doses of an opioid (such as fentanyl). The combination appears to increase both the analgesia and the penetration of the block without any obvious drawbacks. Recent evidence suggests that there are no measurable fetal effects of the opioid at doses in current use. Infusion regimes vary considerably but most are based on either 0.1% bupivacaine or 0.2% ropivacaine, each with $1-5\ \mu g\ ml^{-1}$ of fentanyl. Each unit should have a single standard mixture with which all anaesthetists and midwives should be familiar. This mixture is infused at a variable rate up to 15 ml per hour, though occasionally this mixture is given by bolus top-up rather than infusion.

Patient-controlled epidural analgesia (PCEA) is gaining popularity slowly, either as patient-administered boluses alone or as patient-administered boluses to supplement a background infusion.

Complications

Epidural anaesthesia carries a risk of complications, the more major of which are listed in Figure SC5.

(1) **Dural tap** occurs in about 0.5% of obstetric epidurals. Once recognised, the management is straightforward. A working epidural must be established in another space. There should be no bearing down in the second stage of labour and there should be an elective forceps delivery. After delivery an epidural infusion should be set up with 0.9% saline or Hartmann's solution, and 1 litre

- Dural tap
- Intravascular injection
- Intrathecal injection
- Neurological
- Backache
- Pressure areas

Figure SC5 Complications of epidural analgesia

infused over 24 hours. The patient should be reviewed daily by a senior member of staff. If the patient develops a postural occipitofrontal headache then this should initially be treated by encouraging oral fluids and by simple analgesia. Ibuprofen in regular doses is often effective. If the headache becomes incapacitating, an epidural blood patch should be offered. If accepted, this should be carried out with the minimum of delay. Infection or pyrexia will contraindicate the technique. Under aseptic conditions a new epidural puncture is carried out and up to 20 ml of the patient's blood is injected into the epidural space. Further blood is sent for culture. To reduce the already small risk of epidural infection, some units advocate the systemic administration of a broad-spectrum antibiotic before the blood is taken. A blood patch is usually successful in alleviating the headache.

(2) **Intravascular injection.** While proper use of test doses will identify intrathecal and intravascular injections at that stage, epidural catheters can migrate into vessels or across the dura at any stage during the conduct of the technique, and the full dose of local anaesthetic may be inadvertently injected into the circulation. For this reason full resuscitation facilities should be immediately available at all times, and all staff involved, both anaesthetists and midwives, should be prepared for this eventuality.

Injection of local anaesthetic into the epidural veins may only cause paraesthesia of the tongue and lips but can also cause sudden loss of consciousness as the local anaesthetic agent affects the brain. The effect is usually temporary, but in the case of bupivacaine may be prolonged. The airway and respiration must be adequately maintained, and tracheal intubation and controlled ventilation may be necessary. Once this has been achieved the circulation must be supported by fluids, vasopressors and cardiac massage if appropriate.

(3) **Intrathecal injection.** The effects of intrathecal injection may be slower in onset but no less of a problem than intravascular injection. Progressive rising paralysis of the whole body, including the muscles of respiration, occurs, accompanied by significant falls in blood pressure. The feature which distinguishes intrathecal injection from massive epidural is the onset of cranial nerve effects, particularly facial paralysis, trigeminal anaesthesia and rapid loss of consciousness. As with intravenous injection, the airway must be addressed first, followed by the circulation, as detailed above.

These rare but major problems are the reason for direct observation of the patient for 20 minutes after an epidural injection or top-up.

(4) Neurological complications of epidural analgesia are extremely rare and usually relate to cauda equina syndrome if there has been local neural toxicity by either too high a concentration of epinephrine in the injected drug or, more likely, the wrong drug administered. The majority of neurological complications following childbirth are related not to epidurals but to the management of labour, particularly where a large fetus has become obstructed in the second stage of labour for a prolonged time. This scenario results in compression of the roots and trunks of the lumbosacral plexus within the pelvis, especially L1 as it passes over the brim of the true pelvis. The most common defects subsequently are foot drop (lateral peroneal nerve), sciatic palsies or femoral nerve palsies.

(5) Backache. Epidural analgesia in labour has developed a reputation for causing low-grade but persistent backache after delivery, which is probably related not to epidural analgesia itself but to the management of the back in labour. In the absence of pain sensation, proprioception and muscle tone to protect the joints and ligaments of the back, there is a possibility of musculoskeletal strain.

(6) Pressure sores are not usually associated with young women, but the lack of sensation and motor block provided by epidural analgesia prevent the patient moving during labour. Patients should be encouraged to move regularly to prevent pressure sores developing, particularly over the sacrum.

Operative anaesthesia

Anaesthesia for operative surgery in obstetrics falls into two main areas. First, operative delivery, for example Caesarean section (the most common) and forceps procedures. Second, post-delivery procedures such as retained placenta. Both groups are amenable to being carried out under regional or general anaesthesia. In the case of retained placenta, before considering a regional technique (such as spinal anaesthesia) which removes sympathetic tone and causes profound vasodilatation, it is essential to accurately assess blood loss and restore circulating volume.

Regional anaesthesia

Central neural blockade for operative obstetric anaesthesia requires a different approach to the provision of analgesia in labour. In labour the only essential feature is analgesia – motor block is a distinct disadvantage. For obstetric surgery, including forceps delivery, removal of retained placenta and Caesarean section, complete anaesthesia of the relevant area is necessary. In labour the highest dermatome required is T10, whereas for Caesarean section the upper limit needs to be a minimum of T6, though there is still some debate about whether it should be even higher than this to adequately cover the variable innervation of the peritoneum. The dose of local anaesthetic agent necessary to achieve this at term is only about two-thirds of that required in the non-pregnant patient for a comparable result.

For obstetric surgery an epidural catheter is inserted in the usual way and, after a test dose, a main dose of local anaesthetic agent is given. This may be given as one dose or in divided doses. The local anaesthetic agent of choice should ensure rapid onset of an intense block with a duration of action in excess of 1 hour. Bupivacaine 0.5% up to 30 ml (with or without adrenaline) or 20 ml lidocaine 2% with epinephrine usually produce satisfactory blockade.

Spinal anaesthesia for obstetrics offers advantages over epidural anaesthesia because of speed of onset and intensity of block, but disadvantages because of severity and speed of onset of hypotension and the less adjustable nature of the technique. The major disadvantage of spinal anaesthesia in obstetric anaesthesia has always been the incidence of post-dural puncture headache (PDPH). This has been significantly reduced by the use of solid-tipped needles with side holes such as the Sprotte and Whitacre point needles. The only spinal solutions with current product licences are 0.5% hyperbaric bupivacaine and 0.5% plain levobupivacaine. This latter solution is slightly hypobaric. Hyperbaric solutions of 0.5% ropivacaine are being investigated with a view to commercial availability.

The prevention and management of hypotension as a result of central neural blockade falls into two areas: volume loading and vasopressors. Volume loading before the administration of the block requires administration of 500–1000 ml of crystalloid solution or 500 ml colloid solution. Traditionally ephedrine has also been used in small intravenous doses (3 mg) to correct hypotension. Ephedrine crosses the placental barrier and may thus cause a fetal tachycardia.

In the preoperative period the patient should be warned that regional anaesthesia may not give total loss of sensation but that general anaesthesia can be offered if necessary. This is an increasing field of complaint and litigation.

There is increasing use of combined spinal–epidural anaesthesia for operative delivery. This provides the speed of onset and intensity of spinal anaesthesia with the adjustability and duration of epidural anaesthesia.

General anaesthesia

Obstetric general anaesthesia is usually considered to be one of the higher-risk subspecialties of anaesthesia because of the potential for urgency, uncontrolled bleeding and inhalation of gastric contents. In fact, as a cause of maternal mortality, anaesthesia ranks very low, on a par with amniotic fluid embolism and ruptured thoracic aneurysm. This low mortality is not a reason for complacency, but a result of sustained work in eliminating the main causes of anaesthetic-related problems by intensive training in managing difficult intubation, and universal antacid prophylaxis.

As a rule of thumb, there is no such thing as a pregnant woman with an empty stomach. The gastric contents also tend to be more acid than in the non-pregnant woman. Progesterone-induced relaxation of the lower oesophageal sphincter, along with the higher intra-abdominal pressure in late pregnancy, tends to encourage the regurgitation and aspiration of gastric contents into the trachea. While Mendelson actually described obstruction to respiration by solid matter, the aspiration of liquid and the resulting chemical pneumonitis are usually called Mendelson's syndrome. Acid aspiration in pregnancy causes a gross chemical pneumonitis, which distinguishes it from the aspiration pneumonia of the non-pregnant. Routine antacid prophylaxis in the delivery suite reduces both the volume and the acidity of gastric contents. Common regimes involve administration of regular oral H_2 receptor antagonists to all admissions to the delivery suite and 0.3 molar sodium citrate solution when a decision is made to proceed to surgery. Variations on this theme include the administration of intravenous ranitidine and metoclopramide, the latter to encourage gastric emptying, although this effect is difficult to show and variable. Magnesium trisilicate mixture is little used now because it is particulate and does not mix well with gastric contents.

In the second and third trimesters of pregnancy tracheal intubation is considered mandatory because of the potential for acid aspiration. For the same reasons rapid sequence induction (RSI) with cricoid pressure is also necessary. The hormonal changes of pregnancy, as pertaining to intestinal function, remain for some 48 hours post partum and so it is wise to apply RSI for up to a week after delivery. The standard general anaesthetic technique involves a wedge under the right buttock to displace the uterus from the inferior vena cava, rapid sequence induction with thiopental and suxamethonium (propofol has no licence for use in late pregnancy). Tracheal intubation should be followed by controlled ventilation of the lungs with 50–70% nitrous oxide and a volatile agent of choice. Suitable muscle relaxants include atracurium and vecuronium. Mivacurium should be used with care because of the reduced activity of plasma cholinesterase in late pregnancy, which may delay its offset. At the end of the procedure the tracheal tube should be removed with the patient in the lateral position, head down. Extubation should be considered only after the return of protective reflexes.

Tracheal intubation in the pregnant woman can be notoriously difficult. The anatomy of the chest changes in pregnancy, with an increase in functional residual capacity (FRC) giving an impression of hyperinflation. This is combined with an increase in the size of the breasts and an apparent shortening of the neck (because of the increase in FRC). Note that the majority of pregnant women have a full set of natural teeth.

Pre-eclampsia may cause laryngeal oedema, and it is now recognised that the Mallampati score may change as labour progresses, causing further difficulties. Endotracheal tube size should be reduced in expectation of difficulty. While the laryngeal mask does not provide sufficient barrier to gastric contents for routine use, in a case of difficult tracheal intubation it may have a role (See Section 1, Chapter 2).

Equipment for the management of difficult intubation must be available at all times and within arm's reach whenever obstetric anaesthesia is practised. Desirable equipment includes a range of laryngoscope blades and handles, including a polio blade, a variety of tube sizes down to 6.0 mm, and stylets and bougies to aid intubation. Where death has occurred after difficult or failed intubation the cause has not been the failure to intubate but the failure to oxygenate the patient between attempts. **This point cannot be emphasised enough**.

Accidental awareness is more commonly encountered in obstetric general anaesthesia than in any other specialty. The cause is usually either failure to introduce sufficiently high concentrations of vapour early enough, before the brain concentration of the induction agent begins to fall, or failure to maintain sufficiently high concentrations of vapour and nitrous oxide throughout the procedure.

When to consider a patient pregnant

As a general rule, the risks of acid aspiration begin to outweigh the risks of tracheal intubation at about 16 weeks gestation, and from this time onwards the patient should be considered as an obstetric problem. The hormonal changes of pregnancy fade rapidly after delivery, along with the effects on gastric function, and so it is probably safe to revert to non-pregnancy anaesthetic techniques at about 1 week post partum.

The paediatric patient

This section is predominantly concerned with children of 20 kg in weight or greater. In practice, this will usually equate with an age of about 5 years.

Assessment

Preoperative assessment in children should be as rigorous as in adults, and questions should be addressed to the child even though the parents may answer for them. Most children are healthy but chronic conditions such as asthma, multiple allergies, congenital heart disease and systemic conditions (such as muscular dystrophy) may also be encountered. The presence of one congenital abnormality should stimulate the search for others. Chromosomal abnormalities may be linked particularly with congenital heart disease. Except for true emergency surgery, children with colds or upper respiratory tract infections should have their surgery cancelled and rescheduled to a later date. The inflamed airway is exquisitely sensitive to any kind of manipulation, resulting in laryngeal spasm. Laryngeal spasm in children is particularly dangerous because of the rapid onset of severe desaturation, made more marked by their higher metabolic rate.

There is no universally good premedicant for children. Trimeprazine makes many children irritable and uncontrollable in an unpredictable way, and the injectable premedicants are probably better avoided because of the distress caused by the injection. Day-case admission can result in insufficient time for anxiolytic premedication to have effect (and the use of sedatives in day surgery may be undesirable). All children should have topical local anaesthetic cream or gel applied to the proposed venepuncture site at least 1 hour before anaesthesia. Drug doses in children should always be calculated on a weight-related basis, a calculation which will give an approximation of the required dose. If dilution of a drug is proposed then each syringe should be labelled with the drug name and concentration. Ambiguity must be avoided at all costs.

Equipment

Anaesthetic equipment for patients under 20 kg body weight is quite specialised, and there is no gradation to adult equipment. For all paediatric patients the breathing system dead space and resistance should be kept to a minimum by avoiding catheter mounts, angle pieces and valves. Controlled ventilation may be preferable because of the inevitable increase in dead space after induction of anaesthesia and the increased work of breathing. The Mapleson E or F system is preferable for patients less than 20 kg but can also be used for heavier patients if the volume of the expiratory limb is more than the calculated tidal volume and the fresh gas flow for spontaneous ventilation is more than 2.5 times minute volume. Tidal volume approximates to 8 ml kg^{-1} in the child, and a respiratory rate of about 20 per minute is usual. If ventilation is to be controlled then a minute volume divider type of ventilator should only be used for tidal volume settings greater than 300 ml. The reason for this is that below this the ventilator becomes inaccurate in delivery because of the higher proportion of compressible volume related to total tidal volume. For required tidal volumes less than 300 ml either a 'T piece occluder' type system should be used, or a Mapleson D with a ventilator such as the Nuffield Anaesthesia Ventilator Series 200.

If tracheal intubation is proposed then account should be taken of the increased resistance to breathing that this introduces. The resistance to flow in a tube is inversely related to the fourth power of the radius, and so halving the diameter will increase resistance by 16 times. Any tracheal tube will have a smaller internal diameter than the natural airway, particularly if the tube is cuffed. Unless there is a risk of tracheal soiling, uncuffed tubes are preferable because of the larger internal diameter that this allows. The anatomy of the child larynx is different from the adult (Figure SC6). In consequence, the use of cuffed tubes in the under-10 age group renders the subglottic region vulnerable to oedema, particularly if an overly large tube is introduced with force. Even small amounts of secretion in a tracheal tube will significantly increase the resistance to gas flow.

Fluid therapy

Intravenous fluids in children should be given via a burette giving set or a volume controlled pump and should always be calculated on a weight related basis. A minimum of 2 ml kg^{-1} per hour should be given to those not receiving oral fluids. Blood replacement can be very difficult to calculate, and is based on replacing loss for loss when 10% blood volume has been spilt. Losses are assessed by swab weighing and accurate suction measurement. Blood volume may be estimated as 80 ml kg^{-1} in small children, falling to 70 ml kg^{-1} in adults. Blood loss of 8 ml kg^{-1} will, therefore, need replacing during surgery.

Analgesia

Postoperative analgesia should not be withheld because the dose calculations are inconvenient. Much of the surgery carried out on children lends itself very well to regional

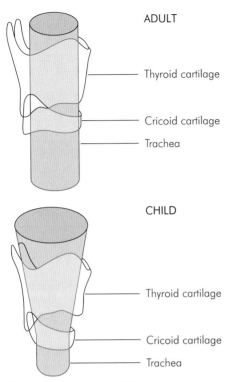

ADULT

—— Thyroid cartilage

—— Cricoid cartilage

—— Trachea

CHILD

—— Thyroid cartilage

—— Cricoid cartilage

—— Trachea

Figure SC6 Anatomy of the infant larynx

anaesthesia when used to supplement light general anaesthesia, and this method provides very high-quality early postoperative analgesia. Although intramuscular opioids remain popular, there are many other routes of administration for analgesic drugs. Most children over 6 years of age can use PCA to advantage, using skills learned at computer controls. Subcutaneous infusions of opioids may be useful, and oral preparations (such as Oramorph®) should not be forgotten. Rectal administration of non-steroidal agents (such as diclofenac) is rapidly gaining ground.

Specialist surgery
General and urological surgery
Elective general and urological surgery in childhood tends to be restricted to herniotomy, orchidopexy and circumcision, all of which can be carried out on a day-case basis with a combination of general and regional anaesthesia. Appendicectomy is another frequent operation in children and is always an inpatient (emergency or urgent) procedure. Groin incisions can be covered very well by inguinal field blockade, while penile block is particularly good for circumcision. In contrast, the more widespread and bilateral anaesthesia of a caudal block may restrict mobility, particularly in larger children. Oral analgesia should be given before the effect of the local anaesthetic wears off. For appendicectomy, a rapid sequence induction technique should be used. Wound infiltration with local anaesthetic provides some postoperative pain relief. While some of these children are relatively well, others are pyrexial and toxic, particularly if the diagnosis is made late. These latter need to be managed very carefully and their state of hydration properly assessed and corrected in the preoperative period.

Orthopaedic surgery
Much of the orthopaedic surgery in this age group is the result of trauma. A full skeletal survey should be carried out so that other injuries are not missed, particularly head injuries and cervical spine injuries. Blood loss and analgesia requirements should receive particular attention before anaesthesia. After trauma, patients are usually assumed to have a full stomach and should be managed as such, with preoxygenation and rapid sequence induction techniques. Postoperative analgesia for fractures and soft tissue injuries is best provided by regional anaesthesia, although there is some debate about the development of compartment syndrome being masked if there are forearm or lower leg fractures. Elective orthopaedic procedures in children aged 5 years and over differ little in their anaesthesia requirements from those in adults.

ENT and dental surgery
The core of both ENT and dental anaesthesia is the problem of the shared airway. In both types of surgery the anaesthetist and the surgeon need good access to a clear airway kept free of debris and blood. This has resulted in the development of special equipment and techniques for this situation.

In the main, dental surgery in children is restricted to simple exodontia. Historically the main indication was caries; with improvements in dental hygiene and fluoridation of water the reason has changed but the procedure has not. Currently children lose teeth not because of caries but because of crowding within the mouth. Until the conclusions of the Poswillo report (Poswillo 1990) were applied, this procedure tended to be carried out in general dental surgeries with little or no monitoring equipment and minimal facilities. The report concluded that whenever and wherever dental anaesthesia were carried out the equipment and monitoring should be to the same standard as in the best-equipped hospital operating theatres. Consequently, dental extraction under general anaesthesia is now carried out in very few practices, all of which are licensed and carry the full range of monitoring and resuscitation equipment.

Unless there are medical reasons for inpatient surgery, dental extraction is always carried out on a 'walk in, walk out' basis. The day-case rules should be applied rigidly. Preoperative assessment is carried out as usual, with particular reference to fasting and respiratory conditions (such as asthma). There is little opportunity for preoperative investigation or correction of abnormalities. Induction of anaesthesia may be intravenous or inhalational, but venous access should be obtained in all cases. Care should be taken with intravenous drugs because of the risks of unrecognised fainting on induction, leading to hypotension and cerebral vascular insufficiency. Inhalational induction is well tolerated in children, particularly if halothane (or the newer agent, sevoflurane) is used and a good rapport is obtained between anaesthetist and patient. The standard method involves 30–40% oxygen in nitrous oxide with sevoflurane, introduced via a nasal mask. Once the mouth can be opened without resistance a pack is inserted by the surgeon which should separate the mouth from the pharynx. The teeth are then removed. The anaesthetist must maintain the airway, ensure oxygenation and anaesthesia and monitor the patient. Once the teeth have been removed and the mouth cleared of debris the inhaled anaesthetic agents are turned off and 100% oxygen administered until the child is awake. Recovery should be in the lateral position so that blood and debris are not inhaled. Debate has continued about whether the sitting or the supine position is better or safer. The supine position avoids unrecognised major falls in blood pressure but encourages regurgitation, whereas the sitting position discourages regurgitation but increases the likelihood of unrecognised fainting on induction.

The majority of older children will accept dental extraction with local anaesthesia but if extractions are proposed in more than two quadrants of the mouth then it is unwise to do this all at one sitting because of the inevitable risk of total anaesthesia of the tongue and palate leading to obstruction or aspiration.

General anaesthesia may be necessary for conservative dentistry in those with severe learning difficulties. This may be a prolonged procedure involving multiple restorations and should be carried out with the airway protected by either an endotracheal tube or a laryngeal mask and an absorbent pack in place. Dental drills have an incorporated water spray, which can precipitate laryngeal spasm in the unprotected airway.

ENT surgery requires a shared airway, typical procedures being tonsillectomy and adenoidectomy, where the surgeon is both operating in the airway and causing bleeding from it. Adenoidectomy in isolation requires the airway to be maintained via the mouth, either by tracheal tube or by laryngeal mask. Suction clearance of the mouth at the end of the procedure should be carried out under direct vision. Tonsillectomy in isolation may be carried out using either a nasotracheal tube or, as suggested recently, a laryngeal mask airway – although this remains controversial against securing the airway with endotracheal intubation (oral or nasal). Suction at the end must again be carried out under direct vision, but gently, so as not to disturb the tonsillar bed. In both of these cases postoperative analgesia should be provided parenterally before the recovery phase. There are advocates of both spontaneous and controlled ventilation for these procedures. Anaesthesia for myringotomy or suction clearance of the ears can be relatively simple, intravenous or inhalational induction with face mask or laryngeal mask for airway maintenance.

Ophthalmic surgery

Ophthalmic surgery in the over-5s is usually for squint surgery or penetrating eye injury, probing and syringing of lachrymal ducts being confined to younger children.

Squint surgery is usually carried out as a day case, though the facility for overnight stay should always be available. Preoperative assessment should be as rigorous as for any other form of surgery. Induction of anaesthesia should include a weight-related dose of a vagolytic drug such as glycopyrrolate to prevent the severe bradycardia which results from even gentle traction on the extraocular muscles. Induction may be by the inhaled or intravenous route. Squint correction causes the same airway access problems for the anaesthetist as other head and neck surgery. The choice of tracheal intubation or laryngeal mask airway is largely a matter of personal preference, though tracheal tubes cause much more emergence laryngospasm than do laryngeal mask airways. Ventilation may be controlled or spontaneous. Postoperative analgesia may be provided by topical local anaesthetic agents, systemic opioids or NSAIDs.

- Arterial PCO_2
- Arterial PO_2
- Cerebral perfusion pressure
- Intracranial pressure
- Temperature
- Drugs

Figure SC7 Factors affecting cerebral blood flow

The head-injured patient

Applied physiology

The skull is a closed box containing brain tissue, extracellular fluid, CSF and blood. In the presence of space-occupying lesions, tumour, blood clot or oedema, for example, the fixed volume of contents increases at the expense of the rest. Early in the disease process, when the incremental change in volume is still small, any sudden increase in pressure can be compensated for by changes in CSF or blood volume, cushioning the effect of the insult. Later, in the presence of a larger space-occupying lesion, the compliance of the intracranial contents is reduced and so the pressure change is unbuffered and there may be damage to tissue, either directly, by distortion of nerve tracts, or by secondary reductions in blood flow.

In the normal (uninjured) brain cerebral blood flow (CBF) is affected by several factors (Figure SC7).

Arterial PCO_2

A relatively linear response exists between $PaCO_2$ values of 2.6 and 10.7 kPa. At the lower end of this range CBF will be half normal, and correspondingly double at the higher end. Reduced $PaCO_2$ decreases both cerebral blood flow and intracranial pressure (ICP), mediated by CSF pH. After a step change in $PaCO_2$, the CSF bicarbonate concentration returns to normal over the next 24 hours, and the ICP and CBF return to normal even if the change in $PaCO_2$ is maintained. Hyperventilation can, therefore, only be used in the short term to reduce ICP.

Arterial PO_2

A small increase in CBF occurs with the administration of 100% oxygen. Hypoxia on the other hand, if severe ($PaO_2 < 6$ kPa), will result in greatly increased CBF.

Cerebral perfusion pressure

Cerebral perfusion pressure (CPP) is calculated as the mean arterial pressure (MAP) minus (ICP + CVP). Autoregulation maintains steady CBF between CPP values of 50 and 150 mmHg.

Intracranial pressure

Raised ICP will obviously reduce CBF, and raised venous pressure secondarily raises ICP, with the same net result. Sudden rises in venous pressure during coughing or straining may cause serious falls in CBF, putting cerebral perfusion at risk in the compromised brain.

Temperature

Hypothermia reduces both CBF and the cerebral metabolic rate for oxygen. Similarly, rises in temperature increase CBF and oxygen consumption.

Drugs

The anaesthetic induction agents, with the exception of ketamine, reduce CBF and cerebral metabolism. Ketamine and the inhalational agents cause rises in CBF via a vasodilator effect, with consequent increases in ICP. This can be mitigated to some extent by hyperventilation.

Management of head injury

Head injury should be considered significant if there has been certain loss of consciousness (however brief). Blood or CSF in the ear canal or nose imply skull fracture with the accompanying risk of meningitis due to the ingress of pathogens. In closed head injury, even of a relatively minor nature, there is a variable amount of oedema and cerebral contusion, which increases the volume of the intracranial contents, displacing both CSF and blood volume and reducing compliance. Extra- and subdural haematomata also behave as large space-occupying lesions, causing compression and distortion of the brain. Functional disabilities may be seen at an early stage. These include unsteadiness of gait, disorientation, irritability, nausea and vomiting. As the oedema or space occupation increases or becomes more widespread, the compliance is reduced further and cerebral blood flow is compromised, causing hypoxic damage to brain tissue. Cerebral blood flow depends on the cerebral perfusion pressure, which in turn depends on the relationship between mean arterial blood pressure and intracranial pressure. As intracranial pressure increases so CBF falls. The standard international assessment of cerebral function is the Glasgow coma scale (GCS) (Figure SC8). This is a very useful indicator but should not be taken in isolation. The best response in each category gives a maximum score of 15, indicating minimal injury, while the minimum score is 3, indicating a very poor state with a very poor outcome. Trends in GCS are more valuable than single estimations.

Category	Score
Best performance	
Eye opening	
spontaneous	4
to speech	3
to pain	2
nil	1
Verbal response	
oriented	5
confused	4
inappropriate	3
incomprehensible	2
nil	1
Motor response	
obeys commands	6
localising	5
withdrawing	4
flexing	3
extending	2
nil	1

Figure SC8 Glasgow coma scale

The crux of immediate management in head injury is to avoid secondary injury. The primary injury has already occurred, and any damage done will be largely irreversible. Oedema develops around the injury site and secondary injury must be avoided by reducing ICP (especially avoiding dramatic rises in ICP) and preventing hypoxic damage. The main decision to be made is whether the patient requires tracheal intubation – for control of ICP, for surgery to other parts of the body, for investigations such as CT scanning or for transport to other facilities. In general, a GCS less than 8 indicates the need for major intervention and intensive care management. In addition to the GCS, the pattern of respiration, pulse and blood pressure should be taken into consideration. Spontaneous hyperventilation indicates significantly raised ICP, as does arterial hypertension accompanied by bradycardia. Control of ICP is of the utmost importance. Uncontrollable confusion and irritability may indicate significant brain injury, and indicates the need for intervention. Indications for intubation after head injury are listed in Figure SC9.

- Coma – not obeying commands, not speaking, no eye opening, i.e. GCS ≤ 8
- Significantly deteriorating conscious level (i.e. fall in motor score of two points or more)
- Loss of protective laryngeal reflexes
- Hypoxaemia ($PaO_2 < 13$ kPa on oxygen)
- Hypercarbia ($PaCO_2 > 6$ kPa)
- Spontaneous hyperventilation causing $PaCO_2 < 4.0$ kPa
- Bilateral fractured mandible
- Copious bleeding into the mouth (e.g. from skull-base fracture)
- Seizures

An intubated patient should be ventilated with muscle relaxation, and should receive appropriate sedation and analgesia. Aim for a $PaO_2 > 13$ kPa, $PaCO_2$ 4.0–4.5 kPa unless there is clinical or radiological evidence of raised intracranial pressure, when more aggressive hyperventilation is justified to a $PaCO_2$ of not less than 4 kPa. If hyperventilation is used the FiO_2 should be increased.

Association of Anaesthetists of Great Britain and Ireland. *Recommendations for the Safe Transfer of Patients with Brain Injury.* London: AAGBI, 2006.

Figure SC9 Indications for intubation and ventilation for transfer after brain injury

Practical technique

By and large, secondary brain injury may be avoided by good oxygenation and airway management and by avoiding rises in ICP, particularly as a result of an unmodified pressor response to intubation. Although it might appear that unconscious patients do not need to be anaesthetised before intubation, this is not so. In this particular situation induction agents are used not primarily for the abolition of consciousness but to reduce ICP before intubation. Intubation without previous pharmacological reduction of ICP or without modification of the pressor response may cause more damage than the original injury and should be avoided at all costs. The sympathoadrenal response to intubation may be minimised by the administration of an adequate dose of induction agent accompanied by an opioid agent such as alfentanil. The appropriate muscle relaxant to use for intubation is potentially controversial. Rapid intubation is desirable but suxamethonium can cause a significant rise in ICP. This is certainly the case in the normal brain, but recent work suggests that it may not be the case in the injured (and therefore less compliant) brain. The rise in ICP may be an effect of the drug itself rather than the fasciculations it causes. The non-depolarising relaxants are, therefore, preferable in terms of ICP management, but this ignores the fact that many head-injured patients have full stomachs and a soiled airway, or are vomiting because of their raised ICP. A possible solution lies in the administration of a large dose of a non-depolarising relaxant such as vecuronium, given after careful preoxygenation and the application of cricoid pressure. The fasciculations of suxamethonium may be modified or abolished by pre-curarisation with a small dose of a non-depolarising relaxant (such as 20 mg gallamine) or by pretreatment with 0.1 mg kg^{-1} suxamethonium, both of which may inhibit intubating conditions. The risk of aspiration must be carefully weighed against any minor advantage in ICP control.

Subsequently, ventilation of the lungs must be maintained by face mask or laryngeal mask airway until the relaxant reaches maximum clinical effect, so as to avoid coughing and movement, which will increase the intracranial pressure even more than intubation itself. Once intubation has been safely achieved the pressor response to the presence of the tube must also be modified to control ICP. This can be achieved by adequate sedation or general anaesthesia with controlled ventilation and moderate hyperventilation. Inhalational agents should be avoided because of their cerebral vasodilator effect and anaesthesia maintained by repeated bolus or infusions of intravenous agents. If possible, fluid loading should be restricted or avoided. Excessive crystalloid resuscitation may increase cerebral oedema. Intravenous mannitol (as 10 or 20 g boluses) may reduce cerebral oedema to some extent but should not be given unless a urinary catheter is in situ, because the stimulation from a full bladder may increase ICP and also anaesthetic dose requirements.

Monitoring should conform to the accepted minimum monitoring standards and should include non-invasive blood pressure, pulse oximetry and end-tidal CO_2 analysis. Blood loss from scalp wounds may be significant in itself and should not be forgotten.

Transfer of the head-injured patient

Head-injured patients and those with suspected intracranial haemorrhage may require transfer between hospitals either for CT scanning or for definitive management of their injuries. This can be a difficult and dangerous enterprise and should be carried out with the greatest of care. Facilities in ambulances, helicopters and scanning rooms are limited, as is space, but nevertheless the management of the airway and ICP must take precedence over speed or convenience. The patient must be stabilised before transfer. The escort must be capable of managing the predictable eventualities – re-intubation, hypertension, hypotension – and thus must take with them sufficient equipment, drugs and fluids to maintain anaesthesia and relaxation. Ambulances should be able to travel quickly but smoothly, without the severe shocks of fast travel. Monitoring should include automatic blood pressure, pulse oximetry and preferably end-tidal CO_2 measurement. For CT scanning, there must be appropriate equipment in the scanning room. An anaesthetic machine with automatic ventilator, piped gases and full monitoring are essential. Figure SC10 gives a useful checklist for transfer of a head-injured patient.

The day-case patient

Day-stay surgery implies that the patient's admission to the hospital is scheduled, and that admission and discharge are planned for the same day. In practice this usually means that admissions in the morning are discharged at midday while midday admissions are discharged in the early evening and the facility then closed overnight.

For the patient, this means the shortest possible time away from the work or home environment and as little disruption as possible to social circumstances.

Anaesthesia and surgery are major insults to the patient's physiology, however minor they may appear, and thus there must be rigorous policies and protocols for the day surgery unit, with patients carefully selected with regard to fitness and type of surgery.

The criteria to be applied fall into several categories:
- Social circumstances
- Surgical procedure
- Medical fitness
- Anaesthetic technique
- Admission facilities

Social circumstances

The patient's social circumstances must provide a safe environment for the postoperative care of a recently anaesthetised patient, even if the procedure has been carried out under local anaesthetic or sedation only. For the first 24 hours after anaesthesia, there must be a responsible adult present on the premises to care for the patient and to manage untoward events. The patient must be brought to, and taken from, hospital by a responsible adult. He or she must live within easy travelling distance of the hospital in case of urgent readmission (this is usually taken as

System	Checklist
Respiration	$PaO_2 > 13$ kPa?
	$PaCO_2 < 5$ kPa?
	Airway clear?
	Airway protected adequately?
	Intubation and ventilation required?
Circulation	BP mean > 80 mmHg? (adults)
	Pulse < 100 per minute? (adults)
	Peripheral perfusion?
	Two reliable large IV cannulae in situ?
	Estimated blood loss already replaced?
	Arterial line?
	Central venous access if appropriate?
Head injury	GCS?
	GCS trend? (improving/deteriorating)
	Focal signs?
	Skull fracture?
	Seizures controlled?
	Raised ICP appropriately managed?
Other injuries	Cervical spine injury (cervical spine protection), chest injury, fractured ribs, pneumothorax excluded?
	Intrathoracic, intra-abdominal bleed?
	Pelvic, long bone fracture?
	Extracranial injuries splinted?
Escort	Doctor and escort adequately experienced?
	Instructed about this case?
	Adequate equipment and drugs?
	Can use equipment and drugs?
	Sufficient oxygen supplies?
	Case notes and x rays?
	Transfer documentation prepared?
	Where to go in the neurosurgical unit?
	Telephone numbers programmed into mobile phone?
	Mobile phone battery fully charged?
	Name and bleep number of receiving doctor?
	Money in case of emergencies?

Association of Anaesthetists of Great Britain and Ireland. *Recommendations for the Safe Transfer of Patients with Brain Injury* London: AAGBI, 2006.

Figure SC10 Transfer checklist for neurosurgical patients

within 30 minutes' travelling time). Patients must not go home by public transport, and preferably not by taxi. If these criteria cannot be fulfilled then the surgery must be carried out on an inpatient basis. If the patient arrives for day surgery without these criteria being satisfied then the operation should be cancelled and admission reorganised. Part of the admission process must be to check that these criteria have been satisfied.

Specific advice should be given to each patient concerning postoperative welfare. The patient must be told to avoid alcohol for 24 hours postoperatively, because the depressant effect of alcohol acts synergistically with the residual anaesthetic drugs and, especially if barbiturate anaesthetics are used, may cause unconsciousness. Patients must be told not to drive vehicles or operate machinery, because their physical and mental reactions may not be good enough to keep them out of danger. Car insurance may be invalidated by driving under the residual influence of anaesthetics, and the police may charge the driver with driving under the influence of drugs. They must not cook or be involved in baby care. Lifetime or important decisions should not be made in the postoperative period, because patients may be residually disinhibited.

Preoperatively the day-case patient must be told these rules in front of a witness, or must sign a form to say that they have been read while not under the influence of anaesthetic drugs. The responsible escorting adult must also understand these rules.

Surgical procedure

The types of surgery suitable for day-case work include those with only minor disturbances of nutrition, which last only a short time (usually taken to be less than 45 minutes of anaesthesia) and which do not usually require opioid analgesia afterwards. Surgery where significant blood loss is predicted, or where the abdomen is electively opened, is not suitable (except for minor laparoscopic surgery). Surgery where there will be major limitation of mobility is not suitable. Unilateral inguinal hernia repair may be suitable (especially if local anaesthesia is employed), but bilateral repair is not. Surgery should only be carried out by surgeons experienced in the procedure in question. Figure SC11 indicates some procedures that may be suitable for day-case work, other factors being satisfied.

Medical fitness

Patients must be ASA P1 or P2 (see Section 1, Chapter 1: Figure PR2) and between the ages of 16 and 65. Patients outside this age range may be acceptable subject to special

General surgery	Unilateral hernia repair
	Unilateral varicose veins (not prone)
	Sebaceous cysts
	Small benign breast lumps
	Child circumcision
Urology	Cystoscopy (± biopsy)
	Diathermy to small bladder tumours
	Hydrocoele
	Varicocoele
	Vasectomy
Gynaecology	Diagnostic laparoscopy
	Laparoscopic test of tubal patency
	Termination of pregnancy
Ophthalmology	Probing of tear ducts
	Cataract surgery (rigid application of other criteria)
	Squint surgery (single eye)
Orthopaedics	Arthroscopy (minor arthroscopic surgery)
	Joint/back manipulation
Oral surgery	Removal of third molars
ENT	Myringotomy
	Antral washout
	Nasal polypectomy
	Nasal septoplasty
	Direct laryngoscopy and pharyngoscopy
Haematology	Blood sampling and chemotherapy

Figure SC11 Operations suitable for day stay

arrangements between the anaesthetist and the surgeon. If it is planned to carry out surgery on small children (3 years old or more in a district general hospital) organisationally it is better to arrange a full list of children with a paediatric trained nurse in attendance rather than to have children interspersed within an adult list (Department of Health 1991). Patients over 65 may be acceptable if they are otherwise healthy. Drug-controlled diabetic patients are never suitable for day-case surgery. Essential hypertension is not necessarily a contraindication provided control is good. Cardiovascular diseases such as angina, cardiac failure or arrhythmias are unacceptable. Controlled atrial fibrillation may be an exception to this if stable and treated.

Obesity is not acceptable (criteria differ, but body weight >100 kg or body mass index >30 may be taken as exclusion guidelines). These rules apply to regional anaesthesia and general anaesthesia equally.

Anaesthetic technique
Intraoperative
Anaesthesia should be restricted to simple techniques with proven good recovery characteristics, particularly in terms of postoperative nausea and vomiting and analgesia. Techniques that employ regional analgesia are particularly suitable, provided that mobility is not restricted by the local block. Spinal anaesthesia and femoral nerve blockade are considered unsuitable because of the major inhibition of mobility that results. Caudal analgesia is acceptable in small children, but for circumcision a penile block provides good postoperative analgesia without motor effects. Spinal anaesthesia in ambulatory young people is notorious for post-dural puncture headache and for postural hypotension and should be avoided. Elective tracheal intubation should be avoided because of the risk of laryngeal oedema (and major nasal haemorrhage if nasal intubation is employed), but, having said that, it has been in routine use for day-stay removal of third molar teeth for many years. This latter situation is changing with the increasing use of the laryngeal mask airway. Elective controlled ventilation used to be considered as a contraindication to day surgery until the advent of mivacurium, which is short acting and does not need reversal. The use of reversal drugs may reduce the likelihood of patient discharge because of their autonomic and central nervous effects. The laryngeal mask makes day-case controlled ventilation feasible where it would not otherwise be so. Thiopental is not a suitable induction agent for day-case general anaesthesia, whereas propofol is indicated because of the relatively rapid recovery without significant hangover.

Postoperative
Pain should be controlled by the use of regional anaesthetic techniques with the addition of non-steroidal anti-inflammatory drugs (NSAIDs) if suitable. Rectal diclofenac is in widespread use but should be discussed with the patient preoperatively. Account must be taken of the fact that local anaesthesia will wear off after several hours.

The patient should be encouraged to take moderate analgesics before the effect of the local anaesthetic wears off, and should be discharged with a suitable supply to take home.

Admission facilities

Wherever surgery is carried out on a day-stay basis there must always be the facility to admit the patient overnight. If that facility does not exist, either because there are no inpatient beds available or because the day unit is a remote site, then surgery should not proceed.

The usual anaesthetic reasons for overnight admission following day surgery are nausea and vomiting or pain requiring opioid analgesia. Complications of surgery are a common reason for admission, as is prolonged surgery with consequent slow postoperative recovery, usually because the criteria for day surgery have been breached, either by unsuitable surgery or unsuitable surgeon. Records should be kept of the reasons for refusal of day-case surgery and the incidence and reasons for unplanned postoperative admission.

The obese patient

Obesity can be defined as a body mass index (BMI) of more than 30. The BMI is calculated by dividing the weight (kg) by the square of the height (m^2).

Applied physiology

Oxygen consumption and the work of breathing are increased, while chest compliance and functional residual capacity are reduced. Tidal volume and closing volume may overlap while conscious, resulting in poor aeration and a tendency to hypoxia even at rest. These factors increase shunting and the incidence of hypoxia and, when FRC is reduced by anaesthesia or positional changes on the operating table, shunting is further increased. Hypoxia is commonly seen because of these changes, and because of the tendency for the diaphragm to be elevated by pressure from abdominal wall fat. Postoperative hypoxia is particularly frequently encountered and, because of the failure to adequately expand the chest, the incidence of atelectasis and hypostatic infection increases.

Blood volume and cardiac output are increased, increasing cardiac work. There is also a tendency to coronary artery disease that is exacerbated by lack of exercise. The increase in both intra-abdominal and abdominal wall fat increases the intra-abdominal pressure, raising the incidence of functional and anatomical hiatus hernia. The resting volume of gastric juice is also increased, as is its acidity. The increase in intra-abdominal pressure reduces venous return from the legs, predisposing to DVT and pulmonary embolism. There is a higher incidence of wound infection and wound dehiscence. Surgical access can be difficult because of the distribution of fat.

Anaesthesia

For the anaesthetist there are often anatomical problems in establishing venous access, particularly if central venous access is needed. Airway maintenance may be difficult because of the tendency to a short fat neck and, in females, protruding breasts. Intubation may also be difficult, and preoxygenation is recommended. Chest compliance is reduced and so the work of ventilation increases, sometimes to the extent that mechanical ventilators may be unable to generate the inflation pressure necessary to achieve adequate tidal volumes. This can also be a problem if a laryngeal mask airway is used because the inflation pressure may exceed the LMA leak pressure. The high inflation pressures necessary will further reduce venous return, and falls in cardiac output may be significant.

Non-invasive blood pressure measurements may give erroneous readings if the cuff size is not chosen correctly. A cuff that is relatively too small will give falsely high readings. Regional anaesthetic techniques may be more difficult because of difficult nerve location and loss of landmarks, and extra-long needles may be necessary. There is more fat in the epidural space and so **smaller** doses of local anaesthetic agents may produce the same effect as in the normal patient. Placing epidural and spinal needles can be particularly difficult because of the increased distance between skin and landmarks. The sitting position may help because the skin and bone midlines may come into opposition whereas in the lateral position these may be some distance apart, making the technique impossible. Finding bony landmarks with a standard hypodermic needle before inserting the epidural needle will improve the chances of success.

All induction agents and vapours are fat-soluble, and a significant proportion of the cardiac output supplies fat, so these drugs are diverted from the brain and into fat stores, increasing the requirement for induction agents and slowing the rise in brain concentration, which tends to increase the incidence of awareness. Similarly, emergence may be slower because of the slower leaching of agents from the fat stores. This latter causes obese patients to be exposed to volatile agents for longer, thus increasing their biotransformation.

The metabolically compromised patient

Liver disease

Applied physiology

The liver is the largest organ in the body, receiving 30% of cardiac output. The majority of nutritional, haematological and detoxification metabolism occurs in the liver, including the breakdown or excretion of many anaesthetic drugs. Other physiological roles of the liver include the manufacture of proteins, lipoproteins and carbohydrates, including the clotting factors and the proteins to which most anaesthetic drugs are bound. Globulins are not produced in the liver. The liver also acts as a store for vitamins, minerals and carbohydrates. In the presence of significant liver disease, all these processes become disturbed.

Different conditions cause differing patterns of dysfunction. Excessive red cell turnover causes jaundice by overloading the pathways of haem breakdown even though other liver functions may remain relatively normal. Obstructive and cholestatic jaundice causes major disruption to metabolic pathways and to the absorption of fats and fat-soluble vitamins, causing further problems. Hepatocellular dysfunction may be toxic or infective in origin but will result in the same picture of unconjugated bilirubinaemia, fat malabsorption and metabolic disturbance. In the end stage of hepatic failure, virtually all the body's metabolic processes are disturbed. Clinical features include clotting failure, coma from ammonia toxicity because of disturbed protein metabolism, hypoglycaemia because of poor glycogen metabolism, water overload and major electrolyte imbalance. There is usually portal hypertension, which causes the formation of collateral circulation including oesophageal varices. If these bleed, then the sudden high protein meal provided by enteral haemoglobin may precipitate hepatic coma in an otherwise compensated patient, a desperate situation which may be irretrievable. Anaesthesia in liver failure is, therefore, not for the inexperienced.

Assessment of patients with liver disease

Full haematological and biochemical screening results should be available to supplement clinical evaluation of the patient. Absorption of vitamin K from the gut depends entirely on the presence of bile salts, and so the synthesis of prothrombin and other clotting factors, which depend on vitamin K, are sensitive barometers of liver function. Albumin has a long plasma half-life and so is an indicator of more chronic disease, when its value will be lowered. Transaminases are released from damaged hepatocytes, but as these enzymes are also present in other tissues this cannot be taken as specific to liver function (which also applies to alkaline phosphatase). Conjugated bilirubinaemia suggests obstructive jaundice whereas unconjugated bilirubinaemia suggests a prehepatic or hepatic cause. In the presence of established liver disease, anaesthetic agents and techniques must be chosen with care and with due consideration for disturbed metabolism, pharmacokinetics, and water and electrolyte balance.

Drugs

Benzodiazepines have a prolonged and more intense effect than usual, and thus should be avoided as premedicants and induction agents. Opioids have a greatly prolonged effect. The metabolism of the barbiturate induction agents is prolonged, but as their effect as induction agents is not terminated by metabolism but by redistribution this is relatively academic except in severe disease, where minimum doses should be used. Etomidate behaves similarly. While suxamethonium is not specifically contraindicated, its effect may be prolonged by reduced plasma cholinesterase activity (which also applies to mivacurium). The behaviour of the other non-depolarising muscle relaxants is largely dependent on protein binding and excretion. All these agents are highly bound to plasma proteins, and so in the hypoproteinaemia of liver disease they will have a higher unbound fraction and a greater effect for the same dose. Although the majority of excretion of pancuronium is by the renal route, reduced biliary excretion may prolong their effect. In the case of atracurium or cisatracurium, much of the breakdown is via non-specific plasma esterases and so subject to prolonged effect in liver disease. In severe hepatic dysfunction the spontaneous degradation which these drugs also undergo may be disturbed by acid–base changes. Patients with severe liver disease tend to be water-overloaded because of secondary hyperaldosteronism, and the volumes of distribution of all drugs will be affected. Liver function has little effect on the choice of anaesthetic vapours. The use of halothane is not contraindicated unless by other considerations, although sevoflurane is the more popular choice.

Local anaesthetic agents may have delayed excretion, though not a prolonged anaesthetic effect. Regional anaesthetic techniques may be contraindicated by abnormal clotting.

Fluids

Fluid and electrolyte balance must be meticulous, and blood glucose monitored frequently because of disturbed glycogen metabolism in the later stages of the disease.

Techniques

Standard general anaesthetic techniques may be used with care in liver disease. Peripheral and central regional anaesthesia, including epidural and spinal techniques, are acceptable unless the INR is greater than 1.5. Renal function is often disturbed in obstructive jaundice and is always affected in hepatic failure. Urine output must be encouraged to avoid the onset of renal failure in the postoperative period. Preoperative infusion of mannitol in the jaundiced patient may help to avoid hepatorenal syndrome: 500 ml mannitol 20% is appropriate.

Repeat anaesthesia

Patients may require repeat anaesthesia, either fortuitously or during a planned course of treatment, and over a short or longer time scale.

The main considerations at preoperative assessment for repeat anaesthesia are to identify if possible the anaesthetic technique used, the drugs involved and any related problems. Problems of particular interest are nausea and vomiting, difficult airway management, difficult intubation, drug reactions and the use of halothane.

Derangement of liver function following halothane exposure shows two clinical pictures. In the first instance a mild and transient disturbance in liver function is seen, and this may be accompanied by mild pyrexia. Resolution is seen within a few days without permanent sequelae. It is suggested that the mechanism underlying this mild picture is the result of the phase 1 transformation products of halothane reacting directly with hepatic macromolecules to cause tissue necrosis. In the second instance massive and fulminant hepatic necrosis occurs. Although rare, mortality is in the region of 40–70%. It is thought that the underlying mechanism of this process is the formation of a hapten–protein complex resulting in immune-mediated destruction of liver tissue. The hapten is likely to be a halothane metabolite; tri-fluroacetyl halide is the most likely culprit.

The Committee on Safety of Medicines (CSM) recommendations for repeated use of halothane are that it should not be used within 3 months of a previous administration unless there is an overwhelming clinical reason for the second use, and that it should not be used if there was unexplained pyrexia or jaundice within 1 week after a previous exposure.

As there are alternative vapours and techniques easily available, and halothane is falling into disuse, many anaesthetists avoid it within a 3-month period unless there is a good clinical reason for second exposure, such as the need for inhalational induction. Even this is being overtaken with the introduction of sevoflurane, which is almost as good as halothane when used for inhalational induction.

Even though a patient may be a regular patient it is important to go through a full preoperative assessment each time because there is always the possibility of new intercurrent disease, particularly in the elderly. Notice should be taken of any problems encountered by previous anaesthetists and patients should be asked when their last anaesthetic was. The vapour used should be noted and avoided in repeat if necessary.

Renal disease
Applied physiology

The kidneys excrete water, electrolytes, water-soluble drugs and water-soluble products of metabolism. Plasma electrolytes, urea and creatinine provide an indication of renal function. While the plasma urea also depends on liver function, the creatinine concentration also depends on the level of protein metabolism in the body. For the plasma creatinine to rise, renal function must be < 30% of normal. As renal function is reduced below this the creatinine and urea will rise, as will the plasma potassium concentration. Water is retained, and the production of new red cells is depressed by reductions in erythropoietin secretion. Acidosis develops, compensated by respiratory alkalosis and cardiac output increases. In established chronic renal failure the haemoglobin may fall to 5–6 g dl^{-1} with a creatinine concentration >700 mmol l^{-1} and potassium >6 mmol l^{-1}. In the early stages of the disease some improvement may be possible by correction of the precipitating cause and by careful attention to fluid and electrolyte balance. One of the more common causes of chronic renal impairment is obstructive uropathy, and the simple expedient of indwelling urinary catheterisation may return the patient to a relatively normal biochemical state.

Patients in renal failure (even if mild) should not be transfused to correct their anaemia unless there is a situation of acute blood loss. To do so will precipitate cardiac failure by volume overload and will suppress the production of normal red cells. Owing to changes in 2,3-DPG concentration, stored red cells do not carry oxygen at their full capacity for some 24 hours post transfusion, and so the effect of transfusion can be a reduction of oxygen delivery to the tissues.

Drugs and techniques

In choosing anaesthetic drugs and techniques, care should be taken to avoid those drugs that are excreted solely through the kidney. Fortunately, all of the induction agents undergo redistribution and biotransformation to inactive products before excretion. Renal impairment may delay the excretion of the opioids and prolong their action. Suxamethonium should be avoided, as it causes the release of potassium from muscle cells and may precipitate cardiac arrhythmias in an already hyperkalaemic patient. The volume of distribution of the non-depolarising relaxants may be increased, reducing their effect while their breakdown and excretion are reduced. Mivacurium, atracurium and cisatracurium may have a relatively normal duration of action, altered only by acidosis. Pancuronium and vecuronium should be used with great care because they are largely excreted unchanged in the urine.

Renal impairment has little bearing on the choice of anaesthetic vapours, though there is a theoretical risk of additional renal toxicity if enflurane or isoflurane are used in high concentration for prolonged periods, as fluoride ion is released during their metabolism and high concentrations of fluoride are known to be nephrotoxic. Aminoglycoside antibiotics should be used with extreme care in renal impairment, as they are renally excreted and both nephrotoxic and ototoxic at the high and sustained levels which are found if normal doses are given to patients with impaired excretion. Attention to fluid and electrolyte balance must be rigorous, replacing only that which has been lost and avoiding potassium-containing fluids. Occasionally a patient may present who maintains renal function only if they have a high urine output, or with a high-output type of renal failure. These patients must not be fluid-restricted in the preoperative period.

Venous access must be considered very carefully in patients likely to need dialysis as chronic fistula or shunt formation may be necessary. It is better to preserve the vessels in one arm if possible. If a fistula is already present then this limb should be avoided at all costs and the limb protected from pressure during surgery. Regional anaesthesia is useful in the renally impaired patient provided that there are no other contraindications. The choice of airway maintenance technique will depend on the proposed surgery.

Diabetes mellitus

Diabetes mellitus is the most common endocrine disorder, and one of the more common coexisting conditions in patients presenting for surgery.

Complications

The complications of diabetes are listed in Figure SC12.

Patients with diabetes may present for incidental surgery or for surgery related to their diabetes, particularly

- Nephropathy
- Peripheral neuropathy
- Autonomic neuropathy
- Cerebral vascular disease
- Coronary artery disease
- Peripheral vascular disease
- Retinopathy
- Lipoatrophy
- Fetal macrosomia
- Hypoglycaemia
- Hyperglycaemia
- Ketoacidosis
- Lactic acidosis
- Obesity
- Infection
- Wound infection
- Delayed healing

Figure SC12 Complications of diabetes

abscesses, wound debridement, amputation of toes, feet or limbs, and cataract surgery, although diabetic patients do not have a higher incidence of cataracts, simply an earlier presentation of the condition. Whether the surgery is incidental or not, and whether the diabetes is insulin- or non-insulin-dependent, there is an interaction between the surgical insult and the diabetes that needs to be properly managed to maintain stability and avoid further complications of both the diabetes and the surgery. Inadequately managed diabetes can result in hyper- or hypoglycaemia, ketoacidosis, wound infection and delayed healing. Occasionally the surgical condition can result in instability and toxic confusion, which will, of course, make the diabetes more unstable and worsen the surgical condition. Patients should not be presented for anaesthesia unless their diabetes is under reasonable control with blood glucose between 3 and 10 mmol l^{-1} during the preoperative fasting period. Any patient whose blood glucose is outside this range should have the surgery postponed until the situation has been corrected, unless the surgical condition is a true emergency. Similarly, any tendency to acidosis or ketosis and any coexisting electrolyte disturbance must be fully corrected before anaesthesia. Unfortunately, there are many patients with gangrene or infection of ischaemic tissue whose diabetes will not come into adequate control until debridement has been carried out. This should not prevent the attempt being made. Patients presented for elective surgery should be seen by a physician with a special interest in diabetes before the day of operation so that their diabetes is under optimal control.

Effect of complications on anaesthesia

Nephropathy causes hypertension and electrolyte disturbances, particularly of potassium and creatinine. These disturbances are a reflection of renal function and give some indication of the adequacy of fluid and electrolyte homeostasis and drug excretion.

Neuropathy. Diabetic peripheral neuropathy is unpredictable in both distribution and effect. This may make the testing of peripheral nerve blocks more difficult. Autonomic neuropathy is not usually formally sought, the test being a formal Valsalva manoeuvre, but it is probably present in a large number of diabetics. The heart may be partly denervated, and so variations in heart rate may not follow the expected patterns. Similarly the peripheral autonomic responses may not be adequate to prevent variations in blood pressure. Gastrointestinal autonomic neuropathy may delay gastric emptying, increasing the likelihood of regurgitation.

Vascular disease. Diabetic vascular disease tends to involve small rather than large vessels, and though there may be no obvious major coronary or cerebral vessel disease, as a general rule it should be assumed that anyone who has peripheral vascular disease also has central and coronary vascular disease. As it is mostly small vessels that are affected, the fall in blood pressure associated with regional or central nerve blockade tends not to be so manifest.

Pregnancy. Diabetic management in pregnancy can be very difficult, with significant increases in insulin requirement during the pregnancy and major, sudden falls in requirement in the puerperium. Diabetics tend to have large immature babies that may need forceps delivery or Caesarean section. All pregnant diabetics should be managed by a competent physician in addition to their obstetrician. Gestational diabetes may also need careful management to prevent complications.

Management

Diabetes may be controlled by diet, oral therapy or insulin, depending on severity. Both oral therapy and some of the insulins may last more than 24 hours from the last dose. This must be borne in mind when preparing patients for surgery. The metabolic disturbances of diabetes may take the form of hypo- or hyperglycaemia, ketoacidosis or lactic acidosis. Surgery tends to produce a slight hyperglycaemia as a normal 'stress' response.

Whichever diabetic management protocol is followed, it must be a straightforward regimen so that problems are avoided while being flexible enough to cope with major and minor surgery, and with both elective and emergency surgery. A suitable management plan is shown in Figure SC13, with adjustments for various situations. Surgery with no significant disturbance of physiology, lifestyle or nutrition may be considered a minor disturbance, the disturbances lasting less than 24 hours. Major disturbance involves substantial disturbance of physiology, lifestyle or nutrition for more than 24 hours.

Infective risk groups

The major risk to healthcare workers is represented by the blood-borne viruses, a group which contains hepatitis A, B and C as well as human immunodeficiency virus (HIV), though the prion diseases have stimulated considerable interest.

Prion diseases

The prion diseases are a group of transmissible neurodegenerative diseases also known as the transmissible spongiform encephalopathies (TSE). While their clinical pictures vary, their common feature is the deposition of an abnormal prion protein in the brain, causing neuronal dysfunction and cell death. All of these diseases are inevitably fatal. Their incubation periods may be very prolonged. Currently there are two animal and seven human prion diseases recognised (Figure SC14). There are no serological tests which can identify this infection during the incubation period, and there is no identifiable immune response.

These diseases have stimulated much scientific interest because the transmissible agent is non-bacterial and non-viral. It appears that the transmissible agent is the protein itself. Despite species differences in the protein, cross-species transmission has been recognised both in the laboratory and in the food chain, leading to much media attention in the 1990s and major changes in animal husbandry.

Prion protein is a membrane-associated glycoprotein normally present in the animal brain. Its function is not known. The disease process is triggered by a replication of this protein leading to deposition of an abnormal form of the protein. The difference between the normal and abnormal forms is in the tertiary structure rather than the amino acid sequence. How the disease is triggered is not known.

Different routes of inoculation vary in their efficiency of transmission. The intracerebral route is the most efficient, with intravenous, intraperitoneal and oral each less efficient. Because of the differences between prion proteins of different species, there is also a species barrier of variable efficiency. Transmission by any route between species

Elective surgery

Ideally all diabetic patients will have been assessed by a physician before admission and brought into adequate control.

Diet-controlled

Minor disturbance

May be suitable for day-case admission. No specific treatment regimen. Blood glucose result available one hour preoperatively. Return to usual diet same day.

Major disturbance

No specific treatment regimen. Blood glucose result available one hour preoperatively. Return to usual diet as soon as surgery allows.

Tablet-controlled

Minor disturbance

Not suitable for day-case surgery. Admit at least the day prior to surgery. No diabetic tablets the day prior to or the day of surgery. Blood glucose and electrolyte results available one hour prior to surgery. Test glucose four-hourly until discharge. Return to normal tablet regimen the day after surgery. Dextrose infusion necessary only if glucose result less than 4 mmol l^{-1}.

Major disturbance

Admit 48 hours preoperatively for stabilisation on insulin infusion regimen (for 24 hours prior to surgery). No oral hypoglycaemics the day prior to or the day of surgery. Two-hourly glucose estimation until stable. Infusion regimen to continue until normal oral intake resumes, then return to oral diabetic therapy for at least 48 hours before discharge. Monitor glucose four-hourly thereafter.

Insulin-controlled

Minor disturbance

Not suitable for day-case surgery. Admit the day before surgery. Half usual dose of short-acting insulin the evening before surgery.

Morning operation – Fast from midnight for a morning list. No insulin in the morning. Blood glucose result one hour preoperatively. The evening after surgery give one-third dose of short-acting insulin with supper. Check blood glucose three hours after supper. Return to usual treatment the day after surgery.

Afternoon operation – Fast from 08:00 for an afternoon list. Half dose of short-acting insulin with light breakfast. Start slow infusion of 5% dextrose (four hours per half-litre). Check blood glucose two-hourly after breakfast. Half dose of short-acting insulin with supper. Check glucose three hours after this. Return to usual treatment the day after surgery.

Major disturbance

Admit 48 hours preoperatively for stabilisation on insulin infusion regimen. Monitor glucose two-hourly in the first 24 hours of the regimen. Continue insulin infusion regimen until full oral intake is resumed. Return to normal treatment for at least 36 hours before discharge. Monitor glucose four-hourly.

Emergency surgery

Diet-controlled

Minor disturbance

Check blood glucose. Return to usual diet same day if possible.

Major disturbance

Check blood glucose prior to operation. Check fasting glucose daily until return to full oral intake. Insulin intervention may be necessary depending on result. Return to usual diet before discharge.

Figure SC13 Management of diabetes

Emergency surgery (*cont.*)
Tablet-controlled
Minor disturbance
Dextrose infusion from time of admission. Check blood glucose prior to operation. Check fasting glucose daily until return to full oral intake. Insulin intervention may be necessary depending on result. Return to usual diet before discharge.

Major disturbance
Commence on insulin infusion regimen after admission and continue until full oral intake re-established, then return to tablets. Check blood glucose two-hourly until on full oral intake. Discharge 48 hours after tablets recommenced, if stable.

Insulin-controlled
Minor disturbance
Insulin infusion regimen from admission. Check blood glucose two-hourly. Return to usual insulin doses only when on full oral intake. Stabilise before discharge.

Major disturbance
Insulin infusion regimen from admission. Continue infusion until re-established on full oral intake then return to usual doses. Stabilise on usual doses for 48 hours before discharge.

Insulin infusion regimen
Laboratory blood sugar and electrolytes before starting regimen. Dextrose 5% 1000 ml eight-hourly by pump (125 ml per hour). Soluble insulin 60 units in 60 ml saline via syringe pump at a rate determined by sliding scale. Two-hourly glucose evaluation.

Blood glucose		Insulin rate
<5	mmol l^{-1}	zero
5–10	mmolw l^{-1}	1 unit per hour
10–15	mmol l^{-1}	2 units per hour
15–20	mmol l^{-1}	3 units per hour
>20	mmol l^{-1}	5 units per hour

Note: Potassium should be added to the infusion bag according to pre-infusion value and twice daily electrolyte results.

Figure SC13 (*Cont.*)

is unpredictable but does occur, both in the laboratory and in nature.

After ingestion, the agent replicates in the lymphoreticular system before entering the spinal cord and brain, possibly via the autonomic nerves. Before the onset of clinical disease, the neural and lymphoreticular tissues may contain high concentrations of the infective agent. This is a major concern both in the food industry and in medicine, because of the possibilities of transmission from food animals to humans by ingestion and between humans by surgical instruments, grafts, blood transfusion and organ transplants.

The human prion protein gene is situated on chromosome 20. There is a polymorphic region at codon 129 that expresses either methionine or valine. Homozygosity for

Human	Animal
Sporadic Creutzfeldt–Jakob disease	Scrapie (sheep)
Familial Creutzfeldt–Jakob disease	Bovine spongiform encephalopathy (cattle)
Iatrogenic Creutzfeldt–Jakob disease	
Variant Creutzfeldt–Jakob disease	
Kuru	
Familial fatal insomnia	
Gerstmann–Sträussler–Scheinker syndrome	

Figure SC14 Types of prion disease

methionine at this codon increases susceptibility to sporadic CJD. Variations in other codons within this area also seem to increase susceptibility to other prion diseases.

Sporadic CJD has a worldwide distribution at an incidence of about 1 in 1 000 000. It tends to be a disease of late middle age, presenting with a rapidly progressing dementia with cerebellar ataxia, myoclonus and rigidity. Mean survival is about 4 months from onset. As it is sporadic, it is suggested that this is the result of a spontaneous mutation in the prion protein which then becomes a template for self-replication.

Iatrogenic CJD follows medical interventions where infected material from one patient is implanted into another. Transmission has occurred following corneal grafts, dura mater grafts and use of human-derived pituitary growth hormone. It has also occurred where surgical instruments used on the brain of a CJD-affected patient have subsequently been used on another patient. The high density of abnormal prion protein in the tonsils and appendix of affected patients has caused concern about the possibility of transmission unless disposable instruments (both surgical and anaesthetic) are used. Unfortunately, when disposable instruments were substituted for reusable instruments in tonsillectomy, the postoperative mortality increased because of an increase in the occurrence of secondary haemorrhage. The current situation is that tonsillectomy is carried out with reusable instruments but only if the surgeon believes that the surgery is strictly necessary.

Familial CJD: The concept of a familial transmissible disease may seem paradoxical. There is a higher than normal incidence of CJD in Slovakia and in Libyan-born Israelis. These populations are highly inbred and may have an excessive dietary exposure to scrapie-affected sheep, these factors acting as multipliers of the abnormal protein genes.

Gerstmann–Sträussler–Scheinker syndrome (GSS) and **fatal familial insomnia** (FFI) are also familial but very rare prion diseases. There seem to be more than 20 mutations of the prion protein gene in GSS and a mutation at codon 178 in FFI. This is believed to lead to an instability of the protein structure.

Variant CJD was first described in 1996 following a cluster of cases whose neuropathology was dissimilar to sporadic CJD. The mean age at onset in vCJD is 29 years, in contrast to 66 years in sCJD. Variant CJD tends to present with psychiatric disorders which then progress to ataxia, dementia and choreiform movements. The duration of decline is considerably longer than for sCJD: up to 18 months. There are also histological differences. The suggestion that vCJD is a variety of BSE that has crossed species is supported by the consistent clinical and pathological picture, the time relationship between the appearance of vCJD as a new disease and the epidemic of bovine spongiform encephalitis (BSE) in the late 1980s and early 1990s, and experimental transmission studies. There are about 20 new cases per year in the United Kingdom. The number of infected but non-clinical cases is unknown. A study of 8318 postoperative routine tonsil and appendix specimens revealed only one affected specimen. If this is representative of the population as a whole, this would imply a total case load of between 30 and 54 000 cases in the UK.

Kuru was first shown to be a prion disease in 1966. Before that time kuru was endemic in the Fore region of Papua New Guinea and was a major cause of death in the affected population. This population practised ritual cannibalism. The women and children tended to consume internal organs and brain, and were the most likely to be affected. Ritual cannibalism ceased in 1960 and the incidence of kuru has declined since.

The appearance of variant CJD has highlighted deficiencies in the cleaning, disinfection and sterilisation procedures used for reusable surgical instruments. Washing by hand (as previously used) does not remove protein deposits from the micropits found in metal surgical instruments. The prion protein is also resistant to the usual chemicals used in the disinfection process, even those that disrupt nucleic acids, and so every hospital sterilisation unit has been upgraded to new standards. Hand washing of instruments has now been replaced by aggressive mechanical washing at high temperatures, followed by full-cycle autoclaving. It is not yet known if this is adequate. Recently, a debate has started over the use of disposable laryngoscope blades, which are deemed to avoid the inevitable (but small) risk of prion transmission due to lymphocyte contamination of blades after laryngoscopy.

Hepatitis A

The hepatitis A virus is a common infection acquired by close contact with infected persons or by food contamination, particularly sewage-contaminated water and shellfish. The incubation period is 2–7 weeks. Carriers have not been reported.

There is a prodromal 'flu-like' illness with marked myalgia proceeding to hepatocellular jaundice which resolves spontaneously without chronic damage.

Hepatitis B

Infection with the hepatitis B virus is much more serious than hepatitis A in that hepatic failure is more common, chronic damage is frequent, the disease is endemic in many parts of the world and some 10% of all those infected will become chronic carriers. The infection may be acquired by vertical transmission from mother to child in utero, or in childhood, or by heterosexual or homosexual contact or direct inoculation of body fluids. The virus is highly infective in small inoculates, unlike HIV. In countries with adequate blood transfusion services this route of transmission is now rare.

The prodromal illness may be severe, with arthralgia and urticaria followed by hepatocellular jaundice. The illness is not usually severe, and the majority of patients clear the virus within a few weeks. All healthcare workers should be immunised against this condition, though occasionally the immunisation may have to be repeated several times.

Hepatitis C

Hepatitis C is indistinguishable from the other viral hepatitides except on serological testing. The usual route of transmission is parenteral inoculation, with large inoculates required to stimulate the infection. Until recently, transfusion of blood and blood products was the major route of infection, which suggests that there must be a pool of chronic carriers in the community. Blood products can now be screened for this infection, but there must be a large number of previously transfused patients who carry the disease. Up to 40% of those infected will develop progressive chronic liver disease.

HIV/AIDS

Infection with the human immunodeficiency virus was only recognised in 1983, but there must have been numerous unrecognised cases before that. The virus is delicate, easily destroyed and has low infectivity. The main routes of transmission are by promiscuous sexual activity (both heterosexual and homosexual) and by the sharing of injection equipment. Many haemophiliacs have been infected by pooled blood transfusion products which were drawn from an infected community before the problem was recognised. Needlestick injury is not a major route of infection except in the case of a large inoculate or frequent small inoculation from an infected population, such as when performing surgery in sub-Saharan Africa. HIV and hepatitis B frequently occur together, particularly in prostitutes and in the homosexual and drug-abusing communities.

Estimates of the prevalence of HIV and AIDS suggest that there are about 38 million people infected worldwide, with between 60 000 and 90 000 cases in the United Kingdom.

The Centers for Disease Control classification of HIV infection recognises four stages of disease, which may overlap:

(1) Acute seroconversion illness, a flu-like illness that usually occurs within 3 months of infection. There is a high viral load but patients tend to remain asymptomatic.
(2) Asymptomatic infection. 10% progress to AIDS within 2–3 years, while the remainder progress to AIDS later, with a median of 10 years.
(3) Persistent generalised lymphadenopathy.
(4) Symptomatic HIV infection.

HIV is one of a family of retroviruses, which have reverse transcriptase as part of their make-up. This enzyme allows the viral RNA to be transcribed into DNA, which is then incorporated into the host cell genome. This virus preferentially infects T-helper lymphocytes, destroying them progressively and leading to a susceptibility to opportunistic infections.

Therapy using combinations of non-nucleoside reverse transcriptase inhibitors (NNRTI; e.g. nevaripine), nucleoside analogue reverse transcriptase inhibitors (NRTI; e.g. zidovudine) and protease inhibitors (PI; e.g. saquinavir) has significantly improved the outcome for infected people. A typical regimen may involve three drugs, but the complex patterns of administration and the high incidence of side effects tend to reduce compliance.

Preoperative assessment of HIV-infected patients should be as thorough as for any other patient. In particular, HIV-infected patients may have respiratory infections with *Pneumocystis*, *Aspergillus*, herpes, cytomegalovirus, *Mycobacterium* or *Candida*. They may have cardiac valvular infections and vegetations, particularly if they are also intravenous drug users. Chronic diarrhoea may be caused by CMV, *Cryptosporidium* or *Candida*. The neurological complications of HIV include aseptic meningitis, herpes encephalitis, polyneuropathy or HIV-related dementia. Kaposi's sarcoma, a skin malignancy, is diagnostic of HIV infection.

The depression of cellular immunity that occurs after general anaesthesia appears to be transient in these patients and causes no obvious deterioration in their condition. Regional anaesthesia is not contraindicated by HIV alone.

HIV-infected patients may require periods of intensive care, often because of respiratory failure as a consequence of *Pneumocystis carinii* infection. Aggressive antibiotic and antiretroviral therapy during mechanical ventilation brings surprisingly good results.

Precautions

Hepatitis B and C may cause chronic liver damage, and due account should be taken of liver function in those patients known to be carriers or known to have had B or C hepatitis. Hepatitis A does not produce chronic sequelae but may present for surgery during the active or prodromal phases of the disease, and again liver function should be tested and the anaesthetic managed accordingly. The AIDS-related conditions may be of interest to the anaesthetist when the patient presents for surgery, but the possibilities are so broad that each must be taken on its merits. Patients may present for lymph node biopsy. Unfortunately, the majority of people infected with hepatitis B, C and HIV are asymptomatic and not known to the medical community. While precautions against cross-infection are usually taken in those patients known to be infected, it is more logical to take precautions in all patients and assume that every patient is potentially infectious. It is thus wise for anaesthetists to develop the habit of wearing gloves and eye protection in all cases. Contaminated needles should **never** be re-sheathed, but disposed of immediately in sharps disposal containers. Syringes should not be transferred from one patient to another, and the person using sharps should dispose of them to reduce the number of staff potentially exposed. All cuts and abrasions on both staff and patients should be covered with waterproof dressings, and all spillages of body fluids should be cleaned immediately with a viricidal solution.

In anaesthetising patients known to have one of the HIV-related syndromes, extreme care should be taken to avoid introducing infections into the patient, who has a life-threatening immune deficiency akin to immunosuppressed leukaemics or transplant recipients. This involves effective skin disinfection before venepuncture and full aseptic technique for other invasive procedures. All other equipment used should be either disposable single-use or have been autoclaved and be re-autoclaved as soon as possible after the event. Figure SC15 details recommended precautions to prevent occupational transmission of HIV from patients to healthcare workers.

Risk	Precaution
Hand contact with body fluids	Wear gloves
Blood splashes	Wear apron/mask/goggles
Needle stick injury	Dispose of sharps into safe container
	Do not pass to another person
Exposed skin lesion	Cover with waterproof dressing
Salivary contact	Minimise handling of used airway equipment
	Sterilise after use
Contaminated equipment	Sterilise as per local policy

Figure SC15 Prevention of occupational transmission of HIV

Needlestick injury

Although great care is taken to avoid needlestick injury, inevitably occasional accidental inoculation can occur. Following injury the puncture site should be encouraged to bleed vigorously and thoroughly washed with soap and water. Eye splashes should be rinsed with sterile eye-wash or water.

Occupational exposure must be reported and recorded in an accident book. Each unit may have a different protocol for this, but most require attendance at A&E. Blood should be taken from the victim, and in high-risk scenarios from the patient (after appropriate consent). If, after consideration of the relative risk (taking into account HIV and hepatitis status), prophylaxis is considered desirable this should be instituted. Triple therapy is usual: this comprises three antiviral drugs, a combination of protease inhibitors and nucleoside analogue reverse transcriptase inhibitors. Counselling should be made available through the occupational health department.

Latex allergy

Allergy to natural rubber latex is an increasing problem for healthcare workers, who may have to carry out procedures on patients who react to latex or who may themselves develop reactions to latex. The reactions tend to fall into two groups, either skin contact or anaphylactic in type. Both are serious problems, and no distinction should be made between them. Natural latex contains a variety of highly allergenic proteins, which cause reaction by repeated exposure and hypersensitivity. Continued exposure increases the severity of the reaction. It is interesting that there are reports of cross-reactions to similar proteins in fruits such as banana, avocado and kiwifruit as well as nuts.

If a patient reports possible latex allergy, skin testing by dermatologists is possible, but it is time-consuming and potentially dangerous – so it may be wise to accept the report at face value and treat such patients as if they are positive.

Perioperative care

For planned surgery the patient should be first on a morning operating list, to avoid the possibility of latex particles being in the operating theatre atmosphere. All staff should be familiar with the local latex allergy policy and aware of their responsibilities. Traffic in the room should be kept to a minimum.

All staff should wear non-latex gloves.

If possible all anaesthetic breathing system tubing should be made of plastics or man-made rubbers such as neoprene. If it is not possible to replace this tubing then it should be covered with stockinet gauze to prevent transfer of particles from the rubber to the patient by staff handling the exposed rubber. Similarly blood pressure cuff bladders and tubing should be covered so that there is no contact with the patient. All breathing systems should have a bacterial filter at the patient end to prevent latex particles entering the patient's airway. For airway maintenance PVC tracheal tubes and laryngeal mask airways are acceptable, as they do not contain latex. Face masks should be made of plastic. IV cannulae are usually latex-free, though it is always wise to check beforehand.

Syringes should be checked for latex, though most modern syringes are latex-free and labelled as such. Standard blood-giving sets contain latex in the injection port at the cannula connection. These should be avoided. Even supposedly latex-free fluid-giving sets may contain latex in injection ports. These should be removed, but if this is not possible, should not be used as injection ports because of the possibility of coring and embolising particles of latex. A three-way tap is preferable.

Equipment for local and regional anaesthesia does not usually contain latex, but each anaesthetic department should identify which products are latex-free and keep a stock of these products.

Note that the rubber seals on drug ampoules do not contain latex.

An anaphylaxis pack should be available in the operating theatre while a latex-allergic patient is present. The patient should be anaesthetised in the operating theatre and recover in the same room rather than being transferred to a recovery room where the atmosphere is less well controlled.

Each anaesthetic and operating theatre department should develop a policy on the management of latex allergy and a box containing latex-free equipment. All staff should familiarise themselves with both of these.

Jehovah's Witnesses

In general, a patient's religious beliefs have little impact on the conduct of anaesthesia, though there may be dignity and dietary issues, and issues around the care of the dying and the newly dead.

In the case of Jehovah's Witnesses there are a number of issues around consent for administration of blood and blood products and transplantation. This becomes more complex where children are involved. The Association of Anaesthetists of Great Britain and Ireland (2005) has produced a booklet which gives a very good summary of the situation and is recommended reading for all anaesthetists. In general it may be safer to ask the patient and their religious advisors about specific issues rather than making assumptions that may be in error. Interviews are best conducted on a one-to-one basis rather than having the advisors in the room. This may avoid any suggestion of coercion by the advisor.

Infusion or reinfusion of blood is not usually acceptable once that blood has left the circulation, even if it is the patient's own blood. For some patients the cell-saver systems in use for major joint replacement may be acceptable. Reinfusion from cardiopulmonary bypass machines may be acceptable provided the blood does not come to a standstill. In general, stored blood or blood products are not acceptable, though if the patient will die without, they may be acceptable.

Preoperative iron therapy is acceptable, though in the presence of a normal haemoglobin concentration it will make little difference. Erythropoietin may be acceptable if it is the recombinant rather than the human-derived form.

In children there are complex legal issues concerning the child's autonomy. This has been complicated rather than clarified by the Children Act. Children who are able to understand the need for surgery and the possible risks and outcomes are autonomous and capable of making their own decisions regarding blood and blood products, regardless of the views of the parents. Otherwise, the physician has a duty of care to the patient and, in the situation where the child will die without transfusion, the doctor may override the views of the parents. In the elective situation it may be wise to consult the hospital legal department. These situations are relatively uncommon.

In general, Jehovah's Witnesses are willing to donate or receive almost any other type of transplant, though there should always be discussion on an individual case basis, especially if blood or blood products may be involved.

Magnetic resonance imaging

Imaging methods such as CT (computerised tomography) and MRI (magnetic resonance imaging) have specific requirements for anaesthesia. The need for anaesthetic input arises from the need for a patient to remain motionless during the scan. This is primarily a problem in children and in the case of head injury in adults too. General anaesthesia or sedation may be necessary. The radiology department has the problem of being a site remote from the rest of anaesthetic activity, and space is often an additional safetyw issue.

In MRI the strong magnetic field (1–3 teslar) means that any equipment within the scanning room must be free of ferromagnetic metals and unaffected by the magnetic field. The MRI room itself is noisy, and the long-term effects of very strong magnetic field exposure are not known. The patient would usually be stabilised on sedation or anaesthesia outside the room and then transferred into the scanner. The patient is then monitored at a distance. A secure airway (endotracheal tube) is strongly recommended, as a poorly functioning LMA will be difficult to identify. Breathing circuits may be very long, resulting in increased resistance to breathing and increased compliance of the tubing. Elective ventilation may therefore be worthwhile, and it has the additional advantage of giving controlled apnoea for the purpose of improved scan quality. Gas-sampling tubes of a similar length lead to some mixing within the tube and a significant delay to the signal. The physics of MRI is covered in Section 4, Chapter 1.

References and further reading

Association of Anaesthetists of Great Britain and Ireland. *HIV and Other Blood Borne Viruses: Guidance for Anaesthetists*. London: AAGBI, 1992.

Association of Anaesthetists of Great Britain and Ireland. *Day Surgery*, 2nd edn. London: AAGBI, 2005.

Association of Anaesthetists of Great Britain and Ireland. *Management of Anaesthesia for Jehovah's Witnesses*, 2nd edn. London: AAGBI, 2005.

Association of Anaesthetists of Great Britain and Ireland. *Recommendations for the Safe Transfer of Patients with Brain Injury*. London: AAGBI, 2006.

Department of Health. *Welfare of Children and Young People in Hospital*. London: HMSO, 1991.

Melzack R, Wall PD. Pain mechanism: a new theory. *Science* 1965; **150**: 971–9.

Michenfelder JD. *Anaesthesia and the Brain*. Edinburgh: Churchill Livingstone, 1988.

Poswillo DE (chairman). *General Anaesthesia, Sedation and Resuscitation in Dentistry*. Report of an Expert Working Party. Standing Dental Advisory Committee, 1990.

Report on Confidential Enquiries into Maternal Deaths in the United Kingdom. The series. London: HMSO.

Steward DJ, Lerman J. *Manual of Paediatric Anaesthesia*, 5th edn. Edinburgh: Churchill Livingstone, 2001.

CHAPTER 6

The surgical insult

C. A. Pinnock and R. M. Haden

GENERAL SURGERY
Laparotomy
Head and neck surgery
Rectum and anus
Laparoscopic cholecystectomy

UROLOGICAL SURGERY
Transurethral resection of the prostate (TURP)
Radical prostatectomy
Cystectomy
Transurethral resection of bladder tumour (TURBT)
Nephrectomy
Percutaneous nephrolithotomy (PCNL)
Transvaginal tension-free tape (TVT)

ORTHOPAEDIC SURGERY
Joint replacement surgery
Laminectomy
Fractured neck of femur

GYNAECOLOGICAL SURGERY
Hysterectomy
Laparoscopy
Evacuation and termination (ERPC/STOP)

EAR, NOSE AND THROAT SURGERY
Laryngoscopy
Tonsillectomy
Middle ear surgery
Tracheostomy

OPHTHALMIC SURGERY
Cataract surgery
Squint surgery
Retinal surgery
Penetrating eye injury
Dacryocystorhinostomy (DCR)

ORAL AND MAXILLOFACIAL SURGERY
Dental extraction
Fractured mandible
Fractured zygoma
Fractured maxilla

Surgery of any kind represents a traumatic insult to the body and is accompanied by a verifiable stress response dependent on the magnitude of the insult. While the general principles of broad-based anaesthesia have been covered in Section 1, Chapters 2, 3 and 4, the purpose of this chapter is to alert the reader to operative procedures that have specific problems or caveats associated with them. For reasons of space, only the more frequently encountered operations have been included.

General surgery

Laparotomy

The majority of patients requiring laparotomy will present an aspiration risk, and therefore require rapid sequence induction and subsequent muscular relaxation with controlled ventilation. In the case of a perforated viscus (duodenal ulcer, for example) electrolyte imbalance, dehydration and cardiovascular instability make for a high-risk procedure. The presence of faecal soiling of the peritoneum is a particularly bad prognostic indicator. Anastomosis of the bowel requires special consideration. Survival of anastomoses is maximised if the blood supply to the joined section is not compromised in any way. In practice, this requires the avoidance of reversal drugs (and therefore a careful choice of relaxant and its dose) and the use of epidural anaesthesia, usually combined with general anaesthesia if there are no contraindicating factors to the technique (such as poor haemodynamic resuscitation). Epidural anaesthesia provides better postoperative pain relief than patient-controlled analgesia (PCA), which is important in the avoidance of pneumonia after upper abdominal incisions. Extubation of patients following a surgical procedure that has involved handling of the bowel should be left until the protective reflexes have returned, as the risk of regurgitation is ever-present. In cases of intestinal obstruction, the use of nitrous oxide may cause the bowel to enlarge dramatically, making it difficult for the surgeon to close the abdomen.

Fundamentals of Anaesthesia, 3rd edition, ed. Tim Smith, Colin Pinnock and Ted Lin. Published by Cambridge University Press. © Cambridge University Press 2008.

Head and neck surgery

Surgery to the head and neck, whether thyroid, parathyroid or salivary glands are the target, encompasses the same basic principles. Airway security is of paramount importance and the likely situation is one of obscuration of the patient and breathing circuitry with head towels, making intubation and subsequent controlled ventilation preferable to the use of the laryngeal mask airway, although this device is in use. Avoidance of coughing is important and adequate muscular relaxation and depth of anaesthesia will ensure that this complication does not arise. Spontaneous respiration is not recommended. In the case of thyroid surgery adequate assessment of the airway is necessary if there is any degree of goitre. Parathyroidectomy can be a prolonged procedure, in which case warming precautions (mattress and fluids) should be used. Patients covered with head towels require suitable eye protection to avoid corneal damage.

Rectum and anus

Surgery to the rectum and anus (e.g. manual dilatation of the anus and haemorrhoidectomy) is highly stimulating and requires adequate depth of anaesthesia to prevent the development of hypertension, tachycardia and laryngeal spasm. Caudal anaesthesia is appropriate in this situation but may be technically difficult in adults. Pilonidal sinus deserves special mention. Many of these patients are obese and for reasons of surgical access require placing in the prone position. Airway security is best achieved by endotracheal intubation followed by controlled ventilation, and eye protection should be employed. Caudal anaesthesia is contraindicated in the presence of active infection close to the site of injection.

Laparoscopic cholecystectomy

While the recovery from laparoscopic cholecystectomy is both quicker and less problematic than from the traditional open operation, the procedure itself carries a considerably greater physiological insult and greater morbidity. Patients who are fit for the open procedure may not be fit for a laparoscopic procedure. The abdomen is filled to high pressure with carbon dioxide and the patient is required to be positioned in a steep head-up position with left rotation. The diaphragm therefore becomes splinted and the lungs compressed, widening the carina and moving it to a higher position in the chest. A properly placed tracheal tube may enter a main bronchus once the abdomen is inflated. The heart may be rotated from its usual position, distorting the great vessels. The venous return from the lower half of the body is compromised by the intra-abdominal pressure and position. Hypertension is induced by the absorption of carbon dioxide. These factors combine to produce a patient with poor venous return, low cardiac output and high systemic resistance, a recipe for significant cardiac strain even in the absence of coronary artery disease. The increased intragastric pressure encourages regurgitation. Peritoneal stretching can also induce severe vagal bradycardia. The standard anaesthetic technique for this procedure is a controlled ventilation technique via a tracheal tube. A dose of a vagolytic drug may be given before the start of surgery in order to avoid the vagal bradycardia of peritoneal stretching. Postoperative analgesia with systemic opioids and non-steroidal anti-inflammatory drugs (NSAIDs) is usually sufficient, though the pneumoperitoneum causes shoulder pain which may be resistant to opioids until the carbon dioxide has been absorbed. There is a risk that laparoscopic procedures may be converted to open procedures if the anatomy is difficult or if bleeding becomes a problem.

Laparoscopic techniques are increasingly being used to assist in major surgery, to reduce the size of the surgical incision. While this may be carried out by traditional laparoscopy, in some techniques an artificial cavity is created within the preperitoneal or retroperitoneal space. These procedures may be more prolonged than traditional open surgery, and carry a risk of significant surgical emphysema or gas embolism. They may be accompanied by significant postoperative pain, although this is usually short-lived.

Urological surgery

Transurethral resection of the prostate (TURP)

Open prostatectomy has become a very infrequent procedure, the majority being undertaken as transurethral resection of the prostate (TURP). Prostatic hypertrophy, whether benign or malignant, is one of the conditions of the ageing population and tends to coincide with other conditions of the ageing population – ischaemic heart disease, hypertension, diabetes and respiratory disease – which must all be taken into account in planning anaesthesia. Patients requiring prostatectomy may have disturbed plasma electrolytes because of chronic back pressure on the kidneys. This situation may improve with good preoperative drainage by urethral or suprapubic catheterisation, but the electrolyte results rarely return to normal, and thus mild elevations of urea or creatinine values are common. Urethral instrumentation is notorious for causing gram negative septicaemia, and so patients with indwelling catheters or those known to have pre-existing infection should have their operations covered by a renal function related dose of a suitable antibiotic, such as gentamicin. Blood loss in prostatectomy is related to resection time rather than size of the prostate, and is generally accepted to be less if spinal anaesthesia is used rather than general anaesthesia. This also has the advantage that any catheter manipulations or bladder washouts necessary in the immediate postoperative period will be covered by the residual effects of the anaesthetic. Spinal anaesthesia has advantages in those with pre-existing respiratory disease, though its use in the presence of ischaemic heart disease is more contentious. Prolonged surgery with continuous irrigation can cause dramatic falls in the patient's temperature, which can only be partly corrected by warming the irrigation and intravenous fluids. Blankets covering the upper body may also help, but the majority of re-warming must be done in the postoperative period. Blood loss at prostatectomy can be difficult to assess, though a variety of methods are available. The lithotomy position tends to increase peripheral resistance until the patient is returned to the supine position, when there is a major fall in peripheral resistance often accompanied by a fall in arterial pressure – which should, therefore, be measured and corrected before transfer from the operating theatre into recovery.

A possible complication of this procedure is the TUR syndrome (Figure SI1).

Radical prostatectomy

Radical prostatectomy has become common for younger, fitter men with prostate-confined cancer. This is a major undertaking and is not the same operation as a retropubic prostatectomy.

This operation involves a laparotomy-type incision, often a head-down or 'arched back' position, and a potential for major blood loss. It may be a prolonged procedure. General anaesthesia with epidural analgesia would be the norm. Airway maintenance is usually with a tracheal tube, and invasive monitoring is common. Management of the circulation can be difficult if the patient is placed in the 'arched back' position because of venous pooling in the legs and in the upper body, with reduced cardiac output as a consequence. Postoperative admission to a high dependency unit is usual.

Cystectomy

Urinary cystectomy is a major procedure involving removal of the bladder and prostate (in men) and formation of a urinary diversion by implantation of the ureters into an

- Endoscopic surgery requires continuous irrigation with a solution of glycine (1.5% in water). At 200 mOsm l^{-1} this is the minimum non-haemolysing concentration. This solution is deliberately non-electrolytic so that the diathermy current is applied to the tissue rather than being dissipated in the fluid.
- If significant volumes of this solution get into either the general circulation or the tissues, from where it is absorbed, then there may be serious fluid and electrolyte disturbances.
- The most obvious are water excess and hyponatraemia. Cerebral oedema develops, leading to confusion, hypertension and bradycardia, though loss of consciousness or convulsions is not uncommon. Respiratory distress accompanied by hypoxia (because of interstitial pulmonary oedema) and cardiac effects such as rhythm and contractility changes may also be seen.
- Glycine is an inhibitory neurotransmitter and can lead to temporary blindness. It has an intravascular half-life of 85 minutes, and breakdown products include oxalate and ammonia. The plasma sodium concentration may fall to extreme levels: below 100 mmol l^{-1} is not unknown.
- If the irrigation fluid is in the tissues or free in the peritoneal cavity then laparotomy for drainage may be the only possible method of treatment. Emergency anaesthesia in this situation is fraught with difficulties, but it is one of those occasions when the patient must be accepted as they are, without any attempt to improve the situation in the preoperative period. General anaesthesia employing intubation and controlled ventilation is the first choice.
- A glycine solution containing 1% ethanol is now available. The use of breath alcohol estimations can give an estimate of fluid absorption during the procedure, and this technique is gaining popularity for resectoscopic surgery.

Figure SI1   TUR syndrome

isolated loop of small bowel. Anaesthesia for this would normally involve general anaesthesia with tracheal intubation, epidural analgesia and invasive monitoring, followed by admission to an intensive care bed. There is a potential for significant blood loss. Once the ureters have been disconnected from the bladder, blood loss and urine output may be difficult to assess because the urine drains into the abdominal cavity and is removed by suction along with any blood loss. Again, this procedure is often carried out in the 'arched back' position. The surgery may be prolonged, with its attendant problems.

Transurethral resection of bladder tumour (TURBT)

Bladder tumours are not usually large and rarely result in major blood loss. Occasionally patients will be anaemic at presentation from frank blood loss over a period of time. Anaemia should be corrected. Use of diathermy in the bladder can stimulate the obturator nerve, which is close by in the pelvis, lateral to the bladder. This causes mass movement of the patient's legs, which can result in perforation of the bladder and vascular or bowel damage by the resectoscope. This situation can only be prevented by using muscular relaxation and controlled ventilation. Good relaxation is also necessary for adequate bimanual surgical assessment of the tumour and the bladder, and anaesthesia should not be terminated until this is complete. Patients with bladder tumours become regular attenders, and so at each attendance the anaesthetist must establish the time since the last general anaesthetic, which agents were used and the patient's response to them. As time passes new medical conditions may appear or pre-existing conditions deteriorate, so a full preoperative assessment should be carried out at each admission.

A possible complication of this procedure is the TUR syndrome (Figure SI1).

Nephrectomy

Nephrectomy for benign disease is usually carried out through a loin incision, whereas if malignancy is involved (including ureteric disease) the operation is generally performed through a laparotomy. The essential difference is the position of the patient, supine for laparotomy but in the lateral position for the loin approach. When in the lateral position the operating table may be arched to increase the distance between the rib cage and the pelvis to improve surgical access. This may cause kinking of the great vessels in the abdomen. In both positions there may be significant blood loss because of damage to renal vessels close to the aorta or inferior vena cava. In left-sided operations the diaphragm and pleura are in danger, and the anaesthetist should be prepared to deal with pneumothorax.

The vessels of the dependent arm may be partly occluded in this position, and therefore all monitoring and infusions should be on the upper arm. Loin incisions are particularly painful postoperatively because of their proximity to the ribcage. Continuous epidural analgesia is particularly effective for both types of incision. Pyeloplasty is usually carried out in the lateral position through a loin incision and the above comments apply.

Percutaneous nephrolithotomy (PCNL)

Percutaneous nephrolithotomy is an endoscopic procedure to remove stones from the kidney without open surgery. The patient is placed prone. A large needle is passed under x ray control into the relevant renal calyx and a large-bore cannula passed along the track. The endoscope is then passed through this cannula accompanied by continuous irrigation with glycine or saline, depending upon the method used to extract the stones. Saline is used with electrohydraulic lithotripsy whereas glycine or saline may be used with the lithoclast.

PCNL can take several hours, and it therefore becomes difficult to maintain patient temperature throughout, particularly with the use of large volumes of irrigant. There can be considerable blood loss and significant absorption of irrigating solution causing facial and cerebral oedema. If glycine is used there may be features of the TUR syndrome (Figure SI1). Severe pain is the norm in the immediate postoperative period. Standard anaesthetic techniques for this involve tracheal intubation, controlled ventilation and epidural analgesia for postoperative pain relief. The epidural dressing must be waterproof and be placed away from the operative puncture site. The usual precautions are necessary for the prone position, particularly eye protection and padding of pressure points. Care should be exercised in the tension of any bandage used to tie in the tracheal tube, as the facial oedema may cause this to cut into the patient, increasing the possibility of a restricted cerebral vascular supply. This procedure can be a major physiological strain on patients with ischaemic heart disease. It carries a significant mortality. The patients should be admitted to a high dependency unit for the immediate postoperative period, though the less healthy patients may require the full facilities of an intensive care unit on a planned basis.

Transvaginal tension-free tape (TVT)

Transvaginal tension-free tape support of the bladder neck is a relatively new procedure for stress incontinence. It is often performed using spinal anaesthesia because of the surgeon's need to adjust the tension of the buttressing tape to the minimum (which prevents leakage). This involves the patient either coughing or straining part way through the procedure, and thus it is necessary to limit the level of block to no higher than the T10 dermatome so that some power remains in the abdominal musculature. This is difficult to achieve in a predictable way. Some practitioners are using propofol and remifentanil infusion techniques, awakening the patient when required. Obviously this requires acceptable analgesia, for which local anaesthetic infiltration is used.

Orthopaedic surgery

Joint replacement surgery

The most frequently performed operations in this category are hip and knee arthroplasty. Total hip replacement may be carried out under epidural, spinal or general anaesthesia. Peripheral nerve blockade may be useful for postoperative analgesia (e.g. paravascular '3 in 1', iliac crest and lumbar plexus block) but the hip joint is not easy to denervate in this manner due to its multiple nerve supply. Hip replacement may be carried out in the supine or lateral positions, and it is essential, especially in this relatively older patient group, that great care is taken in positioning the patient and protecting any potential pressure areas (see Section 1, Chapter 3 for other positioning guidance). Revision surgery and bone grafting to the acetabulum complicate the procedure greatly and add to the likelihood of extensive blood loss and the need for close haemodynamic monitoring.

The most major incident to anticipate is cement reaction, which generally occurs with cementing of the femoral, rather than the acetabular, prosthesis. Various mechanisms have been suggested as implicated in cement reactions, and these are listed in Figure SI2. The clinical picture is one of hypotension accompanied by falling oxygen saturation which usually reverts over a 10–20 minute time course. Increase of inspired oxygen and circulatory support may become necessary. It is important that fluid balance is adequate before the cementing of the femoral component. Measures which have been used to reduce the likelihood of cement reaction include distal bone plug in the shaft to

Pulmonary embolisation	Marrow
	Fat
	Cement
	Air
Methylmethacrylate absorption	
Pressurisation of femoral cavity	
Heat from cement reaction within femoral cavity	

Figure SI2 Mechanisms of cement reaction

limit the spread of cement, venting of the shaft to reduce pressure and air trapping, and waiting for the mixture to be relatively non-viscous before insertion to reduce the likelihood of monomer absorption. Although less common, a similar reaction may be seen after cemented humeral prostheses.

Anaesthesia for total knee arthroplasty is broadly similar but does not show the same picture of cement reaction unless extra-long femoral components are used after extensive reaming. Femoral and sciatic blockade may be used for analgesia or operation, and in general techniques of anaesthesia are as for hip arthroplasty. The use of a tourniquet restricts blood loss intraoperatively, but postoperative losses may be brisk. After release of the tourniquet metabolic products are released into the circulation, representing an acid load which may cause temporary acidosis and a rise in end-tidal carbon dioxide. Bilateral joint replacements are severe surgical insults that should not be undertaken lightly.

Laminectomy

The primary requirement of back surgery is the prone or knee–chest position. Adequate eye care is important, and there is no substitute for endotracheal intubation (possibly with an armoured tube) and controlled ventilation using individual drugs of choice. The patient's arms must be carefully and symmetrically moved when turning into the prone position to avoid shoulder dislocation, and pressure points should be padded. A suitable support should be employed to avoid abdominal compression, which will both embarrass ventilation and cause venous congestion in the epidural plexus. The Montreal mattress and Toronto frame are frequently used.

Fractured neck of femur

There are several operations for the treatment of fractured neck of femur (dynamic hip screw, cannulated screws, etc.), depending on the precise site of the break. The majority of patients presenting for this procedure are elderly and frail, and may be the victims of severe polypharmacy. A picture of dehydration and cardiac decompensation is frequently seen. As the operation is urgent rather than emergency, attention should be paid to the correction of those features that can be improved (uncontrolled atrial fibrillation and electrolyte imbalance, to name but two).

Spinal anaesthesia is the most commonly employed technique for this procedure, although care must be taken to ensure adequate fluid resuscitation otherwise severe hypotension may result from sympathetic blockade of the lower limbs. Turning the patient for spinal insertion may necessitate analgesia (particularly in the case of heavy solutions when the injured leg will be underneath) and small incremental doses of IV ketamine with or without midazolam are frequently used. Epidural and general anaesthesia may also be used, and although the mortality from general anaesthesia is higher in the short term, there is very little difference after three months or so have elapsed, when death rates from all techniques approximate. Mortality is lowest where surgery is carried out within 24–48 hours of admission.

Gynaecological surgery

Hysterectomy

Hysterectomy may be undertaken by abdominal or vaginal route. Abdominal hysterectomy equates to a laparotomy in its anaesthesia requirements, although the use of a low transverse incision has encouraged the use of the laryngeal mask airway instead of endotracheal intubation (assuming no other contraindications, such as morbid obesity). Muscular relaxation and controlled ventilation are usually required, with volatile agent and opioid of choice. Postoperative pain relief may be delivered by the use of epidural infusions or PCA. The combination of PCA with a rectally administered NSAID (such as diclofenac 100 mg) is widespread. Rectal administration of NSAIDs in gynaecological surgery is especially indicated, as the high concentrations of the drug which are found in the pelvic venous plexus after absorption ensure delivery to the surgical field. Vaginal hysterectomy is less of an insult than abdominal hysterectomy but has broadly similar anaesthesia requirements. Caudal injection of local anaesthetic agents provides a degree of postoperative analgesia, although it is unlikely that the level of block from this technique will reach sufficient height to be fully effective (T10); therefore, additional analgesia should be provided. If rectal drug administration after pelvic floor repair is desired, this is best administered by the operating surgeon after completion, when the suppository can be gently inserted without damage to the suture line.

Transcervical resection of endometrium (TCRE) and microwave endometrial ablation (MEA) are starting to replace hysterectomy as a treatment for uncomplicated menorrhagia. In TCRE a resectoscope is inserted through the cervix, after which endometrium is resected by laser or diathermy under direct vision. Fluid irrigation of the uterus is necessary in the same way as for TUR. The irrigating solution is isotonic glycine, and the problems of absorption are identical to those of TUR syndrome

(Figure SI1). The use of irrigating solutions containing 1% alcohol is recommended, as absorption can be monitored by the measurement of breath alcohol using a suitable meter and normogram tables. TCRE is not accompanied by significant postoperative discomfort. In terms of anaesthetic requirement, MEA varies little from dilatation and curettage (D&C). General anaesthesia with spontaneous ventilation via a face mask or laryngeal mask is therefore adequate.

Laparoscopy

Laparoscopy involves the inflation of the abdomen with carbon dioxide before the insertion of an endoscope to examine the abdominal contents. The degree of inflation of the abdomen varies greatly between surgeons. Although the procedure is possible with the patient breathing spontaneously, this is not recommended and controlled ventilation with muscular relaxation is the norm (suitable agents being mivacurium and atracurium). Use of the laryngeal mask airway is common but not universal. The procedure is usually of short duration and not accompanied by great postoperative discomfort except in the case of sterilisation or other tubal surgery, where the presence of occluding clips on the Fallopian tubes may precipitate spasm. In this situation opioid drugs may be needed postoperatively, although NSAIDs are probably a better first-line treatment (especially if a day-case patient). The most alarming problem during laparoscopy is that of a severe bradycardia which may be precipitated on inflating the abdomen. Vagolytic drugs should be always at hand, and if necessary the abdomen should be deflated until the heart rate stabilises. Asystolic arrest has been reported. Laparoscopy may be used to confirm the diagnosis of ectopic pregnancy. The patient must be carefully assessed to ensure that there is no great degree of concealed blood loss. The onset of muscle relaxation under anaesthesia in a patient with a bleeding ectopic pregnancy can result in sudden, massive haemorrhage, in which case aggressive fluid replacement and urgent laparotomy are required. Large-scale blood replacement should always be followed by haematological assessment of coagulation and appropriate remedial therapy.

Evacuation and termination (ERPC/STOP)

Evacuation of retained products of conception (ERPC) and suction termination of pregnancy (STOP) are similar in their anaesthesia requirements. As the volatile anaesthetic agents have a relaxant effect on the uterus, their use is associated with increased blood loss, although this may not reach clinical significance. For this reason a technique of intermittent (or infused) induction agent is usual. Propofol with or without supplemental opioid agent is popular for what is a short, minimally disruptive procedure. Patients requiring ERPC should be assessed for preoperative blood loss and resuscitated as necessary. The use of oxytocic agents during anaesthesia for STOP is occasionally accompanied by untoward effects (peripheral vasoconstriction, for example).

Ear, nose and throat surgery

Laryngoscopy

Direct laryngoscopy and its variants (which may include the use of lasers in the airway) demand special techniques of airway management because the surgeon works directly in the airway and needs access to the larynx. Specially designed small tracheal tubes, tubes with a cuff and an insufflation port or special laser-proof tubes are available, and all have their uses. Because of the difficulties of maintaining spontaneous or controlled ventilation under these circumstances, the usual techniques involve a total intravenous technique with controlled ventilation using an insufflation device such as the Sanders injector or high-frequency jet ventilator. If lasers are to be used in the airway then great care must be taken to isolate the trachea below the tube cuff from the airway above the cuff, because any backwash of gas containing oxygen might result in an explosion or fire when the laser is next fired. Nitrous oxide is flammable.

Tonsillectomy

Anaesthesia for tonsillectomy with or without adenoidectomy requires defence of the shared airway from blood and debris. This necessarily involves endotracheal intubation after induction, which may be gaseous or IV. If an uncuffed tube is used in the child patient, a suitable pack (ribbon gauze, for example) should be placed around the laryngeal additus to protect the larynx from contamination of blood and saliva. Use of a Boyle–Davis gag will prevent compression of the tube during surgical positioning. Having decided upon intubation, controlled ventilation should be used, and commonly a non-depolarising relaxant, opioid, vapour combination is used for the maintenance of anaesthesia. Extubation should be undertaken in the head-down lateral position after adequate pharyngeal suction. There are two choices for timing of this event: while the patient is still deep, or after protective reflexes have returned. The latter is more common today. Blood loss should be particularly carefully assessed in young children. The potential for transmission of prion disease

by surgical and anaesthetic instruments is discussed in Section 1, Chapter 5.

Post-tonsillectomy haemorrhage is a specific problem that requires mention. Following post-tonsillectomy haemorrhage, the patient will usually be pale, tachycardic and sweaty. Intravenous resuscitation is essential before induction, and two different techniques of anaesthesia have been recommended. In both situations the patient should be placed head-down, in left lateral position, with suction to hand. Following preparation of all equipment a choice may be made between intravenous or gaseous induction. In the first instance after the usual RSI precautions (pre-oxygenation, cricoid pressure) a cautious dose of induction agent is given, followed by suxamethonium and securement of the airway by endotracheal intubation. Alternatively, a gaseous induction of vapour and oxygen may be employed, using suction as necessary and enough time to achieve a plane of anaesthesia deep enough to permit laryngoscopy and intubation. Maintenance and extubation are as described above. Some authorities recommend the emptying of swallowed blood from the stomach with a nasogastric tube before extubation, which would appear a wise counsel.

Middle ear surgery

Middle ear surgery has one main requirement which differentiates it from other surgical procedures. This is the need to control blood loss in order to provide the surgeon with the best possible view down the microscope. In practice, 'smooth' anaesthesia is desirable (for example no coughing or straining) and a relaxant, opioid, vapour technique is usually employed after intubation with an armoured endotracheal tube. Lidocaine spray to the larynx has been advocated before intubation to reduce the response to the presence of the tube, as has the use of alfentanil with induction. Arterial hypotension is often requested, and provided there are no contraindications this may be achieved by the use of sodium nitroprusside by controlled infusion or beta-blockade (esmolol is a suitable choice). Inspired oxygen concentration should be increased and a slight head-up tilt will reduce bleeding by aiding venous drainage. It has been suggested that avoidance of nitrous oxide is beneficial to avoid pressure rises in the middle ear as it diffuses in. Oxygen–air mixtures are, therefore, recommended in this situation. An anti-emetic agent should be administered during the procedure, as nausea from disturbance of labyrinthine function is frequent and postoperative vomiting is particularly undesirable.

Tracheostomy

The majority of elective tracheostomies are performed on intensive care patients following long-term oral intubation. In this instance anaesthesia is usually maintained by the use of opioid agents with or without volatile supplementation and muscle relaxants as required to facilitate controlled ventilation. The critical element of the procedure is to avoid completely withdrawing the existing endotracheal tube before the surgeon has gained control of the airway with the tracheostomy tube and secured it in place. If this is not achievable, the original tube can be re-advanced and oxygenation maintained. If the endotracheal tube has been removed without securing the tracheostomy tube correctly, a potentially dangerous situation develops which may be fatal. Transfer of connecting tubing from old to new tube should be as quick as possible to avoid desaturation. Emergency tracheostomy is a difficult and hazardous procedure best performed under local anaesthesia.

Ophthalmic surgery

Cataract surgery

Cataracts may be congenital, traumatic, steroid- or radiation-induced, or degenerative. In degenerative cataracts there will also be other medical conditions associated with ageing. While diabetics have no more cataracts than the general population, they tend to present earlier and so there seems to be a preponderance of diabetic patients presenting for cataract surgery. Steroid-induced cataracts present in patients taking long-term steroids for other conditions, particularly eczema or asthma, which should be taken into account. Cataract surgery demands a still eye with low intraocular pressure. This can usually be achieved by smooth anaesthesia with muscle relaxation and controlled ventilation to achieve mild hypocapnia, whether via a tracheal tube or a laryngeal mask, though the latter is preferable because of the lack of intubation pressor response or laryngeal spasm and coughing on extubation. There is a fashion for local anaesthesia for cataract surgery despite this having a higher failure rate, more complications and less predictable reduction of intraocular pressure. Patients who cannot lie flat without coughing or distress, or who cannot communicate because of language, deafness or dementia cannot safely have their cataract surgery under local anaesthesia. They may or may not be fit for general anaesthesia.

Squint surgery

The majority of patients for squint surgery are children, though occasional adults may present for cosmetic corrections. This operation is difficult to carry out with local anaesthesia because of the age of the patient and the manipulations necessary in the orbit. General anaesthesia should be carried out with the airway maintained by either a laryngeal mask or tracheal tube. There is little to choose between spontaneous and controlled ventilation. All patients having squint surgery should receive a weight-related dose of a vagolytic such as glycopyrrolate to obtund the oculo-cardiac reflex, which can cause severe bradycardia on traction of the extraocular muscles. This is much easier to prevent than treat. Tracheal tubes in small children restrict the cross-sectional area of the airway with a consequent increase in resistance to gas flow (resistance is inversely proportional to the 4th power of the radius). After extubation, the smallest amount of laryngeal or tracheal oedema can cause major falls in oxygen saturation. Laryngeal spasm at extubation causes sudden dramatic falls in saturation and the facilities for re-intubation with a muscle relaxant should be immediately to hand. Waiting for the spasm to break is a recipe for disaster. The tracheal tube used during the surgery should not be disposed of until the patient leaves the recovery room.

Retinal surgery

Retinal detachments present sporadically, but are not usually so urgent that they have to be done immediately on presentation. The patients are often hypertensive, though whether this is cause or effect is debatable. The surgery may be prolonged and is often carried out in semi-darkness. In this situation too soft an eye may be a disadvantage in that the low intraocular pressure may cause further tearing of the retina. Controlled ventilation is advantageous due to the duration of the surgery. A vagolytic agent should be given to prevent the oculo-cardiac reflex during surgical manipulation of the globe. The oculo-cardiac reflex also occurs during exenteration or enucleation. Occasionally the surgeon may wish to introduce a gas bubble between the vitreous and retina to tamponade the retina. If this is planned then nitrous oxide should be avoided or turned off as soon as the decision is made. Nitrous oxide diffuses into closed gas-filled spaces and increases the volume of the bubble or, if the area has low compliance, the pressure will rise. While this may be acceptable during the procedure, it will diffuse out in the postoperative period and the pressure or volume will reduce, reducing the tamponade effect.

Penetrating eye injury

Penetrating eye injuries may require induction of anaesthesia in the presence of a potentially full stomach.

Unfortunately, suxamethonium causes a significant rise in intraocular pressure, which may cause further damage, especially if there is already vitreous loss or the lens is disrupted. An alternative is a rapid sequence induction using a generous dose of a rapid onset non-depolarising relaxant instead of suxamethonium. Vecuronium or rocuronium are suitable choices. Rocuronium at 1.5 mg kg^{-1} gives equivalent intubating conditions to suxamethonium. It should be noted, however, that this dose ($3 \times ED_{95}$) may last up to 1 hour. If the penetration of the globe has been with metallic fragments then the search for these may involve magnets or repeated x rays, which can require multiple changes of position or prolonged surgery.

Dacryocystorhinostomy (DCR)

Dacryocystorhinostomy is a potentially bloody procedure usually requiring an anaesthetic technique designed to reduce blood loss. The patient is usually placed with the table head up to improve venous drainage. A vasoconstrictor is introduced inside the nose to reduce mucosal bleeding. The blood pressure is often lowered to further reduce bleeding. Hypotension may be achieved by increasing the inspired concentration of anaesthetic vapour, or by introducing agents which cause peripheral vasodilatation such as trimetaphan or sodium nitroprusside. Trimetaphan is a ganglion-blocking drug and its use causes the pupils to become fixed and dilated. These agents must be used with extreme caution. Mild hyperventilation will also help to reduce the blood pressure. The airway is usually maintained with a tracheal tube, though the laryngeal mask will avoid the pressor response to the presence of the tube and so may avoid the need for active reduction of blood pressure. A pharyngeal pack is essential to absorb blood that trickles down from the nasopharynx.

Oral and maxillofacial surgery

Dental extraction

Simple dental extraction demands good control of a shared airway and a degree of understanding between anaesthetist and dentist. Dental extraction should be carried out with the same standard of equipment and monitoring as in the best hospital operating theatres, including ECG, oximetry, NIBP and expired gas analysis. The majority of dental extractions are carried out on a day-case basis unless there is significant coexisting disease. There is still some debate as to whether the sitting position or the supine position is better, both have advantages and disadvantages. The supine position provides some protection against fainting

on induction of anaesthesia, a potentially dangerous event, while encouraging regurgitation of stomach contents.

Induction of anaesthesia may be by inhalation or intravenous injection, but in both cases venous access should be obtained first. The sudden falls in blood pressure associated with propofol tend to limit its use in the dental chair, particularly in the sitting position.

There is no need for intravenous opioids, and simple analgesics are adequate in the postoperative period. Many children prefer inhalational induction, which should be with halothane or sevoflurane in a nitrous oxide/oxygen mixture. Isoflurane has too pungent a smell and enflurane causes too much coughing and salivation to be useful. Desflurane also carries a significant incidence of airway irritation. Inhalation induction and maintenance are carried out using a nasal mask. Once adequate anaesthesia has been established, the mouth is opened and a pack inserted between the mouth cavity and the pharynx, separating the nasal airway from the oral airway. In this way, the extraction can be carried out without dilution of the anaesthetic gases by mouth breathing, and the airway can be maintained without contamination by blood and debris. Recovery should be in the lateral position, preferably head down.

Removal of wisdom teeth

Surgical removal of wisdom teeth demands that the surgeon has good access to the mouth cavity while the airway is protected from debris, water and blood. This is usually achieved by nasal intubation and use of a pharyngeal pack. The reinforced laryngeal mask is also used by experienced anaesthetists. Nasal intubation can cause significant bleeding and pharyngeal tears. An accidental pharyngeal mucosal tear must be recognised and treated with a broad spectrum antibiotic to avoid major infective complications (including potential mediastinitis). The anaesthetist must choose between spontaneous and controlled ventilation. If spontaneous ventilation is used then there is a high incidence of cardiac arrhythmia, particularly with halothane. Most of the disturbances resolve with emergence from anaesthesia and require no intervention. Care must be taken to remove the pharyngeal pack at the end of the procedure. Recovery should be in the lateral position with observation of blood loss and postoperative pain relief provided by NSAIDs.

Fractured mandible

Surgical treatment of a fractured mandible involves stabilisation of the fracture against the mandible itself or against the maxilla via the upper teeth. The fracture may be plated, in which case the airway at the end of the procedure is clear, or the mandible may be wired to the upper teeth, in which case the mouth is closed at the end. It can be difficult to establish at the beginning of the procedure which situation will pertain at the end. Provided that the mouth can be opened before anaesthesia is induced, an IV induction may be used, followed by nasal intubation and a pharyngeal pack. Ventilation may be controlled or spontaneous but with due consideration for the duration of surgery and the recovery phase. An anti-emetic should be given before the end of the procedure because vomiting in a semiconscious patient with a closed mouth is disastrous. The pack must be removed before the end of the surgery. Spontaneous respiration must be re-established in the operating theatre, following which the tube must not be removed until the patient is conscious and can maintain their own airway. The tracheal tube used must be retained until the patient leaves the recovery room. If the mouth is wired closed then a pair of wire cutters must go with the patient wherever they are while in hospital in case the wires need to be cut in an emergency. NSAIDs are suitable for postoperative analgesia. The opioids are less suitable because of their sedative effects. There is a case to be made for patients with wired jaws to be nursed on an HDU or ICU overnight for airway observation.

Fractured zygoma

Fracture of the zygoma indicates that severe trauma has taken place, and the preoperative assessment should take into account the possibility of closed head injury. The fracture is usually reduced via an incision above the temporal hair line and so the anaesthetist must be remote from the head. IV induction should be used, followed by controlled or spontaneous ventilation via an oral tracheal tube or a reinforced laryngeal mask airway. Whichever the airway device, it must be securely fixed, because there may be significant head movement during the reduction. There is always the possibility of further open surgery if the initial manipulation fails.

Fractured maxilla

Anaesthesia for fractured maxilla is not for the inexperienced. The fracture indicates severe trauma, and preoperative assessment should take into account the possibility of closed head injury. The combination of significant head injury and maxillary fracture is an indication for tracheostomy as part of the surgical procedure, as is fracture of both maxilla and mandible together. The sur-

gical procedure may involve stabilisation of the maxilla against the mandible or the skull, either of which will cause airway management problems. A compromised airway is an indication for inhalation induction followed by an 'exploratory' laryngoscopy before a muscle relaxant is given. An oral tracheal tube may be used unless the mouth is to be wired closed, in which case an oral tube will suffice while a tracheostomy is performed. Nasal tubes should not be used because of the displacement of the maxilla, usually backward. Ventilation should be controlled and the anaesthetic machine placed remotely. Access to the head is difficult, particularly at the end of the procedure if a 'halo' device is used to fix the maxilla to the skull. The patient should be nursed on an ICU/HDU after surgery.

Trismus

Fractures of the mandible and infection or haematoma in the mouth can cause significant swelling, inflammation of the tissues and spasm of the muscles of mastication, resulting in an inability to open the mouth adequately. The spasm may or may not relax after induction of anaesthesia. In this situation, intravenous induction can prove rapidly fatal because the patency of the airway is only maintained by muscle power, which is lost on induction of anaesthesia. If at this point it proves impossible to open the mouth or maintain the airway then the patient will die of hypoxia unless a cricothyrotomy is performed immediately. The presence of trismus, for whatever reason, demands inhalational induction. If, during the induction, the airway becomes compromised, then the anaesthetic may be terminated without risk to the patient and consciousness restored. Alternatives must then be considered with the patient awake. Tracheostomy under local anaesthesia is one option. If the inhalational anaesthetic proceeds without difficulty then the degree of trismus can be assessed whilst the patient is unconscious, with a view to tracheal intubation or laryngeal mask airway placement. Muscle relaxants should not be used unless a good view of the glottis has been obtained under anaesthesia. Blind nasal intubation has no place in this scenario because of the risk of torrential haemorrhage in an uncontrollable airway and because success is not guaranteed.

References and further reading

Williamson KM, Mushambi MC. Complications of hysteroscopic treatment of menorrhagia. *Br J Anaesth* 1996; **77**: 305–8.

Yentis SM, Hirsch NP, Smith GB. *Anaesthesia and Intensive Care A–Z*, 3rd edn. Oxford: Butterworth-Heinemann, 2004.

CHAPTER 7

Regional anaesthesia and analgesia

H. B. J. Fischer

Regional anaesthesia has its origins in 1884, 38 years after the discovery of general anaesthesia, when Carl Koller instilled a solution of cocaine into a patient's eye and performed glaucoma surgery 'under local'. This landmark discovery led to an explosion of interest in blocking nerve conduction as surgeons looked for less dangerous alternatives to the general anaesthetic techniques then available.

General principles of management

Several important factors, common to all major regional anaesthesia techniques, require consideration to minimise risks and promote high standards of patient care.

Patient preparation

Preoperative preparation of the patient for regional anaesthesia should fulfil the same standards of care as for general anaesthesia because regional anaesthesia should not be regarded as a shortcut for high-risk patients. A full explanation of the intended block should cover the conduct of the injection, patient management during surgery and recovery from the effects of the block. The advantages to patient, surgeon and anaesthetist may be discussed. The more common side effects that may be experienced should be outlined and the patient offered the choice of whether to remain fully conscious during surgery, have a sedative premedication or intravenous sedation during the procedure. Major complications of regional anaesthesia are rare (less than 1%). Contraindications to regional anaesthesia are also relatively uncommon, and are shown in Figure RA1.

Performing the block

Major regional anaesthetic techniques require formal sterile procedures, especially central nerve blocks, where meningitis and epidural abscess are rare but definite risks. All regional anaesthesia techniques have associated complications, and local anaesthetic drugs have potentially toxic properties. Airway and resuscitation skills are, therefore, essential to the practice of regional anaesthesia. Figure RA2 describes the general requirements for successful practice.

Perioperative management

During performance of the block verbal contact with the patient should be maintained to offer reassurance and explanation of the unfolding events. Staff within the operating theatre must be aware of the impact of their noise and activity on the patient. Patients who have received premedication or intravenous sedation often sleep during surgery once the block is fully established and the initial surge of activity during preparation for surgery has subsided. Occasional verbal contact should still be maintained as part of the routine monitoring of the patient. Central neural blocks have the potential to cause hypotension due to peripheral vasodilatation and reduced venous return. Hypotension responds to changes in posture. Slight head-down tilt with elevation of the legs will restore venous return, and intravenous fluids may be required. Bradycardia should be treated with appropriate vagolytic therapy (for example glycopyrrolate 200–400 μg IV) and vasopressors may be necessary if hypotension does not respond

Fundamentals of Anaesthesia, 3rd edition, ed. Tim Smith, Colin Pinnock and Ted Lin. Published by Cambridge University Press. © Cambridge University Press 2008.

to the above measures. Ephedrine in 3 mg intravenous aliquots is most commonly used as it has both vasopressor and chronotropic effects without increasing myocardial oxygen requirements excessively.

The patient will be unable to protect anaesthetised limbs from pressure or extremes of posture and, if the procedure is prolonged, may become distressed by being unable to change position. It is therefore important to protect the anaesthetised parts of the body and to maintain a comfortable posture for the patient. Postoperatively, the affected limbs need protection from injury and pressure, and patients should be mobilised with care to guard against postural hypotension until the effects of the block have worn off.

- Patient refusal despite adequate explanation
- Uncooperative patient (obtunded conscious, for example)
- Anticoagulation or coagulopathy
- Untreated hypovolaemia (particularly applies to spinal anaesthesia)
- Major infection
- Trauma or burns over injection site
- Raised intracranial pressure (particularly central blockade)

Figure RA1 Contraindications to regional anaesthesia

- Secure intravenous access
- Full resuscitation apparatus
- Adequate patient monitoring equipment
- Ability to administer general anaesthesia rapidly
- Fully trained anaesthetic assistance
- Suitable sterile packs (reusable or disposable)
- A full range of sterile needles and other necessary equipment
- Adequate space to maintain sterility
- Surroundings that offer privacy, good lighting and warmth

Figure RA2 Requirements for performing major regional anaesthesia techniques

Central neural blockade

There are three neuraxial techniques in common use, and their terminology can confuse because terms are used interchangeably. **Spinal** (synonym: intrathecal or subarachnoid), **epidural** (synonym: extradural or peridural) and **caudal** (synonym: sacral epidural) are the preferred terms for anaesthesia and analgesia within the boundaries of the spinal column.

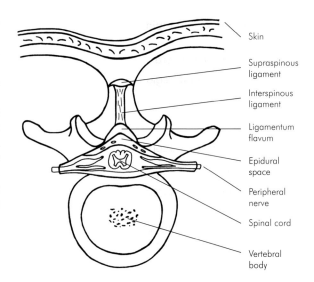

Figure RA3 Cross section of the lumbar spine at L1

Spinal anaesthesia
Indications
Spinal anaesthesia is used for a wide variety of both elective and emergency surgical procedures below the level of the umbilicus. For surgery above the umbilicus, high spinals are now rarely used because of associated difficulties of maintaining spontaneous ventilation and abolishing the painful stimuli from traction on the peritoneum and pressure on the diaphragm.

Anatomy
Spinal anaesthesia requires the injection of a small volume of local anaesthetic agent directly into the cerebrospinal fluid (CSF) in the lumbar region, below the level of L1/2, where the spinal cord ends. Figure RA3 shows the typical anatomy of the lumbar spine in cross section.

The meninges surround the spinal cord from the foramen magnum as far down as the second sacral segment (S2). The dura mater is a tough fibro-elastic membrane, beneath which lies the delicate arachnoid mater. The dura mater invests the spinal cord and the spinal nerve roots, forming the dural cuffs which extend laterally as far as the intervertebral foraminae. Although the arachnoid is attached to the dura there is a potential space between the layers (the subdural space) and inadvertent injection into this space is a recognised complication of both spinal and epidural injections. The pia mater is a delicate vascular layer closely adherent to the spinal cord. Lateral projections of the pia form the dentate ligaments, which attach

Total volume (brain and spinal cord) approximately 130 ml

Volume around spinal cord approximately 35 ml

CSF pressure in lumbar region   6–10 cmH$_2$O
                                  (lateral position)

                                  20–25 cmH$_2$O
                                  (sitting)

Hydrogen ion concentration 40–45 nmol l^{-1}

Protein content 20–40 mg l^{-1}

Figure RA4 Composition of CSF

to the dura and stabilise the spinal cord. The filum terminale is the caudal extension of the pia that anchors the spinal cord and dura to the periosteum of the coccyx. There are 31 pairs of spinal nerves (8 cervical, 12 thoracic, 5 lumbar, 5 sacral, 1 coccygeal) arising from the spinal cord, which extends from the foramen magnum to the L1/2 vertebral level. Below this level, the lumbar and sacral nerves form the cauda equina, which offers a large surface area of nerve roots covered only by the pia mater and accounts for the sensitivity of these nerves to local anaesthetic agents administered centrally.

Physiology
CSF is a clear fluid with a mean specific gravity of 1.006 at 37 °C, which is actively secreted by the choroid plexi in the lateral and fourth ventricles at a rate of up to 500 ml per day. There is no active flow, movement occurring by diffusion and changes in posture. Absorption occurs (at equilibrium with production) via the arachnoid villi of the major cerebral sinuses. The typical composition of CSF is shown in Figure RA4. A number of factors affect the spread of local anaesthetic within the CSF, and these are listed in Figure RA5.

The maximal spread, duration and quality of the block is mostly influenced by the posture of the patient during and immediately after the injection and the density of the solution. The ratio of the density of the solution to that of CSF is expressed as baricity (where isobaricity = 1.0). If the injection is made at the L3/4 interspace with the patient in the left lateral position and the patient is then immediately turned supine, hypo- and hyperbaric solutions produce different effects due to their distribution patterns. Hypobaric solutions are not commonly available in the UK now but have been used traditionally for lower abdominal and lower extremity surgery as they tend to be restricted to the top of the lumbar lordosis when

Major influence
- Baricity of solution
- Posture of patient
- Volume of solution
- Mass of drug injected
- Volume of CSF

Minor influence
- Intervertebral level of injection
- Height of patient
- Age of patient
- Weight of patient
- Speed of injection
- Induced turbulence (barbotage)
- Posture

Figure RA5 Factors influencing intrathecal spread of solutions

the patient lies supine. With the use of head-up tilt, the height of the block can be encouraged in a cephalad direction but at the expense of a patchy quality of anaesthesia and an unpredictable height. Head-down tilt will restrict the caudad limit of the block. Isobaric solutions are not influenced by posture and may be expected to produce a block influenced more by level of injection and volume. Commercially produced bupivacaine (normally described as isobaric) is slightly hypobaric (0.999) at body temperature and can produce unpredictable results with changing posture. Hyperbaric bupivacaine is the most commonly used drug for spinal anaesthesia in the UK at present. As hyperbaric solutions are hypertonic they remain affected by posture for up to 30 minutes after injection and so sensory levels may change within that time. This explains why so-called saddle blocks and unilateral spinals can rarely, if ever, be achieved with hyperbaric solutions.

The effects of a spinal anaesthetic on the physiology of the major organ systems are related primarily to the height of the block. Specific organ systems affected are detailed below.

Nervous system
As a rule there is total neural blockade caudad to the injection site while cephalad to it the concentration of local anaesthetic decreases, producing a differential nerve block of the sensory, motor and autonomic fibres. Sympathetic fibres are most sensitive and may be blocked two to six segments higher than sensory fibres, which in turn may be blocked a few segments higher than the associated motor block.

Respiratory system

Below the thoracic nerves, spinal anaesthesia has no clinical effect on respiratory function but as the intercostal nerves become progressively blocked, active expiratory mechanics are impaired, producing a reduction in vital capacity and expiratory reserve volume. Tidal volume and other inspiratory mechanics remain normal due to increased diaphragm movement. Patients may complain of dyspnoea and may lose the ability to cough effectively. If there is exceptional cephalad spread and the cervical nerves become affected, apnoea due to phrenic nerve blockade can occur.

Cardiovascular system

Progressive blockade of the thoracolumbar sympathetic outflow produces increasing vasodilatation of the resistance and capacitance vessels and a reduction of 15–18% in systemic vascular resistance. If the cardiac output is maintained, there will be a similar fall in mean arterial pressure. If, however, the cardiac output falls due to a reduction in preload (for example due to hypovolaemia or a reduction in venous return due to postural changes) then hypotension may develop rapidly, especially if the block reaches the cardioaccelerator fibres above the level of T4/5, when a reflex bradycardia may occur. Above the level of the block there is usually compensatory vasoconstriction, but this is not sufficient to prevent significant falls in arterial pressure if the block is extensive.

Gastrointestinal system

Sympathetic blockade allows vagal parasympathetic activity to predominate. Gastric emptying and peristalsis continue, sphincters relax and the bowel is generally contracted. This may preclude the use of central blockade in patients with obstructed bowel, at least until the obstruction has been relieved. However, the incidence of postoperative ileus is reduced by spinal and epidural blockade, and this is one of their main benefits. Nausea and vomiting can occur as a result of the unopposed vagal activity, if the peritoneal contents are stimulated in the awake patient.

Equipment

Spinal anaesthesia requires specialised needles and introducers in addition to the general equipment necessary for central nerve blocks (Figure RA6). There is an inevitable incidence of post-dural puncture headache (PDPH) with spinal anaesthesia, ranging from 0.2% to 24%, and many designs of needle have been introduced to try and reduce this problem. Currently the lowest incidence of PDPH is

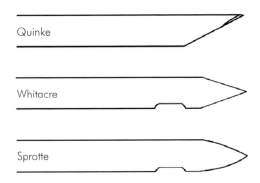

Figure RA6 Tip design of spinal needles

associated with very narrow-gauge, short-bevel needles (26–29 G) and 24 G pencil-point Whitacre tip designs, or the more specialised Sprotte designs with a large side-opening hole. The narrow gauge and relatively blunt tips of these needles necessitate insertion through a properly designed introducer, which should be closely matched to the type of spinal needle being used, to avoid tip damage.

Technique

Successful spinal anaesthesia depends on a reliable lumbar puncture technique. First establish venous access with a wide-bore cannula and then position the patient either in the lateral position with the spine flexed maximally to open up the gaps between the vertebral spines or in the sitting position with the feet placed on a low stool at the side of the bed and the elbows resting on the thighs (Figure RA7). Each position has drawbacks and advantages, and the choice is usually made on personal preference. In either case, a skilled assistant is necessary to position the patient correctly, maintain and support the posture and establish a rapport with them during the conduct of the block.

A line joining both iliac crests (Tuffier's line) passes across the spine of L4 and is a reliable landmark for locating the L3/4 interspace, which is usually easily defined and is the one most often used. The technique for spinal anaesthesia is described in Figure RA8.

Note that 22 G needles are robust enough to be used in patients with calcified ligaments or other anatomical difficulties, and they are recommended for elderly patients, where these problems are more common and the risk of PDPH is very low. If an introducer is required, it should be inserted into the deep layers of the interspinous ligament, so that the needle has only a short distance to travel. Narrow gauge needles may deviate or be damaged by the ligamentum flavum, calcified ligaments or osteophytes and also will give little feedback. After performing the block the blood pressure, pulse rate and ECG should be monitored, as the onset of sympathetic nerve blockade is quite rapid. When using 3 ml bupivacaine 0.5% in 8% glucose (so-called hyperbaric solution), motor and sensory loss will be apparent within a few minutes but the block may not be fully complete for up to 25 minutes. Sensory block

Degree of motor block	Bromage criterion	% score
(1) No block	Full flexion of knees and feet	0
(2) Partial block	Just able to flex knees plus full flexion of feet	33
(3) Almost complete	Unable to flex knees, some foot flexion still	66
(4) Complete	Unable to move legs or feet	100

Figure RA9 The Bromage motor block scale (1965)

Operation site	Block level	Drug volume (hyperbaric bupivacaine 0.5%)
Perianal	L 4/5	2.5 ml
Urogenital	T 10	2.75–3.0 ml
Lower abdominal	T 6/7	3.0–3.25 ml

Figure RA10 Drug doses in spinal anaesthesia

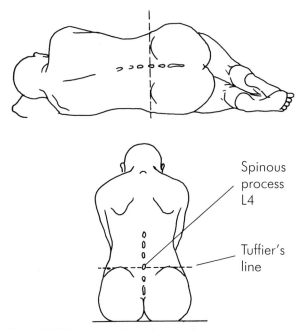

Figure RA7 Patient positions for spinal anaesthesia

Sterilise the skin over the lumbar spine with a spirit-based antiseptic and raise a skin weal with lidocaine 1% over the appropriate interspace. Inject 2–3 ml more lidocaine into the subcutaneous tissue. Anchor the skin over the interspace by pressing the non-dominant index finger on the spine of the cephalad vertebra and insert the needle or introducer in the midline at 90 degrees to the skin. Feedback from the needle tip will monitor the progress of the needle through the supraspinous and interspinous ligaments, the ligamentum flavum and sometimes the dura mater. If bone is contacted, withdraw the needle to the subcutaneous tissue and redirect slightly cephalad in the first instance. Puncture of the dura is usually obvious, and when the stylet is removed CSF should flow freely.

Figure RA8 The technique for spinal anaesthesia

can be tested using a blunt pinprick or loss of temperature sensation with an alcohol swab. Dermatomes should be tested bilaterally starting in the dermatome nearest to the level of injection. Motor loss is usually estimated using the Bromage scale (Figure RA9).

Normally, the whole procedure is conducted with the patient conscious or lightly premedicated, so as to maintain verbal contact and cooperation. If turning the patient is likely to be painful (for example those with fractured neck of femur) then intravenous ketamine 0.5 mg kg^{-1} may be administered to provide analgesia during insertion of the spinal.

Drugs, doses and volumes

Figure RA10 gives a guide to drug administration for various operative sites, based on a fit adult of normal stature (70 kg); smaller volumes may be necessary for higher-risk patients. Hyperbaric bupivacaine 0.5% gives a reliable surgical block for 2–3 hours. Plain 'isobaric' bupivacaine 0.5% 3–4 ml is also commonly used but is less reliable above T10. Lidocaine 5% in 8% glucose is sometimes indicated for short-duration blocks; 2.5–3.0 ml lasts up to 1 hour at T10 and up to 2 hours in the lower limbs.

Complications

Some complications (hypotension, urinary retention, bradycardia) are actually physiological consequences of central neural blockade and should not represent a clinical problem if correctly managed. If management is inappropriate, secondary effects such as nausea and vomiting, faintness or vasovagal loss of consciousness may follow. Total spinal blockade requires urgent supportive mangement, which may include leg elevation, ventilatory support including intubation, IV fluids and vasopressors.

Headache

Loss of CSF through the dural puncture site will produce a low-pressure headache due to traction on the cranial meninges. The main characteristics of a spinal headache are that it is minimal when lying flat, is severe when sitting up or standing, occurs in the occipital and bifrontal distribution and may be worsened by coughing or straining. In severe cases the traction may produce cranial nerve symptoms with alterations in vision and hearing. Onset is usually within 24 hours of the injection, and the majority of PDPH diminishes rapidly with rest, oral analgesia and adequate hydration and should resolve within 7 days. Occasionally more invasive treatment is required in high-risk groups such as pregnant women and after puncture with large-bore needles. An epidural blood patch, in which 20–30 ml of the patient's blood is withdrawn from a vein under the strictest sterile precautions and injected through an epidural needle placed as close to the level of the dural puncture as possible, is very effective at relieving a PDPH, with >90% success with the first injection. Other causes of headache should be considered before ascribing the cause to the spinal and a careful history of events should be elicited, as headaches are a very frequent complaint after surgery.

Neurological sequelae

Temporary symptoms of paraesthesia, hypoaesthesia and motor weakness may follow spinal anaesthesia but are not necessarily the result of trauma to a spinal nerve root. These symptoms occur from pressure, surgical trauma or stretching of the root or peripheral nerve, and the great majority resolve spontaneously within a few weeks. Serious, permanent neurological damage is extremely rare (less than 1/10 000) but in view of the serious consequences of such an event, any neurological sequelae should be formally examined by a neurologist with experience of this type of damage as soon as the problem arises. Other rare causes of neurological damage include brain damage and anterior spinal artery syndrome due to excessive and

Surgery
- Thoracic
- Pulmonary
- Cardiac
- Vascular
- Abdominal
- Gastrointestinal
- Gynaecological
- Urological
- Orthopaedic and trauma

Acute pain relief
- Postoperative analgesia
- Trauma
- Miscellaneous (pancreatitis, ischaemic pain)

Chronic pain states
- Chronic benign pain
- Cancer pain

Figure RA11 Indications for epidural anaesthesia and analgesia

prolonged hypotension, infection (meningitis and epidural abscess), arachnoiditis and cauda equina syndrome (both associated with the injection of incorrect solutions), and are usually the result of a failure of technique.

Epidural anaesthesia
Indications

Surgery can be undertaken within the abdomen and the lower limbs using an epidural as the sole anaesthetic technique, but it is more usual to combine epidural anaesthesia and a light general anaesthetic. Epidural infusions are now extensively used for acute and chronic pain relief (Figure RA11).

The salient significant differences between spinal and epidural approaches are summarised in Figure RA12.

The differences in Figure RA12 apply to single-shot, local anaesthetic blocks. The addition of adjuvant drugs (such as opioids or α_2 agonists) can alter the characteristics of each technique. For epidural administration it is customary to insert a catheter to allow top-up doses or prolonged infusions, whereas spinal catheters are not commonplace. Combined spinal and epidural (CSE) anaesthesia is increasingly used, especially for obstetric surgery, to utilise the benefits of both techniques (Carrie 1990). Surgical block can be rapidly established with a small dose of spinal bupivacaine (2–2.5 ml hyperbaric solution) followed by the slower onset of a low-dose epidural, which can be used to extend operating time and postoperative analgesia.

	Spinal	Epidural
Onset	2–5 minutes	20–30 minutes
Duration	2–3 hours (single shot)	3–5 hours
Drug volume	2.5–4 ml	20–30 ml
Quality of block	Rapid surgical anaesthesia	May be inadequate in some dermatomes

Figure RA12 Differences between spinal and epidural techniques

In summary, spinals provide rapid-onset, short-duration surgical anaesthesia below the umbilicus with small doses of drug. Epidurals have a slower onset time, require large doses of drug and produce less dense surgical anaesthesia but can be used more flexibly in the lumbar and thoracic regions, and their duration may be extended to days or weeks for analgesia by the insertion of a catheter.

Anatomy

The anatomy of the epidural space is described in Section 1 Chapter 5 (pages 80–81). Refer also to Figure RA3.

Physiology

The effects of epidural anaesthesia on the major organ systems are similar to those of spinal anaesthesia, with the height of the block being the major determinant. In a patient with compromised cardiovascular or respiratory reserve, the slower onset of epidural blockade gives more time to manage the onset of hypotension and other side effects, although against this advantage must be weighed the risks of the need for a much larger dose of local anaesthetic drug. The spread of local anaesthetic solution within the epidural space and thus the ultimate height of block is determined by a number of factors (Figure RA13).

Equipment

In addition to the equipment necessary for spinal anaesthesia (see previously) a suitable epidural pack will be required. There are several commercial packs readily available, and most contain a loss-of-resistance syringe, Tuohy needle, catheter and bacterial filter.

Technique

The practical technique of lumbar midline approach to the epidural space is described in Figure RA14.

The description in Figure RA14 relates to loss of resistance to air. There are advocates for the use of saline, and each technique has its own benefits and drawbacks. These are summarised in Figure RA15.

Only 3 ml air or saline (or less) should be injected in order to minimise bubble formation, dilution of local anaesthetic and confusion with CSF. In distinguishing saline from CSF, saline should be cold on the skin compared with CSF, and CSF will show positive for glucose on proprietary stick testing.

Drugs, doses and volumes
Injection of the local anaesthetic agent
Single-shot technique. A test dose through the needle of 3 ml lidocaine 2% plus epinephrine 1:200 000 may detect

Factors	Comment
Drug mass	Drug mass is critical, and more important than either volume or concentration.
Drug volume	For a given drug mass, larger volume gives more spread than a small volume.
Site of injection	The epidural space increases in volume in a caudal direction. Thus a given volume will spread further in the cervical > thoracic > lumbar > sacral.
	Onset is fastest and the block most intense in the dermatomes nearest the site of injection.
Age	A given volume spreads further with increasing age over 40 years.
Raised abdominal pressure	Smaller volumes may be needed in pregnancy and morbid obesity.
Patient position	Prolonged sitting position may reduce upward spread. Earlier onset of block in dependent side.
Injection technique	Slow 'unfractionated' injection of dose through needle gives fewer incomplete blocks than 'fractionated' or incremental doses.

Figure RA13 Factors affecting spread of epidural solutions

The Tuohy needle, the loss of resistance syringe, the catheter and filter must be examined and prepared for use. Connect the filter and catheter and fill with saline to ensure free passage of solution. Position the patient in either the lateral or sitting position as for a spinal injection and identify the appropriate vertebral interspace. Sterilise and drape the area, raise a skin weal with lidocaine 1% and anchor the skin over the cephalad spine of the interspace with the non-dominant index finger. Insert a 21 G hypodermic needle at right angles to the skin exactly in the midline of the interspace to inject more local anaesthetic into the interspinous ligaments and identify the route of the Tuohy needle. Insert the Tuohy needle in the direction indicated by the hypodermic needle. The needle will pass easily through the superficial layers, but as it passes through the supraspinous and interspinous ligaments resistance will become more obvious. If the needle strikes bone, withdraw it slightly and re-angle slightly cephalad but still in the midline. At this point remove the trochar and attach the loss of resistance syringe filled with air or saline as required. Carefully advance the needle and syringe combination through the deep layers of the interspinous ligament and into the ligamentum flavum. Constantly check for loss of resistance as the needle is advanced through the ligament, which is 3–5 mm thick in the midline. As the tip of the needle enters the epidural space, there will be a simultaneous loss of resistance in the syringe, an audible 'click' and a tactile feeling of the needle advancing more easily, which requires great control to prevent sudden advancement within the epidural space. Immobilise the Tuohy needle once the loss of resistance occurs, carefully remove the syringe and check that no blood or CSF drains from the needle. CSF will normally emerge from a Tuohy needle with sufficient volume and velocity to leave no doubt as to its identity.

Figure RA14 The technique for epidural insertion

Air	Saline
Requires LOR syringe	Ordinary syringe
Intermittent testing and movement of needle	Continuous pressure on plunger and movement of needle
Easy to learn	More difficult to learn
Air bubbles may form space and expand with N_2O	Saline may be confused with CSF

Figure RA15 Loss of resistance (LOR) to air or saline

Catheter techniques. The initial dose of local anaesthetic agent may be administered via the needle followed by insertion of a catheter for subsequent top-up doses. This method dilates the epidural space, allows easier insertion of the catheter, and produces a more rapid onset of anaesthesia and fewer missed segments. Alternatively, the catheter is inserted immediately loss of resistance is confirmed, the test dose administered and the main dose given in incremental doses via the catheter. Figure RA16 shows some indicative dosing requirements for a fit adult male with the injection made at L3/4. Lidocaine is usually used with 1:200 000 epinephrine to reduce absorption and prolong duration. Bupivacaine 0.75% offers the same duration as 0.5% solution but gives a better quality sensory and motor block.

Whichever method of epidural injection is used, the ECG, heart rate, oxygen saturation and blood pressure must be monitored frequently as the block develops over 15–20 minutes. The development of segmental sensory loss should be followed by testing of dermatomal levels as for a spinal block.

Complications

Complications of epidural block are similar to those of a spinal block, but there is a difference of severity and incidence for each of the following complications.

Post-dural puncture headache

This complication of accidental dural puncture carries a higher risk of headache developing and the headache is more severe due to the larger hole made in the dura. In non-obstetric patients about half of those who have a dural puncture will develop a headache severe enough to require a blood patch, but in the obstetric population over 90% of sufferers will require one.

inadvertent spinal or intravascular injection, denoted by the rapid onset of a spinal block or a sudden tachycardia (although there is an incidence of false negative test doses). The local anaesthetic agent may be injected slowly over 2 minutes in 5 ml aliquots to allow for detection of signs of impending toxicity.

Block height	Drug and volume			Duration
Lumbosacral (L1–S5 approx)	Lidocaine	2.0%	20–25 ml	2–3 h
	Bupivacaine	0.5%	18–20 ml	4–6 h
	Bupivacaine (racemic or levo)	0.75%	10–15 ml	4–6 h
	Ropivacaine	7.5 mg ml^{-1}	20–25 ml	4–6 h
Thoracolumbar (T5–L4/5 approx)	Lidocaine	2.0%	25–30 ml	2–3 h
	Bupivacaine	0.5%	20–25 ml	4–6 h
	Bupivacaine (racemic or levo)	0.75%	15–20 ml	4–6 h
	Ropivacaine	7.5 mg ml^{-1}	15–25 ml	4–6 h

Figure RA16 Drug doses in epidural anaesthesia

Cause	Notes
Needle track pain	Localised and temporary
Postural	Extremes of posture during surgery or labour
Drug or additive	2-Chloroprocaine and EDTA
Epidural abscess or haematoma	Rare but important to treat
Recurrence of previous low back pain	

Figure RA17 Causes of back pain after epidural or spinal block

Patient factors	Technique factors
Spinal abnormalities	Technical difficulty
Age over 70 years	Repeated attempts
Female	Traumatic puncture
Anticoagulant therapy	Catheter placement
Coagulopathy	Catheter removal

Figure RA18 Risk factors for spinal haematoma after CNB

Back pain
Back pain is sometimes reported after epidural (and spinal) anaesthesia, and it may be related to several causes (Figure RA17).

Epidural haematoma
Although reported after diagnostic lumbar puncture, haematoma formation is excessively rare after spinal and epidural anaesthesia. The majority of reported cases occur in patients with a coagulopathy or anticoagulant treatment. Current knowledge suggests that it is safe to use spinal and epidural techniques in patients receiving prophylactic heparinisation for surgery. If there is doubt then the guidance shown in Figure RA19 may help decide if it is safe to proceed with a central block. The same criteria apply to removing as well as inserting an epidural catheter.

Thromboprophylaxis and central nerve blocks
There are several million central nerve blocks (CNB) carried out in Europe each year. The majority of these patients receive either unfractionated heparin (UFH) or low molecular weight heparin (LMWH) preoperatively. Despite such high numbers there has hitherto been a wide discrepancy between countries in guidelines for the use of thromboprophylaxis when central nerve blocks are desirable. The maximum probable incidence of spinal haematoma following CNB in patients without risk factors is 1/320 000 for spinals and 1/200 000 for epidurals. The maximum risk accompanies epidural catheterisation, and the minimum is associated with single-shot spinal techniques with fine gauge needles. Around 75% of significant spinal haematomas are associated with 'bloody taps' or bleeding diathesis. It is thought that 50% of significant haematomas are associated with catheter removal. Risk factors for spinal haematoma after CNB are summarised in Figure RA18. The European Society for Regional Anaesthesia (ESRA) has recommended good-practice guidelines for thromboprophylaxis and CNB, and these are given in Figure RA19.

Caudal anaesthesia
Indications
The caudal route for injection of local anaesthetic agents provides a way of administering a sacral epidural. There are multiple indications for the use of caudal anaesthesia, listed in Figure RA20.

UFH

Prophylactic doses

Extensive experience within Europe. No appreciable risk if interval of approximately 4 hours between a dose of 5000 units of UFH and insertion of CNB or removal of catheter or 1 hour interval after insertion of CNB (or removal of catheter) before next dose is given.

Therapeutic doses

For vascular or cardiac surgery. Start IV infusion 1 hour after CNB and maintain PTT at 1.5 times normal. Remove catheter 4 hours after stopping infusion and check for normal PTT, ACT and platelet count.

LMWH

For prophylaxis (up to 40 mg enoxaparin/day) no increase in risk compared to UFH provided there are no additional risk factors and there is a 10–12 hour interval between the last dose of LMWH and CNB (or removal of catheter).

There should then be a 6–8 hour interval before the next dose. Therefore a once-daily dosage regimen is preferable.

Antiplatelet agents (aspirin, NSAIDs)

Very few case reports of problems in the absence of other risk factors.

Beware the use of concurrent therapy – dextrans, anticoagulants, heparin.

If time allows, stop therapy 1–3 days pre-op for NSAIDs and 3 days or more for aspirin, ticlopidine and other antiplatelet drugs.

Otherwise, measure platelets, careful visual inspection and bleeding history. There are no universally accepted tests for adequate platelet function.

Oral anticoagulants

Therapeutic levels of coumarins are an absolute contraindication.

Stop agent, convert to heparin, monitor INR and prothrombin time (factor VII, but II and X also affected).

If INR exceeds 1.5, proceed with caution (spinal rather than epidural). Beware catheter removal.

Figure RA19 ESRA good practice guidelines for thromboprophylaxis and CNB

Adult
- Surgery
  - anorectal
  - gynaecology
  - orthopaedic surgery
- Obstetric
  - episiotomy
  - removal of placenta
- Chronic pain
  - coccydynia
  - spinal manipulation

Paediatric
- Major abdominal and orthopaedic surgery
- Inguinal hernia repair
- Surgery to genitalia

Figure RA20 Indications for caudal anaesthesia

Anatomy

The normal anatomy of the sacrum is subject to great variation in the extent to which the laminae of the five sacral vertebrae fuse in the midline to form the sacral canal. The sacral hiatus normally results from the failure of the laminae of S4 and S5 to fuse, but it can vary in size from complete absence (approximately 5% of the population) to complete bifida of the sacrum. The dural sac ends at the S2 level in adults, a level which approximates to a line drawn between the posterior superior iliac spines. In pre-adolescent children there is a predictable relationship between age, volume of injection and height of block (Schulte-Steinburg & Ralhfs 1977), but pubertal growth changes the volume and shape of the sacral canal and this relationship is lost in adults.

Physiology

The effect of caudal anaesthesia is limited to the lumbar and sacral nerves, and therefore there will be less effect on cardiovascular, respiratory and gastrointestinal performance than with other epidural techniques. Motor weakness is limited to the legs, and sensory loss is usually subumbilical. Autonomic disturbance is limited to bladder and anorectal dysfunction as both sympathetic and pelvic parasympathetic outflow is blocked.

Equipment

A 22 G short bevel needle should be used for adults and larger children and a 23 G hypodermic needle for smaller children and babies. For prolonged anaesthesia and postoperative analgesia in children, continuous caudal

Place the patient in the lateral position as for a spinal or lumbar epidural. Note that the posterior superior iliac spines and the sacral hiatus form an equilateral triangle (Figure RA22). Use the index finger of the non-dominant hand to palpate the sacral cornuae either side of the hiatus, which normally feels like a small depression between the bony landmarks. With the hiatus located, sterilise and prepare the area and insert the needle at an angle of about 60 degrees to the skin through the subcutaneous tissues. The sacrococcygeal membrane is tough and offers obvious resistance to the needle; once through the membrane, re-angle the needle to 20–30 degrees (Figure RA23) and carefully advance the needle a few millimetres, ensuring that it remains in free space. If it strikes bone or will not advance freely, withdraw slightly and reposition the needle or begin the whole procedure again. Do not advance the needle more than a few millimetres within the sacral canal, especially in children, because the dural sac extends beyond S2 in some individuals. Aspirate to check for blood and CSF and then slowly inject 3 ml of chosen solution to test for low resistance to injection. If this feels normal and there is no subcutaneous swelling denoting needle misplacement in the superficial tissues, slowly inject the main dose, with frequent aspiration checks.

Figure RA21 The technique of caudal anaesthesia

epidurals, employing a 20 G epidural catheter inserted through an 18 G Tuohy needle, are becoming popular.

Technique
It is most common to administer a caudal after inducing general anaesthesia. The practical technique is described in Figure RA21.

Drugs, doses and volumes
Paediatric. The linear relationship between age, volume and segmental spread is utilised in a number of formulae. The best known is that of Armitage (1979), and this is shown in Figure RA24.

If the volume of bupivacaine used exceeds 20 ml, motor blockade can be minimised by using bupivacaine 0.19% (dilute 3 parts bupivacaine 0.25% with one part normal saline) and use the calculated volume as in Figure RA24. Lidocaine 1% in the same volumes gives analgesia for 3–4 hours compared with 6–8 hours for bupivacaine.

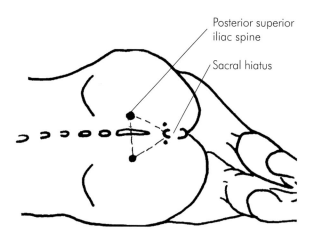

Figure RA22 Patient position for caudal anaesthesia

Adults. 25–30 ml bupivacaine 0.5% provides 6–8 hours of subumbilical analgesia with a variable degree of segmental spread and motor blockade. If analgesia is necessary only within the sacral nerves, 20 ml is sufficient.

Complications
Incorrect needle placement is the commonest problem of the technique, and is usually a matter of difficulty palpating landmarks. If the needle is too superficial, then the only adverse effect is a subcutaneous injection and a failed block. If the needle is inserted too deeply, it can pass through the sacrococcygeal joint into the pelvic cavity and thus the viscera, risking contamination of the epidural space. In pregnant patients there are reports of the needle entering the birth canal and damaging the foetal head. Intravascular injection is a risk due to the rich plexus of veins within the sacral canal. If the marrow of the sacral vertebra is cannulated and the dose injected, rapid systemic absorption can occur. Infection from a dirty technique in a potentially unsterile area is a constant risk. Dural puncture is an uncommon but important complication because of the potentially large volume of local anaesthetic solution that can be inadvertently injected intrathecally.

Peripheral nerve blockade
There are several peripheral nerve blocks that have an important role in providing anaesthesia and postoperative analgesia for surgery of the upper and lower extremities and the body surface (Pinnock et al. 1996). A select few are detailed below.

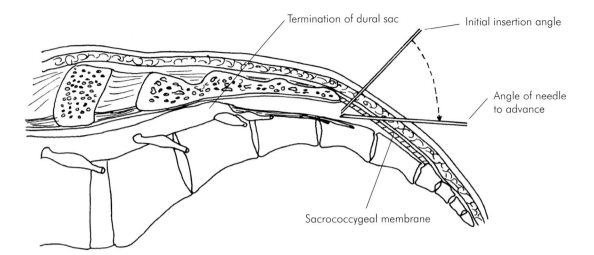

Figure RA23 Needle angulation for caudal anaesthesia

Block height	Volume (ml kg^{-1})
Lumbosacral	0.5
Thoracolumbar	1.0
Mid thoracic	1.25

Figure RA24 Drug doses for paediatric caudal block (bupivacaine 0.25%)

Brachial plexus block
Indications
Brachial plexus anaesthesia is indicated for a wide variety of surgical procedures and for the management of acute and chronic pain (Figure RA25).

Anatomy
The anatomy of the brachial plexus is described in Section 1, Chapter 10. The important practical feature is the fascia that invests the plexus from its origins at the

Indication	Notes
Trauma and orthopaedic surgery fracture manipulation or fixation joint replacement soft tissue trauma	Possibility of compartment syndrome with closed trauma
Vascular and reconstructive surgery shunt formation plastic reconstruction microvascular surgery	Prolonged sympathetic blockade improves blood flow to critical perfusion areas
Acute pain postoperative analgesia continuous passive movement (after joint surgery)	Up to 24 h analgesia with bupivacaine 0.75%
Chronic pain reflex sympathetic dystrophy terminal cancer pain	Catheter insertion into sheath allows prolonged infusions

Figure RA25 Indications for brachial plexus blockade

cervical roots between the middle and anterior scalene muscles to the five terminal nerves at the mid-humeral level. Blockade of the brachial plexus is theoretically possible with entry into this fascia at any level, although the resulting block will vary according to the volume and subsequent spread of solution. There are several techniques described in the literature, but the three most common are the **interscalene** (which blocks at the level of the five cervical roots), the **supraclavicular** (which blocks at the level of the three trunks) and the **axillary** (which blocks at the level of the five terminal nerves). Only the supraclavicular and the axillary are described below, as the interscalene is technically more demanding.

Equipment

For single-shot injections, a short bevel 22 G, 3.5 cm regional block needle is ideal as it relays considerable information to the user about the tissue layers, particularly the sheath itself. The tactile response from the needle plus the frequent paraesthesiae when the needle is correctly placed should ensure a high success rate (>85%). Experienced clinicians use a peripheral nerve stimulator to confirm accurate needle placement, and this is a useful adjunct to teaching blocks or performing them in sedated or anaesthetised patients. To ensure that the needle is not displaced by manipulating or changing the syringes during injection, the 'immobile needle' concept (Winnie 1969) uses a short (10–15 cm) extension set from the needle to the syringe. This allows the operator to carefully control the needle while an assistant makes the injection or changes the syringes.

Techniques

The axillary approach is the easiest technique to learn, and carries the lowest risk of serious complications. The practical technique is described in Figure RA26, and patient position is shown in Figure RA27.

Note: the needle may enter the axillary artery, in which case apply gentle aspiration and continue to slowly advance the needle through the posterior wall of the artery until blood can no longer be aspirated. At this point the patient may experience parasthesiae within the distribution of the radial nerve, and after careful negative aspiration the injection can be completed – the transarterial approach. Firm digital pressure must be maintained for several minutes if the artery is punctured. In a fit adult, 40 ml local anaesthetic will usually produce an effective brachial plexus block, but it may not uniformly block all five terminal nerves because of variable spread within the sheath. Thus a partial block

Position the patient supine with the shoulder abducted to 90 degrees and the elbow flexed to 90 degrees (Figure RA27). Identify the lateral border of the pectoralis major and palpate the axillary arterial pulse at this level on the medial surface of the arm. Follow the pulsation proximal into the axilla to identify where the pulse is most obvious, and raise a skin weal with a 25 G needle and 1–2 ml of local anaesthetic over this point. Fix the artery with the non-dominant index finger and insert a 22 G short bevel, 3.5 cm needle either above or below the index finger aiming towards the pulse, at a depth of 1–2 cm. In a normal adult arm there will be resistance from the fascial sheath followed by a distinct 'pop' and the patient may experience parasthesiae in the distribution of the ulnar nerve. The needle should be immobilised at this stage and the injection made after negative aspiration. Digital pressure applied distal to the needle during the injection and maintained while the needle is removed and the arm adducted after injection will encourage proximal spread of solution.

Figure RA26 The technique of axillary approach to the brachial plexus

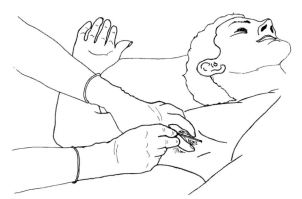

Figure RA27 Patient position for axillary brachial plexus block

may occur with a nerve territory being missed (usually the musculocutaneous) rather than a dermatomal pattern of failure as would be the case with an interscalene block, where the injection is made at the level of the roots. With a supraclavicular block, partial failure is manifested as both a dermatomal (C8/T1) and nerve territory (median or ulnar) failure, because the inferior trunk is the most likely to be missed.

Position the patient supine with the head supported by a single pillow and turned slightly away from the side to be blocked and the arm extended downwards, beside the thigh, to depress the clavicle (Figure RA29). If the muscular landmarks are difficult to identify, ask the patient to lift his or her head slightly off the pillow to throw the muscle into relief; the interscalene groove can be highlighted by vigorous sniffing. Trace the interscalene groove distally with the non-dominant index finger until the pulsation of the subclavian artery is palpable – usually about 1 cm behind the midpoint of the clavicle. Raise a skin weal of local anaesthetic at this point and then insert a 22 G short bevel 3.5 cm needle parallel to the neck in the horizontal plane towards the pulse of the subclavian artery. It is not crucial to feel the arterial pulse, if the groove can be identified accurately. Advance the needle until the sheath is detected at a depth of about 1–2 cm as an increased resistance with a distinct 'pop' when the needle penetrates. The patient may experience parasthesiae in the distribution of the superior trunk (C5/6, median, musculocutaneous or radial nerves). Aspirate to ensure that the needle has not entered the subclavian artery and slowly make the injection. If arterial blood is aspirated, carefully withdraw the needle a few millimetres until aspiration is negative; the needle will still be within the fascial sheath and the injection can be made as normal. Digital pressure proximal to the needle insertion will encourage distal spread as the large volume is injected.

Figure RA28 The technique of subclavian perivascular brachial plexus block

The supraclavicular approach. There is a variety of techniques described, but the subclavian perivascular approach (Winnie & Collins 1964) is very successful and deservedly popular. A line drawn from the cricoid cartilage laterally across the sternomastoid muscle meets the posterior border of that muscle at the point where the interscalene groove emerges from under the sternomastoid, running caudally between the anterior and middle scalenus muscles laterally towards the midpoint of the posterior border of the clavicle, providing useful landmarks. The practical technique is described in Figure RA28, and patient position is shown in Figure RA29.

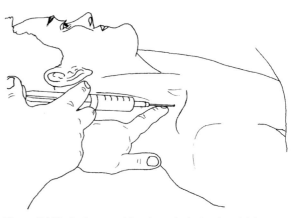

Figure RA29 Patient position for subclavian brachial plexus block

Drug	Volume	Duration
Lidocaine 1.5% + epinephrine	40–50 ml	3–4 h
Bupivacaine 0.5% (racemic or levo)	35–40 ml	9–11 h
Ropivacaine 0.5%	35–40 ml	9–11 h

Figure RA30 Drug doses and duration for brachial plexus block

Drugs, doses and volumes

Figure RA30 illustrates the drugs, volumes and average duration of block for surgical anaesthesia with respect to axillary and supraclavicular approaches to brachial plexus block. Although the relatively large volumes indicated may be above data sheet maxima, they are more effective than smaller volumes, widely used, and known to be safe due to the low rates of systemic absorption from the brachial plexus sheath. Regard should always be paid to maximum doses of local anaesthetic agent when calculated on a body weight basis. For axillary block the technique will be most effective in the medial aspect of the upper arm, forearm and hand, whereas for supraclavicular block distribution is fairly uniform below the shoulder but may be less dense in the ulnar aspect of the hand.

Complications

Some complications may be considered as inevitable side effects of a successful block whereas others are potentially dangerous (Figure RA31).

Axillary
- Haematoma
- Vascular damage

Supraclavicular
- Phrenic nerve block
- Horner's syndrome
- Recurrent laryngeal nerve block

Pneumothorax

Figure RA31 Complications of brachial plexus block

Femoral nerve block
Indications
The femoral nerve is normally blocked in combination with the sciatic, obturator and lateral cutaneous nerves, as appropriate, to ensure an adequate block for the proposed site of surgery. The main indication is for major orthopaedic procedures of the lower limb, especially surgery to the femur and knee joint. Postoperative analgesia following a total knee replacement or cruciate ligament reconstruction can be impressive, as a single-shot femoral nerve block may last up to 24 hours if bupivacaine 0.75% is used.

Anatomy
The femoral nerve is the largest branch of the lumbar plexus and enters the thigh lateral to the femoral artery in its own fascial sheath (Figure RA32). It can be discretely blocked as a single nerve using 10 ml solution but a large volume (20–30 ml) produces, in effect, a distal approach to the

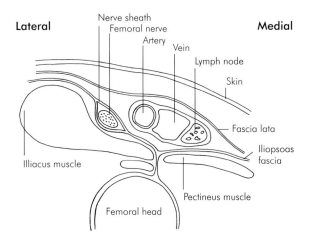

Figure RA32 Anatomy of the femoral nerve in cross section

Position the patient supine and identify the inguinal ligament and the femoral arterial pulse immediately distal to it. The point of injection should be 1 cm lateral to the pulsation and 1–2 cm distal to the inguinal ligament. Having raised a skin weal of lidocaine, insert a 22 G short bevel regional block needle at about 45 degrees, aiming cephalad. A distinct pop as the needle pierces the fascia lata may be felt, followed by a secondary pop as it enters the nerve sheath. Parasthesiae in the distribution of the femoral or saphenous nerves indicates close proximity to the nerve. After aspiration, slowly inject the chosen volume. In anaesthetised patients, a peripheral nerve stimulator will aid accurate location.

Figure RA33 The technique of femoral nerve block

Drug	Volume	Duration
Bupivacaine 0.5% (racemic or levo)	15 ml	12–18 h
Bupivacaine 0.75%	12 ml	18–24 h
Bupivacaine 0.5% (racemic or levo) (for '3 in 1')	20–30 ml	8–12 h

Figure RA34 Drug doses for femoral nerve block

lumbar plexus which also blocks the obturator nerve and lateral cutaneous nerve of the thigh, the so-called '3 in 1' block (Winnie et al. 1973), although there is some uncertainty whether all three nerves are reliably blocked with this approach.

Technique
The practical technique of femoral nerve blockade is given in Figure RA33.

Drugs, doses and volumes
Figure RA34 shows the duration of a single-shot femoral nerve block using a long-acting local anaesthetic solution. Duration can be extended by the insertion of a catheter into the femoral nerve sheath for continuous infusion.

Complications
The only significant complication of femoral nerve block is the accidental injection of local anaesthetic into the femoral

vessels, which are immediately adjacent to the nerve. Attention to detail when performing the block and careful aspiration prior to injection will prevent this avoidable complication. The limb will be anaesthetic for many hours and it must, therefore, be protected from pressure sores and prolonged immobility.

Ankle block
Indications
The nerve supply to the foot can be blocked at the ankle to provide surgical anaesthesia and postoperative pain relief for any operation performed distal to the malleoli. The main indications are orthopaedic and trauma surgery to the forefoot and digits. Surgery such as correction of hallux valgus is very painful and ankle blocks, using bupivacaine 0.5%, can provide 18–24 hours analgesia. Although it is usual to perform a combination of blocks at the ankle under light general anaesthesia, it is possible to use the technique in conscious patients. The practical techniques are described in Figure RA35.

Anatomy
The five nerves which supply the foot and the ankle are the terminal branches of the femoral and sciatic nerves. The saphenous nerve is the terminal branch of the femoral nerve and supplies the skin over the medial malleolus and a variable amount of the medial border of the foot. It passes anterior to the medial malleolus, accompanied by the saphenous vein. The other nerves are branches of the sciatic nerve, which divides into the common peroneal and tibial nerves within the popliteal fossa. The deep and superficial peroneal nerves emerge onto the dorsum of the foot at the level of the extensor skin crease between the pulse of the dorsalis pedis and the tendon of extensor hallucis longus. The deep peroneal nerve supplies the deep structures of the dorsum of the foot and the skin of the first webspace only; the superficial peroneal nerve supplies the skin of the dorsum of the foot and the lateral three webspaces. The tibial nerve runs in a sulcus behind the medial malleolus, deep to the medial collateral ligament of the ankle, accompanied by the corresponding tibial vessels, and divides into medial and lateral plantar nerves which supply the sole of the foot and the deep plantar structures. The sural nerve runs subcutaneously between the lateral malleolus and the calcaneus to supply the lateral border of the foot.

Tibial nerve
Palpate the lower border of the medial malleolus and the medial surface of the calcaneal tuberosity. At the midpoint of a line between these two bony landmarks insert a 23 G needle at 90 degrees to the skin until it just touches the periosteum of the calcaneus just below the sustentaculum tali, which can be felt as a crescent-shaped protuberance on the calcaneus. Withdraw the needle 1–2 mm, aspirate and slowly inject 5–6 ml. If the injection is in the correct plane, deep to the medical collateral ligament, the local anaesthetic will spread proximally and distally along the course of the tibial nerve.

Deep peroneal nerve
Position the foot at right angles to the tibia and palpate the pulse of dorsalis pedis. Identify the tendon of extensor hallucis longus by moving the great toe and insert a 23 G needle between these two landmarks at 45 degrees to the skin until contact is made with the distal end of the tibia. Withdraw the needle 1–2 mm, aspirate and slowly inject 4–5 ml of local anaesthetic.

Superficial peroneal nerve
Withdraw the needle into the subcutaneous tissue having completed the deep peroneal injection, and realign it, aiming towards the lateral border of the foot. Advance the needle slowly and inject 4–5 ml of local anaesthetic subcutaneously to produce a weal of local anaesthetic extending laterally across the dorsum of the foot. This weal can be gently massaged to spread it further laterally.

Sural nerve
Palpate the lower border of the lateral malleolus and the lateral aspect of the calcaneal tuberosity and make a subcutaneous injection of 5 ml of local anaesthetic between these two points.

Saphenous nerve
Identify the saphenous vein, if possible, anterior and proximal to the medial malleolus, and inject a subcutaneous weal of 3–4 ml of local anaesthetic around the vein, using a 23 G needle. Take care to avoid intravenous injection and trauma to the vein.

Figure RA35 The technique of ankle block

Drugs, doses and volumes

Bupivacaine 0.5% will provide surgical anaesthesia for 3–4 hours and 12–18 hours analgesia, although up to 24 hours is possible. For minor surgery, especially in ambulant patients, lidocaine 2% will provide 1–2 hours surgical anaesthesia and 4–6 hours analgesia. Each nerve requires approximately 5–6 ml; thus the total volume used depends on the number of nerves blocked, although a maximum of 20 ml is recommended.

Complications

The main complications of these nerve blocks are the potential for intravascular injection or vascular trauma, as all the injections are made into neurovascular bundles (except the sural nerve). However, the volumes of local anaesthetic are small, the needle used should be no larger than 23 gauge, and aspirating the needle before each injection will minimise the risk.

Many patients will be mobilised soon after surgery, and they must be supervised and non-weight bearing whilst the blocks are still working because they will have no sensory or proprioceptive awareness in the sole of the foot if the tibial nerve has been blocked.

Inguinal field block
Indications

Inguinal field block in combination with light general anaesthesia is ideally suited to day case repair of a hernia. The technique offers rapid recovery from anaesthesia and postoperative analgesia lasting for 6–8 hours. If the surgery is to be performed using local anaesthesia as a sole technique, a larger volume of more dilute local anaesthetic is preferable, and the surgeon may need to reinforce the anaesthesia by direct infiltration of the deeper structures within the inguinal canal. The technique of inguinal field block is detailed in Figure RA36.

Anatomy

The anatomy of the inguinal region is described in Chapter 1, Section 10 (page 196).

Drugs, doses and volumes

Bupivacaine 0.5% with epinephrine 1:200 000 to a total of 30 ml for supplementation of light general anaesthesia will provide up to 8 hours postoperative analgesia. For local anaesthesia as a sole technique, 50 ml prilocaine 1% is suitable, but only 2–3 hours postoperative analgesia will result.

Lie the patient in the supine position and identify the anterior superior iliac spine (ASIS) and the pubic tubercle – the bony landmarks which define the two injection points. The top injection point will be 1 cm medial and 2 cm caudal to the ASIS. Make a skin weal of lidocaine at this point and insert a 22 G short bevel regional block needle, at right angles to the skin, directly downwards through the skin and subcutaneous tissue. At a depth of 1–2 cm (more in obese patients), the needle will encounter the external oblique aponeurosis, which will offer marked resistance to penetration. Move the needle from side to side in a horizontal plane and a distinct scratching over the surface of the aponeurosis will be felt. The iliohypogastric nerve (T12/L1) lies just deep to the aponeurosis, so once the needle penetrates it, immobilise the needle and inject 5 ml of local anaesthetic. Carefully advance the needle another 0.5–1 cm to penetrate the internal oblique muscle (there is often a slight loss of resistance as the needle leaves the inner surface of the muscle) and inject a further 5 ml of solution to block the ilioinguinal nerve (T12/L1), immediately deep to the muscle. Withdraw the needle to the subcutaneous tissues and infiltrate a subcutaneous, fan-shaped area, using 10 ml of solution to block the terminal fibres of the subcostal nerve (T12).

The second part of the injection should be made over the pubic tubercle. Insert the needle directly down to the tubercle and inject 5 ml of solution around the external inguinal ring to anaesthetise the genitofemoral nerve (L1/2). Make a second fan-shaped subcutaneous infiltration to block any fibres that may cross the midline.

Figure RA36 The technique of inguinal field block

Complications

There are few important complications, as the technique is mainly one of infiltration together with the discrete blockade of three small peripheral nerves. From the first point of injection, puncture of the peritoneum and viscera is possible if a long needle is used. Inadvertent intravascular injection is always a possibility with the second point of injection, especially the femoral vessels. It is also possible to block the femoral nerve from the same point and the patient may complain of pain in the hernia site and a numb, heavy leg.

Penile block

Indications

The main indication for penile block is for postoperative analgesia for adult and paediatric male circumcision, although any surgery on the shaft of the penis will benefit. Analgesia is comparable with that produced by a caudal block and avoids the motor and sensory effects on the legs and the autonomic dysfunction of bladder and bowel control. There are no major complications provided that epinephrine or other vasoconstrictors are not used and intravascular injection is avoided.

Anatomy

The shaft and glans of the penis are supplied by a pair of nerves (the dorsal penile nerves) which are terminal branches of the pudendal nerve (S2, 3, 4). The paired nerves emerge beneath the inferior surface of the pubic symphysis separated by the suspensory ligament and deep to Buck's fascia (the fascial sheath surrounding the corpora cavernosa). The perineal nerves (from the other branch of the pudendal nerve) which innervate the anterior part of the scrotum and the midline ventral surface of the penis need to be blocked for complete penile analgesia.

Technique

The technique of penile nerve block is given in Figure RA37. It is customary to perform this block on anaesthetised or sedated patients.

Drugs, doses and volumes

Avoid local anaesthetic solutions that contain epinephrine. Bupivacaine 0.5% will provide 6–8 hours postoperative analgesia following circumcision. 10 ml is sufficient for an adult; children need 3–6 ml according to body weight and size. Limit total dose of bupivacaine to 2 mg kg^{-1} body weight.

Local anaesthesia of the upper airway

The mucosal surfaces of the mouth, oropharnyx, glottis and larynx may be anaesthetised by a combination of topical anaesthesia and discrete nerve blocks.

Indications

Intubation of the trachea in patients with difficult airway due to trauma or disease.

Palpate the inferior edge of the pubic symphysis with the non-dominant index finger and insert a 21 G (adult) or 23 G (paediatric) needle at about 45 degrees until it contacts the pubis or passes just caudad to it. If the needle contacts the pubis, re-angle it to walk it off the inferior edge and through Buck's fascia, which may be detectable as a slight resistance to the needle. After careful aspiration, make a single injection in the midline (both dorsal nerves may be reliably blocked by a single injection). In an adult, inject 7 ml and then inject a further 3 ml as a subcutaneous weal across the midline of the ventral surface of the penis at its junction with the scrotum, starting approximately 1 cm lateral to the midline raphe and finishing 1 cm lateral on the other side. It is important to keep the needle subcutaneous while making this injection as the urethra is superficial at this point. In children the volume needs to be reduced pro rata according to body weight and penile size.

Figure RA37 The technique of penile block

Anatomy

The nerve supply of the airway comes from three sources. The trigeminal nerve supplies the nasopharnyx, palate (V2) and anterior aspect of tongue (V3). The glossopharyngeal nerve supplies the oropharynx, posterior aspect of tongue and soft palate. The vagus nerve gives off two nerves – the superior laryngeal and recurrent laryngeal nerves – which supply motor and sensory fibres to the airway below the epiglottis. The superior laryngeal nerve emerges beneath the inferior edge of the greater cornu of the hyoid before it divides into the internal and external branches.

Technique

The technique of local anaesthesia of the upper airway comprises three parts, topical anaesthesia, superior laryngeal nerve block and transtracheal anaesthesia. Practical details are given in Figure RA38.

Intravenous regional anaesthesia (IVRA)

The technique in current use differs from the original description of August Bier in 1908, although it is often called 'Bier's block'. Bier placed two tourniquets on the forearm and injected procaine directly into a vein isolated

To topically anaesthetise the mouth and oropharynx, sit the patient up with the mouth open maximally and spray four metered puffs of lidocaine (10 mg per spray) onto the tongue and wait a few minutes for it to take effect. Depress the tongue and spray a further four puffs onto the posterior part of the tongue and pharynx. Although the superior laryngeal nerve can be topically anaesthetised by placing a pledget soaked in lidocaine 2% into each pyriform fossa with Krause forceps, once the mouth and tongue are blocked, it is more usually blocked discretely as follows. Place the patient supine with the head extended and palpate the hyoid bone just cephalad to the thyroid cartilage. Displace the hyoid slightly towards the side to be blocked and insert a 25 G, 2.5 cm needle just under the inferior border of the hyoid and inject 2–3 ml of lidocaine 1%, moving the needle gently in and out through the thyrohyoid membrane (Figure RA39). Repeat on the other side. To complete the airway anaesthesia, with the patient in the same position as above, palpate the inferior border of the thyroid cartilage and, having first anaesthetised the skin, insert a 21 G, 2.5 cm needle through the cricothyroid membrane into the lumen of the trachea. Ensure that air is freely aspirable and then rapidly inject 3–4 ml of lidocaine 2%. This will precipitate brisk coughing, which spreads the local anaesthetic throughout the trachea and up into the larynx and vocal cords (Figure RA40). Total dose of lidocaine in an average 70 kg adult should not exceed 200 mg.

Figure RA38 The technique of local anaesthesia of the airway

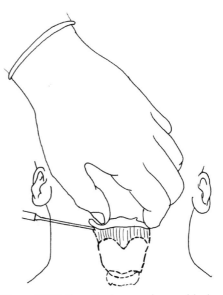

Figure RA39 Superior laryngeal nerve block

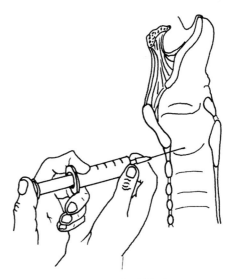

Figure RA40 Transtracheal block

by surgical cut-down. Although a two-tourniquet technique has been re-evaluated recently, one tourniquet is used in modern practice.

Indications
Any surgery lasting less than 1 hour below the level of the elbow in the arm or the ankle in the leg.

Equipment
The tourniquet used must be properly maintained with regular calibration of the pressure gauge and must be of an approved design. Sphygmomanometer cuffs should never be used. Specially designed double cuff tourniquets are available: these allow the proximal cuff to be blown up while the block is established, and then the distal cuff is inflated over anaesthetised skin for use during surgery and the proximal one deflated. This improves comfort during prolonged procedures, but the patient may still experience deep pain from ischaemic muscle.

Technique
The practical technique for performing IVRA is shown in Figure RA41.

Place an intravenous cannula in the dorsum of both hands, one for injection of the local anaesthetic and the other to allow for drug and fluid requirements during surgery. Wrap a layer of wool padding around the upper arm and place the tourniquet over the padding, ensuring that it is of the correct dimensions for the limb and properly secured. Elevate the limb and use a compression bandage to exsanguinate it or simply compress the axillary artery and keep the arm elevated for three minutes. Inflate the tourniquet to 100 mmHg above the patient's systolic blood pressure, remove the compression bandage and observe the arm for one minute to ensure that the veins remain empty. If blood begins to flow under the tourniquet the procedure should be repeated, using a pressure 150 mmHg above systolic, or an alternative anaesthetic technique considered. Inject the local anaesthetic solution slowly (20 ml per minute) to avoid high intravenous pressures which could force it under the tourniquet.

Figure RA41 The technique of performing IVRA

Analgesia will be complete within 15 minutes using prilocaine 0.5%. The cuff should remain inflated for at least 20 minutes, after which time deflation of the cuff and systemic release of the local anaesthetic drug should not cause untoward reactions, although occasionally some transient minor systemic symptoms such as light-headedness or tinnitus are reported. IVRA in the leg is not practical if the cuff has to be placed around the thigh, as inflation pressures of 300–400 mmHg above systolic and very large volumes of local anaesthetic are required. If the surgery is limited to below the ankle, however, then a cuff around the calf is possible, using pressures and drug volumes similar to those in the arm, although exsanguination may not be ideal as the lower leg has a two-bone compartment and vessels between the tibia and fibula will not be compressed. There is also a risk of damage to the peroneal nerve in the region of the head of the fibula if a high tourniquet is applied.

Drugs, doses and volumes

The local anaesthetic agent currently licensed for IVRA is prilocaine 0.5%. For an adult male, 60 ml 0.5% (300 mg) produces good sensory and motor block and is well within the maximum recommended dose of 600 mg.

References and further reading

Armitage EN. Caudal block in children. *Anaesthesia* 1979; **34**: 396.

Bromage PR. A comparison of the hydrochloride and carbon dioxide salts of lidocaine and prilocaine in epidural analgesia. *Acta Anaesthsiol Scand Suppl* 1965; **16**: 55–69.

Brown DL. *Regional Anesthesia and Analgesia.* Philadelphia, PA: Saunders, 1996.

Carrie LES. Extradural, spinal or combined block for obstetric surgical anaesthesia. *Br J Anaesth* 1990; **65**: 225–33.

Greene NM. Distribution of local anaesthetic solutions within the subarachnoid space. *Anesth Analg* 1985; **64**: 715–30.

Pinnock CA, Fischer HBJ, Jones RP. *Peripheral Nerve Blockade.* Edinburgh: Churchill Livingstone, 1996.

Schulte-Steinburg O, Ralhfs VW. Spread of extradural analgesia following caudal injection in children: a statistical study. *Br J Anaesth* 1977; **49**: 1027–34.

Winnie AP. An 'immobile needle' for nerve blocks. *Anesthesiology* 1969; **31**: 577–8.

Winnie AP, Collins V. The subclavian perivascular technique of brachial plexus anesthesia. *Anesthesiology* 1964; **25**: 353–63.

Winnie AP, Rammamurthy S, Durrani A. The inguinal paravascular technic of lumbar plexus anesthesia: the '3 in 1' block. *Anesth Analg* 1973; **52**: 989–96.

CHAPTER 8

Principles of resuscitation

A. J. Stronach

Cardiorespiratory arrest

The contents of this chapter are firmly linked to the teaching and algorithms of the Resuscitation Council (UK) (2005) and the European Resuscitation Council (2005). The current guidelines are evidence-based and were published after representatives from the world's major resuscitation organisations met and reviewed scientific evidence and audit data accrued since the year 2000. From this meeting the 2005 International Consensus on Cardiopulmonary Resuscitation and Emergency Cardiovascular Care Science with Treatment Recommendations (International Liaison Committee on Resuscitation 2005) were published. This is the evidence on which the current guidelines are based.

Causes

A person suffers a cardiorespiratory arrest either because of a primary cardiac problem or secondary to non-cardiac causes. The majority of cardiac arrests occurring outside hospital are from ventricular fibrillation (VF) in adults due to myocardial ischaemia arising from pre-existing ischaemic heart disease (IHD). Other cardiac conditions which may lead to cardiorespiratory arrest include valvular heart disease, cardiomyopathy, myocarditis, endocarditis

and conduction defects, e.g. Wolff–Parkinson–White syndrome or prolonged atrioventricular (AV) block.

An important secondary cause of cardiorespiratory arrest is uncorrected hypoxia resulting from airway obstruction. Hypoxia leads to myocardial failure, which is compounded by the resulting hypercarbia and acidosis. A bradycardia will develop, and this will be followed by an asystolic cardiac arrest unless the airway obstruction is cleared. Some causes of airway obstruction are listed in Figure RS1.

Other non-cardiac causes of cardiac arrest include:
- Hypothermia
- Intracerebral haemorrhage
- Mechanical
  - massive pulmonary thromboembolism or air embolism
  - tension pneumothorax
  - pneumopericardium
  - cardiac tamponade
  - hypovolaemia
- Poisoning

Despite trained cardiac arrest teams being present and readily available to manage cardiac arrests in hospital, less than 20% of patients who suffer an in-hospital cardiac

Fundamentals of Anaesthesia, 3rd edition, ed. Tim Smith, Colin Pinnock and Ted Lin. Published by Cambridge University Press. © Cambridge University Press 2008.

Cause	Nature of obstruction
Coma	Tongue displacement
Anaphylaxis	Tongue, oropharyngeal and laryngeal oedema, bronchospasm, pulmonary oedema
Foreign body	Oropharyngeal, laryngeal, tracheal and bronchial obstruction, bronchospasm
Trauma	Oropharyngeal and laryngeal damage
Infection	Oropharyngeal, laryngeal and pulmonary oedema
Asthma	Bronchospasm
Irritants/poisons/ burns/smoke inhalation	Tongue/oropharyngeal/ laryngeal oedema, laryngeal/bronchospasm, pulmonary oedema
Near-drowning	Pulmonary oedema
Neurogenic shock	Pulmonary oedema
Aspiration	Pulmonary oedema

Adapted from European Resuscitation Council. European Resuscitation Council Guidelines for Resuscitation 2005. *Resuscitation* 2005; **67** (Suppl.1): S1–S190 (Figure 4.3: Causes of Airway Obstruction).

Figure RS1 Causes of airway obstruction

arrest will survive to go home. Most of those who do survive are in cardiac monitored beds and are rapidly resuscitated from VF secondary to myocardial ischaemia.

Most unmonitored patients who suffer cardiac arrest have shown evidence of hypoxia and hypotension for several hours prior to their arrest, which either goes unnoticed or is poorly treated. The presenting rhythm at these cardiac arrests is usually pulseless electrical activity (PEA) or asystole, and the outcome is poor. It is therefore imperative that, as well as being able to recognise a patient who is having a cardiorespiratory arrest, systems are put in place to allow early identification and management of those patients who if left untreated will deteriorate and suffer a cardiorespiratory arrest.

Recognition

Previous guidelines recommended palpating for the presence of a pulse to diagnose a cardiorespiratory arrest. Checking for a carotid pulse, whether by trained healthcare professionals or by lay rescuers, has been shown to be not only time-consuming but also an inaccurate method of confirming either the presence or absence of circulation. The guidelines now advise that an unconscious, unresponsive patient who is not moving and not breathing normally is diagnosed as having a cardiorespiratory arrest. Agonal breathing, which is seen as occasional gasps, slow, laboured or noisy breathing, is a common sign in the early stages of cardiac arrest and should be recognised as a sign of cardiac arrest and not mistaken for normal breathing. There is, however, no evidence to suggest that checking for an unresponsive patient who is not breathing normally is necessarily diagnostically superior to feeling for a carotid pulse.

As well as being able to recognise patients who have suffered a cardiorespiratory arrest, it is important to identify acutely ill patients whose condition is deteriorating, since cardiac arrest in this group of patients is often predictable and may be preventable. Early-warning scoring systems such as MEWS (modified early warning system) and PARS (patient at risk score) have been established in many hospitals for several years. These scoring systems use data obtained from regularly monitoring the vital signs in patients, so that appropriate help is called for at an early stage. Effective treatment can then be started to prevent further deterioration. Such systems, however, rely on the accuracy of recorded physiological parameters, which are not always recorded either regularly or accurately on general wards.

The most important determinant of survival at a cardiac arrest is the presence of someone who is trained, willing, able and equipped to act in an emergency. In some hospitals medical emergency teams, made up of medical and nursing staff from critical care and medical backgrounds, have replaced cardiac arrest teams. These have been established to respond not only to cardiac arrests but also to patients with acute physiological deterioration (Figure RS2). It is now recognised that medical emergencies, and not only cardiorespiratory arrests, need the presence of appropriately trained personnel.

Cardiopulmonary resuscitation

Although cardiopulmonary resuscitation (CPR) is traditionally divided into basic life support (BLS) and advanced life support (ALS), this division is arbitrary when cardiac arrests occur in hospital. The immediate response will depend both on the skills of the initial rescuer and on the equipment available. The aim of effective CPR is to

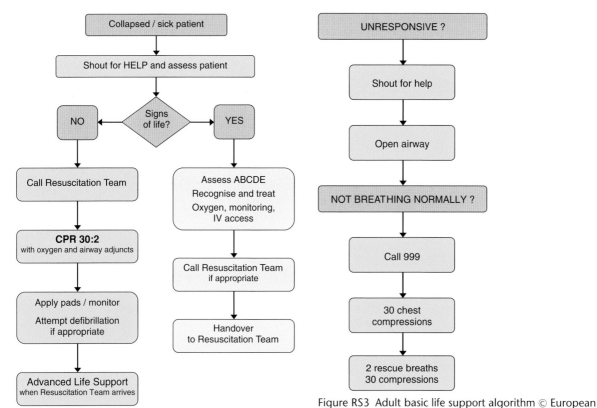

Figure RS2 Algorithm for in-hospital resuscitation © European Resuscitation Council (2005) and Resuscitation Council (UK) (2005)

Figure RS3 Adult basic life support algorithm © European Resuscitation Council (2005) and Resuscitation Council (UK) (2005)

restore a spontaneous circulation to the patient as soon as possible. Although in most circumstances it is possible to support ventilation for prolonged periods effectively, there is no equivalent method of providing circulatory support without a heart beating in an effective rhythm producing cardiac output.

Basic life support

Basic life support (BLS), strictly defined, is the maintenance of a clear airway while supporting ventilation and circulation without the use of specialist equipment other than a protective airway device, e.g. a pocket mask. The current guidelines place a greater emphasis on good-quality chest compressions with minimal interruptions, as there is evidence that this is associated with improved survival.

The recommendation of a specific cardiac compression: ventilation ratio is a compromise between the need to generate forward blood flow and the need to supply oxygen to the lungs to optimise oxygen delivery to the brain and

other vital organs. A 30 : 2 ratio is recommended, taking into account evidence available to optimise outcomes during CPR. The guidelines have also been simplified to aid learning and retention of BLS skills.

The adult BLS algorithm is as shown in Figure RS3. Before approaching a collapsed person a priority is to ensure both personal safety and that of bystanders. Although this is more important outside hospital, there are still safety issues to be considered within the hospital environment. Check for a response by shaking the person's shoulders gently and asking loudly 'are you alright?' If there is no response, shout for help and turn the patient onto his or her back (except in pregnancy: see Resuscitation of the pregnant patient, below), and commence BLS.

Airway

The maintenance of a patent airway during the management of a cardiorespiratory arrest is imperative. In an unconscious patient the tongue falls backwards and the airway is obstructed at the oropharyngeal level. Three simple airway manoeuvres, head tilt, chin lift and jaw thrust, can all be used to open the airway. In a patient who is still making respiratory effort, this may prevent the patient from deteriorating and suffering a cardiorespiratory arrest. The **head tilt**, which flexes the lower cervical spine while extending the head at the atlanto-occipital joint, and the **chin lift** may be sufficient to open an obstructed airway. If not, a **jaw thrust** may be added to further displace the tongue forwards.

In trauma cases where there is a suspected cervical spine injury manual in-line traction must be applied and jaw thrust/chin lift techniques used to open the airway. If still unable to adequately clear the airway a gentle head tilt may be added. Although all these airway manoeuvres are associated with some cervical spine movement, the maintenance of an open airway is the overriding priority. The complication of damage to spinal cord from excessive head tilt has never been reported in cases where cervical spine injury has been suspected.

Look in the mouth to check for any obvious obstruction and use a finger sweep to clear any visible foreign body present within the oropharynx. Then, taking no longer than 10 seconds, **look** for chest moments, **listen** for breath sounds, and **feel** for air movement. If the respiratory pattern is not normal and the patient is unresponsive, call for help and start cardiac compressions. Only those experienced in clinical assessment should check for the presence of circulation by palpating for the carotid pulse.

Circulation

Chest compressions must be started with the patient placed in a supine position on a firm surface. The correct hand position for cardiac compressions is found by placing the heel of the dominant hand in the centre of the chest between the nipples. The heel of other hand is then placed on top and the fingers interlocked, ensuring that pressure is applied over the sternum and not the ribs or abdomen. The rescuer positions him- or herself vertically above the patient's chest and with straight arms applies compressions to a depth of 4–5 centimetres and at a rate of 100–120 compressions per minute.

The time taken for compression and release should be equal. After each compression all pressure on the chest must be released without losing contact between hands and sternum. If chest recoil is not complete it may lead to significantly increased intrathoracic pressure, decreased venous return and decreased coronary and cerebral perfusion.

Properly executed cardiac compressions are tiring, and there is evidence that the quality of chest compressions deteriorates as the rescuer tires. If there is more than one rescuer present, change the person performing cardiac compressions every two minutes.

Cardiac compressions generate forward blood flow by increasing intrathoracic pressure and directly compressing the heart. Although the mean carotid arterial pressure, even with good-quality cardiac compressions, seldom exceeds 40 mmHg, it provides a small but critical blood flow to the brain and myocardium.

During a VF arrest, blood continues to flow into and dilate the right ventricle. Early CPR prevents the right ventricle dilating and thereby increases the likelihood that a defibrillatory shock will terminate VF and enable the heart to resume an effective rhythm. It may also prevent an initial rhythm of VF deteriorating to asystole. With the evidence that a patient stands the best chance of survival if rapidly resuscitated from VF, automated external defibrillators (AED) are being introduced widely in public places as well as becoming standard equipment on many hospital wards. For in-hospital cardiac arrests the use of an AED is an integral part of BLS.

Allowance has now been made in the guidelines for the rescuer who is unable or unwilling to perform mouth-to-mouth ventilation. Chest compressions alone are recommended in this situation. This will only be effective for the first few minutes, and then only in cases of non-hypoxic cardiac arrests, as within 4–6 minutes all oxygen stores are depleted. It is not recommended as standard management.

Rescue breathing

Expired air ventilation is the standard method used for rescue breathing in BLS, and produces an inspired oxygen content of 16–17%. Using chin lift/head tilt and/or jaw thrust manoeuvres, the airway is opened while the rescuer takes a normal breath. If a pocket mask is not readily available, the soft part of the nose is closed by pinching between the index finger and thumb and the rescuer's lips are placed round the patient's mouth, making sure that a good seal is achieved before expiration. As well as mouth-to-mouth and mouth-to-nose ventilation, if the mouth is clenched shut or is badly injured, mouth-to-tracheal stoma ventilation is effective. The chest must be observed to rise and fall during each rescue breath.

Each rescue breath is given over one second (not two seconds as previously recommended), at a rate of 10–12 breaths per minute, to produce tidal volumes of about 500 ml. This not only limits interruptions to cardiac compressions but also causes significantly less gastric distension. Gastric distension splints the diaphragm and interferes with ventilation as well as increasing the risk of aspiration. Large tidal volumes also increase intrathoracic pressure, decreasing coronary and cerebral perfusion, and in animals they have been shown to reduce the chance of successful return of spontaneous circulation. Oxygenation is not impaired by the use of smaller tidal volumes, and the resulting hypercarbia and acidosis has not been shown to adversely affect outcome.

If cardiac output and normal respiration are re-established, the patient should be turned into the recovery position. This is a stable lateral position, with the head dependent and no pressure on the chest to impair breathing. With increasing levels of obesity, the ease of turning the patient should be balanced against the risks of injury to the rescuer, and the risks associated with leaving the victim supine.

Special situations
Foreign-body airway obstruction
Choking in adults tends to occur when eating, and should be promptly recognised and treated (Figure RS4). If it is not, and the victim's airway is severely compromised, his or her condition will rapidly deteriorate to a cardiorespiratory arrest. If there is mild respiratory distress, characterised by the ability to speak, breathe and cough, the victim should be encouraged to cough to clear the obstruction.

If there is severe airway obstruction the victim will be unable to speak, breathe or cough. If the victim remains conscious, stand to one side slightly behind him or her and, while supporting the chest with one hand, lean the victim forwards so that the obstructing object when dislodged comes out of the mouth. Immediately give up to five back blows between the shoulder blades with the heel of your hand. The aim is to dislodge the foreign body with each blow, rather than to give all five.

If this fails to relieve the airway obstruction, give up to five abdominal thrusts. Stand behind the victim, with both arms around the upper part of the abdomen, between the umbilicus and xiphisternum. Clench your fist and, while holding this with your other hand, pull sharply inwards and upwards. Repeat the abdominal thrust manoeuvre up to five times. There is no evidence to suggest which method should be used first. If the obstruction is still not relieved,

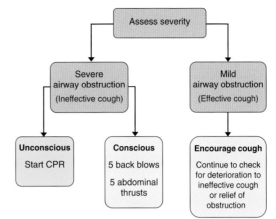

Figure RS4 Adult choking algorithm © European Resuscitation Council (2005) and Resuscitation Council (UK) (2005)

continue alternating five back blows with five abdominal thrusts.

If the patient is initially unconscious or loses consciousness at any time, support the victim carefully to the ground, call for help and start BLS (Figure RS3).

Cardiorespiratory arrest secondary to hypoxia
In cases of identifiable asphyxia, e.g. drowning, trauma and intoxication, the victim should receive one minute of CPR before a single rescuer calls for help. Five initial rescue breaths are given before starting chest compressions.

Advanced life support
Advanced life support (ALS) is a continuum of BLS and involves the use of extra equipment to aid resuscitation attempts. The adult ALS algorithm (Figure RS5) provides a standardised approach to the treatment of all adult patients presenting in cardiac arrest.

Arrhythmias associated with a cardiac arrest are divided into two groups: shockable rhythms (ventricular fibrillation (VF) and ventricular tachycardia (VT)) and non-shockable rhythms (asystole and pulseless electrical activity (PEA)). The principal difference in the management of these arrhythmias is the need for early defibrillation in patients with VF/VT. Subsequent actions, including advanced airway management, ventilation, good-quality chest compressions, venous access and administration of epinephrine, are common to both groups.

During CPR it is imperative that repeated attempts are made to identify and treat potentially reversible causes. For

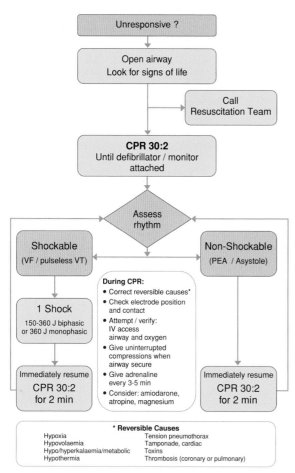

Figure RS5 Adult advanced life support algorithm
© European Resuscitation Council (2005) and
Resuscitation Council (UK) (2005)

ease of memory, these have been divided into groups of conditions beginning with the letter H or T. Those beginning with H are hypoxia, hypovolaemia, hyperkalaemia, hypokalaemia, hypocalcaemia (and other metabolic disorders including acidaemia) and hypothermia. Those beginning with T are tension pneumothorax, cardiac tamponade, toxins and thromboembolic causes.

Airway

Even when correctly performed by experienced personnel, the simple airway manoeuvres as taught in BLS do not always allow maintenance of a clear airway. The use of mechanical aids should help, although if they are used by inadequately trained personnel there may be increased

complications without any improvement in airway management.

Forceps or suction are used to remove any foreign material visible in the oropharynx.

Pharyngeal airways, inserted by either the oral or the nasal route, overcome the backward displacement of the soft palate and tongue. The oral airway can only be used in unconscious patients and must be removed if there is gagging or retching. The cuffed oropharyngeal airway (COPA) may be a useful airway device to improve bag-mask ventilation. The nasopharyngeal airway is used in situations where the mouth cannot be opened, but it must be inserted gently as there is a risk of haemorrhage. In most cases the benefit of improved airway patency outweighs this risk.

A laryngeal mask airway (LMA) is relatively easy to insert and provides more efficient ventilation than standard bag-mask ventilation. Cardiac compressions still need to be interrupted to enable adequate ventilation without an excessive air leak. The LMA only offers partial airway protection during CPR, but there have been very few case reports of aspiration in this situation.

A combitube is a double-lumen tube. It is inserted blindly over the tongue and provides a route for ventilation whether it has been inserted into the trachea or the oesophagus. Care must be taken to ensure that the correct port is used for ventilation. Although relatively easy to insert it is used rarely because of concerns of inadvertent oesophageal ventilation.

Endotracheal intubation remains the gold standard in airway management during CPR. It protects the airway from aspiration, prevents gastric distension, allows suction of airway secretions, provides a route for drug administration and allows cardiac compressions to continue uninterrupted during ventilation. Disadvantages include a comparatively high failure rate when performed by non-anaesthetists, risk of a misplaced tube, and prolonged periods of time without cardiac compressions while attempts are made to intubate. Endotracheal intubation should therefore only be attempted by trained personnel, taking no longer than 30 seconds to complete the process. Correct placement of the endotracheal tube must be confirmed, as with intubation in theatre.

A needle or surgical cricothyroidotomy can be lifesaving in the 'can't intubate, can't ventilate' scenario when there is extensive facial trauma or laryngeal obstruction secondary to oedema or foreign-body ingestion. Percutaneous or surgical tracheostomies are not recommended in this emergency situation as they take too long to perform.

Ventilation

As in BLS, inspiratory time for ventilation should be limited to one second, producing a tidal volume of about 500 ml at a rate of 10–12 breaths per minute. This allows adequate ventilation without excessive interruptions to cardiac compressions. Although expired air ventilation provides effective ventilation, an inspired oxygen concentration of only 16–17% can be achieved. A self-inflating bag will deliver 21% oxygen, and this can be increased to 45% if oxygen is attached directly to the bag. With the addition of a reservoir system and oxygen at 15 l per minute, an inspired oxygen concentration exceeding 85% can be achieved.

To effectively ventilate a patient with a bag-mask technique is difficult, and meticulous attention must be paid to maintaining an open airway while observing the rise and fall of the chest. Even if skilled in airway management, bag-mask ventilation is often a two-person technique.

Circulation

When an unmonitored patient suffers a cardiac arrest, initial attention should be focused on providing good-quality chest compressions as described for BLS (cardiac compressions : ventilation ratio 30 : 2). As soon as a defibrillator arrives the cardiac rhythm must be monitored and the appropriate limb of the ALS algorithm (Figure RS5) followed, depending on the diagnosis.

Shockable rhythms (VF/VT)

The most common presenting rhythm at a cardiac arrest is VF. If VF is present for more than a few minutes the myocardium is depleted of oxygen and metabolic substrates. A brief period of chest compressions before defibrillation will deliver small amounts of oxygen and energy substrates and increase the probability of restoring a perfusing rhythm after shock delivery. Early defibrillation has been shown to improve the chances of survival in VF/VT arrests.

Once VF or pulseless VT has been diagnosed, defibrillation should be attempted as soon as possible (see Figure RS5 for recommended shock energies). CPR should then immediately be resumed and continued for two minutes before reassessing the rhythm. If VT/VF persists give a second shock and restart CPR immediately. Continue for a further two minutes before pausing to reassess the rhythm. If VT/VF persists, give epinephrine 1 mg intravenously (IV) followed by a third shock. Restart CPR and continue for a further two minutes before pausing to reassess the

rhythm. If VT/VF is still present give amiodarone 300 mg IV followed by a fourth shock. Again restart CPR and continue for a further two minutes before reassessing the rhythm. On subsequent cycles, if VT/VF persists, give epinephrine 1 mg IV immediately before alternate shocks (every 3–5 minutes) and further shocks at two-minute intervals.

If at any time organised electrical activity is seen when checking the rhythm, check for a pulse. If there is no pulse present, change to the non-shockable limb of the algorithm, and similarly if the rhythm deteriorates to asystole.

Fine VF is very difficult to distinguish from asystole, and is unlikely to be shocked into a perfusing rhythm. Start CPR, which may improve the amplitude and frequency of VF and the chances of successful defibrillation.

A precordial thump is now recommended only in the case of a witnessed cardiac arrest when a defibrillator is not immediately available. Although a precordial thump may convert VT to sinus rhythm, and has been reported to convert VF into sinus rhythm if given within 10 seconds of a VF arrest, rare adverse effects have also been reported. These include rate acceleration of VT, conversion of VT to VF, complete heart block and asystole.

A precordial thump is performed by using the ulnar edge of a tightly clenched fist, to deliver a sharp impact to the lower half of the sternum from a height of about 20 cm. The fist should immediately be retracted to create an impulse-like stimulus. The mechanical energy of the thump is converted to electrical energy, which may be sufficient to achieve defibrillation.

Electrical defibrillation

Electrical defibrillation is the passage of an electrical current across the myocardium that is of sufficient magnitude to depolarise a critical mass of myocardium. If the heart is still viable, normal pacemakers will take over and produce coordinated electrical activity, which will restore spontaneous circulation. The optimum energy to use is that which achieves defibrillation of a critical mass of myocardium while causing minimal myocardial damage. Transthoracic impedance, typically 70–80 Ω in adults, is at its lowest at the end of expiration, and defibrillation should be attempted at this point of the respiratory cycle. Shaving a hairy chest may also further reduce impedance by improving contact between pad/paddle and skin.

Manual paddles may still be used, but are being replaced in many hospitals by self-adhesive pads, which allow defibrillation from a safe distance. Pads or paddles can be placed in the anteroapical position, with the right sternal pad to the right of the sternum below the clavicle and the apical pad in the mid-axillary line in the V6 ECG electrode position. An alternative position is to place pads/paddles anteroposteriorly, which may provide more effective defibrillation. However, this must be balanced against the difficulty in applying the posterior pad/paddle to an unconscious patient.

ALS guidelines now advise a single shock protocol (Figure RS5), and not three stacked shocks as previously recommended. The stacked shock protocol led to significant periods of time without cardiac compressions, which has been shown to be detrimental to a patient's chances of survival. Defibrillator technology has also advanced, and newer defibrillators now produce biphasic waveforms, which are more efficient than the monophasic waveforms produced by older defibrillators. The success of the first shock from a biphasic defibrillator now exceeds 90%, and failure to terminate VF/VT indicates the need for further CPR to improve myocardial oxygenation rather than the need for further shocks. Biphasic devices produce either truncated exponential waveforms or rectilinear biphasic waveforms, and these require different energy levels for defibrillation. Manufacturers should display an effective waveform energy range on the biphasic device, but if unsure use 200 J for the first shock.

Even if defibrillation is successful, it is very rare for a pulse to become palpable immediately after defibrillation, and CPR must therefore be restarted immediately after delivery of a shock. If a perfusing rhythm has not been restored, this avoids a further interruption of CPR. If a perfusing rhythm has been restored, CPR is not detrimental and will not precipitate further episodes of VF/VT. If the shock has converted VF/VT into asystole, then a further period of CPR may induce VF, which has a better prognosis.

Non-shockable rhythms (pulseless electrical activity and asystole)

Pulseless electrical activity (PEA) is when cardiac electrical activity is present but there are no palpable pulses. A PEA arrest resulting from primary myocardial pump failure carries a very poor prognosis. However, it is often secondary to potentially reversible causes, listed in Figure RS5, and if these are rapidly identified and appropriately treated, PEA is often survivable.

When **PEA** is diagnosed CPR must be started immediately according to the ALS algorithm, and when IV access is achieved 1 mg of epinephrine (IV) should be given. If the initial heart rate is less than 60 beats per minute give

3 mg of atropine. Continue CPR at a ratio of 30 : 2 until the airway is secured with an endotracheal tube, and then continue cardiac compressions uninterrupted with a ventilation rate of 10 breaths per minute. After two minutes of CPR recheck the rhythm, and if an organised rhythm is present also check for a pulse. If PEA persists, continue with two-minute cycles of CPR, giving further epinephrine 1 mg IV on alternate cycles (every 3–5 minutes). Repeated attempts should be made to identify and treat any potentially reversible causes.

As soon as **asystole** is diagnosed start CPR immediately. While continuing CPR, check that all monitoring devices are correctly attached and there is not a disconnection producing an apparent asystolic trace. Establish IV access, give 1 mg of epinephrine (IV), 3 mg of atropine (IV) and continue with CPR for two minutes, before rechecking the rhythm. If asystole persists, the airway should be secured and CPR continued in accordance with the ALS algorithm (Figure RS5). Epinephrine (1 mg IV boluses) should be given every 3–5 minutes. During rhythm checks the ECG should carefully be scrutinised for the presence of P waves: if present, pacing may restore a perfusing rhythm.

If at any time the rhythm changes to VF/VT then the shockable limb of the ALS algorithm should be followed.

Drug usage

The most common route for drug administration during a cardiorespiratory arrest is via a peripheral IV cannula. It is relatively quick and easy to establish, when compared with central venous access, and is safer. When drugs are given peripherally each dose should be flushed with 10–20 ml of saline and the limb elevated for 10–20 seconds to facilitate drug delivery. If a CVP line is present it should be used in preference to peripheral lines as higher peak drug concentrations are achieved and drug circulation times are shorter. However, to insert a central venous line at the time of a cardiac arrest is time-consuming, which necessitates time without chest compressions, and is associated with a high risk of complications. It is not recommended as standard treatment. The intraosseous (IO) route, although traditionally described in children, can also be considered in adults.

If unable to establish IV access, in an intubated patient, the tracheal route can also be used to administer some drugs. Plasma concentrations achieved from tracheal administration of drugs are extremely variable and unpredictable, and larger doses of the drug, 3–10 times the IV dose, are used. Dilute the drug to at least 10 ml with sterile water, not saline, as this may achieve better absorption.

Epinephrine

Epinephrine 1 mg IV is the vasopressor of choice in all forms of cardiac arrest. It has potent alpha effects, causing widespread vasoconstriction and increasing coronary and cerebral perfusion pressure. Its beneficial beta-adrenergic effects are increased coronary and cerebral blood flow through inotropic and chronotropic actions. However, some of these beneficial beta effects may be offset by increased myocardial oxygen consumption and increased ventricular arrhythmogenicity.

Vasopressin

A recent meta-analysis (Aung & Htay 2005) has shown no statistical difference, in terms of return of spontaneous circulation, between the use of vasopressin and epinephrine. Vasopressin is a naturally occurring antidiuretic hormone and has powerful vasoconstrictor effects through its action on smooth muscle V1 receptors. There is insufficient evidence to recommend a change to the use of vasopressin as a first-line vasopressor in cases of cardiac arrest.

Atropine

A single dose of atropine 3 mg IV, which will provide maximum vagal blockade, may theoretically reverse asystole that is precipitated or exacerbated by excessive vagal tone.

Amiodarone

Amiodarone is a membrane-stabilising antiarrhythmic drug that increases the duration of both the action potential and refractory period in atrial and ventricular myocardium, as well as slowing atrioventricular conduction. It has mild negative inotropic actions and causes peripheral vasodilatation.

Amiodarone is used in shock-refractory VF/VT. If VF/VT persists after three shocks, 300 mg amiodarone IV should be given. A further dose of 150 mg followed by an infusion of 900 mg over 24 hours is then recommended. It is also indicated in haemodynamically stable VT.

Lidocaine

Lidocaine's position as the first-line antiarrhythmic drug has now been superseded by amiodarone. Lidocaine has a membrane-stabilising action and increases the refractory period. It can be used in a dose of 1 mg kg^{-1} in shock-refractory VF/VT if amiodarone is not readily available. It should not be used if amiodarone has already been given.

Sodium bicarbonate

The routine use of sodium bicarbonate during a cardiac arrest is not recommended. The best treatment for an acidosis resulting from cardiorespiratory arrest is good-quality CPR and a rapid return of spontaneous circulation. Bicarbonate has a number of adverse effects, including the exacerbation of intracellular acidosis, a negative inotropic effect on ischaemic myocardium, a large sodium load, and the shift of the oxygen dissociation curve to the left, which further inhibits release of oxygen to tissues.

The use of 50 mmol of sodium bicarbonate is indicated if the cardiac arrest is associated with hyperkalaemia or tricyclic antidepressant overdose, or in patients with pre-existing metabolic acidosis. The use of bicarbonate when the arterial pH is less than 7.1 remains controversial. The dose of bicarbonate may be repeated if necessary according to the patient's clinical condition and repeated blood gas analysis.

Arterial blood gases do not accurately reflect acid–base status of tissues during a cardiorespiratory arrest. There is a rapid accumulation of carbon dioxide and lactic acid due to poor tissue perfusion and a marked arteriovenous difference in pH. Theoretically a mixed venous gas, or venous gas taken from a central line, will provide a closer estimate of tissue acid–base status.

Calcium

Calcium has a vital role in cellular mechanisms underlying myocardial contraction. It is indicated in PEA secondary to hyperkalaemia, hypocalcaemia, overdose of calcium blocking drugs and overdose of magnesium. The initial dose is 10 ml of 10% calcium chloride (6.8 mmol Ca^{2+}).

Calcium should be used cautiously, as high levels are harmful to ischaemic myocardium and may impair cerebral recovery. It may also slow the heart and cause arrhythmias. Calcium must not be given simultaneously with bicarbonate through the same IV access.

Magnesium

Magnesium (4 ml of 50% solution; 8 mmol) should be given for refractory VF when there is any suspicion of hypomagnesaemia, e.g. patients on potassium-losing diuretics. It should also be considered in torsades de pointes and digoxin toxicity.

Aminophylline

Aminophylline is a phosphodiesterase inhibitor which has chronotropic and inotropic actions. It may be used in asystolic cardiac arrest or peri-arrest bradycardia which is refractory to atropine.

Fibrinolytics

Fibrinolytics should be considered in patients with proven or suspected pulmonary embolism. There is insufficient evidence to recommend its use in cardiac arrest from other causes.

Complications of CPR

Iatrogenic complications of CPR are relatively common, and some of these may pose problems in the post-resuscitation period. However, since the alternative to CPR is death, CPR can be justified in most circumstances provided that care is taken to minimise the risks both to the patient and to the rescuer.

Frequent complications of chest compressions include rib and sternal fractures, and less commonly visceral and cardiac trauma. Poor airway management may lead to aspiration of gastric contents or unrecognised oesophageal intubation.

Other post-resuscitation problems, not necessarily resulting from substandard CPR, include pulmonary oedema, recurrent cardiac arrest, cardiogenic shock, multiple organ dysfunction and adverse neurological outcome (see below).

Complications associated with defibrillator use

A clear 'stand back' command should be given prior to defibrillation to avoid accidental defibrillation of a member of the resuscitation team.

There have been several reports of burns to patients through the incorrect use of defibrillator paddles. Poor contact between defibrillator paddles/pads and the patient's chest increases transthoracic impedance, which causes arcing of current and burns to the patient. Manual metal paddles must always be used with conduction gel or gel pads to reduce this risk, and this may be further reduced by the use of self-adhesive pads. Excessively hairy patients may need to be shaved to ensure good paddle/pad contact prior to defibrillation. GTN patches must also be removed before defibrillation.

Sparks from poorly applied defibrillator paddles/pads may cause a fire in an oxygen-rich environment. Risks of fire from oxygen during defibrillation may be minimised by the following strategies. If using bag-mask ventilation the oxygen mask should be moved to a distance of at least one metre from the patient's chest during defibrillation. Leave a ventilation bag attached to an endotracheal tube provided the oxygen source is more than one metre away. In the critical care/theatre setting the ventilator should be left connected to the patient.

Transmission of infection

There have been isolated reports of rescuers becoming infected with tuberculosis and severe acute respiratory syndrome (SARS) from patients during CPR. The transmission of HIV through CPR has never been reported. Universal safety precautions should be taken when dealing with patients known to have serious infections, e.g. tuberculosis, HIV, hepatitis B virus or SARS.

Neurological injury

Although not entirely preventable, poor neurological outcome may be minimised by meticulous care in the immediate post-resuscitation period. Ideally the patient should be transferred to a critical care setting, where he or she may require a period of intubation, sedation and controlled ventilation to optimise oxygenation and maintain normocarbia. Invasive monitoring, inotropes, vasodilators and diuretics may be required to optimise the patient haemodynamically. Insulin should be given to ensure tight glycaemic control, and hyperthermia should be treated aggressively with antipyretics. There is some evidence emerging that a period of active cooling to induce therapeutic hypothermia, 32–34 °C for 12–24 hours after the arrest, may improve neurological outcome, particularly when the presenting rhythm is VF. Seizures should be controlled by the use of anticonvulsants, e.g. benzodiazepines, phenytoin and/or barbiturates.

Management of life-threatening peri-arrest arrhythmias

Life-threatening peri-arrest arrhythmias can be divided into two broad groups, those that are stable and can be treated with antiarrhythmic drugs, and those that are unstable and need immediate cardioversion or pacing. In general the action of drugs is slower and less reliable than electricity. All antiarrhythmic treatments – physical manoeuvres, drugs and electrical cardioversion – can also be pro-arrhythmogenic, and antiarrhythmic drugs may cause myocardial depression and hypotension. Initial management is to assess the patient, give oxygen, gain IV access, record a 12-lead ECG (Figure RS6) and correct any

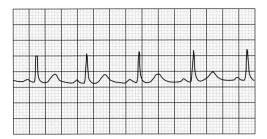

Normal

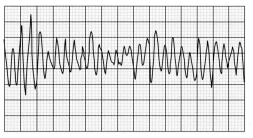

Ventricular fibrillation

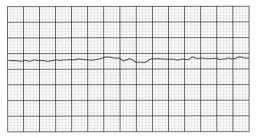

Asystole

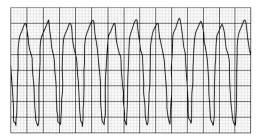

Broad complex tachycardia

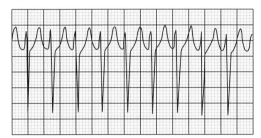

Narrow complex tachycardia

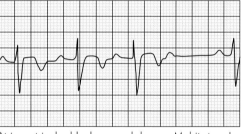

Atrioventricular block, second degree, Mobitz type I (Wenkebach)

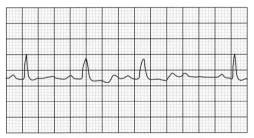
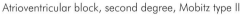
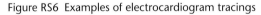

Atrioventricular block, second degree, Mobitz type II

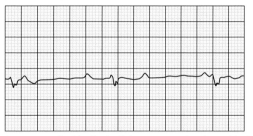

Atrioventricular block, third degree, complete heart block

Figure RS6 Examples of electrocardiogram tracings

electrolyte abnormalities, particularly potassium, magnesium and calcium.

Signs of an unstable arrhythmia include pallor, sweating, impaired conscious level and hypotension. These all reflect an inadequate cardiac output. Chest pain, secondary to myocardial ischaemia, is often precipitated by excessive heart rates. Similarly, low heart rates may not be tolerated in patients with poor cardiac reserve. Signs of heart failure, i.e. pulmonary oedema, raised jugular venous pressure and hepatic engorgement, may also be present.

If appropriate, give oxygen, cannulate a vein, and record a 12-lead ECG

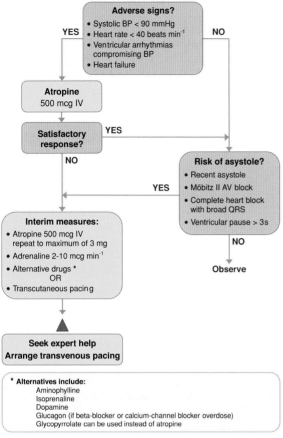

Adverse signs?
- Systolic BP < 90 mmHg
- Heart rate < 40 beats min^{-1}
- Ventricular arrhythmias compromising BP
- Heart failure

YES   NO

Atropine
500 mcg IV

Satisfactory response?   YES

NO

Risk of asystole?
- Recent asystole
- Möbitz II AV block
- Complete heart block with broad QRS
- Ventricular pause > 3s

YES

Interim measures:
- Atropine 500 mcg IV repeat to maximum of 3 mg
- Adrenaline 2-10 mcg min^{-1}
- Alternative drugs *
  OR
- Transcutaneous pacing

NO

Observe

**Seek expert help
Arrange transvenous pacing**

* **Alternatives include:**
  Aminophylline
  Isoprenaline
  Dopamine
  Glucagon (if beta-blocker or calcium-channel blocker overdose)
  Glycopyrrolate can be used instead of atropine

Figure RS7 Bradycardia algorithm (includes rate inappropriately slow for haemodynamic state) © European Resuscitation Council (2005) and Resuscitation Council (UK) (2005)

Bradycardias

A bradycardia is defined as a heart rate of less than 40, or a heart rate of less than 60 in a haemodynamically compromised patient. In a symptomatic patient give atropine 500 µg IV, and if the patient remains symptomatic, repeat this dose every 3–5 minutes up to a maximum of 3 g. If there has been a calcium antagonist or beta-blocker overdose consider using glucagon (Figure RS7).

If the patient is at risk of developing asystole, transvenous pacing may be required. Risk factors for a bradycardia deteriorating to asystole include a recent episode of asystole, Mobitz type II AV block, third-degree (complete) heart block (Figure RS6), or ventricular standstill of more than three seconds. Complete heart block with narrow complexes may not require immediate pacing, as AV junctional ectopic pacemakers can provide a reasonable and stable cardiac output.

Transvenous pacing is the definitive treatment, but if the expertise is not readily available, patients may be managed temporarily with either transcutaneous pacing or an epinephrine infusion in the range of 2–10 µg per minute. If there is no pacing equipment immediately available, fist pacing may be attempted. Apply serial rhythmic blows with a closed fist over the left sternal edge to pace the heart at physiological rate of 50–70 times a minute.

Tachycardias

Guidelines for the management of tachycardias are now contained in a single algorithm that includes treatment of narrow complex tachycardias, broad complex tachycardias and atrial fibrillation (Figure RS8). In an unstable patient, electrical cardioversion should be attempted immediately. The shock must be synchronised to occur with the R wave of the electrocardiogram. If not, and it is delivered during a relatively refractory portion of the cardiac cycle, VF may be induced. A starting energy level of 120–150 J biphasic (200 J monophasic) should be used, except in atrial flutter and other narrow complex tachycardias, which will often cardiovert at lower energy levels (70–120 J biphasic, 100 J monophasic). Although electrical cardioversion is effective it does not prevent the occurrence of subsequent arrhythmias, which should be treated with drugs.

Tachycardias are relatively common in the critically ill patient. As well as treating the arrhythmia, if the patient is clinically compromised, the underlying illness (e.g. sepsis) must also be treated. In patients with normal hearts, adverse signs are unlikely to occur with heart rates of less than 150 per minute.

Broad complex tachycardia

A broad complex tachycardia has a QRS complex greater than 0.12 seconds. They are usually ventricular in origin, but can also be supraventricular with aberrant conduction. If the patient is unstable, treat with electrical cardioversion.

If stable, determine whether the arrhythmia is regular or irregular.
- A **regular** broad complex tachycardia is likely to be VT or a supraventricular rhythm with bundle branch block. Treat with amiodarone 300 mg IV followed by 900 mg over 24 hours. If the arrhythmia is known to be supraventricular, treat as a narrow complex tachycardia.

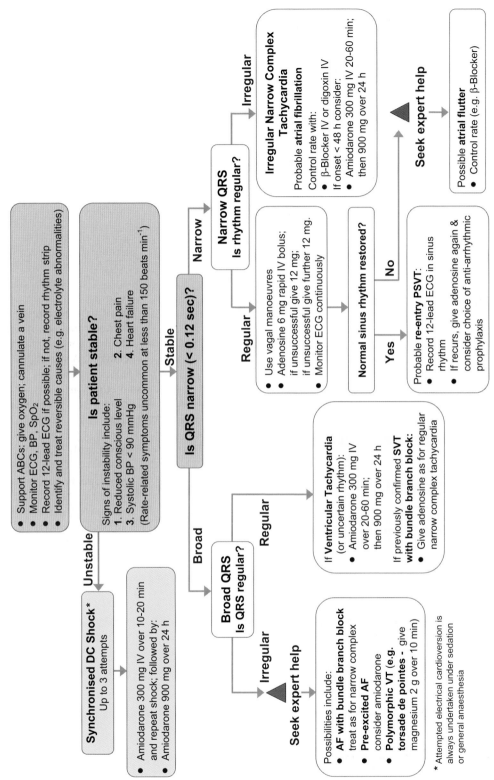

Figure RS8 Tachycardia algorithm (with pulse) © European Resuscitation Council (2005) and Resuscitation Council (UK) (2005)

- An **irregular** broad complex tachycardia is most likely to be atrial fibrillation with bundle branch block, and should be treated as narrow complex atrial fibrillation.

Other possible causes for broad complex tachycardias include atrial fibrillation with ventricular pre-excitation, i.e. patients with Wolff–Parkinson–White (WPW) syndrome, or torsades de pointes (polymorphic VT). In a stable patient who is known to have WPW, the use of amiodarone is probably safe. Adenosine, digoxin, verapamil and diltiazem must be avoided, as these drugs block the AV node and will cause a relative increase in pre-excitation. If possible, expert cardiological advice should be sought in the assessment and management of these patients. Electrical cardioversion remains the safest option for the treatment of the unstable patient.

Torsades de pointes is treated by stopping all drugs known to prolong the QT interval and correcting electrolyte abnormalities. Magnesium sulphate (2 g IV over 10 minutes) should also be given. Expert help is often required to manage these patients, who may require ventricular pacing. If the patient's condition deteriorates proceed to synchronised electrical cardioversion or, if the patient is pulseless, commence the ALS algorithm (Figure RS5).

Narrow complex tachycardia

A narrow complex tachycardia has a QRS interval of less than 0.12 seconds. Sinus tachycardia is a common physiological response to exercise or anxiety and is also seen in patients who are anaemic, in pain, pyrexial or shocked. The management of the tachycardia in these cases is by treating the cause.

Other causes of a regular narrow complex tachycardia include:

- AV nodal re-entry tachycardia (AVNRT). This is the commonest type of paroxysmal supraventricular tachycardia (PSVT). It is often seen in people without any heart disease, and is usually benign. It is a regular narrow complex tachycardia with P waves often not visible.
- AV re-entry tachycardia (AVRT). This occurs in patients with WPW, and is usually benign unless there is coexisting structural heart disease. Again it is a regular narrow complex tachycardia, with P waves often not visible.
- Atrial flutter with regular AV conduction. This usually presents as a 2 : 1 block and produces a tachycardia with a rate of 150 beats per minute. Flutter waves may be difficult to see.

An unstable patient presenting with a **regular** narrow complex tachycardia should be treated with electrical cardioversion. If this is not immediately available, adenosine should be given as a first-line treatment.

A stable patient presenting with a regular narrow complex tachycardia should initially be treated by vagal manoeuvres such as carotid sinus massage or the Valsalva manoeuvre, as these will terminate up to a quarter of episodes of PSVT. Carotid sinus massage should be avoided in the elderly, especially if a carotid bruit is present, as it may dislodge an atheromatous plaque and cause a stroke.

If the tachycardia persists and is not atrial flutter, 6 mg of adenosine should be given as an IV bolus, followed by a 12 mg bolus if no response. A further 12 mg bolus of adenosine may be given if the tachycardia persists. Vagal manoeuvres or adenosine will terminate almost all AVNRTs or AVRTs within seconds, and therefore failure to convert suggests an atrial tachycardia such as atrial flutter. If adenosine is contraindicated, or fails to terminate a narrow complex tachycardia, without first demonstrating it as atrial flutter, give a calcium-channel blocker, e.g. verapamil 2.5–5 mg IV over two minutes. Atrial flutter should be treated by rate control with a beta-blocker.

An **irregular** narrow complex tachycardia is most likely to be atrial fibrillation (AF) with an uncontrolled ventricular response, but may also be atrial flutter with variable block. If the patient is unstable, synchronised electrical cardioversion should be used to treat the arrhythmia.

In a stable patient, treatment options include:

- Rate control by drug therapy. Drugs used to control the heart rate include beta-blockers, digoxin, magnesium, calcium antagonists or a combination of these.
- Rhythm control by amiodarone to encourage cardioversion. Amiodarone is given as a 300 mg IV bolus, followed by 900 mg IV over 24 hours.
- Rhythm control by electrical cardioversion. This is more likely to restore sinus rhythm than chemical cardioversion.
- Treatment to prevent complications. Patients who are in AF are at risk of atrial thrombus formation and should be anticoagulated.

Resuscitation of the pregnant patient

Although there are two potential patients, the best chance of fetal survival is the prompt management of the critically ill mother. It is essential, therefore, that when dealing with a cardiorespiratory arrest in a pregnant patient there is early involvement of a senior obstetrician and neonatologist. A decision to perform a perimortem Caesarean section must be taken early during the resuscitation attempt. If the gestational age of the fetus is more than 24–25 weeks a Caesarean section must definitely be performed, as it may save the life of both mother and baby. If the gestational age is 20–23 weeks a Caesarean section will improve the chances of survival of the mother and should therefore be performed, even though the baby is highly unlikely to survive.

Prompt delivery of the fetus of more than 20 weeks gestation, ideally within five minutes of the cardiac arrest, relieves aortocaval compression and improves thoracic compliance. This increases the efficiency of both chest compressions and ventilation, and improves the chances of survival of both baby and mother.

There are a number of factors that tip the balance of resuscitating the pregnant patient towards non-survival when compared with a non-pregnant patient of similar age. Airway management is made more difficult by the presence of laryngeal oedema and obesity. Other physiological changes of pregnancy predispose a pregnant patient to a greater risk of aspiration owing to the incompetence of the gastroesophageal sphincter and increased intragastric pressure. In addition, the maintenance of adequate oxygenation through ventilation is made more difficult by increased oxygen demand, decreased chest compliance and a reduced functional residual capacity.

Causes

The incidence of cardiac arrests occurring during late pregnancy is 1 in 30 000. Indirect deaths from medical conditions exacerbated by pregnancy are much more frequent than deaths from conditions that arise as a result of pregnancy itself. Causes of cardiorespiratory arrest that also occur in non-pregnant women of a similar age group include acute coronary syndromes, often in patients with pre-existing IHD, congenital heart disease, anaphylaxis, trauma and drug overdose.

Additional causes related to the pregnancy itself are:
- Haemorrhage
- Hypertensive disease of pregnancy
- Peripartum cardiomyopathy
- Amniotic fluid embolism
- Pulmonary embolism

As in the non-pregnant patient, common and reversible causes of cardiorespiratory arrest should be promptly recognised and treated during CPR.

Basic life support

BLS should be performed in accordance with the standard adult algorithm (Figure RS3). However, there are a number of issues which make the resuscitation attempt more difficult in the pregnant patient.

- The **airway** will need to be managed with the patient in the semi-lateral position in order to avoid aortocaval syndrome. Pregnant patients are at an increased risk of aspiration, and cricoid pressure should be applied as soon as expertise is available. The patient should be intubated as soon as possible.
- Rescue **breathing** is more difficult as there is reduced chest compliance secondary to flaring of the ribs, splinting of the diaphragm by abdominal contents and the presence of hypertrophied breasts.
- The hand position for **cardiac compressions** should be moved up the sternum, as the diaphragm is displaced upwards by the abdominal contents. Aortocaval compression, a risk from about 20 weeks gestation, must be avoided by lateral displacement of the uterus. To achieve this, the patient can be tilted onto the rescuer's knees, or purpose-made wedges or pillows may be used. Effective forces for chest compression can still be generated up to a 30-degree tilt. Manual displacement of the uterus may also be performed.

Advanced life support

ALS is performed in accordance with the standard adult algorithm (Figure RS5).

Factors which make airway management more difficult in the pregnant patient include the presence of full dentition, hypertrophied breasts, obesity and laryngeal oedema. Tracheal intubation should be carried out as soon as possible. A smaller size of endotracheal tube may be needed and a polio blade required to facilitate access.

It is more difficult to apply paddles/pads for defibrillation owing to the presence of hypertrophied breasts and obesity. There is no evidence of adverse effects of defibrillation to the fetus, and standard energy levels for adults should be used.

Tachyarrhythmias secondary to bupivacaine toxicity are often intractable and are best treated with defibrillation. Cardiac massage may have to be sustained for long periods of time, up to an hour, as bupivacaine is highly tissue-bound and defibrillation may not be successful until some recovery of the myocardium has occurred.

Drug usage

Drugs should be used in accordance with ALS recommendations.

Magnesium sulphate is increasingly used in the management of pre-eclampsia and eclampsia, and if high magnesium concentrations are thought to have contributed to the cardiac arrest then calcium chloride or calcium gluconate should be given intravenously.

Resuscitation of infants and children

There remains little scientific evidence looking specifically at resuscitation in infants and children, and much of the evidence used in producing the following guidelines has been extrapolated from adult studies. The guidelines have been simplified so that there is now a single cardiac compression : ventilation ratio (15 : 2) for all infants and children regardless of age. When a child reaches puberty the adult resuscitation guidelines should be used.

For the guidelines that follow the definition of an infant is a child of less than one year, and a child is from the age of one year until puberty.

Causes

Cardiac arrests tend to occur less commonly in children than in adults, and the aetiology is usually different. They are usually secondary to either respiratory or circulatory failure, rather than originating from a primary cardiac problem. The presenting rhythm is usually a severe bradycardia or asystole resulting from hypoxia. Causes of secondary cardiac arrest in children include trauma, drowning and poisoning.

Primary cardiac arrests resulting in VF are relatively rare, comprising 7–15% of all paediatric arrests. VF tends not to be seen in children unless they are known to have heart disease, and more often occurs in hospitals on critical care units and cardiac wards. In a previously normal child who presents with VF/VT, hypothermia, drug effects and electrolyte disturbances must be considered.

Basic life support

If only the adult BLS algorithm is known, it can be used in children, but the paediatric BLS algorithm has certain modifications which make it more suitable for this age group (Figure RS9).

Confirm that a cardiac arrest has occurred, by gently stimulating the child and asking loudly 'are you alright?' Do not shake the child if a cervical spine injury is suspected. For the single rescuer, one minute of CPR is recommended before calling for help, as the cardiac arrest is more likely to be secondary to hypoxia and this may rapidly respond to rescue breathing. Five initial rescue breaths should be given before starting cardiac compressions. However, if a

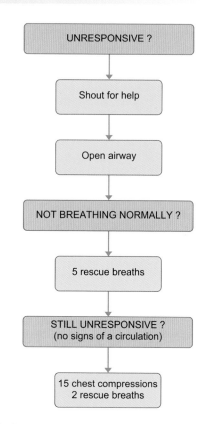

Figure RS9 Paediatric BLS algorithm © European Resuscitation Council (2005) and Resuscitation Council (UK) (2005)

sudden collapse is witnessed, it is more likely to be due to a primary cardiac arrhythmia, and defibrillation takes priority.

Airway

Simple manoeuvres should be used to open the airway. Place a hand on the child's forehead and gently tilt the head back while performing a chin lift. An infant's airway should be managed in the neutral position, although a gentle head tilt manoeuvre may be required to achieve this owing to the relatively large occiput. Care must be taken when positioning fingers so as not to compress the soft tissues, as this may cause airway obstruction. If unable to clear the airway by these manoeuvres alone, the jaw thrust may also be used in children.

Breathing

Assess whether the child or infant is breathing normally by looking for chest movements, listening at the nose and mouth for breath sounds, and feeling for air movement. This assessment should last no longer than 10 seconds.

If the child or infant is not breathing normally, or is only taking infrequent irregular breaths, then rescue breathing should be commenced immediately, and five breaths should be given consecutively. For a child, mouth-to-mouth or mouth-to-nose rescue breathing may be used. In infants, a technique of mouth to mouth-and-nose rescue breathing may be required. Inflation should last for 1–1.5 seconds and the chest observed to rise and fall.

If, despite optimal positioning and having cleared the mouth of any obvious obstructions, adequate rescue breathing is not achieved, move straight on to cardiac compressions.

Circulation

As in adults, signs of circulation include movement, coughing or normal breathing. If confident to do so, check for a pulse, but take no longer than 10 seconds. In a child the carotid pulse should be used for assessment, and in infants the brachial pulse. If circulation is present continue rescue breathing only. If there are no signs of circulation or the pulse rate is less than 60 with poor perfusion, rescue breathing should be combined with cardiac compressions.

Cardiac compressions should compress the chest by approximately one-third of its depth at a rate of 100 compressions per minute. The correct ratio of cardiac compressions : rescue breaths is 15 : 2 for two rescuers, but if alone use the adult ratio of 30 : 2. The advice is to push hard, push fast, minimise interruptions and allow for full chest recoil.

To locate the correct position for hand placement in children, identify the xiphisternum and place the hands one finger's breadth above this. Depending on the size of the child one or two hands may be used. It is important that the pressure is applied over the lower third of the sternum and not the ribs.

In infants either two fingertips may be used to apply cardiac compressions or, when two or more rescuers are present, the two-thumb encircling technique. The two-thumb encircling technique has been shown to produce higher coronary perfusion pressures, as the correct depth and force of compressions are more consistently achieved. However, for the single rescuer it is difficult to swap from

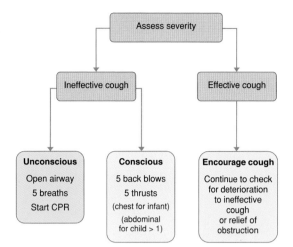

Figure RS10 Paediatric foreign-body airway obstruction algorithm © European Resuscitation Council (2005) and Resuscitation Council (UK) (2005)

cardiac compressions to rescue breathing, so the two-finger technique is preferable.

Once spontaneous circulation and ventilation is established the child must be placed in the recovery position.

Foreign-body airway obstruction

The majority of choking episodes in children and infants are witnessed and occur during play or eating. The child or infant is usually conscious in the initial stages, but if the obstruction is not rapidly cleared, cardiac arrest secondary to hypoxia will ensue. Choking, which occurs suddenly, must be differentiated from other causes of upper airway obstruction in children and infants, such as laryngitis, epiglottitis and croup, in which they are systemically ill and require different management.

The management of choking in children (Figure RS10) is very similar to that in adults. If the victim is conscious and coughing then further coughing should be encouraged. If there is an inadequate cough, and the child remains conscious, then back blows followed by abdominal thrusts should be used to attempt to dislodge the foreign body. In infants, chest thrusts should be used in place of abdominal thrusts. These are similar to chest compressions, but sharper in nature and delivered at slower rate. Abdominal thrusts should not be used to treat choking in infants because the more horizontal position of their ribs leaves the upper abdominal viscera more exposed to trauma.

All these manoeuvres create an 'artificial cough' with the aim of increasing intrathoracic pressure and dislodging

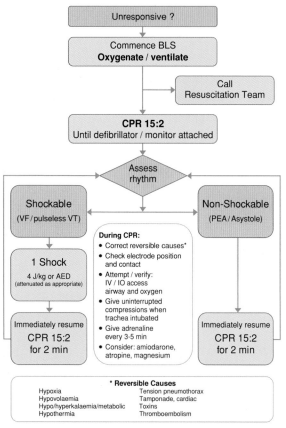

Figure RS11 Paediatric ALS algorithm © European Resuscitation Council (2005) and Resuscitation Council (UK) (2005)

the foreign body. The head of the patient should be kept dependent. Obviously the position used will depend on the size of both the child and the rescuer.

If at any time the child becomes unconscious, commence the paediatric BLS algorithm (Figure RS9).

Advanced life support

As in the adult ALS guidelines, the emphasis for paediatric ALS is continuous cardiac compressions, minimising the 'time off chest' for assessment of cardiac rhythm, defibrillation and endotracheal intubation. The paediatric ALS algorithm (Figure RS11) provides a standardised approach for the treatment of a cardiac arrest in infants and children. During resuscitation attempts reversible causes should be identified and treated as soon as possible.

Airway

Simple oropharyngeal or nasopharyngeal airways, or LMAs, may be used in children. Although they provide

a clear airway for ventilation they do not protect against aspiration or inadvertent gastric distension. Endotracheal intubation remains the airway of choice as it ensures a secure protected airway and, once the patient is intubated, cardiac compressions can be performed continuously.

Traditionally uncuffed endotracheal tubes have been used in children below the age of puberty. There is some evidence that there is no greater risk of complications when cuffed tubes are used in preference to uncuffed tubes even in young children (Cox 2005). A smaller size of cuffed tube may need to be used, and meticulous care must be taken when inflating cuffs since excessive pressures will lead to ischaemic necrosis of surrounding laryngeal tissues and stenosis.

Ventilation

100% oxygen should be used for ventilation during resuscitation. Ventilation should be performed at a rate of 12–20 breaths per minute, and the ideal tidal volume should achieve a modest chest wall rise.

Circulation

Assess the patient for signs of spontaneous circulation, and monitor the cardiac rhythm using either cardiac electrodes in the standard positions or paediatric defibrillator paddles/pads placed just below the right clavicle and at the left anterior axillary line. In small children and infants, placing the paddles/pads front and back may be more appropriate. The cardiac rhythm will determine which limb of the ALS algorithm to follow.

Cardiac compressions should be performed as described for BLS. The person performing cardiac compressions should be changed after every two-minute cycle, as the quality of compressions will decrease with fatigue.

Non-shockable rhythms (asystole or PEA)

Asystole and PEA should be managed according to the non-shockable limb of the paediatric ALS algorithm (Figure RS11) with repeated doses of epinephrine (10 µg kg^{-1} IV or IO) every 3–5 minutes.

Shockable rhythms (VF/VT)

VF and VT should be managed according to the shockable limb of the paediatric ALS algorithm (Figure RS11). The recommendation for the use of a single-shock protocol is based on extrapolated evidence from adult studies. The optimum energy for safe and effective defibrillation in children is unknown, but relatively high energies are known to cause less myocardial damage in children than in adults. The use of biphasic defibrillation is more effective and causes less post-shock myocardial dysfunction. The recommended energy level for defibrillation in children is a non-escalating level of 4 J kg^{-1} (both for monophasic and biphasic defibrillators).

If using an AED device, purpose-made paediatric pads are available which attenuate the output of the machine to 50–75 J. These should be used in children aged one to eight years. Above the age of eight use the adult energy levels. AEDs are not recommended for use in infants.

Once VF or VT is identified, attempt defibrillation as soon as possible and then continue with CPR for two minutes before rechecking the rhythm. If VF/VT persists give a further shock at the same energy level. Again resume CPR for a further two minutes, prior to reassessing the rhythm. If VF/VT continues, epinephrine (10 μg kg^{-1} IV or IO) should be given immediately before the third shock. Again resume CPR for two minutes prior to assessing the rhythm, and if VF/VT persists give amiodarone (5 mg kg^{-1} IV or IO) before the fourth shock.

If VF/VT continues, two-minute cycles of CPR should be performed, pausing only briefly to assess the rhythm. Epinephrine should be given on alternate cycles.

Drug usage

IV access for fluid and drug administration can be very difficult to establish in small children. If not rapidly achieved, insert an IO needle into the proximal tibia to provide vascular access. When using the IO route for drug administration each dose of drug should be followed by a bolus of normal saline to disperse the drug beyond the marrow cavity into the central circulation. In an intubated patient, if unable to achieve IV or IO access, epinephrine, lidocaine, atropine, naloxone and vasopressin may all be given via the endotracheal route.

Since hypovolaemia is a potentially reversible cause of cardiac arrest, unless there are obvious signs of volume overload volume expansion is always indicated. A 20 ml kg^{-1} bolus of an isotonic saline solution should be given, and repeated as necessary. The use of dextrose-based solutions should be avoided, unless there is hypoglycaemia, since it leads to hyponatraemia and hyperglycaemia, which are both associated with poor neurological outcomes after cardiac arrest.

Epinephrine

The use of epinephrine in paediatric cardiac arrest improves coronary and cerebral perfusion due to its potent alpha- and beta-adrenergic actions. The recommended dose in children and infants is 10 μg kg^{-1} (IV/IO) or 100 μg kg^{-1} (via the tracheal route). The use of epinephrine

via the endotracheal route should be avoided if possible, since lower plasma epinephrine concentrations are achieved and these may produce transient beta effects such as hypotension and reduced coronary artery perfusion pressure. The use of higher doses of epinephrine has not been shown to improve either survival or neurological outcome in children and is no longer recommended. The exception to this is if the cardiac arrest was secondary to beta-blocker overdose.

Amiodarone

Amiodarone is now the antiarrhythmic drug of choice in the management of persistent VT/VF. An initial 5 μg kg^{-1} IV/IO bolus should be used. When given via a peripheral vein, amiodarone causes thrombophlebitis and should therefore be flushed through with either dextrose or saline. As in adults, lidocaine is only recommended when amiodarone is unavailable.

Atropine

Since bradycardia and asystole are often secondary to hypoxia, the use of atropine is only recommended if the arrhythmia is unresponsive to ventilation with 100% oxygen and circulatory support. The dose of atropine is 20 μg kg^{-1} (max 600 μg), with a minimum recommended dose of 100 μg in order to avoid its paradoxical effects at low doses.

Sodium bicarbonate

The routine use of sodium bicarbonate during a cardiac arrest is not recommended (see drug usage in adult guidelines). The best treatment of acidosis developing during a cardiac arrest is good-quality cardiac compressions and ventilation. A dose of 1–2 ml kg^{-1} of 8.4% solution (IV or IO) is recommended if there is hyperkalaemia or arrhythmia secondary to tricyclic antidepressant overdose.

Ethical considerations in CPR

The issues that surround ethical decision making during cardiorespiratory resuscitation all relate to life-and-death decisions and the appropriateness of either starting or continuing resuscitation attempts. These decisions are often emotive and distressing, but this does not mean that they ought not to be made. It should be remembered that 70–90% of resuscitation attempts are unsuccessful, and therefore death is inevitable in the majority of cases.

The concept of CPR was originally introduced in the 1960s as a treatment for sudden unexpected deaths, but over the next two decades it evolved to be used for the majority of patients who suffered a cardiorespiratory arrest in hospital. Over the last 20 years guidelines have been developed to enable decisions to be made to stop or withhold resuscitation when inappropriate (BMA 2002). There continues, however, to be a lot of misunderstanding surrounding do-not-attempt-resuscitation (DNAR) orders. A DNAR order simply means that if a patient suffers a cardiorespiratory arrest, cardiac compressions, ventilation or defibrillation should not be attempted. DNAR does not mean 'for no treatment', and all other supportive care should be continued until it is decided that active treatment is inappropriate. At this time there should be a move from aggressive active care towards palliative care. Good communication and documentation of discussions is paramount when making DNAR and limitation of treatment decisions.

Justification of resuscitation

In order to justify resuscitation attempts, CPR must provide an overall benefit to the patient. This is the prolongation of life with a quality that is of value to the patient. For most people, as a minimum, this will be considered to be a life with awareness of their surroundings as well as the ability to interact with others and experience relationships. DNAR decisions are influenced by individual, cultural and religious factors.

There are a number of situations in which CPR will offer no benefit to the patient and should be considered futile. Examples include patients with metastatic malignant disease, those who are already showing signs of irreversible death, and patients who are in a critical care setting with deteriorating vital organ function despite being on maximal therapy, e.g. progressive septic or cardiogenic shock.

Whose decision?

As with any other medical decision, a competent patient who is fully informed has the right to refuse an attempt at resuscitation. Similarly, an advance directive should be considered legally binding.

Ultimately a decision to withhold or stop resuscitation is a medical decision. DNAR orders should be written by a senior doctor, but this should only be done after wide consultation with other healthcare professionals involved in the patient's care. In most cases the patient should also be involved in the decision-making process. If the patient is not competent, relatives should be approached to gain information about the patient's values and what the patient would have wanted to happen in this situation. The families must not be made to feel that they have made the decision. It must also be remembered that not all families will have

the patient's best interests at heart, and they may well have a vested interest in the patient's death or continued existence.

Although a competent patient may refuse resuscitation, he or she cannot demand an inappropriate treatment, and this includes a resuscitation attempt which is deemed to be futile. Where a patient is demanding an inappropriate resuscitation attempt, a second opinion or consultation with a clinical ethics forum should be sought. Application to the courts should be a last resort. There is no ethical imperative requiring a doctor to perform medical procedures in the absence of any medical benefit.

Withholding and withdrawing resuscitation

If there is any uncertainty as to the appropriateness of a resuscitation attempt, then CPR should be started immediately. There is no ethical difference between stopping a resuscitation attempt that has started and withholding resuscitation in the first place. Starting resuscitation allows for information to be gathered to aid decision making.

There are many factors to consider when deciding whether to abandon a resuscitation attempt. These include the medical history of the patient as well as the progress of the resuscitation attempt, e.g. the likely time gap between the cardiac arrest and the start of CPR and the duration of the resuscitation attempt. The longer the resuscitation attempt continues, the smaller the chance of the patient surviving either neurologically intact or to discharge from hospital. The duration of any individual resuscitation attempt is a matter of clinical judgement by the doctors present at the time. If VF persists and it was considered appropriate to start resuscitation, then it is probably worth continuing all the time the patient remains in VF/VT. For a non-VF/VT arrest, if at 20 minutes there continues to be asystole, and no reversible causes have been identified, then to continue CPR is probably futile.

When all the relevant information has been gathered, if it is found there is no justification to continue with resuscitation, CPR should be stopped.

DNAR orders in patients presenting for surgery

A DNAR order in a patient presenting for surgery is not a contraindication to proceeding with surgery. However, discussion needs to take place between the anaesthetist, the surgeon and the patient before surgery in order to clarify the goals and limitations of the proposed treatment. During anaesthesia and surgery there are often periods of increased cardiorespiratory instability, and there needs to be clear documentation regarding which interventions are appropriate. Clearly tracheal intubation, ventilation and the use of vasopressors may be needed, but it may still be felt that electrical cardioversion and cardiac compressions are inappropriate. In some cases, it may be appropriate to suspend the DNAR order, but this should only be taken after full discussion with the patient and surgeon regarding prognosis. General assumptions cannot be made in this situation, and decisions will need to be made on an individual patient basis.

Relatives' presence during resuscitation attempts

The concept of relatives being present during resuscitation attempts was first introduced during the 1980s, mainly in the case of paediatric resuscitation. Subsequent surveys showed that the majority of relatives found the experience of great value, and were the circumstances to be repeated they would wish to be present again. They found it gave them a realistic view of resuscitation, and they could see that everything was being done for their child. It also helped them come to terms with the reality of death and eased the bereavement period.

However, for this to work there must be a dedicated member of staff with the sole responsibility of looking after the relatives and explaining the events of the resuscitation attempt. The relatives must not be allowed to impede resuscitation, and may have to be removed if they do. The attempt must be well run, under good leadership, and the resuscitation team must be comfortable with the concept of family members being present.

The doctor in charge decides when to stop the resuscitation effort, not the patient's family, and this must be expressed with sensitivity and understanding.

References and further reading

Aung K, Htay T. Vasopressin for cardiac arrest: a systematic review and meta-analysis. *Arch Intern Med* 2005; **165**: 17–24.

British Medical Association, Resuscitation Council (UK), Royal College of Nursing. *Decisions Relating to Cardiopulmonary Resuscitation*. London: BMA, 2002.

Cox RG. *Should cuffed endotracheal tubes be used routinely in children? Can J Anaesth* 2005; **52**: 669–74.

European Resuscitation Council. European Resuscitation Council Guidelines for Resuscitation 2005. *Resuscitation* 2005; **67** (Suppl.1): S1–S190.

International Liaison Committee on Resuscitation. Proceedings of the 2005 International Consensus on Cardiopulmonary Resuscitation and Emergency Cardiovascular Care Science with Treatment Recommendations. *Resuscitation* 2005; **67**: 157–341.

Resuscitation Council (UK). *Resuscitation Guidelines 2005*. London: Resuscitation Council, 2005.

CHAPTER 9
Major trauma

J. P. Nolan

PATHOPHYSIOLOGY OF TRAUMA AND HYPOVOLAEMIA
Physiological responses to haemorrhage
Systemic inflammatory response syndrome

ASSESSMENT AND MANAGEMENT OF THE TRAUMA PATIENT
Prehospital phase
Preparation for resuscitation
Primary survey and resuscitation
Secondary survey

MEDICAL HISTORY

ANALGESIA
Systemic analgesia
Local and regional analgesia

MANAGEMENT OF BURNS

ANAESTHESIA FOR PATIENTS WITH SEVERE TRAUMA
Induction of anaesthesia
Intraoperative management

TECHNIQUES
Cannulation of major vessels for resuscitation and monitoring
Chest drainage

In the United Kingdom, trauma kills 14 500 people annually and is the commonest cause of death in those under 40 years. The advanced trauma life support (ATLS) course (American College of Surgeons Committee on Trauma 2004) provides a basic framework onto which hospital specialists can build their individual skills. The ATLS course focuses on the initial management of patients with major injuries during the so-called 'golden hour'. The golden hour reflects the importance of timely treatment. A severely injured patient who is hypoxic, in haemorrhagic shock, or who has an expanding intracranial haematoma, for example, will need rapid, effective resuscitation. The aim is to restore cellular oxygenation before the onset of irreversible shock.

Pathophysiology of trauma and hypovolaemia

Several mechanisms are involved in the development of cellular injury after severe trauma. The commonest is haemorrhage, causing circulatory failure with poor tissue perfusion and generalised hypoxia (hypovolaemic shock). Myocardial trauma may cause cardiogenic shock, while spinal cord trauma may cause neurogenic shock. Severe trauma is a potent cause of the systemic inflammatory response syndrome (SIRS) and this may progress to the multiple organ dysfunction syndrome (MODS) and multiple organ failure.

Physiological responses to haemorrhage

Trauma compromises tissue oxygenation because haemorrhage reduces oxygen delivery and tissue injury and inflammation increase oxygen consumption.

Compensatory responses to haemorrhage are categorised into immediate, early and late. The loss of blood volume is detected by low-pressure stretch receptors in the atria and arterial baroreceptors in the aorta and carotid artery. Efferents from the vasomotor centre trigger an increase in catecholamines, which causes arteriolar constriction, venoconstriction and tachycardia. Early compensatory mechanisms (5–60 minutes) include movement of fluid from the interstitium to the intravascular space and mobilisation of intracellular fluid. Long-term compensation to haemorrhage is by several mechanisms: reduced glomerular filtration rate, salt and water reabsorption (aldosterone and vasopressin), thirst, and increased erythropoiesis.

Hypovolaemic shock can be conveniently divided into four classes according to the percentage of the total blood volume lost, and the associated symptoms and signs (Figure TT1). Blood loss of 15–30% of the total blood volume will typically be associated with a tachycardia

Fundamentals of Anaesthesia, 3rd edition, ed. Tim Smith, Colin Pinnock and Ted Lin. Published by Cambridge University Press. © Cambridge University Press 2008.

	Class 1	Class 2	Class 3	Class 4
Blood loss (% of TBV)	<15%	15–30%	30–40%	>40%
Blood loss per 70 kg (ml)	750	750–1500	1500–2000	>2000
Systolic BP	Normal	Normal	Reduced	Very low
Diastolic BP	Normal	Raised	Reduced	Very low
Heart rate	<100	>100	>120	>140
Respiratory rate	14–20	20–30	30–40	30–40
Urine output (ml h^{-1})	>30	20–30	10–20	0
Mental state	Alert	Anxious or aggressive	Confused	Drowsy or unconscious

Figure TT1 A classification of haemorrhagic shock

>100 bpm and reduced pulse pressure; the increase in diastolic pressure reflects peripheral vasoconstriction. A decrease in systolic pressure suggests a loss of >30% of total blood volume (approximately 1500 ml in a 70 kg adult). Pure haemorrhage without the presence of significant tissue injury may not cause this typical pattern of a stepwise increase in heart rate. Occasionally, the heart rate may remain relatively low until the onset of cardiovascular collapse (Thomas & Dixon 2004).

Haemorrhagic shock causes a significant lactic acidosis: once the mitochondrial PO$_2$ is less than 2 mmHg oxidative phosphorylation is inhibited and pyruvate is unable to enter the Krebs cycle. Instead, pyruvate undergoes anaerobic metabolism in the cytoplasm, a process that is relatively inefficient for adenosine triphosphate (ATP) generation. ATP depletion causes cell membrane pump failure and cell death. Resuscitation must restore oxygen delivery rapidly if irreversible haemorrhagic shock and death of the patient is to be prevented.

Systemic inflammatory response syndrome

Crushed and wounded tissues activate complement which in turn triggers a cascade of inflammatory mediators (C3a, C5a, tumour necrosis factor α (TNF-α), interleukin 1 (IL-1), IL-6 and IL-8). Thus, severe trauma is a potent cause of the systemic inflammatory response syndrome. The diagnostic features of SIRS (Bone 1992) are summarised in Figure TT2. The extent of the inflammatory response to trauma in individuals is influenced significantly by genetic polymorphisms (Cobb & O'Keefe 2004).

In response to trauma, large numbers of polymorphonuclear neutrophils (PMNs) are released from human bone marrow. Depending on the presence of various modulators, the PMNs adhere tightly to endothelium and migrate into the surrounding parenchyma, where they are activated to release superoxide anion (O$_2^-$) and elastase (Roumen et al. 1995). This inflammatory response plays a key role in the development of acute respiratory distress syndrome (ARDS) and MODS (Goris 1996, Saadia & Lipman 1996, Lee et al. 2001, Giannoudis 2003). The metabolic response to severe trauma is biphasic. SIRS occurs during the initial 3–5 days; during this phase, a second insult (or hit), such as surgery, may provoke an exaggerated inflammatory response. Up to 50% of the patients developing organ failure early after trauma do so in the absence of bacterial infection. The initial phase is followed by a period (perhaps 10–14 days) of immunosuppression, when the patient is prone to infection. Multiple organ failure can occur during either of these of these phases.

SIRS is manifested by two or more of the following conditions:
- Temperature > 38 °C or <36 °C
- Heart rate > 90 beats min^{-1}
- Respiratory rate > 20 breaths min^{-1} or PaCO$_2$ < 4.3 kPa
- WBC >12 000 cells mm^{-3}, < 4000 cells mm^{-3}, or >10% immature (band) forms

Figure TT2 The systemic inflammatory response syndrome (SIRS)

Assessment and management of the trauma patient

Prehospital phase

In the United Kingdom, prehospital management of severely injured patients is performed mainly by paramedics. These personnel are trained in tracheal intubation, intravenous cannulation, fluid resuscitation, the provision of analgesia and spinal immobilisation. Paramedics are trained to minimise on-scene time; a prolonged time to definitive care will increase mortality. Unless the patient is trapped, on-scene interventions should be restricted to control of the airway and ventilation, and stabilisation of the spine. The receiving hospital should be given advanced warning of the impending admission of a severely injured patient. Ambulance personnel should be able to communicate directly with emergency department staff via a talk-through link. Concise and essential information on the patient's condition and estimated time of arrival must be given. Emergency department staff can then decide whether to alert the trauma team.

Preparation for resuscitation

With advance warning, medical and nursing staff can prepare a resuscitation bay in readiness for the patient's arrival. This will include running through drip sets, turning on fluid warmers, and drawing up anaesthetic drugs. Members of the resuscitation team should put on protective clothing comprising gloves, plastic aprons and eye protection. The relevant nurses and doctors should be assigned tasks before the patient arrives. In hospitals with formal trauma teams, the roles of individual team members are usually well established (Figure TT3). The team leader should be a suitably experienced doctor from one of the relevant specialties, e.g. emergency medicine, anaesthesia, general surgery or orthopaedic surgery. The role of the team leader is particularly important, and has been defined comprehensively by a British Trauma Society Standards Working Party (Oakley 1994; Figure TT4). These standards represent the ideal and are probably achievable only by hospitals with relatively large trauma units. In the UK, advanced airway management has traditionally been undertaken by anaesthetists; however, some emergency physicians have now acquired the appropriate training and experience to take on this role.

Primary survey and resuscitation

The initial management of the trauma patient is considered in four phases:

- Primary survey
- Resuscitation
- Secondary survey
- Definitive care

Although the first two phases are listed consecutively, they are performed simultaneously. The secondary survey, or

Team leader	Primary and secondary surveys, coordination of team, overall responsibility for the patient while in the A&E department
Doctor 1 & Nurse 1	Airway, ventilation, central venous access, difficult peripheral access, fluid balance, analgesia
Doctor 2 & Nurse 2	All other procedures, chest drain, fracture splintage, urethral catheter
Nurse 3	Measure vital signs, record data, remove clothes, assist other team members
Radiographer	Chest and pelvis x rays, other x rays as requested by team leader
Porter	Take samples to pathology labs, retrieve urgent blood from blood bank

Figure TT3 Composition and role of a typical trauma team

head-to-toe examination of the patient, is not started until the patient has been adequately resuscitated. The aim of the primary survey is to look sequentially for immediately life-threatening injuries, in the order that they are most likely to kill the patient. The correct sequence is:

(1) Airway with cervical spine control
(2) Breathing
(3) Circulation and haemorrhage control
(4) Disability – a rapid assessment of neurological function
(5) Exposure – while considering the environment, and preventing hypothermia

If life-threatening problems are detected, treat them immediately (resuscitate) before proceeding to the next step of the primary survey.

Airway and cervical spine

The first priority during the resuscitation of any severely injured patient is to ensure a clear airway and maintain adequate oxygenation. Place a pulse oximeter probe on the patient's finger. Knowing the patient's arterial blood oxygen saturation is very valuable, although sometimes peripheral vasoconstriction will make it impossible to

- To offer advice to any hospital wishing to discuss or refer a patient, and to accept appropriate referrals
- To obtain a history from prehospital personnel (for direct admissions) or from the referring doctor and medical escort (for transferred patients)
- To examine the patient (performing a primary and secondary survey)
- To establish the priorities for investigation and intervention
- To coordinate the trauma team
- To maintain an overview, avoiding undue involvement in practical procedures, but intervening appropriately in critical situations
- To supervise the administration of fluids, blood and blood products
- To provide analgesia
- To request and interpret investigations in conjunction with other team members
- To consult with or refer to other specialists where appropriate, indicating any perceived needs for urgent intervention
- To supervise spinal precautions
- To supervise the patient during transfer within the hospital and during imaging procedures
- To coordinate the assignment of the consultant responsible for continuing care
- To arrange transfer to the operating room, intensive care unit, or other ward area (or to another hospital when indicated), and to provide a detailed handover to their staff
- To review the patient subsequently to help maintain continuity
- To inform the family
- To excuse the trauma team members at the end of the resuscitation, and to debrief the team after difficult cases
- To make a detailed note in the patient's records, to record agreed information for audit, and to provide a brief report for the referring hospital

Figure TT4 The role of the trauma team leader

obtain a reliable reading. If the airway is obstructed, immediate basic manoeuvres such as suction, chin lift and jaw thrust may clear it temporarily. A soft nasopharyngeal airway (size 6.0–7.0 mm) may be particularly useful in the semiconscious patient who will not tolerate a Guedel airway. Give high-concentration oxygen to every patient with multiple injuries. In the unintubated, spontaneously

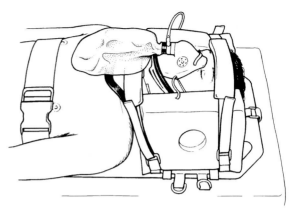

Figure TT5 Cervical spine immobilisation with semi-rigid collar, lateral blocks and spine board

breathing patient this is provided with a mask and reservoir bag ($FiO_2 = 0.85$).

Care of the cervical spine
Every patient sustaining significant blunt trauma, particularly above the clavicles, should be assumed to have a cervical spine injury until proven otherwise. Such patients should have their cervical spines immobilised at the accident scene. The most effective method comprises a combination of an appropriately sized semi-rigid cervical collar, lateral supports and straps (Figure TT5). Undertake all airway manoeuvres carefully without moving the neck (Nolan & Parr 1997). Significant subluxation of the cervical spine can occur during aggressive chin lift or jaw thrust despite the presence of an appropriate collar. Mask ventilation can displace the cervical spine as much as oral intubation. Manual in-line stabilisation of the neck will minimise movement of the cervical spine during oral intubation, but take care to avoid excessive traction, which may distract a cervical fracture. In the resuscitation room, the cervical spine cannot be deemed undamaged until the patient has been examined by an experienced clinician and/or appropriate radiological procedures have been completed. A reliable clinical examination cannot be obtained if the patient has sustained a significant closed head injury, is intoxicated, or has a reduced conscious level from any other cause (Hoffman *et al.* 2000).

Advanced airway management
In the unconscious patient, or in the presence of haemorrhage from maxillofacial injuries, for example, the airway

must be secured by placing a cuffed tube in the trachea. Other reasons for intubating the trauma patient during the resuscitation phase are to optimise oxygen delivery and to enable appropriate procedures to be performed on unco-operative patients. The choice of technique for intubating a patient with a suspected or confirmed cervical spine injury will depend on the indication and on the skill and experience of the individual clinician. If performed with care, tracheal intubation of a patient with a cervical spine injury carries relatively little risk (McLeod & Calder 2000). Occasionally, awake fibreoptic intubation may be appropriate, but this will take much longer to achieve and is rarely applicable in the resuscitation phase. Do not attempt blind nasal intubation.

The technique of choice for emergency intubation of a patient with a potential cervical spine injury is direct laryngoscopy and oral intubation with manual in-line stabilisation of the cervical spine, following a period of pre-oxygenation, intravenous induction of anaesthesia, paralysis with suxamethonium and application of cricoid pressure. Manual in-line stabilisation reduces neck movement during intubation, but care must be taken to avoid excessive axial traction. An assistant kneels at the head of the patient and to one side to leave room for the intubator. The assistant holds the patient's head firmly down on the trolley by grasping the mastoid processes. The tape, lateral blocks and front of the collar are removed. The front of a single-piece collar can be folded under the patient's shoulder, leaving the posterior portion of the collar in situ behind the head. Do not attempt laryngoscopy and intubation with the collar in place – it will make it very difficult to get an adequate view of the larynx. Placing the patient's head and neck in neutral alignment will make the view at laryngoscopy worse; in this position the view of the larynx will be grade 3 or worse in approximately 20% of patients (Nolan & Wilson 1993). Intubation will be aided greatly by the use of a gum-elastic bougie. Another very useful instrument to use in these circumstances is the McCoy levering laryngoscope: it reduces the incidence of grade 3 or worse views to 5%. If intubation of the patient proves impossible the airway should be secured by surgical cricothyroidotomy. A laryngeal mask may provide a temporary airway, but does not guarantee protection against aspiration. The ProSeal LMA is probably better under these circumstances (Cook *et al.* 2005, Cook & Hommers 2006). The intubating laryngeal mask has the advantage that it can be inserted easily with the head and neck in the neutral position and in >95% of cases it will enable tracheal intubation, but it is a more complex technique. The Combitube is popular in

some parts of Europe and offers some protection against aspiration. The laryngeal tube has yet to be evaluated in the trauma patient population.

Needle cricothyroidotomy, with a 14 G cannula followed by jet insufflation of oxygen from a high pressure source (400 kPa), is an alternative method of providing temporary oxygenation but as with the LMA, will not protect against aspiration. Standard cannulae may kink and become obstructed so try to use a device manufactured specifically for needle cricothyroidotomy.

Breathing

Look and listen to the chest to confirm that both sides are being ventilated adequately and measure the respiratory rate. The following chest injuries are immediately life-threatening and must be diagnosed and treated in the primary survey:

- Tension pneumothorax
- Open pneumothorax
- Flail chest
- Massive haemothorax
- Cardiac tamponade

Tension pneumothorax

Reduced chest movement, reduced breath sounds and a resonant percussion note on the affected side, along with respiratory distress, hypotension and tachycardia, indicate a tension pneumothorax. Deviation of the trachea to the opposite side is a late sign, and neck veins may not be distended in the presence of hypovolaemia. Treatment is immediate decompression with a large cannula placed in the 2nd intercostal space, in the mid-clavicular line on the affected side. Once intravenous access has been obtained, insert a large chest drain (32 F) in the 5th intercostal space in the anterior axillary line, and connect to an underwater seal drain.

Open pneumothorax

Cover an open pneumothorax with an occlusive dressing and seal on three sides: the unsealed side should act as a flutter valve. Insert a chest drain away from the wound in the same hemithorax.

Flail chest

Multiple fractures in adjacent ribs will cause a segment of the chest wall to lose bony continuity with the thoracic cage. This flail segment will move paradoxically with inspiration. The immediately life-threatening problem is the underlying lung contusion, which can cause severe hypoxia. The patient must be given effective analgesia, and a thoracic epidural is ideal (see below). Assisted ventilation, via a tracheal tube or by a non-invasive technique, is required if hypoxia persists despite supplemental oxygen.

Massive haemothorax

A massive haemothorax is defined as more than 1500 ml blood in a hemithorax, and it will cause reduced chest movement, a dull percussion note and hypoxaemia. Start fluid resuscitation and insert a chest drain. The patient is likely to require a thoracotomy if blood loss from the chest drain exceeds 200 ml per hour, but this decision will depend also on the patient's general physiological state.

Cardiac tamponade

Whilst not a disorder of breathing, it is logical to consider the possibility of cardiac tamponade while examining the chest, particularly if the patient has sustained a penetrating injury to the chest or upper abdomen. Distended neck veins in the presence of hypotension are suggestive of cardiac tamponade, although after rapid volume resuscitation myocardial contusion will also present in this way. If the appropriate expertise is available, ultrasound examination in the resuscitation room is the best way to make the diagnosis. If ultrasound is unavailable and cardiac tamponade is suspected, and the patient is deteriorating despite all resuscitative efforts, pericardiocentesis should be attempted and is occasionally successful. In the presence of a suitably experienced surgeon, thoracotomy and pericardiotomy is the more effective procedure.

Circulation

Control any major external haemorrhage with direct pressure. Rapidly assess the patient's haemodynamic state and attach ECG leads. Until proven otherwise, hypotension should be assumed to be caused by hypovolaemia. Less likely causes include myocardial contusion, cardiac tamponade, tension pneumothorax, neurogenic shock and sepsis.

Intravenous access

Insert two short, large-bore intravenous cannulae (14 gauge or larger) into a peripheral vein. Most anaesthetists are confident in inserting central lines but this may not be easy in the hypovolaemic patient and there is a risk of creating a pneumothorax. The femoral vein provides a good route for a large-bore cannula. In the hypovolaemic patient, central venous pressure monitoring will be required after the initial fluid challenge. The intraosseous route (usually via the proximal tibia) is useful in children but will not enable flow rates high enough for effective fluid resuscitation in adults. Obtain a sample for arterial blood gas analysis at this stage. Severely injured patients will have a marked base deficit, and its correction will help to confirm adequate resuscitation. Insert an arterial cannula for continuous direct blood pressure monitoring.

Fluids

A crystalloid or colloid provides the initial fluid challenge. Despite a wealth of literature on the subject, and conclusions from extensive reviews, which of these is used initially does not matter, as long as an appropriate volume is given. There is a trend toward increasing use of crystalloids in the UK. A recent randomised controlled trial of albumin versus saline in critically ill patients supports the use of crystalloids in trauma patients (Finfer et al. 2004). The volume status of the patient is best determined by observing the change in vital signs after a reasonably large fluid challenge (such as 2 litres of crystalloid or 1 litre of colloid). Failure to improve the vital signs suggests exsanguinating haemorrhage, and the need for immediate surgical intervention and transfusion of blood (a full cross-match will take 45 minutes, group confirmed blood can be issued in 10 minutes, and group O blood can be obtained immediately). A transient response to this fluid challenge suggests that the patient may have lost 20–40% of circulating blood volume and has ongoing bleeding; he or she will require immediate surgical assessment and is likely to need blood. A sustained reduction in heart rate and increase in blood pressure implies only moderate blood loss (<20% blood volume).

In the absence of obvious external haemorrhage, the likely sources of severe haemorrhage are the chest, abdomen or pelvis. Explore these possibilities and treat them during the primary survey. Careful examination of the chest should exclude massive haemothorax. Obvious abdominal distension mandates a laparotomy, while an equivocal abdominal examination is an indication for computerised tomograpy (CT) or ultrasound (see under secondary survey, below). A severely disrupted pelvis may be detected by springing the iliac crests. This assessment should be made only once; repeated attempts will exacerbate bleeding from large pelvic vessels. The pelvis should be 'closed' immediately by the application of an external fixator, which will reduce the bleeding.

Fluid warming

Warm all intravenous fluids. A high-capacity fluid warmer will be required to cope with the rapid infusion rates used during trauma patient resuscitation. Hypothermia (core temperature less than 35 °C) is a serious complication of severe trauma and haemorrhage and is an independent predictor of mortality. Hypothermia has several adverse effects (Sessler 2001):

- It causes a gradual decline in heart rate and cardiac output while increasing the propensity for myocardial dysrhythmias. One study has shown an increase in the incidence of morbid cardiac events in mildly hypothermic patients undergoing a variety of surgical procedures.
- The oxyhaemoglobin dissociation curve is shifted to the left by a decrease in temperature, thus impairing peripheral oxygen delivery in the hypovolaemic patient at a time when it is needed most.
- Shivering may compound the lactic acidosis that typically accompanies hypovolaemia, and this may be further aggravated by a decreased metabolic clearance of lactic acid by the liver.
- Hypothermia contributes to the coagulopathy accompanying massive transfusion. The likely mechanisms involved include retarding the function of enzymes in the clotting cascade, enhanced plasma fibrinolytic activity, and reduced platelet aggregation.
- Mild hypothermia in the perioperative period increases the incidence of wound infection.

Resuscitation end points

Simply returning the heart rate, blood pressure and urine output to normal does not represent a suitable resuscitation end point for the trauma patient (Moore *et al.* 2004). Plasma lactate and base deficit are better end points to use.

Hypotensive resuscitation

Recent evidence from several animal studies and one human study has suggested that in some circumstances aggressive fluid resuscitation, before surgical control of the bleeding, may be detrimental to the trauma patient (Roberts *et al.* 2001). In the presence of active bleeding, increasing the blood pressure with fluid accelerates the loss of red blood cells and may hamper clotting mechanisms. However, older patients and those with a significant head injury will require fluid resuscitation to restore vital organ perfusion. The balance is between the risk of inducing organ ischaemia and the risk of accelerating haemorrhage.

Disability

Record the size of the pupils and their reaction to light, and rapidly assess the Glasgow coma scale (GCS) score, which is described in Section 1, Chapter 5 (Figure SC8). If the patient requires urgent induction of anaesthesia and intubation, a quick neurological assessment should be performed first.

Exposure and environmental control

It is likely that the patient's clothes will have been removed by this stage. If not, undress him or her completely and apply a forced-air warming blanket to keep the patient warm.

Tubes

Insert a urinary catheter: urine output is an excellent indicator of the adequacy of resuscitation. Before inserting the catheter, check for indications of a ruptured urethra such as scrotal haematoma, blood at the meatus or a high prostate. If any of these signs are present, ask a urologist to assess the patient – the specialist may make one attempt to gently insert a urethral catheter before using the suprapubic route. Insert a gastric tube to drain the stomach contents and reduce the risk of aspiration. If there is any suspicion of a basal skull fracture, use the orogastric route, which eliminates the possibility of passing a nasogastric tube through a basal skull fracture and into the brain.

X rays

Chest and pelvic x rays will be required for all patients sustaining significant blunt trauma. These films must be taken in the resuscitation room and should be obtained as soon as possible, but without interrupting the resuscitation process. If the x ray equipment is mounted on an overhead gantry and members of the trauma team are wearing lead coats, it should be possible to get these x rays during the resuscitation phase. A lateral x ray of the cervical spine will not change the patient's management at this stage: a cervical spine injury is assumed until a reliable clinical examination has been performed and/or adequate radiological investigations are completed.

Secondary survey

Do not undertake the detailed head-to-toe survey until resuscitation is well under way and the patient's vital signs are stable. Re-evaluate the patient continually, so that ongoing bleeding is detected early. Patients with exsanguinating haemorrhage may need a laparotomy as part of the resuscitation phase. They should be transferred directly to the operating theatre; the secondary survey is postponed until the completion of life-saving surgery. Alert staff in the operating theatre and ICU as soon as any severely injured patient is admitted to the resuscitation room. The objectives of the secondary survey are: to examine the patient from head to toe and front to back; to take a complete medical history; to gather all clinical, laboratory and radiological information; and to devise a management plan.

Head

Inspect and feel the scalp for lacerations, haematomas or depressed fractures. Look for evidence of a basal skull fracture:

- Panda (raccoon) eyes
- Battle's sign (bruising over the mastoid process)
- Subhyaloid haemorrhage
- Scleral haemorrhage without a posterior margin
- Haemotympanum
- CSF rhinorrhoea and otorrhoea

Brain injury can be divided into primary and secondary groups. Primary injury (concussion, contusion, and laceration) occurs at the moment of impact and, other than preventative strategies, there is nothing that can be done about it. Secondary brain injury is compounded by hypoxia, hypercarbia and hypotension. These factors can be prevented or rapidly treated. Guidelines for the management of severe head injury have been published by the European Brain Injury Consortium (Maas *et al.* 1997) and the Brain Trauma Foundation (Bullock *et al.* 1996). Goals include a mean blood pressure of at least 90 mmHg, $SaO_2 > 95\%$ and, if mechanically ventilated, a $PaCO_2$ of approximately 4.5 kPa. Guidelines have also been published by the National Institute for Clinical Excellence (NICE, 2003).

The conscious level is assessed using the GCS, which is reliable and reproducible. As the GCS is a dynamic measurement, the trend of conscious level change is more important than one static reading. Record the pupillary response and the presence of any lateralising signs. A dilated pupil in a patient in coma can be caused by pressure on the occulomotor nerve from a displaced medial temporal

Immediately
- Coma – not obeying commands, not speaking, not eye opening (that is, GCS $\leq$ 8).
- Loss of protective laryngeal reflexes
- Ventilatory insufficiency as judged by blood gases: hypoxaemia ($PaO_2 < 9$ kPa on air or <13 kPa on oxygen) or hypercarbia ($PaCO_2 > 6$ kPa).
- Spontaneous hyperventilation (causing $PaCO_2 < 3.5$ kPa)
- Respiratory arrhythmia

Before transfer of the patient to the regional neurosurgical unit
- Significantly deteriorating conscious level, even if not coma
- Bilateral fractured mandible
- Copious bleeding into mouth (for example, from skull base fracture)
- Seizures

Figure TT6 Indications for intubation and ventilation after head injury

lobe, and is a sign of ipsilateral haematoma or brain injury. A haematoma pressing on the motor cortex usually causes contralateral motor weakness. However, it may be of such a size that the whole hemisphere is shifted, pressing the opposite cerebral peduncle against the edge of tentorium. This will cause ipsilateral weakness, although its clinical detection is masked because the patient will be deeply comatose.

Indications for intubation and ventilation after head injury are listed in Figure TT6 (National Institute for Clinical Excellence 2003).

Unless they are conscious and cooperative, trauma patients requiring a CT scan are normally intubated and ventilated for at least the duration of the scan. Depending on the results of the CT scan, these patients are often sedated and mechanically ventilated for at least 24 hours even if their pre-induction GCS was greater than 9.

Indications for urgent CT scan after head injury have also been defined by NICE (National Institute for Clinical Excellence 2003), and are shown in Figure TT7.

Referral to the regional neurosurgical unit is indicated for:

- All patients with an intracranial mass
- Primary brain injury requiring ventilation
- Compound depressed skull fracture
- Persistent CSF leak

Immediate CT scan
- GCS < 13 at any point since the injury
- GCS = 13 or 14 at 2 hours after the injury
- Suspected open or depressed skull fracture
- Any sign of basal skull fracture (haemotympanum, 'panda' eyes, cerebrospinal fluid otorrhoea, Battle's sign)
- Post-traumatic seizure
- Focal neurological deficit
- More than one episode of vomiting (clinical judgement should be used regarding the cause of vomiting in those aged 12 years or younger, and whether imaging is necessary)
- Amnesia for greater than 30 minutes of events before impact. The assessment of amnesia will not be possible in pre-verbal children and is unlikely to be possible in any child aged under 5 years.

Immediate CT scan if the patient has experienced some loss of consciousness or amnesia since the injury
- Age ≥ 65 years
- Coagulopathy (history of bleeding, clotting disorder, current treatment with warfarin)
- Dangerous mechanism of injury (a pedestrian struck by a motor vehicle, an occupant ejected from a motor vehicle or a fall from a height of greater than 1 metre or five stairs). A lower threshold for height of falls should be used when dealing with infants and young children (that is, aged under 5 years).

Figure TT7 Indications for head CT scan after head injury

- Penetrating skull injury
- Patients deteriorating rapidly with signs of an intracranial mass lesion

Mannitol 0.5–1.0 g kg^{-1} may be considered after discussion with the neurosurgeon; it can reduce intracranial pressure and will buy time before surgery.

Face and neck
Palpate the face and look for steps around the orbital margins and along the zygoma. Check for mobile segments in the mid-face or mandible. While an assistant maintains the head and neck in neutral alignment, inspect the neck for swelling or lacerations. Carefully palpate the cervical spinous processes for tenderness or deformities. In the patient who is awake, alert, sober, neurologically normal

and without distracting injuries, the cervical spine may be cleared if there is no pain at rest and, subsequently, on flexion and extension (Hoffman *et al.* 2000). All other patients will require lateral, AP and open-mouth x rays of the cervical spine, or helical CT scans with reconstruction. If the cervical spine cannot be seen clearly on plain x rays, down to the junction of the 7th cervical (C7) and 1st thoracic (T1) vertebrae, a CT scan of that area will be required.

Interpretation of cervical spine x rays is notoriously difficult. Alignment can be checked by identifying the four lordotic curves on the lateral x ray: the anterior vertebral line, the anterior spinal canal, the posterior spinal canal, and the spinous process tips. Widening of the prevertebral space may be another indication of cervical spine injury. X rays show the resting position and not the dynamics of the injury. Apparently normal cervical x rays alone do not 'clear' the cervical spine; they must be accompanied by a reliable clinical examination. Thus, a sensible approach to the resuscitation of trauma patients with known mechanisms of injury is to initially treat all of them as if they had an unstable cervical spine injury, even if the initial plain films are normal. The use of appropriate x rays and targeted CT scanning may enable the cervical spine to be cleared in due course. CT scanning of the entire cervical spine with 3D reconstruction is now the standard technique for clearing the cervical spine in patients with multiple injuries, especially those who are unconscious (Morris & McCoy 2004, Morris & Mullan 2004, Brohi *et al.* 2005).

Thorax
There are six potentially life-threatening injuries (two contusions and four 'ruptures') that can be identified by careful examination of the chest during the secondary survey:
- Pulmonary contusion
- Cardiac contusion
- Aortic rupture (blunt aortic injury)
- Ruptured diaphragm
- Oesophageal rupture
- Rupture of the tracheobronchial tree

Pulmonary contusion
Inspect the chest for signs of considerable decelerating forces, such as seat belt bruising. Even in the absence of rib fractures, pulmonary contusion is the commonest potentially lethal chest injury. Young adults and children have compliant ribs and considerable energy can be transmitted to the lungs in the absence of rib fractures. The earliest indication of pulmonary contusion is hypoxaemia (reduced PaO_2/FiO_2 ratio). The chest radiograph will show

patchy infiltrates over the affected area but it may be normal initially. Increasing the F_IO_2 alone may provide sufficient oxygenation but, failing that, the patient may require continuous positive airway pressure (CPAP) by face mask, or tracheal intubation and positive pressure ventilation. Check the ventilator settings continually. Use a small tidal volume (5–7 ml kg^{-1}) and keep the peak inspiratory pressure below 35 cm H$_2$O to minimise volutrauma and barotrauma. While avoiding hypoxaemia, try to keep the F_IO_2 less than 0.5. These ventilation strategies have probably contributed to the recent reduction in trauma-associated ARDS (Navarrete-Navarro et al. 2001). The patient with chest trauma requires appropriate fluid resuscitation, but fluid overload will worsen lung contusion.

Cardiac contusion

Consider cardiac contusion in any patient with severe blunt chest trauma, particularly those with sternal fractures. Cardiac arrhythmias and ST changes on the ECG may indicate contusion, but these signs are very non-specific. Elevated creatine kinase isoenzymes are equally insensitive for diagnosing myocardial contusion; plasma troponin may be slightly better. An elevated CVP in the presence of hypotension will be the earliest indication of myocardial dysfunction secondary to severe cardiac contusion, but cardiac tamponade must be excluded. Most clinicians will use echocardiography to confirm the diagnosis of cardiac contusion. The right ventricle is most frequently injured, as it is predominantly an anterior structure. Patients with severe cardiac contusion tend to have other serious injuries that will mandate their admission to an intensive care unit. Thus the decision to admit a patient to ICU rarely depends on the diagnosis of cardiac contusion alone. The severely contused myocardium is likely to require inotropic support.

Blunt aortic injury

The thoracic aorta is at risk in any patient subjected to a significant decelerating force, e.g., a fall from a height or a high-speed road traffic crash. Only 10–15% of these patients will reach hospital alive and of these survivors, untreated, two-thirds will die of delayed rupture within 2 weeks. The commonest site for aortic injury is at the aortic isthmus, just distal to the origin of the left subclavian artery at the level of the ligamentum arteriosum. Deceleration produces huge shear forces at this site because the relatively mobile aortic arch travels forward relative to the fixed descending aorta. The tear in the intima and media may involve either part or all of the circumference of the aorta, and in survivors the haematoma is contained by an intact aortic adventitia and mediastinal pleura. Patients sustaining traumatic aortic rupture usually have multiple injuries and may be hypotensive at presentation. However, upper extremity hypertension is present in 40% of cases as the haematoma compresses the true lumen, causing a 'pseudo-coarctation'. The supine chest radiograph will show a widened mediastinum in the vast majority of cases. Although this is a sensitive sign of aortic rupture, it is not very specific. An erect chest radiograph provides a clearer view of the thoracic aorta (Figure TT8). Other signs suggesting possible rupture of the aorta are listed in Figure TT9.

If the chest radiograph is equivocal, further investigation will be required. Helical CT scan is as good as arteriography for delineating aortic injury, and a number of centres are now using transoesophageal echocardiography to diagnose traumatic aortic ruptures. If a rupture of the thoracic aorta is suspected, maintain the blood pressure at 80–100 mmHg systolic (using a beta-blocker such as esmolol) to reduce the risk of further dissection or rupture. Pure vasodilators, such as sodium nitroprusside (SNP), increase the pulse pressure and will not reduce the shear forces on the aortic wall. When bleeding from other injuries has been controlled, transfer the patient to the nearest cardiothoracic unit.

Rupture of the diaphragm

Rupture of the diaphragm occurs in about 5% of patients sustaining severe blunt trauma to the trunk. It can be difficult to diagnose initially, particularly when other severe injuries dominate the patient's management, and consequently the diagnosis is often made late. Approximately 75% of ruptures occur on the left side. The stomach or colon commonly herniates into the chest, and strangulation of these organs is a significant complication. Signs and symptoms detected during the secondary survey may include diminished breath sounds on the ipsilateral side, pain in the chest and abdomen, and respiratory distress. Diagnosis can be made on a plain radiograph (elevated hemidiaphragm, gas bubbles above the diaphragm, shift of the mediastinum to the opposite side, nasogastric tube in the chest). The diagnosis can be confirmed by instilling contrast media through the nasogastric tube and repeating the radiographic examination. If chest radiography is indeterminate, CT with thin cuts and reformatted images will usually provide the definite answer. Once the patient has been stabilised, the diaphragm will require surgical repair.

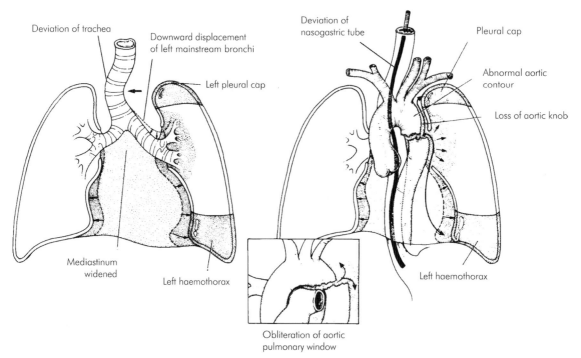

Figure TT8 Radiological features of traumatic aortic rupture

- Widening of the mediastinum
- Pleural capping
- Left haemothorax
- Deviation of the trachea to the right
- Depression of the left mainstem bronchus
- Loss of the aortic knob
- Deviation of the nasogastric tube to the right
- Fractures of the upper three ribs (although disputed recently)
- Fracture of the thoracic spine

Figure TT9 Signs associated with traumatic rupture of the aorta

Oesophageal rupture

A severe blow to the upper abdomen may result in a torn lower oesophagus, as gastric contents are forcefully ejected. The conscious patient will complain of severe chest and abdominal pain, and mediastinal air may be visible on the chest x ray. Gastric contents may appear in the chest drain. The diagnosis is confirmed by contrast study of the oesophagus or endoscopy. Urgent surgery is essential, since accompanying mediastinitis carries a high mortality.

Tracheobronchial injury

Laryngeal fractures are, fortunately, rare. Signs of laryngeal injury include hoarseness, subcutaneous emphysema, and palpable fracture crepitus. Total airway obstruction or severe respiratory distress will have been managed by intubation or surgical airway during the primary survey and resuscitation phases. This is the one situation where tracheostomy, rather than cricothyroidotomy, is indicated. Less severe laryngeal injuries may be assessed by CT before any appropriate surgery. Transections of the trachea or bronchi proximal to the pleural reflection cause massive mediastinal and cervical emphysema. Injuries distal to the pleural sheath lead to pneumothoraces. Typically, these will not resolve after chest drainage, since the bronchopleural fistula causes a large air leak. Most bronchial injuries occur within 2.5 cm of the carina and the diagnosis is confirmed by bronchoscopy. Tracheobronchial injuries require urgent repair through a thoracotomy.

Abdomen

A thorough examination of the whole abdomen is required. The priority is to determine quickly the need for laparotomy and not to spend considerable time trying to define precisely which viscus is injured. Inspect the abdomen for bruising, lacerations and distension. Careful palpation may reveal tenderness. A rectal examination is performed to assess sphincter tone and to exclude the presence of pelvic fracture or a high prostate. If abdominal examination is unreliable, exclusion of intra-abdominal injury will require CT scan, ultrasound or, rarely now, diagnostic peritoneal lavage (DPL). Modern multi-slice helical CT scanners are very fast, which makes CT scanning the technique of choice in severe trauma. In experienced hands, ultrasound has sensitivity, specificity and accuracy comparable to DPL, and it can be undertaken at the bedside. In the UK, 24-hour access to an experienced ultrasonographer may be a problem. Some trauma surgeons and emergency physicians are now using ultrasound themselves to evaluate trauma patients rapidly. Focused assessment with sonography for trauma (FAST) involves scanning four distinct regions identified as the four Ps: pericardial, perihepatic, perisplenic and pelvic. While ultrasound and DPL are good for detecting blood, CT will provide information on specific organ injury; however, CT may miss some gastrointestinal, diaphragmatic and pancreatic injuries.

In patients with multiple injuries the practice of 'damage control' surgery is in vogue. This emphasises rapid but definitive haemostasis, closure of all hollow viscus injuries or performing only essential bowel resections, and delaying the more standard reconstruction until after the patient has been stabilised and all physiological parameters have been corrected (Shapiro 2000, Parr & Alabdi 2004).

Major pelvic trauma resulting in exsanguinating haemorrhage should be dealt with during the resuscitative phase.

Extremities

Inspect all limbs for bruising, wounds and deformities, and examine for vascular and neurological defects. Correct any neurovascular impairment by realignment of any deformity and splintage of the limb.

Spinal column

A detailed neurological examination at this stage should detect any motor or sensory deficits. The patient will need to be log rolled to enable a thorough inspection and palpation of the whole length of the spine. A safe log roll requires a total of five people: three to control and turn the patient's body, one to maintain the cervical spine in neutral alignment with the rest of the body, and one to examine the spine. The person controlling the cervical spine should command the team.

In the patient with multiple injuries who requires CT scans of at least the chest and abdomen, reconstruction of these images in the sagittal plane will provide 'scanograms' of the thoracolumbar spine. These provide more information on alignment than lateral and AP x rays, and can be used instead of the latter to 'clear' the thoracolumbar spine (Hauser *et al.* 2003).

Medical history

Obtain a medical history from the patient, relatives and/or the ambulance crew. A useful mnemonic is:

A Allergies
M Medications
P Past medical history
L Last meal
E Event leading to the injury and the environment

It is possible that a patient's pre-existing medical problem contributed to or precipitated an accident, e.g. myocardial infarction while driving a car.

The paramedics will be able to give invaluable information about the mechanism of injury. The speed of a road traffic crash and the direction of impact will dictate the likely injury patterns.

Analgesia

Systemic analgesia

Give effective analgesia as soon as practically possible. If the patient needs surgery imminently, then immediate induction of general anaesthesia is a logical and very effective solution to the patient's pain. If not, titrate intravenous opioid (e.g., fentanyl or morphine) to the desired affect. Head-injured patients will require adequate pain relief for any other injuries. **Careful** titration of intravenous morphine or fentanyl will provide effective pain relief without serious respiratory depression. There is no role for intramuscular codeine in trauma patients.

Non-steroidal anti-inflammatory drugs (NSAIDs) provide moderate analgesia but are relatively contraindicated in patients with hypovolaemia; these patients depend on renal prostaglandins to maintain renal blood flow. In normovolaemic trauma patients, use of NSAIDs may reduce the need for opioids.

Local and regional analgesia

Local anaesthetic blocks are ideal in the acute trauma patient. Unfortunately, there are relatively few blocks that

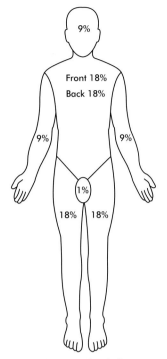

Figure TT10 Rule of nines

humidified high-concentration oxygen to all patients suspected of having thermal or smoke injury to the respiratory tract. Undertake arterial blood gas analysis and measure the carboxyhaemoglobin concentration. Consider the need for early intubation in the presence of any of the following:

- Altered consciousness
- Direct burns to the face or oropharynx
- Hoarseness or stridor
- Soot in the nostrils or sputum
- Expiratory rhonchi
- Dysphagia
- Drooling and dribbling saliva

Having established intravenous access, start fluid resuscitation and cover burnt areas with cling film. The simple 'rule of nines' (Figure TT10) enables an approximate calculation of the surface area of the burn, which is determined more precisely later using a Lund and Browder chart (Figure TT11). Most burns centres are now using crystalloid for initial fluid resuscitation. Give 2–4 ml of crystalloid per kilogram body weight per percent burn area in the first 24 hours. Give one half of this fluid in the first eight hours, and the remainder over the next 16 hours. The exact volume of fluid given depends on vital signs, central venous pressure and urine output. Patients with full-thickness burns of >10% of the body surface area will probably require blood. Patients with severe burns need potent analgesia, which is best given by carefully titrating intravenous opioids.

are both simple and effective. One of these is the femoral nerve block for a fracture of the femoral shaft.

Regional analgesia has a useful role in some acute trauma patients. Exclude hypovolaemia and coagulopathy before attempting epidural or spinal analgesia in the acute trauma patient. In patients with multiple rib fractures, including flail segments, a thoracic epidural will provide excellent analgesia. This will help the patient to tolerate physiotherapy and to maintain adequate ventilation. All these factors help to reduce the requirement for intubation and mechanical ventilation. A lumbar epidural will benefit patients with lower limb injuries and, assuming there are no contraindications, this can be placed intraoperatively.

Management of burns

The standard 'ABC' principles apply to treating patients with severe burns. Patients with severe burns should be stabilised and transferred to the nearest burns centre. The patient with a thermal injury to the respiratory tract may develop airway obstruction rapidly from the oedema. Give

Anaesthesia for patients with severe trauma

Induction of anaesthesia

A smooth induction of anaesthesia and neuromuscular blockade provides optimal conditions for intubating high-risk trauma patients. All anaesthetic induction drugs are vasodilators and respiratory depressants and have the potential to produce or worsen hypotension. There is no evidence that the choice of induction drug alters survival in major trauma patients. Their appropriate use during resuscitation involves a careful assessment of the clinical situation and a thorough knowledge of their clinical pharmacology. The safest strategy is for the anaesthetist to use drugs with which he or she is familiar: the trauma resuscitation room is not the place for experimentation. Anaesthetic requirement is assessed individually, and the risk of awareness kept to a minimum. Severely injured

CHART FOR ESTIMATING SEVERITY OF BURN WOUND

NAME _____ WARD _____ NUMBER _____ DATE _____

AGE _____ ADMISSION WEIGHT _____

LUND AND BROWDER CHARTS

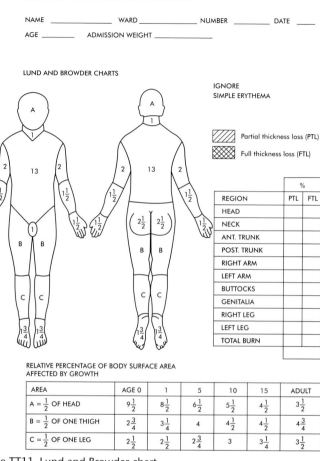

IGNORE
SIMPLE ERYTHEMA

Partial thickness loss (PTL)

Full thickness loss (FTL)

REGION	%	
	PTL	FTL
HEAD		
NECK		
ANT. TRUNK		
POST. TRUNK		
RIGHT ARM		
LEFT ARM		
BUTTOCKS		
GENITALIA		
RIGHT LEG		
LEFT LEG		
TOTAL BURN		

RELATIVE PERCENTAGE OF BODY SURFACE AREA
AFFECTED BY GROWTH

AREA	AGE 0	1	5	10	15	ADULT
A = $\frac{1}{2}$ OF HEAD	$9\frac{1}{2}$	$8\frac{1}{2}$	$6\frac{1}{2}$	$5\frac{1}{2}$	$4\frac{1}{2}$	$3\frac{1}{2}$
B = $\frac{1}{2}$ OF ONE THIGH	$2\frac{3}{4}$	$3\frac{1}{4}$	4	$4\frac{1}{2}$	$4\frac{1}{2}$	$4\frac{3}{4}$
C = $\frac{1}{2}$ OF ONE LEG	$2\frac{1}{2}$	$2\frac{1}{2}$	$2\frac{3}{4}$	3	$3\frac{1}{4}$	$3\frac{1}{2}$

Figure TT11 Lund and Browder chart

patients requiring intubation fall generally into one of three groups:

(a) Stable and adequately resuscitated. These patients should receive a standard or slightly reduced dose of induction drug.

(b) Unstable or inadequately resuscitated but require immediate intubation. These patients should receive a reduced, titrated dose of induction drug.

(c) In extremis – severely obtunded and hypotensive. Induction drugs would be inappropriate, but muscle relaxants may be used to facilitate intubation. Give anaesthetic and analgesic drugs as soon as adequate cerebral perfusion is achieved.

Suxamethonium retains its status as the neuromuscular blocker with the fastest onset of action, and remains the most popular relaxant for intubation of the acute trauma patient. In the presence of adequate anaesthesia, suxamethonium does not increase intracranial pressure in severe head-injured patients. Rocuronium is almost as fast in onset and is favoured by some trauma anaesthetists. Contrary to more traditional opinions, the longer duration of action in comparison with suxamethonium may be an advantage during trauma patient resuscitation.

Intraoperative management

The following considerations are of relevance to the anaesthetist during surgery for the severely injured patient:

• Prolonged surgery. The patient will be at risk from pressure areas and from heat loss. Anaesthetists (and surgeons) should rotate to avoid exhaustion. Avoid nitrous oxide in those cases expected to last more than 6 hours.

- Fluid loss. Be prepared for heavy blood and 'third space' losses. The combination of hypothermia and massive transfusion will cause profound coagulopathy. Expect to see a significant metabolic acidosis in patients with major injuries. This needs frequent monitoring (arterial blood gases) and correction with fluids and inotropes, as appropriate. Massive haemorrhage is treated with blood, FFP, platelets and cryoprecipitate guided by coagulation tests and clinical evidence of coagulopathy. Consider the use of recombinant factor VIIa if coagulopathy persists despite adequate treatment with other blood products (Boffard *et al.* 2005).
- Multiple surgical teams. It is more efficient if surgical teams from different specialties are able to work simultaneously; however, this may severely restrict the space available to the anaesthetist!
- Acute lung injury. Trauma patients are at significant risk of hypoxia from acute lung injury. This may be secondary to direct pulmonary contusion or to fat embolism from orthopaedic injuries. Advanced ventilatory modes may be required to maintain appropriate oxygenation.

Techniques

Cannulation of major vessels for resuscitation and monitoring

Cannulation of the femoral vein

In hypovolaemic patients in whom percutaneous access to arm veins is impossible, a useful alternative is the femoral vein. This large vein is consistently located directly medial to the femoral artery in the groin, and as long as the artery is palpable the vein is normally easily cannulated using a Seldinger technique. A pulmonary artery introducer sheath (8.5 F internal diameter) will enable very high fluid flows.

Cannulation of the subclavian vein

Central venous cannulation can be difficult in the hypovolaemic patient. The major complications are pneumothorax and accidental arterial puncture. Significant air emboli are very rare. In the blunt trauma patient, internal jugular venous cannulation is not recommended because most approaches to this vein require turning of

- Position the patient slightly head-down (keeping the head and neck in neutral alignment) and clean the skin overlying the chosen site
- Infiltrate with local anaesthetic if appropriate
- Using a thin-walled needle attached to a 10 ml syringe, puncture the skin just below the midpoint of the clavicle and, keeping the needle very close to the underside of the clavicle, advance toward the suprasternal notch while aspirating on the syringe
- Once blood can be aspirated freely, detach the syringe and feed in the guide wire for about 15 cm
- Remove the needle, taking care not to displace the wire
- Make a small incision in the skin adjacent to the wire and insert the dilator over the wire
- Remove the dilator, leaving the wire in situ, and finally insert the introducer sheath over the wire
- Remove the wire and attach the intravenous giving set to the introducer sheath
- Suture the sheath in position and cover with a sterile dressing

Figure TT12 Subclavian vein cannulation

the patient's head, and this cannot be done unless the cervical spine has been cleared. Subclavian cannulation can be performed while the patient's cervical collar is on and with the head and neck in neutral alignment. If an 8.5 F introducer sheath is used it will enable rapid flow and the ability to monitor central venous pressure. If a chest drain has been inserted, use the same side for subclavian access unless a major vascular injury is suspected. The practical technique is given in Figure TT12.

Chest drainage

A tension pneumothorax should be immediately decompressed by insertion of a cannula through the second intercostal space in the mid-clavicular line. A chest drain is then inserted. Other indications for chest drainage in the trauma patient are simple pneumothorax, haemothorax, and rib fractures in a patient requiring positive pressure ventilation. Do not use a trochar for chest drain insertion: it can cause serious lacerations of the lung and pulmonary vessels. The practical technique is given in Figure TT13.

- Place the patient supine with the ipsilateral arm at right angles to the chest
- The insertion point is in the 5th intercostal space (nipple level) in the anterior axillary line
- Infiltrate down to the upper border of the rib with 1% lidocaine
- Make a 3 cm incision along the upper border of the 5th rib
- Using Kelly's forceps, bluntly dissect down into the pleural cavity
- Insert a finger into the pleural cavity and sweep around to ensure that the lung is clear of the chest wall
- Select a large chest drain (32–36 F), remove the trochar, and insert the Kelly's forceps through the distal side hole
- Insert the chest drain into the pleural cavity using the forceps as a guide
- Suture the chest drain securely to the skin and connect it to an underwater drainage system
- Obtain a chest x ray to check for lung expansion and tube position
- Leave the drain in situ until the lung is re-expanded and drainage of fluid and/or air has stopped
- Do not clamp chest drains in a patient receiving positive pressure ventilation – the intrapleural pressure is always positive and the patient can be transported safely as long the drains are not moved above the level of the chest

Figure TT13 Insertion of chest drain

References and further reading

American College of Surgeons Committee on Trauma. *Advanced Trauma Life Support for Doctors. Student Course Manual.* Chicago: American College of Surgeons, 2004.

Boffard KD, Riou B, Warren B, *et al.* Recombinant factor VIIa as adjunctive therapy for bleeding control in severely injured trauma patients: two parallel randomized, placebo-controlled, double-blind clinical trials. *J Trauma* 2005; **59**: 8–15; discussion 15–18.

Bone RC, Balk RA, Cerra FB, *et al.* Definitions for sepsis and organ failure and guidelines for the use of innovative therapies in sepsis. The ACCP/SCCM Consensus Conference Committee. American College of Chest Physicians/Society of Critical Care Medicine. *Chest* 1992; **101**: 1644–55.

Brohi K, Healy M, Fotheringham T, *et al.* Helical computed tomographic scanning for the evaluation of the cervical spine in the unconscious, intubated trauma patient. *J Trauma* 2005; **58**: 897–901.

Bullock R, Chesnut RM, Clifton G, *et al.* Guidelines for the management of severe head injury. Brain Trauma Foundation. *Eur J Emerg Med* 1996; **3**: 109–27.

Cobb JP, O'Keefe GE. Injury research in the genomic era. *Lancet* 2004; **363**: 2076–83.

Cook TM, Hommers C. New airways for resuscitation? *Resuscitation* 2006; **69**: 371–87.

Cook TM, Lee G, Nolan JP. The ProSeal™ laryngeal mask airway: a review of the literature. *Can J Anaesth* 2005; **52**: 739–60.

Finfer S, Bellomo R, Boyce N, *et al.* A comparison of albumin and saline for fluid resuscitation in the intensive care unit. *N Engl J Med* 2004; **350**: 2247–56.

Giannoudis PV. Current concepts of the inflammatory response after major trauma: an update. *Injury* 2003; **34**: 397–404.

Goris RJ. MODS/SIRS: result of an overwhelming inflammatory response? *World J Surg* 1996; **20**: 418–21.

Hauser CJ, Visvikis G, Hinrichs C, *et al.* Prospective validation of computed tomographic screening of the thoracolumbar spine in trauma. *J Trauma* 2003; **55**: 228–34; discussion 234–5.

Hoffman JR, Mower WR, Wolfson AB, Todd KH, Zucker MI. Validity of a set of clinical criteria to rule out injury to the cervical spine in patients with blunt trauma. National Emergency X-Radiography Utilization Study Group. *N Engl J Med* 2000; **343**: 94–9.

Lee CC, Marill KA, Carter WA, Crupi RS. A current concept of trauma-induced multiorgan failure. *Ann Emerg Med* 2001; **38**: 170–6.

Maas AI, Dearden M, Teasdale GM, *et al.* EBIC-guidelines for management of severe head injury in adults. European Brain Injury Consortium. *Acta Neurochir (Wien)* 1997; **139**: 286–94.

McLeod AD, Calder I. Spinal cord injury and direct laryngoscopy: the legend lives on. *Br J Anaesth* 2000; **84**: 705–9.

Moore FA, McKinley BA, Moore EE. The next generation in shock resuscitation. *Lancet* 2004; **363**: 1988–96.

Morris CG, McCoy E. Clearing the cervical spine in unconscious polytrauma victims, balancing risks and effective screening. *Anaesthesia* 2004; **59**: 464–82.

Morris CG, Mullan B. Clearing the cervical spine after polytrauma: implementing unified management for unconscious victims in the intensive care unit. *Anaesthesia* 2004; **59**: 755–61.

National Institute for Clinical Excellence. *Head Injury: Triage, Assessment, Investigation and Early Management of Head Injury in Infants, Children and Adults.* London: NICE, 2003.

Navarrete-Navarro P, Rodriguez A, Reynolds N, *et al.* Acute respiratory distress syndrome among trauma patients: trends in ICU mortality, risk factors, complications and resource utilization. *Intensive Care Med* 2001; **27**: 1133–40.

Nolan JP, Parr MJA. Aspects of resuscitation in trauma. *Br J Anaesth* 1997; **79**: 226–40.

Nolan JP, Wilson ME. Orotracheal intubation in patients with potential cervical spine injuries: an indication for the gum elastic bougie. *Anaesthesia* 1993; **48**: 630–3.

Oakley PA. Setting and living up to national standards for the care of the injured. British Trauma Society. *Injury* 1994; **25**: 595–604.

Parr MJ, Alabdi T. Damage control surgery and intensive care. *Injury* 2004; **35**: 713–22.

Roberts I, Evans P, Bunn F, Kwan I, Crowhurst E. Is the normalisation of blood pressure in bleeding trauma patients harmful? *Lancet* 2001; **357**: 385–7.

Roumen RM, Redl H, Schlag G, *et al.* Inflammatory mediators in relation to the development of multiple organ failure in patients after severe blunt trauma. *Crit Care Med* 1995; **23**: 474–80.

Saadia R, Lipman J. Multiple organ failure after trauma. *BMJ* 1996; **313**: 573–4.

Sessler DI. Complications and treatment of mild hypothermia. *Anesthesiology* 2001; **95**: 531–43.

Shapiro MB, Jenkins DH, Schwab CW, Rotondo MF. Damage control: collective review. *J Trauma* 2000; **49**: 969–78.

Thomas I, Dixon J. Bradycardia in acute haemorrhage. *BMJ* 2004; **328**: 451–3.

CHAPTER 10

Clinical anatomy

C. A. Pinnock and R. P. Jones

RESPIRATORY SYSTEM
Mouth
Nose
Pharynx
Larynx
Trachea
Bronchial tree
Lungs

PLEURA AND MEDIASTINUM
Pleura
Mediastinum
Diaphragm
Heart

NERVOUS SYSTEM
Spinal cord
Spinal meninges
Spinal nerves
Peripheral nerves
Autonomic nervous system
Cranial nerves

VERTEBRAL COLUMN

SPECIAL ZONES
Thoracic inlet
Intercostal spaces
Abdominal wall
Inguinal canal
Antecubital fossa
Orbit
Base of the skull

Respiratory system

Mouth

Structure

The mouth (Figure CA1) extends from the lips to the isthmus of the fauces. It contains the tongue, alveolar arches that comprise the gums and teeth and the openings of the salivary glands. The mouth may be divided into two sections, the vestibule and the cavity proper.

The vestibule is a slit-like cavity bounded externally by cheeks and lips. The gingivae and teeth provide the boundary to the mouth cavity proper. The mucous membrane is stratified squamous epithelium and the opening of the parotid duct lies just above the second molar crown.

The oral cavity proper is limited by the maxilla anteriorly and laterally. It is roofed by the hard and soft palates. The floor of the cavity mainly consists of the tongue. Posteriorly the oropharyngeal isthmus separates the oral cavity from the oropharynx. The lining consists of mucous membrane, which is stratified squamous epithelium with mucous glands beneath.

Teeth
Structure

Each tooth has a crown, a neck and roots that penetrate the alveolar bone. The central cavity of the tooth is filled with pulp and surrounded by dentine. At the crown the dentine is covered by enamel whereas the dentine of the root is covered by cementum. Within the alveolar socket the periodontal membrane fixes the tooth in position.

Nerve supply

The teeth of the upper jaw are supplied by the anterior and posterior superior alveolar nerves whereas the teeth of the lower jaw are supplied by the inferior alveolar nerve.

The nerve supply of the gums is different for labial and lingual surfaces. The gums of the upper jaw receive supply to the labial surface via the infraorbital and posterior superior alveolar nerves and supply to the lingual surface via the nasopalatine and greater palatine nerves. The gums of the lower jaw receive supply to the labial surface via the

Fundamentals of Anaesthesia, 3rd edition, ed. Tim Smith, Colin Pinnock and Ted Lin. Published by Cambridge University Press. © Cambridge University Press 2008.

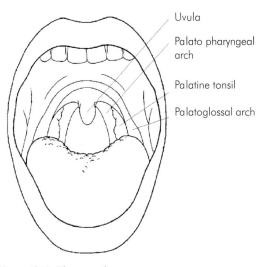

Uvula

Palato pharyngeal arch

Palatine tonsil

Palatoglossal arch

Figure CA1 The mouth

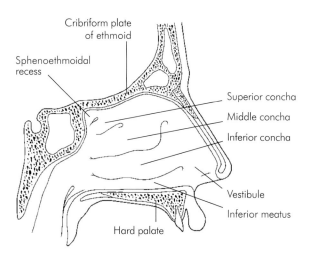

Cribriform plate
of ethmoid

Sphenoethmoidal
recess

Superior concha

Middle concha

Inferior concha

Vestibule

Inferior meatus

Hard palate

Figure CA2 The lateral wall of the left nasal cavity

mental and buccal surfaces. The lingual nerve supplies the lingual surface of the gums of the lower jaw.

Tongue
Structure
The tongue is a muscular structure occupying most of the mouth. It is attached to the mandible and the hyoid bone and rests on the geniohyoid and mylohyoid muscles. A V-shaped groove separates the tongue into an anterior two thirds and a posterior one third.

Muscles
The tongue has both intrinsic and extrinsic muscles. The intrinsic muscles are arranged in vertical, horizontal and transverse bundles and mainly act to change the shape of the tongue. The extrinsic muscles are genioglossus, hyoglossus, styloglossus and palatoglossus. The extrinsic muscles move the tongue. Palatoglossus is supplied by the pharyngeal plexus (vagus) whereas all the other muscles are supplied by cranial nerve IX.

Nerve supply
The lingual nerve supplies the mucous membrane of the anterior two thirds. Taste fibres leave the lingual nerve in the chorda tympani and pass via the facial nerve to the nucleus of the tractus solitarius.

The glossopharyngeal nerve transmits taste and general sensation from the posterior third of the tongue.

The salivary glands receive efferent parasympathetic supply from the superior salivary nucleus in the pons.

Blood supply
The tongue is supplied by the lingual artery and drains via the deep lingual vein into the internal jugular vein.

Lymphatic drainage
The tip of the tongue drains into the submental nodes, the sides into the submandibular glands and the posterior third into the retropharyngeal and jugulodigastric nodes.

Nose
Structure
The nose may be divided into the external nose, which is made up of bone and cartilage, and the nasal cavities. The nasal septum divides the nasal cavity into two separate areas which open anteriorly through the nares and posteriorly through the choanae. The dilated area just within the external nose is termed the vestibule. Each nasal cavity has a roof, floor and two walls.

The roof is made of the nasal cartilages, nasal bones and frontal bones, the cribriform plate of the ethmoid and the body of the sphenoid. It is arched anteroposteriorly.

The floor is concave and consists of the horizontal plate of the palatine bone and the palatine process of the maxilla.

The medial wall is the nasal septum, made of septal cartilage with a contribution from the ethmoid and vomer.

The lateral wall has a bony framework which mainly comprises the ethmoidal labyrinth, the maxilla and the perpendicular plate of the palatine bone. The surface area is increased by the presence of three conchae: superior, inferior and middle, each of which overlies a meatus (Figure CA2).

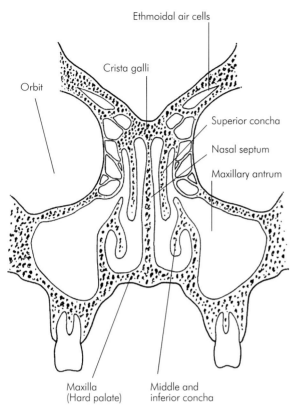

Figure CA3 Coronal section of the nose and maxillary sinus

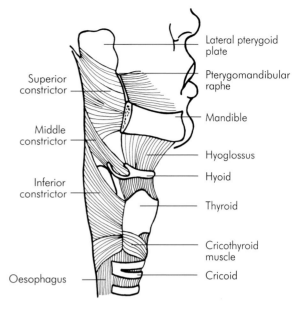

Figure CA4 The pharynx

The paranasal sinuses and the nasolacrimal duct open onto the lateral wall through orifices. The sphenoid sinus opens into the sphenoethmoidal recess. The middle ethmoidal cells cause a bulge in the middle meatus, onto which they open. This is the bulla ethmoidalis. Below the bulla a semicircular groove, the hiatus semilunaris, has the openings of the frontal, ethmoidal and maxillary sinuses (Figure CA3).

The nose is lined by vascular mucoperiosteum. Apart from the superior concha and its immediate surrounding area, which is covered by yellow olfactory epithelium, the nose is surfaced by respiratory epithelium.

Blood supply

The ophthalmic and maxillary arteries supply the nose. Venous drainage is provided by the facial vein and pterygoid venous plexus.

Nerve supply

The specialised olfactory zone is supplied by the olfactory nerve. The first and second divisions of the trigeminal nerve provide general sensation.

The septum is mainly supplied by the nasopalatine branch of the maxillary nerve.

The lateral wall is supplied by the lateral posterior superior nasal nerve, the anterior superior alveolar nerve and the nasociliary nerve. All are branches of the maxillary nerve.

The floor is supplied by the anterior superior alveolar nerve and the greater palatine nerve.

Lymphatic drainage

The anterior nasal cavity drains into the submandibular nodes, and the posterior into the retropharyngeal lymph nodes.

Pharynx
Structure

The pharynx (Figure CA4) is basically a wide muscular tube forming the common upper pathway of alimentary and respiratory tracts. It extends from the base of the skull to the level of C6. The pharynx lies posterior to, and communicates with, the nose, mouth and larynx. This relationship divides the pharynx into three sections: naso-, oro- and laryngopharynx. The posterior surface of the pharynx lies on the prevertebral fascia and cervical vertebrae. The pharynx has four coats:

(1) **Mucous coat**. The mucosa is stratified squamous epithelium, excepting the nasopharynx, where the lining is ciliated, columnar epithelium.

(2) **Fibrous coat**. This is generally thin, but becomes condensed to form the capsule of the tonsil.

(3) **Muscular coat**. This comprises the three constrictor muscles – superior, middle and inferior – plus stylopharyngeus, salpingopharyngeus and palatopharyngeus. The constrictor muscles have an extensive bilateral origin from mandible, hyoid and larynx. Each constrictor spreads out from its anterior attachment to pass posteriorly, joining in the midline raphe. The superior constrictor arises from the pterygoid plate, the pterygoid hamulus, the pterygomandibular raphe and the inner aspect of the mandible. The middle constrictor arises from the stylohyoid ligament, and the greater and lesser horns of the hyoid. The inferior constrictor is the largest muscle of the three, arising from the thyroid cartilage, cricoid cartilage and the tendinous arch of cricothyroid. Functionally the muscle has two parts, with different muscle fibre orientation. It is between the two that the formation of a pharyngeal pouch may occur.

(4) **Fascial coat**. The buccopharyngeal fascia forms the thin fibrous coat of the pharynx.

Nasopharynx

The nasopharynx communicates with the oropharynx through the pharyngeal isthmus. The Eustachian tube opens into the nasopharynx just below the inferior nasal concha. The adenoids (nasopharyngeal tonsil) lie on the roof and posterior wall of the nasopharynx. The adenoid is a collection of lymphoid tissue covered by ciliated epithelium positioned against the superior constrictor. The sphenoid sinus lies posterior and slightly above the nasopharynx, separating it from the sella turcica.

Oropharynx

Anteriorly the oropharynx communicates with the oral cavity via the faucial isthmus. It extends to the level of the upper border of the epiglottis, where it becomes continuous with the laryngopharynx. The lateral wall of the faucial isthmus contains palatopharyngeus and palatoglossus lying within folds of mucous membrane; these are the arches of the fauces. The palatine tonsils are collections of lymphoid tissue lying on the pillars of the fauces.

Laryngopharynx

The laryngopharynx extends between the tip of the epiglottis and the lower border of the cricoid cartilage (C6).

Anteriorly the opening of the larynx presents together with the posterior surfaces of the arytenoid and cricoid cartilages. The recesses on each side of the larynx formed by its posterior bulging into the laryngopharynx are the piriform fossae. These are famous as the resting place of stray fish bones and other similar items.

Blood supply

The pharynx receives arterial supply from the ascending pharyngeal, superior thyroid, lingual, facial and maxillary vessels. Venous drainage is provided by the internal jugular vein via the pharyngeal plexus.

Nerve supply

This is mainly from the pharyngeal plexus, which lies on the surface of the middle constrictor muscle. The plexus is formed by three main components:

(1) Sensory fibres in the pharyngeal branches of the glossopharyngeal (CN IX) and vagus (CN X) nerves.

(2) Motor fibres from the nucleus ambiguus travelling in the pharyngeal branch of the vagus supply all muscles except stylopharyngeus (which has its motor supply via the glossopharyngeal).

(3) Branches from the cervical sympathetic chain.

An additional sensory supply to the nasopharynx is provided by the pharyngeal branch of the maxillary nerve. The laryngopharynx receives sensory branches from the internal and recurrent laryngeal nerves. Note that the tonsil has a threefold nerve supply: glossopharyngeal nerve via the pharyngeal plexus, posterior palatine branch of the maxillary nerve, fibres from the lingual branch of the mandibular nerve.

Lymphatic drainage

The nasopharynx drains into the retropharyngeal lymph nodes, and the remainder of the pharynx into the deep cervical chain.

Larynx
Structure

The larynx (Figures CA5–CA9) is a functional sphincter at the beginning of the respiratory tree to protect the trachea from foreign bodies. It is lined by ciliated columnar epithelium and consists of a framework of cartilages linked together by ligaments which are moved by a series of muscles.

Cartilages of the larynx

There are four cartilages of importance:

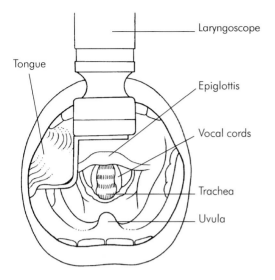

Figure CA5 Larynx, direct laryngoscopic view

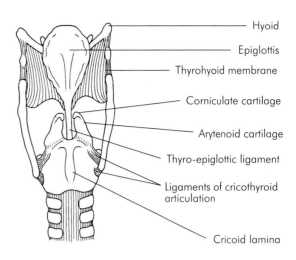

Figure CA7 Larynx, posterior view

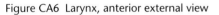

Figure CA6 Larynx, anterior external view

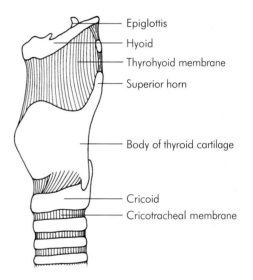

Figure CA8 Larynx, lateral view

(1) The **thyroid cartilage** is said to be shaped like a shield. It consists of two plates that join in the midline inferiorly to form the thyroid notch (Adam's apple). Each plate has a superior and inferior horn or cornua at the upper and lower limit of its posterior border, respectively. The inferior horn articulates with the cricoid cartilage.

(2) The **cricoid cartilage** is shaped like a signet ring, with the large laminal portion being posterior. Each lateral surface features a facet that articulates with the

inferior horn of the thyroid cartilage. The upper border of the lamina has an articular facet for the arytenoid cartilage.

(3) There is a pair of **arytenoid cartilages**, each shaped like a triple-sided pyramid possessing medial, posterior and anterolateral surfaces. Each arytenoid cartilage projects anteriorly as the vocal process and in a similar fashion laterally as the muscular process. The posterior and lateral cricoarytenoid muscles are inserted into the muscular process.

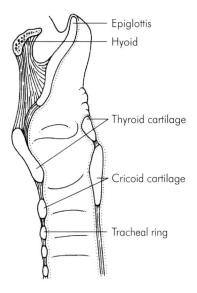

Figure CA9 Larynx, sectional view

(Labels: Epiglottis, Hyoid, Thyroid cartilage, Cricoid cartilage, Tracheal ring)

(4) The **epiglottis** is a leaf-shaped cartilage. It has a lower tapered end which is joined to the thyroid cartilage by the thyroepiglottic ligament. The free upper end is broader and projects superiorly behind the tongue. The lowest part of the anterior surface of the epiglottis is attached to the hyoid by the hyoepiglottic ligament. Two other minor cartilages are the corniculate and the cuneiform.

Ligaments of the larynx

The ligaments of the larynx may be divided into extrinsic and intrinsic.

Extrinsic ligaments are the thyrohyoid membrane, cricotracheal, cricothyroid, and hyoepiglottic ligaments.

- The thyrohyoid membrane joins the upper border of the thyroid cartilage and the hyoid. The membrane is pierced by two important structures: the internal branch of the superior laryngeal nerve and the superior laryngeal artery.
- The cricotracheal ligament joins the first ring of the trachea to the cricoid cartilage.
- The cricothyroid ligament joins the cricoid cartilage to the thyroid cartilage.
- The hyoepiglottic ligament joins the epiglottis to the body of the hyoid.

The intrinsic ligaments of the larynx are of minor importance, being the capsules of the small synovial joints between cricoid and arytenoids. The larynx possesses a fibrous internal framework which is composed of the quadrangular membrane, the cricovocal membrane and the vocal ligament (which is strictly a thickened upper border of the cricovocal membrane) providing the framework of the true vocal cord.

Muscles of the larynx

There are three extrinsic muscles of the larynx and six intrinsic ones.

Extrinsic group:

(1) The **sternothyroid** arises from the manubrium to insert into the lamina of the thyroid cartilage. It is a depressor of the larynx.
(2) The **thyrohyoid** arises from the oblique line of the thyroid lamina to insert onto the greater horn of the hyoid. It is an elevator of the larynx.
(3) The **inferior constrictor** is a constrictor of the pharynx (see above).

Intrinsic group. These are paired, with the exception of the transverse arytenoid:

(1) The **cricothyroid** arises from the anterior surface of the arch of the cricoid cartilage to insert on the inferior horn and adjacent lower border of the thyroid cartilage. Contraction of the muscle approximates the cricoid and thyroid cartilages causing tilting of the cricoid. The antero-posterior diameter of the glottis is thus increased. The net result is an increase in the tension of the vocal cords.
(2) The **posterior cricoarytenoid** arises from the posterior surface of the lamina of the cricoid cartilage to insert on the muscular surface of the arytenoid. Contraction of the muscle externally rotates the arytenoid and by doing so abducts the vocal cord.
(3) The **lateral cricoarytenoid** arises from the outer lateral arch of the cricoid cartilage to insert into the muscular process of the arytenoid. Contraction of the muscle internally rotates the arytenoid which results in vocal cord adduction and closure, therefore, of the glottis.
(4) The **transverse arytenoid** (or interarytenoid) is attached to the posterior surfaces of both arytenoids. Contraction of the muscle increases tension between the two arytenoids and causes constriction of the glottis by narrowing of its posterior section.
(5) The **aryepiglottic** is a continuation of the oblique fibres of the transverse arytenoid lying within the

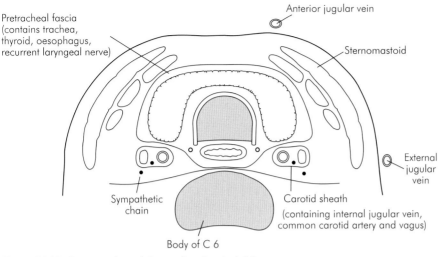

Pretracheal fascia (contains trachea, thyroid, oesophagus, recurrent laryngeal nerve)

Anterior jugular vein

Sternomastoid

External jugular vein

Sympathetic chain

Carotid sheath (containing internal jugular vein, common carotid artery and vagus)

Body of C 6

Figure CA10 Cross section of the neck at level of C6

aryepiglottic fold. The only action of the muscle is to cause a minor constriction of the laryngeal inlet.

(6) The **thyroarytenoid** arises from the junction of the two laminae of the thyroid cartilage and is inserted into the anterolateral surface of the arytenoid. Contraction of the muscle pulls the arytenoid anteriorly which results in vocal cord relaxation. Some fibres of the thyroarytenoid are inserted into the vocal cord to make the vocalis muscle. This may have a role in adjusting cord tension.

Blood supply

The larynx receives arterial supply from the laryngeal branches of the superior and inferior thyroid arteries. The respective veins provide venous drainage.

Nerve supply

The mucous membrane of the larynx above the vocal cords is supplied by the internal laryngeal nerve, that below by the recurrent laryngeal nerve. All muscles of the larynx are supplied by the recurrent laryngeal nerve **except for** the cricothyroid, which is supplied by the superior (also known as external) laryngeal nerve.

Lymphatic drainage

Most lymphatic drainage passes to the deep cervical chain. A small amount of lymph from the anterior and inferior areas of the larynx passes to the prelaryngeal and pretracheal nodes.

Trachea
Structure

The trachea descends from the lower border of the cricoid cartilage (C6) to terminate at its bifurcation into the two main bronchi at the sternal angle (T4). The length of the adult trachea varies between 10 and 15 cm. The walls of the trachea are formed of fibrous tissue reinforced by 15–20 incomplete cartilaginous rings. Internally the trachea is lined by respiratory epithelium. The trachea may be divided into two portions, that in the neck and that in the thorax.

Relations in the neck

The trachea lies in the midline, anterior to the oesophagus with the recurrent laryngeal nerve residing in a lateral position in a groove between the two. In front of the trachea lie the cervical fascia, infrahyoid muscles, isthmus of the thyroid gland and the jugular venous arch. Laterally lie the lobes of the thyroid gland, carotid sheath and the inferior thyroid artery. The relationships of the trachea at level C6 are shown in Figure CA10.

Relations in the thorax

The trachea is traversed anteriorly by two major vascular structures, the brachiocephalic artery and the left brachiocephalic vein. To the left lie the common carotid and subclavian arteries and the aortic arch. To the right lie the right branch of the vagus, azygos vein and mediastinal pleura. The carina is situated anteriorly to the oesophagus behind the bifurcation of the pulmonary trunk.

Blood supply

Arterial supply is from the inferior thyroid artery, and venous drainage via the inferior thyroid veins.

Nerve supply

Recurrent laryngeal branch of the vagus, with an additional sympathetic contribution from the middle cervical ganglion.

Lymphatic drainage

Drainage flows to the deep cervical, pretracheal and paratracheal lymph nodes.

Bronchial tree

The bronchial tree consists of extrapulmonary bronchi and intrapulmonary bronchi.

Extrapulmonary bronchi

At the carina, the two main bronchi arise. The right main bronchus is shorter, wider and more upright than the left. The right pulmonary artery and azygos vein are intimately related to the right main bronchus. The left main bronchus passes under the aortic arch anterior to the oesophagus, thoracic duct and descending aorta. The structure of the extrapulmonary bronchi is very similar to that of the trachea.

Intrapulmonary bronchi

Branching of the intrapulmonary bronchi gives rise to functional units – the bronchopleural segments. The right upper lobe bronchus arises from the right main bronchus just before the hilus and on entering the lung tissue it divides into apical, anterior and posterior segmental bronchi. The middle lobe bronchus arises from the right bronchus below the upper lobe bronchus and subsequently divides into the medial and lateral segmental bronchi. The continuing portion of the right bronchus runs to the lower lobe and divides into apical, anterior, medial, lateral and posterior basal segmental bronchi.

The left upper lobe bronchus arises from the left main bronchus within the lung and divides into five segmental bronchi, the superior and inferior of which supply the lingula. The continuing portion of the left bronchus runs to the lower lobe and then divides also into five segmental bronchi. Nomenclature here is as for the right side (Figure CA11).

The successive divisions of the bronchial tree may be simplified as follows:
- Main bronchus
- Segmental bronchus
- Bronchioli
- Respiratory bronchioli
- Alveolar ducts
- Atria
- Alveolar sacs
- Alveoli

Microstructure of the bronchial tree

The epithelium of the large bronchi has several layers. The basal layer sits on a basal membrane, the intermediate layer consists of spindle cells, and the superficial layer consists of ciliated columnar epithelium with occasional mucus-secreting goblet cells. As the bronchi divide and become narrower the epithelium changes to ciliated cuboidal with few goblet cells. The epithelium in the alveoli is only 0.2 microns thick and the blood–air interface consists of capillary wall, capillary basement membrane, alveolar basement membrane and alveolar epithelium. Interspersed with the flattened epithelial cells are larger cells with vacuoles. These are type II pneumocytes, which secrete surfactant.

The submucous layer of the bronchial tree consists of an elastic layer of longitudinal fibres and a deeper unstriped muscle coat.

Lungs

Structure

Each lung lies in its own pleural sac, which is attached to the mediastinum at the hilus. The lung has an apex in the root of the neck and a base that rests on the diaphragm. The left lung has an indentation on its anterior surface, which is the cardiac notch. Deep fissures divide the lungs into lobes. The oblique fissure divides the left lung into upper and lower lobes. The right lung is divided into upper, middle and lower lobes by the oblique and horizontal fissures. The lingula represents the rudimentary middle lobe of the left lung. Each lung has a hilus containing a main bronchus, pulmonary artery, pulmonary veins, pulmonary nerve plexus and lymph nodes surrounded by a collar of pleura.

Blood supply

Lung tissue is directly supplied by the bronchial branches of the descending aorta. Venous drainage is by the bronchial veins, which feed into the azygos vein. As regards oxygenation, poorly oxygenated blood travels to the alveoli via the

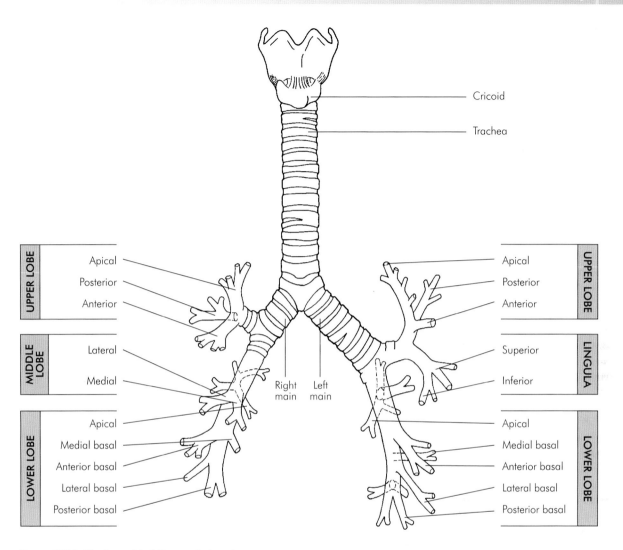

Figure CA11 The bronchi of the respiratory tree

pulmonary artery and returns ultimately to the pulmonary veins. See cardiac section, below, for details.

Nerve supply

There is direct parasympathetic supply via the vagus nerve, and sympathetic fibres from the thoracic sympathetic chain. Both travel in the pulmonary plexus. Sensory fibres arise from the vagus.

Lymphatic drainage

Most drainage is by way of the subpleural lymphatic plexus and the deep bronchial plexus, both of which drain to the bronchopulmonary nodes and thence to the mediastinal lymph trunks.

Pleura and mediastinum

Pleura

Structure

The pleura is a twin-walled serous-lined sac. The two layers are termed visceral and parietal. The visceral pleura invests the lung tissue and the parietal pleura invests the diaphragm, chest wall, apex of the thorax and the mediastinum. The upper limit of the pleura is about 3 cm above the midpoint of the clavicle. From here the lines of pleural reflections pass behind the sternoclavicular joints to meet in the midline at the level of the second costal cartilage. At the level of the fourth costal cartilage the lines deviate from each other. On the left the line of reflection deviates laterally, descending along the lateral margin of the sternum as far as the sixth costal cartilage. On the right the line continues vertically downwards. At the level of the sixth costal cartilage both lines of reflection pass to the eighth rib in the mid-clavicular line and then to the tenth rib in the mid-axillary line and finally on to the twelfth rib in the paravertebral line.

Blood supply

The pleura receives a supply of arterial and venous vessels from the organs which it covers.

Nerve supply

The visceral pleura has no sensory supply but the parietal pleura is supplied by fibres from all subjacent tissue.

Lymphatic drainage

The visceral pleura initially drains to the superficial plexus of the lung and thence to the hilar nodes. The parietal pleura drains into parasternal, diaphragmatic and posterior mediastinal nodes.

Mediastinum

The mediastinum is the area lying between the pleural sacs. The pericardium makes an artificial division into four regions. The middle mediastinum is the space occupied by the pericardium and its contents; the anterior mediastinum lies between the middle mediastinum and the sternum; the posterior mediastinum is that space between the pericardium and diaphragm; the superior mediastinum lies between the pericardium below and thoracic inlet above.

Diaphragm

A major muscle of respiration, the diaphragm is a musculotendinous septum between thorax and abdomen. It comprises a central tendinous portion and a peripheral muscular portion. The attachments of the diaphragm are **central** and **peripheral** (Figures CA12, CA13).

- **Central attachment.** The fibres of the tendinous section are concentrated into a trilobed central tendon, which blends superiorly with the fibrous pericardium.
- **Peripheral attachment.** A complex arrangement consisting of attachments to the crura, medial, median and lateral arcuate ligaments, costal margin and the xiphoid.

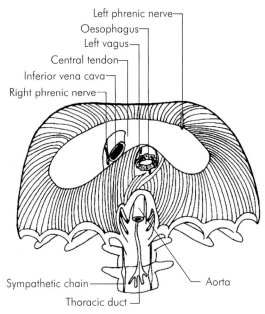
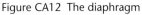

Left phrenic nerve
Oesophagus
Left vagus
Central tendon
Inferior vena cava
Right phrenic nerve
Sympathetic chain
Aorta
Thoracic duct

Figure CA12 The diaphragm

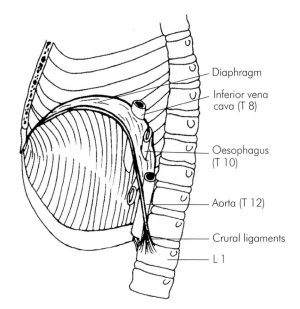

Diaphragm
Inferior vena cava (T 8)
Oesophagus (T 10)
Aorta (T 12)
Crural ligaments
L 1

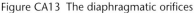

Figure CA13 The diaphragmatic orifices

Diaphragmatic foramina

- The inferior vena cava passes through the diaphragm within the central tendon to the right side at the level of T8. This foramen also transmits the right phrenic nerve.

- The oesophagus passes through the diaphragm to the left of the midline at the level of T10. This foramen also transmits the vagi.
- The aorta passes through the diaphragm behind the median arcuate ligament at T12. The thoracic duct and azygos vein also pass through this foramen.
- The left phrenic nerve pierces the left dome of the diaphragm.

Relations
The heart and lungs within their respective sacs lie above. Inferiorly, on the right are the liver and the right kidney, and on the left are the fundus of the stomach, the spleen and the left kidney.

Nerve supply
The diaphragm is supplied by two phrenic nerves (C3, 4, 5).

Heart
Structure
The heart is a muscular pump consisting of four chambers delineated by the coronary and interventricular sulci. The heart lies within the pericardial sac, effectively suspended by the great vessels. Its shape is said to be that of an irregular cone with a base and an apex, lying obliquely across the middle mediastinum. The base is posterior facing and mainly consists of left atrium. The apex represents the tip of the left ventricle. The anterior surface is formed by the right ventricle (Figure CA14).

Chambers of the heart
(1) **Right atrium**. The superior vena cava enters the right atrium in its superoposterior part. The inferior vena cava and coronary sinus enter the right atrium inferiorly and the anterior cardiac vein enters the chamber anteriorly. A vertical ridge runs between the venae cavae and this is termed the crista terminalis. The openings of both inferior vena cava and coronary sinus are guarded by vestigial valves. An oval depression on the surface of the atrial septum, the fossa ovalis, marks the site of the fetal foramen ovale.
(2) **Right ventricle**. The right ventricle communicates with the right atrium by way of the tricuspid valve, which possesses three cusps, medial, anterior and inferior. The pulmonary trunk communicates with the right ventricle by way of the pulmonary valve, which also has three cusps, posterior, right anterior and left anterior. A division between inflow and

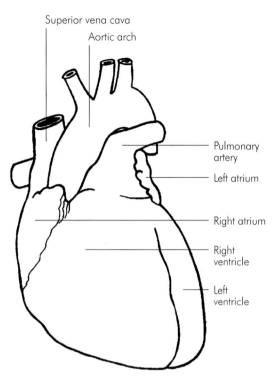

Figure CA14 Chambers of the heart

outflow tracts is provided by the infundibulo-ventricular crest, a muscular ridge. Trabeculae on the wall project papillary muscles which attach to the tricuspid valve by way of chordae tendinae.
(3) **Left atrium**. The left atrium is a rectangular chamber behind the right atrium. Superiorly a small projection arises on the left of the pulmonary trunk, the left auricle. Four pulmonary veins enter the chamber posteriorly by way of valveless orifices. On the septal surface a shallow depression corresponds to the fossa ovalis of the right atrium.
(4) **Left ventricle**. The left ventricle communicates with the left atrium via the mitral valve, which has two cusps, anterior and posterior, connected by chordae tendinae to papillary muscles. The origin of the aorta is defended by the aortic valve, which has three cusps, right and left posterior and anterior, above which lie the aortic sinuses. The right coronary artery arises from the anterior sinus and the left from the left posterior sinus. The wall of the left ventricle is ridged by thick trabeculae carnae.

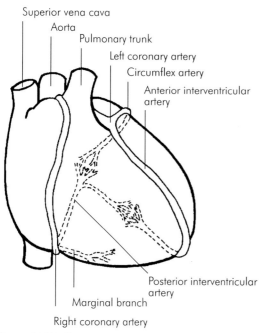

Figure CA15 The coronary arteries

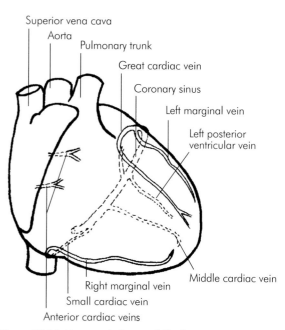

Figure CA16 Venous drainage of the heart

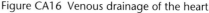

Conducting system

The conducting system of the heart is provided by specialised cardiac muscle tissue within the sinoatrial (SA) and atrioventricular (AV) nodes and the bundle branch system of Purkinje fibres. The SA node consists of an area of conducting tissue in the wall of the right atrium at the upper end of the crista terminalis and to the right of the opening of the superior vena cava. The SA node transmits impulses through the atrial wall to the AV node, which is a similar structure in the septal wall of the right atrium above the opening of the coronary sinus.

The AV node gives rise to the AV bundle (the bundle of His) which descends across the interventricular septum to divide into right and left branches. The branches ramify into a subendocardial plexus in the ventricular wall.

Nerve supply

The nerve supply of the heart arises from the vagus, which provides cardio-inhibitory fibres, and the cervical and upper thoracic sympathetic ganglia, which provide cardio-acceleratory fibres via the superficial and deep cardiac plexi.

Blood supply

The heart receives arterial blood from right and left coronary arteries (Figure CA15).

The right coronary artery arises from the anterior aortic sinus, passing forward between the right atrium and pulmonary trunk to then run in the right coronary sulcus to anastomose with the left coronary artery. The branches are as follows:
(1) Atrial branches
(2) Ventricular branches
(3) Marginal artery
(4) Posterior interventricular artery

The left coronary artery arises from the left posterior aortic sinus to pass between the left atrium and pulmonary trunk to run in the left coronary sulcus and then anastomose with the right coronary artery as described above. The branches are as follows:
(1) Atrial branches
(2) Ventricular branches
(3) Anterior interventricular artery
(4) Circumflex artery (sourcing marginal artery)

The sinuses of Valsalva are small outpocketings of the aortic wall in proximity to the coronary ostia. They produce small eddy currents which prevent the aortic valve cusps from obscuring the coronary ostia.

The venous drainage of the heart is complex (Figure CA16). The majority of the venous drainage is provided by veins accompanying the coronary arteries, which

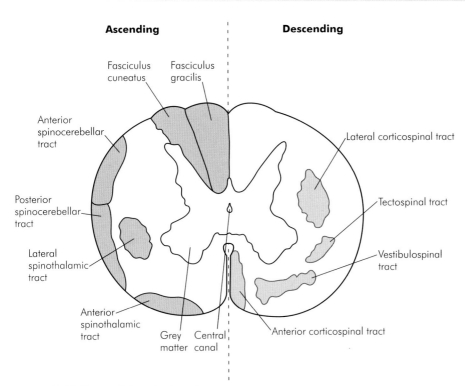

Ascending   **Descending**

Fasciculus cuneatus   Fasciculus gracilis

Anterior spinocerebellar tract

Lateral corticospinal tract

Posterior spinocerebellar tract

Tectospinal tract

Lateral spinothalamic tract

Vestibulospinal tract

Anterior spinothalamic tract   Grey matter   Central canal

Anterior corticospinal tract

Figure CA17 Tracts of the spinal cord

then open directly into the right atrium. Some venous blood drains directly into the cavity via the venae cordis minimae, very small veins. The anterior cardiac vein crosses the atrioventricular groove and opens into the right atrium. The remainder of the venous drainage is provided by the coronary sinus, which has the following tributaries:
(1) Great cardiac vein
(2) Middle cardiac vein
(3) Small cardiac vein
(4) Oblique vein
(5) Left posterior ventricular vein

Lymphatic drainage
Lymphatic drainage of the heart passes to the tracheo-bronchial lymph nodes.

Pericardium
The pericardium is a fibroserous membrane that surrounds the heart and great vessels. There are two layers, an outer fibrous pericardium and an inner serous pericardium.

The serous pericardium has the form of a closed sac in which the heart is invaginated. It has visceral and parietal layers. The fibrous pericardium exists as a strong sac containing the heart itself and the accompanying serous pericardium.

Nervous system
Spinal cord
The spinal cord in the adult human is approximately 45 cm long. It is said to be cylindrical in shape, although flattened in the anteroposterior diameter. Above, the spinal cord is continuous with the brain stem, and below it tapers into the conus medullaris, which is attached to the coccyx by the filum terminale. The cord usually ends at the level of L1/2, although there is great variation in this.

Macroscopically the cord has slight grooves on its anterior and posterior surfaces, the anterior median fissure and posterior median sulcus respectively. In transverse section a central canal can be seen with an H-shaped area of grey matter composed of nerve cells surrounded by white matter composed of nerve fibres (Figure CA17). The grey matter is divided by virtue of its H shape into two anterior horns (carrying the anterior columns) and two posterior horns (carrying the posterior columns), the two being cross-linked by the transverse comissure, which corresponds to the cross-bar of the H shape. The white matter is largely composed of medullated cells in a longitudinal orientation, which are classified according to their relationship to the grey matter into posterior, anterior and lateral white columns.

Ascending tracts of the cord

(1) The posterior white column transmits fine touch sensation and proprioception. The two fasciculi (medial and lateral) connect to their respective cuneate and gracile nuclei in the medulla. The fibres then cross in the medullary decussation to reach the sensory cortex via the thalamus.

(2) The lateral white column carries the lateral spinothalamic tract, which conveys pain and temperature sensation. The cell bodies lie in the posterior horn of the opposite side and fibres then cross in the anterior white commissure to ascend to the thalamus.

(3) The anterior and posterior spinocerebellar tracts ascend in the lateral column. Proprioception sensation is transmitted through these tracts, without crossing, to the cerebellum.

Descending tracts of the cord

(1) The pyramidal tract is the major motor pathway of the cord. It lies in the posterior part of the lateral white column. The tract arises from the pyramidal cells in the motor cortex to cross in the medulla and descend in the pyramidal tract of the contralateral side. At each segmental level fibres pass to the anterior horn of the same side to make the link between upper and lower motor neurones.

(2) The direct pyramidal tract is a minor tract running close to the anterior median fissure. Fibres descend from the motor cortex without crossing, in contrast to the pyramidal tract. At each segmental level fibres cross to the opposite anterior horn.

Blood supply

The spinal cord receives arterial supply from the anterior and posterior spinal arteries, with additional contributions from spinal branches of the vertebral, intercostal, lumbar and sacral arteries. Radicular arteries serve to reinforce the anterior spinal arterial supply and in the low thoracic or high lumbar level one of these is large and supplies most of the lower two-thirds of the cord: this is the arteria radicularis magna. Venous drainage is by way of a complex of anterior and posterior spinal veins which drain into segmental veins and thence to the azygos, lumbar and sacral veins according to level.

Spinal meninges

There are three layers covering the spinal cord: the dura, arachnoid and pia mater.

Dura mater

The dura mater consists of two layers. On the surface of the brain the layers are separated by the cerebral venous sinuses. On the surface of the spinal cord the inner dural layer is densely fibrous and the outer layer less so. The outer or endosteal layer ends at the foramen magnum, where it blends with the periosteum of the skull. Most commonly the dural sac ends within the sacrum at the level of S2. It may however, terminate as high as L5. The attachments of the dura are as follows:

(1) Superiorly: the edges of the foramen magnum, bodies of C2 and C3 vertebrae

(2) Anteriorly: posterior longitudinal ligament

(3) Laterally: a sheath along the dorsal and ventral nerve roots

(4) Inferiorly: the filum terminale

The anatomy of the epidural space is detailed in Section 1, Chapter 5 (pages 80–81).

Arachnoid mater

The arachnoid mater is a delicate membrane closely applied to the dura mater. In some areas the arachnoid herniates the dura mater to form the arachnoid villi, which have a major role in the circulation of CSF. The cerebral layer of arachnoid loosely invests the brain and only dips into the main longitudinal fissure between the cerebral hemispheres.

Pia mater

The pia mater is the innermost layer of the three and is closely applied to the surface of the brain and spinal cord. The pia extends into all the sulci of the brain and invests both cranial and spinal nerves, their roots and the filum terminale. In the roof of the third and fourth ventricles and the medial wall of the lateral ventricles the two layers of the pia fuse and form the choroid plexuses. Anteriorly the spinal pia mater is thickened to form the linea splendens, and on each side of the spinal cord a serrated fold of pia is termed the ligamentum denticulatum, which pierces the arachnoid to attach to dura, thus stabilising the cord within its dural sheath.

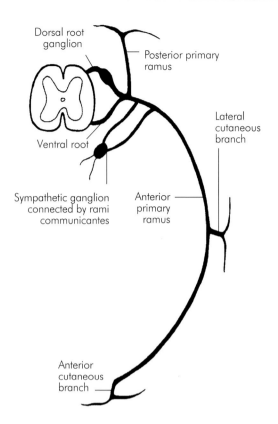

Figure CA18 A typical spinal nerve

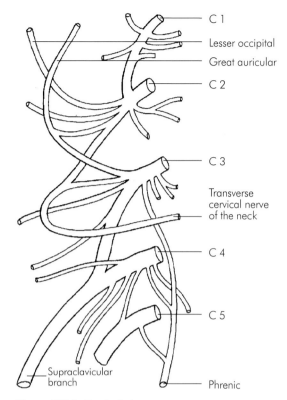

Figure CA19 Cervical plexus

Spinal nerves

There are 31 pairs of spinal nerves (8 cervical, 12 thoracic, 5 lumbar, 5 sacral, 1 coccygeal) formed in the vertebral canal by the union of ventral and dorsal nerve roots. The ventral roots transmit efferent motor impulses from the cord and the dorsal roots transmit sensory information to the cord. The cell bodies of the sensory fibres are grouped in a ganglion on the dorsal root. When each nerve leaves the vertebral canal it divides into anterior (ventral) and posterior (dorsal) rami.

In most regions adjacent ventral rami connect to form major plexuses: cervical, brachial and lumbosacral. In the thoracic region the ventral rami become intercostal and subcostal nerves. Dorsal rami pass posteriorly to divide into medial and lateral branches to supply the muscles and skin of the posterior aspect of the body (Figure CA18).

There is a wide variation in the dermatomes corresponding to the spinal nerves; relatively consistent landmarks are nipple at T4/5 and umbilicus at T10.

Peripheral nerves

The **cervical plexus** and its branches are shown in Figure CA19. The nerves of the upper limb derive from the **brachial plexus**. The branches and relationships of the brachial plexus are shown in Figures CA20 and CA21. The nerves of the leg derive from the **lumbosacral plexus** (Figures CA22, CA23).

The sciatic nerve is the largest nerve in the body. It is derived from the roots of L4,5 S1,2,3 on the anterior surface of piriformis and descends through the greater sciatic foramen to run posteriorly within the thigh. On approaching the popliteal fossa it divides into tibial and common peroneal branches.

The tibial nerve is a terminal branch of the sciatic. It descends through the popliteal fossa through the flexor compartment to the level of the medial malleolus, where it gives rise to medial and lateral plantar nerves.

The common peroneal nerve descends laterally in the popliteal fossa, passing into peroneus longus, where it divides into superficial and deep peroneal nerves. The sural nerve arises from the common peroneal high in

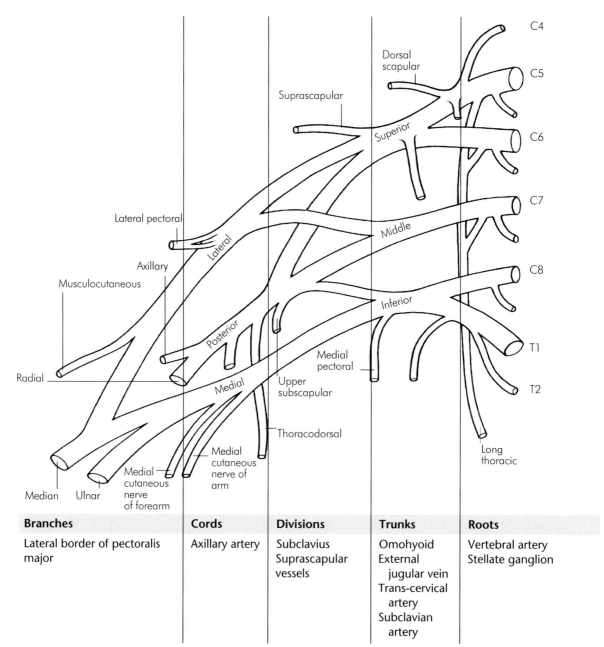

Figure CA20 Brachial plexus: relationships

Branches	Cords	Divisions	Trunks	Roots
Lateral border of pectoralis major	Axillary artery	Subclavius Suprascapular vessels	Omohyoid External jugular vein Trans-cervical artery Subclavian artery	Vertebral artery Stellate ganglion

the popliteal fossa before passing to lie behind the lateral malleolus.

The obturator nerve is a branch of the lumbosacral plexus which descends medial to psoas and runs along the lateral pelvic wall, after which it enters the thigh through the obturator foramen to divide into anterior and posterior branches.

The femoral nerve arises from the roots of L2,3,4 and descends in the pelvis in the groove between psoas and iliacus to enter the thigh deep to the inguinal ligament. It

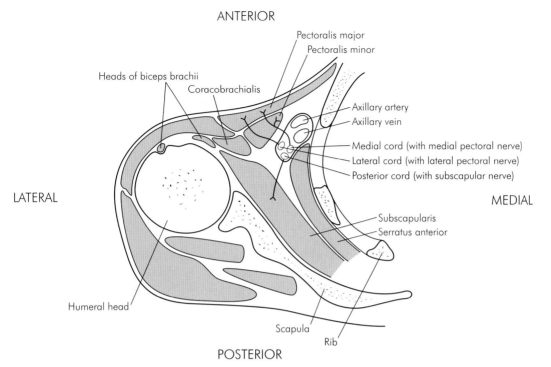

ANTERIOR

Pectoralis major
Pectoralis minor

Heads of biceps brachii
Coracobrachialis

Axillary artery
Axillary vein
Medial cord (with medial pectoral nerve)
Lateral cord (with lateral pectoral nerve)
Posterior cord (with subscapular nerve)

LATERAL

MEDIAL

Subscapularis
Serratus anterior

Humeral head

Scapula
Rib

POSTERIOR

Figure CA21 Relationships of the cords of the brachial plexus in the axilla

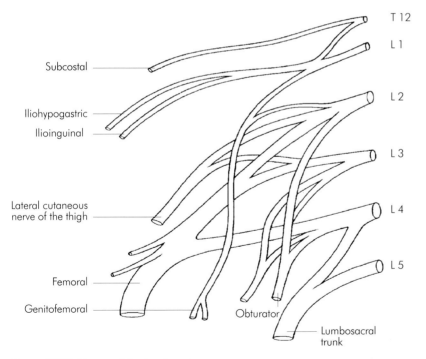

T 12
L 1

Subcostal

L 2

Iliohypogastric
Ilioinguinal

L 3

Lateral cutaneous
nerve of the thigh

L 4

L 5

Femoral

Genitofemoral

Obturator

Lumbosacral
trunk

Figure CA22 Nerves of the lumbar plexus

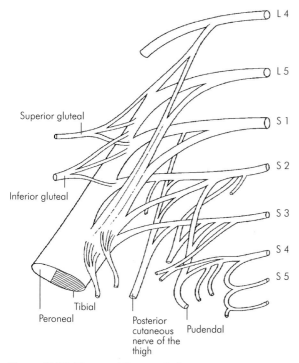

Figure CA23 Nerves of the sacral plexus

divides into anterior, medial and muscular branches and also the important saphenous branch, which emerges from sartorius to run medially in proximity with the saphenous nerve. For detail of the nerves of the foot see Section 1, Chapter 7.

Autonomic nervous system
The autonomic nervous system consists of two complementary components, the sympathetic and parasympathetic nervous systems, whose fibres arise from the neurones of the visceral columns of the brain and spinal cord. Fibres synapse with peripheral ganglia before reaching their target organs.

Sympathetic nervous system
From T1 to L2 each ventral ramus gives a bundle of myelinated preganglionic fibres (white rami communicantes) to form the sympathetic trunk. Each ventral ramus receives a bundle of unmyelinated postganglionic fibres from the sympathetic trunk (grey rami communicantes). The ganglia of the sympathetic system lie in two trunks either side of the vertebral column. There are 3 cervical, 12 thoracic, 5 lumbar and 5 sacral ganglia.

Parasympathetic nervous system
The system is formed by preganglionic fibres from the following cranial nerves: oculomotor, facial, glossopharyngeal and vagus and a sacral component comprising preganglionic fibres from S2,3,4. This is known as the craniosacral outflow. Although the ganglia of the parasympathetic system are usually ill-defined and close to their target organs, the cranial nerves involved have anatomically discrete identifiable ganglia. Postganglionic parasympathetic fibres are short and unmyelinated.

Cranial nerves
Olfactory (I)
The fibres of the olfactory nerve are actually the central processes of the olfactory cells rather than peripheral processes of a central group of ganglion cells.

The nerve fibres originate in the bipolar olfactory cells of the nasal mucosa and subsequently join to form approximately 20 bundles which pass through the cribriform plate of the ethmoid to terminate by synapsing with mitral cells in the olfactory bulb. Axons pass back from the mitral cells to the cortex of the uncus, whereupon the final path becomes uncertain.

Optic (II)
Embryologically the optic nerve is part of the forebrain. Fibres originate in the ganglionic layer of the retina, from which axons converge on the optic disc, piercing the sclera to form the optic nerve. The nerve runs posteriorly through the orbit and optic canal into the middle cranial fossa, where it joins its partner from the contralateral side to form the optic chiasm. In the chiasm the fibres from the medial half of the retina cross to the opposite side while fibres from the lateral side of the retina pass in the optic tract of the same side. The optic tract passes backward to the lateral geniculate body of the thalamus and thence to the occipital visual cortex.

Oculomotor (III)
The oculomotor nerve has both somatic motor and parasympathetic motor fibres. The somatic fibres supply the muscles of the eye excepting superior oblique (VI) and lateral rectus (IV). The parasympathetic fibres synapse within the ciliary ganglion and supply the sphincter pupillae and ciliary muscles. The nerve arises in the upper midbrain, where the nuclei lie within the periaqueductal grey matter. Fibres pass forwards through the midbrain, exiting between the cerebral peduncles. Passing forwards, the nerve pierces dura mater to run in the lateral wall

of the cavernous sinus, after which it divides into superior and inferior branches. The superior branch passes through the superior orbital fissure to supply superior rectus and levator palpebrae superioris. The inferior division passes through the tendinous ring to supply medial rectus, inferior rectus and inferior oblique.

Trochlear (IV)

The trochlear nerve provides motor supply to the superior oblique muscle. It arises from a nucleus in the periaqueductal grey matter of the lower midbrain. Fibres pass dorsally around the cerebral aqueduct to decussate with the nerve of the opposite side, then passing forward through posterior and middle cranial fossae to enter the orbit via the superior orbital fissure. In the middle cranial fossa the trochlear nerve pierces the dura and runs in the lateral wall of the cavernous sinus in a similar manner to the oculomotor nerve, which is slightly more medially placed.

Trigeminal (V)

The trigeminal nerve is the principal sensory nerve of the face, nose and mouth. It also supplies motor fibres to the muscles of mastication. The nerve has three sensory nuclei, spinal, mesencephalic and superior (in the pons), and one motor (also in the pons). The nerve originates in the pons as a major sensory and more minor motor root. It passes forward to the trigeminal ganglion, which is situated on the petrous temporal bone. The three divisions, ophthalmic, maxillary and mandibular, emerge from the anterior border of the ganglion. The motor root bypasses the ganglion to rejoin the mandibular nerve later.

Ophthalmic division: passes forward on the lateral wall of the cavernous sinus (below oculomotor and trochlear nerves) and divides into three branches: lacrimal, frontal and nasociliary. The branches of the nasociliary nerve are the anterior ethmoidal, posterior ethmoidal, infratrochlear and long ciliary nerves.

Maxillary division: runs along the inferior border of the cavernous sinus below the ophthalmic nerve and leaves the skull via the foramen rotundum. After traversing the pterygopalatine fossa the nerve is termed the infra orbital nerve and it emerges through the infra-orbital foramen to supply adjacent areas of the face. Fibres pass to the pterygopalatine ganglion and the maxillary nerve has the following branches: zygomatic, posterior superior alveolar and infra orbital which themselves branch into smaller nerves.

Mandibular division: sensory to the lower third of the face, the anterior two-thirds of the tongue and floor of the mouth. The mandibular nerve carries the motor supply to the muscles of mastication, tensor tympani, tensor palati, mylohyoid and the anterior belly of the digastric muscle.

The motor and sensory components pass separately through the foramen ovale and then join into a short trunk which lies on the tensor palati muscle. At this point the middle meningeal artery lies posterior to the nerve and the otic ganglion is medial to it. The sensory branches are as follows: meningeal, buccal, auriculotemporal, inferior alveolar and lingual.

Abducent (VI)

The nucleus of the abducent nerve resides in the lower pons. It leaves the inferior border of the pons to pass forward through the cavernous sinus, lying lateral to the internal carotid artery and medial to cranial nerves II, IV and V. The nerve enters the orbit to pierce lateral rectus, which it supplies.

Facial (VII)

The facial nerve has a mixed function. It supplies motor fibres to the muscles of facial expression, parasympathetic secretomotor fibres to the submandibular and sublingual salivary glands and taste sensation from the anterior two-thirds of the tongue. There are three respective nuclei in the pons for these three functions. The fibres associated with taste pass to the geniculate ganglion and thence to the nucleus of the tractus solitarius, from which they then cross to the opposite lateral nucleus of the thalamus, ending in the sensory cortex. The secretomotor fibres arise in the superior salivary nucleus in the pons, close to the motor nucleus. The motor nucleus lies within the reticular formation of the lower pons. The nerve leaves the pons to run laterally in conjunction with the vestibulocochlear nerve though the internal auditory meatus to the facial ganglion, where it takes a sharp posterior turn to pass downwards through the stylomastoid foramen. Just before this point it gives off the chorda tympani, which later joins the lingual nerve to supply taste sensation to the anterior two-thirds of the tongue. After emerging from the stylomastoid foramen the facial nerve is entirely motor and has the following branches: posterior auricular, digastric and stylohyoid.

Vestibulocochlear (VIII)

Within the auditory nerve are two types of fibre, vestibular and cochlear, hence its alternative name. The nerve is formed in the internal meatus and then passes medially to join the brain stem at the cerebromedullary angle. Cochlear fibres arising from the bipolar spiral ganglion cells of the cochlea pass to the dorsal and ventral cochlear nuclei in the upper medulla. Efferent fibres cross to the opposite side to form the auditory striae in the floor of the fourth ventricle, those from the ventral nucleus particularly forming the trapezoid body in the pons. Fibres ascend from the trapezoid body in the lateral lemniscus to reach the medial geniculate body, and thence to the auditory cortex. Vestibular fibres arising from the semicircular ducts, saccule and utricle pass to the vestibular ganglion in the internal meatus and ultimately terminate in the vestibular nuclei in the floor of the fourth ventricle. Efferent fibres travel to the cerebellum in the inferior cerebellar peduncle and there are other vestibular connections to the nuclei of cranial nerves II, IV, VI and XI via the medial longitudinal bundle.

Glossopharyngeal (IX)

The glossopharyngeal nerve provides sensation to the pharynx, tonsil and posterior one-third of the tongue (including taste), motor supply to stylopharyngeus and secretomotor innervation to the parotid gland. The carotid branch of the glossopharyngeal supplies the carotid body and carotid sinus. Four nuclei correspond to the various roles of the nerve in the following way. The rostral part of the nucleus ambiguus (strictly vagus) is the nucleus of the motor path to stylopharyngeus. The inferior salivary nucleus supplies the secretomotor fibres to the parotid. The nucleus of the tractus solitarius (shared with fibres of VII and X) receives the taste fibres. General sensory fibres terminate in the dorsal sensory nucleus of the vagus. The roots of the glossopharyngeal leave the medulla just lateral to the olive. The nerve passes through the jugular foramen and pierces the pharyngeal wall between superior and middle constrictor muscles. There are two main branches, the tympanic branch and the carotid branch, which is of importance as it supplies the carotid sinus and carotid body.

Vagus (X)

The vagus nerve is the longest and most widely distributed of the cranial nerves. The vagus provides motor, sensory and secretomotor supply. It provides motor innervation to the larynx, bronchial muscles, gastrointestinal tract and the heart (through cardio-inhibitory fibres). Sensory supply is distributed to the dura mater, respiratory tract, gastrointestinal tract and heart. The vagus also provides secretomotor innervation to the bronchial mucus glands and gastrointestinal tract. The vagus has three nuclei. The dorsal nucleus of the vagus is a mixed motor and sensory centre situated below the floor of the fourth ventricle. The nucleus ambiguus is a motor nucleus situated within the reticular formation of the medulla. The third nucleus is the nucleus of the tractus solitarius, which is concerned with taste sensation. It is situated in the central grey matter of the medulla. The vagus emerges from the medulla lateral to the olive as a group of rootlets, then leaves the skull through the jugular foramen as a single trunk. At the level of the base of skull the vagus has two ganglia, the superior and inferior sensory ganglia. Below the inferior ganglion the vagus receives a communication from the accessory nerve representing its cranial root. The nerve descends through the neck to reach the thorax, where it is joined by its contralateral partner in the oesophageal plexus to form anterior and posterior vagal trunks, which travel asymmetrically through the thorax and abdomen, providing extensive visceral innervation en route.

Accessory (XI)

The accessory nerve provides the motor supply to sternomastoid and trapezius muscles. The nerve has two roots, a small cranial root travelling by way of the vagus and a larger spinal root from nuclei in the upper five cervical segments of the spinal cord. The nerve arises in the vertebral canal and ascends through the foramen magnum into the posterior cranial fossa. It leaves the skull by way of the jugular foramen and passes anterior to the internal jugular vein into the body of sternomastoid. Subsequently the nerve crosses the posterior triangle of the neck to pierce trapezius.

Hypoglossal (XII)

The hypoglossal nerve provides motor supply to all the intrinsic and extrinsic muscles of the tongue except palatoglossus. The nerve has its nucleus in the floor of the fourth ventricle and arises as a series of rootlets which leave the medulla between pyramid and olive. After uniting into one trunk the nerve leaves the skull by the hypoglossal canal. The nerve passes downwards between the internal carotid artery and jugular vein to the level of the angle of the jaw, where it loops over the lingual artery before reaching hyoglossus and genioglossus and terminating in direct motor innervation of the muscles of the tongue. The hypoglossal nerve receives some fibres from the ventral ramus of C1 at the level of the base of skull. The majority of these fibres pass into the descendens hypoglossi, which descends as a discrete branch, being joined by the descendens cervicalis (made up of fibres from C2 and C3) to form the ansa hypoglossi, which supplies omohyoid, sternothyroid and geniohyoid.

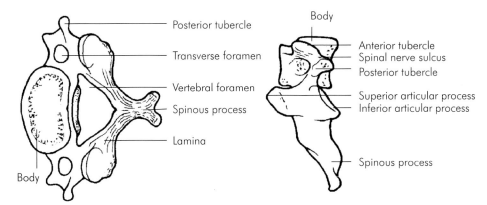

Figure CA24 Cervical vertebra, superior and lateral views

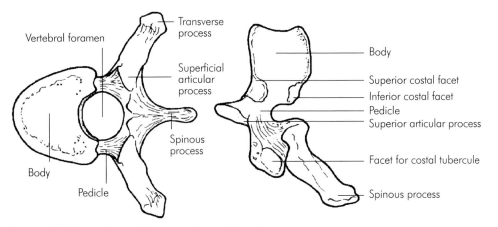

Figure CA25 Thoracic vertebra, superior and lateral views

Vertebral column

There are seven cervical vertebrae, the atlas, axis and the similar C3–7. There are 12 thoracic vertebrae and five lumbar vertebrae. Five fused sacral segments form the sacrum, and the coccyx has four fused segments. Structures of typical vertebrae are shown in Figures CA24–CA27.

Special zones

Thoracic inlet

The thoracic inlet slopes downwards and forwards, making an angle of 60° to the horizontal. It is approximately 10 cm wide and 5 cm from front to back.

The thoracic inlet (Figure CA28) is bounded posteriorly by the first thoracic vertebra, anteriorly by the manubrium and first rib, and laterally by the costal cartilage. The shape of the inlet is said to be kidney-shaped, because of the protrusion of the body of T1 into what would otherwise be an oval. The thoracic inlet transmits the trachea, oesophagus, large vascular trunks (brachiocephalic, left carotid and left subclavian arteries and brachiocephalic vein), vagi, thoracic duct, phrenic nerves and cervical sympathetic chain.

The first rib (Figure CA29) is short, wide and flattened. It lies in an oblique plane. The first rib has a rounded head with a facet that articulates with the body of T1, a long neck and a tubercle that articulates with the transverse process of T1. The inferior surface of the rib is smooth and lies on the pleura. The scalene tubercle on the medial border of the rib indicates the attachment of the scalenus anterior muscle. Anteriorly the upper surface of the first rib gives attachment to the costoclavicular

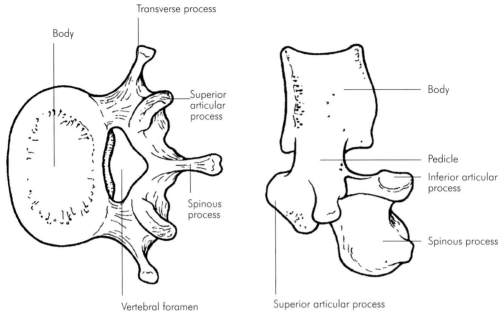

Figure CA26 Lumbar vertebra, superior and lateral views

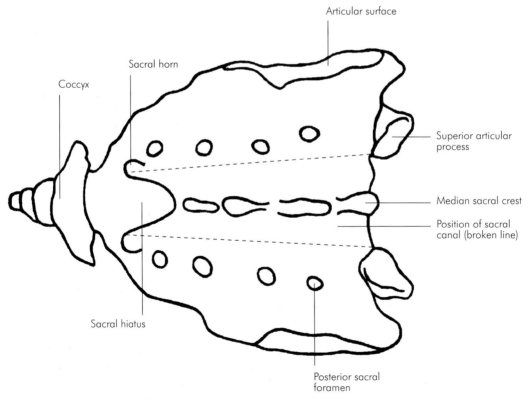

Figure CA27 Sacrum, posterior view

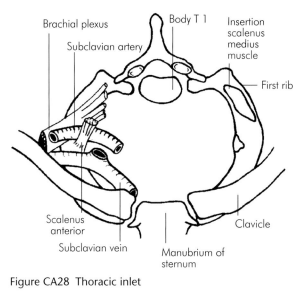

Figure CA28 Thoracic inlet

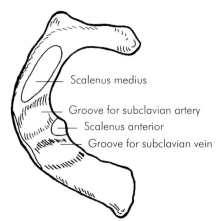

Figure CA29 Surface markings of the first rib (superior view)

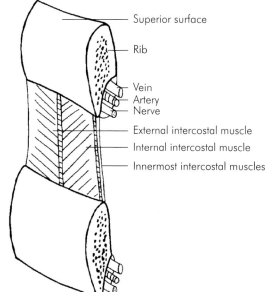

Figure CA30 Intercostal space

ligament and subclavius muscle. Between the pleura and the neck of the rib lie the sympathetic trunk, the large branch of the anterior primary ramus of T1 passing to the brachial plexus and the superior intercostal vessels. The inner margin of the first rib gives attachment to the suprapleural membrane (Sibson's fascia), which joins the transverse process of C7.

Intercostal spaces

The intercostal spaces are bounded by their related ribs and costal cartilages. They contain the intercostal muscles, vessels and nerves. Deep to the intercostal spaces lies the pleura. The intercostal muscles are arranged as follows: the external intercostal muscle descends in an oblique manner forwards from the lower border of the rib above to the upper border of the rib below. The internal intercostal muscle is an incomplete sheet between the ribs and the pleura which attaches to the sternum, costal cartilages and ribs. Additionally, there is an innermost layer of muscles that is incomplete and consists of sternocostalis, the intracostals and subcostals. The contents of the intercostal space are the components of the neurovascular bundle. These (from top to bottom) are the posterior intercostal vein, the posterior intercostal artery and the intercostal nerve. The neurovascular bundle is protected by the costal groove of the upper rib, as shown in Figure CA30.

Abdominal wall
Structure

The most important muscle of the abdominal wall is the rectus abdominus. This is inserted into the pubic symphysis over a 3 cm wide area and inserts onto the 5th, 6th and 7th costal cartilages. The muscle generally is marked by three fibrous intersections on its anterior surface. Rectus abdominus lies within a sheath – the rectus sheath, formed by a split in the aponeurosis of internal oblique. The rectus sheath is reinforced posteriorly by the aponeurosis of transversus abdominus and anteriorly by the aponeurosis of external oblique. At its uppermost extremity the rectus lies directly on the costal cartilages, because neither internal oblique nor transversus abdominus extend superiorly to this level. Below the arcuate line of Douglas (halfway between umbilicus and pubis) the aponeuroses of external oblique, internal oblique and transversus abdominus pass anterior to the rectus itself, which therefore rests on transversalis fascia, fat and peritoneum. Fusion of the aponeuroses of the rectus sheath in the midline forms the linea alba, which extends from the xiphoid to the pubis.

Blood supply

There is a substantial and varied blood supply to the abdominal wall. Of particular importance are the superior and inferior epigastric vessels. The surface marking of these vessels is represented by a line from the femoral pulse in the groin to a point just lateral to the umbilicus.

Nerve supply

The anterior primary rami of T7–L1 supply the anterior abdominal wall. The intercostal nerves (T7–11) and the subcostal nerve (T12) enter the abdominal wall between the interdigitations of the diaphragm, eventually piercing the rectus abdominus to supply the skin. The first lumbar nerve, in contrast, divides anterior to the quadratus lumborum muscle into the iliohypogastric and ilioinguinal nerves. The iliohypogastric nerve pierces internal oblique close to the anterior superior iliac spine and then runs deep to external oblique to supply the skin of the suprapubic area. The ilioinguinal nerve pierces internal oblique and traverses the inguinal canal. It emerges through the external ring (or occasionally through the aponeurosis of external oblique to supply a variable area of the genitalia and upper thigh). There is no deep fascia over the abdominal wall, but the superficial fatty tissue may be termed Camper's and Scarpa's fascia (the latter being deeper, although there is no real distinction between the two).

Useful landmarks of the abdominal wall include the xiphoid–T9, and the umbilicus–L4.

Inguinal canal

The inguinal canal (Figure CA31) is an obliquely angled path through the anterior abdominal wall. It extends from the deep ring, which is a weakness in the transversalis fascia at the midpoint of the inguinal ligament, to the superficial ring, which is a deficiency in the aponeurosis of external oblique situated superomedial to the pubic tubercle. The

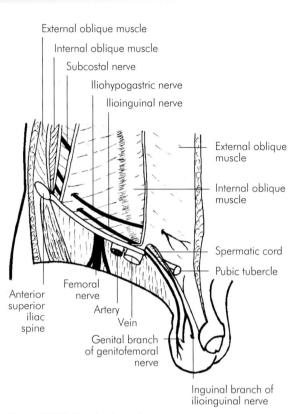

Figure CA31 Inguinal canal

inguinal canal is approximately 5 cm long and has the following boundaries:
(1) Anterior wall: external oblique aponeurosis, reinforced laterally by internal oblique
(2) Posterior wall: transversalis fascia, reinforced medially by the conjoint tendon
(3) Floor: edge of the inguinal ligament
(4) Roof: internal oblique, becoming conjoint tendon laterally

Contents: inferior epigastric artery, spermatic cord, round ligament and fat.

Antecubital fossa

The antecubital fossa is a triangle bounded inferomedially by pronator teres, inferolaterally by brachioradialis and superiorly by a line passing through the medial and lateral condyles of the humerus. The roof of the antecubital fossa consists of deep fascia, which is reinforced by the bicipital aponeurosis. On the deep fascia lie the median cubital vein and medial cutaneous nerve of the forearm.

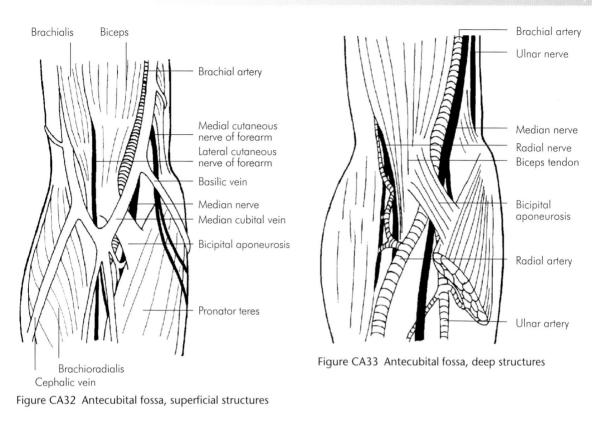

Figure CA32 Antecubital fossa, superficial structures

Figure CA33 Antecubital fossa, deep structures

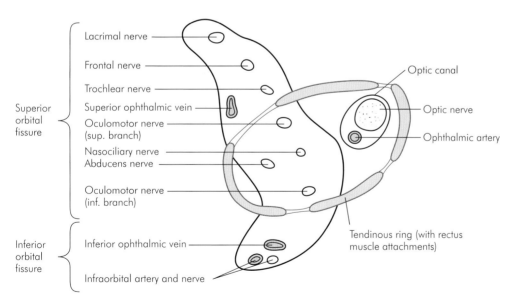

Figure CA34 Structures passing through the orbital fissures

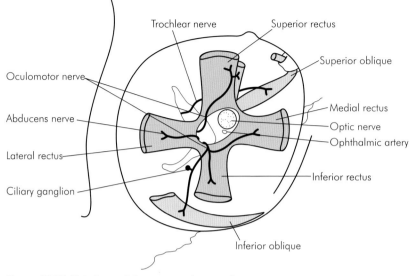

Figure CA35 Relations of the extraocular muscles

Lateral structures include the cephalic vein and lateral cutaneous nerve of the forearm, and medially lies the basilic vein. Within the antecubital fossa from medial to lateral lie the median nerve, brachial artery, tendon of biceps and the radial nerve (Figures CA32, CA33).

Orbit
Orbital cavity

The orbital cavities lie within the facial skeleton. They are broadly pyramidal in shape and contain the globes, muscles, nerves, vessels and fat.

The roof of the orbit is mainly formed by the frontal bone but the posterior portion is derived from the greater wing of the sphenoid. It separates the orbit from the anterior cranial fossa. The floor is composed of the maxilla and zygoma, with the maxillary air sinus lying beneath. The lateral wall is formed by the greater wing of the sphenoid and the zygomatic bone. The lateral wall separates the orbit from the temporal fossa. The medial wall has several components: from anterior to posterior these are the frontal process of the maxilla, the lacrimal bone, the orbital plate of the ethmoid and the sphenoid bone.

The orbit contains three posterior openings. The optic canal opens into the apex of the orbit and transmits the optic nerve together with its meninges and the ophthalmic artery. The superior orbital fissure lies between the greater and lesser wings of the sphenoid. The inferior orbital fissure lies between the floor and lateral wall. It opens into the pterygopalatine fossa medially and the infratemporal fossa laterally. The relationships of both fissures are shown in Figure CA34.

For the structure of the globe itself, see Section 2, Chapter 9.

Extraocular muscles

There are four rectus muscles: superior, inferior, medial and lateral. Anteriorly these muscles pass forward to attach to the sclera at the equator of the globe. Posteriorly they attach to a common tendinous ring around the optic canal and the medial end of the superior orbital fissure.

The superior oblique muscle is attached posteriorly to the common tendinous ring. The muscle passes forward around a cartilaginous 'pulley' (the trochlea) to travel backwards and laterally before inserting into the sclera behind the equator.

The inferior oblique is attached posteriorly to the floor of the orbit. It passes backwards and laterally below the inferior rectus muscle to attach to the sclera behind the equator. The lateral rectus muscle is supplied by the abducent nerve (VI), the superior oblique by the trochlear nerve (IV) and all the others by the oculomotor nerve (III). The relationships of the extraocular muscles are shown in Figure CA35.

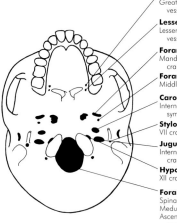

Greater palatine foramen
Greater palatine nerve and vessels

Lesser palatine foramen
Lesser palatine nerve and vessels

Foramen ovale
Mandibular division of V cranial nerve

Foramen spinosum
Middle meningeal artery

Carotid canal
Internal carotid artery and sympathetic fibres

Stylomastoid foramen
VII cranial nerve

Jugular foramen
Internal jugular vein IX X XI cranial nerves

Hypoglossal canal
XII cranial nerve

Foramen magnum
Spinal cord
Medulla junction
Ascending spinal portion XI cranial nerve
Spinal and vertebral arteries
Branches of C1–C3 spinal nerves

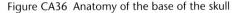

Figure CA36 Anatomy of the base of the skull

Blood supply

The ophthalmic artery is a branch of the internal carotid. It arises in the middle cranial fossa and enters the orbit through the optic canal, lying inferior to the optic nerve. Branches include the central artery of the retina, ciliary branches, muscular branches and small branches which accompany the nerves within the orbit.

The venous drainage of the orbit occurs via the superior and inferior ophthalmic veins, which pass through the superior orbital fissure to empty into the cavernous sinus.

Base of the skull

The base of the skull contains various foramina which transmit contents of anatomical interest. These are illustrated in Figure CA36.

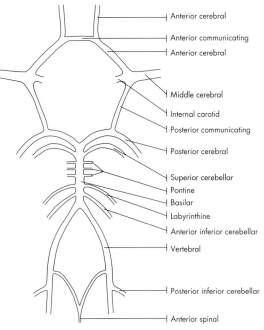

Anterior cerebral

Anterior communicating

Anterior cerebral

Middle cerebral

Internal carotid

Posterior communicating

Posterior cerebral

Superior cerebellar

Pontine

Basilar

Labyrinthine

Anterior inferior cerebellar

Vertebral

Posterior inferior cerebellar

Anterior spinal

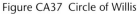

Figure CA37 Circle of Willis

Cerebral circulation

The anatomy of the arterial supply to the brain (the circle of Willis) described on p 321 is shown in Figure CA37.

References and further reading

Ellis H, Feldman S, Harrop-Griffiths AW. *Anatomy for Anaesthetists*, 8th ed. Oxford: Blackwell, 2003.

Erdmann A. *Concise Anatomy for Anaesthesia*. London: Greenwich Medical Media, 2001.

CHAPTER **1**

Cellular physiology

E. S. Lin

ORGANISATION AND CONTROL
Metabolism and metabolic control
Cell function and control
Organ systems and homeostatic control

CELL STRUCTURE
Basic cell morphology

CELL MEMBRANE
Membrane functions
Membrane structure
Integral membrane proteins
Membrane transport of substances
Membrane transport mechanisms

CELL NUCLEUS
Nucleus and nucleolus
Nucleic acids
Protein synthesis

CELL COMMUNICATION
Chemical messengers
Receptors
Membrane signal transduction
Second chemical messengers

AGEING
Ageing and dyshomeostasis
Theories of ageing

Organisation and control

The physiology of the body divides itself into different levels of functional organisation. Natural boundaries define three major levels, those of metabolism, cellular function and organ systems. The control mechanisms at each level form an essential part of the physiology, and direct function towards the ultimate goal of homeostasis. Homeostasis can be defined as maintenance of the composition and properties of extracellular fluid.

Metabolism and metabolic control

Metabolism is a global term encapsulating the mass of biochemical pathways that form the chemical machine providing energy and materials for the maintenance of life. These pathways are controlled at a biochemical level by various factors that determine the rate of metabolic reactions, including:

- Chemical parameters affecting reaction rates, e.g. concentration of reactants, temperature, activation energy requirements, presence of catalysts
- Enzyme concentration and activity. Factors affecting the rate of enzyme-mediated reactions include substrate concentration, presence of cofactors or coenzymes, and activation or inhibition by reaction

products (see allosteric and covalent modulation, below)
- The law of mass action and feedback control

At a systemic level metabolism is controlled largely by the endocrine hormones. These substances produce broad physiological changes in the body by exerting multiple effects on cell biochemistry. Some examples of the cellular metabolic effects of hormones are given in Figure PG1.

Cell function and control

Cell function involves both intra- and extracellular processes.

Intracellular functions

Intracellular functions include:
- Maintaining the internal milieu
- Reproducing DNA
- Production of RNA
- Repairing cell structures
- Synthesis of substances for export
- Metabolism of imported substances
- Production of chemical energy
- Cell motility

Fundamentals of Anaesthesia, 3rd edition, ed. Tim Smith, Colin Pinnock and Ted Lin. Published by Cambridge University Press. © Cambridge University Press 2008.

Hormone	Gland	Metabolic effects
Insulin	Beta cells in the islets of Langerhans	↑ glycolysis ↑ glycogen synthesis ↑ protein synthesis ↑ triacylglycerol synthesis ↑ fatty acid synthesis ↓ glycogenolysis ↓ ketone formation ↓ breakdown of triglycerides
Glucagon	Alpha cells in the islets of Langerhans	↑ glycogenolysis ↑ ketone formation ↑ gluconeogenesis
Epinephrine	Adrenal medulla	↑ glycogenolysis ↑ gluconeogenesis ↑ lipolysis
Cortisol	Adrenal cortex	↑ gluconeogenesis ↑ lipolysis ↑ protein catabolism ↓ DNA synthesis
Growth hormone	Anterior pituitary	↑ gluconeogenesis ↑ lipolysis
Thyroid hormone	Thyroid	*Normal concentrations* ↑ RNA synthesis ↑ protein synthesis *High concentrations* ↑ basal metabolic rate ↓ protein synthesis uncouples oxidative phosphorylation

Figure PG1 Hormone effects on cell metabolism

These functions are highly dependent on the intracellular milieu, which is in turn determined by the composition and properties of the extracellular fluid. Therefore intracellular control mechanisms are directed to maintaining these environments.

Intracellular control

Control of intracellular processes is achieved by various molecular mechanisms. All of the above intracellular functions are influenced by chemical messengers. Chemical signals are received at the extracellular membrane surface via molecular messengers. Often, second chemical messengers are activated at the inner surface of the cell membrane, and these mediate intracellular changes. Intracellular control mechanisms include:

- Activation or inhibition of enzymes
- Regulation of gene expression
- Changes in membrane permeability
- Regulation of membrane receptor activity
- Changes in membrane potential

Extracellular functions

Extracellular functions involve interaction and communication with other cells. This interaction may occur via mechanical, chemical or electrical mechanisms. The most common form of intercellular communication is via chemical messenger. Common groups of messengers are neurotransmitters, neurohormones, endocrine hormones and paracrine secretions.

Cell interactions can result in different types of response. Cells interacting with other cells in the immediate vicinity can produce local homeostatic responses such as an inflammatory response triggered by tissue injury. Coordinated functioning of masses of similar cells can result in specialised tissue or visceral activity such as myocardial contraction or gut peristalsis. Finally, interaction may occur with remote cells, as occurs in the systemic effects of hormones or systemic responses of the immune system. Intercellular communication mechanisms are discussed in more detail below.

Local homeostatic responses

Local homeostatic responses involve the secretion of chemical messengers by cells in the immediate vicinity of the target cell (paracrine secretion). Alternatively, messengers may be secreted by a cell to act on itself (autocrine secretion). An example of such a local response is the inflammatory response in the case of injury, when local metabolites are released to increase blood flow to the injured tissues.

A group of paracrine agents commonly encountered is the eicosanoids, which are derivatives of arachidonic acid. These include prostaglandins, prostacyclin, leukotrienes and thromboxanes. These agents exert a wide spectrum of effects in many physiological processes including blood coagulation, smooth muscle contraction, pain mechanisms and local inflammatory responses.

Organ systeme and homeostatic control

Organ systems and their control mechanisms provide the macroscopic means of controlling homeostasis and interfacing the body with its external environment. The traditionally described systems, such as the cardiovascular, respiratory and neurological systems, all exert their control over the body's physiology by well-recognised mechanisms.

Negative feedback system

The most common homeostatic control mechanism is the negative feedback system. A negative feedback system operates to maintain a constant output parameter or steady state, even if the output parameter is disturbed by an applied stimulus. When the steady state is disturbed the system first detects the change in the output parameter. It then produces an opposite polarity signal (negative feedback signal) proportional to the output deviation, and feeds this signal back to the input of the system. This feedback signal changes the input, and thus acts to correct the output deviation (Figure PG2).

A simple physiological example of a negative feedback system is illustrated by the gamma efferent system controlling resting length in skeletal muscle to maintain posture. Here the output parameter is muscle stretch and the input is the gamma efferent signal to the muscle. When stretch

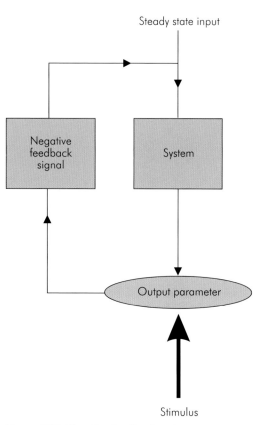

Figure PG2 Negative feedback system

is increased, the displacement is detected by the muscle spindles, which feed back a signal to produce an increase in gamma efferent signal strength. This increases muscle tone, thus acting to correct the original stretch or stimulus. Such a response is referred to as a reflex and describes the events in the simple 'knee jerk'.

The analogous homeostatic reflex is designed to maintain a given physiological parameter at a constant value or in a steady state. The physiological parameter may be a variable such as mean arterial blood pressure, which rests normally at its operating point. When a change occurs in the blood pressure, the change is detected by a baroreceptor that relays a signal to an integrating centre (vasomotor centre of the medulla). The integrating centre then transmits a signal to an effector (vascular smooth muscle), which exerts a response to oppose the original change.

Positive feedback system

Positive feedback systems are also used for physiological control, although in these cases the system is not used

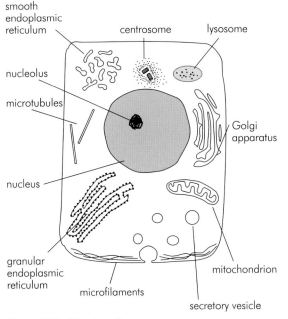

smooth endoplasmic reticulum

centrosome

lysosome

nucleolus

microtubules

Golgi apparatus

nucleus

granular endoplasmic reticulum

microfilaments

mitochondrion

secretory vesicle

Figure PG3 A basic cell

to control a specific physiological parameter, but rather to produce a systemic response directed towards maintaining homeostasis. In such a system there is no polarity change in the feedback signal, and thus, instead of opposing the detected physiological change, the feedback signal acts to increase the deviation. This produces a cascade effect that can be identified in certain physiological responses, such as the coagulation cascade during blood clot formation.

Cell structure

Cellular function is reflected by cell structure. In broad terms, a cell consists of the cell plasma membrane, the cytosol, intracellular organelles and the nucleus.

Basic cell morphology

A basic cell is illustrated in Figure PG3. The outer cell membrane surrounds various functional structures or organelles, the largest of which is the nucleus. The medium surrounding the nucleus is the cytoplasm.

Cytoplasm

'Cytoplasm' is used to describe all intracellular contents outside the nucleus. It consists of the organelles and the cytosol.

Cytosol

Cytosol refers to the intracelluar fluid containing proteins and electrolytes. Intracellular fluid forms 40% of body weight and possesses an electrolyte composition, which is discussed in Section 2, Chapter 2 (pages 226–7).

Organelles

A summary of the organelles and their functions is shown in Figure PG4.

Cytoskeleton

This system of microscopic fibres maintains the cell structure and enables cell movement to occur. Its main components are:

- Microtubules – 25 nm diameter structures with 5 nm thick walls. Tubule length is a dynamic balance between assembly (at the positive end) and disassembly (at the negative end) of protein subunits
- Muscle thick filaments – composed of myosin 15 nm in diameter
- Intermediate filaments – solid fibres about 10 nm in diameter
- Microfilaments – solid fibres about 5 nm in diameter made of polymerised actin

Cellular motion, shape changes and ciliary or flagellar movement all involve molecular motor mechanisms based on the action of ATPases. These form moving flexible cross-bridges between cytoskeletal components and membranes or organelles. The actin–myosin mechanism responsible for muscle contraction is a molecular motor mechanism that occurs universally in other cells. Other examples of molecular motors include dynamin and kinesin, which act on microtubules.

Mitochondria

These are sausage-shaped structures with outer and inner membranes. Their main function is to produce chemical energy in the form of ATP by oxidative phosphorylation. The inner membrane is folded to form cristae, which are studded with units containing the oxidative phosphorylating and ATP-synthesising enzymes (Figure PG5). The matrix contains enzymes required to drive the citric acid cycle, which in turn provides the substrate for oxidative phosphorylation. Mitochondria also contain a small amount of DNA, which is solely of maternal origin.

Endoplasmic reticulum (ER)

This membranous structure is composed of complex folds and tubules. In its granular form, ribosomes are attached

Cytoskeleton	Maintains the structure of the cell
Membrane	Container for cell, nucleus and other organelles
	Structural support and control of environment on either side
Mitochondria	Energy source for the cell generating ATP via oxidative phosphorylation
Nucleus	Contains the genetic material in the form of chromosomes
	The central site of cell division or mitosis
	Nucleolus synthesises ribosomes
Centrosome	Formation of mitotic spindle in cell division
Endoplasmic reticulum (ER)	Rough (granular) ER has ribosomes attached and is responsible for protein synthesis
	Smooth (agranular) ER is the site of steroid synthesis and detoxification
Ribosome	The actual site of protein synthesis in the ER, or may occur free in cytoplasm
Golgi apparatus	Processes proteins for secretion from cell
Lysosomes	Breakdown and elimination of intracellular debris or exogenous substances
Peroxisomes	Catalyse various anabolic and catabolic reactions, e.g. breakdown of long chain fatty acids
Cilia	Used by the cell to propel mucus or other substances over exposed mucosal surfaces

Figure PG4 Intracellular organelles and their functions

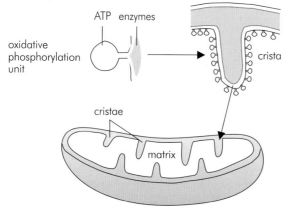

Figure PG5 Mitochondrion structure

to the cytoplasmic surfaces and are the primary site for protein synthesis in the cell. Agranular ER is free from ribosomes and is the site of steroid synthesis and detoxification.

Ribosomes
Ribosomes are about 32 nm in diameter with large and small subunits. They are composed of 65% RNA and 35% protein, and are the sites of protein synthesis. Free ribosomes exist in the cytoplasm and synthesise haemoglobin, peroxisomal and mitochondrial proteins.

Centrosome
This is composed of two centrioles at right angles to each other. The centrioles are cylindrical structures in which nine triplets of microtubules form the walls. A cylinder of pericentriolar material surrounds these structures. The whole structure is situated near the nucleus and is activated at the start of mitosis. Initially the centrioles replicate, and then the centriole pairs separate to form the mitotic spindle.

Golgi apparatus
This consists of flattened membranous sacs or cisterns that are stacked together to form a polarised structure with cis and trans ends, separated by a middle region. The Golgi apparatus prepares proteins for secretion (via exocytosis) by receiving the proteins from the ER at the cis side, coding them for destination and finally producing secretory granules or vesicles at the trans side (Figure PG6).

Intercellular connections
The organisation of cells into tissues involves the formation of specialised junctions between the cells. Three basic types of junction are described (Figure PG7).

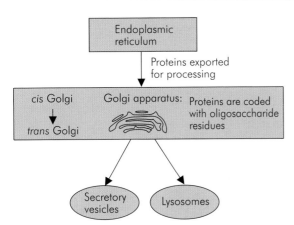

Figure PG6 Golgi apparatus and protein processing

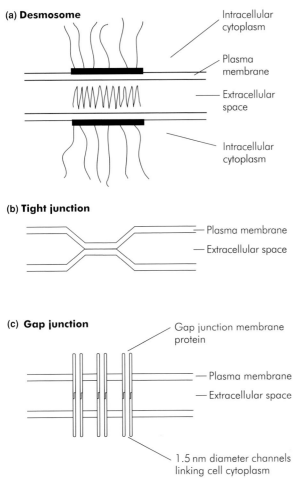

Figure PG7 Intercellular connections

- Desmosomes – disc-shaped junctions that provide mechanical bonding between cells subject to stress (e.g. epithelium, skin)
- Tight junctions – circumferential junctions that seal the extracellular space between epithelial cells, preventing the passage of molecules between cells
- Gap junctions – small channels (diameter 1.5 nm) that allow transfer of small ions and molecules between cells

Cilia

These projections on the luminal surface of epithelial cells are motile processes that move secretions and other substances across the surface of the cell. They are composed of nine pairs of microtubules arranged circumferentially around a central pair of microtubules. Each cilium is attached to a basal granule that has a structure similar to that of a centriole. Ciliary movement is produced by molecular motor mechanisms that cause the microtubules to slide relative to each other.

Cell membrane

Membrane functions

Membranes surround all cells and the majority of intracellular organelles. The cell membrane has a primary function of controlling the passage of substances across it to maintain the intracellular environment, which is an essential requirement for cellular metabolism. Controlling the movement of ions across the membrane also establishes ion concentration gradients and electrical potential differences (membrane potential) across the membrane, which enable cells to perform specialised functions. A summary of cell membrane functions is as follows:

- Regulation of the passage of substances across it for intracellular homeostasis
- Establishment of ion concentration gradients (K^+ and Na^+)
- Establishment of membrane potential
- Container for cell contents
- Anchorage for cytoskeleton
- Structural function for tissues acting as a site for intercellular connections
- Communication via chemical messengers
- Communication via action potentials

Membrane structure

Cell membranes are based on a double phospholipid layer structure. The phospholipid molecules are amphipathic,

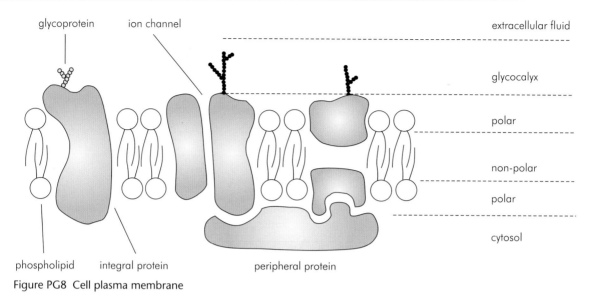

Figure PG8 Cell plasma membrane

with one end charged and the other non-polar. The membrane is formed by a double layer of these amphipathic molecules with the polar ends orientated outwards. This double layer is interrupted by integral membrane protein molecules, which often span the membrane completely and are referred to as transmembrane proteins. Membrane proteins and lipids may possess polysaccharide chains attached to their extracellular surface, which appears as a fuzzy coat visible on electron microscopy, known as the glycocalyx (Figure PG8).

Integral membrane proteins

Integral membrane proteins have various functions. Some form controllable channels for the passage of ions or water. Another group transmits chemical signals across the cell membrane by acting as active carriers. More recently, cell adhesion molecules have been identified that determine the cell's ability to attach to basal laminae and to other cells. Types of integral membrane proteins include:

- Ion channels
- Transport carriers
- Cell adhesion molecules
- Second messenger enzymes
- G proteins

Peripheral membrane proteins are located on the cytoplasmic membrane surface, where they are attached to polar regions of the integral membrane proteins. These peripheral proteins are associated with cell motility and shape.

Cell adhesion molecules (CAM)

This is a large group of membrane proteins with several subdivisions and a wide range of functions. Their primary properties form the basis for cells to adhere either to other cells (to other CAMs) or to the extracellular matrix (i.e. collagen and glycoprotein elements in connective tissue). These adhesive properties are rapidly controllable and may also be linked to signal transduction by the same molecules. The scope of CAM function thus extends well beyond a simple structural role, and involves both normal and pathological processes. Some of the processes involving adhesion molecules are:

- Transduction of signals controlling differentiation, gene expression and motility
- Programmed assembly of cells to form the complex architecture of individual tissues
- Morphogenesis of embryological tissues and organs
- Formation of intercellular connections in epithelial tissues
- Adhesion of leukocytes to vascular endothelium
- Enablement of leukocyte motility
- Directing of leukocyte migration in inflammation
- Platelet adhesion in blood coagulation
- Pathogenesis of airway inflammation in asthma
- Epithelial cell adhesion to basement membranes and the pathogenesis of bullous diseases

An outline of the different families of CAMs is summarised in Figure PG9.

Integrins	Platelet adhesion
	Expressed on leukocytes and binds to IgSF (endothelium)
	Leukocyte motility
	Cell-matrix adhesion
Selectins	Expressed on circulating leukocytes
	Stored in endothelial cells and allow rolling of leukocytes
	Stored in platelets
	Leukocyte–endothelial adhesion
Cadherins	Morphogenesis of tissues
	Metastasis of tumours
	Embryological development
Immunoglobulin superfamily (IgSF)	Expressed on endothelium and binds to integrins (leukocytes)
	Expressed on gut mucosa and binds integrins and selectins (lymphocytes)

Figure PG9 Families of cell adhesion molecules and their properties

G proteins

This group of membrane proteins has a high affinity for guanine nucleotides. Over 16 G proteins have been identified, composed of α, β and γ subunits, suggesting the existence of many more. Activation of the G protein enables it to bind guanosine triphosphate (GTP) and interact with an effector protein. The activated G protein then deactivates itself by intrinsic GTPase activity (Figure PG10). This reduces the GTP to GDP, thus deactivating the G protein.

Activation of the G protein system can result in various effects. It can control the release of second messengers via Gs- and Gi-type proteins that have stimulatory or inhibitory effects on enzymes such as adenylyl cyclase. Some G proteins are directly coupled to ion channels, and thus control membrane permeability to ions. Others can increase intracellular calcium concentrations and activate intracellular kinases. The heterogeneous nature of G proteins means that a first messenger common to several tissues can produce a spectrum of different cellular responses according to the tissue targeted. This variability is further increased by the fact that more than one G protein may be activated by a single receptor, and several effector proteins can be coupled to a single G protein.

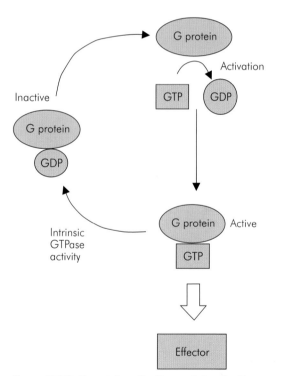

Figure PG10 G protein activation and deactivation

Second messenger enzymes

The production of second messengers – cyclic AMP, cyclic GMP, inositol triphosphate and diacylglycerol – takes place at the cell membrane. The enzymes responsible for their production are adenylyl cyclase, guanylyl cyclase and tyrosine kinase. The activities of these enzymes are controlled by various pathways, which involve both activation and inhibition. Second messenger effects are multiple and widespread intracellularly.

Substance	Size (nm)	Site	Mechanism
Water	0.13	Lipid bilayer	Osmosis
Oxygen	0.12	Lipid bilayer	Diffusion
Nitrogen	0.12	Lipid bilayer	Diffusion
Carbon dioxide	0.12	Lipid bilayer	Diffusion
Sodium ions	0.19	Lipid bilayer	Ion diffusion
		ATPase pump	Active transport
Potassium ions	0.23	Ion channel	Ion diffusion
		ATPase pump	Active transport
Calcium ions	0.17	Ion channel	Ion diffusion
		ATPase pump	Active transport
Urea	0.23	Lipid bilayer	Diffusion
Steroids	<1.0	Lipid bilayer	Diffusion
Fatty acid	<1.0	Lipid bilayer	Diffusion
Glucose	0.38	Transport proteins	Facilitated diffusion
Proteins	>7.5	Vesicles	Exocytosis
			Endocytosis

Figure PG11 Examples of substances transported across membranes

Membrane transport of substances

Cell membranes control the movement of a wide range of particles and substances between the intra- and extracellular spaces. These include gases, ions, water, proteins and intracellular granules or debris. Different components of the membrane are associated with different mechanisms of transport. The phospholipid bilayer areas of the membrane allow diffusion of water, small molecules and lipid-soluble substances. Transmembrane proteins provide active mechanisms for transport and allow ion diffusion via channels. Examples of substances transported across membranes are shown in Figure PG11.

Membrane transport mechanisms

Various mechanisms exist for the transport of substances across the cell membrane. Mechanisms such as diffusion and osmosis are passive and do not require the expenditure of energy. Active transport is mediated by integral membrane proteins and uses energy often in the form of ATP. Membrane transport mechanisms include:
- Diffusion
- Ion channel diffusion
- Facilitated diffusion
- Primary active transport
- Secondary active transport
- Osmosis
- Exo- and endocytosis

Diffusion

This describes the resultant movement of solute molecules due to their random thermal motion. It is a passive process, and net movement of the solute occurs when a concentration gradient is present (from a high to a low concentration). Certain molecules can diffuse across the phospholipid bilayer areas of a cell membrane.

In general, the rate of diffusion through a membrane, Q, is dependent on the concentration gradient ($C_1 - C_2$), the area of membrane exposed, A, the membrane thickness, D, and the permeability constant k_p:

$$Q = k_p A (C_1 - C_2)/D$$

The permeability constant, k_p, depends on the local temperature and the characteristics of the membrane; molecular properties also affect it. The phospholipid bilayers are relatively impermeable to ions and large polar (hydrophilic) molecules, but permeable to small polar molecules and lipophilic substances. Thus, the rate of diffusion across the cell membrane:

- Increases with concentration gradient
- Increases with surface area
- Decreases with membrane thickness
- Increases with temperature
- Increases with lipid solubility
- Decreases with molecular weight
- Decreases with electrical charge of particle

A cell membrane acts as a diffusion barrier to solute molecules and can reduce their rates of diffusion by a factor of between 10^3 and 10^6, compared with free diffusion rates in water.

Osmosis

This term describes the net movement of water molecules due to diffusion between areas of different concentration. Pure water has a molar concentration of 55.5 M. In a solution, the addition of solute reduces the water concentration by replacing some water molecules with a solute molecule (or ion). Thus, a 1 M solution of glucose will have a reduced water concentration of $55.5 - 1 = 54.5$ M. In the case of a solute that dissociates in solution, twice as many particles are formed. Thus, a 1 M solution of NaCl will reduce the water concentration by twice as much, since each molecule of NaCl produces two particles, a sodium ion and a chloride ion. The 1 M solution of NaCl then has a water concentration of $55.5 - 2 = 53.5$ M.

Osmolarity

The concentration of a solution can be expressed in terms of its osmolarity, reflecting the osmotic effect of the solute particles. The osmolarity of the 1 M glucose solution is thus 1 Osm (osmol l^{-1}) while the 1 M NaCl solution has an osmolarity of 2 Osm.

Osmotic pressure

A concentration gradient of water can be produced between two compartments separated by a semipermeable membrane, such as a cell membrane, which is permeable to water but impermeable to solute. In this case, net diffusion of water molecules will occur from the compartment with the lower concentration of solute (higher concentration of water) across the membrane into the higher solute concentration (lower concentration of water). The movement of water into a compartment due to osmosis will have the physical effects of increasing the volume of the compartment and/or increasing the pressure in the compartment. This movement of water can be opposed by an increase in pressure in the compartment. The pressure required to

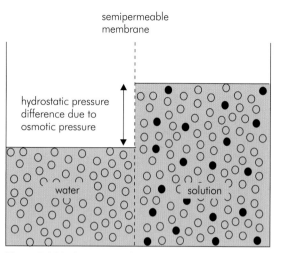

Figure PG12 Osmosis and osmotic pressure

oppose the net movement of water into a solution is the osmotic pressure. This is a property of the solution indirectly reflecting its osmolarity (Figure PG12).

Tonicity

In a cell, changes in volume can be produced according to the osmolarity of the intra- and extracellular fluids. Net movement of water into the cell occurs when the cell is placed in a solution of lower osmolarity (hypotonic), giving rise to swelling and ultimately cell disruption or haemolysis. Placing a cell in a solution of higher osmolarity than the intracellular contents (hypertonic) causes shrinking. Normal extracellular fluid has an osmolarity of 300 mOsm, which is equal to (isotonic) that of the intracellular fluid. Since intra- and extracellular solute concentrations are maintained by the cell membrane permeability properties, no net movement of water occurs into or out of cells and they remain in equilibrium. Hyperosmotic, hypo-osmotic and iso-osmotic describe solution osmolarity irrespective of the membrane permeability to the solute contained. Thus, the tonicity of such a solution may not correspond to its osmolarity.

Ion diffusion

Although the phospholipid bilayer portions of the cell membrane are impermeable to ions, ion channels formed by transmembrane proteins render the cell membrane selectively permeable to Na^+, K^+, Ca^{2+} and Cl^-. The walls of these channels are formed by polypeptide subunits, which may number up to 12 per channel (Figure PG13).

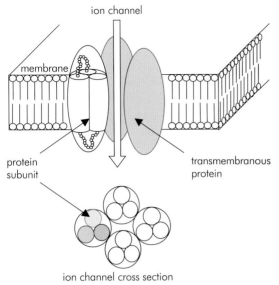

Figure PG13 Ion channel

Rapid changes in ion concentrations (such as in the production of action potentials) are produced by opening and closing the channels (gating) and consequently producing dramatic changes in permeability to a given ion. The gating of ion channels may be controlled by chemical messengers binding to the subunits (ligand gating, e.g. acetyl choline receptors), changes in membrane potential (voltage gating, e.g. Na^+ channel) and stretching of the membrane (mechanical gating). Factors determining permeability of a cell membrane to a given ion are:

- Chemical messenger concentration
- Membrane potential
- Membrane conformation
- Density of specific ion channels

Active transport

Active transport is mediated by integral membrane proteins or carriers that bind a substance on one side of the membrane, undergo a conformational change and then release the substance on the opposite side of the membrane. Carriers may be specific for a given substance (uniport), or they may transport a combination of substances (symport), or finally they may exchange one substance for another (antiport). Factors affecting rate of active transport include:

- Degree of carrier saturation
- Density of carriers on membrane
- The speed of carrier conformational change

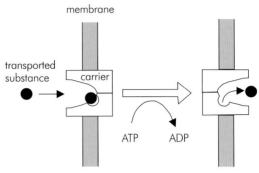

Figure PG14 Primary active transport

Primary active transport

Active transport requires the expenditure of energy, since it usually moves substances against a concentration or electrical potential gradient (i.e. against an electrochemical gradient). In primary active transport, energy is obtained directly from the hydrolysis of ATP and then catalysed by the carrier, which binds the released phosphate (Figure PG14). Phosphorylation of the carrier produces covalent modulation of its structure. $Na^+K^+ATPase$ is an antiport carrier responsible for maintaining transmembrane ion gradients of Na^+ and K^+. This carrier 'pumps' three Na^+ ions out of the cell in exchange for two potassium ions (Figure PG15), both against their respective concentration gradients. Other ion pumps (uniport systems) move calcium ($Ca^{2+}ATPase$) and hydrogen ions ($H^+ATPase$) across cell and organelle membranes against electrochemical gradients.

Secondary active transport

In this process a symport carrier transports a substance and an ion (usually Na^+) together. The carrier possesses two binding sites one for the substance and one for the ion. The substance binds to the first carrier site. The change in carrier conformation required to release the substance on the opposite side of the membrane is then powered by the ion binding to the second site, which produces allosteric modulation of the carrier structure. Since the ion always passes from high to low concentrations, there is no direct energy input required, and the energy for this secondary transport process is ultimately derived from the energy required to maintain the ion concentration gradient. The transported substance can travel in the same direction as the ion (co-transport) or in the opposite direction (counter-transport). An example of such a

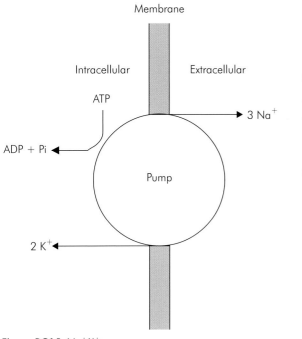

Figure PG15 Na$^+$K$^+$ pump

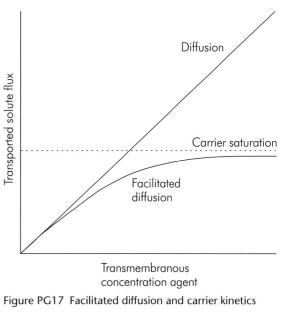

Figure PG17 Facilitated diffusion and carrier kinetics

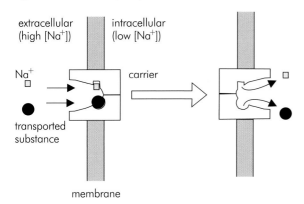

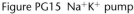

Figure PG16 Secondary active transport

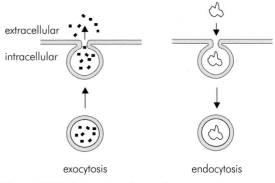

Figure PG18 Exo- and endocytosis

system is the transport of glucose and Na$^+$ in the gut (Figure PG16).

Facilitated diffusion

This is a misnomer, since no diffusive process is involved. Facilitated diffusion describes the transport of a substance from a high to low concentration via a carrier. No energy coupling is required for this process, since movement occurs down the concentration gradient. However, diffusion is not involved, and thus the transport kinetics are

characteristic of carrier-mediated transport (Figure PG17) and carrier saturation occurs. An example of this process is the transport of glucose into the cell, which occurs via a set of four different carriers.

Exo- and endocytosis

This mode of transport does not require substances to pass through the membrane structure, but transports substances contained in membrane-covered vesicles. In endocytosis, extracellular material is absorbed by being packaged into vesicles at the cell membrane. The vesicles are formed by invagination of the membrane. An equivalent process in reverse is exocytosis, which allows the cell to export intracellular substances or debris (Figure PG18).

Cell nucleus

Nucleus and nucleolus

Most cells in the body carry a single nucleus (exceptions are skeletal muscle cells, which are multinucleate, and red blood cells, which are anucleate). The nucleus is surrounded by a double membrane – the nuclear envelope. This envelope is interrupted at intervals by openings – the nuclear pores – that allow the passage of specific proteins into and out of the nucleus.

The most important substances in the nucleus are the nucleic acids deoxyribonucleic acid (DNA) and ribonucleic acid (RNA).

Genetic material is contained as a DNA–protein complex and forms the bulk of the nuclear contents. In addition, there is a dense patch of granules visible under light microscopy known as the nucleolus. The nucleolus is rich in RNA; it synthesises the ribosomal subunits for export to the cytoplasm, where the complete ribosomes are assembled and act as sites for protein synthesis.

Nucleic acids

Nucleic acids are nucleotide polymers. Each nucleotide consists of a purine or pyrimidine base, a sugar (deoxyribose or ribose) and a phosphate group. The DNA molecule is a double helix, each component helix being a chain of nucleotides. DNA nucleotides contain deoxyribose sugar combined with one of the following bases: adenine (A), guanine (G), cytosine (C) and thymine (T). The deoxyribose molecules are linked by phosphate bonds to form the backbone of each spiral, and the spirals are linked via the protruding bases to form the DNA double helix (Figure PG19).

Genetic information is coded linearly along the double helix structure by the sequence of the base pairs. The alphabet for this genetic code is formed by triplets of bases, each triplet coding for an amino acid, e.g. the triplet sequence cytosine–guanine–thymine (CGT) codes for the amino acid alanine. Figure PG20 shows the DNA coding for a small polypeptide.

RNA is a single-stranded nucleotide polymer that differs from DNA in function and structure (Figure PG21). Three types of RNA are recognised: messenger (mRNA), transfer (tRNA) and ribosomal (rRNA). They are all synthesised in the nucleus using DNA as a template, but differ from each other in molecular size and function. The bulk of cellular RNA is rRNA, which together with specific proteins forms the ribosomal subunits; however, its function remains uncertain.

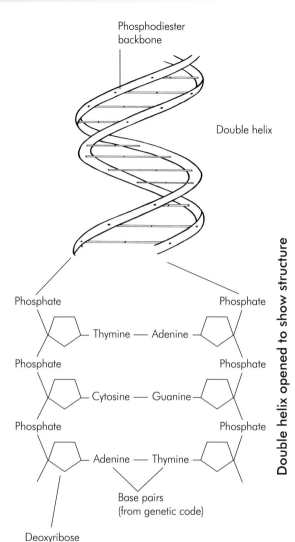

Figure PG19 Double helix of DNA

The human genome

The total genetic material in the nucleus forms a blueprint for the individual and is referred to as the genome. The genetic information is coded into giant molecules of DNA. These DNA molecules form large complexes with proteins, which appear as clumps of stained material, chromatin, under light microscopy. During cell division the chromatin forms paired bodies in the nucleus known as chromosomes. The human genome is contained in 46 chromosomes (23 pairs), each chromosome consisting of a single DNA molecule–protein complex. The genetic coding responsible for producing a single polypeptide is known as

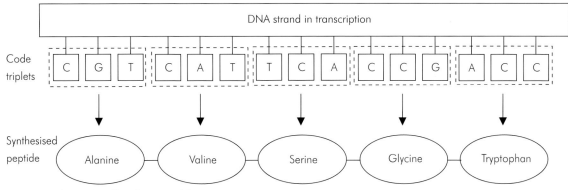

Figure PG20 DNA coding for a peptide

	DNA	mRNA	tRNA
Structure	Double helix	Single strand	Single strand
Nucleotide sugar	Deoxyribose	Ribose	Ribose
Purines	Adenine	Adenine	Adenine
	Guanine	Guanine	Guanine
Pyrimidines	Cytosine	Cytosine	Cytosine
	Thymine	Uracil	Uracil
Number of bases in a molecule	$<10^5$	$<10^3$	80
Function	Stores amino acid sequences for protein synthesis	Transfers amino acid sequence as codons from DNA to ribosomes	Links amino acids to mRNA codons

Figure PG21 Properties of DNA and RNA

a gene, which represents a unit of hereditary information. There are between 50 000 and 100 000 genes in the human genome, which contain 3×10^9 base pairs.

Protein synthesis

The process of synthesising proteins from the genetic information coded on DNA in the nucleus is outlined in Figure PG22. Transcription describes the first stage, in which mRNA is synthesised by RNA polymerase bound to the gene for the protein being synthesised. The mRNA then undergoes post-transcriptional processing. The processed RNA passes from the nucleus into the cytoplasm, where one end binds to the surface of a ribosome. Free amino acids are concentrated around the ribosomal surface, where they are loaded onto tRNA by aminoacyl-tRNA synthetase.

The surface-bound region of the mRNA is the site where the polypeptide is gradually elongated by the addition of amino acids in sequence. It provides two adjacent codons that recognise and bind tRNA by the corresponding anti-codon. The first codon binds tRNA carrying the incomplete peptide chain. The adjacent site binds tRNA carrying the next amino acid in the sequence, which is then added to the chain. The addition of each new amino acid is then completed by a shift of the active region along the mRNA strand by one codon. The cycle can then be repeated to add the next amino acid to the peptide.

Control of protein synthesis

Genes possess different regions, of which only the exons are transcribed to produce mRNA for protein synthesis (Figure PG23). At any given time, only a fraction of the genes in a cell are being transcribed. Control of the transcription process in each gene is exerted via a promoter region to which RNA polymerase binds before

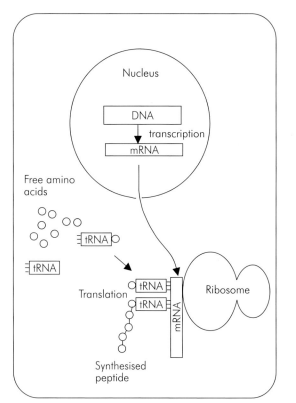

Figure PG22 Protein synthesis

commencing transcription. Control of protein synthesis is exerted via transcription factors that allow RNA polymerase to bind to the promoter site and to commence transcription. These controlling factors may originate from within the same cell, or originate from other cells via the extracellular fluid. A single transcription factor may control transcription for several genes.

Control of the rate of protein synthesis may also be exerted at the translation stage and by controlling the breakdown of mRNA in the cytoplasm.

Cell communication

Intercellular communication is the basic machinery through which homeostatic control is applied. Cells almost always use a chemical messenger to communicate with target cells, which may be local or remote in location. One group of chemical messengers is formed by the neurotransmitters, which are secreted by one neurone to target a neighbouring neurone just a synapse away. On the other hand, a hormone travels in the circulation to target multiple tissues remote from the secreting cells. In general terms, chemical messengers (ligands) are usually received by cell membrane proteins (receptors), and this interaction triggers the required cellular response by various mechanisms.

Chemical messengers

Chemical messengers that reach a target cell in the extracellular fluid, whether via the circulation or through the interstitium, are referred to as first chemical messengers. The action of a first chemical messenger often results in the intracellular release of an active ligand, which is termed a second messenger. Various groups of first messengers are recognised, such as neurotransmitters, neuromuscular transmitters, hormones, paracrine agents and autocrine agents. These are differentiated by their origin, the route travelled by the messengers and the cells targeted. Some examples are shown in Figure PG24.

All chemical messengers or ligands interact with their target cells by binding to receptors and therefore have common properties that determine their performance.

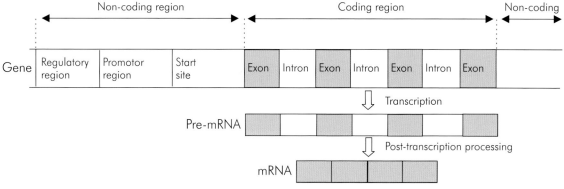

Figure PG23 Gene regions

Messenger	Origin	Route	Target cell
Neurotransmitters norepinephrine acetylcholine serotonin	Neurone	Synapse	Adjacent neurone
Hormones thyroxine insulin cortisol	Gland	Circulation	Multiple tissues
Neurohormones vasopressin oxytocin ACTH TSH	Neurone	Circulation	Multiple tissues Endocrine glands
Neuromuscular transmitter acetylcholine	Neurone	Circulation	Muscle cell
Paracrine agents eicosanoids cytokines	Local cell	Extracellular fluid	Neighbouring cells
Autocrine agent eicosanoids cytokines	Local cell	Extracellular fluid	Cell of origin

Figure PG24 Types of first chemical messenger and their target cells

Properties of a ligand
Ligands show the following properties:
- Affinity – strength of binding with the receptor
- Competition – ability of different ligands to bind to the same receptor
- Agonist activity – ability of a ligand to trigger the cell response
- Antagonist activity – ability of a ligand to bind to a receptor without triggering the cell response, i.e. to block the receptor
- Half-life – time taken for ligand to be metabolised to half its concentration
- Lipid solubility – lipid-insoluble ligands activate receptors at the membrane surface; lipid-soluble ligands activate intracellular or intranuclear receptors

Receptors
'Receptor' refers to the region of a protein molecule that provides a binding site for a ligand. Receptors are usually situated on integral membrane proteins, and are activated by lipid-insoluble messengers at the membrane surface. Lipid-soluble messengers may cross the membrane to activate intracellular receptors. Receptors are not fixed components of the membrane, but are free to change position and to alter in population density.

Receptor properties
The properties of receptors are:
- Specificity – selectivity of a receptor, determining how specifically it binds to a single ligand
- Saturation – percentage of receptors already occupied by a ligand
- Down-regulation – a decrease in the number of receptors available for a given ligand
- Up-regulation – an increase in the number of available receptors for a given ligand
- Sensitivity – responsiveness of a target cell to a given ligand, dependent on the density of receptors
- Supersensitivity – increased sensitivity of a cell as a result of up-regulation

Binding site modulation
The first stage in transduction is the production of a change in shape or modulation of the binding site, when the ligand binds to the receptor. There are two main mechanisms

Allosteric modulation

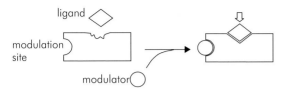

Covalent modulation

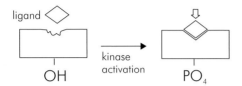

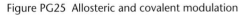

Figure PG25 Allosteric and covalent modulation

by which this occurs, allosteric modulation and covalent modulation (Figure PG25).

Allosteric modulation

In this case the receptor possesses two binding sites, one (the functional site) for the ligand and the other (the regulatory site) for a modulator molecule. Binding of the modulator molecule enables ligand binding to occur at the functional site.

Covalent modulation

This form of modulation requires the attachment of a phosphate group to the receptor (phosphorylation) to enable the functional site to bind the ligand.

Membrane signal transduction

When a ligand binds to a receptor, modulation sets off a sequence of events which can be thought of as transduction of a chemical signal received by the cell. Signal transduction ultimately results in alterations in cell function. These changes can affect:

- Membrane permeability
- Membrane potential
- Membrane transport
- Contractile activity
- Secretory activity
- Protein synthesis

Different mechanisms are activated following modulation of the receptor protein.

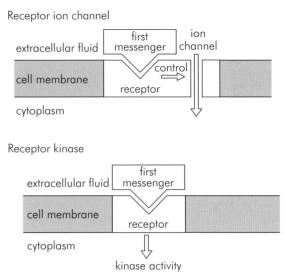

Figure PG26 Signal transduction mechanisms

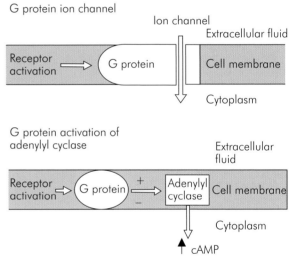

Figure PG27 G protein signal transduction

Membrane signal transduction mechanisms

- Receptors act as ion channels that are opened or closed by ligand binding (Figure PG26).
- Receptors function as protein kinases that are activated on ligand binding (Figure PG26).
- Receptors activate G proteins, which then mediate further actions. These include gating ion channels or releasing second messengers intracellularly (Figure PG27).

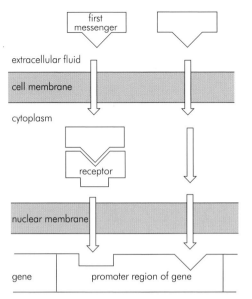

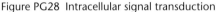

Figure PG28 Intracellular signal transduction

Intracellular transduction

Lipophilic first messengers, such as steroids, can cross the phospholipid bilayer and activate intracellular receptors in the following ways (Figure PG28):

- Ligand crosses cell membrane to form complex with cytosol receptor. This complex moves into nucleus and binds to promoter region of gene.
- Ligand moves across cell and nuclear membranes to form complex with nuclear receptor. This complex binds to promoter region of gene.

Second chemical messengers

This term refers to substances released intracellularly, following G protein activation of effector proteins (enzymes such as adenylyl cyclase and guanylyl cyclase). The second messengers released diffuse through the cytosol and exert wide-ranging effects, usually by activation of a protein kinase (Figure PG29). The kinase in turn activates or inhibits a range of cellular functions by enzyme phosphorylation. This sequence of events can be thought

Second messenger	Precursor or origin	Mediator	Examples of cell functions influenced
Cyclic AMP	ATP	Adenylyl cyclase	Protein synthesis
			Calcium ion transport
			DNA synthesis
			RNA synthesis
			Lipid breakdown
			Glycogen breakdown
			Glycogen synthesis
			Ion channels
			Active transport
Cyclic GMP	GTP	Guanylyl cyclase	Physiology of vision
Inositol triphosphate (IP$_3$)	Phosphotidyl inositol diphosphate (PIP$_2$)	Phospholipase C	Release of calcium from endoplasmic reticulum
Diacylglycerol (DAG)	Phosphatidyl inositol diphosphate (PIP$_2$)	Phospholipase C	Activation of protein kinase C used in membrane protein regulation
Calcium	Entry via calcium channels	G proteins	Activation of protein kinases via calmodulin or directly
	Release from endoplasmic reticulum	G proteins	Skeletal, smooth and cardiac muscle contraction
			Synaptic function
			Protein synthesis

Figure PG29 Second messengers and their functions

of as a cascade triggered by a single messenger. The cascade effectively amplifies and processes the effect of low concentrations of a ligand to produce widespread cellular changes, tailored to the needs of different tissues.

The second messengers cyclic AMP and cyclic GMP are metabolised by phosphodiesterase, which can be inhibited by methylxanthines (caffeine, theophylline). These compounds thus augment the second messenger effects.

Intracellular calcium

The extracellular-to-cytosol concentration gradient of calcium is $>10^4$. Thus calcium enters the cytosol readily via calcium channels that are controlled by ligand or voltage gating. Alternatively, calcium can be released internally from the endoplasmic reticulum, which acts as a store. Active decrease of intracellular calcium levels is mediated by a $Ca^{2+}H^+$ ATPase, a Na^+Ca^{2+} antiport system and reuptake into the endoplasmic reticulum.

Calcium exerts wide-ranging effects intracellularly by binding to a group of proteins including calmodulin, troponin and calbindin.

Calmodulin is one of the most prominent of these proteins, with wide-ranging activation of protein kinases involved in many aspects of cellular function (Figure PG30).

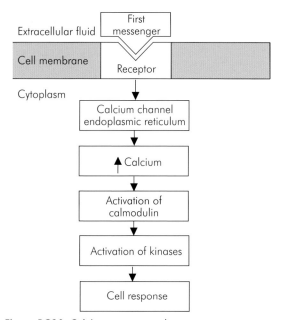

Figure PG30 Calcium as a second messenger

Ageing

Ageing is a physiological process that involves general changes in the body systems that are distinct from the pathological changes associated with disease. These changes are illustrated in Figure PG31, which shows the parameters in relation to those of an equivalent young adult.

The changes usually reflect a decline in function. This functional deterioration occurs in all of the physiological systems, and includes those shown in Figure PG32.

Ageing and dyshomeostasis

The deterioration normally associated with the ageing process leads to a reduction in the effectiveness of homeostatic control mechanisms or dyshomeostasis. This contributes to an increased prevalence of certain conditions with age. These include:

- Dehydration
- Hypokalaemia
- Hyponatraemia
- Ankle oedema
- Diabetes mellitus
- Hypothyroidism
- Hypothermia

Theories of ageing

Three theories on the origins of ageing have been put forward: wear and tear, adaptive evolution and non-adaptive evolution.

Parameter for a 70-year-old male	% of young adult value
Muscle mass	74
Total body water	87
Cardiac output at rest	64
Cardiac reserve	50
PaO$_2$	90
Oxygen consumption at rest	74
Maximal oxygen consumption	65
Renal blood flow	60
Max urine concentration	64
Cerebral blood flow	80

Figure PG31 Changes in physiological parameters due to ageing

System	Change due to ageing
Cardiovascular	↓ cardiac output and reserve ↓ heart rate ↓ stroke volume ↓ LV compliance
Respiratory	↓ PaO_2 ↓ lung elasticity ↓ chest wall compliance ↓ vital capacity ↑ residual volume
Gastrointestinal	↓ sense of smell and taste ↓ coordination of swallowing and peristaltic reflexes ↓ gastric and pancreatic secretion ↓ large bowel motility
Endocrine	↑ norepinephrine levels ↓ renin and aldosterone levels ↓ carbohydrate tolerance ↑ vasopressin levels ↓ oestrogen in female ↓ testosterone levels in male
Renal	↓ kidney mass ↓ ability to concentrate urine ↓ renal response to vasopressin ↑ prostate mass
CNS	↓ brain mass ↓ acetylcholine activity ↓ cerebral blood flow ↓ short-term memory and learning ability ↑ reaction time
Musculoskeletal	↓ bone and muscle mass ↓ muscle effectiveness
Immunity	↓ cellular and humoral immunity

Figure PG32 Effects of ageing on physiological systems

Wear and tear

This states that the ageing process is a natural deterioration as a result of the continuous functioning of a highly complex organism.

Adaptive evolution

Adaptive evolution suggests that ageing is a genetically programmed termination of life in the interests of evolutionary selection.

Non-adaptive evolution

Non-adaptive evolution suggests that the ageing process has evolved as an optimum balance between the limited energy sources available to the organism and the demands of normal function and repair.

Several cellular mechanisms are associated with ageing. It is unclear at present whether any of these predominate in determining the rate and extent of the process. The more important processes are:

- Accumulation of cells with random DNA mutations
- Increased cross-linking of collagens and proteins by glycosylation
- Accumulation of cytoplasmic lipofuscin granules
- Accumulation of oxidant radicals
- Genetic clock determining the number of cell reduplications
- Pleiotropic genes with 'good' effects early in life and 'bad' effects later in life

In general, it remains fair to say that the ageing process is incompletely understood at present.

CHAPTER 2

Body fluids

J. Skoyles

Fluid compartment volumes

Total body water (TBW)

Water comprises the major part of body weight, forming about 60% of the body weight of a young adult male. This percentage varies with build, sex and age in the following manner:

- TBW in the adult can range from 45% to 75% of body weight. This large variation is the result of individual differences in adipose tissue, which contains relatively little water.
- TBW in the female adult is less than in the male of the same age. In the young adult female TBW only forms about 50% of body weight. This difference between the sexes develops during puberty and decreases in old age due to a reduction in adipose tissue.
- TBW as a proportion of body weight may be as high as 80% in the neonate.

TBW is divided into several fluid compartments (Figure FL1), the main division being between intracellular fluid (ICF) and extracellular fluid (ECF).

The variations of TBW (% body weight) and ECF (% body weight) with age are shown in Figure FL2.

Intracellular fluid (ICF)

The ICF compartment contains about 60% of TBW. The volume of the ICF compartment, including red blood cell contents (2 litres), amounts to about 27 litres. The water content and composition of ICF varies according to the function of the tissue. As noted above, adipose tissue will have much lower water content than lean body tissue, which contains about 70 ml per 100 g water.

Extracellular fluid (ECF)

About one-third of total body water is ECF. Although ECF as a percentage of body weight varies with age (Figure FL2), when expressed as an index of body surface area it remains relatively constant throughout life. The ECF volume to body surface area index is about 7.5 litres per square metre. ECF is composed of several components (Figure FL3).

Plasma

Plasma volume equates to the intravascular component of ECF and amounts to about 5% of body weight. The total blood volume is composed of plasma and the red blood cell volume. Plasma volume (V_{PL}) can be measured using

Fundamentals of Anaesthesia, 3rd edition, ed. Tim Smith, Colin Pinnock and Ted Lin. Published by Cambridge University Press. © Cambridge University Press 2008.

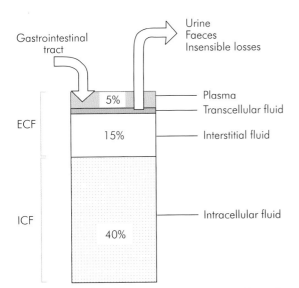

Figure FL1 Body fluid compartments as percentage of body weight

Age	TBW (% body weight)	ECF (% body weight)
Neonate	80	45
6 months	70	35
1 year	60	28
5 years	65	25
Young adult	60	22
Elderly	50	20

Figure FL2 Variation of TBW and ECF with age

a dilution technique. The fractional red blood cell volume is readily available as the haematocrit (%). Given these values, the total blood volume (V_{BL}) can be calculated:

$$V_{PL} = 3.5\,\text{litres}$$
$$\text{Haematocrit (Hct)} = 45\%$$
$$\text{Total blood volume } (V_{BL}) = \frac{V_{PL} \times 100}{(100 - \text{Hct})}$$
$$= 6.4\,\text{litres}$$

Transcellular fluid

The transcellular fluid compartment is composed of fluids that have been secreted but are separated from the plasma by an epithelial layer. These include:
- Cerebrospinal fluid
- Intraocular fluid
- Gastrointestinal fluid

Fluid	% body weight	Volume (litres)
Interstitial fluid	15	10.5
Plasma	5	3.5
Transcellular fluid	1	0.7
Total ECF	21	14.7

Figure FL3 Components of ECF in a 70 kg adult

- Bile
- Pleural, peritoneal and pericardial fluid
- Sweat

The composition of transcellular fluid differs from both plasma and interstitial fluid since it is controlled by the secretory cells.

Measurement of fluid compartment volumes

Compartment volumes are estimated by dilutional techniques. In these methods, an indicator dye that is freely distributed (but contained) within the compartment being estimated is injected into the compartment. The mass of indicator used and the concentration in the fluid are measured. Then the size of the compartment can be determined using the formula:

Volume of compartment
$$= \frac{\text{mass of indicator}}{\text{concentration in compartment}}$$

In reality, this method calculates the volume of distribution of the injected indicator. The mass of indicator must be corrected for excretion and metabolism during the time allowed for distribution.

Indicator methods used to estimate the volume of various compartments are summarised in Figure FL4.

Solutions and semipermeable membranes

Concentration of a solution

The concentration of a solution is usually expressed in terms of the amount of solute present in a given amount of solvent. In the body, concentrations can be varied in fluid compartments by the movement of solute or solvent (water) into a compartment. The concentrations of various substances can be critical for normal function (e.g. extracellular potassium). Several units are used to express concentration, and the following definitions should be noted.

Compartment	Indicator	Comments
Total body water (TBW)	Antipyrine D_2O	Tendency to underestimate uniform distribution
Extracellular fluid (ECF)	Radioisotopes of Na^+, Br^-, Cl^-	These enter cells and so overestimate
	Saccharides (mannitol, inulin)	Incomplete distribution and so underestimate
Plasma volume (V_{PL})	Radioisotope ^{131}I albumin	Total blood volume (V_{BL}) may be derived from V_{PL} and haematocrit (Hct)
Red cell volume (V_{RBC})	Red cells tagged with radioisotope ^{51}Cr	Measures fraction of red blood cells tagged to determine V_{RBC} Measures concentration of tagged cells to determine V_{BL}
Intracellular fluid (ICF)		Derived from: ICF = TBW − ECF
Interstitial fluid volume (V_{INT})		Derived from: V_{INT} = ECF − VPL

Figure FL4 Measurement of fluid compartment volumes

Amount of solute

A given amount of any substance can simply be measured by its mass (g, kg). In chemical reactions, it is more useful to use the unit *moles*, since this relates to the number of molecules present:

$$1 \text{ mole (mol)} = \text{gram molecular weight}$$
$$1 \text{ millimole (mmol)} = (\text{gram molecular weight}) 10^{-3}$$
$$1 \text{ micromole (μmol)} = (\text{gram molecular weight}) 10^{-6}$$
$$1 \text{ mole contains } 6.0247 \times 10^{23} \text{ molecules (Avogadro's number)}$$

Chemical and electrochemical activity of a solution

The effects exerted by a solution are related to concentration. This is most commonly expressed as mass per unit volume ($mg\ ml^{-1}$, $g\ l^{-1}$, $kg\ m^{-3}$). However, the chemical and electrochemical activity of a solution is more closely related to the number of molecules present in a given amount of solution. Concentration of a solution is thus better expressed in terms of its molarity or its molality:

- **Molarity** – moles of solute per litre of solution (solute plus water) ($mol\ l^{-1}$)
- **Molality** – moles of solute per kg of solvent (water) ($mol\ kg^{-1}\ H_2O$)

Interpretation of laboratory values depends on how electrolyte concentrations are indexed (with reference to either litres of plasma water or total plasma volume). The latter includes the volume of proteins, about 7% of total plasma volume, as 93% of plasma volume is water. It follows that laboratory values expressed as $mmol\ l^{-1}$ plasma water will be greater than results expressed as $mmol\ l^{-1}$ plasma volume. This discrepancy will be increased when plasma volume is occupied by other particles, such as in hyperlipidaemia.

Equivalent weight

Chemical reactions between elements occur with fixed proportions of different elements by weight. A gram equivalent weight can be defined for each element. This is the weight of an element that reacts with 8.000 g O_2. An electrical equivalent weight can also be defined for an ion, which is equal to the atomic weight divided by its valency. Thus, the electrical equivalent weight of Na^+ (atomic weight = 23) is 23/1 = 23, while the electrical equivalent weight of Ca^{2+} (atomic weight = 40) is 40/2 = 20. The concentration of a solution may thus be measured in terms of its *normality*, where a normal solution (1 N solution) contains 1 g equivalent solute per litre solution.

Membranes separating fluid compartments

Membranes separate the fluid compartments of the body. They differ widely in structure and function. The membrane separating the ICF and ECF compartments is the plasma membrane surrounding cells, a complex structure based on a biphospholipid structure, with highly active functions determining membrane permeability to different particle species, and hence maintaining significant differences between the compositions of ICF and ECF. The membrane separating interstitial fluid from intravascular fluid is the capillary wall, in which the permeability to water and solutes is mainly dependent on passive mechanisms. The movement of both solutes and water across these membranes determines the composition of fluid in the different compartments.

Movement of water across a membrane

The membranes separating the fluid compartments generally allow the free passage of water, but not solutes, across them. Such membranes are known as semipermeable membranes. If a semipermeable membrane separates two aqueous solutions of different concentrations, water molecules will diffuse across the membrane to equalise the concentrations. *Osmosis* describes this diffusion process. The solutions on each side of the membrane do not have to be of identical solutes, since the osmotic activity of the solutes is dependent on the number and not the type of free particles in solution.

Osmotic pressure

The osmotic activity of solute particles in an aqueous solution can be visualised as exerting an *osmotic pressure*, which would potentially draw water into the solution. This can be demonstrated as a hydrostatic pressure difference between two compartments separated by a semipermeable membrane, one containing solution and the other containing water alone. Osmotic pressure can thus be defined as the pressure required to prevent osmosis when the solution is separated from pure solvent by a semipermeable membrane (Figure FL5).

Calculation of osmotic pressure from molality of a solution

The osmotic pressure of a solution can be calculated from the solution molality. In a dilute solution, with a solute which does not dissociate or associate, osmotic pressure (π) is dependent on temperature and molal concentration. This can be expressed as:

$\pi \propto$ absolute temperature (T) at a given concentration.
Also, $\pi \propto$ absolute concentration (C) at a given temperature.

van't Hoff equation for osmotic pressure

In 1877, van't Hoff noted the similarity of behaviour between dilute solutions and gases. Combining the two relations above gives the van't Hoff equation for the

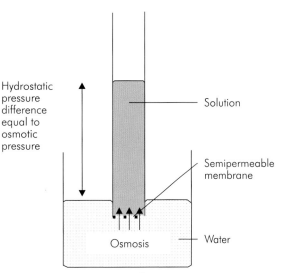

Figure FL5 Demonstration of osmotic pressure

osmotic pressure exerted by a dilute solution as:

osmotic pressure (π) = RTC (pascals),

where:

R = universal gas constant (= 8.32 J/K)
T = absolute temperature (K)
C = osmolality (mOsm kg^{-1}H$_2$O)

This can be applied to find the osmotic pressure of plasma at body temperature (T = 307 K, C = 290 mOsm kg^{-1} H$_2$O), thus:

Osmotic pressure of plasma = 8.32 × 307 × 290 Pa
= 740729.6 Pa
= 740.7 kPa

The osmole

The concentration of solute particles in solution can be expressed in osmoles (Osm), to reflect the osmotic activity of the solution, where:

1 osmole = amount of solute that exerts an osmotic pressure of 1 atm when placed in 22.4 litres of solution at 0 °C

For a substance that does not associate or dissociate in solution (e.g. glucose),

1 osmole = 1 mole

For a substance which dissociates into two osmotically active particles (e.g. NaCl $\rightarrow$ Na$^+$ + Cl$^-$),

1 osmole = 1 mole/2

For a substance that dissociates into three osmotically active particles (e.g. CaCl$_2$ $\rightarrow$ Ca^{2+} + 2 Cl$^-$), then

1 osmole = 1 mole/3

Osmolality and osmolarity of a solution

Osmolarity is the concentration of a solution expressed in osmoles of solute per litre of solution (solute plus water). The units of osmolarity are thus osmoles per litre (Osm l^{-1}) or milliosmoles per litre (mOsm l^{-1})

Osmolality is the concentration of a solution expressed as osmoles of solute per kg solvent (water alone). The units of osmolality are thus osmoles per kg water (Osm kg^{-1} H$_2$O) or milliosmoles per kg water (mOsm kg^{-1} H$_2$O). Osmolality is thus independent of temperature and the volume occupied by the solute. Note particularly:

- As osmolality is independent of temperature, and independent of the volume taken up by the solutes within the solution, it is the preferred term in most physiological applications.
- Equivalent osmolal (or osmolar) concentrations will exert the same osmotic pressures, even though the molality (or molarity) of the solutions may differ.

The molality of a solution can be converted to its osmolality by multiplying molality by the number of discrete solute particles formed when a molecule of solute is in solution (e.g. for CaCl$_2$ solutions multiply by 3).

Osmolality of body fluids

The osmolality of a body fluid is usually higher than its osmolarity because of protein and lipid content, which occupy a small but finite volume. In practice this difference is insignificant except in cases of gross hyperproteinaemia or hyperlipidaemia.

Plasma osmolality ranges from 280 to 295 mOsm kg^{-1} H$_2$O, and is maintained constant at about 290 mOsm kg^{-1} H$_2$O throughout the body. The similar osmolality of all major body fluids is due to the free permeability to water of the endothelium and plasma membranes, which separate the various fluid compartments. The distribution and number of osmotically active particles contained by each primarily determine the size of these compartments.

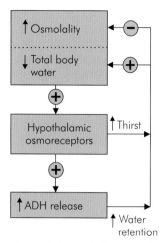

Figure FL6 Regulation of body fluid osmolality

Regulation of body fluid osmolality

The regulation of body fluid osmolality is inextricably linked to the control of total body water (TBW). It involves the secretion of vasopressin (antidiuretic hormone, ADH) in response to an increase in osmolality or a decrease in TBW. Although osmoreceptors appear sensitive enough to respond to small changes in osmolality, their response can be overridden by the haemodynamic response to changes in effective circulating volume. An outline of these responses is shown in Figure FL6.

Measurement of osmolality

The osmolality of a solution can be estimated in practice by measuring depression of freezing point of the solution, when compared with the pure solvent. This depression of freezing point depends on the number and not the type of particle in solution. A solution of 1mOsm kg^{-1} H$_2$O freezes at $-1.86\,^\circ$C. Normal plasma freezes at $-0.54\,^\circ$C. This, therefore, corresponds to a plasma osmolality as determined by the relationship:

$$\text{Plasma osmolality} = \frac{0.54}{1.86} \times 10^3 \text{mOsm kg}^{-1}\text{ H}_2\text{O}$$
$$= 290 \text{ mOsm kg}^{-1}\text{ H}_2\text{O}$$

Estimation of osmolality from solute concentration

Plasma osmolality can also be estimated from the molality of the major solutes: sodium, chloride, urea and glucose:

$$\text{Plasma osmolality} = 2 \times [\text{Na}^+] + [\text{glucose}] + [\text{urea}]$$
$$= 2 \times 140 + 5.0 + 5.0$$
$$= 290 \text{ mOsm kg}^{-1}\text{ H}_2\text{O}$$

Similarly the osmolality of IV solutions can also be estimated from their concentration. Thus, for normal saline:

$$0.9\% \text{ NaCl} = 9\,\text{g}\,\text{l}^{-1} = 9\,\text{g}\,\text{kg}^{-1}\,H_2O$$
$$= 9/(23 + 35.5) \times 10^3\,\text{mmol}\,\text{kg}^{-1}\,H_2O$$
$$= (154\,\text{Na}^+ + 154\,\text{Cl}^-)\,\text{mOsm}\,\text{kg}^{-1}\,H_2O$$
$$= 308\,\text{mOsm}\,\text{kg}^{-1}\,H_2O$$

Tonicity of a solution

Solutions with different osmolalities separated by a semipermeable membrane can result in significant physiological effects due to the passage of water from the lower osmolality side to the higher osmolality side. An example is provided by the swelling and haemolysis of red blood cells placed in water, which occurs due to the movement of water into the red blood cells.

Tonicity describes the relative osmolality between two fluid compartments. Thus, if one compartment contains solution of lower osmolality, it is hypotonic compared with the higher osmolality compartment. Similarly, the higher osmolality compartment is hypertonic relative to the lower osmolality side. This terminology is most commonly applied to the ECF surrounding cells, e.g. plasma around red blood cells.

- Isotonicity describes a solution within which cells can be suspended without a change in cell volume.
- Cells placed in a hypertonic solution will shrink in volume.
- Cells placed in a hypotonic solution will swell in volume.
- A 0.9% solution of NaCl is approximately isotonic (308 mOsm kg^{-1} H$_2$O).

Plasma colloid osmotic pressure

The plasma proteins, albumin and globulins do not normally pass out of the capillaries into the interstitium since they are reflected by the capillary endothelium. The retained plasma proteins raise the plasma osmotic pressure above that of the interstitial fluid by an amount referred to as the *colloid osmotic pressure* (or oncotic pressure). Quantitatively, the most important protein contributing to the colloid osmotic pressure is albumin which is responsible for up to 75% of the total 25 mmHg colloid osmotic pressure.

Distribution of a solute across a membrane

Solute particles are distributed between fluid compartments according to the permeability of the separating membrane to each type of particle. Both passive and active mechanisms determine the movement of solutes across a membrane. Active processes such as carrier proteins or ion channels selectively transport or allow the diffusion of substances across a membrane. Passive movement of particles can occur through *pores* or *fenestrations*, or even through the membrane, depending on lipid solubility.

The distribution of different solute particles across cell plasma membranes is determined by their complex functions and structure. The mechanisms involved are both active and passive.

Movement of solute across a capillary wall generally occurs in the filtrate as it passes from the capillary lumen into the interstitium. Large protein molecules remain in the capillary plasma unable to be filtered out because of their size. This capillary filtration process, and the balance of forces (Starling forces) driving it, is described in Section 2, Chapter 6 (pages 308–9).

The structure of capillaries and the composition of fluid passing across the capillary walls differs between tissues. These differences reflect the variation in function between vessels such as glomerular capillaries in the kidneys, and capillaries found, for example, in skeletal muscle.

The main transport mechanisms involved across capillary endothelium are:

- Filtration, which describes the action of hydrostatic pressure forcing fluid out of the capillaries. It is opposed by the plasma colloid osmotic pressure.
- Diffusion, which is the passive movement of substances under the influence of concentration gradients, and occurs through fenestrations and intercellular junctions. The main diffusion barrier is the basement membrane.
- Transcytosis, which is the active transfer of substance by endocytosis from the capillary lumen, followed by exocytosis out of the endothelial cells. It only represents a small fraction of the total transport across capillary endothelium.

Gibbs–Donnan effect

Passive movement of solute particles usually occurs under the influence of a chemical concentration or electrical gradient. Consider the case of two compartments (A and B) each containing NaCl but separated by a semipermeable membrane. The diffusion of Na$^+$ and Cl$^-$ occurs between the compartments to equalise chemical concentration gradients and to maintain electrical neutrality on either side of the membrane (Figure FL7a).

(a)

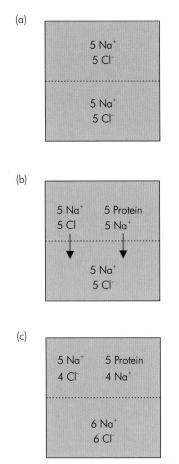

(b)

(c)

Figure FL7 Gibbs–Donnan equilibrium

If protein is trapped in one of the compartments it can affect the distribution of the diffusible ions by the Gibbs–Donnan effect. This occurs due to the negative charge on protein molecules, which acts by holding Na^+ back on one side of the membrane to preserve electroneutrality in the compartment (Figure FL7b). The chemical gradient of Na^+ across the membrane will then redistribute Na^+ (followed by Cl^- to preserve electroneutrality) between the compartments until an equilibrium is reached (Figure FL7c), when:

$$[cation]_A \times [anion]_A = [cation]_B \times [anion]_B$$
$$[Na^+]_A \times [Cl^-]_A = [Na^+]_B \times [Cl^-]_B$$
$$9 \times 4 = 6 \times 6$$

This mechanism is referred to as the Gibbs–Donnan effect and, in vivo, affects the distributions of Na^+ and Cl^- between the intravascular and interstitial compartments in the body.

In this situation the Gibbs–Donnan effect gives rise to:
- Unequal distributions of diffusible ions, Na^+ and Cl^-, between intravascular and interstitial compartments
- Higher Na^+ concentration in the protein-containing plasma compartment and higher Cl^- concentration in the interstitial compartment
- A small electrical potential difference across the membrane

The Gibbs–Donnan effect is significant in the distribution of diffusible ions across a largely passive semipermeable membrane such as capillary endothelium separating intravascular and interstitial compartments.

The Gibbs–Donnan equilibrium described above results when the diffusion of the ions down their chemical concentration gradients is balanced by the electrostatic attraction of the protein molecules trapped in one compartment of the model. This balance between chemical and electrostatic forces produces an electrical potential difference across the membrane. The magnitude of this potential difference can be calculated using the Nernst equation and is dependent on the ratio of the diffusible ion concentrations on either side of the membrane at equilibrium. Thus, applying the Nernst equation to a capillary wall:

$$\text{capillary wall potential} = \frac{RT}{FZ_{Na}} \times \log_e \frac{[Na^+]_{INT}}{[Na^+]_C}$$
$$= 62 \times (145/153)$$
$$= -3.24 \, mV$$

Thus there is a potential difference across the capillary wall of about 3 mV, the endothelial surface being negative with respect to the interstitium.

Composition of body fluids

The compositions of the major body fluids – plasma, interstitial and intracellular – are shown in Figure FL8.

Intracellular fluid

ICF composition varies according to cell function. There are general differences between ICF and interstitial fluid. These include low intracellular Na^+, Cl^- and HCO_3^- concentrations compared with the extracellular values. The predominant cation is K^+, and the organic phosphates and proteins are the principal intracellular anions.

The composition of ICF is maintained largely by the cell plasma membrane in a stable but dynamic state of flux. Membrane transport occurs by passive mechanisms

Substance	Plasma	Interstitial fluid	Intracellular fluid
Cations			
Na^+	153	145	10
K^+	4.3	4.1	159
Ca^{2+}	2.7	2.4	<1
Mg^{2+}	1.1	1	40
Total	161.1	152.5	209
Anions			
Cl^-	112	117	3
HCO_3^-	25.8	27.1	7
Proteins	15.1	<0.1	45
Others	8.2	8.4	154
Total	161.1	152.5	209

Figure FL8 Compositions of plasma, interstitial fluid and intracellular fluid (mmol l^{-1})

Plasma protein group	Name
Proteolytic systems	Kinins
Carrier proteins	Albumin
	Haptoglobulin
	Transferrin
	Ceruloplasmin
	Pre-albumin
	Transcortin
	Transcobalamin
Protease inhibitors	α_1-antitrypsin
	α_2-macroglobulin
	Antithrombin III
Acute phase proteins	Interleukin 1
	Tumour necrosis factor
	C-reactive protein
Immunoglobulins	IgG, IgA, IgM, IgD, IgE

Figure FL9 Plasma proteins

such as diffusion and osmosis, which do not require energy expenditure, as well as active transport.

Interstitial fluid

The composition of interstitial fluid is dependent on the filtration of plasma through the capillary wall. This is largely a passive process driven by the balance of hydrostatic and colloid osmotic pressures. The diffusible ions are, therefore, of approximately equal concentrations in plasma and interstitial fluid. The retention of protein in the capillaries, however, results in a small discrepancy due to the Gibbs–Donnan effect.

Plasma

The distinguishing component in plasma is the retained plasma protein. There is a total protein content in plasma of about 7 g per 100 ml. The various plasma proteins are outlined in Figure FL9.

Albumin

Albumin accounts for 60% of plasma protein. One of its main functions is to act as a transport protein binding free fatty acids and bilirubin. It is also the principal component responsible for plasma colloid osmotic pressure. Of plasma albumin, 5% circulates through the interstitial fluid compartment each hour, while 60% of the total mass of

albumin is actually extravascular. The intravascular half-life of albumin is 19 days.

Immunoglobulins

Immunoglobulins form about 20% of plasma proteins and are split into five groups, each with differing functions and structures. IgG, IgD and IgE are monomers with molecular weights between 150 000 and 190 000 daltons; IgA is secreted as a dimer with a molecular weight of 400 000; IgM is a pentamer with a molecular weight of 900 000. IgM immunoglobulin is completely confined to the intravascular space.

Transcellular fluids

Some of the transcellular fluids differ considerably from plasma in composition. Excessive losses of different transcellular fluids can give rise to significant water and electrolyte disturbances, when disease is present. Some examples of transcellular fluid composition are given in Figure FL10.

Disorders of water and electrolyte balance

Sodium and water

The regulation of total body sodium is inextricably linked to the loss or retention of water, and disturbances in total body sodium content will thus be compensated for by changes in total body water. Similarly compensation for

Substance (mmol l^{-1})	Saliva	Gastric juice	Bile	Sweat
Na^+	33	60	149	45
K^+	20	9	5	5
Cl^-	34	84	101	58
HCO_3^-	0	0	45	0
pH	6.6	3	8	5.2

Figure FL10 Composition of some transcellular fluids

a disturbance of TBW will include readjustment of body sodium levels.

Disturbances of total body water
Some examples of body water disturbances are outlined in Figure FL11.

Abnormalities of plasma sodium
Although total body sodium and total body water are different physiological entities, they are interdependent, so that a disturbance in one quantity will activate compensatory mechanisms which affect both. In practice, they are not readily measured and the clinical management of sodium/water disturbances often relies on the measurement of plasma sodium levels and osmolalities.

Hypernatraemia
Hypernatraemia occurs when plasma sodium is >145 mmol l^{-1}. It often presents with an altered sensorium, this being dependent on the speed of plasma sodium change and plasma osmolality. Coma ensues at plasma osmolalities >350 mOsm kg^{-1} H_2O. Hypernatraemia may occur with decreased or increased ECF volume (ECFV) and increased or decreased total body sodium, depending on the cause

Cause	ECFV	Total body free water	Total body sodium
Diuresis, vomiting, pyrexia	Low	↓↓	↓
Over-transfusion with hypertonic sodium solutions	High	↑	↑↑

Figure FL12 Features of hypernatraemia

of the original disturbance (Figure FL12). Thus the clinical signs and symptoms accompanying hypernatraemia may reflect hypervolaemia or hypovolaemia. Where hypovolaemia is present, sodium deficit can be replaced relatively rapidly compared with the replacement of free water. Free water deficits should be replaced gradually to avoid an increased risk of cerebral oedema.

Hyponatraemia
Hyponatraemia occurs when plasma sodium is <135 mmol l^{-1}. There are different clinical syndromes associated with hyponatraemia, depending on the underlying cause (Figure FL13).
- Hyponatraemia will be associated with water intoxication, which is described above, and is due to excessive water intake or excessive water retention due to inappropriate vasopressin secretion.
- Hypervolaemia will accompany hyponatraemia when the primary disturbance is an increase in TBW, and regulatory mechanisms attempt to maintain plasma osmolality by sodium retention.
- Hypovolaemia and hyponatraemia occur when the primary disturbance is an excessive loss of water and sodium with inappropriate (hypotonic fluids) and inadequate resuscitation.

Condition	Definition	Cause
Dehydration	A decrease in TBW with or without a loss of sodium	↓ intake, e.g. nil by mouth, dysphagia ↑ insensible loss, e.g. pyrexia, hyperhidrosis, hyperventilation
Water deficiency	A decrease in TBW without a comparable decrease in body sodium	↑ urinary loss, e.g. diabetes insipidus, diabetes mellitus ↑ gastrointestinal losses, e.g. vomiting, diarrhoea
Water intoxication	An increase in TBW without a comparable increase in body sodium	Renal failure, inappropriate vasopressin secretion, hepatic failure, IV infusion of dextrose

Figure FL11 Disturbances of total body water (TBW)

Cause	ECFV	Total body free water	Total body sodium	Urinary sodium
Cardiac failure, renal failure, hepatic failure, TUR syndrome	High	↑↑↑	↑	<20 mmol l^{-1}
Inappropriate vasopressin secretion	Normal ECFV, plasma osmolality <290 mOsm kg^{-1} H$_2$O	↑	→	<20 mmol l^{-1}, urine osmolality >100 mOsm kg^{-1} H$_2$O
Adrenal failure	Low	↓	↓↓↓	>20 mmol l^{-1}

Figure FL13 Features of hyponatraemia

Clinical signs and symptoms of hyponatraemia are those of hypovolaemia or hypervolaemia, depending on the underlying disturbance. Central signs range from mild lethargy to seizures and respiratory arrest. Rapid correction can lead to central pontine myelinolysis.

Potassium

Potassium is the main intracellular cation and plays an important role intracellularly in protein synthesis, acid–base balance and maintaining osmolality. Although extracellular concentrations are comparatively low, extracellular levels are also important because they affect membrane potentials and plasma acid–base balance. Some details of potassium excess (hyperkalaemia) and potassium deficit (hypokalaemia) are outlined in Figure FL14.

Calcium

Calcium is quantitatively the most common mineral in the body, with a total body content of about 1200 g. Of calcium, >99% is in bone, the remainder being in body fluids partially ionised and partially protein-bound. Ionised calcium is important as a cofactor, particularly in the coagulation cascade. Calcium is central in maintaining excitability of the myocardium, skeletal muscle, smooth muscle and nerves. It also has a significant role in the regulation of membrane permeability. See Figure FL14 for some details of calcium imbalance.

Magnesium

The total body content of magnesium is about 25 g, of which one-half is contained in bone and teeth. The normal plasma levels are about 1.1 mmol l^{-1}. The most important function of magnesium systemically is its role as a cofactor, since it is essential for the activity of all kinases. These enzymes catalyse phosphorylation reactions by ATP.

Since this is the main mechanism for the transfer of chemical energy in intermediate metabolism, magnesium plays a key role in functions such as muscle contraction as well as pathways such as glycolysis. Regulation of magnesium levels in the body is not clear but may involve parathormone and aldosterone. Figure FL14 details the effects of magnesium imbalance.

Special fluids

Lymph and the lymphatic system

The lymphatics are a system of blind-ending tubules with endothelium similar to blood capillaries. There is neither basement membrane nor intercellular gaps, and pinocytosis makes the vessels permeable to proteins. Lymph nodes are encapsulated collections of specialised tissue situated along the course of the lymphatic vessels. They are populated by phagocytic cells lining medullary and cortical sinuses. These engulf bacteria so that under normal conditions the lymph exiting the nodes is sterile.

Ultimately two main vessels, the right lymphatic and thoracic duct, drain into the subclavian veins. The 24-hour production of lymph is 2–4 litres. The low resistance of the lymphatic branching system, the presence of valves and positive intrathoracic pressures promote forward flow. There is also a high resistance to returning to the interstitial space.

The lymphatic capillaries supplement the venous capillaries in the drainage of tissue fluid. Lymph pumps augment fluid removal. These take the form of adjacent arteriolar pulsations compressing and dilating the lymph vessels, as is found in skeletal muscle. Excessive accumulation of tissue fluid is oedema. Other functions of the lymphatics include the return and absorption of nutrients. Plasma lipids are transported as lipoproteins and neutral fat as chylomicrons, and concentrations vary with

Disorder	Cause	Symptoms and signs
Hypokalaemia	Acute – administration of insulin and glucose, familial periodic paralysis, vomiting, diarrhoea	Tachycardia, extrasystoles, cardiac dilatation
	Chronic – dietary insufficiency, malabsorption, diuretics, hyperaldosteronism, Cushing's syndrome	Weakness, hypotonia and paralysis of muscle, metabolic alkalosis
Hyperkalaemia	Renal failure, Addison's disease, iatrogenic (spironolactone, administration of potassium supplements)	Cardiac arrhythmias, heart block, cardiac arrest in diastole
		Weakness, numbness paraesthesiae, listlessness, confusion
Hypocalcaemia	Hypoparathyroidism, post-thyroidectomy, vitamin D deficiency, renal failure, hyperventilation	Tetany, convulsions, cataracts, ectopic calcification in CNS
Hypercalcaemia	Hyperparathyroidism, malignancy, sarcoidosis, multiple myeloma, vitamin D toxicity, milk-alkali syndrome	Nephrolithiasis, personality changes, muscle weakness and atrophy, abdominal discomfort, corneal calcification
Hypomagnesaemia	Diarrhoea, malabsorption, hyperaldosteronism	'Calcium-resistant' tetany, muscular weakness, depression, irritability, convulsions
Hypermagnesaemia	Renal failure, iatrogenic administration	Prolonged AV and intraventricular conduction rates

Figure FL14 Disorders of potassium, calcium and magnesium balance

dietary intake. Chylomicrons are small fat globules comprising lipid and protein that are created by the intestinal mucosa.

Lymph has the following features:

- Protein content is lower than plasma and depends on the drained organ.
- Contains all coagulation factors, especially hepatic lymph.
- Antibodies are found in high concentrations.
- Electrolyte composition is similar to plasma.
- Lymphocytes are common, red cells and platelets are rare.

Cerebrospinal fluid (CSF)

About 150 ml cerebrospinal fluid surrounds the structures of the CNS and fills the cerebral ventricles. This fluid is continually produced at 600 ml per 24 hours, it circulates and is reabsorbed into the cerebrovenous system. The majority of CSF (70%) is produced by the choroid plexuses within the cerebral ventricles; the remaining 30% is produced in the endothelium of cerebral capillaries. The choroid plexuses are networks of cerebral blood vessels exposed to the cerebrospinal fluid in the third and lateral ventricles. They produce the CSF by modified ultrafiltration from the plexus capillaries into the ventricles. The filtration barrier consists of capillary endothelium, basement membrane and choroid epithelium, which also actively modifies the composition of the CSF produced.

Circulation of CSF

The CSF flows through the lateral ventricles to the brain stem, where it passes via the third and fourth ventricles, aided by ciliated ependymal cells, which line the ventricles. From the fourth ventricle the CSF exits to the subarachnoid space via the lateral foramina of Luschka and the median foramen of Magendie. It then circulates around the brainstem, brain and spinal cord in the subarachnoid space, finally to be reabsorbed by arachnoid villi in the venous sinuses of the skull. The rate of reabsorption is

Substance		CSF	Plasma
Protein	(g l^{-1})	0.3	70
HCO$_3^1$	(mmol l^{-1})	23	25
Glucose	(mmol l^{-1})	4.8	8
Na$^+$	(mmol l^{-1})	147	150
K$^+$	(mmol l^{-1})	2.9	4.6
Cl$^-$	(mmol l^{-1})	112	100
pH		7.32	7.4
Osmolality	(mOsm kg^{-1} H$_2$O)	290	290
PCO$_2$	(kPa)	6.6	5.3

Figure FL15 Concentrations of major substances in CSF and plasma

proportional to CSF outflow pressure. This is normally 11.2 cmH$_2$O. Reabsorption ceases if it is <7 cmH$_2$O.

Composition of CSF
As noted, the filtration process producing the CSF in the choroid plexuses is ultrafiltration, which is modified (by active secretion) by the ependymal cells. The concentrations of the major constituents in CSF are given in Figure FL15.

Functions of CSF
The main functions of CSF are:
- Providing buoyancy and protection
- Ionic homeostasis
- Respiratory control

Ionic homeostasis
The ionic composition of interstitial fluid in the CNS is tightly controlled. Both the CSF and the cerebral capillaries contribute to the formation of interstitial fluid. CSF is in free communication with the interstitial fluid in the brain and has the same composition, but there can be a significant time lag in the equilibration of changes between CSF and interstitial fluid. The formation of interstitial fluid and the CSF occurs across a blood–brain barrier located in the cerebral capillaries and the choroid plexuses respectively. This barrier separates the cerebral circulation from the cerebral tissue and serves several functions, which are to:
- Provide tight control over ion concentrations in the CNS
- Protect the brain from transient changes in plasma glucose
- Protect the brain from endogenous and exogenous toxins
- Prevent the release of central neurotransmitters into the systemic circulation

CNS chemoreceptor respiratory control
The central chemoreceptors involved in respiratory control are situated on the ventral surface of the medulla and the floor of the fourth ventricle. The chemoreceptors are bathed in interstitial fluid, which as noted is in communication with the CSF, as well as being formed by cerebral capillaries. The blood–brain barrier is freely permeable to CO$_2$ but relatively impermeable to H$^+$ and HCO$_3^-$. Thus, CO$_2$ diffuses across into the CSF and interstitial fluid in proportion to arterial PCO$_2$. The low protein concentration in CSF and interstitial fluid limits its buffering capacity, and pH changes are greater than those in plasma for a given change in PCO$_2$.

The initial response to increasing plasma PCO$_2$ is formation of H$^+$ and HCO$_3^-$ in the epithelial cells, catalysed by carbonic anhydrase. Compensation then takes place through the secretion of HCO$_3^-$ buffering CSF and interstitial pH. The concentration of HCO$_3^-$ in CSF and cerebral interstitial fluid is always lower than in plasma, because of the lack of protein buffering in these fluids. The chemoreceptor response to H$^+$ is to stimulate hyperventilation.

Intraocular fluid
Aqueous and vitreous humour are formed from plasma. Aqueous is a plasma diasylate with a continuous hourly turnover and provides the metabolic and respiratory substrate for the anterior chamber. Specialised cells in the ciliary body actively secrete aqueous humour. The principal route of drainage is via the canal of Schlemm. Production and drainage maintains intraocular pressure at 15–18 mmHg. Vitreous humour in the posterior chamber contains the gelatine-like protein vitrein.

Pleural fluid
Capillaries on the surface of highly vascular visceral and parietal pleurae form a thin lubricating layer of fluid. The forces of ultrafiltration and reabsorption apply as in the formation of any transcellular fluid discussed above. The hydrostatic pressure in pulmonary capillaries is low compared with a high plasma colloid pressure. The Starling shifts are in favour of reabsorption, leaving a thin intrapleural layer of fluid.

CHAPTER 3
Haematology and immunology

J. R. Neilson and J. K. Wood

Red blood cells

Red blood cells (erythrocytes) provide the system for oxygen delivery from the lungs to the tissues, and evolution has produced a very specialised cell for this purpose. The erythrocyte lacks organelles and a nucleus and is no more than a membrane enclosing a solution of protein and electrolytes. Over 95% of the protein content is the oxygen transport protein haemoglobin, the remainder being enzymes required to maintain haemoglobin in a functional, reduced state and enzymes for glycolysis. The biconcave shape of erythrocytes increases the surface-area-to-volume ratio, making gas exchange more efficient, and also makes the cell more deformable (compared with a sphere) and therefore more able to navigate the microvasculature. Under normal circumstances the average survival of erythrocytes is 120 days.

Haemopoiesis starts in the yolk sac in the 2-week-old embryo. At 6 weeks the liver, and to a lesser extent the spleen, start to produce haemopoietic cells and by 12–16 weeks the liver is the main haemopoietic tissue. The bone marrow starts to produce blood cells at 20 weeks. At birth haemopoietic (red) marrow occupies all bones.

Fat gradually replaces the red marrow until in adults red marrow is confined to the axial skeleton only.

Manufacture of erythrocytes (erythropoiesis) occurs predominantly in the bone marrow from the seventh month of gestation. A homeostatic mechanism ensures that under physiological conditions the rate of production equals the rate of destruction, but at the same time there is a capability to respond to demands such as hypoxia, haemorrhage or haemolysis by increasing production. Erythropoietin (EPO) is a glycoprotein produced mainly in the kidney but also in the liver. It is one of the most important erythropoietic stimuli. Specialised cells in the renal and hepatic parenchyma have been shown to manufacture EPO. In the kidney, the cells are located outside the tubular basement membrane mainly in the inner cortex and outer medulla. Serum levels increase in response to hypoxia, anaemia and increased metabolism (due to effects of corticosteriods, androgens, thyroxine and growth hormone). The bone marrow is among the most highly proliferative tissues in the body and therefore requires an uninterrupted supply of nutrients. Those particularly needed for erythropoiesis include iron (for haem), vitamin B_{12}, folate and

Fundamentals of Anaesthesia, 3rd edition, ed. Tim Smith, Colin Pinnock and Ted Lin. Published by Cambridge University Press. © Cambridge University Press 2008.

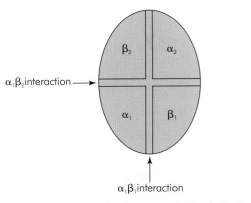

Figure HA1 Relationship between globin chains in haemoglobin

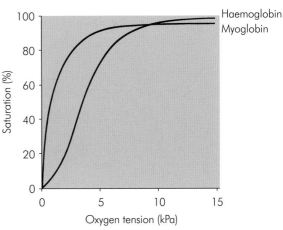

Figure HA2 Oxygen–haemoglobin dissociation curve

pyridoxine (for DNA synthesis), riboflavin, vitamin E and copper.

Haemoglobin

Eighteen times more energy is available if glucose is metabolised aerobically than anaerobically. Hence, the transition to aerobic life was a major step in evolutionary terms. The acquisition of oxygen-carrying molecules became necessary to overcome the relative insolubility of oxygen in water. The oxygen carriers in vertebrates are haemoglobin and myoglobin. Haemoglobin increases the oxygen-carrying capacity of 1 litre of blood more than 50-fold, and it also is involved in the transport of CO_2 and hydrogen ions (H^+). Myoglobin is present in skeletal muscle and serves as an oxygen store, releasing oxygen when needed.

Structure and function of haemoglobin

The haemoglobin A molecule has four polypeptide chains (two α and two β chains), each of which has a covalently bound haem group consisting of a porphyrin ring with a central iron atom in the ferrous (Fe^{2+}) state. A single oxygen molecule can bind to the central iron atom of each haem group. The cross-links between the polypeptide chains consist of non-covalent electrostatic interactions (salt links). There are two distinct types of salt link in the haemoglobin molecule (Figure HA1).

The breathing molecule

The haemoglobin molecule is said to 'breathe' during oxygen uptake and release. Deoxyhaemoglobin is in the taut (T) configuration while the binding of oxygen produces a more relaxed (R) configuration by breaking salt links in the $\alpha_1\beta_2$ and $\alpha_2\beta_1$ interactions. The first oxygen molecule binds relatively weakly to haemoglobin, since more salt links must be broken (and therefore more energy is required) compared with the subsequent two oxygen molecules, and less energy still is required for the binding of the fourth oxygen molecule. This sequential increase in oxygen affinity explains the sigmoid shape of the oxygen dissociation curve of haemoglobin (Figure HA2). Myoglobin, being a single chain molecule, has a hyperbolic-shaped oxygen dissociation curve.

Effect of CO_2, H^+ and 2,3-DPG

CO_2 binds to the terminal amino groups of haemoglobin as bicarbonate, which is formed in the red cell by the action of carbonic anhydrase:

$$CO_2 + H_2O \rightleftharpoons HCO_3^- + H^+$$

This lowers the oxygen affinity of haemoglobin, shifting the oxygen dissociation curve to the right. Much of the hydrogen ion generated by this reaction is taken up by deoxyhaemoglobin, which has a higher affinity for H^+ than oxyhaemoglobin:

$$HbO_2 + H^+ \rightleftharpoons HbH^+ + O_2$$

Hence, under acid conditions the equilibrium between deoxy- and oxyhaemoglobin shifts in favour of deoxyhaemoglobin – this is called the 'Bohr effect'. Acidic conditions, therefore, reduce the oxygen affinity of haemoglobin and shift the oxygen dissociation curve to the right. In the highly oxygenated environment of the alveolar capillaries of the lungs the above reactions are reversed.

2,3-Diphosphoglycerate (2,3-DPG) is produced in a side reaction of the Embden–Meyerhof pathway. Binding to haemoglobin in the ratio of one molecule of 2,3-DPG per tetramer, it reduces the oxygen affinity of haemoglobin 26-fold (oxygen dissociation curve moves to the right). In the absence of 2,3-DPG, haemoglobin would unload little oxygen in the capillaries.

Part of the 'storage lesion' of blood for transfusion is a fall in 2,3-DPG levels to about 30% of normal after 3 weeks storage in whole blood in CPD-A medium (citrate-phosphate-dextrose-adenine). This is improved with storage in plasma-reduced blood in SAGM (saline-adenine-glucose-mannitol). The clinical significance of the low 2,3-DPG is only likely to be of importance in recipients with severe anaemia or cardiac ischaemia. 2,3-DPG levels are restored to at least 50% of normal in 24 hours and 95% of normal at 72 hours after transfusion.

An increase in body temperature is capable of shifting the oxygen dissociation curve to the right and is an appropriate response to exercise. The converse is also true, but in hypothermic individuals the oxygen requirement also falls.

Genetic control of haemoglobin synthesis and the haemoglobinopathies

The genes for the α-globins are located on the short arm of chromosome 16. The order of the genes on the chromosome is determined when they appear during development. There are also pseudogenes that during evolution have acquired mutations and are not expressed. After 8 weeks of embryonic development there are two functional α-chain genes per chromosome (α_1 and α_2), which are normally expressed equally. Hence there are four functioning α genes in each erythroid precursor.

The β-globin gene cluster is located on the short arm of chromosome 11, and there is a single pseudogene in this cluster (ψ β). While there are two genes controlling expression of γ chains (γ G and γ A), which are present in foetal haemoglobin, there is only a single functional β-chain gene per chromosome. Alteration of the coding regions (exons) of the globin genes is likely to alter the amino acid sequence of the corresponding globin chain and the end result is a haemoglobinopathy (e.g. sickle cell disease). On the other hand, if there is lack of expression of a globin chain as a result of deletion or mutation at critical control regions (e.g. RNA splice sites) then a thalassaemia results. Although sickle cell and thalassaemia are the two most common anomalies of haemoglobin, there are other abnormal forms.

Sickle cell disease
Pathophysiology

Sickle cell disease is a result of a single DNA base change (adenine to thymine) which results in the substitution of valine for glutamic acid at position 6 of the β-globin chain. Sickle haemoglobin (HbS) polymerises into microfibrils (crystals) in the deoxygenated state. It is thought that the formation of parallel HbS microfibrils causes red cell membrane damage, which results in the classical sickle cell deformity. The effect of this is to shorten the survival of sickle red cells (to 5–15 days in homozygous sickle cell disease), causing haemolytic anaemia. In addition, the deformed red cells are more rigid and less capable of passing through the microcirculation. The result is obstruction, clinically manifest as 'crises', e.g. bone pain, pulmonary syndrome and stroke.

The rate of polymerisation of HbS is related to the 50th power of its concentration. Polymerisation is also affected by the presence of other haemoglobin types, which may inhibit this process to varying degrees. Haemoglobin C and D are not sickling haemoglobins, but inhibit the sickling of HbS much less than HbA and HbF. Hence, persons with double heterozygosity for HbS and HbC or HbD have a sickling disorder, whereas heterozygotes for HbS do not.

Sickle cell disease exists widely throughout Africa and in parts of Asia, the Arabian peninsula and southern Europe. The high prevalence of this debilitating disease is a result of balanced polymorphism driven by the relative resistance of heterozygotes to malaria. The majority of sickle cell disease seen in the UK is found in African-Caribbean populations in large cities, where up to 10% of individuals carry the β^S gene. In Africa this may be as high as 45%.

Clinical features: sickle trait

Sufferers of sickle trait have normal growth, development, exercise tolerance and life expectancy. Black American football players, for example, have the same prevalence of sickle trait as the general population. There are rare reports of high-altitude splenic infarction, though it must be stressed that most persons with sickle trait tolerate high altitude with impunity.

Clinical features: sickle cell disease

The clinical features of sickle cell disease can be summarised as follows:

- Anaemia – universal. Most patients have a haemoglobin level between 5 and 10 g dl^{-1}. It is generally well tolerated and does not require therapy.

- Vaso-occlusive (painful) crises – the most common manifestation that brings the patient into hospital contact. There is sudden onset of severe pain, usually in bones and joints, which reflects bone marrow ischaemia due to sickling in the bone marrow sinusoids. It may be precipitated by infection or exposure to cold, although often no precipitant can be identified. Abdominal crises may present as an acute abdomen and can be difficult to distinguish from biliary colic. The absence of bowel sounds, however, should alert the physician to a disorder requiring surgical intervention.
- Acute chest syndrome – features include pleuritic chest pain, fever, tachypnoea, pulmonary infiltrates and leucocytosis. It is difficult to distinguish infection, infarction due to sickling and pulmonary embolism. Hypoxia is common and ventilatory support is sometimes needed.
- Stroke – perhaps the most important complication, with the majority occurring in children. Infarction is the usual pathology.
- In children – aplastic crises (parvovirus), splenic sequestration (major cause of death in children under 2 years old), dactylitis, delayed growth and development.
- Long-term complications in adults – include cholelithiasis, sickle retinopathy, leg ulcers (more common in the tropics), renal impairment and chronic bone damage from recurrent crises.

Diagnosis
Some other haemoglobin types may mimic sickle cell disease. To obtain an exact diagnosis, haemoglobin electrophoresis should be performed.

Management
Ideally all patients should be managed in centres with experience in managing haemoglobinopathies. Management of specific problems is as follows:
- Vaso-occlusive crises – adequate and prompt pain relief is essential. Opioids are often required. Adequate hydration is essential. Broad-spectrum antibiotics should be given if infection is suspected. Hypoxia is the only proven indication for oxygen therapy.
- Surgery – to reduce the risk of acute chest syndrome, patients with sickle cell disease should be transfused to reduce the HbS level to about 30% and to raise the $Hb > 10$ g dl^{-1} before major surgery. Transfusion for minor procedures (e.g. myringotomy) is not indicated.

- Pregnancy – transfusion therapy during pregnancy reduces the incidence of painful crises but has not been shown to alter pregnancy outcome.
- Prophylaxis – penicillin V 250–500 mg bd (important in hyposplenic status). Vaccination against pneumococcus, *Haemophilus influenzae* and meningococcus is recommended.

Thalassaemias
The thalassaemias are genetic disorders of globin chain synthesis (α or β). The genetic lesion results in failure of expression of the globin chain gene involved. In the α thalassaemias gene deletion is the usual mechanism, and in the β thalassaemias gene mutation resulting in abnormal processing is most often responsible. Heterozygotes are said to have thalassaemia trait and are asymptomatic but may have characteristic blood count abnormalities.

Alpha thalassaemia
In α thalassaemias there is reduced or absent α-chain synthesis. It is critical in the understanding of these disorders to recall that there are two α-chain genes on each chromosome and, therefore, four genes in any diploid cell. Either one gene is deleted on the same chromosome (α^+) or both are (α^0). The homozygous condition in which no α chains are produced (—/— or $\alpha^0\alpha^0$) is not compatible with life, the fetus being stillborn at 28–40 weeks or surviving a few hours after birth. It is termed the Hb Barts–Hydrops syndrome.

Alpha thalassaemia trait
This may be suspected in persons having thalassaemic indices (MCH < 27 pg, low MCV, raised RBC) with normal HbA_2 level and who are iron-replete.

Beta thalassaemia
In β thalassaemia there is reduced or absent β-chain synthesis. Each diploid cell has two β-chain genes. Mutation is the usual abnormality at the DNA level, which results in transcriptional dysfunction, RNA processing error or non-functional mRNA. This can result in either reduced β-chain production from that gene (β^+) or absent production (β^0). Each racial group affected has its own repertoire of mutations. Affected populations originate from the Mediterranean, Indian subcontinent or Southeast Asia.

Homozygous β thalassaemia – thalassaemia major (Cooley's anaemia)

There is absent or greatly reduced β-chain synthesis. This becomes apparent with the natural fall in fetal haemoglobin ($\alpha_2\gamma_2$) levels due to the switch from γ to β chain production. The infant presents with anaemia during the first 6 months of life. If transfusion therapy is not instituted then the infant may demonstrate the typical thalassaemic facies (frontal bossing, maxillary hyperplasia). With transfusion therapy there is normal development for the first decade, but iron overload then becomes clinically apparent in the absence of chelation therapy (desferrioxamine) and death occurs in the second or third decade. Chelation is usually started in infancy, and with good compliance patients can expect to live well into their 30s and perhaps longer. In a select group of children bone marrow transplantation is an option, but not without risk of transplant-related death.

Beta thalassaemia trait

This is asymptomatic with a thalassaemic blood picture. The HbA$_2$ ($\alpha_2\delta_2$) level is elevated due to a relative reduction in β-chain synthesis with normal δ-chain synthesis. Iron deficiency can reduce HbA$_2$ levels into the normal range, and therefore HbA$_2$ should be measured for diagnostic purposes when the individual is iron-replete.

Transfusion medicine

Transfusion medicine involves the procurement, processing, testing and administration of blood and its components. It is also concerned with the prevention, investigation and treatment of transfusion-related complications.

To many disciplines this translates into the provision of safe red cells for transfusion as soon as possible. While emphasis is rightly placed on virological safety, the important objective of serological compatibility is the responsibility of the laboratory and clinicians, and deaths still occur as a result of ABO incompatability, most often as a result of clerical error. The blood group systems were recognised following a reaction between the recipient's serum and donor red cells. Historically, this occurred in vitro and/or in vivo as a transfusion reaction or haemolytic disease of the newborn (HDN), such reactions being simple antibody–antigen reactions. If the particular antibody is able to fix complement (IgM, IgG), then lysis occurs. If this occurs in vivo, an immediate (intravascular) haemolytic transfusion reaction occurs.

Blood group	Naturally occurring antibodies (IgM)	UK (%)
O	Anti-A, anti-B	47
A	Anti-B	42
B	Anti-A	8
AB	None	3

Figure HA3 Relative frequencies of ABO groups

ABO system

The ABO system is the most important because of the presence of naturally occurring IgM antibodies to groups A and B in subjects lacking these antigens. These antibodies are active at 37 °C and readily cause immediate haemolytic transfusion reactions in ABO incompatibility. They are not present at birth, and are thought to arise after exposure to foreign antigens in infancy. Figure HA3 gives the frequencies of the ABO groups in the UK. Among blood group A and AB individuals approximately one-quarter have a lower density of A antigen on the surface of the red cells, and such subjects are referred to as A$_2$ and A$_2$B (the rest are A$_1$/A$_1$B). Some A$_2$ and A$_2$B people have low levels of anti-A$_1$ in their serum, though this is rarely of clinical significance as it is not active at 37 °C.

The majority (80%) of individuals can secrete ABO substances in their saliva and other bodily secretions. Persons who are group O and are secretors secrete a precursor substance (H) in the saliva, group A secretors secrete A and H, and so on.

Rhesus system

This is the second most important system, not because of naturally occurring antibodies as in the ABO system, but because Rhesus D (Rh D) antibodies are readily formed when blood from a Rh D-positive donor is infused into a Rh D-negative recipient or when a Rh D-negative mother bears a Rh D-positive infant. These antibodies are IgG and can, therefore, cross the placenta to cause haemolytic disease of the newborn (HDN).

Alongside the D antigen there are four other Rh antigens of importance – C, c, E, e – although a total of 48 Rh antigens have been described. The antigens C and c are allelic, as are E and e. There is no d antigen; the letter is used to indicate a lack of D antigen. D is the most important of the Rh antigens as it is more than 20 times more immunogenic than c, the next most important antigen. Because of the Rh D testing of all donors and recipients, and immuno-prophylaxis with anti-D during pregnancy and at delivery, the relative frequency of anti-D compared with other Rh antibodies has declined significantly in recent years. Red cell units are still labelled Rh D-positive or negative, but a proportion will also have a Rh genotype label. The reason for this is to indicate a lack of certain antigens (c and e in the examples given); these units are, therefore, suitable for patients whose serum contains the corresponding antibodies. Numerous other red cell antigens also exist.

Group and screen

It is of critical importance that blood samples for compatibility testing are correctly identified. The ABO and Rh D groups are established by using monoclonal typing reagents (anti-A, anti-B, anti-A+B and anti-D). In ABO grouping, the reverse group is also performed by mixing the patient's serum with A_1 and B red cells. Then an antibody screen is performed. The patient's serum is tested against red cells that between them carry the antigens listed above. If there is a positive reaction in the antibody screen, then the antibody is identified by testing the patient's serum against a panel of red cells. This is done either in the hospital blood bank or at the regional transfusion centre. Once an alloantibody is identified, appropriate red cell units, lacking the red cell antigen, are selected.

Red cell selection and cross-matching

If a red cell alloantibody is detected then blood should be selected that is known to be negative for that antigen and is ABO- and Rh-compatible. A cross-match follows, where the patient's serum is tested against red cells from the units to be transfused. If the cross-match is negative, then a compatibility label, giving patient details, is attached to the unit and the blood and a compatibility report issued.

Emergency situations

If the situation is life-threatening then group O blood is issued. If the patient is a premenopausal female, O Rh D-negative must be issued. There is generally a shortage of O Rh D-negative blood due to high demand for universal usage in emergency situations. Usually, there is sufficient time to perform ABO and Rh D groups on the patient sample by rapid techniques and to do an immediate spin cross-match before issue. This may take 10–15 minutes. An antibody screen is then performed by the laboratory retrospectively. A label stating that standard pre-transfusion testing has not been performed is attached to the blood bag. In massive transfusion, where one blood volume has been given within 24 hours, ABO- and Rh D-compatible blood can be issued without further serological testing, provided no alloantibodies were present by earlier testing.

Transfusion reactions

Immediate and life-threatening reactions

Immediate haemolytic transfusion reactions

Most often due to ABO incompatability arising from clerical error. Less commonly, due to antibodies against Rh D, Duffy, Kidd and Kell antigens. The antibodies (IgM, IgG1 and IgG3) fix complement and this causes intravascular haemolysis. Features include pain at infusion site, chest and back pain, hypotension, DIC, haemoglobinuria. The mortality rate is 10%.

Bacterial contamination

This is rare but is usually fatal if red cells are contaminated. One of the most frequent organisms responsible is *Yersinia enterocolitica*. There is rapid development of septic shock and collapse. The contaminated blood may be clotted or have a purple discoloration. Platelets can sometimes be contaminated with bacteria, most often gram-positive organisms such as *Staphylococcus epidermidis*. This relates to storage of platelets at 22 °C.

Life-threatening reactions associated with dyspnoea

Anaphylaxis

Anaphylaxis is rare but may be fatal. It is most often related to IgA deficiency in the recipient associated with complement-fixing anti-IgA.

Transfusion-related acute lung injury (TRALI)

This is rare. It is due to anti-leukocyte antibodies in donor plasma, and most often seen associated with fresh frozen plasma (FFP). Hypoxia develops during or in the hours following transfusion. There are associated bilateral lung infiltrates radiographically. This syndrome is easily confused with ARDS, and in the critical care setting TRALI may be overlooked as a cause of this clinical picture. Respiratory support is often required and IV methylprednisolone should be given. In contrast with ARDS, recovery is usual within 48 hours. Recurrence is not a problem as the antibodies existed in the **donor** plasma.

Congestive cardiac failure (usually LVF)

This is a common adverse effect of transfusion in the elderly, and can be late in onset. Patients with ischaemic heart disease are most at risk. It can be avoided by prophylactic diuretics and transfusion of only two units a day by slow infusion – one unit in 3 hours.

Non-life-threatening transfusion reactions
Febrile non-haemolytic transfusion reactions (FNHTR)

This is the most common type of transfusion reaction. It is due to recipient anti-leukocyte antibodies. These may be acquired following pregnancy or after transfusion of cellular blood components. The patient may experience a rigor, but temperature may rise without one. There are no signs or symptoms to suggest a haemolytic reaction, but severe FNHTRs may be associated with moderate hypotension, nausea, vomiting, cyanosis and collapse. If FNHTRs have already been experienced, further reactions can be prevented by paracetamol before transfusion. Leucodepletion of blood components may be indicated if reactions persist despite this measure. Primary prevention of FNHTR by leucodepletion is appropriate in some situations, e.g. aplastic anaemia, renal transplant candidates, transfusion-dependent patients.

Urticarial reactions

Urticarial reactions to donor plasma proteins may be treated with antihistamines. If there are repeated reactions unresponsive to antihistamines, washed red cells should be given.

Delayed haemolytic transfusion reactions

These occur in patients who have been transfused previously or have had a previous pregnancy, and who have developed a red cell antibody, the titre of which has fallen to undetectable levels. Re-exposure to the corresponding antigen in a later transfusion results in a secondary immune response and haemolysis of the transfused cells. IgG antibodies are generally responsible and haemolysis is generally extravascular, though occasionally can be intravascular.

Clinical features include fever and a fall in haemoglobin level associated with jaundice between 4 and 14 days following transfusion. If the haemolysis is intravascular, then there may be haemoglobinuria. The clinical severity is related to the volume of incompatible blood transfused. Diagnosis requires a positive direct antiglobulin test and the demonstration of an alloantibody either in the serum or in a red cell eluate, which is antibody eluted from the red blood cells.

- Bone marrow failure – if this is reversible (e.g. after chemotherapy), prophylaxis to maintain platelets $>10 \times 10^9 \; l^{-1}$ is appropriate. In chronic bone marrow failure platelets are generally given if the patient is haemorrhagic
- Platelet function disorders – very occasionally required prior to surgery
- Massive blood transfusion – clinically significant dilutional thrombocytopenia occurs after the transfusion of about 1.5 blood volumes. The platelet count should be maintained $>50 \times 10^9 \; l^{-1}$
- Cardiopulmonary bypass surgery – platelet functional abnormalities and thrombocytopenia are common in this situation. Platelet transfusion should be reserved for patients with non-surgical bleeding. Prophylaxis is not indicated
- Disseminated intravascular coagulation (DIC) – in acute DIC with haemorrhage and thrombocytopenia. Fibrin degradation products (FDPs) impair platelet function. In the absence of bleeding and in chronic DIC platelet transfusion is not indicated
- Prior to surgery and invasive procedures – platelet count should be raised to $50 \times 10^9 \; l^{-1}$. For operations on critical sites (e.g. brain and eye) the platelet count should be raised to $100 \times 10^9 \; l^{-1}$

Note that a 'standard dose' of platelets in an adult may be considered as 4 units m^{-2}.

Figure HA4 Indications for the use of platelet concentrates

Use of blood components

Guidelines are available for the use of platelets and fresh frozen plasma (FFP). Figures HA4–HA6 give indications for the use of platelets, FFP and cryoprecipitate respectively.

Haemostasis

The arrest of bleeding following an injury is a rapid and complex process that involves changes in the involved vessel (smooth muscle constricts and the endothelium becomes procoagulant), platelets (become activated and aggregate) and plasma (fibrin formation). Simultaneous inhibitory mechanisms ensure these processes are confined to the site of injury and do not propagate to, or occur in, normal vasculature. Subsequently, the removal of the clot (fibrinolysis) occurs as part of tissue remodelling. Although there

- Replacement of single coagulation factor deficiencies where a specific concentrate is not available
- Immediate reversal of warfarin effect – but in life-threatening bleeding due to warfarin prothrombinase complex concentrates (PCC = intermediate purity factor IX) and factor VII concentrates are indicated, together with vitamin K (5 mg IV)
- DIC if there is haemorrhage and coagulation abnormality – if there is no haemorrhage or the condition is chronic FFP is not indicated
- Thrombotic thrombocytopenic purpura – a rare disorder which is treated with plasmapheresis using cryoprecipitate-poor FFP
- Massive transfusion if there are abnormal coagulation tests (PT and/or APTT ratio $\geq$ 1.5) and fibrinogen >1.5 g l^{-1} (if <1.5 g l^{-1} cryoprecipitate indicated). Coagulation tests need to be repeated frequently to assess the need for further components
- Liver disease – if there is bleeding or prior to surgery/procedures if the PT ratio is prolonged $\geq$1.5
- Cardiopulmonary bypass if there is non-surgical bleeding and a coagulation abnormality with normal platelet count and function

Note that a 'standard' dose of FFP in an adult may be considered as 4 units.

Figure HA5 Indications for the use of fresh frozen plasma

---

are newer theories of the mechanism of clot formation, the classical division into intrinsic and extrinsic systems still has validity and aids understanding.

Abnormal coagulation tests are among the commonest reasons for seeking haematological advice, both inside and outside normal working hours. In many cases, the underlying coagulation abnormality and its treatment can be deduced from a basic knowledge of the coagulation mechanism. The classical theory of blood coagulation that describes intrinsic and extrinsic systems is particularly useful for understanding in vitro coagulation tests. More modern theories have managed to explain some of the apparent paradoxes of the classical theory, such as why haemophiliacs bleed and patients with factor XII deficiency do not.

The coagulation cascade is shown in Figure HA7. Such cascade reactions allow for considerable amplification as well as many opportunities for control of the process.

- Emergency treatment of haemophilia and von Willebrand's disease when specific concentrates are not available and on the advice of a haematologist
- Dysfibrinogenaemia associated with bleeding
- Massive transfusion if the fibrinogen level is <1.5 g l^{-1}
- DIC if there is bleeding and the fibrinogen level is <1.5 g l^{-1}
- Bleeding associated with renal failure
- Bleeding following thrombolytic therapy. Inhibitors of fibrinolysis (e.g. tranexamic acid) may also be required if the situation is life-threatening, but may result in the formation of large clots at the site of bleeding

Note that a 'standard' dose of cryoprecipitate in an adult may be considered as 10–15 units.

Figure HA6 Indications for the use of cryoprecipitate

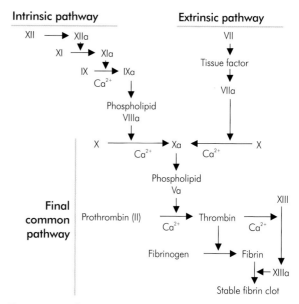

Figure HA7 Classical coagulation cascade

Extrinsic pathway

The extrinsic pathway is so called because to activate coagulation via this pathway a substance (i.e. tissue factor) which is normally present outside the vascular system is required. Tissue factor is a ubiquitous lipoprotein found in particularly high concentrations in placenta, brain and lung. It is also found in monocytes and endothelial cells but is only expressed when these cells are activated, e.g. by endotoxin.

- Oral anticoagulant drug administration
- Liver disease, hepatocellular (decreased production of factors II and VII), obstructive (decreased absorption of vitamin K)
- Vitamin K deficiency
- Disseminated intravascular coagulation
- Hypofibrinogenaemia
- Massive transfusion
- Inherited deficiency of factor VII, X or V
- Heparin

Figure HA8 Causes of a prolonged prothrombin time

Tissue factor is not an enzyme, but a cofactor serving to increase the catalytic activity of factors VII and VIIa in the cleavage of factors X–Xa.

Prothrombin time (PT)

This tests the integrity of the extrinsic pathway. A source of tissue factor (thromboplastin) is added to citrated plasma, calcium chloride is then added to overcome the anticoagulant effect of citrate, and the time taken for a clot to form is measured. Thromboplastin is usually derived from rabbit brain or lung but recently recombinant human thromboplastins have become available. In some laboratories the PT is expressed as an INR (international normalised ratio), which is a device to standardise the PT between laboratories for the purpose of monitoring anticoagulation with coumarins. The INR is the ratio of the PT to mean normal PT, raised to the power of the ISI (international sensitivity index) of the thromboplastin used in the system. Since sensitive thromboplastins (ISI close to 1.0) are usually used in the UK the INR often approximates to the PT ratio. The commonest causes of a prolonged PT are given in Figure HA8.

Intrinsic pathway

The intrinsic pathway was thought to activate blood coagulation by involving only substances present in the plasma. Initiation of coagulation via this pathway requires 'contact activation'. This occurs when prekallikrein (PK) and factors XII and XI are activated in the presence of high molecular weight kininogen (HMWK) on exposure to certain surfaces: in vivo to negatively charged surfaces such as collagen, in vitro to glass or kaolin (Figure HA9). The sequential activation of factors XI and IX then occurs, culminating in the activation of factor X by factor IX with factor VIII as a cofactor.

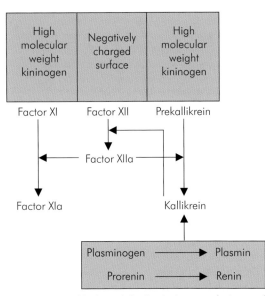

Figure HA9 Initiation of the intrinsic coagulation pathway

Activated partial thromboplastin time (APTT)

This was designed to assess the potential of the intrinsic pathway. It is also known as the PTTK (partial thromboplastin time with kaolin) and the KCCT (kaolin cephalin clotting time). The plasma is pre-incubated with kaolin and phospholipid to activate the contact factors, calcium chloride is then added and the time recorded for a clot to form. The sensitivities of different phospholipid reagents to deficiencies of the clinically important factors (VIII and IX) in the intrinsic pathway vary. APTT is used to monitor heparin therapy; unfortunately, it has not yet been possible to standardise these reagents for the monitoring of heparins in the same way that thromboplastins have been for oral anticoagulant control, making local derivation of therapeutic ranges for heparin necessary. The most frequent causes of a prolonged APTT are shown in Figure HA10.

Final common pathway

The final common pathway sees the conversion of prothrombin to thrombin by factor Xa with factor Va as a cofactor. Thrombin has a central role in coagulation. Critically it cleaves fibrinogen to form fibrin monomers that then spontaneously aggregate to form fibrin strands that are subsequently cross-linked by factor XIIa, resulting in a stable clot. Factor XII is activated by thrombin, as are the cofactors factor V and VIII. Thrombin induces platelet aggregation and, by combining with thrombomodulin,

- Heparin therapy
- Sample contamination by heparin, e.g. by taking sample from a line through which heparin has been administered (including 'Hepflush')
- Liver disease
- Disseminated intravascular coagulation
- Hypofibrinogenaemia
- Massive transfusion
- Coagulation inhibitor, e.g. lupus anticoagulant, acquired factor VIII inhibitor
- Inherited deficiency of factors xl, VIII, IX, x, PK or HMWK

Figure HA10 Causes of a prolonged APTT

- Hypofibrinogenaemia
  - Disseminated intravascular coagulation
  - Fibrinolytic therapy
  - Massive transfusion
  - Inherited deficiency (rare)
- Dysfibrinogenaemia (abnormal fibrinogen molecule)
  - Inherited (rare)
  - Acquired (liver disease most common cause)
- Raised FDP levels – DIC or liver disease
- Heparin

Figure HA11 Causes of a prolonged TT

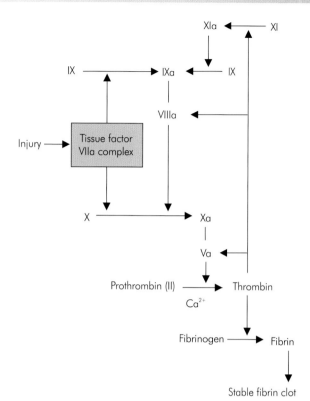

Figure HA12 A revised coagulation hypothesis

activates protein C, an anticoagulant protein, which results in the inactivation of factors V and VIII.

Deficiency of factors X, V, II and fibrinogen causes prolongation of both the PT and the APTT. Hence the function of the final common pathway can be monitored by using both tests. In reality, since isolated deficiency of factors X or V is rare, the commonest reason for prolongation of both tests in a patient not receiving oral anticoagulants is hypofibrinogenaemia.

Thrombin time (TT)

The TT tests the key reaction in the coagulation cascade: the conversion of fibrinogen to fibrin. Conceptually it is the simplest of all the coagulation tests as it consists of simply adding a solution of thrombin to platelet-poor plasma and measuring the time taken for a clot to form; the addition of calcium is not necessary. TT is very sensitive to low levels of heparin, this probably being the most common reason for a prolonged TT; other reasons are shown in

Figure HA11. In many laboratories the TT is not performed as part of a routine coagulation screen, and instead the fibrinogen is measured. This can be done in an assay based loosely on the TT (Clauss method), but increasingly with the introduction of automation into the coagulation laboratory, fibrinogen is estimated during the performance of the PT by optometrical analysis of clot formation.

A revised view of in vivo coagulation (Figure HA12) takes into account the paradoxes offered by the above scheme. For example, while patients severely deficient in factors VIII and IX (haemophiliacs) bleed spontaneously, those with factor XII, PK or HMWK deficiency do not have a bleeding diathesis but do have considerably prolonged APTTs. So it is clear that the classical cascade theory is important as a means of understanding what is occurring in the screening coagulation tests, but comprehension of in vivo coagulation requires alternative explanations.

It is important to realise that coagulation reactions occur on surfaces, e.g. platelets, activated endothelium and subendothelial collagen. When coagulation is initiated thrombin is formed in the absence of activated factors

V and VIII, and trace amounts of thrombin then activate factors V and VIII. These are large molecules that act as cofactors in their respective reactions and localise reactions to surfaces. The overall result is an increase by many thousand-fold in the efficiency of the coagulation mechanism.

It is tissue factor that initiates coagulation in vivo by forming a complex with factor VIIa and then activating factor X (it is not clear how factor VII is activated). However, this complex also activates factor IX, which is a significant departure from the classical hypothesis. The importance of this is only realised upon activation of factors V and VIII: the predominant action of factor VIIa/TF becomes activation of factor IX, and massive amplification of the coagulation mechanism then occurs via two highly efficient reactions, resulting in thrombin formation. Factor VIIa/TF complex is quickly inhibited by tissue factor pathway inhibitor, so factor Xa generation must occur via factor VIIIa/IXa. This is augmented by factor XIa, which is activated by thrombin, this being a late step in the pathway. The critical roles of factors XIa and VIIIa in this scheme are demonstrated by the severity of the bleeding when these factors are deficient. Contact activation has no place in coagulation in vivo.

Natural inhibitors of coagulation

The cascade structure of the coagulation system ensures very rapid activation of coagulation, for example, it has been estimated that 10 ml plasma can generate sufficient thrombin to clot all the body's fibrinogen in 30 s; clearly this may be deleterious, so equally powerful inhibitors of coagulation in the plasma ensure that the haemostatic response is confined to the vicinity of the platelet plug and vascular injury. Tissue factor pathway inhibitor has already been mentioned, but there are two other broad groups of coagulation inhibitors: serine protease inhibitors, the most important of which is anti-thrombin (previously called anti-thrombin III), and the coagulation co-factor (VIIIa and Va) inhibitors which are proteins C and S.

Antithrombin

Antithrombin complexes with the serine protease coagulation factors (thrombin, Xa, XIIa, XIa, and IXa but not VIIa) and inactivates them. The resulting inhibitor–protease complex is rapidly removed by the liver. The affinity for thrombin is highest, followed by factor Xa. Heparin binds to antithrombin and induces a 2300-fold increase

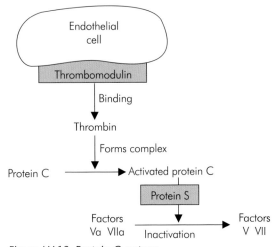

Figure HA13 Protein C system

in thrombin inactivation. Endothelial glycosaminoglycans act in a similar fashion. Reduction in plasma antithrombin levels results in a tendency to venous thrombosis.

Other serine protease inhibitors include heparin cofactor II, α_1-antitrypsin, C_1 esterase inhibitor, α_2-antiplasmin and α_2-macroglobulin. Deficiency of these inhibitors has not been clearly associated with thrombosis.

Protein C system

The protein C system is responsible for the inactivation of the activated cofactors Va and VIIIa. Protein C and S are vitamin K-dependent factors. The system is represented in Figure HA13.

Thrombin behaves as an anticoagulant when it binds to thrombomodulin, which is present on the endothelial surface. The resulting complex activates protein C, which in the presence of protein S inactivates factors Va and VIIIa by cleavage. Thus thrombosis is prevented from propagating along normal vessels close to a point of injury.

Reduced plasma levels of protein C and S are associated with thrombosis and can be inherited in an autosomal dominant fashion. Deficiency of thrombomodulin has not been described, and probably results in non-viability. The most common inherited cause of a thrombotic tendency is a mutation of factor V (factor V Leiden) which alters the activated protein C (APC) cleavage site. This results in reduced APC-induced cleavage and is demonstrated in vitro by the APC resistance (APCR) test. This is an autosomal dominant trait.

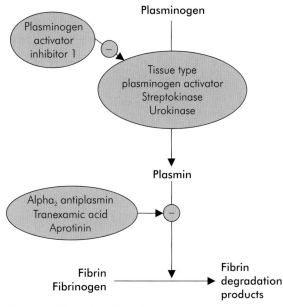

Figure HA14 Fibrinolytic system

- Coagulation factors – V, X, protein S
- Adhesive proteins – von Willebrand's factor, fibrinogen, fibronectin, vitronectin
- Growth factors
  ○ platelet-derived growth factor (PDGF)
  ○ platelet factor 4 (PF4)
  ○ β-thromboglobulin

Figure HA15 Contents of platelet alpha granules

a volume of 5–8 fl (fl is the abbreviation for the SI unit femtolitre, l^{-15}: see Section 4, Chapter 1, Figure PH21). The normal life span of a platelet is between 8 and 14 days. They contain granules of which the most numerous are α granules (the contents of which are listed in Figure HA15). Dense bodies are less numerous but are of importance as their deficiency (storage pool disease) can result in significant haemorrhage. Dense bodies contain platelet nucleotides (ADP, ATP, 5-HT).

Platelets function by adhesion to sites of injury. They change shape and release their granules and then aggregate together to form the platelet plug. They also provide the surfaces that enhance the coagulation reaction, and growth factors contained in the α granules stimulate tissue repair. Global platelet function can be tested by measuring the bleeding time, which is best performed by experienced laboratory staff using the template method (normal <9 min). It should be remembered that thrombocytopenia results in prolongation of the bleeding time. Qualitative platelet defects can be assessed by platelet aggregometry to various stimuli.

Fibrinolysis

A scheme for the fibrinolytic system is shown in Figure HA14. Intrinsic activation of fibrinolysis, via kallikrein, is possible but the physiological relevance is uncertain. Tissue-type plasminogen activators (t-PA) are of greatest importance. t-PA is synthesised by endothelial cells; its release is stimulated by venous occlusion, thrombin, epinephrine, vasopressin and strenuous exercise. Its biological activity increases dramatically when bound to fibrin.

In vivo activity of the fibrinolytic system is routinely assessed in clinical situations by measuring fibrin degradation products (FDPs), which usually include the products of fibrinogen degradation and therefore do not rely on the presence of fibrin. D-dimers, on the other hand, are only produced by digestion of cross-linked fibrin and are therefore a more specific indicator of fibrinolysis which has been exploited recently in the assessment of suspected pulmonary embolism.

Platelets

Platelets are responsible for forming the primary haemostatic plug following injury. They are produced in the bone marrow by the cytoplasmic budding of megakaryocytes. They are biconvex discs with a diameter of 2–4 μm and

Platelet adhesion

Blood vessel injury results in exposure of subendothelial collagen and microfibrils. Larger von Willebrand's factor (vWF) molecules bind to the microfibrils and platelets adhere to the vWF via platelet glycoprotein 1b. Following this, the glycoprotein IIb–IIIa complex becomes exposed, which increases adhesion (and is also involved in aggregation).

Platelet shape change

This occurs within seconds of adhesion. The platelet becomes more spherical and spiky, which enhances interaction between platelets. The platelet granules migrate towards the surface.

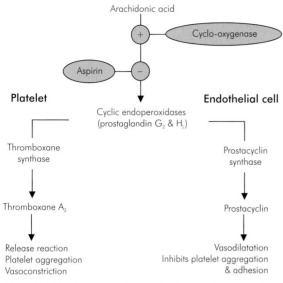

Figure HA16 Prostaglandin metabolism in platelet and endothelial cell

Platelet release reaction

This follows immediately and involves the release of the contents of platelet granules. It is sustained for several minutes. Thus coagulation factors, adhesive proteins, growth factors and nucleotides are delivered to the site of injury.

Platelet aggregation

At the site of injury ADP is released from damaged cells and, following platelet release reaction, this binds to platelets and exposes the GP IIb–IIIa complex. Fibrinogen binds to this receptor, and as it is a dimeric molecule is capable of forming bridges between platelets. The other main physiological inducer of platelet aggregation is thromboxane A_2, which is a product of arachidonic acid metabolism in the platelet.

Prostaglandin metabolism in platelets

This is a critical part of platelet activation, because blocking it (with aspirin) prevents the release reaction. Arachidonic acid is released from membrane phospholipid by phospholipase A_2. Prostaglandin metabolism in the platelet and endothelial cell is shown in Figure HA16.

von Willebrand's factor

von Willebrand's factor consists of large molecules (multimers) made up of a variable number of subunits. It is produced in endothelial cells and megakaryocytes, then stored in Weibel–Palade bodies of endothelial cells and α granules of platelets. The main function of vWF is in platelet adhesion; however, it also acts as a carrier of factor VIII. vWF deficiency results in the most common inherited bleeding tendency – von Willebrand's disease, which is estimated to occur in up to 1% of the population. It is most commonly a mild quantitative (type 1) deficiency, but type 2 (qualitative) and type 3 (severe quantitative) also occur. Deficiency of vWF produces two haemostatic defects – a prolonged bleeding time due to failure of platelet adhesion and a coagulation defect due to reduced levels of factor VIII.

The immune system

Mononuclear phagocyte system

Previously referred to as the reticuloendothelial system when endothelial cells, fibroblasts and granulocytes were included, the mononuclear phagocyte system is composed of cells derived from the bone marrow.

It has been demonstrated that the cells of the mononuclear phagocyte system can be generated from bone marrow stem cells or from peripheral blood monocytes. The two main types of cells are:

- Professional phagocytes
- Antigen-presenting cells (APCs)

Figure HA17 lists the cells of the mononuclear phagocyte system.

Phagocytic function

Human monocyte/macrophages have specific receptors on their surface that allow them to bind to microorganisms. These include the mannosyl–fucosyl receptors (MFRs) which bind to microbial saccharides and a lipopolysaccharide binding protein (LBP) which binds gram-negative bacteria. Once bound, the microbes are ingested to form a phagosome. Lysosomes then merge with the phagosome, and the micro-organism is killed and digested. The lysosome contents include proteolytic enzymes, peroxidase, elastase and collagenase. The exact enzymes present vary according to the type of macrophage, e.g. peritoneal macrophages are peroxidase-negative. The presence of complement receptors on macrophages and neutrophils improves phagocytic efficiency if micro-organisms are opsonised (coated) with complement. Fcγ receptors are present on the surface of monocyte/macrophages and bind the Fc portion of IgG, which also serves as an opsonin. There are three types of receptor: FcγRI, FcγRII and FcγRIII, which have high,

- Professional phagocytes
  - Circulating monocytes
  - Kupffer cells (liver)
  - Mesangial macrophage (kidney)
  - Alveolar macrophage (lung)
  - Serosal macrophage (pleura, peritoneum)
  - Splenic sinus macrophage
  - Lymph node sinus macrophage

- Antigen-presenting cells
  - Langerhans cells (skin)
  - Interdigitating cells (lymph node)
  - Follicular dendritic cells (lymph node, thymus)
  - Macrophages

Figure HA17 Cells of the mononuclear phagocyte system

intermediate and low affinity for the Fc portion of IgG and probably have different functions, e.g. triggering extracellular killing, opsonisation and phagocytosis. Phagocytosis also occurs by receptor-independent mechanisms.

Antigen presentation

Macrophages are capable of presenting antigen to T lymphocytes but there are also other specialised cells for this purpose. Foreign protein is digested into small peptides that are processed and expressed on the cell surface in conjunction with HLA class II molecules, which are found only on antigen-presenting cells (APCs) and B lymphocytes. The specialist APCs have many fine, long projections (dendrites) which maximise the surface area over which interaction with T cells can occur. They are found in the T-cell-rich areas of lymphoid tissue. Other cell types, when stimulated, can function as antigen-presenting cells, and these include endothelial and epithelial cells. Here antigen is presented in association with major histocompatibility (MHC) molecules, which are present on the surface of all nucleated cells.

Interaction between antigen-presenting cells and T lymphocytes

Linear peptide fragments bind to the peptide groove of MHC molecules in the rough endoplasmic reticulum of antigen-presenting cells and then these molecules are expressed on the cell surface. Only a minority of peptide fragments from a protein antigen (from any source) are capable of being processed in this way.

The antigen is 'recognised' by specific T helper cells (TH). The T-cell receptor (TCR) binds to the antigen–MHC molecule complex. Further molecular interactions

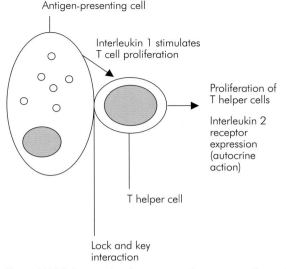

Figure HA18 Interaction between antigen-presenting cell and T helper cell

occur once the cells are brought into close proximity by this interaction (Figure HA18). The result is an exchange of cytokines including interleukin 1 (IL-1), produced by macrophages, which stimulates TH proliferation and expression of interleukin 2 (IL-2) receptors on TH cells. Activation of T cells also results in the production of interferon γ, which stimulates the expression of MHC molecules on macrophages, producing positive feedback.

These processes are the first events following challenge by a new antigen, and the development of an effective immune response depends on the production, by proliferation, of adequate numbers of TH cells. An immune response follows, and this can be antibody-mediated (a B-lymphocyte function) or cell-mediated (a T-cell and macrophage function).

Antibody-mediated response

Antigen binds to the surface immunoglobulin of specific B lymphocytes. It is processed and expressed in association with MHC molecules. The B cell is now capable of interacting with specific TH cells, which will have been activated by interaction with APCs. This B–T interaction results in delivery of stimulatory cytokines by the TH cells, and the result is the proliferation and then differentiation of B cells to produce plasma cells and then antibody (Figure HA19). B cells can also be activated by interacting with antigen

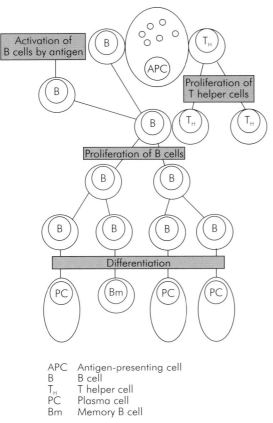

APC	Antigen-presenting cell
B	B cell
T$_H$	T helper cell
PC	Plasma cell
Bm	Memory B cell

Figure HA19 B-cell activation and interaction with T cells

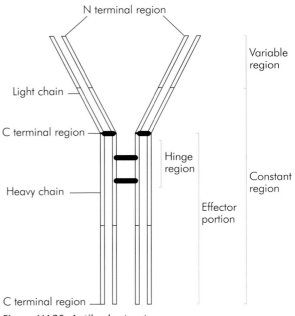

Figure HA20 Antibody structure

presented by APCs, with subsequent proliferation and differentiation signals coming from T$_H$ cells. A proportion of B cells, rather than differentiating to form plasma cells, enter a resting phase to become memory B cells (B$_M$). Similarly a subpopulation of the stimulated T$_H$ population will become memory T$_H$ cells.

Antibody structure, subtypes and diversity

Immunoglobulins are composed of four peptide chains – two heavy chains (IgH) and two light chains (Figure HA20). There are five structural heavy chain variants to produce IgG, IgM, IgA, IgD and IgE. IgM is pentameric and IgA dimeric. There are two structural light chain variants – κ and λ. Most of the molecule consists of framework on which the highly variable antigen binding site is located. Diversity of antigen binding sites is achieved by immunoglobulin gene rearrangement at the DNA level

where a variable gene (V, one of several hundred), joining gene (J, one of six) and diversity gene (D, one of 30) are combined to produce a unique gene in each developing B cell, which then produces the unique antigen binding site. More refinement is achieved with point mutation of the VDJ recombination, and this may occur during B-cell activation and proliferation. Subsequently the best antigen–antibody matches selectively proliferate, enhancing the overall response. The relatively frequent occurrence of recombinational inaccuracy of the VDJ adds a further mechanism of diversity generation.

Primary and secondary antibody responses

Following an initial antigen challenge there is a lag phase where no antibody is detectable. Then there is a logarithmic increase in antibody levels to a plateau, and there follows a decline to low or undetectable levels. Such a primary response consists predominantly of IgM, with IgG present but appearing slightly later. If the individual is challenged again, then there is a shorter lag phase before antibody is detected, the rise in antibody titre is up to 10 times greater than in the primary response, the plateau is more prolonged and the decline is slow. The secondary response consists almost entirely of IgG and the affinity of the antibodies is greater, a process called antibody maturation.

A typical example of primary and secondary antibody responses occurs with a delayed haemolytic transfusion reaction. Initial exposure to the foreign red cell antigen results in no clinical effects, but low-level antibody is produced and subsequently declines. Antibody screening after the decline may miss a low-level antibody, but should the individual be exposed to the antigen again, a brisk secondary response occurs which results in the destruction of the antibody-coated transfused red cells by the mononuclear phagocyte system. Clinically this is apparent after 4–14 days when the patient presents with anaemia, fever and jaundice.

Cell-mediated immunity
T-cell-independent mechanisms
The two T-cell-independent mechanisms are phagocytosis and cytokine release.

- Phagocytosis – macrophages and granulocytes are capable of migrating to sites of infection stimulated by chemotactic components released by micro-organisms. They can then bind, engulf and kill pathogens, utilising oxidant free radicals and peroxides.
- Cytokine release – cytokines are peptide or glycopeptide mediators released from stimulated cells. Examples include the interleukins (lymphokines), interferons, colony stimulating factors (CSFs) and tumour necrosis factor (TNF). Macrophages release TNF in response to micro-organisms and are an important part of the inflammatory response (below). TNF also enhances granulocyte and macrophage microbicidal capacity.

T-cell-dependent mechanisms
Cytotoxic T cells (Tc)
A subpopulation of peripheral blood lymphocytes forms cytotoxic T cells (Tc). These recognise antigen when presented in association with the relevant MHC molecules. It is thought that Tc cells are important in recognising and destroying virus-infected cells.

The antigen associated with an MHC molecule is recognised by the T-cell receptor (TCR) in the same way that Th cells recognise antigen presented by APCs. The TCR is analogous to the immunoglobulin molecule expressed on the surface of B cells in that diversity is generated by similar mechanisms.

Other cytotoxic cells
- Natural killer cells (NK cells) do not have rearranged TCR genes. It is thought that they recognise tumour-associated antigens. They also have Fc receptors on their surface and can destroy antibody-coated cells.
- Lymphokine-activated killer cells (LAK cells) are formed by the culture of peripheral lymphocytes in IL-2. Enhanced tumour killing results. It is thought that LAK cells are activated NK cells.
- Antibody-dependent cell-mediated cytotoxicity (ADCC) requires effector cells to have an Fc receptor. Antibody-coated cells are thus recognised and destroyed. Cells capable of such killing are Tc cells, NK cells, mononuclear phagocytes and granulocytes.

The role of Th cells in cell-mediated immunity is very important, as Th cells provide cytokines necessary for activation and proliferation.

The inflammatory response
The clinical signs of inflammation are heat, redness, swelling, pain, and reduced function. Inflammation is a response to injury or invasion by pathogens. Three fundamental events are involved:

- Hyperaemia – there is an increase in blood supply to the affected area. This is a result of arteriolar relaxation.
- Exudation – there is an increase in capillary permeability resulting from retraction of endothelial cells. Larger molecules are allowed to pass across the endothelium, and thus plasma enzyme systems reach the site of inflammation.
- Emigration of leucocytes – initially phagocytes and then lymphocytes migrate between endothelial cells into the surrounding tissues along chemotactic gradients.

Pathologically inflammation is diagnosed when there are increased numbers of granulocytes, macrophages and lymphocytes in a tissue section.

Mediators of inflammation
The kinin system
The products of this system mediate the immediate vasoactive response (Figure HA21).

Histamine and leukotrienes (B_4 and D_4)
These are released by basophils and their tissue equivalent, mast cells, after stimulation by microbes, and result in increased vascular permeability. Leukotrienes together with neutrophil chemotactic factor (also produced by mast cells) stimulate the migration of granulocytes to sites of

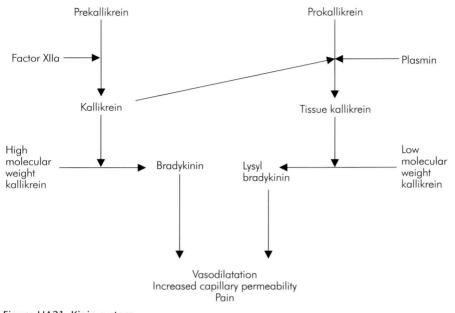

Figure HA21 Kinin system

invasion or injury. Leukotrienes are products of arachidonic acid metabolism via the lipoxygenase pathway.

Neutrophil adhesion and migration across the endothelium

Under normal, steady-state conditions, while leucocytes flow in close proximity to the endothelium they do not adhere to it. At sites of inflammation, endothelial cells become activated by mediators such as TNF-α, and one of the effects of this is adhesion molecule synthesis and expression on the surface of endothelial cells. One of the first to be expressed is E-selectin (4–12 hours); later intercellular adhesion molecule 1 (ICAM-1) is produced.

Neutrophils, upon stimulation by inflammatory mediators, express preformed adhesion molecules such as LFA-1 and CR3. The result is neutrophil adhesion. The neutrophil then, attracted by chemotactic agents, migrates between endothelial cells and along the subendothelial matrix of collagen, laminin, etc., using different adhesion molecules, to sites of injury. Lymphocytes and macrophages migrate in a similar way, but later than neutrophils.

Once present at the site of injury, neutrophils release mediators including platelet activating factor (PAF), which stimulates mediator release from platelets and increases vascular permeability and smooth muscle contraction. PAF also activates other neutrophils. Macrophages and monocytes also migrate along the same chemotactic gradients and engulf microbes, as well as presenting antigens to T and B lymphocytes as described above. Mononuclear cells and lymphocytes release cytokines.

Tumour necrosis factor

TNF is a mediator of inflammation released by macrophages and lymphocytes in the presence of bacterial pathogens. It activates endothelial cells and enhances phagocytic function. Activated endothelium becomes procoagulant, adhesive, more permeable and produces increased nitric oxide, resulting in smooth muscle relaxation and vasodilatation. TNF and nitric oxide are important mediators of septic shock.

Complement

Complement components C3a and C5a are inflammatory mediators, and their production is described below. Both stimulate mast cell de-granulation and smooth muscle contraction. C5a also increases capillary permeability, activates neutrophils and stimulates phagocyte chemotaxis.

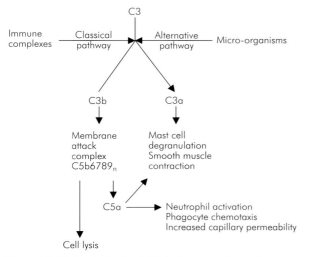

Figure HA22 Central role of C3 in the complement pathway

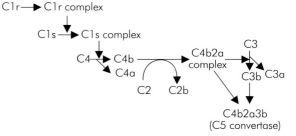

Figure HA23 Classical complement pathway

Classical pathway

The classical complement pathway (Figure HA23) forms part of the specific immune response. C1q can bind to the Fc regions of aggregates of IgG1 or IgG3 molecules bound to antigen (immune complexes). C1q also attaches to single antigen-bound IgM molecules, which are by nature pentameric. C1r and C1s are also components of the C1 complex. Binding of C1q leads to conformation change in the C1 complex resulting in auto-activation of C1r, which in turn activates C1s. The next step is activation of C4 with the production of C4b, which avidly binds surface carbohydrates or proteins: thus complement activation is localised to a surface. As with the coagulation cascade, the large number of steps ensures amplification and offers opportunity for regulation. The C4b2a complex catalyses the central step, the cleavage of C3.

Inhibitors of the classical pathway help ensure localisation of complement activation. C1 inhibitor in the serum inactivates C1r and C1s. Complement control proteins (such as decay accelerating factor) are present on the surface of cells and interfere with the C4b–C2 interaction, preventing complement activation and damage to nearby normal cells.

Alternative pathway

The alternative pathway (Figure HA24) is a non-specific immune function and relies on continual low-level complement activation. This is achieved by hydrolysis of C3 to form C3i, which in the presence of magnesium is able to associate with Factor B. The C3iB complex is then itself cleaved by Factor D to form C3iBb and Ba. C3iBb is able to act as a C3 convertase (i.e. catalyses C3 $\leftrightarrow$ C3b + C3a). The above reactions occur in the fluid phase but C3b attaches itself to any adjacent surface. Autologous cells can inactivate C3b. The surfaces of micro-organisms, however, stabilise C3b and facilitate C3 binding to factor B and,

Other plasma enzyme systems are also involved in inflammation, namely the coagulation cascade and the fibrinolytic system. FDPs are capable of increasing vascular permeability and stimulating neutrophil and macrophage chemotaxis.

The complement cascade

'Complement', coined by Ehrlich, refers to the activity in serum which when combined with antibody results in the lysis of bacteria. It has since been realised that complement performs three major functions:

- Opsonisation (coating) of bacteria and immune complexes
- Activation and attraction (chemotaxis) of phagocytes
- Lysis of target cells

There are many proteins involved in the complement system, and a detailed account of all of these is not appropriate here. An outline of complement activation is given in the classical and alternative pathways below. The central event of the complement pathway is the cleavage of C3 to form C3b and C3a (Figure HA22). C3b attaches to micro-organisms or immune complexes and acts as a site of membrane attack complex formation. It also acts as an opsonin. The small peptide cleaved from C3, C3a, stimulates mast cell degranulation and smooth muscle contraction.

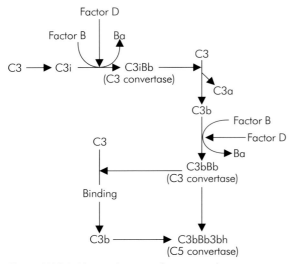

Figure HA24 Alternative complement pathway

as above, factor D cleaves the resulting complex to form C3bBb and Ba. C3bBb is a C3 convertase and also combines to C3b to act as a C5 convertase, which initiates membrane attack complex formation. Here again is a system in which a large number of reaction steps occurring on a surface produces considerable amplification. Bacteria with surface-bound C3b, C3i or C4b (which implies immunoglobulin binding also) are said to be opsonised, and are readily phagocytosed by neutrophils or macrophages. This is initiated by binding to complement receptors on the phagocyte's surface. Otherwise lysis may occur, as outlined below.

Formation of the membrane attack complex

This is the final common pathway of complement activation. The first step is cleavage of C5 to C5a (a mediator of inflammation) and C5b. C5b can then aggregate with C6 and C7 to produce C5b67 which, being hydrophobic, attaches to plasma membranes. C8 then binds to a site on C5b and penetrates the membrane. The resulting C5b678 complex polymerises a number of C9 molecules to form the membrane attack complex (C5b6789n), which is essentially a pore in the cell membrane; lysis is thus produced.

Once the C5b67 complex is formed it can attach to any nearby membrane and produce lysis – this is sometimes called 'the innocent bystander' effect. This is prevented in the fluid phase by proteins such as vitronectin

inactivating this complex. On cell membranes a protein (MIRL = membrane inhibitor of reactive lysis) performs a similar function against membrane attack complex.

Hypersensitivity

Hypersensitivity occurs when an otherwise beneficial immune response is inappropriate or exaggerated, resulting in tissue damage. It occurs on re-exposure to the antigen concerned, and the damage may be due to one or more of four mechanisms – referred to as type I, II, III and IV hypersensitivity.

Type I

Type I hypersensitivity, also referred to as immediate hypersensitivity, is an IgE-mediated response. IgE is synthesised by specific B cells, with APC and Th cells critically involved as described above. IgE is released and binds to tissue mast cells via their Fc receptors. If the antigen is subsequently encountered it binds to the mast-cell-bound IgE, and this stimulates mast cell degranulation and release of preformed mediators (Figure HA25). The clinical effects depend on the site where the antigen is encountered. In the skin eczema or urticaria will result; if the antigen is inhaled asthma occurs; in the nasal passages allergic rhinitis (hay fever) develops.

In severe cases the reaction can be generalised, producing anaphylactic shock. The mechanism is the same but there is widespread mediator release. This occurs most commonly on exposure to certain drugs or foods (e.g. penicillin, peanuts) in response to insect stings (e.g. bee and wasp) and on exposure to blood components (e.g. plasma in an IgA-deficient individual). This response should be distinguished from the anaphylactoid reaction that can be induced by certain drugs (e.g. codeine and morphine) which act on mast cells directly and not via IgE.

Type II

This occurs when IgG and/or IgM molecules interact with complement to produce target cell damage. An example of this is Goodpasture's syndrome, where an anti-basement membrane immunoglobulin is produced. This together with complement is deposited on the glomerular and pulmonary basement membranes, and neutrophils attach via their Fc and complement receptors. As they are unable to phagocytose, they discharge their lysosomal contents, which results in damage to the basement membrane. The

Mediator	Action
Histamine	Vasodilatation
	Increases vascular permeability, smooth muscle contraction
Platelet activating factor (PAF)	Platelet degranulation and aggregation leading to microthrombi formation & neutrophil chemotaxis
Tryptase	Protease acting to cleave C3 to C3a and C3b
Kininogenase	Activates kinin system
Cytokines, e.g. IL-5, TNF-α, IL-8	Granulocyte chemotaxis including eosinophils & basophils
Leukotriene B$_4$	Basophil chemotaxis
Leukotriene C$_4$ & D$_4$	Smooth muscle contraction
	Mucosal oedema
	Increased mucus secretion

Figure HA25 Mediators released by tissue mast cells and their actions

clinical effects are renal failure and pulmonary haemorrhage. Autoimmune haemolytic anaemia and myasthenia gravis are further examples of type II hypersensitivity reactions.

Type III
This is a result of the production of large quantities of immune complex that cannot be adequately cleared by the mononuclear phagocyte system. There is often widespread deposition of these immune complexes that activate complement via the classical pathway. There are numerous diseases that are immune-complex-related (Figure HA26), and their clinical features reflect the sites of deposition.

Type IV
Type IV hypersensitivity reactions are produced by cell-mediated mechanisms and generally take >12 hours to develop. Previously called delayed hypersensitivity, three types are described:
- Contact hypersensitivity, which is a cutaneous reaction, maximal at 48–72 hours. Most commonly

- Infections
  ○ Bacterial endocarditis
  ○ Hepatitis B
  ○ Dengue fever
- Autoimmune diseases
  ○ Rheumatoid arthritis
  ○ SLE
  ○ Polyarteritis nodosa and microscopic polyarteritis
  ○ Polymyositis
  ○ Cutaneous vasculitis
  ○ Fibrosing alveolitis
  ○ Cryoglobulinaemia

Figure HA26 Examples of immune-complex-related diseases

this is in response to a hapten, which is a molecule too small to induce an immune response. Instead, it combines with normal proteins to produce a neo-antigen. Examples include metals such as nickel and chromate. Antigen is presented to Langerhans cells, which interact with sensitised TH cells, and these then release cytokines, activating keratinocytes that release further cytokines to produce the eczematous lesions.
- Tuberculin-type hypersensitivity, which is maximal at 48–72 hours, is the reaction that occurs after intradermal injection of tuberculin. The antigen-presenting cells are thought to be predominantly macrophages. The cells responsible for the reaction are TH and TC cells, macrophages and monocytes. Granuloma formation may follow due to persistence of antigen.
- Granulomatous hypersensitivity is most important clinically because it is responsible for diseases such as tuberculosis, leprosy, schistosomiasis, leishmaniasis and sarcoidosis. Again, TH cells are critical in the production of these reactions, which result from a continuous antigen stimulus or where macrophages are unable to destroy the antigen. The result is granuloma formation in the presence of antigen.

References and further reading
British Committee for Standards in Haematology. Guidelines for the use of platelet transfusions. *Br J Haematol* 2003; **122**: 10–23.

British Committee for Standards in Haematology. Guidelines for the use of fresh-frozen plasma, cryoprecipitate and cryosupernatant. *Br J Haematol* 2004; **126**: 11–28.

Goodnight SC, Hathaway WE. *Disorders of Hemostasis and Thrombosis: a Clinical Guide*, 2nd edn. New York, NY: McGraw-Hill, 2001.

Greer JP, Foerster J, Lukens JN, *et al.* (eds.). *Wintrobe's Clinical Hematology*, 11th edn. Philadelphia: Lippincott Williams & Wilkins, 2003.

Hoffbrand AV, Catovsky D, Tuddenham EGD (eds.). *Postgraduate Haematology*, 5th edn. Oxford: Blackwell, 2005.

Klein HG, Anstee DJ. *Mollison's Blood Transfusion in Clinical Medicine*, 11th edn. Oxford: Blackwell, 2005.

McClelland B (ed.). *Handbook of Transfusion Medicine*, 4th edn. London: HMSO, 2007.

Roitt I, Brostoff J, Male D (eds.). *Immunology*, 6th edn. Edinburgh: Mosby, 2001.

CHAPTER 4

Muscle physiology

I. T. Campbell and D. Liu

Skeletal muscle

Skeletal muscle fibres are attached to bone by tendons of strong connective tissue. The proximal attachment is known as the 'origin' and the distal attachment is the 'insertion', the two being connected by the muscle 'belly'. The precise shape and distribution of a muscle, or muscle group, about a joint depends on its particular function. In summary, the functions of skeletal muscle are to provide:

- A mechanical response to environmental stimuli
- A short-term store of glycogen and glucose
- A long-term metabolic reserve of protein for gluconeogenesis

Microscopic structure
Muscle cell

Muscle cells or fibres are quite large: they are typically about 100 μm in diameter, and may run the full length of the muscle. They are multinucleated, are surrounded by a membrane, the endomysium, and are bound into fasciculi. These fasciculi are surrounded by the perimysium, and combine to make up the whole muscle. This, in turn, is covered by connective tissue sheet, the epimysium (Figure MP1).

Myofibril

The muscle cells or fibres are made up of myofibrils enclosed by the cell membrane (sarcolemma). The myofibrils consist of two types of myofilaments. There are thick filaments composed of myosin and thin filaments that are made up of actin.

Sarcomere

The myofibril is made up of basic contractile units called sarcomeres. The microscopic appearance of the sarcomere identifies various regions, which are known by letters (Figure MP2).

The sarcomere is composed principally of myosin filaments and actin filaments. The myosin filaments occupy the central part of the sarcomere and comprise the A band. The A band is transected by the M line, which keeps the myosin filaments in side-by-side alignment. The myosin filaments interdigitate with the thin actin filaments whose ends are joined to the Z line or disc which maintains their spatial arrangement. The area of myosin filaments in the middle of the sarcomere not overlapped by actin filaments is known as the H zone. A cross section of the sarcomere in areas where the two types of filament overlap shows that the two types of filament are arranged in a hexagonal pattern (Figure MP3). The myoplasm between the filaments contains glycogen, myoglobin, the enzymes involved in glycolysis and mitochondria.

Myofilaments
Thin myofilament

The thin actin filament is a helical structure composed of two chains of actin molecules wound around each other. It is about 5.5 nm in diameter, and the two chains are structured so that they make a half turn of the helix every 35–37 nm. A long, thin fibrous protein, tropomyosin, lies between the two strands of actin. Associated with the tropomyosin at each half turn of the actin/tropomyosin

Fundamentals of Anaesthesia, 3rd edition, ed. Tim Smith, Colin Pinnock and Ted Lin. Published by Cambridge University Press. © Cambridge University Press 2008.

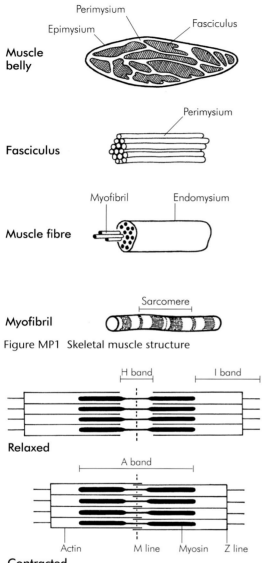

Figure MP1 Skeletal muscle structure

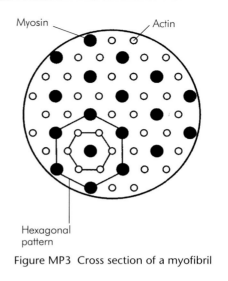

Figure MP3 Cross section of a myofibril

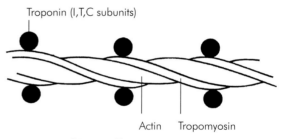

Figure MP4 Thin myofilament

Figure MP2 Structure of sarcomere

strand is a protein complex called troponin consisting of three subunits: troponin I, troponin T and troponin C (Figure MP4).

Thick myofilament

The thick myosin filament is made up of myosin molecules that consist of two parts, a rod-shaped 'tail' section and a head portion consisting of two globular heads with ATP

and actin binding sites. Associated with each of the heads are two protein molecules called myosin 'light' chains because of their low molecular weight. They have a regulatory function in muscle contraction.

The myosin filaments are packed together with the tail regions making up the structure of the thick filament (Figure MP5). The heads project from the side of the myosin filament in a helical fashion, with one turn of the helix every six molecules, so that the heads project at 60° to each other and at a distance from each other of 14.3 nm. Each myosin filament is constructed of two groups of myosin molecules with their tails abutting. There is thus an area bare of myosin heads, or cross-bridge-free region that constitutes the midpoint of the H zone. The heads are thus at opposite ends of the halves of the myosin filament. The assembled filaments are all held in place by the Z discs, the M line and associated accessory proteins, nebulin and titin.

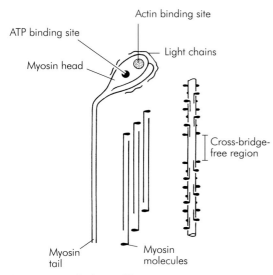

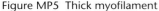

Figure MP5 Thick myofilament

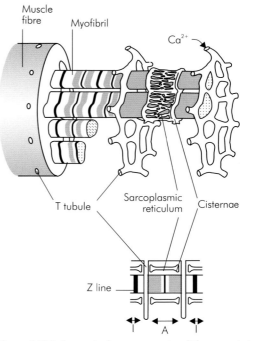

Figure MP6 Separated components of the sarcotubular system

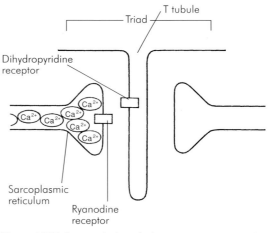

Figure MP7 Sarcotubular triad

Sarcotubular system

The sarcoplasmic reticulum is a network of intracellular membranes and tubules which extends throughout the muscle cell, wrapping itself around the myofibrils. It encloses a space containing calcium ions (Ca^{2+}), which play a key role in the contractile mechanism of muscle. The sarcoplasmic reticulum has enlarged terminal sacs or 'cisternae' which lie close to the T tubules at the A–I junction (Figure MP6). The bulk of the contained Ca^{2+} accumulates within these sacs. The T tubules are essentially a continuation of the extracellular space and conduct the wave of depolarisation along the sarcolemma into the depths of the cell. The combination of a T tubule and two adjoining terminal cisternae on either side is termed a triad (Figure MP7).

Muscle contraction

Muscle contracts by movement of the actin and myosin filaments past each other. The A band (composed of myosin filaments) remains the same size, but the Z lines move inwards and the width of the H zone and the I bands diminish. The distance between the two groups of actin filaments diminishes, and at maximum contraction they overlap.

Myosin–actin interaction

Contraction of a sarcomere is caused by interaction between the myosin and actin filaments. This is a cyclical sequence of events repeatedly triggered by stimulated release of calcium ions. The reaction producing the movement between the filaments occurs between the myosin heads and the actin filaments, and can be referred to as the 'power stroke' (Figure MP8).

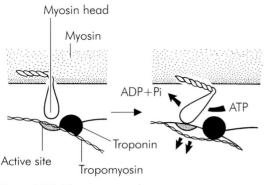

Figure MP8 The power stroke

Myosin–actin power stroke

In the power stroke the myosin heads attach to the actin at 90° and subsequently bend to 45°, producing relative movement between the filaments. The myosin then detaches from the actin and the process starts again. Each power stroke shortens the muscle by about 1%: the thick filaments each have about 500 myosin heads and during a rapid contraction these move at 5/s. This whole process uses energy in the form of ATP and requires the presence of the calcium contained by the sarcoplasmic reticulum. When a myofibril is stimulated Ca^{2+} is released into the myoplasm from the sarcoplasmic reticulum, principally from the terminal cisternae. This binds to the C unit of the troponin regulating complex, which is attached to the tropomyosin. This causes a conformational change in the other subunits of troponin (I and T), which in turn results in movement of the tropomyosin strand within the groove of the actin molecule, revealing active sites on the actin filament to which myosin can attach. When this happens, the power stroke of the myosin head is initiated and the two filaments move past each other.

Myosin–actin contraction cycle

The myosin–actin cycle involves the consumption of energy provided by ATP. In resting muscle a molecule of ATP, split into ADP and inorganic phosphate (Pi), is bound to each myosin head. The cycle of events making up the myosin–actin interaction cycle can be considered in the following stages, the numbers of which refer to Figure MP9:

- Stage 1 – at the completion of the power stroke myosin is still attached to actin. ATP then binds to myosin, causing its release from actin and also release of Ca^{2+}.

- Stage 2 – ATP is hydrolysed, energising myosin, but ADP and Pi remain bound to myosin.
- Stage 3 – in presence of Ca^{2+} and actin, reattachment of the energised myosin head occurs.
- Stage 4 – power stroke occurs as ADP and Pi are released.

Muscle contraction is initiated by the release of calcium ions from the sarcoplasmic reticulum into the myoplasm resulting from depolarisation of the sarcolemma (initiated by the motor nerve) at the motor endplate. The process is termed 'excitation–contraction coupling', and for a nerve stimulus to ensure an adequate release of calcium throughout the whole length and depth of a fibre the process has to be efficient.

Membrane depolarisation is initiated at a motor endplate, and a wave of depolarisation spreads along the sarcolemma in the same way as it does in a peripheral nerve. It is carried into the depths of the fibre by a system of invaginations of sarcolemma found in association with the junction of the A and I bands of the myofibril.

Excitation–contraction coupling

Resting Ca^{2+} concentration in the myoplasm is between 10^{-7} and 10^{-8} mol per litre. The resting state is maintained by the storage of Ca^{2+} in the sarcoplasmic reticulum, where it binds to a specific calcium-binding protein called calsequestrin. Calcium ions are released when the sarcolemma is depolarised and the wave of depolarisation spreads into the depths of the cell via the T tubules. A calcium release channel in the sarcoplasmic reticulum opens and Ca^{2+} passes from the sarcoplasmic reticulum into the myoplasm; myoplasmic Ca^{2+} concentrations increase to 10^{-5} mol l^{-1}. The calcium binding sites on troponin C are occupied and muscle contraction takes place by the mechanisms discussed above.

The Ca^{2+} release channel is also known as the ryanodine receptor (after a plant alkaloid). It has a transmembraneous part and a section that projects into the myoplasm where it bridges the gap between the sarcoplasmic reticulum and the sarcolemma. It also lies close to the dihydropyridine receptor (a slow Ca^{2+} channel) of the T tubular system, and the two proteins may be coupled.

Relaxation occurs when myoplasmic Ca^{2+} falls due to reuptake by the sarcoplasmic reticulum, and this is an energy-consuming process. Troponin C loses its Ca^{2+} and the myosin head detaches from the actin filament. Factors that diminish the reuptake of Ca^{2+}, such as profound fatigue and ischaemia, decrease the ability of the muscle

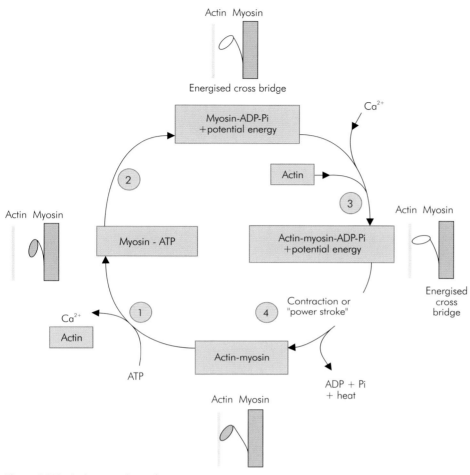

Figure MP9 Actin–myosin cycle

to relax, and it tends towards the rigidity seen in rigor mortis.

Single muscle fibre contraction

A muscle contraction is the result of the combined responses of many individual muscle fibres of different types. It is also the temporal summation of the response of these fibres to multiple action potentials transmitted by the motor nerve. Consider the mechanical response of a single muscle fibre and its response to repeated action potentials. When a muscle contracts, the tension developed varies with time and its length may change depending on the load it is attached to. Three different types of muscle contraction can be described:

- Isometric – a contraction with no change in length
- Isotonic – a contraction with constant load but shortening length
- Lengthening contraction – a contraction in which the external load is greater than the tension developed by the muscle, causing the muscle to increase in length in spite of its contraction

Single fibre twitch

A muscle fibre responds to a single stimulus with a single brief contraction mediated by the release of Ca^{2+}. This is called a twitch. Isometric and isotonic twitches are illustrated in Figure MP10. The following characteristics can be seen:

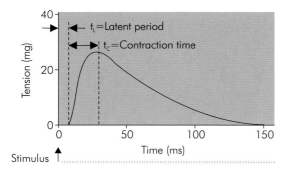

(a) Isometric twitch of single muscle fibre

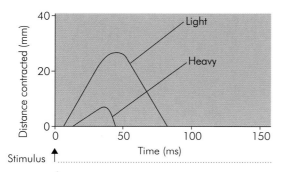

(b) Isotonic twitch of single muscle fibre with
light load and heavy load

Figure MP10 Single fibre twitch response

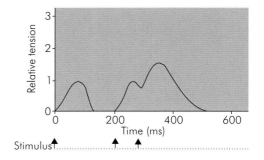

(a) Repeated isometric twitches of single
muscle fibre

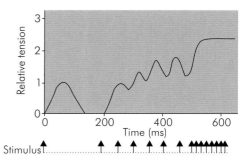

(b) High-frequency twitches of single
muscle fibre giving tetany

Figure MP11 Single fibre repeated twitch response

- There is a latent period between stimulus and onset of developed tension. This varies between fibre types.
- Contraction time is that time between onset of tension development and maximum tension, which differs between fibre types.
- The shortening profile of isotonic contractions depends on the applied load.

Relaxation follows with the immediate reuptake of Ca^{2+} by the sarcoplasmic reticulum. This reuptake starts before maximal contraction has taken place, so the muscle fibre does not develop the strongest force of which it is capable. Muscle tissue has the properties of absolute and relative refractoriness seen in most excitable tissue, but the time periods of de- and repolarisations are shorter than the time usually taken for contraction and relaxation.

Repeated action potentials produce different results according to the interval between stimuli. If a second stimulus comes along before complete reuptake of the Ca^{2+}, it elicits a contraction stronger than the first (Figure MP11a).

A series of stimuli repeated rapidly produces a gradual augmentation of contraction until the tension developed reaches a maximum, which is then sustained. This is called a tetanic contraction, and it is significantly stronger than that produced by a single twitch (Figure MP11b).

Muscle metabolism
Energy for muscle contraction
Adenosine triphosphate (ATP) is the immediate energy source for muscle contraction. There are three main pathways forming ATP for contraction:
- Phosphorylation of ADP by creatine phosphate (CP) – very rapid and occurs at the onset of contraction. It is

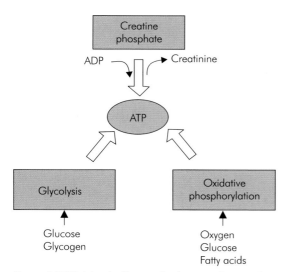

Figure MP12 Metabolism and substrates in muscle contraction

limited by the content of CP in the cell, only lasts a few seconds and lasts until OP and GP can take over.

- Oxidative phosphorylation (OP) in mitochondria – requires oxygen and supplies most of ATP requirements during moderate exercise levels.
- Glycolytic phosphorylation (GP) in the cytoplasm – does not require oxygen and normally only produces small numbers of ATP molecules per mole of glucose, but can produce greater quantities if the enzymes and substrate are available. Glycolytic phosphorylation produces lactic acid and incurs an 'oxygen debt' which may be repaid by a prolonged elevation of oxygen usage after muscle activity has ceased.

The energy sources and substrates used during muscle contraction are summarised in Figure MP12.

Metabolic substrates during contraction

The principal fuel for muscle metabolism is glycogen. The following points summarise substrate utilisation:

- Glycogen mobilisation is stimulated by Ca^{2+} and epinephrine.
- Muscle glycogen only lasts about 10 minutes during moderate exercise.
- For the next 30 minutes, blood glucose and fatty acids provide substrate equally.
- After this, fatty acids become the predominant fuel.

Muscle fibre types

Muscle fibres are classified according to their mechanical performance and their metabolic performance. Mechanical performance is reflected by maximal shortening velocity, which is dependent on the myosin–ATPase activity in the fibre. Metabolic performance is determined by whether ATP formation is mainly oxidative or glycolytic. A high oxidative capacity in a fibre will give it the ability to resist fatigue, since this will avoid the accumulation of an oxygen debt during prolonged contraction. On this basis three main types of fibre may be identified:

- Type I – slow oxidative fibres, red in colour
- Type II – fast glycolytic fibres, white in colour
- Type III – fast oxidative fibres

Type I fibres are metabolically and mechanically relatively slow compared with type II fibres, but they have greater oxidative capacity and are capable of sustained work rates over prolonged periods without incurring a significant oxygen debt. Type II fibres, on the other hand, are fast metabolically and mechanically, and are capable of intense work rates, but only for short periods as they readily accumulate a significant oxygen debt. Functionally, type I fibres predominate in muscles associated with continuous slow sustained contractions, such as the paraspinal muscle columns responsible for maintaining posture. Type II fibres are found mainly in muscles performing short, rapid movements such as the oculomotor muscles and the small muscles of the hand. A comparison of the properties of these muscle fibres is given in Figure MP13.

In practice, few muscles are made up exclusively of red or white fibres. Classically, sprinters have relatively more white fibres and marathon runners relatively more red. With periods of inactivity there is a relative increase in the number of white fibres.

Neuromuscular transmission

Electrical impulses are transmitted from the motor neurone to the muscle by the release of acetylcholine (ACh). This transducer process is similar to that of synaptic transmission. ACh is the only neurotransmitter involved in skeletal neuromuscular transmission. It diffuses across the junctional gap and interacts with specific receptors on the postjunctional membrane of the motor endplates.

Neuromuscular junction (NMJ)

When the motor neurone reaches its termination, it becomes unmyelinated and branches into a number of terminal buttons or endfeet. At the same time the muscle

Property	Type I	Type II	Type III
Colour	Red	White	Red
Diameter	Small	Large	Intermediate
Formation of ATP	Oxidative phosphorylation	Glycolysis	Oxidative phosphorylation
Mitochondria	Many	Few	Many
Glycogen content	Low	High	Intermediate
Glycolytic enzymes	Low	High	Intermediate
Myosin-ATPase activity	Low	High	High
Contraction speed	Slow	Fast	Fast
Myoglobin content	High	Low	High
Fatigue rate	Slow	High	Intermediate
Mitochondria	Many	Few	Many

Figure MP13 Comparison of type I, II and III muscle fibres

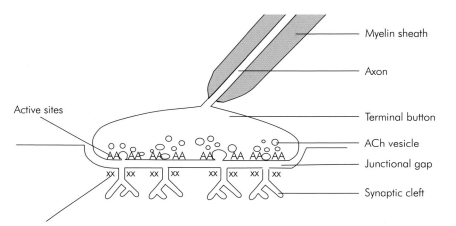

Figure MP14 Structure of the NMJ

membrane, opposite the endfeet, becomes thickened and invaginated to form junctional folds. Between the endfeet and the motor endplate is the junctional gap, structurally similar to the synaptic cleft. The whole structure is known as the NMJ (Figure MP14).

Acetylcholine receptors

ACh receptors in the postjunctional membrane of the motor endplate are of the nicotinic type. A normal neuromuscular endplate on average contains about 50 million ACh receptors. They are situated at the crests of the junctional folds. The nicotinic ACh receptor is a protein with a molecular weight of about 250 000 daltons, and it is made up of five polypeptide subunits: two identical α subunits, one β, one γ (replaced by ϵ in adult mammals) and one δ subunit. Each subunit is encoded by a different gene and has similar overall structure. The five subunits are arranged in a cylindrical fashion surrounding a central funnel-shaped pore, which is the ion channel (Figure MP15). The receptor spans the membrane and possesses both hydrophilic and hydrophobic regions.

When ACh molecules bind to the receptors, they do so by binding onto specific binding sites on the α subunits. As a result, they induce a change in the configuration of the

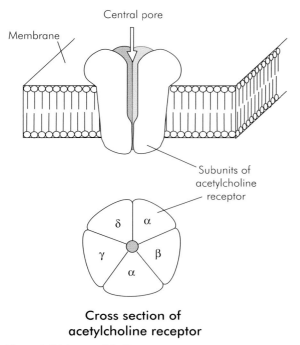

Cross section of
acetylcholine receptor

Figure MP15 Acetylcholine receptor structure

receptor so that the central pore opens, allowing Na^+ and other ions to pass down their concentration and electrical gradients. This sudden influx of Na^+ ions into the cell results in depolarisation.

Acetylcholine synthesis and storage (prejunctional)

Synthesis of acetylcholine involves the reaction of acetyl-coenzyme A (acetyl-CoA) and choline, catalysed by the enzyme choline acetyltransferase. Acetyl-CoA is synthesised in the mitochondria of the axon terminals from pyruvate. About 50% of the choline is derived from the breakdown of ACh; the remainder is extracted from the extracellular fluid by a Na^+-dependent active transport process in the cell membrane which is the rate-limiting step in ACh synthesis. Choline acetyltransferase is originally synthesised on the ribosomes in the cell bodies of motor neurones and transported distally by axoplasmic flow to the nerve terminals, where high concentration can be detected. Enzyme activity is inhibited by acetylcholine but enhanced by nerve stimulation (Figure MP16).

ACh molecules are stored in the vesicles situated in the nerve endings. Each vesicle contains about 4000 molecules of ACh. There appear to be different stores of vesicles that differ in their availability for release, depending on the level of demand (nerve stimulation). Thus there are the readily releasable store (80%) and the stationary store (20%).

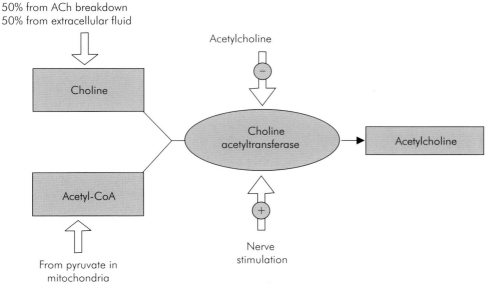

Figure MP16 Acetylcholine synthesis

Mechanism of neuromuscular transmission (junctional)

The vesicles situated in the active zone (that part of the terminal endfoot immediately opposite the junctional folds) spontaneously and randomly fuse with the presynaptic membrane and release ACh molecules into the NMJ. This process is known as exocytosis. Acetylcholine then diffuses across the NMJ and interacts with ACh receptors located on the postsynaptic folds of the muscle membrane. This small spontaneous discharge is only sufficient to produce small transient electrical changes in the postsynaptic membrane known as *miniature endplate potential* or MEPP. However, when the motor neurone is adequately stimulated, action potentials increase the permeability of nerve endings to Ca^{2+} ions. This increase in intracellular Ca^{2+} ion concentration triggers a marked increase in exocytosis of vesicles. This leads to an explosive release of ACh across the junctional gap, increasing the Na^+ and K^+ conductance of the membrane. The sudden influx of Na^+ produces a depolarising potential, known as *endplate potential.*

Acetylcholine inactivation (postjunctional)

For repolarisation to occur, it is necessary to remove ACh rapidly from the junctional gap. ACh is hydrolysed to choline and acetate. This reaction is catalysed by the enzyme acetylcholinesterase, also known as true acetylcholinesterase. This is found specifically at nerve endings, unlike pseudocholinesterase (plasma cholinesterase), which is present in the plasma and is not involved in ACh breakdown at the NMJ.

Action potential generation and transmission in muscle

Each nerve impulse releases about 60 ACh vesicles. This is sufficient to activate about 10 times the number of ACh receptors required to produce a propagatable endplate potential. Thus there is usually a 10-fold safety margin to protect normal neuromuscular transmission.

The electrical events and changes in ion permeability in skeletal muscle induced by the arrival of an action potential are similar to that in nerve tissue. However, the resting membrane potential of skeletal muscle is about -90 mV. The action potential lasts 2–4 ms and is conducted along the muscle fibre at about 5 ms^{-1}.

The potential change at the endplate depolarises the adjacent muscle membrane to its firing level, by transiently increasing Na^+ and K^+ conductance. Action potentials are generated on either side of the endplate and are conducted away from the endplate to the rest of the muscle. The muscle action potential then leads to depolarisation along the T tubules and finally results in muscle contraction.

Central control of muscle tone and movement

Skeletal muscle fibres contract in response to activity in α motor neurones of the anterior horn of the spinal cord. One motor axon innervates a number of fibres, the precise number depending on the task performed by that particular muscle. Muscles controlling fine movement, such as the small muscles of the eye, have fewer fibres per neurone than those with more general functions. In the eye muscles the neurone : fibre ratio is 1 : 15, whereas the anterior tibialis and gastrocnemius have ratios of 1 : 2000.

There is a strict order of recruitment of fibres in a given muscle contraction, and for that particular contraction it is always the same. Oxidative fibres are innervated by the smaller neurones and it is these that are recruited first, the larger neurones and the glycolytic fibres coming in as the size or strength of the muscle contraction increases.

Muscle spindles and the γ-efferent system

Good control of muscle tone and stretch is essential for the maintenance of posture and for accuracy of movements. This control is mediated by stretch receptors in the skeletal muscles, called 'muscle spindles'. These fusiform structures are scattered throughout the fibres of a skeletal muscle. They are small specialised structures composed of 4–20 intrafusal (within-spindle) fibres and are supplied by both sensory (Ia and IIa afferents) and motor (γ-efferent) nerves.

In the control of muscle tone and movement the spindles provide a feedback signal which tends to maintain a skeletal muscle at a desired length, or controls the rate at which a muscle lengthens or shortens. Thus the spindles provide a static signal (via IIa afferents) helping to maintain posture, and a dynamic component (via Ia afferents) controlling the rate of contraction and, hence, smoothness of movements. When the position of a muscle is disturbed by stretching, the spindles are also stretched, which increases their feedback signal to the spinal cord. This increases α motor output and skeletal muscle tone opposing the original disturbance (Figure MP17).

The γ-efferent motor nerves to the spindles pre-tension the intrafusal fibres, which effectively sets their sensitivity. Gamma efferent tone is under the influence of higher centres in the central nervous system such as the cortex, basal ganglia and cerebellum. If γ-efferent tone is high the

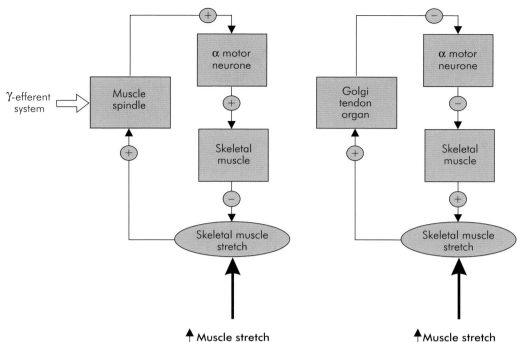

Figure MP17 Muscle control and γ-efferent system

Figure MP18 Golgi tendon organ reflex

spindles are taut and slight disturbances in skeletal muscle length elicit reflex contraction of the skeletal muscle. The skeletal musculature then appears to be clinically hypertonic. This can occur with upper motor neurone lesions such as those following cerebrovascular accidents. When γ-efferent tone is low, muscular hypotonia results, as may occur with some cerebellar lesions.

Golgi tendon organ reflex

Another reflex that modulates contraction and relaxation of skeletal muscles is mediated by the Golgi tendon organs. These are situated in the muscle tendon just adjacent to the muscle fibres. The Golgi tendon organs also respond to muscle stretch but supply a feedback signal (via Ib afferents) to inhibitory neurones in the spinal cord. These neurones synapse with the α motor neurones, inhibiting them and reducing skeletal muscle tone during contraction. The Golgi tendon feedback signal also stimulates antagonist muscles of opposing groups to the inhibited muscle (Figure MP18). The result is to smooth rapid or jerky muscle contraction. If a muscle is subjected to an excessive stretching force the Golgi tendon organ reflex can cause virtual relaxation of the muscle, thus helping to protect it

against mechanical rupture. The Golgi tendon organ reflex is thus an example of a positive feedback loop.

The combination of Golgi tendon organ and muscle spindle activity provides a dynamic balance of two opposing signals, which controls the α motor neurone output. This control has a static component helping to maintain posture and a dynamic component providing smooth and accurate movements.

Smooth muscle

As the name implies, smooth muscles do not possess the cross-striations that are characteristics of the skeletal and cardiac muscles. Smooth muscles are innervated by the autonomic nervous system and thus are not under voluntary control. They play a vital role in the functioning of most hollow viscera and, in particular, the regulation of vascular resistance.

Structure

Each smooth muscle fibre is a spindle-shaped cell consisting of a single nucleus capable of cell division. Cell diameter varies between 2 and 10 μm. Smooth muscle fibre contains myosin, actin and tropomyosin, but unlike in skeletal muscle there is no regular arrangement between these fibrils. There is also an absence of troponin and only a poorly developed sarcoplasmic reticulum. Compared with skeletal muscle, smooth muscle contains only one-third as much myosin but twice as much actin; however, the maximal tension achievable per unit of cross-sectional area by smooth muscles is similar to that of skeletal muscle. Smooth muscles contain only a few mitochondria, and cellular metabolism depends largely on glycolysis.

Types

Based on the electrical characteristics, smooth muscles can generally be divided into two types, single-unit and multi-unit. However, these only represent the two extremes of a spectrum exhibited by smooth muscles.

Single-unit smooth muscles

The membranes can propagate action potentials from cell to cell through low-resistance bridges (or gap junctions) and may exhibit spontaneous action potentials. All muscle fibres may undergo electrical and mechanical activity in a synchronous manner. In other words, the whole muscle responds to stimulation as a single unit. In addition, the contractility of this type of muscle is also influenced by neurohumoral factors. The nerve terminals are often restricted to regions of the muscle that contain the pacemaker cells. By regulating the activity of the pacemaker cells, the activity of the entire muscle can thus be controlled. Single-unit smooth muscles are characteristically found in the gastrointestinal tract, uterus, ureters and small-diameter blood vessels.

Multi-unit smooth muscles

Multi-unit smooth muscles rarely contain gap junctions, compared with single-unit smooth muscles, but are densely innervated by autonomic nerve fibres. Each muscle fibre responds independently of its adjacent fibre, and they therefore behave as independent multiple units. Contractility of the whole muscle depends on the number of muscle fibres activated and on the frequency of nerve stimulation. Spontaneous action potentials do not usually occur in multi-unit smooth muscles. Stretching does not induce contraction in this type of muscle. Examples of this type of muscle can be located in the large airways, most blood vessels, the iris and ciliary body.

Smooth muscle contraction

Action potential will either release Ca^{2+} from the sarcoplasmic reticulum or open up voltage-gated Ca^{2+} channels in the cell membrane. As in the case of striated muscle, the latter may trigger further Ca^{2+} release from the sarcoplasmic reticulum. It is this change in the intracellular Ca^{2+} concentration that plays a pivotal role in the contractile activity of smooth muscle. Unlike skeletal muscle, where calcium binds to troponin, calcium binds to calmodulin in the cytoplasm in smooth muscle. The calmodulin–Ca^{2+} complex then activates myosin light chain kinase, which uses ATP to phosphorylate the myosin cross-bridges. The latter then binds to actin filaments to produce contraction.

In single-unit smooth muscle, the membrane potential is often unstable and recurrent depolarisation leads to continuous, irregular contractions. Because of this instability, there is no constant 'resting' potential. The smooth muscle cell depolarises until it reaches the threshold potential and produces an action potential. During depolarisation, voltage-gated Ca^{2+} channels open, generating calcium action potentials rather than sodium action potentials as in the case of skeletal muscle.

Properties

Certain smooth muscle cells have the propensity to depolarise spontaneously. In the absence of extrinsic neurohumoral stimulation these cells are known as pacemaker cells. The change in membrane potential is known as pacemaker potential. This property is not unique to smooth muscles, occurring also in cardiac pacemaker cells and a few neurones in the central nervous system.

A series of such action potentials may occur, leading to a tonic state of contractile activity. This tonic state is also known as 'smooth muscle tone'.

Property	Single-unit smooth muscle	Multi-unit smooth muscle
Gap junctions	Yes	Few
Pacemaker potentials	Yes	No
Tone	Yes	No
Neuro-control	Yes	Yes
Hormonal control	Yes	Yes
Stretch-induced contraction	Yes	No

Figure MP19 Differences between single-unit and multi-unit smooth muscle

	Skeletal muscle	Cardiac muscle	Smooth muscle
Structure			
Motor endplate	Present	None	None
Mitochondria	Few	Many	Few
Sarcomere	Yes	Yes	None
Sarcoplasmic reticulum	Extensively developed	Well developed	Poorly developed
Syncytium	None	Yes	Yes
Function			
Pacemaker	No	Yes (fast)	Yes (slow)
Response	All or none	All or none	Graded
Tetanic contraction	Yes	No	Yes

Figure MP20 Comparison between skeletal, cardiac and smooth muscle

Stretching of the muscle causes depolarisation and reinforces the existing tone. Stretching opens mechanosensitive ion channels, which may lead to membrane depolarisation and induces contraction. It is this property that is involved in autoregulation of blood flow. However, if the muscle is held at the greater length after stretching, the tension gradually decreases. It can be demonstrated that the tension generated by a particular length of smooth muscle progressively decreases when the muscle is kept stretched. This property is referred to as the plasticity of smooth muscle.

The similarities and differences between single-unit and multi-unit smooth muscle are summarised in Figure MP19.

Extrinsic control

Unlike striated muscle, where contraction is an all-or-none response, in smooth muscle the contractile state is graded according to the concentration of intracellular calcium, which in turn is controlled by graded changes in the membrane potential, not just by action potentials. These graded changes are influenced by extrinsic factors as follows:

- Autonomic nervous system – postganglionic fibres from sympathetic and parasympathetic nerves innervate smooth muscle. A single smooth muscle fibre may be influenced by neurotransmitters from more than one neurone. Both excitatory and inhibitory responses can be elicited, depending not only on the type of neurotransmitter but also on the type of receptors present on the membrane.
- Hormones – the plasma membrane of smooth muscle cells contains receptors for a variety of hormones. Binding of a hormone to the membrane receptors may result in the opening or closure of ion channels. In addition, it may release second messengers that may result in the release of calcium from the sarcoplasmic reticulum. This in turn may increase or decrease contractile activity.
- Local humoral factors – local factors such as paracrine agents, oxygen concentration, pH, osmolarity and ionic composition of the ECF surrounding the smooth muscle may also exert marked influence on the intracellular calcium concentration.

Comparison between skeletal, cardiac and smooth muscle

Although the basic contractile mechanisms of the various types of muscle are based on interaction between myosin and actin filaments, their ultimate physiological functions differ significantly. This variation is reflected in gross as well as microscopic differences between skeletal, cardiac and smooth muscle. Figure MP20 highlights some differences in structure and function between the different types of muscle.

CHAPTER 5

Cardiac physiology

J. L. C. Swanevelder

The heart

The cardiovascular system acts as a transport system for the tissues and has the following functions:
- Supply of oxygen and removal of CO_2
- Delivery of nutrients and removal of metabolic waste products
- Delivery of hormones and vasoactive substances to target cells

The heart is the driving force behind this system, and can be considered a transducer that converts chemical energy into mechanical energy. It consists of a right-sided low-pressure pump and a left-sided high-pressure pump. Each of these pumps is composed of an atrium and a ventricle. The atria prime the ventricles, which in turn eject the cardiac output (CO) into either the pulmonary or the systemic circulation.

Cardiac muscle

Cardiac muscle is striated, the striations being due to the structure of the contractile intracellular myofibrils. The myofibrils are composed of sarcomere units which are identical to those of skeletal muscle, composed of thick and thin filaments arranged to give the characteristic Z line, A band and I band striations. The thick filaments are composed of myosin molecules, whose tails are linked to form the filament leaving the actin binding 'heads' of the molecules free. Each thick filament is surrounded by six thin filaments composed of a double spiral of actin molecules in combination with tropomyosin and troponin. These thin filaments form a hexagonal tube around the thick myosin filament. Contraction of the sarcomere is then produced by a coupling and decoupling reaction between the myosin heads and actin filaments, which results in a 'walking' action of the myosin heads along the thin filaments and causes the thick filaments to slide along the axis

Fundamentals of Anaesthesia, 3rd edition, ed. Tim Smith, Colin Pinnock and Ted Lin. Published by Cambridge University Press. © Cambridge University Press 2008.

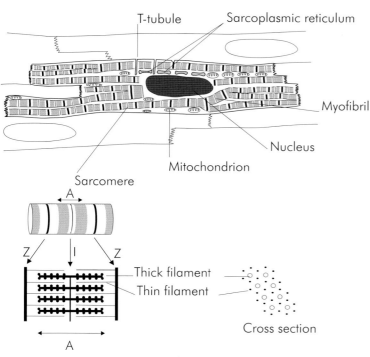

Figure HE1 Cardiac muscle structure

of the actin tubes. The actin–myosin coupling and decoupling reaction lies at the heart of the contractile process and is fuelled by ATP and Ca^{2+}.

Each cardiac muscle cell is surrounded by a cell membrane, the sarcolemma. This forms invaginations penetrating deeply into the cell, which are called transverse or T tubules. These tubules are located at the Z lines and spread the action potential (AP) into the interior of the muscle cell. A system of closed cisterns and tubules, the sarcoplasmic reticulum (SR), surrounds each myofibril, the cisterns being closely related to the T tubules. The SR acts as a reversible intracellular store for calcium ions.

Differences between cardiac muscle and skeletal muscle

Cardiac muscle differs from skeletal muscle in that the individual cells or fibres are tightly coupled, mechanically and electrically, to form a functional syncytium. This is achieved by branching and interdigitation of the cells and specialised end-to-end membrane junctions called intercalated disks. Intercalated disks are located at positions corresponding to Z lines (Figure HE1). Functionally the result is an all-or-nothing contractile response of the myocardium when stimulated. Cardiac muscle is not a true syncytium, as each cardiac muscle cell has a single nucleus and is surrounded by the sarcolemma. A further difference lies in the electrically conductive characteristics of the cardiac muscle fibres, which offer a low resistance to the propagation of AP along the axis of muscle cells due to the intercalated disks. The intercalated disks allow rapid transmission of AP between cells via gap junctions that are composed of connections or open channels connecting the cytosol of adjacent cells. Cardiac muscle cells contain much greater numbers of packed mitochondria and are more richly supplied with capillaries than skeletal muscle, since the myocardium cannot afford to incur an oxygen debt by using anaerobic metabolism.

Excitation–contraction coupling

This term describes the events initially triggered by an AP and which culminate in contraction of a myofibril. Propagation of an AP along the sarcolemma and into the muscle cell through the T-tubule system causes calcium ions (Ca^{2+}) to enter the cell through voltage-dependent channels, receptor-dependent channels and also by passive diffusion across the sarcolemma. This initial rise in

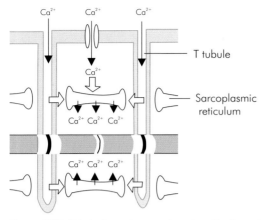

Figure HE2 T tubule and sarcoplasmic reticulum structure

Ca^{2+} triggers further release of Ca^{2+} from the sarcoplasmic reticulum. As a result, intracellular Ca^{2+} levels increase from resting values of 10^{-7} mmol l^{-1} to concentrations of 10^{-4} mmol l^{-1} (Figure HE2). The released calcium acts on the thin filaments, binding to troponin and causing tropomyosin to move and reveal the actin binding sites for the myosin heads. This enables the myosin heads to attach themselves to the actin filaments and contraction commences. Contraction proceeds by a 'walk-along' or 'ratchet' process, in which ATP is hydrolysed to ADP by ATPase in the myosin head. The energy released produces the 'power stroke' that slides the myosin on the actin.

The strength of cardiac muscle contraction is highly dependent on the calcium concentration in the extracellular fluid. At the end of the AP plateau the calcium flow into the cell decreases, and the intracellular Ca^{2+} is actively pumped back into the sarcoplasmic reticulum and T tubules by a Ca^+Mg^+ATPase pump. The chemical interaction between actin and myosin ceases and the muscle relaxes until the next AP.

Cardiac action potentials

An action potential (AP) is a spontaneous depolarisation of the membrane of an excitable cell, usually in response to a stimulus. Two different types of AP are found in the heart: fast and slow responses. In the myocardium two cell types produce fast-response AP: contractile myocardial cells and conduction system cells. Slow-response AP are normally produced by the pacemaker cells in the sinoatrial (SA) node and the atrioventricular (AV) node. These pacemaker cells

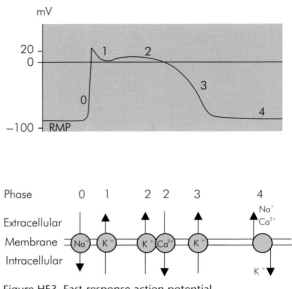

Figure HE3 Fast-response action potential

spontaneously depolarise to produce slow-response AP, exhibiting a property called automaticity.

Fast-response action potentials

The fast-response AP of the cardiac muscle cell can be divided into five distinct phases (Figure HE3):
- Phase 0 – initial rapid depolarisation/upstroke
- Phase 1 – early rapid repolarisation
- Phase 2 – prolonged plateau phase
- Phase 3 – final rapid repolarisation
- Phase 4 – resting membrane potential (RMP)

Resting membrane potential

The RMP is the electrical potential across the cell membrane during diastole and is about −90 mV, the intracellular membrane surface being negative with respect to the extracellular surface. RMP is maintained by the permeability properties of the cell membrane, which retains negative ions in the cell but allows positive ions to diffuse out. The cell membrane is impermeable to negatively charged ions such as proteins, sulphates and phosphates, which, therefore, remain intracellularly. In contrast, membrane permeability to potassium is higher, allowing it to diffuse out of the cell under its concentration gradient of about 30 : 1. Potassium diffuses out of the cell until an equilibrium is reached at which the electrostatic attraction of the retained anions balances the chemical force moving the potassium down its concentration gradient out of the cell. This equilibrium is expressed mathematically by the Nernst equation in the following way:

Electrostatic force = Chemical force

or

$$\text{Equilibrium potential} = \frac{RT}{FZ_K} \times \log_e \frac{[K_O^+]}{[K_I^+]}$$

where

$[K_I^+]$ = potassium concentration inside cell membrane
$[K_O^+]$ = potassium concentration outside cell membrane
R = gas constant
T = absolute temperature
F = Faraday's constant
Z_K = valency of potassium

Thus the membrane potential due to K^+

$$= 62 \times \log_{10} \frac{[K_O^+]}{[K_I^+]}$$

Thus, as RMP is due mainly to the distribution and diffusion of potassium ions (below), it can be said that:

$$RMP = 62 \times \log_{10} \frac{[5]}{[150]}$$
$$= -94\,\text{mV}$$

The intracellular–extracellular concentration gradient of potassium must be maintained if RMP is to stay constant. This is achieved by the active transport of potassium from the extracellular fluid to the intracellular space by a Na^+K^+ATPase pump.

Other ions also contribute to RMP by producing transmembrane potentials due to the balance between chemical and electrostatic forces acting on them. For instance, sodium will diffuse across the cell membrane in the opposite direction to potassium (i.e. extra- to intracellular) because of the normal resting sodium concentration gradient. Accordingly, this movement of sodium into the cell will reduce the membrane potential set up by potassium. However, because membrane permeability to sodium under resting conditions is relatively low, this effect is small, merely reducing the membrane potential by about 4 mV. Similarly, the cell membrane is relatively impermeable to other ions in the resting state, and therefore the RMP is primarily determined by the intra–extracellular distribution of potassium ions.

To summarise, RMP is maintained by three mechanisms:

- Retention of many intracellular anions (proteins, phosphates and sulphates) to which the cell membrane is not permeable.
- The resting cell membrane is almost 100 times more permeable to potassium than to sodium, allowing potassium to flow down its concentration gradient out of the cell while keeping sodium extracellular.
- Maintenance of an intracellular–extracellular concentration gradient for potassium ions by a Na^+K^+ATPase pump. This transports potassium actively into the cell and sodium out of the cell (three Na^+ ions for every two K^+ ions) and is dependent on energy supplied by the hydrolysis of ATP.

The fast-response AP is described by the following phases:

Phase 0 – rapid depolarisation
An AP is produced when an electrical stimulus increases RMP (causes it to become less negative) to a threshold potential (TP). At this value, fast sodium channels open for a very short period and potassium channels close. Sodium rapidly enters the cell under the influence of its concentration gradient and the electrostatic attraction of the intracellular anions, to make the inside positive in comparison with the outside by +20 mV. At the end of this stage, the sodium channels close. This phase coincides with the 'all-or-nothing' depolarisation of the myocardium and the QRS complex of the ECG.

Phase 1 – early rapid repolarisation
This phase describes a brief fall in membrane potential towards zero following the rapid rise in phase 0. This occurs due to the start of potassium flow out of the cell under the positive intracellular electrical gradient and chemical gradients. At the same time slow, L-type, Ca^{2+} channels open, providing a prolonged influx of calcium ions which maintains the positive intracellular charge. There is also movement intracellularly of chloride following sodium into the cell along the electrical gradient. This leads to an initial rapid repolarisation of the cell membrane to just above 0 mV.

Phase 2 – plateau phase
During this phase, the continued influx of calcium via the slow L-type Ca^{2+} channels is balanced by the continued efflux of potassium commenced in phase 1. This maintains the zero or slightly positive membrane potential and corresponds in time with the ST segment of the ECG.

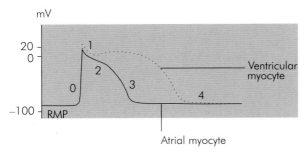

Figure HE4 Atrial and ventricular myocyte action potentials

Phase 3 – final rapid repolarisation

Potassium permeability rapidly increases at this stage and potassium flows out to restore the transmembrane potential to −90 mV. Although repolarisation of the membrane is complete by the end of phase 3, the normal ionic gradients have not yet been re-established across the membrane.

Phase 4 – restoration of ionic concentrations and resting state

During this phase ATPase-dependent ion pumps exchange intracellular sodium and calcium ions for extracellular potassium, thus restoring the resting ionic gradients. When an equilibrium state is reached electrostatic forces equal the chemical forces acting on the different ions and RMP is re-established. This phase corresponds to diastole.

Atrial cell action potentials

Atrial myocyte AP are also of the rapid-response type but vary from the ventricular AP in having a shorter duration plateau (phase 2). This effect is due to a much greater early repolarisation current (phase 1) in the atrial AP than in the ventricular case (Figure HE4).

Excitability of cardiac cells

Excitability describes the ability of cardiac tissue to depolarise to a given electrical stimulus. It is dependent on the difference between RMP and TP, and thus changes in RMP will alter myocardial excitability. When RMP decreases (becomes more negative) this difference becomes greater and the heart becomes less excitable. Similarly, excitability is increased as the difference between RMP and TP decreases. Various factors affect excitability, including:

- Catecholamines
- β blockers
- Local anaesthetic agents
- Plasma electrolyte concentrations

Refractoriness

During rapid depolarisation (phase 0) and the early part of repolarisation (phases 1, 2 and initial part of 3), the cell cannot be depolarised to produce another AP regardless of stimulus strength. The sodium and calcium channels are inactivated and repolarisation must occur before they can open again. This is called the absolute refractory period. During the latter part of phase 3 and early phase 4 a stronger than normal impulse can lead to an AP. This is called the relative refractory period. For the duration of this period the heart is particularly vulnerable because an impulse at this time might produce repetitive, asynchronous depolarisation (e.g. ventricular fibrillation or tachycardia). The absolute and relative refractory periods together form the effective refractory period.

Pacemaker cells

The heart continues to beat after all nerves to it are sectioned. This happens because of the specialised pacemaker tissue (P-cell) that makes up the conduction system of the heart. These cells are found in the SA and AV nodes and also in the His–Purkinje system. Pacemaker cells exhibit automaticity (ability to depolarise spontaneously) and rhythmicity (ability to maintain a regular discharge rate). Normally atrial and ventricular myocardial cells do not have pacemaker ability and they only discharge spontaneously when injured. There are, however, latent pacemakers in other parts of the conduction system that can take over when conduction from the SA and AV nodes is blocked.

Slow-response action potentials

The AP produced when a pacemaker cell depolarises spontaneously is called a slow-response AP (Figure HE5). The most negative potential reached just before depolarisation is called the 'maximum diastolic potential' (MDP), which is only −60 mV compared with the RMP of −90 mV for a myocardial muscle cell. The reason for this is that the pacemaker cell membranes are more permeable to sodium ions in their resting state. Phases can be identified in the slow-response AP which correspond superficially to some phases of the rapid-response, as detailed below, although the underlying events differ.

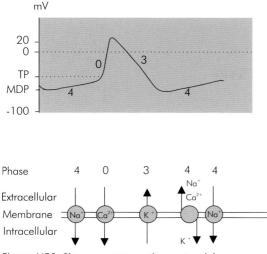

Figure HE5 Slow-response action potential

Phase 4 – restoration of ionic gradients and resting state

Pacemaker cells do not maintain a stable RMP, but instead depolarise spontaneously because of increased membrane permeability to cations during this phase. Sodium and calcium slowly 'leak' into the cell. Although potassium diffuses out simultaneously during this phase the inward 'leak' of sodium predominates to cause the membrane potential to gradually increase until a TP is reached at about -40 mV. This property is called spontaneous diastolic depolarisation or pacemaker automaticity, and is directly related to the positive slope of phase 4.

Phase 0 – rapid depolarisation

Rapid depolarisation occurs at TP and is mainly due to calcium influx through transient (or T-type) Ca^{2+} channels, which are slower than the rapid sodium channels responsible for phase 0 in the myocardial cell AP. The slope of phase 0 is, therefore, less steep than in the rapid AP case. The phase 0 slope in these cells is also reduced because of onset at a less negative transmembrane potential.

Phase 3 – repolarisation

In the slow-response AP, repolarisation is effectively a single-phase equivalent to phase 3 in the rapid-response. Effectively phase 1 is absent and phase 2 is very brief, resulting in the absence of a plateau effect.

Differences between pacemaker and myocardial cell action potential

Pacemaker AP have the following features which differ from those of the myocardial cells:
- Less negative phase 4 membrane potential
- Less negative TP
- Spontaneous depolarisation in phase 4
- Less steep slope in phase 0 (dependence on T-type Ca^{2+} channels)
- Absence of phase 2 (plateau)

Ion channels and action potentials

AP owe their basic characteristics to voltage-controlled changes in membrane permeability to different ions. The main ions concerned are potassium, sodium and calcium, whose membrane permeabilities are dependent on various types of ion diffusion channel. These ion channels have been described in vitro by controlling and varying membrane potentials in different ion solutions, using a technique called 'patch clamping'. Different channels can then be identified by the changes in current produced as the channels open and close according to their control potentials. Some of these channels are outlined in Figure HE6.

Automaticity of pacemaker cells

Automaticity is the ability of pacemaker cells to maintain a spontaneous rhythm, and it depends mainly on the leakage of sodium into the cell in phase 4 of the AP. This occurs via specific sodium channels that are activated when the membrane potential has become hyperpolarised, i.e. reached about -50 mV during repolarisation. These channels then allow an inward hyperpolarisation current (i_f), which commences the spontaneous depolarisation of phase 4. The sodium current (i_f) is aided to a small extent by overlap of the decaying rapid depolarisation calcium current and opposed by extracellular diffusion of potassium. Automaticity is dependent on the slope of phase 4 of the AP, which is influenced by the autonomic system and various drugs.

Pacemaker discharge rate

Pacemaker discharge rate is controlled primarily by the autonomic system. Control is mediated by changes in AP characteristics. The following characteristics are associated with variation of the discharge rate (Figure HE7):
- Slope of phase 4 in AP – an increase in the slope of phase 4 reduces the time to reach TP during spontaneous depolarisation, and thus increases

Action potential	Phase	Ion	Channel/gating mechanism
Rapid response (ventricular)	0	Na^+	Fast channels with 'm' activation and 'h' inactivation gates
	1,2,3	K^+	Transient outward current (i_{to}) channel
	2,3,4	K^+	Inward rectifier K^+ current (i_{K1}) channel
	2,3,4	K^+	Delayed rectifier K^+ current (i_K) channel
	2	Ca^{2+}	Slow (long-lasting, L-type) Ca^{2+} channel blocked by calcium antagonists
Slow response (pacemaker)	0	Ca^{2+}	Transient (T-type) Ca^{2+} channel
	4	Na^+	Specific channels 'leaking' sodium current (i_f) into pacemaker cells

Figure HE6 Voltage-controlled ion channels in action potentials

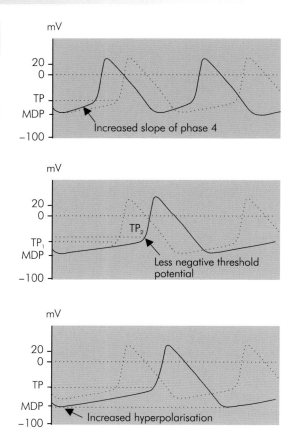

Figure HE7 Changes in pacemaker action potential causing variation of discharge rate

pacemaker rate. Similarly, a decrease in the phase 4 slope results in a slower pacemaker rate. Phase 4 slope can be varied by the autonomic nervous system.

- Threshold potential – if this becomes less negative the pacemaker rate will decrease. Drugs such as quinidine and procainamide have this effect.
- Hyperpolarisation potential – if hyperpolarisation is increased, i.e. the membrane potential becomes more negative, spontaneous discharge will take longer to reach TP during phase 4 and the pacemaker rate will decrease. This occurs with increases in acetylcholine levels.

Conduction system

The conduction system of the heart is composed of specialised cardiac tissues that form the following structures (Figure HE8):

- Sinoatrial (SA) node
- Atrial conduction pathways
- Atrioventricular (AV) node

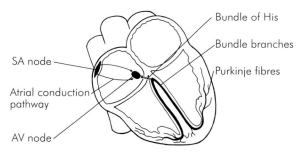

Figure HE8 Anatomy of the conduction system

- Bundle of His
- Bundle branches
- Purkinje fibres

The SA node is the normal cardiac pacemaker, with a resting rate of between 60 and 100 per minute. It is a group of modified myocardial cells located close to the junction of the superior vena cava with the right atrium. Blood supply is usually from a branch of the right coronary artery. Depolarisation spreads from the SA node through the atria and converges on the AV node.

The two atria are electrically separated from the two ventricles except for three internodal communication pathways, the anterior (Bachmann), middle (Wenckebach) and posterior (Thorel) bundles, which connect the SA node to the AV node. The AV node is located in the right posterior part of the right atrium close to the tricuspid valve and the coronary sinus opening. Anomalous accessory pathways (like the bundle of Kent) can sometimes connect the atria directly to the ventricle or other areas of the conducting system and cause a pre-excitation syndrome with arrhythmias. Blood supply to the AV node is also from a branch off the right coronary artery. The AV node is connected to the bundle of His, which distributes the impulse to the ventricles via the left and right bundle branches in the interventricular septum. There is a slight delay (about 0.13 s) of the impulse before it enters the AV node, inside the AV node and in the bundle of His. This delay permits completion of both atrial electrical activation and conduction before ventricular activation is started. The left bundle branch divides into the anterior and posterior fascicles. These bundles and fascicles run subendocardially down the septum and into the Purkinje system, which spreads the impulse to all parts of the ventricular muscle. Conduction velocity through the bundle branches and the Purkinje system is the most rapid of the conduction system. The AP also begins endocardially and spreads out to the outside of the heart. However, repolarisation occurs from the outside to the inside. Ventricular activation is earliest at the apex and latest at the base of the heart, giving it an apical to basal contraction pattern.

Conduction system defects

Defects can arise in any part of the conduction system. Some examples of arrhythmias occurring due to lesions in different parts of the conduction system are shown in Figure HE9.

The electrocardiogram

In an electrophysiological sense the heart consists of two chambers. The two atria function as a single electrophysiological unit and are separated from the biventricular unit by the fibrous AV ring. Electrical communication between these two units is only possible through the specialised conduction system. The main electrical events of the cardiac

Site	Arrhythmia	Features
Sinoatrial node	Sick sinus syndrome	Sinus arrest, sinus bradycardia, tachycardias
Atrial conduction pathways	Wolff–Parkinson–White syndrome	Supraventricular tachycardia
Atrioventricular node	AV junctional rhythm	Bradycardia with abnormal P waves
Bundle of His	Complete (3° block) AV block	Bradycardia with dissociated P waves
Bundle branches	Bundle branch block	abnormal broad QRS complexes (>0.12 s)

Figure HE9 Arrhythmias due to conduction system defects

cycle are the mass de- and repolarisation of the atria and ventricles. These can be thought of as waves of depolarisation (or repolarisation) that propagate through the cardiac tissues. As they propagate they generate potentials that can be sensed by electrodes on the skin surface. The electrocardiogram (ECG) is a recording of the signals picked up by a standard pattern of skin electrodes over the chest. When an electrode detects depolarisation moving towards it, a positive deflection on the ECG is produced. Alternatively, if depolarisation is moving away from the electrode, it produces a negative deflection.

ECG waves and the cardiac cycle

The normal ECG consists of P, QRS, T and U deflections (Figure HE10). Electrical activity precedes corresponding mechanical events during the cardiac cycle as follows:

- The P wave is associated with atrial depolarisation and contraction. The atria repolarise at the same time as ventricular depolarisation; therefore, the atrial repolarisation wave is usually obscured by the prominent QRS complex.
- The PR interval is between the beginning of the P wave and the start of the QRS complex. This represents the time from onset of atrial contraction to the beginning of ventricular contraction. The normal PR interval is about 0.16 s, but it varies with heart rate.

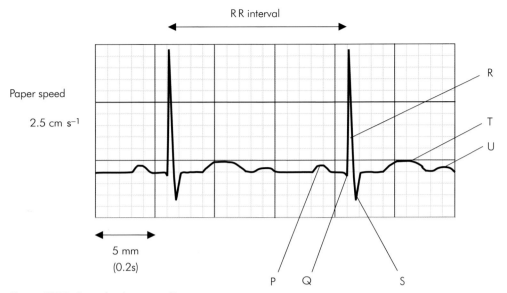

Figure HE10 Sample electrocardiogram trace

- The QRS complex reflects ventricular depolarisation and precedes ventricular contraction. A normal QRS complex has smooth peaks with no notches or slurs and has a duration <0.12 s. The amplitude is dependent on multiple factors including myocardial mass, the cardiac axis, the distance of the sensing electrode from the ventricles and the anatomical orientation of the heart.
- The QT interval lies between the beginning of the Q wave and the end of the T wave. This is about 0.35 s at a normal resting heart rate. The QT interval shortens with tachycardia and lengthens with bradycardia and can be normalised to a heart rate of 60 bpm, by using Bazett's formula for the corrected interval, QTc:

$$QTc = \frac{QT}{\sqrt{RR}}$$

where

RR = interval measured between two R waves.

- The ST segment and T wave are associated with ventricular repolarisation. The ventricles remain contracted until a few milliseconds after repolarisation ends.

- The U wave remains controversial in its origin. It may represent the slow repolarisation of the papillary muscles.

Electrical axis of the heart

Electrical activity in the heart can be represented by a vector, since it possesses both amplitude and direction. A single or resultant vector can be drawn showing the magnitude and direction of the electrical activity in the heart at any instant. This will change continuously throughout the cardiac cycle. Thus, a vector can be drawn to represent maximum electrical activity for any wave of the ECG. During the QRS complex, a maximum vector is normally produced pointing downwards and to the left. This vector reflects peak electrical activity during mass depolarisation of the ventricles, and its direction is referred to as the electrical axis of the heart or the cardiac axis. Various factors may vary the direction of this axis, including the anatomical position of the heart and different pathological conditions (e.g. left ventricular hypertrophy).

ECG leads

An electrical signal is a potential difference detected between two points. In the ECG, signals are recorded between two active surface electrodes or an active electrode and a common or indifferent point. Each signal recorded

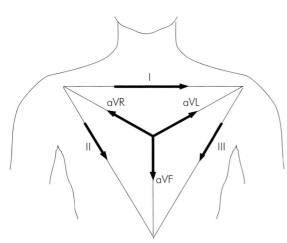

Figure HE11 Einthoven's triangle

is called a lead and may have an amplitude of several milli-volts. There are 12 conventional ECG leads, which may be divided into two main groups:
- Frontal plane leads
- Standard limb leads I, II, III
- Unipolar limb leads aVR, aVL and aVF
- Horizontal plane leads
- Precordial chest leads

Standard limb leads I–III

These leads are recorded with a combination of two active electrodes at a time and are, therefore, bipolar leads. Each signal is recorded in the direction of the sides of an equilateral triangle with an apex on each shoulder and the pubic region, and the heart at its centre. This is called Einthoven's triangle (Figure HE11).
- Lead I – the negative electrode is placed on the right arm and the positive electrode on the left arm.
- Lead II – the negative electrode is placed on the right arm and the positive electrode on the left foot.
- Lead III – the negative electrode is placed on the left arm and the positive electrode on the left foot.

The ECG traces from these three leads are very similar to each other. They all record positive P waves, positive T waves and positive QRS complexes.

Unipolar limb leads aVR, aVL, aVF

Unipolar leads record the difference between an active limb electrode and an indifferent (zero potential) electrode at the centre of Einthoven's triangle (Figure HE11). These signals are of lower amplitude than other leads and require increased amplification (hence referred to as augmented leads):
- aVR – the augmented unipolar right arm lead faces the heart from the right side and is usually orientated to the cavity of the heart. Therefore, all the deflections P, QRS and T are normally negative in this lead.
- aVL – the augmented unipolar left arm lead faces the heart from the left side and is orientated to the anterolateral surface of the left ventricle.
- aVF – the augmented unipolar left leg lead, orientated to the inferior surface of the heart.

Precordial chest leads

These are horizontal-plane, unipolar leads, placed as follows:
- V_1 – fourth intercostal space immediately right of the sternum
- V_2 – fourth intercostal space immediately left of the sternum
- V_3 – exactly halfway between the positions of V_2 and V_4
- V_4 – fifth intercostal space in the mid-clavicular line
- V_5 – same horizontal level as V_4 but on the anterior axillary line
- V_6 – same horizontal level as V_4 and V_5 on the mid-axillary line

Anatomical orientation of ECG electrodes

Although there is considerable variation in the position of the normal heart the atria are usually positioned posteriorly in the chest while the ventricles form the base and anterior surface. The right ventricle is anterolateral to the left ventricle. The ventricles consist of three muscle masses. These are the free walls of the left and right ventricles and the interventricular septum. Electrical activity in the left ventricle and the interventricular septum are predominant. ECG electrodes will pick up signals from the closest structures and those producing the greatest electrical signals. Therefore, ECG signals recorded from the anterior aspect of the heart are mainly due to activity in the interventricular septum, with only a small contribution from the right ventricular wall. Since ECG lead signals reflect activity in different parts of the heart because of their position, they are said to 'look' at different aspects of the heart:
- II, III and aVF look at the inferior surface of the heart.
- I and aVL are orientated towards the superior left lateral wall.

- aVR and V_1 face the cavity of the heart, and the deflections are mainly negative in these leads.
- Leads V_{1-6} are orientated towards the anterior wall. V_1 and V_2 are anterior leads, V_3 and V_4 are septal leads, V_5 and V_6 are lateral leads.
- V_1 and V_2 examine the right ventricle, while V_{4-6} are orientated towards the septum and left ventricle.

There is no lead orientated directly to the posterior wall of the heart.

Calculation of the heart rate

The heart rate (bpm) can be determined from the ECG by measuring the time interval (s) between two successive beats (RR interval), and dividing this into 60 s. Thus:

if RR interval = 0.6 s
$$\text{heart rate} = 60/0.6$$
$$= 100 \text{ bpm}$$

The time scale of the ECG depends on the recording paper speed. Normal paper speed is 2.5 cm s^{-1}, meaning that each large square (5 mm) of the ECG trace represents 0.2 s. In the example shown in Figure HE10, the RR interval is three large squares (15 mm), which is equal to 0.6 s. If the RR interval were to become five large squares (1 s) this would give a heart rate of 60 bpm.

Calculation of the cardiac axis

The direction of the electrical axis of the heart is usually calculated in the frontal plane only, and can be done using two of the frontal ECG leads (these are the standard limb and unipolar limb leads). It is determined as an angle referred to the axes shown in Figure HE12, the normal range lying between 0 and $+90°$.

The cardiac vector, like any vector, can be resolved to give an effect or 'component' in any given direction. The amplitudes of the QRS complexes in the frontal leads represent components of the cardiac vector in the direction of the leads. The cardiac axis can, therefore, be found by the vector summation of any two of these components to find their resultant (here I and aVF are taken for convenience since they lie at 0 and 90° respectively). The direction of the cardiac axis is then given by the angle (θ), of the resultant. A simple algorithm is presented to determine the cardiac axis from I and aVF.

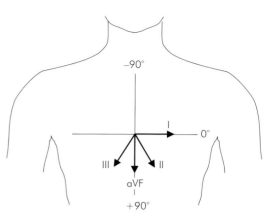

Figure HE12 Reference axes and leads I–III

Calculation algorithm for cardiac axis

An example illustrating the calculation of the cardiac axis from ECG leads I and aVF is shown in Figure HE13. To obtain the axis:

- Determine the amplitudes of the QRS complexes in I and aVF by subtracting the height of the S wave from the height of the R wave in each lead.
- Construct a rectangle with the sides in proportion to the amplitudes of I and aVF. The diagonal then represents the resultant of I and aVF (i.e. the cardiac vector).
- Determine the direction of the cardiac axis from the angle θ by taking the tangent of θ as the ratio of [amplitude of aVF]/[amplitude of I].

Cardiac axis estimation by inspection of standard limb leads

In practice, a rapid estimation of the cardiac axis can be made simply by inspection of the frontal ECG leads. Convenient leads to use are the standard limb leads I, II, III and aVF, which lie at 0, 60, 120 and 90° respectively.

Initially, some basic facts about the relationship between a vector and its components should be noted. The QRS amplitudes in these leads are components of the cardiac vector. The amplitude of a component depends on the angle between the component and the vector it is derived from. As this angle increases the amplitude of the component decreases. Note that:

- For angles $<90°$ the component is positive.
- When the angle between vector and component is zero, i.e. the component is acting in the direction of the vector, the component is maximum and equal to the vector.

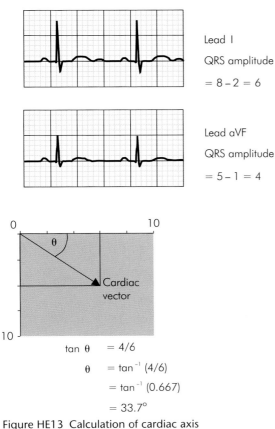

Lead I

QRS amplitude

$= 8 - 2 = 6$

Lead aVF

QRS amplitude

$= 5 - 1 = 4$

$\tan \theta \quad = 4/6$

$\theta \quad = \tan^{-1}(4/6)$

$\quad = \tan^{-1}(0.667)$

$\quad = 33.7°$

Figure HE13 Calculation of cardiac axis

- At 60° the amplitude of the component is half of the vector.
- At 90° the amplitude of the component becomes zero.
- For angles >90° the component becomes negative.

Applying these simple principles will confirm the following estimations. If:
- II = 0, the cardiac axis is at −30° (left axis deviation).
- aVF = 0, the cardiac axis is at 0°.
- I = II, the cardiac axis is at +30°, bisecting the angle between them.
- I and III are each half of II, the cardiac axis is at +60°.
- I = 0, the cardiac axis is at +90°.
- III > II, the cardiac axis is at >90° (right axis deviation).

Monitoring in the operating theatre

During routine non-cardiac surgery standard II and V_5 are usually used as continuous monitoring leads. The P wave is best detected in standard II, which facilitates detection of junctional or ventricular arrhythmias. Chest lead V_5 is most sensitive to ST segment changes and can warn of possible ischaemia. During cardiac surgery all six limb leads are connected for intermittent ST segment examination, and this can increase sensitivity for the detection of ischaemia.

Physiological arrhythmias

A cardiac rhythm is defined by three characteristics:
- The anatomical origin – a description of where the rhythm originates anatomically, e.g. SA node, atria, AV node or ventricles
- The discharge sequence – a description of the pattern of electrical discharge, e.g. sinus rhythm, tachycardia, bradycardia, fibrillation
- The conduction sequence – a description of abnormalities in conduction of the discharge impulses to the myocardium, e.g. 2:1 SA block, complete AV block

Abnormal cardiac rhythms or arrhythmias can arise as a primary or secondary disorder. Acute arrhythmias occurring during the perioperative period can seriously compromise perfusion. An arrhythmia must be correctly diagnosed and the precipitating causes should be removed before treatment is considered. Acute arrhythmias are more likely to be reversible. Chronic arrhythmias are usually disease-related and relatively stable.

Some departures from a perfectly regular cardiac rhythm occur as a result of normal physiological responses, as opposed to having an underlying pathological cause. These are outlined below.

Sinus rhythm

This is the normal rhythm for the heart. All other rhythms are arrhythmias by definition. In the normal adult heart sinus rhythm originates in the SA node, and has a regular pattern of discharge at a resting rate of between 60 and 80 bpm. The conduction sequence occurs on a 1 : 1 basis from SA node to atria to AV node and to the ventricles. The resting rate for neonates varies between 110 and 180 bpm and gradually decreases with increasing age until it reaches the adult rate at about 10 years of age.

Sinus arrhythmia

In healthy young patients with a regular breathing rate, the heart rate increases with inspiration and decreases with expiration. This is a normal finding called sinus arrhythmia. It is caused by an irregular fluctuating discharge of the SA node. During inspiration the stretch receptors in the lungs send impulses via the vagus nerves to inhibit the cardio-inhibitory centre in the medulla oblongata. This stimulates the sinus node, increasing the heart rate. Sinus arrhythmia is characterised by normal PQRST complexes with alternating periods of gradually lengthening and shortening PP intervals.

Sinus bradycardia

This rhythm occurs when the SA node discharges at a rate lower than 60 per minute, with normal PQRST complexes. This is a normal phenomenon in fit young athletes and may also occur during sleep. Sinus bradycardia can be associated with pathological conditions that include myxoedema, uraemia, glaucoma and increased intracranial pressure. Various drugs such as β blockers, digitalis or volatile anaesthetic agents may also cause sinus bradycardia. Occasionally during sinus bradycardia, a ventricular ectopic pacemaker site can take over. This may cause premature ventricular contractions that will usually disappear when the sinus rate speeds up again. When the heart rate goes <40 bpm it is likely to cause hypotension or decreased perfusion, and should be treated immediately with an antimuscarinic drug, β agonist or pacemaker as required.

Sinus tachycardia

Sympathetic stimuli such as emotion, exercise, pain and fever increase the SA discharge rate to >100 per minute, although the PQRST complexes remain normal. It commonly occurs during the perioperative period. Hypovolaemia often causes a sinus tachycardia through the baroreceptor reflex. Certain pathological conditions such as anxiety, thyrotoxicosis, toxaemia and cardiac failure may also cause it. The administration of drugs like epinephrine, atropine, isoprenaline and many others may lead to sinus tachycardia. When the heart rate is >140 bpm there is not enough time for left ventricular filling and the patient becomes haemodynamically compromised. This should be treated initially by removal of the cause, and thereafter pharmacologically.

Effects of electrolyte changes on the ECG

The AP of the heart is dependent upon the sodium and potassium ion distribution across the cell membrane. Electrolyte abnormalities can often produce ECG changes. Some common electrolyte disturbances are described below with their effects on the ECG.

Hypokalaemia

Hypokalaemia makes the RMP of the cardiac muscle fibres more negative. The heart becomes less excitable, but automaticity increases. Moderate hypokalaemia (3–3.5 mmol l^{-1}) causes a prolonged PR interval, flattening of the T wave and a prominent U wave. In severe hypokalaemia (2.5 mmol l^{-1}) ST depression can be seen and late T wave inversion occurs in the precordial leads. The QT interval is often prolonged. None of these changes is exclusively associated with hypokalaemia.

Hyperkalaemia

Hyperkalaemia (>5.5–6 mmol l^{-1}) is a potentially life-threatening condition, especially when the onset is acute. As the extracellular potassium concentration increases, the RMP of the cardiac cell membrane progressively becomes less negative, moving towards TP. Initially this makes the cardiac muscle more excitable. However, a deterioration of the AP also occurs, with a reduction in rapid depolarisation and a loss of the plateau phase. This results in poor contraction of the cardiac muscle. At plasma levels of 6–8 mmol l^{-1}, ventricular tachycardia and fibrillation readily occur. As the RMP approaches the TP (plasma levels >8–10 mmol l^{-1}) the muscle fibres become unexcitable and the heart finally stops in ventricular diastole.

The ECG starts to change when serum potassium level reaches 6.0 mmol l^{-1}. Initially a shortened QT interval and narrow, peaked T wave appears. Further potassium increases produce widening of the QRS complex and PR interval prolongation until the P wave disappears.

Hypocalcaemia

Hypocalcaemia produces a flat, prolonged ST segment and QT interval. Advanced stages of hypocalcaemia may lead to increased ventricular ectopic activity and ventricular tachycardia.

Hypercalcaemia

Hypercalcaemia makes the TP of cardiac muscle fibres less negative, decreases conduction velocity and shortens the refractory period. This increases the likelihood of coupled beats, ventricular tachycardia and ventricular fibrillation.

In acute hyperkalaemia immediate treatment with an IV bolus of calcium opposes the effects of the high potassium levels. At very high calcium levels (animal experiments) the heart will relax less during diastole and will eventually stop in systole (calcium rigor). ECG changes produced by hypercalcaemia are prolongation of the PR interval, widening of the QRS complex and shortening of the QT interval. The T wave is also broadened.

Hypomagnesemia

Hypomagnesemia promotes cell membrane depolarisation and tachyarrhythmias, since magnesium is necessary for the normal functioning of the cardiac cell membrane pump. ECG changes produced by hypomagnesaemia include low-voltage P waves and QRS complexes, prominent U waves and peaked T waves.

Hypermagnesemia

Hypermagnesemia is associated with delayed AV conduction, and therefore presents with a prolonged PR interval, wide QRS complex and T wave elevation at plasma levels >5.0 mmol l^{-1}. Levels >10 mmol l^{-1} may lead to a complete heart block and cardiac arrest.

The cardiac cycle

Each cardiac cycle consists of a period of relaxation (diastole) followed by ventricular contraction (systole). During diastole the ventricles are relaxed to allow filling. In systole the right and left ventricles contract, ejecting blood into the pulmonary and systemic circulations respectively.

Ventricles

The left ventricle pumps blood into the systemic circulation via the aorta. The systemic vascular resistance (SVR) is 5–7 times greater than the pulmonary vascular resistance (PVR). This makes it a high-pressure system (compared with the pulmonary vascular system) which requires a greater mechanical power output from the left ventricle (LV). The free wall of the LV and the interventricular septum form the bulk of the muscle mass in the heart. A normal LV can develop intraventricular pressures up to 300 mmHg. Coronary perfusion to the LV occurs mainly in diastole, when the myocardium is relaxed.

The right ventricle receives blood from the venae cavae and coronary circulation, and pumps it via the pulmonary vasculature into the LV. Since PVR is a fraction of SVR, pulmonary arterial pressures are relatively low and the wall thickness of the right ventricle (RV) is much less than that of the LV. The RV thus resembles a passive conduit rather than a pump. Coronary perfusion to the RV occurs continuously during systole and diastole because of the low intraventricular and intramural pressures.

In spite of the anatomical differences, the mechanical behaviour of the RV and LV is very similar.

The cardiac cycle can be examined in detail by considering the ECG trace, intracardiac pressure and volume curves, and heart valve function (Figure HE14).

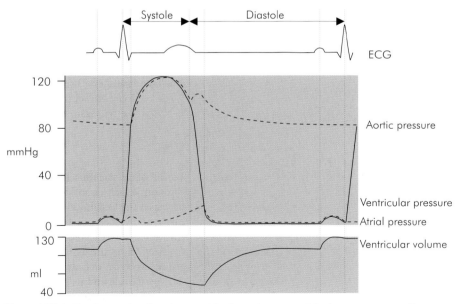

Figure HE14 Cardiac cycle, showing ventricular volume, ventricular pressure, aortic pressure and atrial pressure

Systolic function

Systole can be broken down into the following stages:
- Isovolumetric ventricular contraction
- Ventricular ejection

Systole commences with a period of isovolumetric contraction initiated by the QRS complex of the ECG. During this brief period the volume of the ventricle does not change since both the AV and semilunar valves are closed. Isovolumetric contraction ends when the semilunar valve opens and ejection begins. The events during systole are described below and should be considered along with the ventricular pressure, aortic pressure and ventricular volume curves.

Left ventricular pressure

The QRS complex of the ECG initiates ventricular contraction. As the pressure in the left ventricle increases during isovolumetric contraction, it comes to exceed the pressure in the aorta. At this point the aortic valve opens and ejection begins. The aortic valve opens at about 80 mmHg. Ejection continues as long as ventricular pressure exceeds aortic pressure. The total volume ejected into the aorta is the stroke volume (SV). The ventricular pressure increases initially during ejection, but then starts to decrease as the ventricle relaxes. The gradient between ventricle and aorta starts to reverse at this point, since LV pressure has started to fall but aortic pressure is maintained by the momentum of the last of the ejected blood. When the ventricular to aortic pressure gradient has reversed, the aortic valve closes and isovolumetric relaxation begins. The dicrotic notch on the aortic pressure curve (below) marks this point. The LV pressure normally reaches a systolic maximum of 120 mmHg. At the end of systole the LV pressure is described as the end-systolic pressure and the LV volume is at its smallest (end-systolic volume), about 40–50 ml.

Right ventricular pressure

This follows a similar course to LV pressure. The tricuspid and pulmonary valves dictate events, with ejection occurring into the pulmonary artery. Right ventricular pressure reaches a maximum of about 20–24 mmHg during systole.

Ventricular volume

Diastole commences in the left side of the heart with closure of the aortic valve and relaxation of the left ventricle. Since the mitral and aortic valves are both closed at this time the relaxation is described as isovolumetric. The ventricle contains 40–50 ml blood at this stage (end-systolic volume). Isovolumetric relaxation ends with opening of the mitral valve, when a period of rapid filling of the ventricle begins, which lasts for the first third of diastole. After the initial period of rapid filling follows a period of passive filling called diastasis and flow continues passively into the ventricle, providing up to 75% (60 ml) of the filling volume. During the last third of diastole the P wave of the ECG initiates atrial contraction, which contributes the remaining 25% of filling to give an end-diastolic volume of about 120 ml. The end-diastolic volume of the ventricle is not always 120 ml, but can vary due to changes in venous return to the heart, contractility and heart rate. A similar sequence of events occurs on the right side of the heart, controlled by the pulmonary and tricuspid valves (Figure HE14).

Aortic pressure curve

Ejection of blood into the aorta begins when the aortic valve opens. During ejection the aortic pressure follows the ventricular pressure curve apart from a small pressure gradient. This gradient is about 1–2 mmHg when the aortic valve is normal. As ejection proceeds aortic pressure increases to a maximum (systolic pressure) and starts to fall as the LV relaxes. When the ventricular pressure has fallen below the aortic pressure, the aortic valve closes and ejection ceases. Following closure of the aortic valve, elastic rebound of the aorta walls gives rise to a small hump in the aortic pressure curve forming the dicrotic notch. This notch marks the beginning of diastole. During diastole the aortic pressure gradually falls to a minimum (diastolic pressure), due to the runoff of blood into the systemic circulation.

Atrial pressure

Normally blood fills the right atrium (RA) via the superior and inferior venae cavae, continuously throughout the cardiac cycle. This flow is returned from the peripheral circulation and is called the venous return to the heart. On the left side of the heart, the left atrium (LA) receives blood from the pulmonary vascular bed via the pulmonary veins.

Passive filling of the atria produces RA pressures of 0–2 mmHg and LA pressures of 2–5 mmHg. During diastole atrial pressures follow ventricular pressures since the AV valves are open and the two chambers are joined. Three waves or peaks are produced in the atrial pressure curve during the cycle. At the end of diastole the atria prime the ventricles by contracting and developing pressures between 0 and 5 mmHg. Atrial contraction is shown on the atrial pressure curve as a smooth peak immediately preceding systole, the 'a' wave. As systole begins the AV valves close and a brief period of isovolumetric contraction occurs, producing a second low-pressure peak, the 'c' wave. This is due to the AV valve bulging back into the atrium.

As blood is ejected during systole the atrium continues to fill with the AV valve closed and atrial pressure increases until early diastole when the AV valve opens. At this point rapid filling of the ventricles commences and a sudden fall in atrial pressure follows. This gives rise to the 'v' wave (Figure HE14).

Diastolic function

Diastole can be broken down into the following stages:
- Isovolumetric ventricular relaxation
- Rapid ventricular filling
- Slow ventricular filling (diastasis)
- Atrial contraction

Although diastole appears to be a passive part of the cardiac cycle, it has some important functions:
- Myocardial relaxation – a metabolically active phase. One essential process is the reuptake of calcium by the sarcoplasmic reticulum. Incomplete reuptake leads to diastolic dysfunction due to decreased end-diastolic compliance. The negative slope of the ventricular pressure–time curve during isovolumetric relaxation (termed dP/dt(max)) indicates myocardial relaxation. Increased sympathetic tone or circulating catecholamine levels give rise to an increased dP/dt(max). This is known as positive lusitropy.
- Ventricular filling – provides the volume for the cardiac pump. Most of the ventricular filling occurs during early diastole. There is only a small increase in ventricular volume during diastasis. As the heart rate increases diastasis is shortened first. When the heart rate exceeds about 140 bpm, rapid filling in early diastole becomes compromised and the volume of blood ejected during systole (stroke volume, SV) is significantly decreased.
- Atrial contraction – contributes up to 25% of total ventricular filling in the normal heart. This atrial contribution can become of greater importance in the presence of myocardial ischaemia or ventricular hypertrophy.

- Coronary artery perfusion – the greater part of left coronary blood flow occurs during diastole.

Cardiac valves

The cardiac valves open and close passively in response to the changes in pressure gradient across them. These valves control the sequence of flow between atria and ventricles, and from the ventricles to the pulmonary and systemic circulations. Valve timing in relation to the ventricular pressure curve is shown in Figure HE15.

The AV valves are the mitral and tricuspid valves. These prevent backflow from the ventricles into the atria during systole. The papillary muscles are attached to the AV valves by chordae tendinae. They contract together with the ventricular muscle during systole, but do not help to close the valves. They prevent excessive bulging of the valves into the atria and pull the base of the heart toward the ventricular apex to shorten the longitudinal axis of the ventricle, thus increasing systolic efficiency.

The semilunar (SL) valves are the aortic and pulmonary valves. These prevent backflow from the aorta and pulmonary arteries into the ventricles during diastole. The SL valves function quite differently from the AV valves because they are exposed to higher pressures in the arteries. They are smaller (normal aortic valve area is 2.6–3.5 cm^2 while normal mitral valve area is 4–6 cm^2), and therefore the blood velocity through them is greater.

Disease in the cardiac valves may cause them to leak when they are meant to be closed, thus allowing backflow or regurgitation. This situation leads to inefficiency in producing cardiac output (CO), since the work done by the heart has to increase to compensate for the backflow and yet maintain adequate CO. Mitral and aortic regurgitation are the most common regurgitant lesions.

Alternatively, the orifice of a valve may become narrowed or stenotic. This obstructs the flow of blood through it and requires increased pressure gradients to be generated across the valve to achieve adequate blood flows. In mitral stenosis the valve area can be reduced by >50%. This causes the left atrium to contract more forcefully to maintain ventricular filling. In severe cases a valve area of 1 cm^2 can require the left atrium to produce peak pressures of 25 mmHg to produce normal CO. Aortic stenosis obstructs left ventricular output and increases the workload of the left ventricle. The stenosis can multiply the normal pressure gradient across the aortic valve during systole by 10 times or more. When the aortic valve area

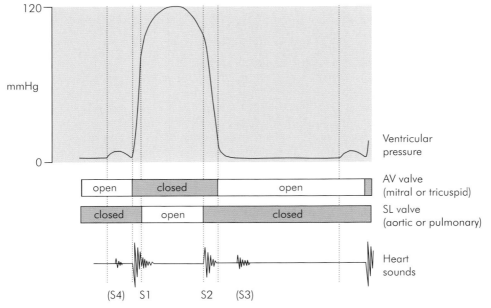

Figure HE15 Heart sounds and timing

decreases by 70% (<0.8 cm^2), the stenosis becomes critical and systolic pressure gradients across the valve of >50 mmHg may be required to produce normal CO.

Differences in timing between left and right sides of the heart

Although the sequence of events on each side of the heart is similar, events occur asynchronously. This disparity in timing reflects differences in anatomy and working pressures between left and right sides of the heart. RA systole precedes LA systole; however, RV contraction starts after LV contraction. In spite of contracting later, the RV starts to eject blood before the LV because pulmonary artery pressure is lower than aortic pressure. Differences of timing also occur in the closure of the heart valves. These differences in valve timing lead to 'splitting' of the heart sounds.

Heart sounds and murmurs

In the normal individual two heart sounds can be heard during each cardiac cycle. They are produced by closure of the valves, which causes the ventricular walls and valve leaflets to vibrate, and also produces turbulence of the interrupted blood flow. The first sound (S1) occurs when the AV valves close at the start of ventricular systole and is best heard over the apex of the heart. The mitral valve normally closes earlier than the tricuspid by 10–30 ms. Thus S1 is split, with the mitral component occurring before the tricuspid component. The second sound (S2) corresponds to closure of the SL valves and is heard at the beginning of diastole. During inspiration the aortic valve closes before the pulmonary valve due to increased venous return, which delays RV ejection. During expiration aortic and pulmonary valve closure is simultaneous, and S2 appears to be a single sound. S2 is louder when the diastolic pressure is elevated in the aorta or pulmonary artery.

Abnormal heart sounds can be heard under pathological conditions. Heart failure can cause a third heart sound (S3) to be heard in mid-diastole. This is due to rapid filling of a dilated non-compliant ventricle following the opening of the AV valves. In conditions where stronger atrial contraction develops to help ventricular filling, a fourth heart sound (S4) may occur immediately before S1 (systole). This is thought to be due to ventricular wall vibration in response to forceful atrial filling.

When the cardiac valves undergo pathological changes abnormal sounds called murmurs can sometimes be heard. Under normal conditions blood flow is not turbulent but remains laminar up to a critical velocity. When blood flows across a narrowed valve, flow velocities are higher and

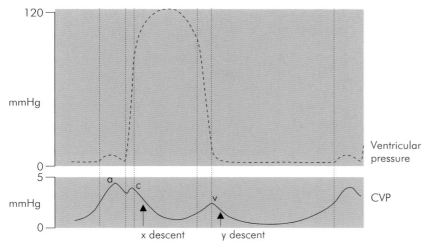

Figure HE16 Central venous pressure waveform

turbulent, giving rise to a murmur. In the case of a 'leaking' or incompetent valve, turbulent regurgitant flow is produced, which also creates a murmur. The most common murmurs occur due to faults in the mitral and aortic valves. The valve involved and the type of lesion (stenotic or regurgitant) can be identified by the timing of the murmur and the site on the chest wall where it is loudest. In normal individuals without cardiac disease (especially children) soft physiological systolic murmurs can often be heard.

Central venous pressure

Central venous pressure (CVP) is usually monitored in the large veins feeding the superior vena cava, i.e. the internal jugular or subclavian veins. The CVP waveform reflects right atrial pressure, and therefore consists of 'a', 'c' and 'v' waves that correspond to atrial contraction, isovolumetric contraction and opening of the tricuspid valve, as described above. There are also two labelled downward deflections, the 'x' and 'y' descents, which occur after the 'c' and 'v' waves respectively (Figure HE16). The 'x' descent reflects the fall in right ventricular pressure when the pulmonary valve opens. The 'y' descent corresponds to the initial drop in atrial pressure caused by rapid ventricular filling when the AV valves open. Various pathological conditions affect mean CVP or alter the CVP waveform. For example, if the timing of atrial and ventricular contraction become dissociated (as in 3° block) the right atrium contracts against a closed tricuspid valve and produces prominent or 'cannon' 'a' waves (Figure HE17).

Factor	Change in CVP
Depleted intravascular volume	↓ mean CVP
Excessive intravascular volume ('overloading' with intravascular fluid)	↑ mean CVP
Cardiac failure	↑ mean CVP
Pericardial tamponade	↑ mean CVP
Bradycardia	More distinct 'a', 'c' and 'v' waves
Tachycardia	Fusion of 'a' and 'c' waves
AV junctional rhythm	Regular cannon 'a' waves
3° AV block	Irregular cannon 'a' waves
Tricuspid regurgitation	Loss of 'c' wave and 'x' descent. Prominent 'v' waves

Figure HE17 Some factors affecting the central venous pressure waveform

The cardiac pump

Ventricular pressure–volume loop

The mechanical performance of the heart as a pump can be summarised using a ventricular pressure–volume (PV) loop. An example for the left ventricle is shown in Figure HE18.

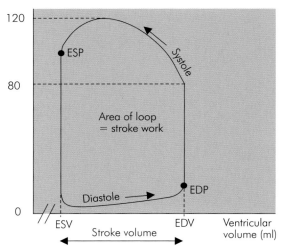

Figure HE18 Pressure–volume loop for left ventricle

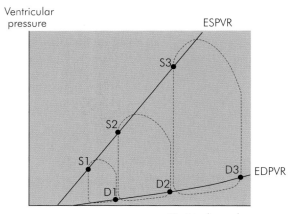

Figure HE19 End-diastolic and end-systolic pressure–volume relationship curves

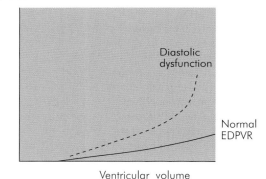

Figure HE20 Effects of diastolic dysfunction on the end-diastolic pressure–volume relationship curve

The cycle starts at the end-diastolic point (EDP). Isovolumetric contraction follows, represented by a vertical ascending segment which ends with the opening of the aortic valve. The ejection phase segment passes across the top of the loop from right to left. Ejection ends at the end-systolic point (ESP) when the aortic valve closes. Isovolumetric relaxation follows next as a vertical descending segment ending when the mitral valve opens. The final lower segment corresponds to ventricular filling and ends when the mitral valve closes at EDP.

The PV loop can be used to derive several parameters reflecting ventricular function including SV, stroke work (SW), end-diastolic volume (EDV) and end-systolic volume (ESV).

End-diastolic pressure–volume relationship

On the ventricular pressure PV loop, the EDP records volume and pressure at the end of diastole. If different PV loops are plotted for a given ventricle, different EDPs are obtained (D1, D2, and D3; Figure HE19).

These points form a PV relationship for the ventricle at end-diastole when plotted. This is called the end-diastolic PV relationship (EDPVR). EDPVR is a useful indicator of diastolic function, and in particular ventricular filling performance, since its gradient is equal to the elastance (or compliance^{-1}) of the ventricle during filling. The steeper this gradient, the lower the compliance of the ventricle during filling. Over the normal range of ventricular filling volumes the EDPVR gradient is approximately linear and the ventricle is relatively compliant. As EDV increases and the ventricle becomes more distended at the end of diastole, the EDPVR gradient becomes steeper, showing a marked decrease in ventricular compliance to filling. Pathological conditions such as ischaemic heart disease and ventricular hypertrophy can shift the EDPVR up and to the left, demonstrating ventricular diastolic dysfunction (Figure HE20).

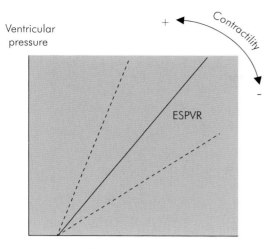

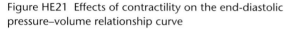

Figure HE21 Effects of contractility on the end-diastolic pressure–volume relationship curve

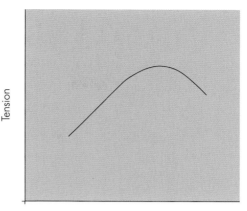

Figure HE22 Frank curve for isolated muscle fibre

End-systolic pressure–volume relationship
The ESP from several ventricular PV loops (S1, S2, S3) may be plotted to give an end-systolic PV curve (Figure HE21). This curve is the ESPVR. The gradient of the ESPVR curve represents the elastance of the contracted ventricle at the end of systole. This is partially dependent on how forcefully the ventricle contracts, and hence is related to ventricular contractility. The ESPVR curve is approximately linear under normal conditions. Increased non-linearity is introduced under ischaemic or hypercontractile conditions and appears as a change in gradient and shift in the curve up or down.

Frank–Starling curve
The function of the heart as a pump is based on cardiac muscle. The contractile properties of cardiac muscle not only provide the engine to drive the cardiac pump but also give the heart an intrinsic ability to adapt its performance to a continually varying venous return. The mechanism underlying this adaptive ability is the Frank–Starling relationship.

The Frank curve
Frank demonstrated in isolated muscle fibre preparations that the tension developed on contraction was dependent on the initial length of the fibre. As initial length increased from resting value, the tension developed during

contraction increased and reached a maximum. Above this, the tension declined as the sarcomeres became overextended (Figure HE22).

The Starling curve
The above property of isolated cardiac muscle fibres can be applied to the muscle fibres in the walls of an intact ventricle, where the length of muscle fibres is related to the volume of the ventricle. In this case the tension per unit cross section (ventricular wall stress, T), developed in the wall during contraction, is dependent on the end-diastolic volume. Laplace's law relates the wall stress to internal pressure in an elastic sphere; thus, the Frank relationship for an isolated muscle fibre translates into a relationship between intraventricular pressure and EDV during isovolumetric contraction. Effectively, the greater the ventricular filling volume, the stronger the contraction of the ventricle – a mechanism that gives the intact heart its built-in ability to adjust to varying levels of venous return.

Starling confirmed in ejecting mammalian hearts that with a constant aortic pressure, an increase in EDV produces a more forceful contraction and an increase in SV.

The Frank–Starling relationship
In the intact heart, a ventricular function curve (the Frank–Starling curve) can be plotted to demonstrate the ability of the ventricle to vary its mechanical output according to its filling volumes. An index of mechanical output (such as SV) can be plotted against a measure of filling pressure (such as CVP) (Figure HE23).

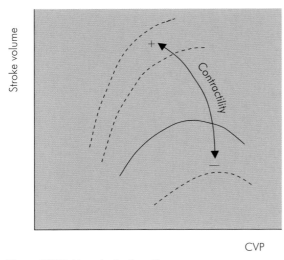

CVP

Figure HE23 Ventricular function curve

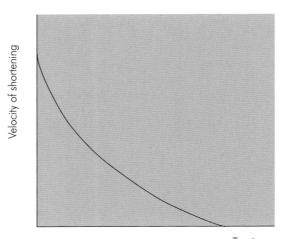

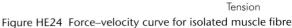

Tension

Figure HE24 Force–velocity curve for isolated muscle fibre

The Frank–Starling curve and cardiac failure

The normal ventricle never fills to an EDV that would place it on the descending limb of the Frank–Starling curve. This is because of a decreased compliance of the ventricle that occurs at high filling pressures. Sarcomere length at optimum filling pressures (about 12 mmHg) is 2.2 µm; however, even if filling pressures are increased four-fold (>50 mmHg) sarcomere length will not increase beyond about 2.6 µm.

If the heart becomes pathologically dilated, as in cardiac failure, ventricular function may then shift to the descending portion of the Frank–Starling curve, and cardiac decompensation ensues. Cardiac function can also deteriorate when factors such as hypoxia, acidosis or β blockers shift the Frank–Starling curve down and to the right, depressing cardiac performance. Alternatively, other factors such as endogenous catecholamines or inotropes can shift the Frank–Starling curve upwards and to the left, enhancing cardiac performance.

Force–velocity curve for cardiac muscle

Starling not only investigated the sarcomere tension–length relationship, but also looked at the interaction between muscle force and velocity. The force–velocity curve demonstrates that the force generated and the velocity of muscle shortening is inversely related. Changes in preload and contractility will influence this relationship by shifting the force–velocity curve (Figure HE24).

Stroke volume and ejection fraction

SV is the volume of blood ejected by the ventricle with a single contraction and can be defined as the difference between the end-diastolic volume and the end-systolic volume in the following equation:

$$SV = EDV - ESV$$

The normal SV is between 70 and 80 ml, and may be normalised to take account of body size by dividing by body surface area (BSA). This gives a stroke index (SI), which for a 70 kg normal person (BSA = 1.7 m^2) is 30–65 ml beat^{-1} m^{-2}. SV can also be given as a percentage of the EDV. It is then called ejection fraction (EF), a formula for which is:

$$\text{Ejection fraction} = \frac{EDV - ESV}{EDV} = \frac{SV}{EDV} \times 100\%$$

The normal EF is about 60–65%, and it is a useful index of ventricular contractility.

Measurement of stroke volume
Ventriculography

This has been the gold standard for measuring ventricular volumes, to which less invasive measurement methods have been compared. However, it is a cumbersome procedure done in the catheter suite and is not appropriate for repeated estimations. Other techniques to measure LV volume and size include computed tomography, magnetic resonance imaging and radionuclide scans, but none is practical in the perioperative setting.

Echocardiography

The end-systolic and end-diastolic areas can be measured by two-dimensional echocardiography to give an estimate of the SV. SV is then multiplied by the heart rate to obtain the CO. This technique is limited by the approximation made to transform the two-dimensional images of the ventricular into volumes.

Transoesophageal echocardiography

A recent development has been the introduction of transoesophageal echocardiography (TOE). Several studies have found a good correlation between left ventricular areas measured by TOE and LV areas or volumes obtained by other techniques. The two-dimensional transgastric short axis view of LV at the level of the papillary muscles reflects LV filling reasonably well. Modern echocardiography includes the automated border detection method that displays the LV area throughout the cardiac cycle, together with the fractional area change (FAC) calculation, where:

$$FAC = \frac{\text{End diastolic area} - \text{End systolic area}}{\text{End diastolic area}}$$

The normal value for FAC varies between 50% and 70%.

Thoracic impedance

A small alternating current of low amplitude and high frequency is introduced between two sets of electrodes around the neck and lower thorax. The resultant electrical impedance between the neck and thoracic electrodes is measured, and represents the transthoracic impedance. Both ventilation and pulsatile blood flow produce changes in thoracic impedance. SV can be estimated by considering the pulsatile cardiac component of the impedance signal only. Cardiac output can then be calculated by measuring the heart rate and taking the product HR × SV. Although this technique is non-invasive and can provide a continuous reading of CO, a significant degree of inaccuracy is present.

Cardiac output

Cardiac output gives a measure of the performance of the heart as a pump. It is defined as the volume of blood pumped by the LV (or RV) per minute, and is equal to the product of the SV and heart rate:

$$CO = SV \times HR$$

With a normal HR = 70–80 bpm and SV = 70–80 ml, the average CO of a 70 kg person varies between 5 and 6 l min^{-1} under resting conditions. To compare patients of different body sizes, CO can be divided by the patient's body surface area to give a normalised parameter called the cardiac index (CI):

$$CI = \frac{CO}{BSA}$$

BSA can be estimated from the height (cm) and weight (kg) of an individual and is quoted in m^2. The average 70 kg adult has a BSA = 1.7 m^2 and a CI = 3–3.5 litres min^{-1} m^{-2}.

When the oxygen demand of the body increases during exercise, the CO of a young, healthy individual can increase up to five-fold. CO should always be evaluated with reference to the oxygen demand at the time.

Cardiac output measurement

In animal models CO can be measured directly by cannulating the aorta, pulmonary artery or any of the great veins and then using an electromagnetic or ultrasonic flowmeter. This is not appropriate in a clinical situation, however, and CO is usually measured by indirect methods. Some current methods of monitoring cardiac output in clinical practice are outlined in Figure HE25.

Indicator dilution techniques

Thermodilution is at present the most commonly used method to measure CO at the bedside. A pulmonary artery catheter (PAC) is inserted, cold saline is injected into the RA, and the change in blood temperature is measured by the PAC thermistor in the pulmonary artery. The cardiac output is calculated using the modified Stewart–Hamilton equation:

$$CO = \frac{V(T_B - T_I) \times K_1 \times K_2}{\int_0^\infty T_B(t)dt}$$

where

V = volume of injectate
T_B = initial blood temperature (°C)
T_I = initial injectate temperature (°C)
K_1 = density constant
K_2 = computation constant

and

$$\int_0^\infty T_B(t)\,dt = \text{integral of blood temperature change}$$

CO is inversely proportional to the area under the temperature–time curve. This technique is popular

Cardiac output (CO) monitor	Method of CO measurement	Advantages	Disadvantages
Pulmonary artery catheter (Swan–Ganz)	Pulmonary artery thermodilution: cold saline bolus injected into PAC, thermodilution principle, measured by thermistor in PAC tip in the pulmonary artery	Continuous PA pressures PACWP measurement Can be used with intra-aortic balloon pump (IABP) Heat dissipation minimised by short travel from injection to catheter tip 'Gold standard' for comparison with newer methods	Invasive – sheath in large vein, catheter through right heart Risk of injury to heart and pulmonary vessels, catheter migration No evident outcome benefit Not continuous
LiDCO	Transpulmonary lithium dilution. Calibration by lithium chloride bolus into CVP or vein while sampling arterial blood past lithium electrode. Continuous CO by arterial wave form analysis	Avoids heat dissipation errors. Uses routine CVP and arterial lines Provides continuous CO Various displays target CO to aid management	Requires 24-hourly calibration No pulmonary artery pressures Not used in patient with IABP Cannot be used in patients on lithium
PiCCO	Transpulmonary thermodilution: cold saline bolus injected into CVP line. Thermistor in femoral a-line. CO by continuous arterial wave form analysis	Arterial line is also used for blood sampling Continuous CO	Arterial line in femoral artery. Errors due to heat dissipation because of trans-pulmonary passage between injection point and thermistor
Pulse contour CO Vigileo	Analysis of arterial waveform characteristics and calculate CO from patient demographic data	Arterial line transducer supplied by manufacturer No calibration input	Uses extrapolation from patient demographic data Dependent on quality of a-line trace No use in patient with IABP
Doppler	Oesophageal or sternal notch Doppler probe. Calculation of CO using Doppler signals and patient demographic data	Does not require vascular access No calibration needed	Consistency of monitoring depends on Doppler trace quality Cannot be used in patient with IABP

Author: R S Pretorius MB ChB MFamMed MMed (Anaes), Consultant Anaesthetist, University Hospitals of Leicester

Figure HE25 Current methods of monitoring cardiac output

because multiple CO estimations can be made at frequent intervals without blood sampling. The accuracy of the technique is influenced by several factors, which include intracardiac shunts, tricuspid regurgitation and positive pressure ventilation.

A modification of this principle is used in the 'continuous' CO monitor. A pulse of electrical current heats up a proximal part of the PAC creating a bolus of warmed blood. The temperature rise is sensed when the warmed blood passes a thermistor in the pulmonary artery. A computer then calculates the 'area under the curve' and, hence, CO.

Dye dilution

This was the most popular technique prior to thermodilution. Indocyanine green is injected into a central vein, while blood is continuously sampled from an arterial cannula. The change in indicator concentration over time is measured, a computer calculates the area under the dye concentration curve, and CO is computed. Unfortunately recirculation and build-up of the indicator results in a high background concentration, which limits the total number of measurements that can be taken. The dye is non-toxic and rapidly removed from circulation by the liver.

Fick method

The Fick principle states that the amount of a substance taken up by an organ (or the whole body) per unit time is equal to the arterial concentration of the substance minus the venous concentration (a–v difference), times the blood flow. This can be applied to the oxygen content of blood to determine CO.

First, the steady-state oxygen content of venous (CvO_2) and arterial blood (CaO_2) are measured. Then oxygen uptake in the lungs is measured over 1 minute ($\dot{V}O_2$). Finally, the Fick principle is applied to calculate the blood flowing in 1 minute:

$$\text{Cardiac output} = \frac{\dot{V}O_2}{(CaO_2 - CvO_2)}$$

Errors in sampling, and the inability to maintain steady-state conditions, limit this technique.

Doppler techniques

Ultrasonic Doppler transducers have been incorporated into pulmonary artery catheters, endotracheal tubes, suprasternal probes and oesophageal probes. These probes can then be used to measure mean blood flow velocity through the aorta or any valve orifice. Using an estimation for the cross-sectional area of flow, the flow velocity–time integral, heart rate and a constant, CO can be calculated.

Control of cardiac pump function

The product of stroke volume (SV) and heart rate (HR) gives cardiac output (CO). The factors determining CO can thus be divided into those affecting HR and those that determine SV. Overall control of CO is a combination of the mechanisms controlling SV and HR. This is illustrated in Figure HE26, and the individual control of SV and HR is considered in detail below.

Stroke volume

Several factors determine SV. The three major determinants of SV are:

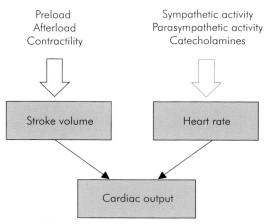

Figure HE26 Control of cardiac output

- Preload
- Afterload
- Contractility

Overall control of SV is summarised in Figure HE27. The above factors are based on physiological concepts arising from the performance of isolated muscle preparations. They have become useful in clinical practice when applied to the intact heart, but are difficult or impractical to measure directly. Hence more easily monitored parameters are used as practical indices. A summary definition for each of the above factors is given, consisting of:
- Physiological definition – a theoretical definition for the parameter
- Physiological index – a measurement from which the physiological definition can be derived
- Practical concept – a description of the parameter suitable for clinical use
- Practical index – a measurement used clinically for the parameter

Preload

In clinical circumstances, 'preload' remains loosely defined and has become synonymous with a range of parameters including CVP, venous return and pulmonary capillary wedge pressure.

A strict definition for preload can be obtained from the Frank relationship between muscle fibre length and developed tension. Here preload is the initial length of the muscle fibre before contraction. In the intact ventricle the preload would, therefore, be equivalent to the end-diastolic volume, since the pre-systolic length of the myocardial fibres will be directly related to EDV. See Figure HE28.

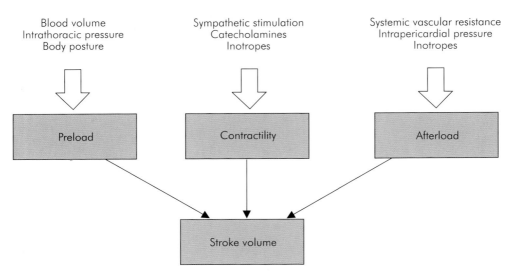

Figure HE27 Control of stroke volume

- Physiological definition – Pre-systolic length of cardiac muscle fibres
- Physiological index – End-diastolic volume
- Practical concept – Filling pressure of ventricles
- Practical index – CVP or PCWP

Various factors affecting EDV include:
  Total blood volume
  Body position
  Intrathoracic and intrapericardial pressures
  Venous tone and compliance
  Pumping action of skeletal muscles
  Synchronous atrial contribution to ventricular filling
  Ventricular end-diastolic compliance

Figure HE28 Summary definition of preload

Measurement of preload

There are no convenient or practical methods of measuring EDV directly. Because of this EDP is often used when assessing the filling conditions of the intact ventricle. EDP is related to EDV by the ventricular end-diastolic PV curve and is sometimes referred to as the 'filling pressure' of the ventricle. EDPVR is approximately linear at normal filling pressures, but the gradient (ventricular elastance = compliance^{-1}) gradually increases as filling pressure increases. EDP is, therefore, only a reasonable index of preload under normal conditions.

In practice, EDP can be estimated on the left side of the heart, by measuring left atrial pressure (LAP), pulmonary capillary wedge pressure (PCWP) or pulmonary artery diastolic pressure (PADP). On the right side, preload is reflected by right atrial pressure (RAP) or central venous pressure. These measurements can be made using a pulmonary artery catheter, but the most common measurements used are CVP and PCWP as indices of right and left preload respectively. Interpretation of these estimates is subject to the following limitations:

- Ventricular compliance may not be normal, as it can be reduced by factors such as myocardial ischaemia, ventricular hypertrophy or pericardial tamponade. In a non-compliant ventricle, higher than normal filling pressures may be required to provide adequate preload.
- The AV valve may be abnormal. The presence of mitral stenosis may require higher than normal filling pressures to achieve adequate preload in the left ventricle.
- Positive intrathoracic pressures can be transmitted through to a pulmonary artery catheter and increase the mean PCWP reading. In the case of a ventilated patient, positive end-expiratory pressure (PEEP) and the inspiratory pressure cycles can affect the PCWP signal.
- Placement of the PAC in the dependent part of the lung can add a hydrostatic pressure component to a PCWP signal.

- Physiological definition – Ventricular wall stress developed during systole
- Physiological index – Systolic ventricular wall stress
- Practical concept – Intraventricular pressure developed during systole
- Practical index – SVR and MAP, PVR and MPAP

Factors which affect afterload include:
 Systemic or pulmonary vascular resistance
 Factors stimulating or depressing cardiac contraction
 Intrathoracic pressure or intrapericardial pressure
 Preload
 Ventricular wall thickness

Figure HE29 Summary definition of afterload

- Increased pulmonary vascular resistance, as in pulmonary hypertension, can lead to higher than normal pulmonary artery diastolic pressure (PADP). This reduces the accuracy of the PADP as an estimate of left-sided preload.

Afterload

In an isolated muscle fibre preparation, afterload is defined as the tension developed during contraction. Thus, afterload is related to the mechanical resistance to shortening of the muscle fibre. In the intact heart, afterload becomes the tension per unit cross section (T), developed in the ventricular wall during systole. This can be related to the intraventricular pressure during systole, by applying Laplace's law for pressure in an elastic sphere as follows:

$$\text{Intraventricular pressure} = \frac{2hT}{r}$$

where

h = ventricular wall thickness
r = radius of the ventricular cavity

Afterload is thus a measure of how forcefully the ventricle contracts during systole to eject blood (Figure HE29).

The normal ventricle has an intrinsic ability to increase its performance in response to increases in afterload, to maintain SV. If the afterload increases suddenly, it causes an initial fall in SV. The ventricle then increases its EDV in response to the change, which in turn restores the SV. This is called the Anrep effect.

Measurement of afterload

Systematic vascular resistance (SVR), SV index and elastance may be used to give an estimate of afterload.

- Arterial pressure or ventricular pressures during systole normally follow each other and are indirect indices of ventricular wall tension. Arterial systolic pressure is often the available measurement, but its accuracy is limited if there is a significant gradient between aorta and ventricle, e.g. as in aortic stenosis.
- Systemic vascular resistance is the most commonly used index of afterload in clinical practice, and can be calculated from mean arterial pressure (MAP), central venous pressure and CO, as follows:

$$\text{SVR} = \frac{\text{MAP} - \text{CVP}}{\text{CO}} \times 80 \, \text{dynes.s cm}^{-5}$$

The normal value for SVR ranges from 900 to 1400 dynes.s cm^{-5}. SVR is not a good estimate of afterload, since it is only one component determining afterload, and does not provide any index of intraventricular pressures generated during systole (i.e. how hard the ventricle is contracting). Clearly, if the ventricle only generates low intraventricular pressures by contracting softly, the afterload is low irrespective of SVR.

In a similar manner the pulmonary vascular resistance (PVR) may be calculated as an index of RV afterload, using mean pulmonary arterial pressure (MPAP), pulmonary capillary wedge pressure and CO:

$$\text{PVR} = \frac{\text{MPAP} - \text{PCWP}}{\text{CO}} \times 80 \, \text{dynes.s cm}^{-5}$$

The normal PVR ranges from 90 to 150 dynes.s cm^{-5}. CO, PAP and PCWP have to be obtained with a PAC to calculate SVR and PVR.

- Systemic vascular impedance is the mechanical property of the vascular system opposing the ejection and flow of blood into it. This is composed of two components. One is the resistive or steady-flow component, which is the SVR (see above). This component is mainly due to the frictional opposition to flow in the vessels. The other component is the reactive or frequency-dependent component, which is due to the compliance of the vessel walls and inertia of the ejected blood. This component is dependent on the pulsatile nature of the flow and rapidity of ejection. A major part of this reactive component is formed by the arterial elastance (Ea).
- Arterial elastance is the inverse of arterial compliance and is a measure of the elastic forces in the arterial system that tend to oppose the ejection of blood into it. Determination of Ea involves plotting a PV curve for the arterial system using different SV and recording

- Physiological definition – Systolic myocardial work done with given pre- and afterload
- Physiological index – Ventricular stroke work index or maximum slope (dP/dt) of ventricular isovolumetric contraction curve
- Practical concept – Ejection fraction for given CVP and MAP
- Practical index – Ejection fraction

Figure HE30 Summary definition of contractility

end-systolic pressures. The slope of the curve then gives the effective elastance (compliance^{-1}) of the arterial system.

Contractility

Contractility is a poorly defined term describing the intrinsic ability of a cardiac muscle fibre to do mechanical work when it contracts with a predefined load and initial degree of stretch. In the intact ventricle contractility reflects the amount of work that can be done for a given pre- and afterload (Figure HE30).

Contractility can be increased by various factors, including:

- Increased serum calcium levels
- Sympathetic stimulation
- Parasympathetic inhibition
- Positive inotropic drugs

Contractility can be decreased by various factors, including:

- Decreased serum calcium levels
- Parasympathetic stimulation
- Sympathetic blockade
- Myocardial ischaemia or infarction
- Hypoxia and acidosis
- Mismatched ventriculoarterial coupling

Measurement of contractility

Contractility is an index of work performance at a given pre- and afterload. Ideally these parameters should be controlled during measurement, which is often impractical. Accordingly, pre- and afterload should be recorded during assessment of contractility. The interpretation of contractility measurements is then made at the given pre- and afterload.

The calculation of ventricular work done during systole requires an integral of the ventricular PV loop area. This is not a practical measurement, but an index loosely reflecting systolic work is stroke work, obtained from the following

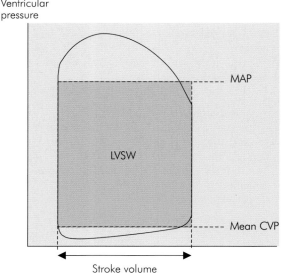

Figure HE31 Left ventricular stroke work estimate for ventricular pressure–volume loop area

product:

SW = (SV) × (mean arterial pressure – filling pressure)

Figure HE31 illustrates how this product approximates to the PV loop area for the left ventricle.

The SV work index (SVWI) is a more useful indicator of contractility. It is calculated by normalising stroke work for body surface area by using stroke index in its calculation. Thus, for the left ventricular stroke work index (LVSWI):

$$LVSWI = \frac{(MAP - PCWP) \times SI}{100} \times 1.36 \text{ g.m m}^{-2}$$

Normal values for LVSWI are 45–60 g.m m^{-2}.

While for the right ventricle (right ventricular stroke work index, RVSWI):

$$RVSWI = \frac{(MPAP - CVP) \times SI}{100} \times 1.36 \text{ g.m m}^{-2}$$

Normal values for RVSWI are 5–10 g.m m^{-2}.

Other measures of contractility include ejection fraction and ventricular function curves.

Ejection fraction (EF) is measured by radionuclide ventriculography or transthoracic echocardiography. It is often derived from the fractional area change (FAC) measurement. EF and FAC are both sensitive to pre- and afterload. These latter parameters should also be evaluated with

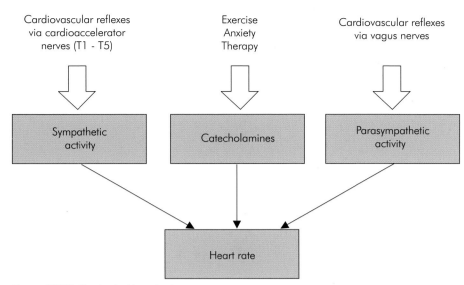

Figure HE32 Control of heart rate

EF or FAC. There is a clear association between EF and prognosis in cardiac patients.

Ventricular function curves can be plotted between an index of ventricular filling (e.g. CVP or PCWP) and an index of ventricular performance (e.g. CO or SV). Factors increasing contractility will shift the curve upwards and to the left while those decreasing contractility will shift it downwards and to the right.

Heart rate

The heart rate (HR) is normally determined by the spontaneous depolarisation rate of the SA node pacemaker cells. The normal heart rate of 60–80 bpm is much slower than the intrinsic rate of the denervated heart (110 bpm). This is because of the dominant parasympathetic tone in the intact cardiovascular system (Figure HE32).

Autonomic control of pacemaker discharge rate

In vivo, control of the pacemaker rate is mediated peripherally via the autonomic nervous system. Central control of pacemaker rate lies in parasympathetic and sympathetic nuclei of the medulla. These are responsible for cardiovascular reflexes, and are influenced by higher centres including the posterior hypothalamus and cortical areas. Relevant autonomic pathways may be categorised as follows:

- Parasympathetic – parasympathetic fibres to the heart originate in the dorsal motor nucleus of the vagus and the nucleus ambiguus in the medulla oblongata. These

parasympathetic fibres travel to the heart via the right and left vagus nerves. During embryological development the right vagus nerve becomes connected to the SA node, while the left vagus supplies the AV node. Vagal stimulation (parasympathetic activity) decreases the slope of phase 4 and also increases hyperpolarisation, thus slowing the heart rate.

- Sympathetic – sympathetic innervation to the heart originates in the sympathetic chain (T1–T5 fibres), passing via the stellate ganglion to all parts of the heart, with a strong representation to the ventricular muscle. The right side distributes to the SA node, while the left side primarily supplies the AV node. Sympathetic activity increases the slope of phase 4, and hence heart rate. This effect occurs in exercise, anxiety and febrile illness.

- Mixed – direct interconnections exist between the parasympathetic and sympathetic cardiac supplies which enable both systems to inhibit each other directly.

Cardiovascular reflexes

Some recognised cardiovascular reflexes controlling heart rate include:

- Lung volume stretch receptor reflex – moderate increases in lung volume increase HR via the vagus nerves.

- Chemoreceptor reflexes – the primary effect of carotid chemoreceptor stimulation is to activate vagal centres in the medulla, giving a decrease in HR. However, this is modified by a secondary effect exerted by concomitant excitation of respiratory centres in the medulla which oppose the primary effect.
- Atrial stretch receptor reflex (Bainbridge reflex) – stimulation of atrial stretch receptors by increases in venous return or blood volume gives rise to acceleration of the HR.
- Baroreceptor reflexes – stimulation of baroreceptors in the aortic arch or carotid sinus, by an increase in blood pressure lead to a decrease in HR. Similarly, a drop in blood pressure causes an increase in HR.

Effects of heart rate on cardiac output

Heart rate affects CO in the following ways:

- An increase in heart rate will lead to a progressive increase in CO up to about 140 bpm. When heart rate increases, SV decreases due to shorter diastolic filling time, but this only becomes significant at higher rates, >140 bpm.
- When HR >150 bpm the decrease in diastolic filling time reduces the CO significantly because it encroaches on rapid filling time. Diastolic time is affected by a tachycardia to a much greater extent than systolic time.
- The Bowditch phenomenon ('Treppe' or staircase effect) is increased inotropy in response to increased chronotropy. This occurs above 40 bpm and is due to the greater availability of intracellular calcium for excitation–contraction coupling which follows the reduced diastolic time available for calcium reuptake (Figure HE33).
- During a tachycardia in a normal heart, EDPVR will move to the left and downwards, i.e. smaller filling volumes at lower EDP. In an ischaemic heart, however, a tachycardia will move EDPVR to the left but upwards, i.e. smaller filling volumes at higher EDP.
- Tachycardia will increase the ventricular end-systolic elastance (Ees) due to the increased contractility.
- A pronounced bradycardia <40 bpm will cause a fall in CO, because the compensatory increase in SV is not enough to make up for the decrease in ejection rate.

Cardiovascular coupling

In clinical practice, assessment of cardiac function often relies on the available measurements of filling pressures

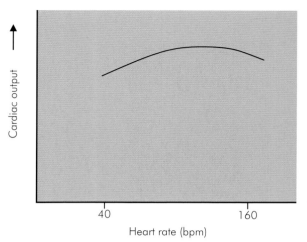

Figure HE33 Treppe or Bowditch effect of heart rate on cardiac output

(CVP and PCWP), arterial pressures (pulmonary and aortic) and CO. These measurements are dependent on two sets of characteristics that reflect:

- Contractile performance of the heart
- Elastance (PV relationship) of the vascular system

Assessing the relative effects of cardiac contractility and vascular system elastance on pressure measurements is important clinically, since it can influence therapeutic decisions.

Interpretation of pressure and CO measurements is aided by a consideration of the interaction or coupling between the heart and the vascular system. This can be performed at the arterial side (ventriculoarterial coupling) for arterial pressures, or on the venous side of the heart (ventriculovenous coupling) for CVP.

Ventriculoarterial coupling

Coupling between the ventricle and arterial system is illustrated by plotting the ventricular elastance and arterial elastance on the same diagram. The ESP (P) then lies at the junction of the curves, which are approximately at right angles to each other. Changes in arterial pressure are reflected by a shift in the position of P. If preload (EDP) is maintained constant, then the direction of displacement of P identifies the degree to which ventricular contractility or arterial elastance is responsible (Figure HE34).

The left ventricle and arterial system can be seen as two elastic chambers with opposing elastances, Ees and Ea respectively. The distribution of blood is determined by

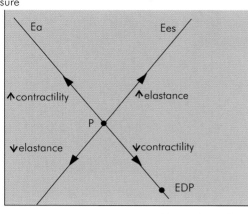

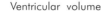

Figure HE34 Ventriculoarterial coupling diagram

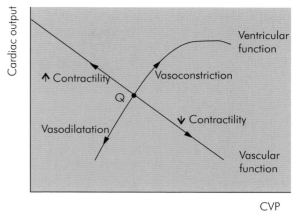

Figure HE35 Ventriculovenous coupling diagram

the individual elastances of the two chambers. Theoretical analysis suggests that the LV will deliver maximal work when Ees = Ea but will work with maximal mechanical efficiency when Ees = 2 × Ea. The implication is that there is an optimum ventriculoarterial coupling ratio for these elastances. If these elastances are mismatched the ventricle may fail, e.g. should the ventricle eject for a prolonged period against a very low afterload.

Ventriculovenous coupling

Description of cardiovascular coupling at the venous side of the heart requires the use of a vascular function curve. This curve describes the changes occurring in CVP as venous return is removed at different rates by the heart. It is obtained by varying the CO and recording the resulting CVP, at constant intravascular volume. The vascular function curve is a pressure–flow relationship at the venous side of the vascular system, dependent on the balance between vascular tone and intravascular volume. Changes in the gradient reflect alterations in vascular tone. Thus, vasodilatation causes a decreased gradient, while an increased gradient is associated with vasoconstriction. Changes in the intercept reflect altered intravascular volume.

A ventriculovenous coupling diagram can be drawn by plotting a vascular function curve and a ventricular function curve on the same axes. The ventricular function curve was described earlier and in Figure HE23. These curves intersect at an operating point (Q). When Q becomes

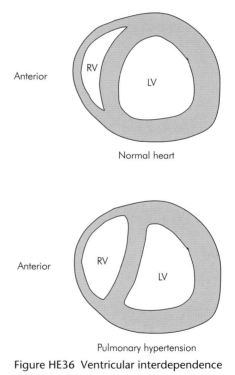

Figure HE36 Ventricular interdependence

displaced by cardiovascular changes, the direction of displacement indicates the relative contributions of vascular tone and ventricular contractility effects to the changes (Figure HE35).

Physiological change	Sign or symptom

Congestion in the pulmonary vascular system	Pulmonary oedema
	  Dyspnoea on exertion
	Orthopnoea
	Paroxysmal nocturnal
	  dyspnoea

Congestion in the systemic vascular system	Dependent oedema
	  (e.g. ankle)
	Hepatomegaly
	Raised jugulovenous
	  pressure

Inadequate systemic circulation	Fatigue Sodium retention Increased intravascular volume

Figure HE37 Signs and symptoms of cardiac failure

Change in heart	Change in physiological index
↓ Ventricular contractility	↓ CO Shift of ventricular function curve down
Ventricular dilatation	↑ CVP ↑ systolic ventricular wall stress ↑ EDV
Ventricular diastolic dysfunction	Shift of EDPVR curve up and left
Altered cardiovascular coupling	Displacement of operating point on ventriculoarterial and ventriculovenous coupling diagrams

Figure HE38 Changes in physiological indices in cardiac failure

Ventricular interdependence

Right and left ventricles are situated inside the same non-compliant pericardium. This means that they are both exposed to the same intrathoracic and intra-alveolar pressures. Changes in volume and pressure of one ventricle will directly affect the other. Normally LV pressure is greater than RV pressure and the interventricular septum bows into the RV. However, the thin free wall of the RV makes it more sensitive to increases in afterload than the LV, and any increase in afterload (e.g. pulmonary hypertension) will lead to dilatation of the RV. Under these circumstances the trans-septal pressure gradient can reverse and the septum can shift to the left, compromising LV filling during diastole. Interaction between the two ventricles occurs during systole and diastole, and is called ventricular interdependence (Figure HE36).

Cardiac failure

Cardiac failure is a state of inadequate circulation due to cardiac dysfunction. The condition manifests itself through two aspects. First, there is a failure to provide adequate arterial pressure and CO ('forward failure') into the systemic circulation. Second, there is a failure to pump away the venous return, which causes congestion in the pulmonary or systemic venous beds ('backward failure').

The course of cardiac failure may be acute or chronic. The commonest cause of acute cardiac failure is myocardial infarction, while chronic failure often arises in ischaemic heart disease, hypertension and valvular disease. In acute cardiac failure hypotension without peripheral oedema may occur. In chronic failure, blood pressure is usually maintained, but signs and symptoms due to congestion develop.

Some of the common signs and symptoms of cardiac failure are shown in Figure HE37. Many of the physiological parameters and indices reflecting aspects of cardiac performance change in cardiac failure. These are outlined in Figure HE38.

CHAPTER 6
Physiology of the circulation

E. S. Lin

Blood vessels

The circulation can be divided into the systemic and the pulmonary circulation. The systemic circulation receives oxygenated blood from the left side of the heart via the aorta and returns desaturated blood to the right side of the heart in the venae cavae. The desaturated blood is delivered to the pulmonary circulation from the right ventricle via the pulmonary artery to be oxygenated and to exchange carbon dioxide. Oxygenated blood is then returned to the left atrium via the pulmonary veins (Figure CR1).

Structure and function

Blood vessel walls are basically structured in three layers. The adventitia is the outer layer and is made up of connective tissue with nerve fibres. The middle layer or media is of varying thickness and contains mainly smooth muscle. The innermost layer is the intima and consists of the endothelium, basement membrane and supporting connective tissue (Figure CR2). The composition of blood vessel walls is mainly a mixture of elastic tissue, fibrous tissue and smooth muscle. This mixture again varies according to the type of vessel. The aorta walls are predominantly elastic and fibrous tissue with little smooth muscle, whereas the vena cava walls consist largely of smooth muscle and fibrous components. The composition of vessel walls reflects their function.

Figure CR3 lists functional aspects relating vessel characteristics to function.

Blood vessel diameter and wall thickness
A major factor determining thickness is mean arterial pressure. Some typical values for vessel diameter, wall thickness and mean arterial pressure are given in Figure CR4.

Blood vessel function
The arteries transport blood under high pressure to the tissues, where they divide into smaller arterioles, which

Fundamentals of Anaesthesia, 3rd edition, ed. Tim Smith, Colin Pinnock and Ted Lin. Published by Cambridge University Press. © Cambridge University Press 2008.

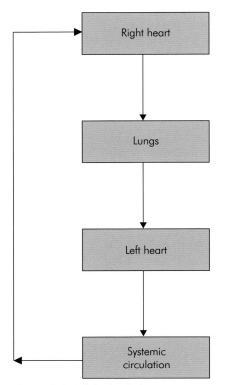

Figure CR1 Adult circulation system

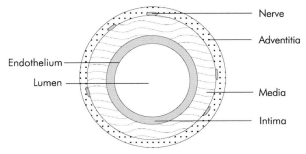

Figure CR2 Blood vessel structure

capillary beds and to store blood volume. The control of regional perfusion is dependent on reflexes and autoregulation, which rely on arteriolar control. The functions of the different types of vessel in the circulatory system are summarised in Figure CR5.

Pressure and flow in the vascular system

Flow and flow velocity

Function of the organ systems depends on the volume of blood flowing per unit time through them, or the volume flow rate. This is often shortened to the term 'flow'. Flow can be measured in millilitres per second (or litres per minute). The total flow through the systemic circulation or the lungs is equal to the cardiac output.

Flow should be differentiated from flow velocity. Flow velocity defines how fast fluid is moving at any given point and has units of centimetres per second. In a blood vessel the flow velocity of blood varies between the centre of the vessel and the vessel wall. If the flow pattern of the blood is described as laminar (i.e. without turbulence) the blood moves smoothly in the direction of the axis of the vessel. The velocity of the blood varies in a predictable

in turn release the blood into capillaries. There the exchange of fluid, nutrients, electrolytes and other substances between the interstitial fluid and the blood take place. The venules collect blood from the capillaries, and join together into veins to transport the blood back to the heart.

Blood vessels also function to smooth the pulsatile pressure waveform in the aorta, to control pressure at the

Characteristic	Functional aspect
Wall thickness	Thick walls provide tensile strength to withstand pressure in arteries
	Thin walls in capillaries allow exchange with interstitial fluid
Elastic component in walls	Smoothing of pulsations, storage of energy to maintain flow in diastole
Smooth muscle component in walls	Control of vessel diameter by autonomic reflex and humoral activity
Fibrous component in walls	Mechanical strength

Figure CR3 Functional aspects of blood vessel wall characteristics

Vessel	Diameter	Wall thickness	Mean pressure (mmHg)
Aorta	25 mm	2 mm	100
Artery	4 mm	1 mm	95
Arteriole	20 μm	6 μm	50
Terminal arteriole	10 μm	2 μm	45
Capillary	8 μm	0.5 μm	30
Venule	20 μm	1 μm	20
Vein	5 mm	0.5 mm	8
Vena cava	30 mm	1.5 mm	3

Figure CR4 Blood vessel diameters and mean pressures

Vessel	Function
Aorta	Storage of energy to maintain delivery in diastole, and damping of pressure pulses
Arteries	Delivery, distribution and damping of pressure waveform
Arterioles	Resistance to control pressure and distribution to capillaries
Capillaries	Microcirculation and exchange
Venules and small veins	Collection
Large veins and venae cavae	Collection, storage capacitance and delivery of venous return (or portal circulations)

Figure CR5 Blood vessels and their functions

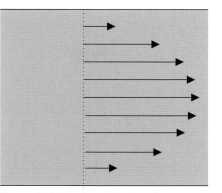

Figure CR6 Physics of laminar flow

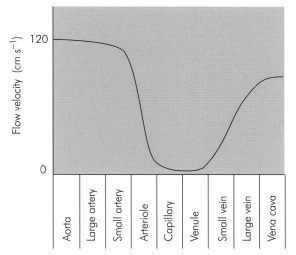

Figure CR7 Flow velocity in different vessels

pattern with maximum velocity in the centre of the vessel and minimum velocity next to the wall, as if the blood is moving in concentric layers (Figure CR6).

Consider a vessel with cross-sectional area A. The mean flow velocity (v) can be taken across the cross section. The flow (Q) is then related to the mean flow velocity (v) by

$$Q = vA$$

This relationship can be applied to the vascular system as a whole, since the number and diameter of any type of blood vessel determines the total cross-sectional area presented to flow at that stage in the vascular system. The greater the total cross-sectional area of any given generation of vessels, the slower the velocity of blood flow through those vessels. The cross-sectional area of the aorta is about 4.5 cm^2 with peak flow velocities of >120 cm s^{-1}. In contrast, the flow velocity in the several billion capillaries of the vascular system is usually between 0 and 1 cm s^{-1} due to a total capillary cross-sectional area of >4500 cm^2 (Figure CR7). These flow velocities reflect the functions of delivery and distribution in the aorta and arteries, as opposed to perfusion and exchange in the capillaries.

In an individual vessel, if the cross-sectional area is reduced by a constriction such as a valve or an atheromatous plaque, the flow velocity increases through the constriction. Such increases in flow velocity can affect the characteristics of the blood flow, making it turbulent and leading to an increased tendency towards thrombus formation. The motion of blood across the stationary surface of the vessel wall produces a viscous drag or

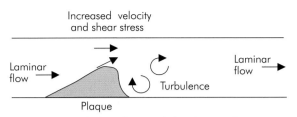

Figure CR8 Turbulent flow and drag in vessels

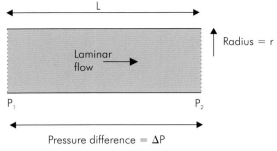

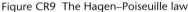

Figure CR9 The Hagen–Poiseuille law

shear stress along the surface of the vessel wall. This shear stress is increased with increased flow velocity, producing a force that tends to pull endothelium and plaques away from the wall, leading to dissection or emboli. Increased flow velocity also produces bruits or murmurs (Figure CR8).

Flow through the systemic circulation

The energy imparted to blood within the circulation by the heart and the elastic recoil of the great vessels causes it to flow through the systemic and pulmonary circulations. There are additional contributions of energy to flow from skeletal muscle contraction and negative intrathoracic pressure during inspiration. These mechanisms create a pressure difference across the vascular system that produces the total flow (cardiac output) through the vascular system. A simple electrical analogy lies in Ohm's law, where a potential difference (V) produces an electrical current (I) through a resistance (R). In this case

$$V = I \times R$$

Thus the pressure difference between mean arterial pressure (MAP) and central venous pressure (CVP) is related to cardiac output (CO) and systemic vascular resistance (SVR) by

$$(MAP) - (CVP) = (CO) \times (SVR)$$

This is often approximated to

$$(MAP) - (CO) \times (SVR)$$

Vascular resistance

'Vascular resistance' is a clinical term used to represent the effect of all the forces opposing blood flow through a vascular bed. It may be applied to the systemic vascular circulation, the pulmonary circulation or a given visceral circulation. The forces opposing blood flow through a vascular system are composed of two main components. First, those which dissipate energy due to frictional effects. This

resistance arises as a result of drag between fluid layers and friction between fluid and vessel walls. The viscosity of the blood is a major determinant of this component of resistance.

The second component of opposing forces arises from the conversion of pump work into stored energy. This occurs when potential energy is stored by the elasticity of distended vessel walls or by gravity as blood is pumped to a greater height within the body. In addition, inertial effects store kinetic energy when blood is accelerated. This component is referred to as the 'reactive' component, and it is dependent on the pulsatile component of the pressure waveform. If the pressure difference applied across a vascular bed were constant the reactive component would be minimal.

In vivo the systemic vascular resistance (SVR) and the pulmonary vascular resistance (PVR) can be estimated using pulmonary artery catheterisation.

Flow in a single vessel

Blood flow through larger vessels (>0.5 mm diameter) can be approximated to the case of an idealised or Newtonian fluid (such as water) flowing though a tube. Under laminar flow conditions with a steady pressure gradient, the flow (Q) between any two points, P_1 and P_2, is dependent on the pressure difference, ΔP, between the points, and inversely dependent on the resistance to flow (R) (Figure CR9):

$$Q = \frac{\Delta P}{R}$$

According to the Hagen–Poiseuille law, which describes laminar flow in tubes, the flow resistance, R, is dependent on the length of the tube and the viscosity of the fluid, but inversely related to the fourth power of the radius. The real situation of blood flowing through a vessel differs from this ideal model in the following respects:

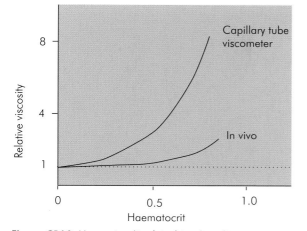
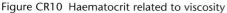

Figure CR10 Haematocrit related to viscosity

- Blood vessels are not uniform in cross section.
- Blood vessel walls are elastic.
- Pressure gradients pushing blood through vessels have a pulsatile component.
- Blood as a fluid behaves differently from a Newtonian fluid due to the cellular components, and its flow properties are not determined solely by viscosity.

Blood viscosity

The rheological properties of blood describe its flow-resistive properties. In a Newtonian fluid these resistive properties are dependent on a constant, the coefficient of viscosity. Blood, however, is a suspension of cells, and although the viscosity can be determined to give an apparent value, this value varies significantly with blood composition and flow conditions. The factors causing this variation in apparent viscosity include:

- Haematocrit – an increase in haematocrit to 0.7 (normal haematocrit = 0.45) can double the apparent viscosity (Figure CR10).
- Diameter of the vessel – apparent blood viscosity can be measured in vitro using a capillary tube viscometer, and decreases as tube diameter decreases to below about 0.3 mm.
- Red blood cell streaming – in smaller-diameter vessels red blood cells stream centrally along the axis of the vessel. This effectively reduces the haematocrit in these vessels. The haematocrit in capillaries may be 25% of the value in larger vessels (Figure CR11).
- In vivo – apparent blood viscosity is lower in vivo than in vitro. At normal haematocrit the in vivo blood

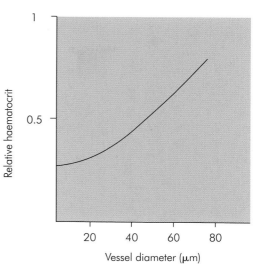

Figure CR11 Haematocrit related to blood vessel size

viscosity may only be half of the equivalent in vitro value.
- Flow velocity – apparent viscosity decreases at higher flow velocities and increases at low flow velocities. This is due to increased red cell aggregation and leucocyte adherence to vessel walls at low flow velocities.

Arterial system

The main function of the arterial system is to distribute and deliver blood to the capillary beds throughout the peripheral vascular system. A secondary arterial function is to convert the high-pressure pulsatile blood flow of the aorta into the low-pressure steady flow of the capillary beds. This modification of the flow and pressure profiles is achieved by the elasticity of the arterial system and is sometimes referred to as hydraulic filtering, or the 'Windkessel' effect (Windkessel – volume of air trapped in a pump reservoir to smooth out pressure variations).

Arterial factors
Flow velocity

In systole, the heart ejects a stroke volume of 70–90 ml blood into the aorta. The heart generates an average flow velocity of 70 cm s^{-1}, with a peak velocity of 120 cm s^{-1}, which makes flow in the aorta turbulent. There is transient backflow at the end of systole until the aortic valve closes. The aorta and arteries distend in systole due to the elasticity of their walls, then subsequent elastic recoil during diastole

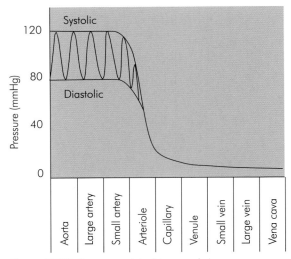

Figure CR12 Pressure related to vessel size

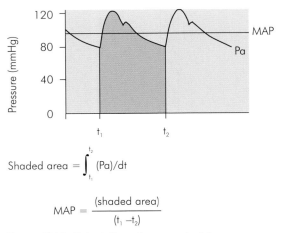

$$\text{Shaded area} = \int_{t_1}^{t_2} (Pa)/dt$$

$$MAP = \frac{(\text{shaded area})}{(t_1 - t_2)}$$

Figure CR13 Calculation of mean arterial pressure

maintains forward flow distally into the peripheral vascular system.

Pressure wave

In the aorta and arteries the pressure is pulsatile. The maximum pressure is the systolic arterial pressure (about 120 mmHg) and the minimum is the diastolic arterial pressure (about 70 mmHg). The difference between diastolic and systolic is the pulse pressure, normally about 50 mmHg.

The aortic pressure wave changes in magnitude and shape occur as it travels through the arterial system. The shape of the pressure wave narrows and high-frequency features such as the incisura (end-systolic notch) become dampened as it moves distally. Initially systolic pressures increase as the pressure waves travel from the aorta distally through the large arteries. At the femoral arteries systolic pressures have risen by 20 mmHg, and by the time pressure waves have reached the foot systolic pressures are 40 mmHg higher than in the aorta. Pressure pulsations begin to become attenuated in the smaller arteries and are finally reduced to a steady pressure with a mean level of 30–35 mmHg by the arterioles, ready for the capillary beds (Figure CR12). The changes in the shape of the pressure waves are mainly due to the viscoelastic properties of the arterial walls. The increases in systolic pressure are thought to be due to factors affecting the propagation of the pressure waves through the vessels, such as reflection, resonance and changes in the velocity of propagation.

Mean arterial pressure

Mean arterial pressure (MAP) is the value obtained when the pressure is averaged over time. It can be obtained from the product of cardiac output and systemic vascular resistance. Since the pressure varies cyclically, MAP can be determined by integrating a pressure signal over the duration of one cycle (this gives the shaded area shown in Figure CR13). The mean pressure is then given by the value of this integral divided by time. An estimate of mean arterial pressure may be made by taking the diastolic plus one-third of the pulse pressure. Thus, for a systolic pressure of 120 mmHg and a diastolic of 70 mmHg, the mean pressure (MAP) is given by

$$MAP \approx 70 + \frac{(120 - 70)}{3}$$
$$= 86.7\,\text{mmHg}.$$

The factors affecting MAP are summarised in Figure CR14.

Compliance

The elasticity of the arterial walls provides an essential mechanism for maintaining forward blood flow during diastole. When the aorta and arteries are distended during systole the elasticity of the walls stores kinetic energy from the ejected blood. This stored energy is then returned in diastole by the recoil of the vessel walls. A useful measure of arterial elasticity is the arterial compliance (Ca). Compliance (as in the respiratory system) is the change in arterial blood volume produced by a unit change in arterial blood pressure. Thus, easily distended arteries have a

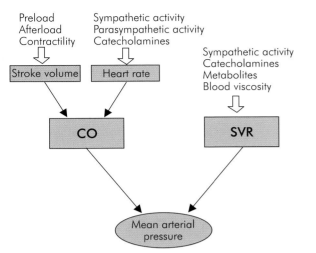

Figure CR14 Factors affecting mean arterial pressure

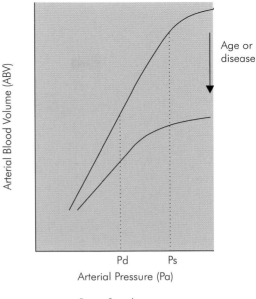

Ps = Systolic pressure
Pd = Diastolic pressure

Figure CR15 Arterial compliance curves

high compliance, and stiff arteries have a low compliance. The reciprocal relationship between Ca and arterial elastance (Ea) should be noted, as Ea is used in describing left-ventricular performance.

Determination of arterial compliance

- In vitro – the pressure–volume curves of post mortem aorta preparations have been plotted for different age groups. This is approximately linear in the young normal subject, the gradient of the curve being equal to Ca. With age the arterial walls increase in stiffness and the gradient decreases to a fraction of its value in young subjects. In addition, the compliance curve becomes curvilinear in the working arterial pressure range (Figure CR15).
- In vivo – the end-systolic points from different ventricular pressure–volume loops can be plotted for a given subject. This gives an arterial elastance curve in which the gradient is equal to Ea.

Determinants of systolic and diastolic pressures

The factors determining systolic and diastolic pressures are summarised in Figure CR16:
- Arterial blood volume (ABV)
- Stroke volume
- Systemic vascular resistance (SVR)
- Arterial compliance (Ca)

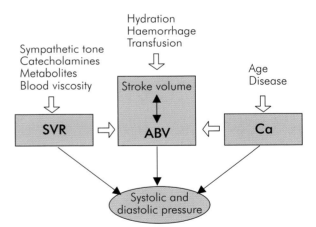

Figure CR16 Factors affecting systolic and diastolic pressure

The arterial system can be visualised as an elastic vessel containing a varying volume of blood. This volume (ABV) varies with the injection of each stroke volume by the left ventricle (LV) and the 'runoff' of blood into the peripheral vessels. The arterial pressure at any instant (Pa) is then dependent on the relationship between ABV, Ca and SVR.

(a) Systole

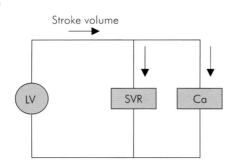

(b) Diastole

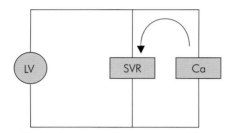

Figure CR17 Circuit demonstrating shunt arterial compliance

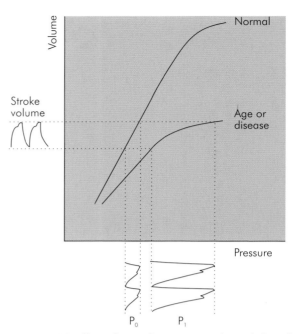

Figure CR18 Effect of compliance on systolic and diastolic pressures

Pa should be differentiated from mean arterial pressure (MAP), which is averaged over time (Figure CR13).

The determination of systolic and diastolic pressures can be examined by extending the electrical circuit analogy used previously to relate MAP to cardiac output and systemic vascular resistance (SVR). Arterial compliance (Ca) is added as a 'shunt' capacitance across SVR to give a parallel resistance–capacitance (RC) circuit (Figure CR17). This is fed by a continual series of current pulses (stroke volumes). Each pulse of current divides between the SVR and Ca. Ca charges to a maximum voltage (systolic pressure) during a current pulse and discharges to a minimum (diastolic pressure) in between pulses. For a given pulse amplitude these maximum and minimum values will be determined by the parallel RC time constant. The effects of SVR and Ca on systolic and diastolic arterial pressures are illustrated by the following notes:

- Ca reduces the peak current through SVR by 'shunting' current away from SVR. Thus, increasing Ca (compliant arteries) leads to reduced systolic pressures.

- Increased Ca also increases the RC time constant, giving a more gradual fall of pressure during diastole and reduced pulse pressures.
- Decreased Ca (stiff arteries) gives reduced shunted current, giving increased peak current through SVR and higher systolic pressures.
- Decreasing Ca also decreases the RC time constant, allowing a more rapid fall in pressure during diastole and increased pulse pressures.
- When arterial compliance is decreased, as with age or disease, the arterial pressure–volume curve becomes non-linear. The effect of this on systolic and diastolic pressures can be seen by comparing the arterial pressure waves produced (P_0 and P_1) by the same stroke volume, using the normal and decreased arterial compliance curves shown in Figure CR18. Projecting the stroke volume variation on the normal compliance curve produces the pressure signal P_0. Repeating this with the decreased compliance curve gives arterial pressure signal P_1. It can be seen that systolic pressure is increased disproportionately compared with diastolic pressure.
- Increased SVR, as occurs in chronic hypertension, produces non-linearity in the pressure–volume curve

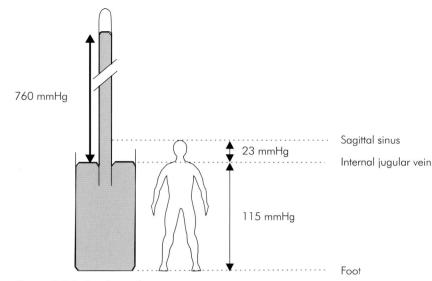

760 mmHg

Sagittal sinus

23 mmHg

Internal jugular vein

115 mmHg

Foot

Figure CR19 Gravity and venous pressure

like the effects of age on the arterial compliance curve. This produces similar increases in systolic and pulse pressures. Increased SVR increases the time constant, slowing the rate of diastolic pressure fall.

Technological factors affecting arterial blood pressure

The value obtained for arterial blood pressure is dependent on the method of measurement and the anatomical site where pressure is sampled. Arterial blood pressure measurements are often made non-invasively using an occluding cuff, as with the sphygmomanometer or oscillotonometer. Alternatively, intra-arterial cannulation may be performed and the arterial pressure measured using a piezoresistive transducer.

Venous system

Venous circulation

Venous blood flow is driven primarily by pressure transmitted from the capillary beds. Venous pressure falls from 15–20 mmHg at the venous end of capillaries to 10–15 mmHg in small veins, and 5–6 mmHg in large extrathoracic veins. Flow in the venules and small veins is continuous. In the great veins, pressure changes due to respiration and the heart beat cause fluctuations in the venous pressure wave. There are three identifiable peaks in the central venous pulse, the 'a', 'c' and 'v' waves, which are related to events in the cardiac cycle. The central venous pulse waveform is described in Section 2, Chapter 5 (page 283).

Other secondary mechanisms also assist venous blood flow back to the heart. These are gravity, the thoracic pump and the muscle pump. Unidirectional venous flow is maintained by the presence of valves in the peripheral veins.

Gravity and the venous system

The pressure in the venous system is largely determined by gravity, since the system can be visualised as a simple manometer (Figure CR19). In the erect position, a hydrostatic gradient is produced from head to toe. The hydrostatic pressure difference between any two points in the venous system can be calculated by taking the product of the difference in height between the points (h), the density of blood ($\rho = 1.050$ g cm^{-3}), and the acceleration due to gravity (g = 980 cm s^{-1}). These figures give a pressure difference equivalent to 0.77 mmHg for every centimetre difference in height.

The venous pressure in the internal jugular vein is normally atmospheric at neck level if the vein is collapsed. Venous pressure above the neck may be less than atmospheric and can be estimated: e.g. 30 cm above the neck (sagittal sinus) venous pressure is less than atmospheric by $30 \times 0.77 = 23$ mmHg.

Similarly in the foot, 150 cm below neck level, venous pressure is greater than atmospheric by $150 \times 0.77 = 115$ mmHg.

Such hydrostatic pressure differences are reduced significantly by the primary and secondary mechanisms outlined above, and by the presence of valves or venous obstruction. Thus, in the foot venous pressures may only be 80 mmHg when standing and decrease further to <30 mmHg when walking.

Jugular venous pressure (JVP)

The superior vena cava (SVC) and internal jugular vein effectively form a manometer connected to the right atrium, and are usually collapsed, being approximately at atmospheric pressure in the neck. In the erect position, the level of blood in the internal jugular vein represents the filling pressure in the right atrium and is not normally visible above the clavicle. The jugular venous pulse may become visible as a pulsatile distension of the internal jugular vein in a reclined or supine position, or when the CVP is increased. The jugular venous pulsations correspond to those of the central venous pulsations as described above. This correlation between jugular venous pulse and central venous pulse is limited if there are any anatomical obstructions to drainage of blood from the superior vena cava.

Cerebral venous pressure and air embolism

In the brain, venous pressure can become sub-atmospheric, since the skull is a rigid container and the cerebral veins are held open by surrounding tissue. These veins are therefore susceptible to air embolism during surgery or if punctured by needles or cannulae open to air. The air embolus forms bubbles that are compressible compared with blood. If a large enough volume (>10 ml) of air becomes trapped in the heart ventricles cardiac output can be reduced significantly with serious effects. Small amounts of air may pass through the heart to become trapped in pulmonary capillaries and be eliminated by diffusion without ill effects. On the other hand a few millilitres of air if shunted into the left ventricle and systemic circulation could have disastrous or even fatal effects. Gas embolism may also occur under positive pressure during laparoscopic surgery.

Thoracic pump

Normal respiration produces cyclical changes in intrathoracic pressure which increase the venous return to the heart. During inspiration intrapleural pressure falls from its resting value of -2 to -6 mmHg. This increase in negative intrathoracic pressure is transmitted to the central veins, reducing CVP and augmenting the pressure gradient between abdomen and thorax, allowing blood to pool in the pulmonary circulation. Central venous blood flow into the thorax may double during inspiration from its resting expiratory level of about 5 ml s^{-1}. Diaphragmatic displacement caudally during inspiration also contributes to increased venous return by increasing intra-abdominal pressure and consequently the abdominothoracic venous pressure gradient. Pooling of blood in the pulmonary circulation during inspiration produces a small decrease in arterial pressure and increase in heart rate. Forced inspiration against a closed glottis (Müller manoeuvre) accentuates these changes.

During expiration, which is normally passive, the diaphragm relaxes, intrapleural pressure returns to resting value, pulmonary blood volume is reduced and blood flow in the large veins decreases. Forced expiration against a closed glottis (Valsalva manoeuvre; see below) can produce positive intrathoracic pressures, with marked changes in heart rate and blood pressure.

Microcirculation and lymphatic system

Structure of a capillary network

Capillaries and venules form an interface with a surface area >6000 m^2 for the exchange of water and solutes between the circulation and tissues. Arterioles feed capillary networks via smaller metarterioles, and the capillaries drain into venules. Metarterioles possess smooth muscle contractile elements in their walls and give rise to capillaries through smooth muscle precapillary sphincters (Figure CR20). While arterioles are supplied by the autonomic system, the innervation of metarterioles and

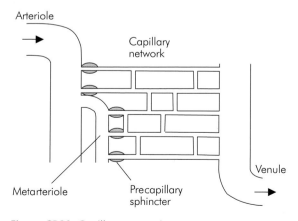

Figure CR20 Capillary network

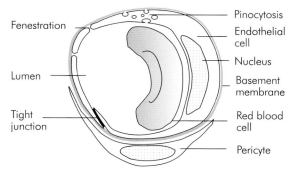

Figure CR21 Capillaries and pericytes

precapillary sphincters is uncertain, and these vessels may only be responsive to local or humoral agents. Capillary blood flow varies according to the activity of the tissue. At rest the majority of capillary beds is collapsed and arteriovenous anastomoses, allowing direct communication between arterioles and venules, shunt blood away from the tissues. These anastomotic channels are widespread in skin and play a prominent role in thermoregulation.

Capillaries and endothelium

Capillaries contain 6% of the circulating blood volume and measure 5 μm in diameter at their arteriolar end, widening to 9 μm at the venous end. These dimensions are comparable with the 7 μm diameter of red blood cells, which decrease in diameter when traversing capillaries. A capillary consists of a tube formed by a single sheet of endothelial cells resting on a basement membrane. Associated with capillaries and venules are interstitial cells called pericytes, akin to renal mesangial cells. These cells release chemicals that mediate capillary permeability and also secrete the basement membrane (Figure CR21).

Capillary exchange

Capillaries have differing structures and permeabilities according to the tissues they serve. Most capillaries comprise a continuous layer of endothelial cells. Intercellular junctions and small pores representing about 0.02% of the capillary surface area permit the diffusion of small molecules <8 nm in size. Larger molecules may cross through cell cytoplasm in vesicles and fat-soluble molecules; water, oxygen and CO_2 pass directly across the cell membrane. Fenestrations, gaps of 20–100 nm diameter, appear in the endothelial cells of endocrine glands, renal glomeruli and intestinal villi to facilitate secretion, filtration and absorption. In the sinusoids of the liver and

in the spleen, the endothelium is discontinuous with gaps of >1000 nm. As a result albumin escapes from hepatic sinusoids much more readily than in other tissues.

In summary, transfer of water and solutes across the endothelium occurs by several mechanisms:

- Diffusion – the main mechanism mediating the exchange of gases, and for the movement of small molecules such as glucose, urea, electrolytes and between circulation and tissues. It occurs at endothelial defects such as pores and fenestrations. Diffusion of gases and lipid-soluble molecules also occurs directly across cell membranes.
- Filtration – the movement of water and small-size solutes across the endothelium under the influence of hydrostatic and osmotic gradients. Transport of substances this way is only a fraction of that occurring by diffusion; however, a significant flow of water circulates between the circulation and interstitial fluid by filtration. About 2% of capillary plasma flow is filtered (20–40 ml min^{-1}).
- Pinocytosis – transports larger (>30 nm) lipid-insoluble molecules across the endothelium. Pinocytotic vesicles form at the cell membrane (endocytosis), migrate across the cell, and expel their contents at the opposite cell membrane (exocytosis). The numbers of pinocytotic vesicles seen varies between tissues, and is greater at the arteriolar end than the venous end of capillaries.
- Direct passage of lipid-soluble compounds and gases occurs by diffusion across cell membranes, through the cells and into the interstitial fluid.

Diffusion across capillary walls

Diffusion is the movement of substances down a concentration gradient. Across the capillary endothelium the diffusion of lipid-insoluble molecules and ions occurs at defects such as intercellular junctions, pores, fenestrations and larger gaps. Gases and lipid-soluble molecules diffuse directly across cell membranes as well as at these endothelial defects. The rate of diffusion of a substance is dependent on concentration gradient ($C_O - C_I$), capillary permeability (k), capillary surface area (A), and capillary wall thickness (D). This is given by Fick's law:

$$\text{Rate of diffusion} = \frac{kA(C_O - C_I)}{D}$$

where

C_O = concentration in the capillary
C_I = concentration in the interstitial fluid

The capillary permeability is a constant combining the various factors that affect the diffusion of different substances, such as:

- Molecular size
- Charge
- Lipid solubility
- Diffusion across membranes as well as pores and fenestrations
- Interactions between solutes

Substances that diffuse readily, such as gases, reach equilibrium close to the proximal end of capillaries, and their exchange rate is said to be 'flow-limited' since it is dependent on the capillary flow rate. In contrast, the movement of substances which diffuse slowly and do not reach equilibrium with the interstitial fluid over the length of the capillary is 'diffusion-limited'. Capillary permeability not only varies between tissues but is also greater at the venous end of the capillaries, and in the venules, than at the proximal end of the capillaries.

Starling forces and filtration

The balance of hydrostatic and colloid osmotic pressures between capillary plasma and interstitial fluid causes fluid to be filtered out of a capillary at the arteriolar end and reabsorbed at the venous end. These forces acting to move fluid in and out of a capillary are sometimes referred to as Starling forces.

In a capillary hydrostatic pressure (P_C) falls from 33 mmHg at the arterial end to 15 mmHg at the venous end. Interstitial hydrostatic pressure (P_{IF}) can vary from 9 to −9 mmHg, depending on the tissue. In solid tissues it is usually near zero or slightly positive (1 mmHg). Loose areolar connective tissue, such as in the epidural space, tends to have a negative hydrostatic pressure.

Colloid osmotic pressure in the capillaries (π_C) is 25 mmHg, while in the interstitial fluid colloid osmotic pressure (π_{IF}) is usually zero. The Starling forces are summarised in Figure CR22.

The pressure acting to force fluid out of the capillary is made up of the hydrostatic pressure in the capillary and the colloid osmotic pressure in the interstitial fluid:

$$\text{Outward pressure} = P_C + \pi_{IF}$$

Similarly the pressure acting to force fluid back into the capillary is made up of the interstitial hydrostatic pressure and the colloid osmotic pressure in the capillary:

$$\text{Inward pressure} = P_{IF} + \pi_C$$

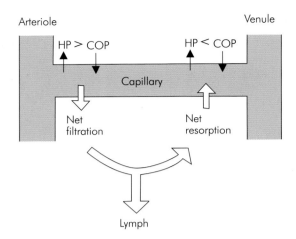

HP = Hydrostatic pressure

COP = Colloid osmotic pressure

Figure CR22 Starling forces

The resultant pressure gradient is the difference between outward and inward pressures (Figure CR22):

$$\text{Pressure gradient} = (P_C + \pi_{IF}) - (P_{IF} + \pi_C)$$

The rate of filtration is proportional to this pressure gradient and is given by

$$\text{Rate of filtration} = [(P_C + \pi_{IF}) - (P_{IF} + \pi_C)] \times K$$

where

K = filtration coefficient of isotonic fluids (i.e. volume rate filtered per unit of pressure) and is about 0.01 ml min^{-1} mmHg^{-1} 100 g^{-1} tissue at 37 °C

Assuming an interstitial hydrostatic pressure (P_{IF}) of 1 mmHg, and an interstitial colloid osmotic pressure (π_{IF}) of zero, it can be seen that at the arterial capillary end

$$\text{Pressure gradient} = 33 - (1 + 25)$$
$$= +7 \text{ mmHg}$$

Therefore, pressure gradient acts outwards, filtering fluid out of the capillary. While at the venous capillary end

$$\text{Pressure gradient} = 15 - (1 + 25)$$
$$= -11 \text{ mmHg}$$

Here the pressure gradient is negative acting inwards, reabsorbing fluid back into the capillary.

Change	Effects
Vasodilatation pressure	↑ proximal capillary hydrostatic pressure ↑ filtration
↑ Intravascular volume	↑ proximal capillary hydrostatic pressure ↑ filtration
Vasoconstriction	↓ proximal capillary hydrostatic pressure ↓ filtration
↓ Intravascular volume	↓ proximal capillary hydrostatic pressure ↓ filtration
Hypoalbuminaemia	↓ capillary colloid osmotic pressure ↑ filtration ↓ reabsorption
↑ Venous pressure	↑ distal capillary hydrostatic pressure ↓ reabsorption

Figure CR23 Factors disturbing capillary filtration equilibrium

The total volume of fluid filtered through the capillaries is dependent on capillary blood flow, but estimates have been made of between 1 and 3 litres per hour. The filtered fluid exceeds the amount of fluid reabsorbed by about 10%, the difference being absorbed by the lymphatic system.

Capillary filtration equilibrium

In a capillary there is normally a dynamic equilibrium between the fluid filtered out, the fluid reabsorbed and the fluid absorbed by lymphatics. Disturbance of this equilibrium either dehydrates tissue or makes it oedematous. The equilibrium can be disturbed by various changes. Some examples are shown in Figure CR23.

The lymphatic system

The functions of the lymphatic system include:
- Drainage of interstitial fluid – the total lymph drainage for an adult is about 2–4 litres per 24 hours.
- Return of 'leaked' protein in the interstitial fluid to the systemic circulation. Lymph from most tissues contains a protein concentration of 20 g l^{-1}.
- Absorption of particles, proteins and other large molecular weight molecules accumulated in inflamed tissues.
- Absorption of protein and fat derived from metabolism and gastrointestinal absorption. The protein concentration is two to three times higher in lymph draining from liver and intestine.

Lymphatic vessels

Lymph flows from lymphatic capillaries, with a single layer of lymphatic endothelial cells, into lymphatic vessels that contain smooth muscle in their walls. This smooth muscle contracts in response to distension by the presence of lymph. Valves within lymph vessels maintain unidirectional flow towards the thoracic ducts, which drain into venous blood at the junction of internal jugular and subclavian veins. External compression from adjacent pulsatile arteries and skeletal muscle contractions augment lymph flow through larger lymphatic vessels.

Tissue oedema

The accumulation of abnormal amounts of interstitial fluid results in tissue swelling and is referred to as oedema. The common mechanisms underlying oedema formation include:
- Increased capillary filtration (raised venous pressure, as in congestive heart failure, incompetent venous valves, venous obstruction)
- Decreased capillary colloid osmotic pressure (hypoalbuminaemia from any cause)
- Increased capillary permeability (inflammation, hypersensitivity, systemic inflammatory response syndrome)
- Decreased lymphatic drainage (lymphatic obstruction by lymphadenopathy, Milroy's disease, filariasis)

Control of the circulation

Control of the circulation ensures that adequate blood flow reaches the tissues to supply their metabolic demands. This is achieved by simultaneous regulation of the cardiac pump and the peripheral vascular system. Pump control varies the cardiac output. Control of the peripheral vascular system regulates the relative intravascular volume that influences venous return to the pump, varies vascular resistance to maintain perfusion pressures, and distributes appropriate flows to the various vascular beds.

Multiple control mechanisms have evolved to regulate the circulation. These may be local (intrinsic) or systemic (extrinsic). Most areas of the peripheral vascular system are under both local and systemic control, but may be dominated by one set of mechanisms more than the other. Circulation in the heart and brain are mainly regulated intrinsically to maintain perfusion independently of systemic disturbances. On the other hand perfusion of the skin and gut are largely controlled extrinsically, increasing the flexibility to maintain vital organ perfusion under adverse conditions.

Resistance vessels and capacitance vessels

Control of the vascular system is mediated via:

- Resistance vessels – these vessels are the arterioles. Increasing or decreasing the tone of the smooth muscle in arterioles (vasoconstriction or vasodilatation) varies the perfusion pressure across a vascular bed. Changes in these vessels also affect flow rates through the capillaries and alter vascular resistance.
- Capacitance vessels – these comprise the venous system. Increasing or decreasing the tone of smooth muscle in the venous system (venoconstriction or venodilatation) varies the relative intravascular volume since the venous system contains >60% of the blood volume. Changes in these vessels have little effect on vascular resistance.

Arterioles

Resistance vessels, or arterioles, possess a high proportion of smooth muscle in their walls. The smooth muscle fibres are arranged circumferentially in the media, and the effect of varying the muscle tone can range from complete obliteration of the vessel lumen to maximal dilatation.

Vascular smooth muscle

Vascular smooth muscle differs from both skeletal muscle and cardiac muscle, both structurally and functionally. Vascular smooth muscle characteristics include:

- Contractions are mediated by actin–myosin interaction dependent on calcium influx, release from the sarcoplasmic reticulum and reuptake. However, actin and myosin filaments are not arranged to give striations.
- Contractions are relatively slow, develop high forces and are maintained for longer durations when compared with striated muscle fibres.
- There are no action potentials generated. Contraction occurs in response to systemic and locally released agents such as catecholamines, acetylcholine and prostaglandins.
- The majority of vascular smooth muscle is innervated by sympathetic fibres that maintain a basal level of vascular tone. Sympathetic stimulation increases vascular resistance.
- The parasympathetic system supplies a small fraction of visceral vessels, which can produce a decrease in vascular resistance when stimulated.

Local mechanisms controlling blood flow
Autoregulation

The blood flow to certain organs (e.g. brain or kidney) is adjusted locally to respond to their activity levels and meet their metabolic demands. This process is known as autoregulation, and it is achieved by various mechanisms. These mechanisms include mechanical responses of smooth muscle, the accumulation of metabolites or products of injury, and the release of factors by the endothelium.

Metabolic regulation

This is the most important control mechanism since it determines the balance of oxygen supply and demand for individual tissues and organs. Exposure of tissue to hypoxia or injury results in the release of factors or accumulation of metabolites, which increase capillary permeability and blood flow. These override central and hormonal control of capillary blood flow. Some examples are:

- Tissue hypoxia or the accumulation of carbon dioxide and hydrogen ions by diffusion around an arteriole causes vasodilatation. Lactic acid, and to a lesser extent pyruvic acid, produced in anaerobic metabolism, vasodilate by reducing tissue pH.
- Adenosine, ATP, ADP and AMP are also strong vasodilators. Adenosine dilates hepatic arteries in response to a fall in flow in the hepatic portal vein.
- The accumulation of potassium and phosphate in exercising muscle augments blood flow to the muscle. This is sometimes referred to as 'active hyperaemia'.

- 'Reactive hyperaemia' occurs when the blood supply to a tissue is occluded, and then the occlusion is released. There follows an immediate vasodilatation and increase in flow to the tissue.
- Local mechanical damage to tissues usually produces localised constriction of vessels associated with serotonin release from platelets at the site of injury.
- An alternative local response to local injury is the 'triple response'. There is an initial red reaction due to arteriolar dilatation caused by the mechanical stimulus. An axon reflex causes a rapid, more widespread brighter red reaction due to further vasodilatation. Later local oedema raises a weal caused by capillary damage.

Mechanical responses of smooth muscle
Myogenic mechanism
Vascular smooth muscle contracts or relaxes in response to changes in transmural pressure. When perfusion pressure in a vessel varies, although blood flow may change initially, the vessel subsequently constricts or dilates in response to the altered transmural pressure, maintaining constant blood flow. Isolated muscle preparations suggest that this local response can maintain constant blood flow over perfusion pressures from 20 to 120 mmHg.

Endothelial mechanism
When flow through a vessel is varied without changes in transmural pressure, increases in flow velocity are associated with dilatation of the vessel. This response may be due to an endothelium-derived factor (e.g. nitric oxide), as it is abolished by removal of the endothelium.

Endothelial factors
Endothelial cells release various local factors that affect blood flow:

- Prostacyclin and thromboxane A_2 – these are arachidonites dependent on the cyclo-oxygenase pathway. Prostacyclin is a vasodilator and inhibits platelet aggregation, while thromboxane A_2 is a vasoconstrictor that promotes platelet aggregation. Regular administration of aspirin causes a predominance of prostacyclin effects, providing prophylaxis against myocardial infarction and stroke.
- Endothelium-derived relaxing factor (EDRF) – original term for nitric oxide (NO), which has been identified as a potent vasodilator. NO is synthesised from arginine by NO synthase and is inactivated by haemoglobin. NO is released from endothelium by multiple factors such as acetylcholine, bradykinin and various polypeptides. Its role is uncertain but it may act locally to maintain perfusion in different parts of the circulation.
- Endothelins – these polypeptides are potent vasoconstrictors that are produced by endothelium throughout the tissues of the body, including the central nervous system, the kidneys and the gut. The endothelins have multiple physiological effects although their exact role remains uncertain. These effects include contraction of vascular smooth muscle, positive inotropy and chronotropy, reduction of glomerular filtration rate, bronchoconstriction and stimulation of cell growth. Three endothelins have been identified – ET-1, ET-2, and ET-3 – together with two G-protein-coupled receptors.

Systemic humoral control of blood flow
Humoral factors affecting the vascular system include both vasodilators and vasoconstrictors. Some examples are shown in Figure CR24.

Catecholamines
Under physiological conditions the most powerful humoral agents affecting the systemic vessels are the catecholamines. Epinephrine is released from the adrenal medulla and exerts its primary effect on cardiac muscle. It also dilates resistance vessels in skeletal muscle via β-adrenergic fibres at low concentrations. At higher concentrations α-adrenergic effects predominate, causing vasoconstriction. Norepinephrine is a powerful vasoconstrictor and is controlled mainly via its release from sympathetic nerve endings as opposed to its release from the adrenal medulla.

Vasopressin
This nine-amino-acid peptide is also called vasopressin (antidiuretic hormone, ADH) because of its primary action in the kidney of causing the retention of free water from the glomerular filtrate in the collecting ducts. In supranormal doses vasopressin increases blood pressure by systemic vasoconstriction. It also stimulates ACTH secretion from the anterior pituitary and promotes glycogenolysis in the liver.

Angiotensin
The juxtaglomerular apparatus of the kidney synthesises and stores renin. Low renal perfusion stimulates the juxtaglomerular apparatus to release rennin, which splits

Action	Agent	Origin
Vasoconstrictors	Norepinephrine	Adrenal medulla, postganglionic nerve endings
	Epinephrine	Adrenal medulla
	Vasopressin	Posterior pituitary
	Angiotensin II	Conversion of angiotensin I in the lung
Vasodilators	Histamine	Mast cells
	Kinins	Pancreas, salivary glands, sweat glands
	Atrial natriuretic peptide (ANP)	Atria
	Vasoactive intestinal peptide (VIP)	Autonomic nerve endings Gastrointestinal tract nerves

Figure CR24 Some endogenous systemic vasoconstrictors and vasodilators

the α_2-globulin angiotensinogen to produce angiotensin I. Angiotensin-converting enzyme (ACE) then cleaves angiotensin I to angiotensin II in the lung. Angiotensin II has central and peripheral vasoconstrictor effects as well as participating in the control of thirst and stimulating the release of aldosterone from the adrenal cortex. Aldosterone increases tubular reabsorption of sodium and, by osmotic effects, water, and stimulates the excretion of potassium and hydrogen ions. Aldosterone also enhances excitability of vascular smooth muscle, augmenting the action of angiotensin II.

Atrial natriuretic peptide (ANP)
This is a 17-amino-acid polypeptide containing a ring formed by a disulphide bond between two cysteine residues. It causes natriuresis, lowers blood pressure and inhibits vasopressin secretion, thus opposing the action of angiotensin II. The rate of release from atrial muscle cells is proportional to the stretch of the atria obtained by changes in central venous pressure.

Kinins
Kinins are peptides originating from the exocrine glands. Bradykinin (9 amino acids) and lysylbradykinin (10 amino acids) are recognised vasodilators. The kinins are formed by kallikreins from protein precursors, and are metabolised by kininases. One kininase is angiotensin-converting enzyme (ACE), which gives this enzyme a pivotal role in the control of blood pressure.

Histamine
This amine is derived from the decarboxylation of histidine, and is produced in the CNS, gastric mucosa and mast cells. Regulation of histamine release is via inhibitory H_1, H_2 and H_3 receptors. Histamine is a potent vasodilator. Hypersensitivity reactions can result in a massive release of histamine, with a disastrous drop in blood pressure due to generalised vasodilatation.

Polypeptides
Other polypeptides have roles in blood pressure control. At cholinergic neurones, vasoactive intestinal peptide causes vasodilatation. Neuropeptide Y causes constriction at sympathetic postganglionic neurones. In association with sensory neurones, substance P causes vasodilatation and increases capillary permeability.

Systemic neurological control of blood flow
All blood vessels except capillaries and venules possess smooth muscle in their walls and are supplied by sympathetic motor fibres. The fibres supplying blood vessels form a plexus in the adventitia, and then extend to the outer layers of smooth muscle cells in the media. These sympathetic fibres possess a normal resting firing rate or tone, which may be increased or decreased. The vascular smooth muscle is innervated by noradrenergic sympathetic fibres, in which increased activity produces vasoconstriction. However, blood vessels in skeletal muscle are also supplied by cholinergic sympathetic fibres, which cause vasodilatation when stimulated. Constriction of arterioles (vasoconstriction) increases systemic vascular resistance, whereas constriction of veins (venoconstriction), especially splanchnic veins, increases the relative intravascular volume, and hence venous return to the heart. Systemic vascular

resistance does not change significantly with venoconstriction when compared with vasoconstriction.

Autonomic reflexes mediate neurological control of the peripheral vascular system. In these reflexes peripheral receptors feed impulses into the vasomotor centres in the CNS via afferent pathways. There the sensory information is used to modulate sympathetic tone, which is relayed back to the peripheral vessels via efferent pathways. Some reflexes are mediated at spinal level while others involve higher centres.

Vasomotor centres in the CNS

The vasomotor centres are areas of the reticular formation in the medulla oblongata and bulbar parts of the pons. The pressor region is located rostrally in the ventrolateral medulla, and provides a tonic output that maintains a background level of vascular smooth muscle tone. When the pressor centre is stimulated it causes increased vasoconstriction, increased heart rate and increased myocardial contractility. The depressor region is caudal and ventromedial to the pressor area. When stimulated, the depressor region decreases blood pressure by inhibiting the pressor area and also inhibiting sympathetic outflow directly at spinal level. Sympathetic tone is, thus, set by the balance between these two centres, which not only respond to afferents from peripheral reflexes, but are also influenced by central chemoreceptors and higher centres in the brain.

The various influences on the vasomotor centres are summarised in Figure CR25.

Efferent pathways

The vasomotor centres project directly to preganglionic neurones in the intermediolateral (IML) grey columns of the spinal cord. There is continuous tonic activity in sympathetic noradrenergic but not cholinergic neurones. Preganglionic fibres pass from the IML columns to the paravertebral sympathetic chain, from which postganglionic fibres carry the sympathetic outflow to the heart, vessels and adrenal medullae.

Afferent pathways

Baroreceptors in the carotid sinuses and chemoreceptors in the carotid bodies feed afferent impulses into the CNS via branches (nerve of Hering) of the glossopharyngeal nerves. Cardiac baroreceptors, aortic arch baroreceptors and aortic body chemoreceptors relay afferent impulses centrally in fibres (cardiac depressor nerves) of the right and left vagus nerves. The nucleus tractus solitarius (NTS) is the sensory nucleus for the glossopharyngeal and vagus nerves,

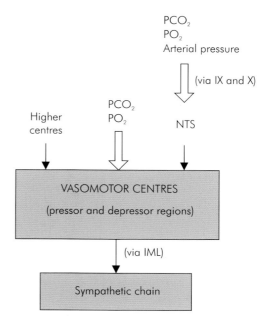

NTS = nucleus tractus solitarius
IML = intermediolateral grey column

Figure CR25 Factors affecting the vasomotor centre

and is located in the dorsomedial medulla. Inhibitory connections pass from the NTS to the pressor centre.

Influence of higher centres on vasomotor tone

The vasomotor centres also respond to higher centres in the brain. These include:

- Hypothalamus – stimulation of the anterior hypothalamus decreases blood pressure and heart rate, while stimulation of the posterolateral hypothalamus increases blood pressure and heart rate. The hypothalamus also controls cutaneous vasodilatation and vasoconstriction in response to environmental or body temperature changes.
- Cerebral cortex – stimulation of the motor and pre-motor areas is associated with increased blood pressure and heart rate.
- Limbic system – emotional stimuli can produce depressor responses such as fainting and blushing.

Baroreceptors

Baroreceptors are irregularly branched and coiled nerve endings located in the walls of the carotid sinus, the aorta and the heart. The carotid sinus is an enlargement of the

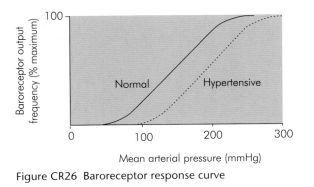

Figure CR26 Baroreceptor response curve

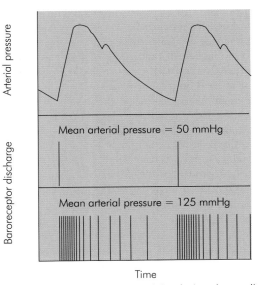

Figure CR27 Baroreceptor activity during the cardiac cycle

internal carotid artery just above its origin. They respond to the degree of stretch in the vessel or heart wall, and hence to the pressure (or more strictly the transmural pressure) in the vessel or heart. When intraluminal pressure increases, wall stretch increases and the frequency of impulses discharged by baroreceptors increases. If stretch decreases, baroreceptor output frequency decreases. The baroreceptor impulses exert an inhibitory influence on the pressor centre, and baroreceptor control thus represents a negative feedback control system to maintain cardiovascular stability. The baroreceptor response curve is sigmoidal but is linear over a pressure range of 80–180 mmHg (Figure CR26).

Baroreceptors respond not only to pressure magnitude but also to rate of change of pressure. The impulse discharge rate is, thus, greater during early systole than diastole. At low pressures there are few discharges during the upstroke of arterial pressure. At higher mean arterial pressures, discharges are present throughout more of the cycle. The frequency remains higher early in the cycle. At very high mean arterial pressures, discharges occur continuously, achieving maximum inhibition of the vasomotor centre (Figure CR27). The effect of this is that baroreceptors respond not only to changes in pressure but also to changes in pulse pressure and heart rate.

Baroreceptors can reset their working range and sensitivity, or are 'adaptive', in response to sustained pressure changes. During chronic hypertension, the baroreceptors adapt to higher pressures and the response curve is shifted to the right. These changes are reversible.

Carotid and aortic baroreceptor reflex

Baroreceptors in the carotid sinus and the arch of the aorta monitor arterial pressure, arterial pulse pressure and heart rate. They play a key role in maintaining cardiovascular homeostasis against acute disturbances as occur in trauma or exercise. Carotid sinus baroreceptors are more sensitive to blood pressure changes than aortic baroreceptors. The carotid baroreceptors also respond to external mechanical stimulation, which increases their firing rate, eliciting an inhibitory vasomotor response. In susceptible individuals this may reduce blood pressure sufficiently to induce syncope. Therapeutically, carotid sinus massage can sometimes be effective in slowing a supraventricular tachycardia.

Cardiopulmonary baroreceptor reflex

Stretch receptors exist in the atria, ventricles and pulmonary vessels. These receptors protect against rapid changes in intravascular volume by varying their tonic discharge, which exerts an inhibitory influence over the medullary pressor centre. They also play a part in controlling heart rate.

There are two types of stretch receptor in the atria. Type A receptors discharge predominantly during atrial systole, while type B discharge during atrial filling, particularly over the later part of diastole. When intravascular volume expands atrial filling is increased, and both A and B receptors are stimulated. The impulses from these receptors are relayed to the medulla by the vagus nerves, which causes inhibition of the pressor centre and stimulation of the sinus node. This results in vasodilatation, a fall in blood pressure, increased renal blood flow, increased urine output, and a rise in heart rate.

Bainbridge reflex

In 1915 the English physiologist F. A. Bainbridge described the reflex increase in heart rate in response to a rapid intravascular infusion of fluid in anaesthetised animals. The receptors are the atrial A and B receptors described above. The afferent limb of the reflex is the vagus nerves, while the efferent limb consists of sympathetic nerves to the sinus node. Heart rate is thus influenced by the two opposing actions of the arterial baroreceptor reflex and the Bainbridge reflex. Whether the heart rate increases or decreases with a sudden increase in intravascular volume is thought to be dependent on the initial heart rate: if it is high it tends to decrease (arterial baroreceptor reflex), while if the initial heart rate is low it tends to increase (Bainbridge reflex).

Pulmonary stretch receptors

Stretch receptors in the lung, although mainly concerned with respiratory control, also inhibit the vasomotor centres when stimulated. Thus, inflation of the lungs results in systemic vasodilatation and a decrease in blood pressure.

Chemoreceptor reflexes

These reflexes are mediated centrally by receptors in the medulla, and peripherally by the carotid and aortic bodies. The chemoreceptors can respond to parameters that reflect hypoxia, hypercapnia, acidaemia or ischaemia. Chemo-receptor reflexes are mainly directed towards respiratory control but do exert some effects over cardiovascular parameters. Afferent pathways are mainly via the glos-sopharyngeal or vagus nerves, although coronary and pulmonary chemoreceptors may also possess sympathetic afferents.

- Peripheral chemoreceptor reflexes – chemoreceptors are in the carotid and aortic bodies. The carotid bodies are small masses of chromaffin tissue situated on the medial aspects of the carotid sinuses, while the aortic bodies are similar organs located over the anterior and posterior aspects of the aortic arch. The chemoreceptors respond primarily to a reduction in arterial oxygen tension (PaO_2), but are also sensitive to a rise in arterial carbon dioxide tension ($PaCO_2$) or a fall in pH. Both respiratory and circulatory centres in the brain stem receive the afferent impulses. The main effects of peripheral chemoreceptor reflexes are on the respiratory centre, but a minor effect is exerted on the pressor centre, with hypoxia and hypercapnia producing increases in blood pressure and a transient bradycardia.

- Central chemoreceptor reflexes – the vasomotor centres as well as other medullary receptors respond to changes in $PaCO_2$ and pH. These central reflexes predominate over the peripheral receptors, stimulating the respiratory centres and causing an increase in pressor tone and decrease in heart rate, following a rise in $PaCO_2$ or a fall in pH. Central chemoreceptors are relatively insensitive to hypoxia, hypoxic reflexes being mediated primarily through the carotid and aortic bodies. Concomitant peripheral vasodilatation often leaves arterial blood pressure unchanged.
- Cushing reflex – a vasomotor centre reflex caused by a direct response of pressor cells to ischaemia. This results in reflex vasoconstriction and decreased heart rate. This increases blood pressure at the expense of cardiac output, but sustains cerebral perfusion pressure.
- The Bezold–Jarisch reflex – a response of coronary artery chemoreceptors to ischaemia causing hypotension and bradycardia but increasing coronary blood flow.
- Pulmonary chemoreceptor reflex – chemoreceptors also exist in the lung, causing apnoea, hypotension and bradycardia when stimulated by ischaemic metabolites.

Pain reflexes

Cutaneous painful stimuli evoke the somatosympathetic reflex. Afferent impulses stimulate the rostral ventrolateral medulla to cause a rise in blood pressure. Prolonged or severe pain may cause vasodilatation and syncope.

Visceral pain often produces a depressor response due to stimulation of vagal or pelvic parasympathetic afferents. In contrast, large bowel has a significant degree of sympathetic innervation and can produce a pressor response when stimulated.

Blood volume

The volume of blood in the body is about 70 ml kg^{-1} in adults and 80 ml kg^{-1} in infants. Various types of blood vessel contain different proportions of the total blood volume. Distribution of blood volume in the vascular system is summarised in Figure CR28.

Central venous pressure and blood volume

The venous system contains about two-thirds of the blood volume, and can be visualised as a 'venous reservoir' supplying blood flow to the heart. Central venous pressure (CVP) is therefore a balance between blood volume, veno-motor tone and the demands of the cardiac pump. At

Location	Volume (%)
Heart	5
Systemic circulation	
Aorta and arteries	11
Capillaries	6
Veins and venules	66
Pulmonary circulation	
Arteries	3
Capillaries	4
Veins and venules	5

Figure CR28 Distribution of blood in the circulatory system

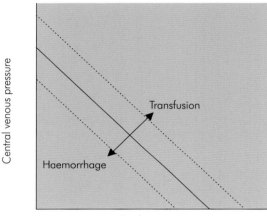

Figure CR29 Vascular function curve

a given blood volume, as cardiac output increases, the rate at which blood is removed from the venous reservoir increases and CVP falls. Similarly, when cardiac output decreases, a rise in CVP is produced. This relationship reflects the passive pressure–volume characteristics of the venous system, and can be described by the vascular function curve (Figure CR29), which plots CVP against cardiac output with a fixed blood volume. Alterations in blood volume, e.g. haemorrhage or transfusion, will shift the vascular function curve up or down.

This relationship should be differentiated from the situation in which blood volume is actively increased to increase cardiac output. This is an application of the Frank–Starling relationship, and is described by a ventricular function curve that plots cardiac output against CVP. A combination of the vascular function curve and the ventricular function curve describes ventriculovenous coupling (see

Section 2, Chapter 5, page 295), which has a potential clinical application in balancing the use of IV infusion and inotropes when optimising cardiac output.

Control of blood volume

The haemodynamic effects of blood volume depend on the volume in the venous reservoir. This is controlled acutely by reflex venoconstriction and redistribution from other areas of the circulatory system. Blood can be diverted from 'reservoirs' such as cutaneous vascular beds, splanchnic vessels and the liver. Longer-term control of blood volume is set by the balance between intravascular fluid and interstitial fluid compartments, fluid intake and renal loss. These mechanisms are illustrated by considering the events occurring in response to haemorrhage.

Circulatory control under special circumstances

Haemorrhage

An acute loss of about 5% or more of the blood volume is accompanied by immediate physiological changes, which can cause a patient to become pale and sweaty with a rapid thready pulse. A rapid respiratory rate and mild cyanosis may also be present. The underlying physiological changes include:

- Decreased systolic and diastolic blood pressures
- Reduced pulse pressure
- Increased heart rate and contractility
- Increased vasoconstriction and venoconstriction
- Diversion of blood centrally from cutaneous, muscular and splanchnic circulations
- Adrenal medulla stimulation with increased circulating catecholamine levels
- Tachypnoea

These initial haemodynamic changes may reverse over about 20 minutes, depending on the extent of the blood loss. If blood loss is excessive, compensatory mechanisms can only produce transient improvement and haemorrhagic shock ensues, with continued haemodynamic deterioration. Compensation for acute blood loss is mediated via a series of mechanisms:

- The baroreceptor reflex gives rise to selective vasoconstriction of arterioles, which increases systemic vascular resistance and preserves cerebral and coronary blood flow.
- Chemoreceptor reflexes augment the baroreceptor reflex, particularly at lower arterial pressures (<60 mmHg), where the baroreceptor response is limited by its threshold effect.

- Cerebral ischaemic response. At mean arterial pressures below 40 mmHg cerebral ischaemia is associated with direct stimulation of the adrenal medulla, augmenting the effects produced by baroreceptor and chemoreceptor reflexes.
- Reabsorption of interstitial fluid – vasoconstriction reduces capillary hydrostatic pressures, which increases net reabsorption of interstitial fluid. About 0.25 ml kg^{-1} tissue fluid can be gained per minute through increased reabsorption. Ultimately fluid is also shifted from the intracellular compartment to the interstitial space, this balance probably being influenced by raised cortisol levels stimulated during haemorrhage.
- Release of catecholamines. Activation of the sympathetic system via the baroreceptor and chemoreceptor reflexes produces stimulation of the adrenal medulla and increased levels of circulating catecholamines.
- Renal conservation of water and salt. Decreased renal perfusion produces secretion of renin from the juxtaglomerular apparatus. The renin converts plasma angiotensinogen to angiotensin I, which in turn becomes angiotensin II, a potent vasoconstrictor. Stimulation of the adrenal cortex also increases aldosterone levels, leading to renal retention of sodium. Reduced intravascular volume decreases firing of atrial stretch receptors and produces increased secretion of vasopressin from the posterior pituitary. This results in the retention of water in the renal collecting ducts. Vasopressin is also a potent vasoconstrictor at higher concentrations. The overall effects are retention of water and sodium, which helps to restore extracellular fluid volume.

Over 6 weeks increased erythropoietin secretion from the kidney stimulates bone marrow to produce more red blood cells and replace haemoglobin lost during haemorrhage.

Valsalva manoeuvre

A. M. Valsalva (1666–1723) was an Italian anatomist who described a manoeuvre for clearing the Eustachian tube. The Valsalva manoeuvre is forced expiration against a closed glottis, and provides a good demonstration of autonomic reflex control of heart rate and blood pressure. The manoeuvre produces a square wave rise in intrathoracic pressure of about 40 mmHg (Figure CR30). The cardiovascular response can be considered in the following stages:

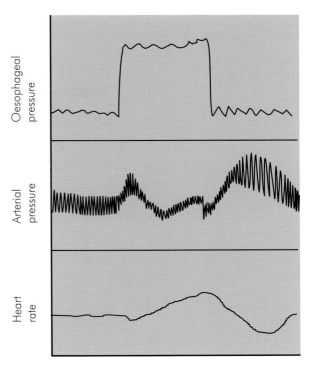

Figure CR30 Valsalva manoeuvre

- Initially there is an immediate increase in arterial blood pressure as the step in intrathoracic pressure is transmitted to the pressure in the aorta. The increased intrathoracic pressure also compresses pulmonary veins, forcing their contents into the left atrium and producing a transient rise in cardiac output.
- The sustained increase in intrathoracic pressure is also accompanied by higher intra-abdominal pressure due to contraction of the abdominal wall muscles. Raised pressure in the abdomen and thorax compresses the venae cavae, reducing the venous return to the right and left sides of the heart. This causes a decrease in arterial and pulse pressures.
- The fall in arterial and pulse pressures results in diminished stimulation of baroreceptors, causing a tachycardia and increased systemic vascular resistance. This restores mean arterial and pulse pressures to about resting values recorded before the manoeuvre.
- Opening the glottis releases the positive intrathoracic pressure, producing a sudden fall in aortic pressure. The resulting drop in arterial pressure is maintained

briefly as blood fills the pulmonary vessels and central veins, rather than providing venous return to the heart. Baroreceptor reflexes again respond to this sudden drop in arterial pressure, and act to restore venous return and cardiac output.

- Finally, as venous return to both sides of the heart increases again, cardiac output is restored, but ejects into a peripheral vascular system already constricted by baroreceptor reflexes. Blood pressure thus overshoots its original resting value, until increased stimulation of baroreceptors causes reflex bradycardia and vasodilatation to restore blood pressure to normal once again.

The events described above occur even after sympathectomy, because reflex activity can still be mediated if the vagus nerves remain intact. However, in the case of autonomic neuropathy, a persisting fall in blood pressure is caused by the high intrathoracic pressure, and there is no reflex tachycardia. Then, on release of the intrathoracic pressure, no overshoot of arterial blood pressure occurs.

Exercise

Exercise activates reflex mechanisms that enhance cardiovascular performance. These include:

- Cerebrocortical activation of the sympathetic system due to anticipation of physical activity. This is sometimes referred to as 'central command'.
- Cardiovascular reflexes due to stimulation of muscle mechanoreceptors during contraction. The afferent limb is via small unmyelinated fibres which relay centrally by unidentified connections, to activate sympathetic fibres to the heart and peripheral vessels.
- Local reflexes stimulated by rapid accumulation of metabolites during muscle contraction.
- Baroreceptor reflexes.

Peripheral chemoreceptors do not play a significant part during exercise, as arterial pH, $PaCO_2$ and PaO_2 remain about normal. In addition to the cardiovascular reflexes outlined above, pulmonary reflexes increase the depth and rate of breathing.

Moderate exercise levels

Prior to commencing exercise, anticipation of activity increases sympathetic discharge and inhibits the parasympathetic system. Mild to moderate degrees of exercise lead to graded changes which:

- Increase cardiovascular performance
- Redistribute blood flow to active areas

Organ system	Blood flow (ml min^{-1})	
	Exercise	Rest
Brain	750	750
Heart	750	250
Skeletal muscle	12 500	1200
Skin	1900	500
Abdominal viscera	600	1400
Kidneys	600	1100
Other	400	600
Total	17 500	5800

Figure CR31 Distribution of blood flow to different organ systems during moderate exercise and rest

- Maintain cerebral blood flow
- Increase oxygen consumption
- Increase the efficiency of oxygen extraction

Regional blood flow during exercise

Blood flow is diverted to active muscle from skin, splanchnic regions, kidneys and inactive muscles. Cutaneous blood flow, although decreased initially, gradually increases during exercise with rising body temperature. As exercise severity increases further and oxygen consumption increases to maximum levels, cutaneous vasoconstriction occurs and blood flow to the skin starts to decrease. Myocardial blood flow increases concomitantly according to metabolic demands. Cerebral blood flow remains unchanged during exercise. These changes in the distribution of blood flow are summarised in Figure CR31.

Skeletal muscle during exercise

Blood flow to the active muscles increases progressively in keeping with the work rate of the tissues. Locally accumulating substances and conditions, such as potassium and adenosine together with a reduction in pH, produce arteriolar dilatation and blood flows up to 20 times resting values. Capillary recruitment increases dramatically. Net movement of fluid into the interstitial compartment occurs and lymph flow increases, aided by muscle contractions. Oxygen extraction can rise by as much as 60 times, outstripping increases in blood flow and leading to greater arteriovenous oxygen differences. This higher degree of extraction is mediated by the right shift in the oxygen–haemoglobin dissociation curve, which is associated with the accumulation of lactic acid, decreased pH, increased $PaCO_2$ and increased temperature.

Cardiac output in exercise

The enhanced cardiac output during exercise is achieved mainly through the heart rate, which follows increased sympathetic and decreased parasympathetic drive of the sinoatrial node. At mild to moderate work rates the heart rate increases proportionately to an appropriate level and is then maintained. As work rate is increased further the heart rate plateaus at about 180 bpm. In trained athletes, cardiac output may increase by seven times resting values, but stroke volume may only increase to twice the resting value.

Venous return and blood volume in exercise

The increase in cardiac output during exercise is accompanied by a commensurate increase in venous return. As a result central venous pressure does not change significantly. Thus the Frank–Starling mechanism does not normally play a major part in increasing stroke volume during moderate exercise. However, when exercise becomes maximal, central venous pressure tends to rise and the Frank–Starling mechanism starts to contribute significantly. The mechanisms augmenting venous return include:

- Increased venomotor tone
- Increased muscle pump activity
- Redirection of blood from cutaneous, renal and splanchnic circulations
- Enhanced thoracic pump action due to increased respiratory rate and tidal volume

Intravascular volume is usually slightly reduced during exercise due to increased insensible losses from the respiratory tract and skin. In addition, there is increased net capillary filtration into the interstitial muscle space. As a result there is often a slight rise in haematocrit during exercise.

Arterial pressure

Both systolic and diastolic blood pressures increase during exercise, although systolic pressure increases relatively more than diastolic. This results in an increased pulse pressure, which is attributed to an increased stroke volume and higher ejection velocity from the left ventricle.

This increased arterial pressure occurs in the face of a decreased systemic vascular resistance (mainly due to vasodilatation in active muscle), and reflects the greatly increased cardiac output (up to seven times resting value).

The sympathetic system is important in maintaining blood pressure during exercise, and if it is compromised by drugs (β blockers) or disease (autonomic neuropathy) effort-induced hypotension or syncope can result. A restricted cardiac output (aortic stenosis) can produce the same effect.

Severe exercise and exhaustion

When exercise is taken to the point of exhaustion, the compensatory reflexes fail and decompensatory changes occur. These include:

- Heart rate rises to plateau of about 180 bpm
- Stroke volume plateaus and may even decrease
- Blood pressure begins to fall
- Dehydration occurs
- Vasoconstriction due to excessive sympathetic activity
- Body temperature continues to rise due to decreased heat loss
- Lactic acid and CO_2 accumulate, giving rise to decreased tissue pH
- Muscle cramps and pain
- Subjective feelings of weariness and lack of drive to continue activity

Special circulations

Cardiac output is distributed between the various organ systems as shown in Figure CR32.

Circulation to the kidneys, lungs and liver are described in Section 2, Chapters 7, 8 and 12 respectively. This section discusses the circulations of the heart, the brain and the fetus.

Coronary circulation

In the root of the aorta, the right coronary artery arises behind the right cusp of the aortic valve, and supplies the right atrium and ventricle. The left coronary artery arises

Organ system	Blood flow (ml min^{-1})	% Cardiac output
Brain	750	13
Heart	250	4
Skeletal muscle	1200	20
Skin	500	9
Abdominal viscera	1400	24
Kidneys	1100	20
Other	600	10
Total	5800	100

Figure CR32 Blood flow to different organ systems at rest

behind the posterior cusp of the aortic valve, and divides close to its origin into circumflex and anterior descending branches, before supplying the left atrium and ventricle. Some overlap of the territory supplied by each main artery usually occurs. Epicardial arteries originate from these main coronary arteries, and branch to form end arteries that penetrate the myocardium. The blood flow through each main artery is equal in 30% of people, but the right coronary artery is dominant in 50%. Two-thirds of coronary blood flow drains into the right atrium via the coronary sinus and anterior coronary veins. The remainder drains directly into the chambers of the heart through small thebesian veins, arteriosinusoidal vessels and arterioluminal vessels. Venous drainage into left-sided chambers constitutes true shunt and makes a small contribution to arterial desaturation.

Coronary blood flow

Total coronary blood flow at rest is about 250 ml per minute. The myocardium normally extracts about 70% of the oxygen content of coronary blood at rest; thus, increasing coronary perfusion is the only way to increase oxygen delivery. At rest the oxygen requirement of the myocardium is 10 ml min^{-1} per 100 g, giving a total basal oxygen requirement of 30 ml min^{-1} for an adult. Cardiac muscle is versatile in its use of substrate, normally using 60% fatty acid and 40% carbohydrate as fuel. It may adapt to use different proportions and include ketone bodies as substrate.

Coronary blood flow and its distribution can be studied using:
- Coronary angiography – radiopaque dye is used to outline coronary vessels and radioactive xenon to quantify regional perfusion.
- Thallium scan – radioactive thallium uptake is used as a marker of regional distribution of perfusion in the myocardium.
- Technetium scan – selective uptake of radioactive technetium marks infarcted areas.

Factors determining coronary blood flow

Since the coronary arteries originate in the root of the aorta, aortic pressure provides the main driving force for coronary blood flow. Normally, this pressure is controlled by baroreceptor reflexes, and regulation of coronary blood flow is thus achieved through coronary vasodilatation or vasoconstriction. Coronary vascular resistance is mainly controlled by local factors. Some of the factors affecting coronary blood flow are detailed below:

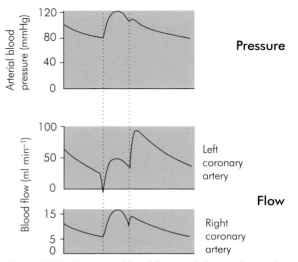

Figure CR33 Coronary blood flow and the cardiac cycle

- Extravascular compression (extracoronary resistance) – this describes the external compression produced by myocardial contraction during the cardiac cycle. Coronary blood flow is reduced to zero in early systole and may even be transiently reversed (Figure CR33). This 'squeezing' effect is greatest at endocardial levels and least towards the epicardium. However, in the normal heart endocardial and epicardial blood flows are about equal in the cardiac cycle. The bulk of coronary blood flow thus occurs during diastole. However, since diastole decreases as heart rate increases, coronary blood flow can become compromised by tachyarrhythmias. Counterpulsation or 'balloon pumping' assists coronary blood flow by inflating an aortic balloon cyclically during diastole.
- Metabolic demands – the correlation between metabolic activity in the heart and coronary blood flow is fixed. Metabolites or an unidentified vasoactive agent act to increase or decrease the oxygen supply if demand is varied. Alternatively, if the oxygen supply is limited cardiac activity adapts. Likely substances responsible for this effect include potassium ions and adenosine.
- Autonomic system – activation of the sympathetic system tends to produce an increase in coronary blood flow. This occurs as a net result of increased metabolic demand in the face of the negative effects of increased contractility and heart rate on coronary blood flow. Under β blockade coronary vessels constrict in

Factor	Effect on coronary vascular resistance
Sympathetic activity	
α receptors	↑
β receptors	↓
Vagal activity	↓
Systolic compression	↑
Coronary perfusion pressure	↑ or ↓
Adenosine	↓
Other metabolic factors	
CO_2, O_2, H^+, K^+	↑ or ↓

Figure CR34 Summary of factors affecting coronary vascular resistance

response to sympathetic stimulation. Stimulation of the vagus nerves produces slight coronary vasodilatation.

- Coronary perfusion pressure (CPP) – this is the pressure across the coronary arteries and equals the difference between aortic pressure and intraventricular pressure. Autoregulation operates over a range of CPP between 60 and 180 mmHg. If CPP changes suddenly, coronary vessels respond by dilating or constricting to dampen dramatic surges or falls in coronary blood flow.

Figure CR34 summarises the factors affecting coronary vascular resistance.

Cardiac ischaemia

When the oxygen demands of the myocardium outstrip the oxygen supply, myocardial dysfunction and tissue damage follow. The oxygen requirements are related to the cardiac work rate, which in turn is dependent on systolic arterial pressure and cardiac output. Oxygen requirements are increased disproportionately by increases in systolic pressure, compared with cardiac output. Thus, if cardiac work is increased by increasing systolic pressure, oxygen requirements are much greater than if the increase in cardiac work were achieved by increasing cardiac output. 'Pressure' work is therefore more expensive than 'volume' work in terms of oxygen consumption. This is a major factor underlying the mortality associated with aortic stenosis. Clinically myocardial ischaemia results in the chest pain of angina pectoris and ultimately the tissue necrosis occurring in myocardial infarction.

Myocardial blood flow may be increased in ischaemic heart disease by:

- Coronary vasodilators (glyceryl trinitrate)
- Coronary thrombus dissolution (streptokinase)
- Coronary angioplasty (dilatation by catheter balloon)
- Coronary bypass graft
- Coronary laser endarterectomy

Cerebral circulation

The left and right carotid arteries join the basilar artery to form the circle of Willis, from which the left and right anterior, middle and posterior cerebral arteries arise. The basilar artery is formed by the anastomosis of the two vertebral arteries. Each carotid artery supplies its own side of the brain, and there is no significant perfusion of the opposite side by a carotid. Cerebral venous drainage is via the internal jugular veins, which are fed by the dural sinuses or directly by cerebral veins.

Brain cells are intolerant of hypoxia and require uninterrupted perfusion. Several seconds of total ischaemia can produce unconsciousness and several minutes may result in irreversible damage. Cerebral vessels are innervated by sympathetic fibres that enter the skull around the carotid arteries. These fibres originate in the superior cervical ganglia. There are also cholinergic fibres from the sphenopalatine ganglia and facial nerve. Cerebral vessels are supplied by sensory fibres originating in the trigeminal ganglia. The stimulation of sensory fibres on vessels by metabolites is thought to cause migraine.

Cerebral blood flow

Mean cerebral blood flow is about 55 ml 100 g^{-1} min^{-1}, and it is maintained within a relatively narrow range compared with other organs. It varies between the anatomical structures of the brain, with grey matter in general receiving more than twice (70 ml 100 g^{-1} min^{-1}) the blood flow of white matter (30 ml 100 g^{-1} min^{-1}).

The brain consumes about 3.5 ml 100 g^{-1} min^{-1} oxygen, leaving the jugular venous blood 65% saturated. Structures such as the colliculi and basal ganglia receive much greater blood flows than the brain stem and cerebellum. Cortical blood flow is dependent on activity, and perfusion of specific areas reaches high levels (>130 ml 100 g^{-1} min^{-1}) when activated.

Cerebral blood flow can be estimated by:

- Kety method – an application of the Fick principle that determines the total cerebral blood flow in ml 100 g^{-1} min^{-1}. Nitrous oxide is used as the transported substance because it has a partition coefficient = 1, which ensures that the brain concentration becomes equal to the jugular venous concentration, after an equilibration time of 10 minutes. A subject breathes 15% nitrous oxide for 10 minutes. The total nitrous oxide transferred to 100 g brain tissue per min (Q) can be determined from the final nitrous oxide content of 100 g of jugular venous blood divided by 10. The average arteriovenous difference (D) in nitrous oxide content per ml is determined from arterial and venous samples during equilibration. The blood flow can then be calculated from the ratio Q/D.

- Scintillography – using radioactive tracers (xenon) to trace regional blood flow.
- SPECT scanning – scintillography enhanced by CT or MRI scanning.
- PET scanning – use of 2-deoxyglucose labelled with a positron emitter.
- Doppler – crude but readily available for clinical use in ICU or operating theatre.

Regulation of cerebral blood flow

Control of cerebral circulation is primarily through autoregulation due to local metabolic factors. Neural control is thought to play a minor role. Total cerebral blood flow is maintained constant over a range of mean arterial pressure and in the face of varying levels of $PaCO_2$ and PaO_2. This is achieved by control of total cerebrovascular resistance and cerebral perfusion pressure (Figure CR35).

Regional cerebral blood flow, on the other hand, is highly variable and varies according to activity and local metabolic factors. The factors affecting total cerebral blood flow include:

- Cerebral perfusion pressure – pressure across the cerebral vessels, given by the difference between mean arterial pressure and (venous pressure + intracranial pressure). Raised intracranial pressure may reduce cerebral perfusion pressure.
- $PaCO_2$ – arterial CO_2 tensions have a marked influence over cerebral blood flow. Low $PaCO_2$ vasoconstricts and raised $PaCO_2$ vasodilates cerebral vessels. Hyperventilation reduces blood volume within the brain and is used to reduce raised intracranial pressure after head injury.
- PaO_2 – low PaO_2 vasodilates and high PaO_2 vasoconstricts, but the effect of oxygen tension on cerebral vessels occurs to a far lesser degree than with $PaCO_2$.
- pH – cerebral vessels are also sensitive to pH independently of $PaCO_2$. A decreased pH causes vasodilatation.
- Metabolites – adenosine and potassium have both been implicated in adjusting local cerebral perfusion. Any event causing decreased PaO_2 or increased oxygen demand produces raised local levels of adenosine in the brain, which are sustained throughout the event. A similar transient rise in potassium ion concentration is also produced. These substances are thought to be instrumental in linking regional blood flow to activity in the brain.

Raised intracranial pressure (ICP)

The skull is a rigid bony enclosure that contains 1400 g brain tissue (80%), 75 ml blood (10%) and 75 ml cerebrospinal fluid (10%). These contents are effectively incompressible; therefore, any increase in one component produces a reciprocal decrease in the others (Monro–Kellie doctrine) and an increase in ICP. Cerebral oedema will thus be accompanied by a reduction in cerebral blood volume and compression of the ventricles. Brain injury secondary to raised ICP occurs when cerebral blood flow is compromised, or when the increase in ICP is asymmetrical and brain shift occurs. Normal ICP is 0–10 mmHg, while >15 mmHg is considered significantly raised. As ICP continues to rise, cerebral blood flow is increasingly reduced and brain tissue becomes ischaemic. Vital centres respond by increasing systemic arterial blood pressure, slowing the heart rate and respiratory rate. The blood pressure response attempts to restore cerebral blood flow by restoring the cerebral perfusion pressure. Ultimately herniation of the cerebellar tonsils through the foramen magnum causes compression of the brainstem and death.

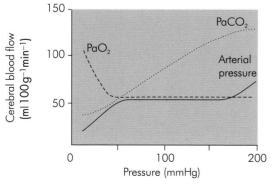

Figure CR35 Autoregulation of cerebral blood flow

Blood–brain barrier

The blood–brain barrier exists between the circulation and the interstitial fluid in the brain. It consists of the ultra-filtration barrier in the choroid plexuses and the barrier around cerebral capillaries. The latter consists of capillary endothelium, basement membrane and a fenestrated layer of astrocyte endfeet. Tight junctions, impermeable to solutes, join capillary endothelial cells and form a basic component of the blood–brain barrier. Water, carbon dioxide and oxygen diffuse freely across the blood–brain barrier, but the transport of glucose, the principal brain substrate, and ionised molecules is controlled. Proteins and some drugs cannot cross the endothelium unless it is inflamed. The blood–brain barrier has the following functions:

- To provide tight control over ionic (H^+, Na^+, K^+, Ca^{2+}, Mg^{2+}) concentrations in the interstitial fluid, because brain cells are extremely sensitive to ion changes
- To protect the brain from transient changes in plasma glucose, the main substrate for the brain
- To protect the brain from endogenous and exogenous toxins in the plasma
- To prevent release of central neurotransmitters into the systemic circulation

Fetal circulation

The fetus and placenta form a unit in which the placenta enables the fetus to exchange carbon dioxide and metabolic waste products for oxygen and nutrients from the maternal circulation. In the fetus the left and right sides of the heart work in parallel, unlike the adult circulation, where the ventricles work in series. The fetal ventricles, acting in parallel, pump blood through the systemic vessels and the placenta, which are also arranged in parallel. The output of the fetal heart is split about 60 : 40, with the majority passing through the placenta, for oxygenation and nutrient–waste exchange (Figure CR36). The oxygenated blood returns from the placenta, about half of it entering the liver with the portal circulation, while the rest joins the inferior vena cava (IVC) directly. IVC blood is therefore relatively well oxygenated and passes back to the heart, where it divides between right and left sides, the majority passing to the left atrium. The right atrium receives superior vena caval blood from the head and upper limbs, which mixes with its portion of the oxygenated IVC blood. The right side of the heart provides two-thirds of the fetal cardiac output, which goes to supply the lower half of the fetus. The blood

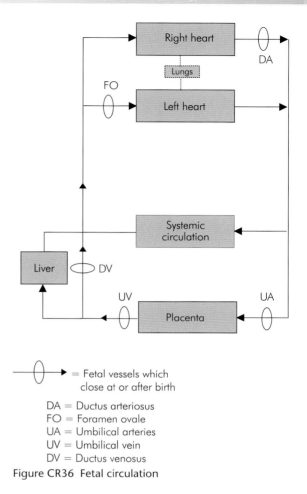

= Fetal vessels which close at or after birth

DA = Ductus arteriosus
FO = Foramen ovale
UA = Umbilical arteries
UV = Umbilical vein
DV = Ductus venosus

Figure CR36 Fetal circulation

filling the left ventricle is nearly all from the IVC, which is therefore better oxygenated than the blood in the right ventricle. The left ventricle output goes to supply the head and upper limbs. The above pattern of fetal circulation is due to the following vascular features in the fetus, which convert to the adult configuration immediately or soon after birth:

- Umbilical arteries – two arteries that arise from the internal iliac arteries and carry 60% of the cardiac output to the placenta.
- Umbilical vein – carries oxygenated blood from the placenta back to the fetal liver and IVC.
- Ductus venosus – splits off 50% of the oxygenated blood from the umbilical vein to bypass the liver and enter the IVC directly.

- Foramen ovale – communication between right and left atria, allowing about two-thirds of the oxygenated IVC blood to pass directly to the left atrium.
- Pulmonary vasculature – fetal lungs are collapsed and have a high pulmonary vascular resistance, allowing only about 10% of the right ventricular output to pass through the lungs.
- Ductus arteriosus – connects pulmonary artery to the aorta, allowing the right ventricular output to bypass the lungs and flow down the aorta to the lower fetal body and placenta.

Changes in fetal circulation at birth

At birth, pulmonary vascular resistance falls markedly as the lungs expand and become aerated. This reduces pulmonary arterial pressures and increases blood flow to the left atrium. Umbilical vessels constrict strongly when exposed to trauma, tension, catecholamines, angiotensin and PaO_2. These stimuli occur at birth and placental circulation ceases, resulting in a rise in systemic vascular resistance and arterial pressure. These changes make left atrial pressure higher than right atrial pressure and tend to close the foramen ovale. The ductus arteriosus closes soon after birth, usually within 48 hours. The mechanism for this closure has not been completely identified, although a

Site	Fetal O_2 saturation
Umbilical vein	80%
IVC/SVC deoxygenated	25%
IVC oxygenated (mixed with placental blood)	67%
Pulmonary artery	52%
Left ventricle	65%
Aorta	62%

Figure CR37 Oxygen saturation in the fetus

high PaO_2 appears to initiate the closure and exposure to a low PaO_2 can reverse the closure in the neonate. Prostaglandins maintain the patency of the ductus arteriosus, and indomethacin may be successful in closing a patent ductus arteriosus in a neonate.

Oxygen saturation in the fetus

The fetal blood is oxygenated from venous pools in the placenta. Thus, oxygen saturations at various points in the fetal circulation are lower than their equivalents in the adult. Some oxygen saturation levels are shown in Figure CR37.

CHAPTER 7

Renal physiology

C. J. Lote

Fundamentals of Anaesthesia, 3rd edition, ed. Tim Smith, Colin Pinnock and Ted Lin. Published by Cambridge University Press. © Cambridge University Press 2008.

Morphology and cellular organisation of the kidney

Each human kidney has 1–1.5 million functional units called nephrons. The nephron is a blind-ended tube, the blind end forming a capsule (Bowman's capsule) around a knot of blood capillaries (the glomerulus). The other parts of the nephron are the proximal tubule, loop of Henle, distal tubule and collecting duct, although in transport terms the nephron has been divided into additional segments (Figure RE1).

The glomeruli, proximal tubules and distal tubules are in the outer part of the kidney, the cortex, whereas the loops of Henle and the collecting ducts extend down into the deeper part, the medulla.

Cortical nephrons possess glomeruli located in the outer two-thirds of the cortex and have very short loops of Henle, which only extend a short distance into the medulla or may not reach the medulla at all. In contrast, nephrons whose glomeruli are in the inner third of the cortex (juxtamedullary nephrons) have long loops of Henle that pass deeply into the medulla. In humans about 15% of nephrons are long-looped, but there are also intermediate types of nephron.

Renal blood supply and vasculature

The kidneys receive 20–25% of the cardiac output but account for only 0.5% of the body weight. Of the blood to the kidney, >90% enters via the renal artery and supplies the renal cortex, which is perfused at about 500 ml $100\,g^{-1}$ tissue min^{-1} (100 times greater than resting muscle blood flow). The remainder of the renal blood supply goes to the capsule and the renal adipose tissue. Some of the cortical blood passes to the medulla; the outer medulla having a blood flow of 100 ml $100\,g^{-1}$ min^{-1}, while the inner medulla receives 20 ml $100\,g^{-1}$ min^{-1}.

Almost all of the blood that enters the kidneys does so at the renal hilum, via the renal artery. The renal artery branches to form several interlobar arteries, which themselves branch to give rise to arcuate (or arciform) arteries, which pass along the boundary between cortex and medulla. From these arcuate arteries, branches travel out at right angles, through the cortex towards the capsule.

These are interlobular arteries, and the afferent arterioles that supply the glomerular capillaries branch off from the interlobular arteries.

The glomerular capillaries are the site of filtration of the blood, the filtrate entering the Bowman's capsule of the nephron. Glomerular capillaries drain into a second arteriole, the efferent arteriole.

Efferent arterioles are portal vessels, since they carry blood from a capillary network directly to a second capillary network. The efferent arterioles from nephrons in the outer two-thirds of the cortex branch to form a dense network of peritubular capillaries, which surround all the cortical tubular elements. The efferent arterioles in the inner one-third of the cortex give rise not only to some peritubular capillaries but also to capillaries that have a hairpin course into and out of the medulla, where they are adjacent to the loops of Henle and collecting tubules. These medullary capillaries are vasa recta (Figure RE1). Vasa recta and peritubular capillaries eventually drain into the renal vein which leaves the kidney at the hilum.

Functions of the renal blood supply

In most organs and tissues of the body, the main purpose of the blood supply is to provide oxygen and to remove CO_2 and other products of metabolism. In the kidney the blood supply not only provides for the metabolic demands of renal tissues but also has to maintain glomerular filtration rate (GFR) and provide oxygen for the active reabsorption of sodium. The kidneys have a very high oxygen consumption, but because of the high blood flow, the arteriovenous oxygen difference across the kidney is small.

The renal cortex receives far more oxygen than it requires, so that the arteriovenous O_2 difference is only 1–2%. However, the medullary blood supply is only just adequate for the oxygen requirements of medullary cells, because the vasa recta arrangement causes oxygen to short-circuit the loops of Henle.

In the cortex, the main function of the blood supply is to provide flow for glomerular filtration and oxygen for sodium reabsorption. Of cortical O_2 consumption, more than 50% is used for sodium reabsorption. If renal blood flow is reduced GFR decreases, together with sodium

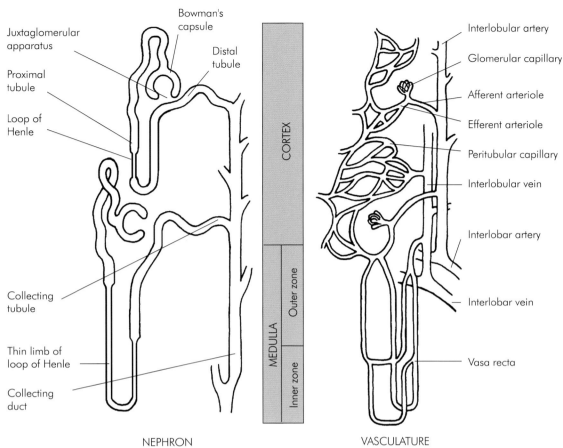

Figure RE1 Anatomy and vasculature of the kidney

reabsorption and oxygen demand. Thus, a reduction in cortical blood flow does not necessarily produce an increase in oxygen uptake and arteriovenous O_2 difference, until the cortical flow is down to about 150 ml 100 g^{-1} tissue min^{-1}.

Renal lymph drainage

Renal lymph vessels begin as blind-ended tubes in the renal cortex (close to the corticomedullary junction) and run parallel to the arcuate veins to leave the kidney at the renal hilum. Other lymph vessels travel towards the cortex and may pass through the capsule. The importance of the renal lymphatic drainage is frequently overlooked, but in fact the volume of lymph draining into the renal hilum per minute is about 0.5 ml – i.e. the kidney produces almost as much lymph per minute as urine. Its function is probably to return protein (reabsorbed from the tubular fluid) to the blood.

Glomerular filtration

The glomerulus

A glomerulus is a knot of capillaries fed by an afferent arteriole and drained by an efferent arteriole. Its function is to produce ultrafiltrate of the plasma. In the central part of the glomerular tuft are irregularly shaped cells, termed mesangial cells. These are phagocytic and may prevent the accumulation, in the basement membrane, of macromolecules that have escaped from the capillaries. The cells may also have a structural role in holding the delicate glomerular structure in position and, in addition, are capable of contraction (i.e. behave like smooth muscle cells) and so may

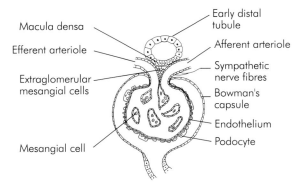

Figure RE2 Structure of the glomerulus

modify the surface area of the glomerular capillaries available for filtration.

Outside the glomerular area, close to the macula densa, are cells identical to mesangial cells, termed extraglomerular mesangial cells, or 'Goormaghtigh cells' (Figure RE2).

The glomerular filter

The glomerular ultrafiltrate forms the basis of the urine ultimately produced by the kidney. In moving from the capillary into the Bowman's capsule, the filtrate must traverse three layers, which are:

- The endothelial cell lining of the glomerular capillaries – in this layer adjacent endothelial cells are in contact with each other, and the cells have many circular fenestrations (pores), with a diameter of about 60 nm. The capillary endothelium acts as a screen to prevent blood cells and platelets from coming into contact with the main filter, which is the basement membrane.
- The glomerular basement membrane – immediately beneath the glomerular endothelium. It forms a continuous layer and is the main filtration barrier allowing the passage of molecules according to their size, shape and charge. It consists of collagen and other glycoproteins, including large amounts of heparan sulphate proteoglycan, with a large number of negative charges.
- The visceral epithelial cells of the Bowman's capsule – the third layer of the filter. These cells are podocytes and have a complex morphology. The cell body has projections (trabeculae) that encircle the basement membrane around the capillary. From the trabeculae, many smaller processes (pedicels) project. Substances passing through the slits (slit pores) between adjacent pedicels must pass close to the surface coating of the

pedicels, and this could influence the filtration behaviour of large charged molecules, since the pedicels are coated with negatively charged sialoglycoproteins. This layer is thought to maintain the basement membrane by the phagocytosis of macromolecules. It may also play a role in permselectivity which supplements that of the basement membrane

Glomerular filtration and the ultrafiltrate

The glomerular filtration rate (GFR) is about 180 litres per day (125 ml min^{-1}). Since the filtrate is derived from plasma, and the average person has only 3 litres of plasma, it follows that this same plasma is filtered (and reabsorbed in the tubules) many times in the course of a day.

Molecular size is the main determinant of whether a substance is filtered or retained in the capillaries. The molecular weight cutoff for the filter is about 70 000 daltons. Plasma albumin, with a molecular weight of 69 000 daltons, passes through the filter in minute quantities (retarded also by its charge, as mentioned above). Smaller molecules pass through the filter more easily, but the filter is freely permeable only to those molecules with a molecular weight below about 7000 daltons (Figure RE3).

Molecular shape and charge also influence filtration, but mainly of large molecules. For example, the rate of filtration of albumin, which has a negative charge, is only about 1/20 that of uncharged dextran molecules of the same molecular weight. This is due to the negative charges of the heparan sulphate proteoglycan in the glomerular basement membrane, and the sialoglycoproteins on the foot processes, which repel anionic macromolecules.

The ultrafiltrate passing into Bowman's capsule from the glomerular capillaries is almost protein-free and contains small molecules and ions in virtually the same concentrations as in the afferent arteriole. Similarly, the efferent arteriolar concentrations of such substances are not significantly altered by the filtration process.

Glomerular filtration forces

The forces determining filtration are similar to those forces determining the formation of tissue fluid through capillaries elsewhere in the body, and depend on the balance between hydrostatic pressure (P_C) and colloid osmotic (π_C) pressure. The balance between P_C and π_C in a normal capillary is shown in Figure RE3a, which illustrates the drop in P_C (solid line) along a capillary from the arteriolar end to the venous end, and also π_C (broken line), which

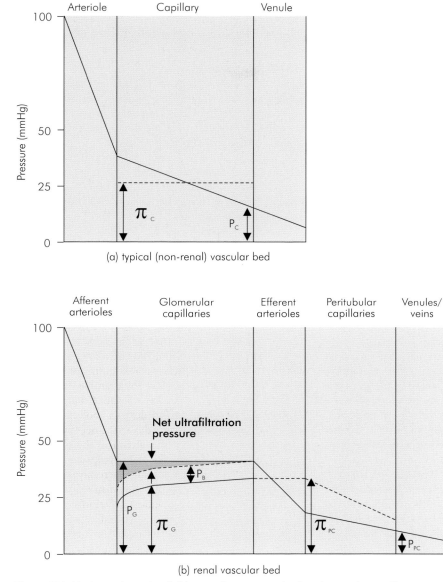

Figure RE3 Hydrostatic and colloid osmotic pressures in the glomerular capillary

remains constant along the length of the capillary. At the arteriolar end, $P_C > \pi_C$, causing fluid to leave the capillary, forming interstitial fluid. At the venous end of the capillary, $\pi_C > P_C$, leading to net tissue fluid reabsorption. There is an approximate balance between the formation and reabsorption of tissue fluid, any excess being drained by lymphatics.

In a glomerulus, the arrangement of the capillaries as portal vessels alters the magnitude of the filtration forces. The presence of a second resistance vessel (the efferent arteriole) following the glomerular capillary bed produces a higher hydrostatic pressure (45 mmHg) than in other capillary beds (32 mmHg). In addition, the fall in pressure along the glomerular capillary length is less marked

(P_G in Figure RE3b). The filtration rate depends on the difference between the forces pushing fluid out of the capillaries (favouring filtration) and forces tending to draw fluid back into the capillaries (opposing filtration). This relationship can be expressed as

GFR $\propto$ Forces favouring filtration
      $-$ Forces opposing filtration

Alternatively put:

$$(P_G + \pi_B) - (P_B + \pi_G)$$

where

P_G = hydrostatic pressure in the glomerular capillaries
P_B = colloid osmotic pressure in Bowman's capsule
π_B = hydrostatic pressure in Bowman's capsule
π_G = colloid osmotic pressure in the glomerular
        capillaries

Since only very small amounts of protein enter the Bowman's capsule, π_B is effectively zero, and therefore it can be said that

GFR $\propto$ $P_G - (P_B + \pi_G)$

At the afferent end of the glomerular capillaries the colloid osmotic pressure, π_G, is initially about 25 mmHg. As the filtration process occurs along the length of the glomerular capillaries, plasma proteins become progressively more concentrated and π_G increases towards the efferent end. Eventually, when π_G reaches about 35 mmHg, the net ultrafiltration pressure is reduced to zero, and there is filtration equilibrium (Figure RE3b).

The permeability of glomerular capillaries is about 100 times greater than the permeability of capillaries elsewhere in the body. There is only a small quantity of protein filtered at the glomerulus, but its loss in the urine would represent a considerable wastage over the course of a day. Essentially, all of the filtered protein (about 30 g per day) is reabsorbed in the proximal tubule and enters the renal lymph vessels.

Filtration coefficient
To evaluate GFR, K_F, the filtration coefficient, must be introduced:

GFR $= K_F(P_G - P_B - \pi_G)$

where

K_F = (glomerular capillary permeability)
      $\times$ (capillary filtration area).

In humans, filtration pressure equilibrium is not quite achieved. A consequence of this disequilibrium is that small changes in K_F have a considerable effect on GFR.

Filtration fraction
Renal blood flow is large in relation to the size of the kidneys (about 1.1 litres per minute), but only a relatively small fraction of this is filtered. Since red blood cells are not filterable, renal plasma flow is the total amount of fluid entering the kidney which is potentially filterable. Renal plasma flow is about 600 ml min^{-1}, of which 120 ml min^{-1} forms the normal GFR. Thus, the filtration fraction is 120/600 or about 20%: i.e. of every 600 ml plasma arriving at the glomeruli, about 480 ml continues into the efferent arterioles.

Glomerular filtration pressure
The net filtration pressure must be sufficient to move plasma out of the glomerular capillary and into the Bowman's capsule. The resulting pressure in the Bowman's capsule must be high enough to overcome the viscosity of the tubular fluid and its friction against the tubule walls, and to maintain the tubules in a patent form against the renal interstitial pressure tending to compress the tubules. Occlusion of the renal blood supply, so that filtration ceases, causes the collapse of the tubular lumina.

Tubuloglomerular feedback
The filtration rate of individual nephrons (the single-nephron GFR, SNGFR) is greater in juxtamedullary nephrons than in cortical nephrons (50 compared with 30 nl min^{-1}). The SNGFR is determined or influenced by the composition of the tubular fluid in the distal nephron, while the concentration itself is influenced by the filtration rate. The mechanism of this tubuloglomerular feedback can be divided into:
- A luminal component, whereby some characteristic of the tubular fluid is recognised by the tubular epithelium
- A mechanism whereby the signal is transmitted to the glomerulus
- An effector mechanism to adjust the rate of glomerular filtration

Such a mechanism can be regarded as preventing the overloading of the reabsorptive capacity of individual nephrons: i.e. if the tubular NaCl load is too high, filtration by that nephron is decreased.

Renal clearance and its applications

Clearance is a key concept whose definition requires emphasis.

Definition of clearance

The clearance of any substance excreted by the kidney is the volume of plasma that is cleared of the substance in unit time. Thus, the units of clearance are those of volume per unit time (usually $ml\ min^{-1}$).

Considering the clearance of a substance x, clearance is given by the formula

$$C_x = \frac{U_x V}{P_x}$$

where

C_x = clearance of x
U_x = urine concentration of x
P_x = plasma concentration of x
V = urine flow ($ml\ min^{-1}$)

In fact, clearance only represents a theoretical volume of plasma, since no aliquot of plasma is completely cleared of any substance during its passage through the kidney. The clearance formula has considerable usefulness for assessing renal function. Clearances of two specific substances, inulin and para-aminohippuric acid (PAH), can be used to measure GFR and the renal plasma flow respectively.

Measurement of clearance

To determine clearance of a substance in practice, the following measurements must be made:
- Plasma concentration of the substance – must either be constant or changing in a predictable way so that an accurate average concentration can be calculated. It therefore follows that clearance measurements are only suitable for average or steady-state determinations of GFR and renal blood flow (RBF), and cannot be used if rapid or transient changes are occurring.
- Urine concentration of the substance – urine flow must be adequate for the assay in the clearance period (which is a minimum of 10–20 minutes).

Inulin clearance: the measurement of GFR

Inulin is a polysaccharide with a molecular weight of about 5500 daltons. It is not a normal constituent of the body, but can be injected (or, usually, infused) intravenously to measure inulin clearance. Inulin is small enough to pass through the glomerular filter without difficulty, but is not reabsorbed, secreted, synthesised or metabolised by the kidney. Thus, all the filtered inulin is excreted and all the inulin that is excreted has entered the urine only by filtration at the glomerulus.

If urinary inulin concentration is U_{in} ($mg\ ml^{-1}$), and urine flow is V ($ml\ min^{-1}$), then the amount of inulin excreted per minute is ($U_{in}V$). This is also the total amount of inulin that enters the nephrons contained in the filtered plasma per minute. The volume of plasma containing this amount of inulin is therefore

$$\frac{U_{in}V\ (mg)}{P_{in}\ (mg\ ml^{-1})}$$

where

P_{in} = plasma concentration of inulin

This volume of plasma is equivalent to the volume cleared of inulin per minute, i.e. the inulin clearance. Thus, the inulin clearance (C_{in}) is equal to GFR. The inulin clearance measurement (and, hence, GFR measurement) is independent of the plasma inulin concentration. For an adult, the normal inulin clearance (GFR) is $125\ ml\ min^{-1}$. From day to day, GFR is remarkably constant in humans. Variations in excretion of water and solutes are much more dependent on changes in tubular reabsorption and secretion than on GFR changes.

If a solute has a clearance value higher than the inulin clearance, then the solute must get into the renal tubules not only by glomerular filtration, but also by tubular secretion (PAH is such a substance: see below). However, if a solute has a clearance value less than that of inulin, there are two possibilities:
- The solute may not be freely filtered at the glomerulus.
- The solute is freely filtered but is then reabsorbed from the tubule.

Creatinine clearance

Because measurements of inulin clearance involve exogenous inulin administration it is rarely used clinically. An alternative way to measure GFR is by using creatinine clearance. Creatinine is a product of muscle metabolism, and as long as the subject remains at rest, the plasma creatinine level stays reasonably constant. Like inulin, it is freely filtered and not reabsorbed, synthesised or metabolised by the kidney, but creatinine is secreted to some extent by the tubules. This tends to make the value for creatinine clearance higher than that for inulin clearance, since the term (U.V) in the formula for clearance is artefactually high. However, as the plasma creatinine assay is not absolutely specific and overestimates the true plasma creatinine concentration, the two errors tend to cancel each other out, and creatinine clearance becomes a reasonable estimate of GFR.

PAH clearance: measurement of renal plasma flow

PAH is one of the groups of organic acids secreted by the proximal tubule. PAH is not only secreted, but also is filtered at the glomerulus. Thus the total amount of PAH excreted is equal to the sum of the amount filtered plus the amount secreted. PAH is almost completely removed from the plasma by the kidneys, even though only a fraction of the plasma is filtered. The clearance of PAH, therefore, provides a measurement of the total renal plasma flow (RPF). (It should be noted that this relationship only holds as long as the tubular maximum, T_m, for the transport of PAH is not exceeded. T_m is reached at a plasma concentration of about 10 mg per 100 ml plasma.) At plasma concentrations <10 mg per 100 ml

PAH delivered to kidneys in plasma
   = PAH excreted in urine

The amount of PAH excreted in the urine is given by

(urinary concentration of PAH) × (urine flow)

which can be expressed as

$U_{PAH} \times V$

where

U_{PAH} = urinary concentration of PAH
  V = urine flow (ml min^{-1})

Also, the PAH delivered to the kidneys is given by

(renal plasma flow) × (plasma concentration of PAH)

which can be expressed as

$RPF \times P_{PAH}$

where

P_{PAH} = plasma concentration of PAH
 RPF = renal plasma flow

Therefore, it follows that

$RPF \times P_{PAH} = U_{PAH} \times V$

So

$$RPF = \frac{U_{PAH} \times V}{P_{PAH}}$$

As can be seen, this is also the clearance formula for PAH. A typical value for RPF is 600 ml min^{-1}.

Calculation of renal blood flow

Given the haematocrit, renal blood flow (RBF) can be obtained. A typical haematocrit is 45%, which means that 45% of the total blood volume is cells, and therefore 55% is plasma. So renal blood flow can be calculated by

$$RBF = \frac{RPF \times 100}{55}$$

which gives about 1091 ml min^{-1}.

The clearance of PAH, although generally used as a measure of renal plasma flow, does not measure the plasma flow exactly, because PAH is not completely cleared from the blood during one passage through the kidney. The PAH extraction is only about 90% complete, because not all of the blood which enters the kidney goes to the glomeruli and tubules. Some goes to the capsule, the perirenal fat and the medulla (the blood in the vasa recta has had some PAH removed by filtration, but is not available for secretion). PAH clearance approximates to cortical plasma flow and is usually called the effective renal plasma flow.

Regulation of renal blood flow and glomerular filtration rate

Autoregulation

Over a wide range of mean arterial pressures (90–200 mmHg) renal blood flow is independent of the perfusion pressure. This is true even if the kidney is denervated. This property is, therefore, termed 'autoregulation' (Figure RE4). GFR also autoregulates. The relationship between blood pressure and renal blood flow demonstrated in Figure RE4 implies that as the perfusion pressure increases, the resistance to flow also increases. Both afferent and efferent arterioles are capable of vasoconstriction. There is still controversy about the mechanisms underlying autoregulation of the kidneys. The most widely accepted explanation is the myogenic theory. According to this, the increase in wall tension of the afferent arterioles, produced by increased perfusion pressure, causes automatic contraction of the smooth muscle fibres in the vessel walls. This increases flow resistance and acts to maintain constant blood flow.

Renal response to increased sympathetic activity

Despite autoregulation, renal haemodynamics vary considerably. Autoregulation means that changes in blood pressure per se in the autoregulatory range have little effect

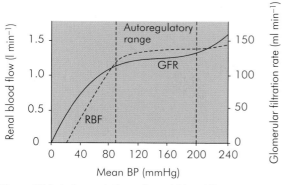

Figure RE4 Autoregulation of renal blood flow

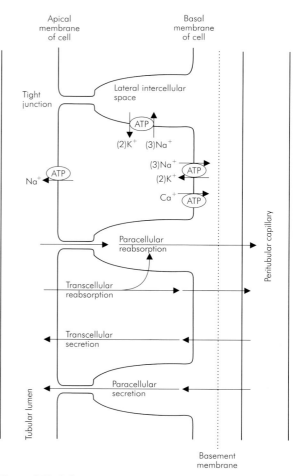

Figure RE5 Solute transport mechanisms in tubular cells

on blood flow, but it does not mean that blood flow is always constant. In many circumstances (e.g. physical or mental stress, haemorrhage), there are increases in the sympathetic nervous activity to the kidney (and to other parts of the body), causing vasoconstriction and, hence, a reduction in renal blood flow, even though the perfusion pressure is still in the autoregulatory range. This suggests that the kidneys play a part in maintaining systemic blood pressure, rather than reacting passively to it.

Other mechanisms include:

- Renal prostaglandin production – renal vasoconstriction in response to renal sympathetic nerve activity is attenuated to some extent by the intrarenal production of vasodilator prostaglandins.
- Angiotensin II – when the renal blood flow is reduced, there is generally an increased filtration fraction, brought about by efferent arteriolar vasoconstriction (mediated by angiotensin II), so that GFR tends to be maintained.
- Tubuloglomerular feedback mechanism – this mechanism may also contribute significantly to renal autoregulation.
- Vasoactive agents – the regulation of GFR also involves other vasoactive agents, which are present within blood vessel walls throughout the body, but may be of particular importance in the kidney, including endothelin (vasoconstrictor) and the vasodilator nitric oxide.

Tubular transport

The final urine that leaves the nephrons to enter the bladder and be excreted is very different from the initial glomerular filtrate, because the composition of the filtrate is modified by selective reabsorption and secretion processes.

Transport of solutes and water across the renal tubular epithelium can occur between the cells (paracellular movement) or through the cells (transcellular movement). Transcellular movement occurs across two cell membranes, the apical and basal membranes of the cell. **Secretion** is movement from the blood, through or between the tubular cells, into the tubular fluid. **Reabsorption** is movement of a substance from the tubular fluid, into or between the tubular cells, and then into the blood. Neither term conveys any information about the nature of the forces causing the movement (Figure RE5).

Primary and secondary active transport

Conventionally, the transport of solutes has been regarded as 'active' if metabolic energy is required, and 'passive' if metabolic energy is not required. This distinction is too simplistic, since many transport processes that do not directly require metabolic energy would nevertheless not occur if metabolic energy were not available.

Primary active transport

This involves the direct coupling of ATP hydrolysis to a transport process in the cell membrane. The most important primary active process in the nephron is the $Na^+K^+ATPase$, located on the basal (and basolateral) side of the cells lining the nephron. The $Na^+K^+ATPase$ accounts for the majority of the oxygen consumption in the kidney and enables the nephrons to reabsorb >99% of the filtered sodium.

Other primary active transport mechanisms in the nephron include a $Ca^{2+}ATPase$, an H^+ (proton)-ATPase, and an $H^+K^+ATPase$ (see Section 2, Chapter 1, page 210).

Secondary active transport

This process uses ionic gradients that have been established across the nephron cell membranes by ATPases, to drive the transport process resulting in secretion or reabsorption of a solute. Although the transport of such solutes is not directly linked to ATP breakdown, nevertheless if primary active transport was not active, then secondary active transport could not occur. The sodium gradient provides the most important driving force for secondary active transport. When the solute that is being transported with Na^+ moves in the same direction as the Na^+ gradient, the process is termed **co-transport**; where the solute is transported against the Na^+ gradient the process is termed **counter-transport** (see Section 2, Chapter 1, pages 210–11).

Ion channels

In addition to ATPases and transporter molecules, epithelial cell membranes also contain proteins that constitute ion 'channels'. There are sodium ion channels in the apical membranes of cells throughout the nephron. These channels are closed by the drug amiloride and opened by a number of hormones. There are also both Cl^- and K^+ channels in the apical membranes. Ion channels allow much faster rates of transport than either ATPases or transporter molecules.

Paracellular movement

This is movement of substances through the spaces between the cells of the nephron. Driving forces for paracellular movement are concentration, osmotic or electrical gradients. Such movements are discussed below in relation to specific substances (Figure RE5).

Water absorption

There is no active water reabsorption. Water reabsorption along the nephron follows solute absorption and can be both trans- and paracellular. It has become clear in recent years that much of the water movement through epithelia is transcellular. This occurs via specific water channels comprising four identical aquaporins (AQP), each having 6 membrane-spanning regions, which form a tube highly permeable to the small water molecule but not to the smaller hydrogen ion. A number of aquaporins have now been identified. Examples of the most important include:

- AQP1 (also called CHIP-28, or 28 kilodalton channel-forming integral protein) is abundant in the apical and basal membranes of renal proximal tubule cells, and the cells of the thin descending limb of Henle, as well as in many extrarenal tissues.
- AQP2 is the vasopressin-sensitive channel.
- AQP3 is in the basolateral membranes of the principal collecting duct principal cells, where it provides an exit route for water, and also in the colon.
- AQP4 is abundant in the brain, and may be important in the hypothalamic osmoreceptor cells, and also in the colon.
- AQP5 is found in the salivary glands.
- AQP6 is located in vesicles within intercalated collecting duct cells.
- AQP7 is found in abundance in the brush border membrane in the proximal convoluted tubule.
- AQP8 exists at low levels within proximal tubules and collecting duct cells, and also within the colon.

The proximal tubule

Morphology of proximal tubule cells

Adjacent proximal tubule cells are in contact with each other at the luminal side (the tight junction), but there are gaps between the cells – lateral intercellular spaces – at the peritubular side (Figure RE5). The luminal surface has a brush border of microvilli, which greatly increases the surface area available for absorption. There are some differences in the transport properties of the early proximal tubule (pars convoluta), compared with later parts (pars convoluta and pars recta), particularly in relation to Cl^- transport.

Sodium reabsorption in the proximal tubule

The proximal tubule is highly permeable to sodium in both directions. Net reabsorption of sodium from the tubule into the peritubular capillaries occurs as a result of the difference between an efflux of sodium from the tubule lumen and a return of sodium back into it. Only about 20% of the sodium efflux from the tubular lumen is ultimately reabsorbed into the peritubular capillaries. Thus the majority of the sodium efflux passes back into the tubular lumen as a backflux. This two-way movement of sodium occurs between the tubular lumen and the tubule cells and is linked with the transport of other substances. Some of the backflux is paracellular.

Sodium entry into tubule cells

The proximal tubule cells have a negative intracellular potential of -70 mV relative to both luminal fluid and peritubular fluid, and the cells have a low intracellular sodium concentration (<30 mmol). So sodium movement from the luminal fluid into the cell is in the direction of a large electrical gradient as well as a chemical concentration gradient. Thus sodium entry into the cell occurs passively. However, this entry of sodium is mediated by carrier proteins that also transport other solutes simultaneously. As noted above, these solutes may be transported with the sodium ions (symport) or in exchange for the sodium (antiport). Many solutes are transported by Na^+-linked symport and antiport. Most of the sodium (80%) entering the tubule cells does so in exchange for H^+ secretion. In turn, H^+ secretion into the tubular lumen leads to the reabsorption of both Cl^- and HCO_3^- (Figure RE6).

Sodium extrusion from tubular cells

The Na^+K^+ATPase pump extrudes sodium from the cells against electrical and chemical gradients. The entry into the cells of potassium ions has little effect on the intracellular K^+ concentration, since K^+ can readily cross cell membranes and so rapidly diffuses out of the cells. The ratio of transport is not 1 : 1; three Na^+ leave for two K^+ ions entering. The active extrusion of sodium from the tubule cells occurs almost entirely across the basolateral and basal surfaces of the cells, and much of this transport is directed into the lateral intercellular spaces.

Reabsorption of other solutes in the proximal tubule

Sodium reabsorption leads to electrical, concentration and osmotic gradients for the reabsorption of such solutes as chloride, potassium and urea, and also for water reabsorption. It is also important for the reabsorption of glucose, amino acids, phosphate and calcium and for the secretion of H^+.

Chloride reabsorption in the proximal tubule

The intracellular electrical potential opposes Cl^- entry into the cells from the tubular lumen. In the early proximal tubule Na^+ absorption is accompanied by HCO_3^- absorption (in the form of CO_2), so that although the tubular osmolality remains similar to that of plasma, the Cl^- concentration is increased. There are two main mechanisms by which Cl^- is absorbed from the tubular lumen into the tubule cells (Figure RE7). These are:

- By antiport in exchange for the secretion of organic anions. The main organic anions involved are bicarbonate (HCO_3^-), formate ($HCOO^-$) and oxalate. In Figure RE7, formate is used as an example. This shows Cl^- reabsorption into tubule cells in exchange for $HCOO^-$, which is secreted back into the tubule. In the lumen the $HCOO^-$ combines with H^+ to form $HCOOH$, which readily diffuses back into the cells. There it dissociates into H^+ and $HCOO^-$. The intracellular H^+ is then antiported back into the tubule in exchange for Na^+, while the $HCOO^-$ drives the antiport of Cl^-. Thus, the net result of the Cl^- and Na^+ antiport systems is the reabsorption of equal amounts of Cl^- and Na^+ from the lumen into the tubular cells.

- In the final two-thirds of the proximal tubule, Cl^- handling differs between superficial nephrons and juxtamedullary ones. In superficial nephrons Cl^- permeability in the late proximal tubule is greater than that for other anions (notably HCO_3^-). Hence Cl^- is reabsorbed from the lumen down its concentration gradient because of the high luminal Cl^- concentration established by HCO_3^- absorption. This occurs mainly by the paracellular route (Figure RE8). Na^+ then follows passively down its electrical gradient. Up to 20% of NaCl reabsorption in the late proximal tubule occurs by this mechanism. In contrast, Cl^- and HCO_3^- permeabilities do not differ in the juxtamedullary nephron tubule.

Glucose

Normally, almost all of the filtered glucose is reabsorbed and a negligible amount is excreted. Since the normal plasma glucose concentration is between 3.3 and 5.5 mmol

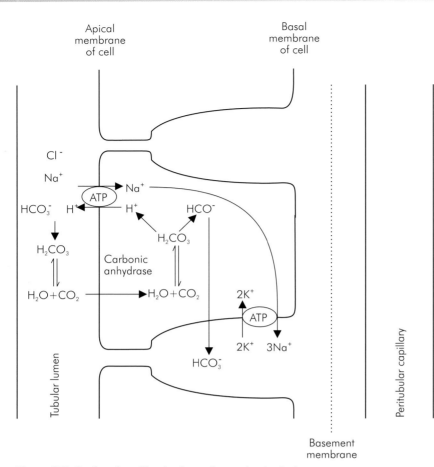

Figure RE6 Sodium handling in the early proximal tubule

per litre (60–100 mg per 100 ml) and GFR is 125 ml per minute, 0.4–0.7 mmol (or 75–125 mg) glucose is reabsorbed every minute. Although most glucose reabsorption occurs in the proximal tubule, more distal parts of the nephron are also capable of reabsorbing glucose. Figure RE9 shows the relationship between filtration, reabsorption and excretion of glucose, and the plasma glucose concentration. The amount of glucose filtered is directly proportional to the plasma glucose concentration. No glucose is excreted in the urine unless the plasma glucose concentration exceeds about 11 mmol l^{-1} (200 mg per 100 ml). At this plasma glucose concentration, those nephrons with the lowest capacity for glucose reabsorption (relative to their filtration rate) reach their glucose reabsorptive rate limit, and glucose begins to be excreted. Further increases in plasma glucose concentration saturate the glucose transport process of an increasing proportion of nephrons until, when the plasma glucose concentration is about 22 mmol l^{-1}, no nephrons can absorb their entire filtered glucose load. The fact that the curves for reabsorption and excretion are 'rounded' indicates the existence of nephron heterogeneity, i.e. that all the nephrons are not identical.

The type of transport process typified by glucose reabsorption is known as T_m-limited transport. 'T_m' means tubular maximum and refers to the maximum tubular transport rate for a particular solute. From Figure RE9, it can be seen that the maximum rate of glucose reabsorption is about 380 mg min^{-1}. This is the T_m for glucose. The most common abnormality of glucose excretion is that caused by a change in the plasma glucose concentration, so that the filtered load is altered: diabetes mellitus is caused by

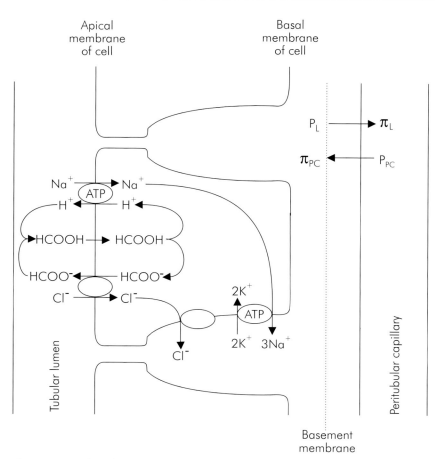

Figure RE7 Sodium handling throughout the proximal tubule

the relative or total absence of the pancreatic hormone, insulin, which regulates the blood glucose concentration. The filtered load of glucose can therefore be far in excess of the reabsorptive capacity of the nephrons, so that glucose is excreted in the urine. This excretion of osmotically active solute causes an osmotic diuresis resulting in water loss from the body and, hence, dehydration and thirst.

Relationship of glucose reabsorption to sodium reabsorption

Proximal tubular glucose absorption is linked to sodium reabsorption. The entry of glucose into the tubular cells is via symport. Symporter carrier proteins that possess both sodium and glucose binding sites transfer sodium ions and glucose molecules simultaneously into the tubular cells.

The movement of sodium occurs down its electrochemical gradient (co-transport), thus providing the energy to transfer glucose against its gradient (counter-transport). Maintenance of the sodium gradient is therefore essential for glucose absorption. This in turn depends on the extrusion of sodium from the proximal tubule cells by the sodium pump.

Note that in the pars convoluta, the stoichiometry of the glucose sodium co-transport is one glucose molecule per sodium ion, but in the pars recta it is one glucose per two sodium ions.

Amino acids

The plasma concentration of amino acids is between 2.5 and 3.5 mmol l^{-1}. Amino acids in the plasma are in a dynamic equilibrium, since they enter the blood from the

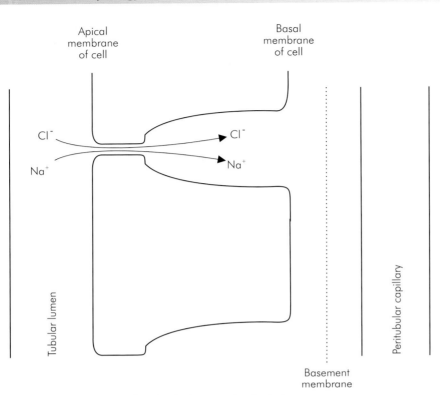

Figure RE8 Sodium handling in the late proximal tubule

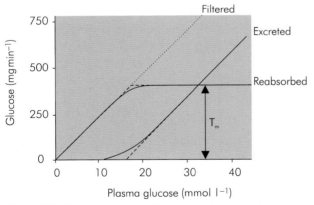

Figure RE9 Glucose transport in the proximal tubule

gut, as products of protein digestion, and are continually being used to restructure the body tissues. Amino acids are readily filtered at the glomeruli, but negligible quantities are excreted, because there are effective T_m-limited transport processes for amino acids in the proximal tubule.

There are several proximal transport processes for amino acid reabsorption coupled with Na^+. These are for:

- Basic amino acids
- Glutamic and aspartic acids
- Neutral amino acids
- Glycine
- Cysteine and cystine
- β and γ amino acids

The functional characteristics of these transport processes are very similar to that for glucose. Amino acid entry into the proximal tubule cells from the lumen is a co-transport process with sodium, the driving force being the sodium gradient.

Phosphate

Phosphate is an essential constituent of the body. Bones and teeth are salts of calcium and phosphate, and the skeleton accounts for about 80% of the body phosphate content. The other 20% is present mainly in intracellular fluid. The extracellular (plasma) phosphate concentration is

1 mmol l^{-1}, and plasma phosphate is freely filtered at the glomerulus. In the nephron, tubular reabsorption and possibly secretion of phosphate occurs. Normally, the urinary phosphate excretion is <20% of the amount filtered, but above a phosphate concentration of about 1.2 mmol l^{-1} increases in filtered phosphate are excreted in the urine, suggesting that there is a T_m for phosphate. Phosphate reabsorption occurs by electroneutral co-transport (i.e. two sodium ions per phosphate ion) across the apical membrane of tubular cells. Two distinct sodium–phosphate transporters are present in the membrane. The rate of phosphate uptake is hormonally regulated, being under the control of PTH (parathyroid hormone) and vitamin D.

Urea

The normal plasma urea concentration is 2.5–7.5 mmol l^{-1}. Only 40–50% of filtered urea is reabsorbed; 50–60% is excreted. Urea is the end product of protein metabolism and clinically is measured as blood urea nitrogen. Because urea is a small molecule, it is reabsorbed in the proximal tubule as a consequence of sodium reabsorption. Thus, as sodium chloride and water are abstracted from the proximal tubule, the urea concentration in the tubular fluid tends to increase and so urea is reabsorbed passively by diffusing down its concentration gradient, out of the tubule. The urea handling of the more distal parts of the nephron plays an important part in the process of concentrating the urine, and is considered later.

Bicarbonate

Normal plasma HCO_3^- concentration is about 25 mmol l^{-1}. Bicarbonate has a key role in acid–base balance, and the kidney contributes to acid–base balance largely by regulating the plasma bicarbonate concentration.

About 90% of the filtered HCO_3^- is reabsorbed in the proximal tubule; the remainder is reabsorbed in the distal tubule and collecting ducts. In the proximal tubule, HCO_3^- reabsorption occurs as a result of H^+ secretion from tubular cells into the lumen. The bicarbonate reabsorption mechanism behaves as if there were a T_m for bicarbonate. However, this apparent T_m can be altered by the rate of H^+ secretion, which is itself loosely dependent on the rate of Na^+ reabsorption.

Water

Water reabsorption occurs in the proximal tubule in the following manner:

- Some 60–70% of the filtered water is reabsorbed in the proximal tubules. About 20% of the reabsorbed water load occurs as a result of the chemical gradient provided by a small degree of hypotonicity (2–5 mOsm l^{-1} lower than plasma) in the tubular lumen, and the increased concentration of Na^+ caused by extrusion into the lateral intercellular spaces.
- A further 40% of the water reabsorbed proximally is attributable to the different permeabilities of anions (primarily Cl^- and HCO_3^-) in superficial nephrons. As described above, tubular Cl^- concentration is increased by the end of the first part of the proximal tubule, due to HCO_3^- reabsorption. In addition, the distal parts of the proximal tubule are more permeable to Cl^- than to other solutes. This causes both Cl^- and water to be reabsorbed in this region.
- The remaining 40% of the total proximal water reabsorption can be attributed to the existence of a hypertonic intermediate compartment – the lateral intercellular spaces

Secretion in the proximal tubule

Tubular secretory mechanisms are very much like tubular reabsorptive mechanisms – the important difference being the direction of transport. Like reabsorptive processes, secretion can be either active or passive – and secretory processes may be gradient time-limited (e.g. the proximal tubule hydrogen secretion) or T_m-limited. There are three proximal tubular secretory mechanisms that have a definite T_m limit. These are for:

- Some organic acids – these include penicillin, chlorothiazide, hippurate, PAH and possibly uric acid
- Some strong organic bases, which include histamine, choline, thiamine, guanidine and probably creatinine
- EDTA (ethylene diamine tetra-acetic acid)

Although most of these substances do not occur endogenously, endogenous organic acids are also transported. There is some anatomical separation of the different secretory processes. Organic acid secretion (and uric acid secretion) takes place in the pars recta, but organic base secretion occurs in the pars convoluta.

When a substance is filtered and actively secreted, the total amount excreted in the urine is greater than the amount filtered due to transport from the peritubular capillaries into the tubular lumen. An example is shown in Figure RE10, illustrating the results of PAH secretion in the proximal tubule. This shows the relationship between

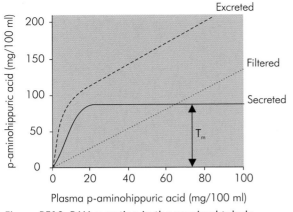

Figure RE10 PAH secretion in the proximal tubule

the plasma concentration of PAH and the rates of filtration, tubular secretion and urinary excretion. For plasma concentrations up to 8 mg per 100 ml, PAH is cleared completely from the peritubular capillaries. For concentrations greater than this the T_m for PAH is exceeded, and excretion rates only increase in step with filtration rates.

The peritubular capillaries

The end result of the transport processes described above is the passage of essentially isotonic fluid from the tubule lumen into the lateral intercellular spaces (LIS). This occurs mainly through tubular cell reabsorption and secretion, but some paracellular movement also occurs into the LIS, but mainly in the late proximal tubule. From here, the NaCl–NaHCO₃ solution can move in two possible directions: either into the peritubular capillaries or back into the tubular lumen.

A proportion of the Na^+ always leaks back, and hence the sodium reabsorption process can be called a 'pump-leak' system (it is also known as a gradient time-limited transport process). The rate of proximal tubular sodium reabsorption can be varied by changes in the rate of backflux into the tubule, as well as by changes in the rate of active sodium extrusion from the cells. The rate of backflux is affected by the rate of uptake from the lateral intercellular spaces into the capillaries. Reabsorption from the tubule is finally completed by the uptake of water and solutes into the peritubular capillaries. The faster the capillary uptake the lower the rate of backflux.

Uptake forces in the peritubular capillaries

The forces governing the movement of fluid across the walls of the peritubular capillaries are Starling forces, i.e.

colloid osmotic pressure (COP) and hydrostatic pressure gradients.

The forces favouring capillary uptake are

(capillary COP) + (LIS hydrostatic pressure)

or

$\pi_{PC} + P_L$

The forces opposing capillary uptake are

(capillary hydrostatic pressure) + (COP in LIS)

or

$P_{PC} + \pi_L$

Therefore, rate of capillary uptake is related to

(forces favouring uptake) − (forces opposing uptake)
$\propto (\pi_{PC} + P_L) - (\pi_L + P_{PC})$

where

π_L and π_{PC} = COPs in LIS and peritubular capillary respectively
P_L and P_{PC} = hydrostatic pressures in LIS and peritubular capillary respectively

Effect of GFR on peritubular fluid uptake

The peritubular capillaries are branches of the efferent arterioles, which in turn arise from the glomerular capillaries. Consequently, the Starling forces in the peritubular capillaries can be modified by the glomerular filtration process. The peritubular capillary COP (π_{PC}) depends on the capillary plasma protein concentration. As plasma proteins are concentrated in the glomerular capillaries by the filtration process, COP in the peritubular capillaries increases with filtration fraction. The peritubular capillary COP is normally high compared with that in the glomerular capillaries, resulting in fluid reabsorption by the peritubular capillaries.

This dependence of π_{PC} on the filtration fraction is a mechanism that automatically adjusts proximal tubular reabsorption to compensate for changes in glomerular filtration. When GFR increases, the forces available to reabsorb the increased volume of filtrate also increase, and vice versa. This glomerulotubular mechanism normally ensures reabsorption of a fixed proportion of the gomerular filtrate by the proximal tubule, i.e. there is constant proximal tubular fractional reabsorption.

However, proximal tubular fractional reabsorption can be altered by other factors, e.g. by alterations in the effective circulating volume. Such alterations are considered later.

The peritubular capillary hydrostatic pressure (P_{PC}) is determined mainly by venous pressure. However, changes in tone of the afferent and efferent glomerular arterioles may also affect P_{PC} by varying the amount of arterial pressure transmitted to the peritubular capillaries.

The loop of Henle

The loop of Henle (LOH) is continuous with the proximal tubule and originates in the renal cortex. It consists of a descending limb that passes into the medulla and loops round to become the ascending limb, which passes back into the cortex. This limb then continues as the distal tubule (Figure RE11).

The fluid entering the LOH is initially isotonic compared with plasma, but after traversing the loop the fluid entering the distal tubule is hypotonic. Thus the tubular fluid is diluted during its passage through the LOH. However, the LOH plays a crucial role in the concentration of urine by functioning as a countercurrent multiplier. The salient process is emphasised below:

The loops of Henle do not concentrate the tubular fluid within them, but manufacture a hypertonic interstitial fluid in the renal medulla. Urine is then concentrated by osmosis from collecting ducts as they pass through the medulla.

The countercurrent mechanism

A proposed mechanism for countercurrent multiplication was described by Wirz, Hargitay and Kuhn in 1951. The hypertonic interstitium is produced by a small osmotic pressure difference between the ascending and descending limbs of the loops (i.e. a small transverse gradient). This small difference is then multiplied into a large longitudinal gradient by the countercurrent arrangement (i.e. flow in opposite directions) in the two adjacent limbs of the loop.

The ascending limb is not uniform in structure, but possesses both a thin and a thick segment. This limb produces an increase in the osmolality of the surrounding interstitium by the extrusion of sodium and accompanying ions. Only the thick segment actively extrudes ions. Both thin and thick segments of the ascending limb are impermeable to water, so that water is unable osmotically to follow the extruded ions. Consequently, the osmolality of the medullary interstitium is increased

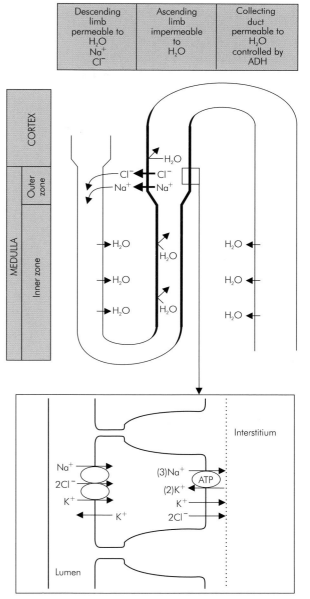

Figure RE11 Sodium and water movement in the loop of Henle

and the osmolality of the fluid in the ascending limb is decreased.

The extrusion process is performed by the tubular cells, which take up ions from the tubular lumen through their apical membrane and extrude ions through their basal

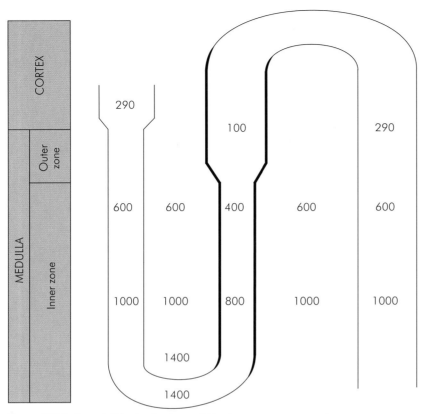

Figure RE12 Osmolalities in the loop of Henle

membrane. The entry of solutes into the cells across the apical membrane involves co-transport of sodium, chloride and potassium, with the stoichiometry of one Na^+, two Cl^- and one K^+, so the process is electrically neutral. The primary active transport on the basal cell membrane is performed by $Na^+K^+ATPase$. This basal membrane transport is also electrically neutral. The thin ascending limb has little $Na^+K^+ATPase$ activity, and thus the thick segment is primarily responsible for the extrusion of sodium. Much of the K^+ leaks back into the tubular lumen, so that it is predominantly NaCl which accumulates in the medullary interstitium. This transport can be inhibited by loop diuretics, such as furosemide and bumetanide.

The descending limb is permeable to water and, to a lesser extent, is also permeable to NaCl. The fluid within the descending limb will therefore come to osmotic equilibrium with the interstitium. In effect, then, one can consider the transport of NaCl out of the ascending limb as being directed into the descending limb.

The sodium extrusion mechanism or 'sodium pump' action in the ascending limb can maintain an osmolality gradient of 200 mOsm kg^{-1} H_2O between the ascending tubular lumen and the interstitium. In effect, since the descending limb is permeable and assumes the same osmolality as the interstitium, the 'sodium pump' can be thought of as maintaining a 200 mOsm kg^{-1} H_2O gradient between the tubular fluid in the adjacent sections of the ascending and descending limbs. The countercurrent arrangement of the limbs will then result in a gradually increasing interstitial (and descending limb) osmolality, as the LOH descends into the renal medulla. In humans the osmolality at the papillary tips may reach 1400 mOsm kg^{-1} H_2O (Figure RE12).

The fluid in the ascending tubule leaving the medulla and entering the cortex is hypotonic to plasma, with an osmolality of about 100 mOsm kg^{-1} H_2O. Thus the ascending limb of the loop of Henle (and its continuation in the cortex as the distal tubule) can be called the 'diluting segment' of the nephron. However, some nephrons possess short loops of Henle, and these are unlikely to lower the osmolality of the ascending limb fluid to 100 mOsm kg^{-1} H_2O.

Long and short loops of Henle

Only 15% of the nephrons (the juxtamedullary nephrons) have long loops of Henle that pass deeply into the medulla. The remaining 85% of nephrons (cortical nephrons) have short loops of Henle that barely reach the medulla, and these nephrons do not make a significant contribution to the manufacture of medullary hypertonicity. However, the collecting tubules of all the nephrons (both cortical and juxtamedullary) pass through the medulla. Thus, only the long-looped nephrons (15% of the total) produce the medullary gradient that concentrates the urine produced by all the nephrons. There are also differences in sodium reabsorption between the long- and short-looped nephrons.

The distal tubule and collecting tubule

The distal tubule

The 'distal tubule', although anatomically defined, is not a distinct section of the nephron in terms of physiological function. Functionally, the distal tubule is a segment of the nephron in which the tubule cells undergo transition from 'ascending limb of Henle type' cells to 'collecting tubule type' cells. The walls of the former cell type have only a very low and essentially constant permeability to water, whereas the 'collecting tubule type' cells have a variable water permeability, which is regulated by the hormone vasopressin (antidiuretic hormone, ADH).

The potential difference across the distal tubular wall varies with distance along the tubule. In the early part, the lumen is positive with respect to the interstitium (as in the ascending limb of Henle), but in the later parts the luminal potential becomes negative and may reach -45 mV. This negative potential is caused by active sodium reabsorption.

The collecting tubules

The collecting tubules have cortical and medullary sections, the two sections having somewhat different properties. Both are relatively impermeable to water, urea and NaCl, but the water permeability is increased by vasopressin. Thus vasopressin leads to urine concentration by permitting the osmotic abstraction of water into the interstitium. Theoretically the urine in the collecting tubule can achieve the same osmolality as the medullary interstitium, but in reality it is usually rather less than this.

Vasopressin also increases the urea permeability of the **medullary** collecting tubules, but has no effect on the urea permeability of the **cortical** collecting tubules. This impermeability of the cortical part of the collecting tubule to urea is one of the factors that make urea so important in the urine concentration mechanism.

Importance of urea in countercurrent multiplication

Previously, the countercurrent multiplication process has only been considered in terms of NaCl transport into the interstitium. However, a considerable fraction of the medullary interstitial osmolality, particularly in the papillary region, is attributable to urea (up to 50%). This high interstitial urea concentration is obtained by diffusion of urea from the medullary collecting tubules, which have an vasopressin-dependent permeability to urea.

The normal plasma concentration of urea is 2.5–7.5 mmol l^{-1}. Urea is freely filterable at the glomerulus, and about 50% of the filtered load is reabsorbed in the proximal tubule. As the tubular fluid passes down the descending limb into the medulla, it passes into the high interstitial urea concentration established by diffusion from the collecting tubules, as described above. The tubular urea concentration thus increases by diffusion from the interstitium in both the descending and ascending limbs, which are permeable to urea.

In the distal and cortical collecting tubules, the urea concentration rises further, as a result of water reabsorption, since these segments are almost impermeable to urea. Initially, when the medullary collecting tubule is reached, the high urea concentration in the tubule causes the diffusion of urea out of the tubule into the interstitium (under the influence of vasopressin), which maintains the high medullary urea concentration. Urea thus recycles between medullary collecting tubule and medullary interstitium via the tubular fluid. This produces a high interstitial urea concentration that helps to increase the final urea concentration in the urine. The maximum attainable urinary osmolality is greater when urea excretion is high because a proportion of this extra urea enters the medullary interstitium.

The role of the vasa recta

In most tissues, the selective permeability of capillaries ensures that the composition of interstitial fluid remains uniform. If medullary capillaries served this purpose, the osmotic gradient built up by the loop of Henle would be dissipated. However, this does not occur, because the hairpin arrangement of the vasa recta enables them to function as countercurrent exchangers (distinguished from countercurrent multipliers by the fact that no energy is necessary). This enables the vasa recta to exchange nutrients for waste products in the renal medulla, without washing away the solutes responsible for medullary hypertonicity.

The vasa recta, like capillaries elsewhere, are permeable to water and solutes. As the descending vasa recta pass into the medulla, water is osmotically abstracted from the capillary blood, into the interstitium, in exchange for solutes (NaCl and urea). More and more water is extracted, as the blood passes further into the medulla, until, at the tip of the loop, the plasma has almost the same osmolality as the surrounding interstitium. This makes the blood very viscous with a high plasma protein concentration. In the ascending vasa recta, the plasma regains water and loses solute.

Since the plasma concentrations of diffusible solutes and plasma osmolality in the vasa recta virtually assume interstitial values, the differences between descending and ascending limbs become very small. Although this minimises transport of water and solutes away from the interstitium, it also makes the exchange of oxygen and CO_2 very inefficient. The renal medulla is, therefore, susceptible to the effects of reduced perfusion.

Renal effects of vasopressin

The main determinant of whether the urine will be copious and dilute, or low in volume and concentrated, is the level of circulating vasopressin. Reabsorption of water in the nephron occurs at several sites. GFR = 180 litres per day. About 70% of this is reabsorbed in the proximal tubule. A further 15% of the glomerular filtrate is reabsorbed by the loop of Henle. This leaves about 23 litres to enter the distal tubules and collecting tubules. It is these 23 litres that are mainly either excreted or reabsorbed, depending on the level of circulating vasopressin.

In the presence of vasopressin, the collecting tubule wall is permeable to water, so the hypertonic medullary interstitium leads to the osmotic abstraction of water from the tubule. Vasopressin also makes the collecting tubules permeable to urea, which leaves the tubule in this region and contributes to the osmolality of the renal medulla. Normal levels of circulating vasopressin produce urine volumes of about 1.5 litres per day, with an osmolality of 300–500 mOsm kg^{-1} H_2O. Vasopressin levels may be increased

to conserve body water, and urine volumes in these circumstances can be as little as 400 ml per day.

In the absence of circulating vasopressin, water reabsorption in the proximal tubule and LOH remains unchanged, since vasopressin does not affect water absorption at these sites. However, the collecting tubules become impermeable to water, and the large volumes entering the medullary collecting tubules pass through and are excreted. In addition, the collecting tubules also become impermeable to urea, preventing the attainment of maximal medullary interstitial osmolality. This in turn also reduces water reabsorption from the descending limb of the loop of Henle. Thus, when no vasopressin is present (diabetes insipidus), urine volume is about 23 litres per day, with an osmolality as low as 60 mOsm kg^{-1} H_2O. Note that adrenal steroids (cortisol) must be present for vasopressin to have its maximum effect on water permeability.

Osmoreceptors and the control of plasma osmolality

Osmoreceptors in the vicinity of the supraoptic and paraventricular areas of the anterior hypothalamus, supplied with blood by the internal carotid artery, regulate the release of the hormone vasopressin. These receptors, and others in the lateral preoptic area of the hypothalamus, also affect thirst. Normal plasma osmolality is associated with a plasma vasopressin concentration of about 4 pg ml^{-1}. Lowering the plasma osmolality reduces vasopressin concentration and raising the plasma osmolality increases the plasma vasopressin concentration. This coupling of the vasopressin-sensitive concentrating mechanism to the precise control of vasopressin release through the osmoreceptors provides a very good regulatory mechanism for plasma osmolality.

Synthesis and storage of vasopressin

Vasopressin is synthesised in the hypothalamus (supraoptic nucleus) as part of a large precursor molecule. After synthesis this is transported to the neurohypophysis (posterior pituitary) within nerve fibres that constitute the hypothalamohypophyseal tract, and it is cleaved progressively as it moves down the axons. In the nerve terminals, vasopressin and neurophysin are stored as insoluble complexes in secretory granules.

Cellular actions of vasopressin controlling water permeability

The renal vasopressin receptors (V_2 receptors) are on the basal membranes of the tubular cells. The V_2 receptor is a G-protein-coupled receptor characterised by seven membrane-spanning regions. Binding of vasopressin to the receptor activates adenylate cyclase, which increases cyclic AMP formation from ATP. The cyclic AMP activates protein kinase, which phosphorylates controlling proteins in water channels (aquaporin 2) close to the apical membrane, which increases water reabsorption from the tubular fluid (see page 339).

Removal of vasopressin from the blood

For precise regulation of plasma osmolality, not only is rapid control of vasopressin release required in response to changes in hydration, but also it is necessary that vasopressin is rapidly removed from the plasma. This removal occurs in the liver and in the kidneys. The kidneys remove about half of the total vasopressin, metabolising the majority and excreting <10% in the urine (plasma half-life of vasopressin is 15 minutes). A number of pharmacological agents may alter vasopressin release and thereby disturb osmoregulation.

Adrenal steroids and the renal response to vasopressin

Adrenal steroids (glucocorticoids) decrease the permeability of the collecting ducts to water. In the absence of adrenal steroids, collecting duct water permeability is above basal level, even if no vasopressin is present. Adrenal insufficiency also impairs the renal response to water loading, i.e. very dilute urine cannot be produced. In adrenal insufficiency the effect of vasopressin on water permeability appears to be reduced.

Regulation of body fluid volume and sodium reabsorption

Regulation of total body fluid volume is dependent on regulation of the extracellular fluid (ECF) volume. Control of ECF volume is mediated by osmoreceptors that affect vasopressin release.

Vasopressin release responds to changes in ECF osmolality and the effective circulating volume (ECV) of blood. The ECV is the component of the ECF that actually perfuses tissues (this may not necessarily be identical to the intravascular volume, since there may be circumstances in which not all of the blood is involved in tissue perfusion). Reflexes controlling the release of vasopressin may be activated by changes in blood pressure, atrial filling, haemorrhage or stress. Thus, a response in vasopressin release takes place within minutes, and acts rapidly to correct a disturbance (Figure RE13).

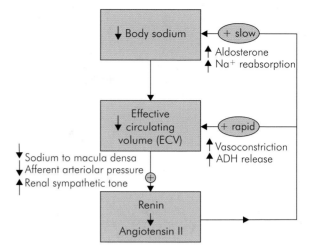

Figure RE13 Regulation of body sodium and extracellular volume

Osmoreceptors respond to changes in ECF osmolality. Since sodium salts are the main osmotically active solutes in the ECF, control of body fluid volume is dependent on the control of body sodium content. Humans can conserve sodium very effectively, and urinary losses can be <1 mmol l^{-1}. However, maximal sodium reabsorption can increase the excretion of K^+ and H^+, and so may disturb acid–base balance. Changes in Na^+ excretion are normally brought about by changes in tubular reabsorption. When disturbances of body fluid osmolality occur, disturbances in body sodium content (and consequently in body fluid volume) may take hours or even days to correct.

Primary control of sodium reabsorption is mediated by the release of the systemic hormones renin, angiotensin and aldosterone. The effects of these hormones are modified by other mechanisms and also depend on changes in ECV. Overall regulation of sodium reabsorption is complex, being influenced by the following factors:
- Systemic hormones
- Starling forces in the peritubular capillaries
- Neurological reflexes
- Renal prostaglandins
- Atrial natriuretic peptide
- Dopamine

Juxtaglomerular apparatus and the macula densa

In a nephron the ascending limb of the loop of Henle re-enters the cortex to become the distal tubule, passing very close to its own Bowman's capsule. At this point it comes into contact with the afferent and efferent arterioles from its own glomerulus. This region of contact is the juxtaglomerular apparatus, and consists of rennin-containing granular cells in the walls of the afferent arterioles, and specialised cells, the macula densa, in the wall of the early distal tubule.

Renin

Renin is an enzyme synthesised and stored in the granular cells of the juxtaglomerular apparatus. It is released into the plasma when the body sodium content decreases. As noted above, body sodium content determines ECV, and it is this relationship that determines renin release. There are three main ways in which decreases in ECV elicit increases in renin release.

Increased sympathetic activity. When there is a reduction of the ECV, decreases in the systemic blood pressure, venous return and cardiac output result. These changes increase sympathetic activity, so increasing arteriolar tone and promoting renin release, via stretch receptor and baroreceptor reflexes. The renin-containing granular cells of the renal afferent arterioles are innervated by sympathetic nerve fibres. Increased sympathetic activity in these causes renin release. This release of renin is mediated by β-adrenoceptors, and is important in maintaining renin release under basal conditions. It is also activated when assuming the upright posture, as well as during sodium depletion.

Decreased wall tension in the afferent arterioles. Decreased renal perfusion pressure in response to reduced ECV leads to increased renin release from the granular cells. The immediate stimulus appears to be arteriolar wall tension and its rate of change (dependent on pulse pressure) at the granular cells. This is known as the afferent arteriolar baroreceptor reflex mechanism. Sympathetic vasoconstriction of the kidney will also increase renin release by this mechanism, since the afferent arteriole is constricted by renal sympathetic nerve activity and this constriction is 'upstream' from the granular cells. This occurs in addition to the release of renin by the β-receptor mechanism.

The macula densa mechanism. A decrease in the delivery of NaCl to the macula densa leads to renin release, but the details of this mechanism are not clear.

Following stimulation of the juxtaglomerular apparatus, renin is released into the blood, where it acts on an α_2-globulin (angiotensinogen) and splits off a decapeptide (angiotensin I). An enzyme on the surface of endothelial cells (converting enzyme) rapidly removes a further two amino acids from angiotensin I, to form the octapeptide, angiotensin II (Figure RE14).

Angiotensin II

A primary action of angiotensin II is its action on the zona glomerulosa of the adrenal cortex to promote the release of aldosterone. Very little aldosterone is stored, but stimulation of its release promotes further aldosterone biosynthesis.

Angiotensin II is an extremely potent vasoconstrictor. Normally this action plays a minor part in the maintenance of systemic blood pressure, but intrarenally this can alter the distribution of glomerular filtration.

A third important role of angiotensin II is its direct effect on proximal tubular sodium reabsorption. Physiological concentrations of angiotensin II increase proximal tubular Na^+ reabsorption. This is mediated by inhibition of adenylate cyclase, which increases Na^+H^+ antiport.

Angiotensin II also inhibits renin release by negative feedback on the juxtaglomerular granular cells, and has various other actions (Figure RE15).

Aldosterone

Aldosterone is an adrenal cortical hormone necessary for normal sodium absorption and excretion. Its role in sodium regulation is exerted more via a permissive action than a controlling action. Changes in plasma aldosterone levels are usually accompanied by parallel changes in vasopressin and form part of the overall mechanism for regulating body fluid volume. The main actions of aldosterone are to promote Na^+ reabsorption from the distal nephron and to promote hydrogen and potassium ion excretion. Actions of aldosterone are summarised in Figure RE15.

Starling forces and proximal tubular sodium reabsorption

When body sodium content changes, the consequent changes in ECV that result automatically adjust proximal tubular Na^+ reabsorption to correct the disturbance.

Reabsorbed sodium chloride and water from the proximal tubule passes to the peritubular capillaries via the lateral intercellular spaces (LIS). The overall rate of reabsorption is determined by the rate of uptake from the LIS into the capillaries. Starling forces govern this uptake, and these are dependent on the hydrostatic pressure and colloid osmotic pressure (COP) in the peritubular capillaries

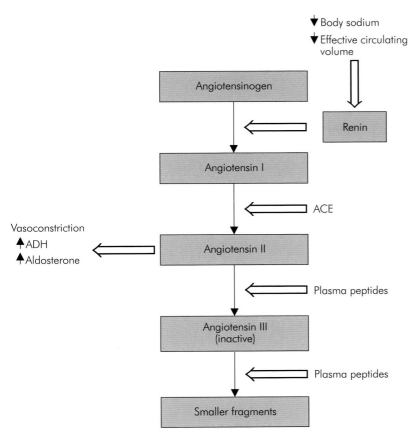

Figure RE14 Renin–angiotensin system

and LIS. The acting Starling forces are summarised by the equation

capillary uptake ∝ forces favouring uptake
              − forces opposing uptake
$$\propto (\pi_{PC} + P_L) - (\pi_L + P_{PC})$$

where

π_{PC} = COP in the peritubular capillaries
π_L = COP in the LIS
P_{PC} = hydrostatic pressure in the peritubular capillaries
P_L = hydrostatic pressure in the LIS

Both P_{PC} and π_{PC} vary with changes in body fluid volume. An increase in body fluid volume results in increased peritubular capillary hydrostatic pressure (P_{PC}) due to an increased venous pressure. At the same time, the plasma proteins are diluted by increased body fluid volume, reducing the capillary COP (π_{PC}). These changes decrease proximal tubular reabsorption of NaCl and water, thus acting to correct the original disturbance.

Long and short loops of Henle in sodium reabsorption

Changes in the proximal reabsorption of sodium affect its delivery to more distal parts of the nephron. Thus, if proximal sodium reabsorption is increased, the distal delivery of sodium to the loop of Henle is decreased. Similarly, if proximal reabsorption is decreased, more sodium is delivered to the LOH.

Consider a disturbance leading to an increase in body sodium and water. From the above discussion this will produce a decrease in proximal sodium reabsorption and an increase in sodium delivered to the ascending LOH. However, in the long LOH, reabsorption from the ascending limb is directly dependent on Na^+ delivery, and hence more Na^+ will be extruded into the interstitium. This

Substance	Actions
Angiotensin II	Stimulates release of aldosterone
	Potent systemic and renal vasoconstrictor
	↑ Na^+ in proximal tubule
	↑ Na^+ in distal tubule
	Stimulates release of vasopressin
	Water retention
	Stimulates thirst
	Inhibits release of renin
Aldosterone	↑ renal Na^+ reabsorption
	↑ renal H^+/K^+ excretion
	↑ Na^+ and K^+ channels in tubule cells
	↑ ATPase synthesis and activity in tubule cells
	↑ gastrointestinal Na^+ reabsorption
	↑ Na^+ reabsorption from sweat glands

Figure RE15 Actions of angiotensin II and aldosterone

would appear to be counterproductive towards correcting the original disturbance of increased body sodium and water. However, nephrons with shorts loops of Henle cannot extrude enough Na^+ from their ascending limbs to reabsorb the entire increased Na^+ load resulting from reduced proximal reabsorption. Thus the final urinary composition of the short-looped nephrons depends on proximal reabsorption to a much greater extent than that of the long-looped nephrons. Effectively the short-looped nephrons can be thought of as 'sodium losing', while the long-looped nephrons are 'sodium retaining' nephrons.

The response to changes in ECV may therefore involve redistribution of the renal blood flow between the two populations of nephrons, to obtain the urine composition that would compensate for the original disturbance in ECV.

Neurological reflexes in the kidney and sodium reabsorption

The nerve supply to the kidney is mainly sympathetic and is controlled by arterial baroreceptors. The sympathetic nerves of the kidney primarily supply the afferent arterioles. Decreased ECV will tend to reduce blood pressure, causing a reflex increase in renal sympathetic activity. Mild stimulation of the renal nerves reduces the blood flow to the superficial short-looped nephrons, and increases blood flow to the juxtamedullary long-looped nephrons, thus tending to conserve sodium. This baroreceptor mechanism also increases proximal tubular Na^+ reabsorption, which conserves sodium. Angiotensin II may mediate this effect, because renal nerve stimulation is known to release renin. This also causes sodium retention by promoting aldosterone release, but, in addition, catecholamines released from the renal sympathetic nerve endings (and from the adrenal medulla) stimulate sodium reabsorption in the proximal tubule by a direct action on sodium transport.

Prostaglandins

In the kidney, there are at least three distinct sites of prostaglandin synthesis:

- The cortex, including arterioles and glomeruli
- Medullary interstitial cells
- Collecting duct epithelial cells

The main prostaglandins synthesised by the kidney are PGE_2, PGI_2, $PGF_{2\alpha}$, PGD_2 and thromboxane A_2 (TXA_2).

Renal prostaglandins are synthesised from arachidonic acid, which is stored esterified in membrane phospholipids. The release of free arachidonic acid occurs enzymatically, and can be inhibited by steroids. Free arachidonic acid is converted by a cyclo-oxygenase enzyme into unstable endoperoxides, which then give rise to the renal prostanoids. The major arachidonate products are PGI_2 (prostacyclin) in the cortex, and PGE_2 in the medulla.

As with other prostaglandins, the renal prostaglandins act locally and have important intrarenal effects. PGE_2 and PGI_2 are produced in increased amounts when renal perfusion is threatened by vasoconstrictors such as norepinephrine, vasopressin and angiotensin II, or when hypotension occurs. These renal prostaglandins are vasodilators that minimise renal vasoconstriction. The use of non-steroidal anti-inflammatory drugs, such as aspirin or indomethacin, can reduce renal prostaglandin synthesis by inhibiting cyclo-oxygenase. This may have no effect on renal blood flow or GFR in normal individuals, but in patients with compromised renal perfusion (e.g. hypotension or receiving vasoconstrictors) these drugs can lead to large falls in GFR.

The anti-vasoconstrictor role of the renal prostaglandins is a cortical effect, and PGI_2 is likely to be the most important prostanoid in this role. Hence decreased ECV leads to increased cortical prostaglandin synthesis.

The medullary prostaglandins (mainly PGE_2) have actions on the renal tubules, predominantly the collecting tubules. Their main actions are natriuretic and diuretic. They also impair the antidiuretic action of vasopressin. These actions may also limit the extent to which Na^+ reabsorption (ATP-dependent) can be stimulated by aldosterone in the renal medulla, and, hence, protect the medullary tubule cells from excessive anoxia during hypovolaemia.

TXA_2, unlike the other renal prostanoids, is a vasoconstrictor. Little TXA_2 is normally produced, but its synthesis increases following prolonged ureteral obstruction.

Atrial natriuretic peptide

Cardiac atrial cells contain granules in which the precursor of α-human atrial natriuretic peptide (ANP) is stored. The atrial genes code for a 'pre-prohormone' with 152 amino acids. The removal of a hydrophobic sequence from the N-terminal end of this leaves the 126 amino acid prohormone. The primary released form of the hormone is α-human ANP (28 amino acids), but smaller fragments have been isolated and similar peptides are released from the brain (brain natriuretic peptide, BNP) and from the kidney itself (renal natriuretic peptide or urodilatin).

ANP can be detected in normal plasma, and increased atrial stretch leads to an increased circulating level of ANP. Many of the effects of ANP are mediated via specific cell surface receptors, which when ANP binds to them elicit an increase in the intracellular level of cyclic guanosine monophosphate (cyclic GMP). The major actions of ANP are:

- Activation of receptors on the inner medullary collecting duct cells, leading to closure of epithelial sodium channels, and inhibition of $Na^+K^+ATPase$, thereby decreasing Na^+ reabsorption at this nephron site
- Inhibition of aldosterone secretion by the zona glomerulosa of the adrenal cortex
- Reduction of renin release, which also causes a reduction in aldosterone secretion
- Vasodilatation, particularly of the afferent arterioles, leading to increased GFR
- Inhibition of vasopressin release by the posterior pituitary

All of these actions contribute to the natriuretic effect of ANP.

Dopamine

The kidneys synthesise dopamine, mostly in the cells of the proximal tubule, and this dopamine synthesis reduces tubular sodium transport, by inhibiting the $Na^+K^+ATPase$ and by decreasing Na^+H^+ antiport activity. Dopamine is also a vasodilator, but the natriuretic effect is mainly due to its tubular action, since dopamine increases sodium excretion even when renal blood flow and GFR are unaffected.

Kinins

Kinins are vasodilator peptides produced from precursor proteins ('kininogens') by the action of the enzyme kallikrein. The effects of renally produced kinins are very similar to those of the prostaglandins: they vasodilate the kidney, antagonise vasopressin-induced increases of urine osmolality and are natriuretic. Their significance in the overall control of sodium excretion is not clear. The haemodynamic effects of kinins are thought to be due to the increased production of nitric oxide.

Natriuretic hormone

There is thought to be an as yet unidentified 'natriuretic hormone', probably of hypothalamic origin, and released during volume expansion or in circumstances where the number of functioning nephrons is reduced, so that the remaining ones must increase the fraction of filtered sodium which they excrete.

Vasopressin in osmotic and volume regulation

There are circumstances in which the maintenance of effective circulating volume is more important to survival than the maintenance of body fluid osmolality. When the effective circulating volume is threatened, volume regulation takes precedence over osmotic regulation.

Changes in effective circulating volume are detected by stretch receptors in atria, and rapidly lead to appropriate alterations in urine flow, which is mediated by changes in vasopressin release (e.g. stretching the left atrial receptors produces a diuresis). These receptors exist in both the venous and arterial sides of the circulatory system. This enables changes in vasopressin secretion to occur in response to both volume and blood pressure changes.

Changes in ECV alter the range of plasma osmolalities over which vasopressin is released (Figure RE16). It can be seen that the normal response curve of vasopressin to plasma osmolality is a straight line. Changes in ECV

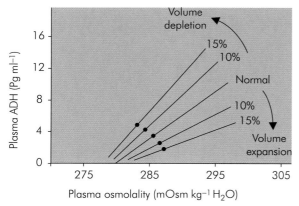

Figure RE16 Vasopressin response to changes in extracellular volume

alter the gradient of this line, which is equivalent to altering the sensitivity of the vasopressin response. Thus, when ECV is decreased, vasopressin levels are higher at a given plasma osmolality, giving rise to retained volume even at the expense of lower than normal osmolality. Under these circumstances of hypovolaemia the vasopressin response is more sensitive. When hypervolaemia is present, the vasopressin response becomes blunted and lower than expected vasopressin levels are found for any given plasma osmolality.

In summary, it can be seen that the regulation of sodium excretion is complex.

Renal regulation of body fluid pH

Normal body fluid pH
The normal blood pH is kept within the range 7.35–7.45, although a range of 7.00–7.80 can be tolerated. Enzyme reactions in the body have a pH optimum, but the pH dependence of such reactions is much less sharply defined than the pH dependence of the whole organism. The pH notation tends to obscure the range of H^+ concentration tolerated, which is broad compared with some other biochemical parameters.

To convert the normal pH range to H^+ concentration values, let concentration of

$$H^+ = [H^+]$$

By definition

$$pH = -\log[H^+]$$

As normal pH = 7.4, therefore

$$-\log[H^+] = 7.4$$
$$[H^+] = \log^{-1}(-7.4)$$
$$= \log^{-1}(-8) \times \log^{-1}(0.6)$$
$$= 10^{-8} \times 3.98$$
$$= 39.8 \times 10^{-9} \, \text{mol} \, l^{-1}$$
$$= 39.8 \, \text{nmol} \, l^{-1}$$

A pH between 7.35 and 7.45 corresponds to an $[H^+]$ range of 45–35 nmol l^{-1}. This means a change of >20% may be tolerated under normal conditions.

Physiological buffers
A buffer solution minimises the change of pH, when acid or base is added to it. Buffer solutions consist of a weak acid and the conjugate base of that acid. Thus, in solution

$$(\text{acid}) \rightleftharpoons (\text{hydrogen ion}) + (\text{conjugate base})$$
$$HA \rightleftharpoons H^+ + A^-$$

When hydrogen ions are added to the buffer solution, the above reaction is driven to the left and the hydrogen ions (H^+) are 'neutralised' by combination with the conjugate base (A^-).

Definition of pK for a buffer
The equilibrium constant (K) for the above dissociation reaction is given by the equation

$$K = \frac{[H^+][A^-]}{HA}$$

and

$$pK = -\log K$$

From the above, and using the definition of pH, it can be seen that pK is the pH at which $[A^-] = [HA]$, i.e. when the weak acid, HA, is half dissociated.

Henderson–Hasselbalch equation
In any buffer system consisting of a dissociating weak acid HA, the pH of the buffer solution is dependent on the ratio of conjugate base concentration $[A^-]$ to undissociated acid concentration $[HA]$.

Rearranging the equation for K from above:

$$[H+] = \frac{K[A^-]}{[HA]}$$

Body compartment	Buffer
Blood	Bicarbonate/CO_2
	Haemoglobin (HHb/Hb$^-$ and HHbO$_2$/HbO$_2$)
	Plasma proteins (H$^+$-protein/protein$^-$)
	Phosphate ($H_2PO_4^-$/HPO_4^{2-})
Extracellular fluid	Bicarbonate/CO_2
	Plasma proteins (H$^+$-protein/protein$^-$)
	Phosphate ($H_2PO_4^-$/HPO_4^{2-})
Intracellular fluid	Plasma proteins (H$^+$–protein/protein–)
	Phosphate ($H_2PO_4^-$/HPO_4^{2-})
	Organic phosphates
	Bicarbonate/CO_2

Figure RE17 Main physiological buffer systems

so

$$\frac{1}{H^+} = \frac{1}{K}\frac{[HA]}{[A^-]}$$

or

$$-\log[H+] = -\log K + \log \frac{[A^-]}{[HA]}$$

therefore

$$pH = pK + \log \frac{[A^-]}{[HA]}$$

which can be expressed as

$$pH = pK + \log \frac{[\text{conjugate base}]}{\text{acid}}$$

which is known as the Henderson–Hasselbalch equation.

Bicarbonate buffer system

In the body fluids there are several buffer systems, summarised in Figure RE17.

Throughout the body fluids, the bicarbonate buffer system is the most important. The reaction sequence for this system is:

$$CO_2 + H_2O \rightleftharpoons H_2CO_3 \rightleftharpoons H^+ + HCO_3^-$$

The importance of the bicarbonate buffer system is due to the ready excretion of CO_2 by the lungs, which eliminates the carbonic acid formed when H$^+$ is neutralised. This is coupled with the continuous maintenance of buffer base levels through reabsorption of bicarbonate in the kidneys.

These actions continually drive the above equations to the left, neutralising H$^+$ as it is produced by intermediate metabolism.

Thus, for the bicarbonate buffer system (pK = 6.3), the Henderson–Hasselbalch equation can be written as follows:

$$pH = 6.3 + \log \frac{[HCO_3^-]}{[H_2CO_3]}$$

[H_2CO_3] is proportional to the PCO_2 (partial pressure of CO_2 in mmHg) and is about 2.0 mmol l^{-1}. Assuming a normal value of [HCO_3^-] = 25 mmol l^{-1}, substitution in the above equation gives:

$$pH = 6.3 + \log \left(\frac{25}{2}\right)$$
$$= 7.39$$

This illustrates how the bicarbonate buffer system determines normal pH for the body fluids, by fixing its [conjugate base] : [acid] ratio. This pH will then determine the [conjugate base] : [acid] ratio for all the other buffer systems in the body.

The bicarbonate system, chemically, is a poor buffer, but physiologically it is extremely effective because of the physiological control over [HCO_3^-] and PCO_2. Since bicarbonate is regulated by the kidneys and PCO_2 by the lungs, it is apparent that pH depends on the activity of both organs.

Renal regulation of plasma bicarbonate concentration

Intermediate metabolism generates a continuous load of H$^+$. This is buffered by the blood buffer systems, which prevent excessive levels of free H$^+$, but become depleted as their base reserves combine with the H$^+$. Thus, the buffer bases need to be constantly regenerated. The most important buffer is bicarbonate, since H$^+$ is readily neutralised by plasma HCO_3^- to give carbonic acid, which is easily excreted as CO_2 in the lungs. The bicarbonate reserve is regenerated continually by the reabsorption process in the kidney. The role of the kidney can thus be seen as the conservation of the remaining HCO_3^- and the generation of additional HCO_3^-.

Renal T_m for bicarbonate

Bicarbonate ion is freely filtered at the glomeruli; hence, the concentration of bicarbonate entering the nephron is 25 mmol l^{-1}.

The kidney behaves as if there is a T_m for bicarbonate reabsorption, with the T_m set close to the amount filtered at the normal plasma concentrations. In fact, the T_m for HCO_3^- is not constant but varies with the rate of H^+ secretion, and also directly with fractional sodium reabsorption. The T_m provides a means of dealing with increases in plasma $[HCO_3^-]$, since an increase will lead to T_m being exceeded and HCO_3^- being excreted until the plasma level reaches normal again.

H^+ and bicarbonate reabsorption

In the proximal tubule 90% of the filtered bicarbonate is reabsorbed from the tubular fluid. This bicarbonate reabsorption is in fact brought about not by the transport of HCO_3^- ions, but by the luminal conversion of HCO_3^- into CO_2. H^+ is secreted from the proximal tubule cell into the lumen, where it associates with HCO_3^- to form H_2CO_3. This carbonic acid dissociates into CO_2 and H_2O. The reaction is catalysed by an enzyme, carbonic anhydrase, which is present in the brush borders of the cells, and so catalyses the luminal reaction without being lost in the urine. The CO_2 so formed can readily diffuse into the tubule cells, where intracellular carbonic anhydrase catalyses the rehydration of CO_2 to H_2CO_3, which dissociates to H^+ and HCO_3^-. The H^+ thus regenerated in the tubular cells is then available for excretion back into the tubule lumen to enable further reabsorption of HCO_3^-. It can, therefore, be claimed that the purpose of H^+ excretion in the kidney is to permit HCO_3^- reabsorption. Under normal circumstances, <0.1% of filtered HCO_3^- is excreted in the final urine.

NaCl and bicarbonate reabsorption

Although the entry of Na^+ into the proximal tubule cells is down the electrochemical gradient, Na^+ entry is coupled to H^+ excretion (via an antiport or counter-transport process) and the transport is electroneutral. In addition, the luminal membrane has a primary H^+ secretory mechanism, using proton ATPase, although this is of little importance in the proximal tubule. However, there is evidence that most apical membrane Na^+ reabsorption is associated with H^+ excretion, which generates CO_2 in the tubular lumen. The CO_2 enters the cells and again forms HCO_3^-, much of which then exchanges with luminal Cl^-, i.e. there is HCO_3^- secretion and Cl^- reabsorption, such that the overall effect is predominantly the reabsorption of NaCl.

Bicarbonate reabsorption in the distal tubule

The acid–base regulating process that occurs in the 'distal tubule' and collecting duct is the same as that in the proximal tubule, being basically HCO_3^- reabsorption and H^+ excretion. The distal nephron processes are, quantitatively, much less important than those in the proximal tubule, since they account for only 10% of the total bicarbonate reabsorption. However, to achieve this, the distal tubule and collecting duct have to secrete H^+ against a much bigger gradient than that in the proximal tubule, and this requires specific mechanisms.

The distal nephron cell types primarily involved in acid–base regulation are the intercalated cells that secrete H^+ across the apical membrane by an H^+ATPase. In addition, there is an H^+K^+ATPase, which pumps H^+ out in exchange for K^+. The linked Na^+H^+ transport of H^+ is of lesser importance in the distal nephron, but does occur in the proximal cells and is one of the means whereby aldosterone enhances H^+ secretion.

H^+ secretion and urinary buffering

In both the proximal tubule and the distal nephron, H^+ secretion is required not only for the reabsorption of filtered HCO_3^- but also to remove H^+ produced in generating additional HCO_3^- to maintain plasma levels. In order for H^+ secretion to occur, there must be some way in which the secreted H^+ can be buffered in the tubular lumen, to provide a continuing gradient for secretion, or at least to prevent the gradient against which secretion is occurring from being too large. It is mainly filtered HCO_3^- which provides this H^+ buffering. However, there are other forms of buffering for the secreted H^+.

Alkaline/acid phosphate as a urinary buffer system

In the plasma there are two phosphate salts, disodium hydrogen phosphate (alkaline phosphate, Na_2HPO_4) and sodium dihydrogen phosphate (acid phosphate, NaH_2PO_4). The ratio of alkaline phosphate to acid phosphate in plasma is about 4 : 1. These phosphate salts form an additional buffer system in the plasma.

Both the acidic and basic forms of phosphate are also filtered at the glomerulus. These then form another system for buffering H^+ in the urine. When H^+ secretion occurs into the tubule, the ratio $[HPO_4^-] : [H_2PO_4^-]$ in the luminal fluid is reduced, i.e. alkaline phosphate is converted into acid phosphate as buffering of the secreted H^+ occurs. Some phosphate buffering takes place in the proximal tubule (since there is a small fall in pH of the tubular fluid proximally), but it takes place mainly in the distal tubule. The $H_2PO_4^-$ constitutes the titratable acidity of the urine.

An important consequence of phosphate buffering in the urine is that secretion levels of H^+ can be maintained. This in turn maintains the levels of HCO_3^- generated intracellularly, since for every H^+ one HCO_3^- is produced, and this HCO_3^- is then available for export to the plasma.

Ammonia excretion

Ammonia is a form of excess nitrogen that is produced as a by-product of protein metabolism in the body. It does not circulate in its free form but forms a buffer system with the ammoniun ion:

$$NH_3 + H^+ \rightleftharpoons NH_4^+$$

The main circulating sources of NH_4^+ are glutamine and glutamic acid. The ultimate fate of NH_4^+ is to be excreted by the kidney either as ammonia or as urea.

NH_4^+ is produced by deamination of glutamine to glutamic acid and to α-ketoglutarate in most parts of the nephron, but mainly in the proximal tubule cells. The NH_4^+ is then excreted into the tubular lumen. Transport of NH_4^+ across cell membranes requires the ammonium ion to split into NH_3, which is freely diffusible, and H^+.

The α-ketoglutarate left behind in the tubule cells reacts with H^+ to form glucose or CO_2, leaving bicarbonate to enter the plasma. Thus the deamination of glutamine produces NH_4^+ and generates bicarbonate for the plasma. If the NH_4^+ were not excreted but remained in the body, then the liver could utilise NH_4^+ and HCO_3^- to produce urea for excretion, but with no gain of HCO_3^-. Thus renal secretion of NH_4^+ also regenerates HCO_3^- for the plasma.

About 50% of the NH_4^+ secreted into the lumen by the proximal tubule cells is reabsorbed by the thick ascending limb of the loop of Henle, and accumulates in the medullary interstitium. This reabsorption occurs by $Na^+/NH_4^+/2\,Cl^-$ co-transport across the apical membrane. The NH_4^+ reabsorption lowers the luminal NH_4^+ concentration, and hence also lowers the luminal NH_3 concentration, which is freely diffusible, as the luminal fluid passes into the distal tubule. This also has the effect of maintaining a higher NH_4^+ concentration in the medullary interstitium, from where the NH_4^+ then passes into the cells of the collecting tubules to be excreted.

NH_4^+ excretion is increased in acidosis because:
- The enzymes in the proximal tubule which deaminate glutamine are stimulated by acidosis.
- NH_3 conversion to NH_4^+ in the collecting tubule is greater if H^+ excretion is greater.
- Increased conversion of NH_3 to NH_4^+ in the collecting duct decreases the concentration of NH_3 in the duct. This increases the diffusion gradient for NH_3, and its rate of removal from the renal medulla.

H^+ secretion in the nephron

The secretion of H^+ in the nephron requires it to combine with ions in the tubular fluid in the following manner:
- Combination of H^+ with HCO_3^- leads to CO_2 absorption by the tubular cells and formation of HCO_3^- intracellularly. This can be viewed as reabsorption of the HCO_3^- from the tubular lumen.
- Combination of H^+ with HPO_4^- or NH_3 leads to formation of HCO_3^- in the tubular cells rather than reabsorption from the tubular lumen. This can be viewed as generation of HCO_3^-.

The H^+ secreted causes the pH of the tubular fluid to fall progressively along the nephron. This fall is small in the proximal tubule (from 7.4 to about 6.9), but the pH may be as low as 4.5 in the collecting duct. Although the urine is usually acidic and can be titrated to determine the 'titratable acidity', this only constitutes a fraction of the total H^+ secreted. This is because

Total H^+ secreted

$$= (H^+ \text{neutralised in } HCO_3^- \text{ reabsorption})$$
$$+ (H^+ \text{combined in } H_2PO_4^- \text{ excretion})$$
$$+ (H^+ \text{combined in } NH_4^+ \text{ excretion})$$

But only the $H2PO_4^-$ excretion is 'titratable acidity'.

Points of emphasis for H^+ secretion in the nephron are:
- H^+ secreted must be combined with anions in the tubular fluid.
- The main anions are HCO_3^-, HPO_4^{2-} and NH_3.
- Combination with HCO_3^- leads to reabsorption of HCO_3^-.
- Combination with HPO_4^{2-} or NH_3 leads to generation of HCO_3^-.

Renal regulation of pH in acid–base balance disturbances

Acid–base disturbances can be divided into disturbances of respiratory origin (respiratory acidosis and alkalosis) and non-respiratory origin (metabolic acidosis and alkalosis). 'Metabolic' refers to acid–base disturbances that affect the bicarbonate buffer system by a means other than an alteration of PCO_2. Metabolic acidosis is by far the most common metabolic disturbance, and is often associated with pathological conditions involving the excess production of acid. Examples of these are diabetic ketoacidosis or septicaemia. Failure to excrete acid, as in renal failure, can also lead to a metabolic acidosis.

In each of the four disturbances, there is initially a change in body fluid pH (i.e. a change in H^+ concentration). However, the buffer and compensatory systems are so effective that this change in pH may be barely measurable.

When changes in extracellular fluid pH occur, there are parallel, although not necessarily identical, changes in intracellular pH. Therefore a change in arterial pH is reflected in the pH of all the cells of the body, including the renal tubule cells. The rate of H^+ secretion from the tubule cells varies inversely with pH (i.e. varies directly with H^+ concentration). This is vital for the compensation for, and correction of, acid–base disturbances.

Compensation and correction in acid–base disturbances

Normal acid–base status comprises not only a pH of 7.4, but also a plasma $[HCO_3^-]$ of about 25 mmol l^{-1} and a PCO_2 of about 40 mmHg. An acid–base disturbance disrupts at least two of these three variables.

Two definitions are important:

- **Compensation** – the restoration of pH towards normal even though $[HCO_3^-]$ and/or PCO_2 are still disturbed
- **Correction** – the restoration of normal pH, $[HCO_3^-]$ and PCO_2

The purpose of homeostatic acid-balance regulating mechanisms is the maintenance of normal pH. The process used for the immediate regulation of pH is adjustment of PCO_2 and $[HCO_3^-]$. The normal levels of these parameters are sacrificed initially to correct for pH disturbances. Ultimately long-term correction requires regeneration of buffer base reserves and secretion of H^+ by the kidneys.

In the following sections, a simplified version of the Henderson–Hasselbalch equation is used to show changes

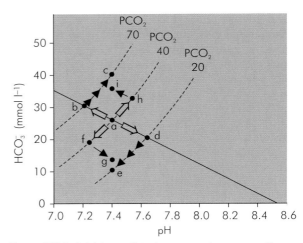

Figure RE18 Acid–base disturbances and compensation

in pH, PCO_2 and HCO_3^-. The simplified form of the Henderson–Hasselbalch equation used is as follows:

$$pH \propto \frac{[HCO_3^-]}{PCO_2}$$

Three types of arrow are used to indicate changes: $\Uparrow$ or $\Downarrow$ are the initial acid–base defect; $\uparrow$ or $\downarrow$ are the consequence of the defect; $\uparrow$ or $\downarrow$ are compensatory changes.

Respiratory acidosis

This is a disturbance of acid–base balance that occurs when the respiratory system is unable to remove sufficient CO_2 from the body, giving rise to higher than normal PCO_2 levels (hypercapnia). This condition might be caused by failure to breathe adequately (hypoventilation) and results in an arterial partial pressure of CO_2 ($PaCO_2$) above 6.0 kPa (45 mmHg). The following reaction becomes displaced to the right by the increased PCO_2:

$$CO_2 + H_2O \rightleftharpoons H_2CO_3 \rightleftharpoons H^+ + HCO_3^-$$

The consequence of this defect is an increased $[H^+]$ (i.e. acidosis – reduced pH), and an increased $[HCO_3^-]$. These changes are illustrated in Figure RE18, which plots the three variables of $[HCO_3^-]$, pH and PCO_2. Normal acid–base status is represented by point a. Respiratory acidosis producing the above disturbances in pH and $[HCO_3^-]$ shifts the acid–base status to b. Inserting these changes into the simplified Henderson–Hasselbalch equation results in

$$\downarrow pH \propto \frac{\uparrow [HCO_3^-]}{\Uparrow PCO_2}$$

A change in $[H^+]$ in the body fluids changes the rate of H^+ secretion from renal tubular cells. In respiratory acidosis, $[H^+]$ is increased; therefore, the rate of H^+ secretion also increases. This increased secretion is sufficient to reabsorb all of the filtered HCO_3^- even though the plasma $[HCO_3^-]$ is raised by the defect and, therefore, the amount of HCO_3^- filtered is increased. In addition, it is also sufficient to generate HCO_3^-, which increases plasma $[HCO_3^-]$ further.

This increased renal H^+ secretion leading to increased plasma $[HCO_3^-]$ is renal compensation for the respiratory acidosis. This compensation is demonstrated in Figure RE18 by a shift of the respiratory acidosis point b to the compensated point c. These compensatory changes can be added to the simplified Henderson–Hasselbalch equation:

$$\downarrow pH\uparrow \propto \frac{\uparrow[HCO_3^-]\downarrow}{\Uparrow pCO_2}$$

Although compensation restores the pH towards normal, PCO_2 remains raised due to the initial defect, and plasma $[HCO_3^-]$ is raised, both as a consequence of the defect and by compensation. To restore normal $[HCO_3^-]$ and PCO_2 would require an alteration in respiration, i.e. correction of the original defect.

Respiratory alkalosis

This is caused by the excessive removal of CO_2 from the body by the respiratory system. This may occur with excessively rapid breathing (hyperventilation). Under these circumstances the $PaCO_2$ falls below 4.6 kPa (35 mmHg). The reaction

$$CO_2 + H_2O \rightleftharpoons H_2CO_3 \rightleftharpoons H^+ + HCO_3^-$$

is displaced to the left by the lowering of PCO_2, and this leads to a decrease in $[H^+]$ (i.e. alkalosis), and a decrease in $[HCO_3^-]$. The changes are illustrated by a shift from the normal status point a to d in Figure RE18.

In the simplified form of the Henderson–Hasselbalch equation:

$$\uparrow pH \propto \frac{\downarrow[HCO_3^-]}{\Downarrow PCO_2}$$

The decreased PCO_2 results in a decreased $[H^+]$ in the renal tubule cells and a reduced rate of H^+ secretion. Thus, although plasma $[HCO_3^-]$ is reduced, which decreases the amount of HCO_3^- filtered by the kidney, the rate of H^+ secretion is insufficient to reabsorb all the filtered bicarbonate, or to generate more bicarbonate. Therefore, HCO_3^- is excreted in the urine, and the plasma $[HCO_3^-]$ falls further.

The reduced H^+ secretion in the renal tubules, leading to HCO_3^- excretion, represents renal compensation for respiratory alkalosis. This compensation is demonstrated by the movement from point d to e in Figure RE18, and can be added to the equation above, resulting in

$$\uparrow pH \sim\downarrow \propto \frac{\downarrow[HCO_3^-]\downarrow}{\Downarrow PCO_2}$$

The renal compensation restores pH towards normal, but lowers the plasma $[HCO_3^-]$ further, even though plasma $[HCO_3^-]$ has already been reduced by the original disturbance. In addition, PCO_2 remains lower than normal. The restoration of normal plasma $[HCO_3^-]$ and PCO_2 levels requires the removal of the respiratory defect, i.e. requires a reduction of ventilation.

The body's mechanisms for control of respiration maintain PCO_2 levels within normal limits ($4.5 < PaCO_2 < 5.5$ kPa). Increase in $PaCO_2$ results in increased $[H^+]$ in body fluid, which stimulates respiration via central and peripheral chemoreceptors. Decreases in $PaCO_2$ decrease ventilation. However, if the PO_2 in the inspired air is below normal, so that PaO_2 falls significantly, then oxygen lack, acting via chemoreceptors in the carotid body, increases ventilation. When this occurs, the $PaCO_2$ falls. This is respiratory alkalosis. Thus hypoxia, leading to increased ventilation, can lead to hypocapnia and respiratory alkalosis. This occurs in normal people when they ascend to a high altitude (>3000 m). Other causes of respiratory alkalosis include hyperventilation.

Metabolic acidosis

Metabolic acidosis is an acidosis that is not caused by a change in the arterial PCO_2. So, in the reaction sequence

$$CO_2 + H_2O \rightleftharpoons H_2CO_3 \rightleftharpoons H^+ + HCO_3$$
$$\nwarrow$$
$$H^+$$

the metabolic acidosis can be regarded as the addition of H^+ to the right of the reaction, so driving it to the left and depleting the plasma HCO_3^- as it does so. The direct loss of HCO_3^- can also cause metabolic acidosis, as can be seen from the Henderson–Hasselbalch equation below. Initially, since respiration is unimpaired, the original disturbance can be assumed to occur at a constant (normal) PCO_2.

Metabolic acidosis is illustrated in Figure RE18 by a shift from normal at point a to f. The simplified

Henderson–Hasselbalch equation becomes

$$\Downarrow pH \propto \frac{\downarrow[HCO_3^-]}{PCO_2}$$

The change in pH, acting on the peripheral chemoreceptors, stimulates respiration so that $PaCO_2$ falls. This is respiratory compensation for metabolic acidosis. However, the lowering of PCO_2 moves the reaction

$$CO_2 + H_2O \rightleftharpoons H_2CO_3 \rightleftharpoons H^+ + HCO_3^-$$

to the left, thus lowering $[H^+]$ and so raising the pH towards normal, but also further lowering the plasma $[HCO_3^-]$. These compensatory changes can be seen by the movement from f to g in Figure RE18, and are added to the simplified Henderson–Hasselbalch equation as follows:

$$\Downarrow pH \uparrow \propto \frac{\downarrow[HCO_3^-]\downarrow}{PCO_2\downarrow}$$

Thus the original disturbance initiates the corrective process to restore pH to normal. This occurs because the increased $[H^+]$ in the blood is reflected in an increased $[H^+]$ in the renal tubular cells. This increases the rate of H^+ secretion, and permits the reabsorption of all the filtered HCO_3^-, particularly as the filtered HCO_3^- load is below normal. In addition, the increased rate of H^+ secretion allows generation of more HCO_3^-, restoring the depleted plasma HCO_3^- reserve and returning pH to normal. The stimulated respiratory drive due to the original disturbed pH can then also be normalised.

It should be noted that in metabolic acidosis there is often nothing wrong with the kidneys. They simply cannot excrete an H^+ load instantaneously. The respiratory compensation, although restoring pH towards normal, also hampers the renal correction of the defect. This is because any decrease in pH also reduces H^+ secretion, and hence reduces renal HCO_3^- reabsorption and regeneration. The exception to this is renal failure, where the kidneys' failure to excrete H^+ is the cause of metabolic acidosis.

Metabolic alkalosis

This is alkalosis that is not caused by a change in the arterial PCO_2. In the reaction sequence

$$CO_2 + H_2O \rightleftharpoons H_2CO_3 \rightleftharpoons H^+ + HCO_3^-$$
$$\searrow \longrightarrow H_2^3O$$
$$OH^-$$

metabolic alkalosis can be regarded as the addition of base (OH^- in the equation, although it can be any H^+ acceptor) to the system. This removes H^+ from the right of the reaction and causes the reaction to move to the right, increasing plasma $[HCO_3^-]$. Initially this can be assumed to occur at a constant (normal) PCO_2, and is shown by a shift from point a to h in Figure RE18. The simplified Henderson–Hasselbalch equation then becomes

$$\Uparrow pH \propto \frac{\uparrow[HCO_3^-]}{PCO_2}$$

The decreased $[H^+]$, acting on chemoreceptors, reduces ventilation and so increases the PCO_2. This is respiratory compensation for metabolic alkalosis. The compensatory changes are illustrated by movement from h to i in Figure RE18, and can be added to the above equation as

$$\Uparrow pH \downarrow \propto \frac{\uparrow[HCO_3^-]\uparrow}{PCO_2\uparrow}$$

The compensation thus reduces the pH, but increases the plasma $[HCO_3^-]$ further, although the effect of respiratory compensation in metabolic alkalosis is normally of very minor importance. Correction of the original disturbance is initiated by the effects of the disturbance itself on renal H^+ secretion. The decreased $[H^+]$ in the body reduces the rate of H^+ secretion, and the increased plasma $[HCO_3^-]$ increases the filtered HCO_3^- load. Thus, H^+ secretion is inadequate to reabsorb all the filtered HCO_3^- or to generate more HCO_3^-. The plasma $[HCO_3^-]$ therefore falls, causing the reaction

$$CO_2 + H_2O \rightleftharpoons H_2CO_3 \rightleftharpoons H^+ + HCO_3^-$$

to move to the right and restoring $[H^+]$ to normal. As in the case of metabolic acidosis, the respiratory compensation hampers the renal correction of the defect. This fact again emphasises that it is the regulation of pH that is all-important, rather than the regulation of $[HCO_3^-]$ or PCO_2 per se.

Micturition

The smooth muscle of the bladder is arranged in spiral, circular and longitudinal bundles. This arrangement forms the detrusor muscle, which is responsible for emptying of the bladder. Two sphincters oppose emptying of the bladder. The first is an incomplete ring of smooth muscle around the urethra – the internal urethral sphincter. The second is a ring of skeletal muscle around the membranous urethra – the external urethral sphincter.

The process of micturition is a spinal reflex that is affected by higher centres. When micturition is initiated, relaxation of the perineal muscles and external urethral sphincter occurs, followed by contraction of the detrusor muscle, which leads to voiding.

The precise mechanism of voluntary micturition remains unclear. Learned ability to exert higher control over the reflex emptying of the bladder when it becomes full is the most likely mechanism.

When the bladder reaches a certain threshold volume (normally about 400 ml) stretch receptors in the bladder wall initiate a voiding reflex. The pelvic nerves constitute the afferent limb of this reflex and the parasympathetic fibres the efferent limb. The threshold for voiding is controlled by the brain stem. A facilitatory area exists in the pons and an inhibitory area in the midbrain. Other cortical areas are also thought to be of importance.

CHAPTER 8

Respiratory physiology

B. L. Appadu and C. D. Hanning

Functional anatomy

The primary function of the respiratory system is the exchange of oxygen and carbon dioxide between the body and the environment. In addition, the lungs also have a metabolic role, act as a filter for small emboli in the circulation, play a part in acid–base balance and contribute to the immune defences of the body. These functions are all reflected in the anatomy of the components of the respiratory system.

Upper airway and larynx

In respiration, the function of the nose, mouth and pharynx is to conduct fresh gas to the larynx, which marks the entrance to the conducting airways. These structures also warm, humidify and filter the gases.

During quiet nasal breathing this section of the airway can provide two-thirds of the total resistance to airflow of the respiratory system. Since the pharynx is a muscular tube without rigid structures to maintain its patency, it can increase the flow resistance considerably, even to the point of total obstruction, depending on the tone of its muscular wall, the associated muscles and the transmural pressure.

The larynx has three main functions:

- Regulation of expiratory airflow (expiratory braking). This is important for vocalisation, coughing and control of end-expiratory lung volume.
- Protection of the lower airway. Vocal cord closure prevents aspiration of foreign material or objects and

Fundamentals of Anaesthesia, 3rd edition, ed. Tim Smith, Colin Pinnock and Ted Lin. Published by Cambridge University Press. © Cambridge University Press 2008.

expiratory braking enables the cough reflex to expel foreign material and secretions.
- Vocalisation.

Conducting airways

The respiratory system is traditionally divided into gas-conducting and gas-exchanging components. The conducting system begins with its smallest cross-sectional area at the level of the larynx. The conducting system begins as the trachea and undergoes irregular dichotomous branching for about 16 generations, forming bronchi and bronchioles (there are seven additional generations which are respiratory airways). The 23 generations are called Weibel's classification, after E. R. Weibel, a contemporary anatomist from Bern in Switzerland.

Adult trachea

This is about 18 mm in diameter and 11 cm in length. The trachea is lined with columnar ciliated epithelium containing many mucus-secreting goblet cells. It also contains a number of receptors that are sensitive to mechanical or chemical stimuli. These mediate respiratory and cough reflexes.

Major bronchi (generations 2–4)

The major bronchi are named after the lobe or segment supplied. Circumferential cartilage rings support them. The right bronchus is wider than the left and leaves the trachea at about 25° from the tracheal axis, while the angle of the left bronchus is about 45°. Inadvertent endobronchial intubation or aspiration of foreign material is, therefore, more likely to occur in the right lung than the left. The right upper lobe bronchus branches posteriorly at about 90° to the right main bronchus. Thus, foreign bodies or fluid aspirated by a supine subject usually enter the right upper lobe.

Small bronchi (generations 5–11)

These are smaller versions of the major bronchi, and their mucosa tends to be more cuboidal than columnar towards the periphery. As the number of bronchi increases, the total cross-sectional area increases markedly, with a reduction in the velocity of gas flow and a decrease in airway resistance.

Bronchioles (generations 12–16)

Bronchioles typically have diameters <1 mm. They are devoid of cartilage and have a high proportion of smooth muscle in their walls in relation to intraluminal diameter. There are three to four bronchiolar generations, the final generation being the terminal bronchioles. Goblet cells are not found in bronchioles, and there is a continued gradual transition from ciliated epithelial cells to cuboidal epithelium.

Respiratory areas of the lung

Gas exchange begins in the smaller bronchioles and extends throughout the succeeding generations of airways to the most peripheral spaces, which are the alveoli.

Respiratory bronchioles (generations 17–19)

These are characterised by intermittent alveolar outpockets. Their cuboidal epithelium is thinning and a muscle layer is still present, forming 'sphincters' around openings to alveoli.

Alveolar ducts and sacs (generations 20–23)

These are formed from the alveoli that line and form their walls. The sacs differ from the ducts in being blind-ended. The alveolus is the basic unit of gas exchange, being a thin-walled pocket, about 0.3 mm in diameter. There are 300 million alveoli, with a total surface area of 50–100 m^2. Three types of cells cover the alveolar surface:
- Type I alveolar cells occupy 80% of the surface for gas exchange. They provide a very thin layer of cytoplasm, spread over a relatively wide area (50 times that of a Type II cell). Type I cells are derived from Type II cells and are highly differentiated and metabolically limited, which makes them susceptible to injury.
- Type II alveolar cells have extensive metabolic and enzymatic capacity and manufacture surfactant. Both type I and II alveolar cells have tight intracellular junctions, providing a relatively impermeable barrier to fluids.
- Type III alveolar cells are alveolar macrophages and form an important part of lung defences. They contain proteolytic enzymes, which may be released during lung injury, thus contributing to pulmonary damage.

Alveoli have holes in their walls called pores of Kohn (8–10 μm in diameter), which permit collateral ventilation between neighbouring alveoli. Similarly, larger-diameter (30 μm) ducts allow collateral ventilation between respiratory bronchioles.

Alveolar–capillary membrane

The alveolar–capillary membrane exists between the alveolar space and the capillary lumen, and consists of alveolar

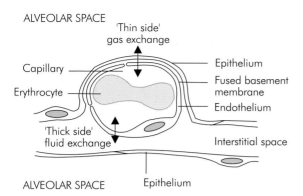

Figure RR1 Alveolar–capillary membrane

epithelium, interstitial tissue and endothelium. This membrane must perform two conflicting functions:
- Gas exchange across the blood–gas barrier
- Fluid exchange between alveolar interstitial tissue and the capillary lumen

In order for these to take place, the capillaries are located asymmetrically in the alveolar walls, which gives them a 'thick side' and a 'thin side'. The 'thick side' is used for fluid exchange with the interstitium, while the 'thin side' forms the blood–gas barrier (Figure RR1).

Blood–gas barrier

This is the barrier between alveolar gas and pulmonary capillary blood, across which gas exchange takes place. It consists of three components:
- Alveolar epithelium, which is a thin layer of type I alveolar cell cytoplasm
- Interstitial tissue, consisting of fused alveolar and endothelial basement membranes
- Pulmonary capillary endothelium

Blood vessels and lymphatics

The lung is divided into lobes, each supplied by its own artery, vein and bronchus. The arterioles form densely packed sheets of capillaries in the walls of the alveoli, thus matching the large ventilated surface area with an equivalent perfused area. Bronchi receive their own blood supply via bronchial arteries originating directly from the aorta.

Lymphatic drainage is important in the lung because of the magnitude of the perfused area and the effect accumulating interstitial fluid would have on gas exchange. Pulmonary lymphatics travel with blood vessels to the hila, ultimately draining into the thoracic duct.

Lung volumes

The lung can be divided into various volumes. These are identified either by measurements made during lung function testing, or according to the function of the lung in gas exchange.

Lung volumes derived from spirometry

During quiet breathing a small volume of gas is moved in and out of the lungs repeatedly. If a maximal inspiration is taken, followed by a maximal expiration, the volume changes occurring can be recorded using a spirometer. Figure RR2 shows a typical spirometer trace of these changes.

Lung volumes vary with age, sex and body size (height more so than weight). The lung volumes are:
- Total lung capacity (TLC) – volume of gas present in the lungs at the end of maximal inspiration
- Tidal volume (V_T) – amount of gas inspired and expired during normal quiet breathing
- Inspiratory reserve volume (IRV) – extra volume of gas that can be inspired over and beyond the normal V_T
- Expiratory reserve volume (ERV) – amount of gas that can be forcefully expired at the end of normal tidal expiration
- Residual volume (RV) – amount of gas remaining in the lungs at the end of a maximum forced expiration
- Vital capacity (VC) – maximal volume of gas which can be expelled after a maximal inspiration
- Functional residual capacity (FRC) – lung volume following expiration during quiet breathing

Some typical values for the above volumes are given in Figure RR3.

Vital capacity

Apart from body size, the major factors that determine VC are the strength of the respiratory muscles, and chest and lung compliance. It is an important clinical measure of respiratory sufficiency, particularly in patients with restrictive diseases. VC < 10 ml kg^{-1} is indicative of impending respiratory failure.

Functional residual capacity

From the spirometry trace in Figure RR2 it can be seen that FRC is the lung volume at the end of normal quiet expiration, and is also equal to the sum of ERV + RV. The thoracic cage normally has a resting volume >FRC, while the normal lung has a volume <FRC. Thus, FRC represents the equilibrium point between the tendency of the lungs to

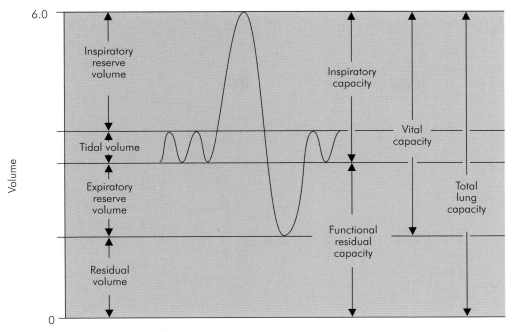

Figure RR2 Spirometer trace of lung volumes

Lung volume	Male	Female
TLC	6000	4200
V_T	500	500
IRV	3300	1900
ERV	1000	700
RV	1200	1100

Figure RR3 Values for lung volumes (ml)

collapse and of the thoracic cage to expand. It is not a fixed volume, and it varies with normal respiration as well as depending on gravity and other factors. FRC is decreased by 20–25% in the supine position and is further decreased by the head-down posture and induction of anaesthesia. Some of the factors affecting FRC are shown in Figure RR4.

Measurement of FRC
Spirometry does not give a value for FRC, nor for TLC and RV. The latter two can be derived if FRC is measured. Two common methods of determining FRC are:
- Helium dilution – used to obtain FRC using a spirometer, and an analyser to measure helium

Factor	Change in FRC
Age	
Posture	
Anaesthesia	
Surgery	
Pulmonary fibrosis	Decreased
Pulmonary oedema	
Obesity	
Abdominal swelling	
Thoracic wall distortion	
Reduced muscle tone	
Positive intrathoracic pressure	
Emphysema	Increased
Asthma	

Figure RR4 Factors affecting FRC

concentration. The subject is connected to the spirometer containing a known volume of fresh gas mixture (V_1) with a known initial concentration of helium (C_1). Normal breathing is allowed to take place through the spirometer until the helium becomes diluted and mixed in the larger combined volume (V_1 + FRC) of the spirometer and the respiratory system of the subject. Oxygen is fed into the spirometer to keep the spirometer reading constant, thus compensating for the difference between oxygen consumption and CO_2 production. Helium is used because it is virtually insoluble and not metabolised. FRC can be derived by measuring final helium concentration (C_2) and using the expression for the amount of helium present before and after as follows:

$$\text{Amount of helium} = V_1 \times C_1 \text{ (before)}$$
$$= (V_1 + FRC) \times C_2 \text{ (after)}$$

- Body plethysmograph – obtains FRC by placing the subject in a closed chamber and measuring the pressure and volume changes occurring when the subject makes an inspiratory effort. Boyle's gas law can be applied before and after the inspiratory effort to derive FRC.

Closing capacity

Closing capacity (CC) is the volume at which airway collapse and closure occurs during expiration. It is important because it can affect gas exchange by virtue of its relationship to FRC. Under normal circumstances FRC is always >CC. However, if FRC decreases or CC increases, for example due to loss of lung elasticity from disease, then airway closure may occur at the end of normal expiration in the dependent areas of the lung. Recent studies have shown that plate-like areas of atelectasis develop in dependent areas of the lungs shortly after induction of anaesthesia. The difference between FRC and CC is also reduced in infants and the elderly.

Dynamic lung volumes

Lung function can also be measured by its dynamic performance during active inflation or deflation. A common test is the recording of expired volumes during forced expiration of a maximal breath. The forced vital capacity (FVC) is the total volume of gas that can be forcibly expired after maximal inspiration. During forced expiration, dynamic compression of the intrathoracic airways occurs, limiting both the rate of expiration and the total amount of gas that can be expelled. The limiting effect may be seen from the expiratory curve of a VC breath, which is linear rather than exponentially declining and is described by the

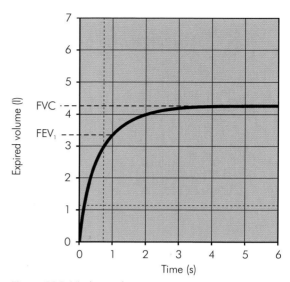

Figure RR5 Vitalograph trace

mid-expiratory flow rate, which applies to the gas volume expired between 25 and 75% of the total ($MEFR_{25-75}$). In clinical practice the volume expired in the first second (FEV_1) is often measured as part of an FVC measurement. The ratio (FEV_1/FVC) can then be derived, which is a useful index of obstructive airways disease. Normally this ratio would be >95%, but it declines with age and 85% may be acceptable in an elderly subject (Figure RR5).

Ventilation

Ventilation describes the process of fresh gas reaching the areas of the lung where gas exchange takes place. Gas exchange is dependent on the volume of gas moved in and out of the lungs per minute. This is referred to as total ventilation (minute ventilation). It is usually measured as the volume of gas expired per minute, and it can be determined for respiratory rate = n breaths per minute and tidal volume = V_T:

$$\text{Total ventilation} = (\text{respiratory rate}) \times (\text{tidal volume})$$
$$= n \times V_T$$

Not all the gas moving in and out of the lungs takes part in gas exchange, since there are two main parts of the lung: **dead space**, which does not take part in gas exchange, and **alveolar space**, in which gas exchange does take place.

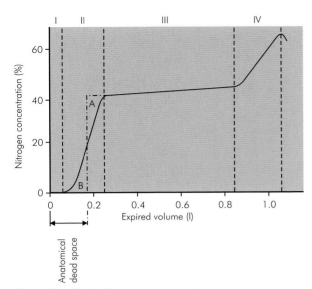

Figure RR6 Fowler's method of dead space measurement

Dead space

Dead space can be subdivided into anatomical dead space, which corresponds to the conducting airways, and alveolar dead space. Alveolar dead space consists of those parts of the lung which are ventilated but not perfused. The sum of the anatomical and alveolar dead space is the physiological dead space.

Anatomical dead space

This is about 2 ml kg^{-1} (150 ml in an adult). Early measurements of the volume were obtained by taking casts of the conducting airways, but it may be measured non-invasively by Fowler's method.

In Fowler's method the patient takes a single VC breath of 100% oxygen and exhales through a rapid nitrogen analyser. Expired N_2 concentration is then plotted against expired volume (Figure RR6). The initial gas from the dead space (phase I) is free of nitrogen, being pure oxygen, and thereafter the nitrogen concentration increases with the introduction of alveolar gas (phase II) until an 'alveolar' plateau is achieved (phase III). The dead space is found by dividing phase II by a vertical line such that area A = area B and measuring the volume from zero.

Anatomical dead space will vary with changes in bronchial muscle tone and also with changes in position of the head and neck or the placing of an endotracheal tube. A functional decrease in anatomical dead space occurs at low V_T, when gas flow in the airways is laminar.

Alveolar dead space

Alveolar volume

Only fresh gas reaching the alveoli takes part in gas exchange. In each breath, only a portion of each V_T will reach the alveoli due to anatomical dead space (V_D). This portion is the alveolar volume (V_A),

e.g. for $V_T = 500$ ml and $V_D = 150$ ml
$$V_A = V_T - V_D$$
$$= 350 \text{ ml}$$

Alveolar ventilation

Alveolar ventilation is the volume of gas per minute reaching the alveolar spaces. It can be calculated from the respiratory rate (n) and alveolar volume (V_A):

e.g. for $V_A = 350$ ml and $n = 15$ breaths min^{-1}
$$\text{alveolar ventilation} = n \times V_A$$
$$= 15 \times 350$$
$$= 5250 \text{ ml min}^{-1}$$

Physiological dead space

Under normal circumstances, physiological dead space differs very little from the anatomical and may be estimated with Bohr's equation.

The total volume of CO_2 expired in one breath (V_TCO_2) may be expressed in two ways.

First, as the product of the alveolar volume and the fractional concentration of CO_2 in the alveolar gas (F_ACO_2):

$$V_TCO_2 = V_A \times F_ACO_2$$

Second, as the product of V_T and the concentration of CO_2 in the mixed expired gas ($F_{\bar{E}}CO_2$):

$$V_TCO_2 = V_T \times F_{\bar{E}}CO_2$$

Thus

$$V_A \times F_ACO_2 = V_T \times F_{\bar{E}}CO_2$$

Substituting, as

$$V_A = V_T - V_D$$

gives

$$(V_T - V_D) \times F_ACO_2 = V_T \times F_{\bar{E}}CO_2$$

Rearrange to give

$$\frac{V_D}{V_T} = \frac{F_ACO_2 - F_{\bar{E}}CO_2}{F_ACO_2}$$

As the barometric pressure is the same for expired gas and alveolar gas, the partial pressures in the alveoli (P_ACO_2) and mixed expired gas ($P\bar{E}CO_2$) may be substituted instead, yielding

$$\frac{V_D}{V_T} = \frac{P_ACO_2 - P\bar{E}CO_2}{P_ACO_2}$$

In practice, $P\bar{E}CO_2$ can be measured from a collection of mixed expired gas in a large bag, and P_ACO_2 may be taken as being equal to P_aCO_2.

Physiological dead space is dependent on both anatomical and alveolar dead space. Anatomical dead space varies as noted above. Alveolar dead space will be increased whenever areas of the lung become better ventilated than perfused.

Respiratory mechanics

The movement of gas in and out of the lungs is a mechanical process, which is dependent on the following factors:

- The respiratory muscles and their actions
- The compliance of the chest wall and the lungs
- The gas flow in the airways

The respiratory muscles and their actions

Respiration can be divided into inspiration and expiration. Inspiration is normally active while expiration is passive.

Inspiration

During inspiration the lungs can be expanded with two degrees of freedom (Figure RR7):

- Displacement of the abdominal contents by contraction of the diaphragm
- Radial expansion of the thoracic cage by the accessory respiratory muscles

Diaphragm

This is the principal muscle of breathing, accounting for about 75% of the air that enters the lungs during spontaneous inspiration. Contraction of the diaphragm moves abdominal contents downward and forward during each inspiration. Two-thirds of the diaphragmatic fibres are slow twitch, making it relatively resistant to fatigue.

Accessory respiratory muscles

These comprise the external intercostal and strap muscles (sternocleidomastoid, anterior serrati, scalenes). During quiet breathing their contribution to inspiration is small. They act mainly to stabilise the upper rib cage

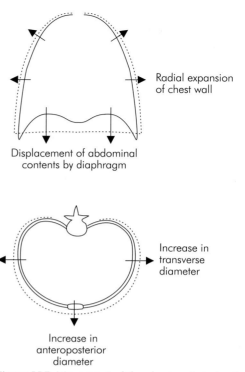

Figure RR7 Movement of the chest wall during inspiration

and preventing indrawing. As respiration deepens, the contribution of these muscles increases by elevating the rib cage and expanding it in the lateral and anteroposterior directions.

Expiration

In contrast with inspiration, the diaphragm relaxes during exhalation and the elastic recoil of the lungs, chest wall and abdominal structures compresses the lungs. Forced expiration for a cough or when airway resistance is increased requires the abdominal muscles and the internal intercostals. Paralysis of abdominal muscles produced by regional anaesthesia does not usually influence alveolar ventilation.

Compliance of the chest wall and lungs

Mechanically the respiratory system consists of two main components, the lungs and thoracic cage (including the diaphragmatic surface), which expand and contract together. Thus, the lungs and chest wall move together as a unit. The lung expands in response to a pressure gradient produced across its surface, called the transpulmonary pressure. The transpulmonary pressure is equal to the difference between the airway pressure in the lungs and the pressure on the lung surface, i.e. in between the lung and chest wall. This pressure is the intrapleural pressure.

Intrapleural pressure

The resting position of the lungs and chest wall occurs at FRC. If isolated, the lungs, being elastic, would collapse to a volume <FRC. However, the isolated thoracic cage would normally have a volume >FRC. Since the chest wall is coupled to the lung surface by the thin layer of intrapleural fluid between parietal and visceral pleura, opposing lung and chest wall recoil forces are in equilibrium at FRC. This produces a pressure of about −0.3 kPa in the pleural space. Normal inspiration reduces intrapleural pressure further to −1.0 kPa, but with forced inspiration it can reach negative pressures of −4.0 kPa or more. Intrapleural pressure may be measured by an intrapleural catheter or from a balloon catheter placed in the mid-oesophagus.

Transpulmonary pressure

Normally, during spontaneous respiration, airway pressures in the lung can be approximated to atmospheric pressure. The pressure on the lung surface is the intrapleural pressure, which may reach −1.0 kPa during inspiration. This is equivalent to a distending transpulmonary pressure of +1.0 kPa.

Lung compliance

The lungs expand in response to the transpulmonary pressures produced by the respiratory muscles. The amount of expansion for a given transpulmonary pressure represents the ease with which the lungs expand. This property is measured by the lung compliance, which is defined by:

$$\text{Lung compliance} = \frac{\text{Change in volume}}{\text{Change in transpulmonary pressure}}$$

A value for compliance can be obtained from the pressure–volume curve for a normal isolated lung undergoing inflation, as shown in Figure RR8. It can be seen that the curve is approximately linear over the 'working range' of the lung centred around FRC. At FRC, lung compliance is about 200 ml cm^{-1} H$_2$O. However, compliance is reduced at high lung volumes because the elastic fibres are fully stretched close to their elastic limit, while at low lung volumes compliance is reduced because airway and alveolar collapse occurs, requiring greater pressures to open up the airways and alveoli. Lung

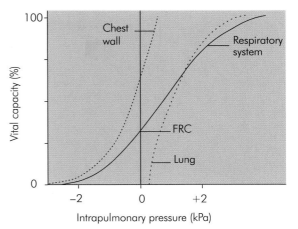

Figure RR8 Lung and chest wall compliance

compliance may also be reduced by other factors (see below).

Chest wall compliance

If a pressure–volume curve is plotted for the isolated thoracic cage (Figure RR8) the chest wall compliance can be obtained from the gradient, and this is also about 200 ml cm^{-1} H$_2$O at FRC. The chest wall compliance can be reduced by disease, as in ankylosing spondylitis, in which the chest wall can become virtually rigid, giving an extremely low compliance value.

Total respiratory system compliance

In the respiratory system the lungs and chest wall move together during inspiration and expiration. The respiratory system compliance is, therefore, the combination of chest wall and lung compliances, e.g. if lung compliance (C_L) = 200 ml cm^{-1} H$_2$O, and chest wall compliance (C_W) = 200 ml cm^{-1} H$_2$O, then respiratory system compliance (C_R) is given by

$$\frac{1}{C_R} = \frac{1}{C_L} + \frac{1}{C_W}$$
$$\frac{1}{C_R} = \frac{1}{200} + \frac{1}{200} = \frac{1}{100}$$
So
$$C_R = 100 \text{ ml cm}^{-1} \text{ H}_2\text{O}$$

The effect of combining lung and chest wall compliances to give the overall respiratory system pressure–volume curve is shown in Figure RR8. Here it can be seen how the respiratory system compliance at FRC (gradient of the curve) is less than the individual gradients for lung or chest wall.

Measurement of respiratory system compliance

Compliance can be obtained from the gradient of a pressure–volume curve plotted for the respiratory system. However, this leads to two different values depending on the measurement technique.

Static compliance

To obtain static compliance a pressure–volume curve is plotted by applying known distending pressures to the respiratory system, and measuring the corresponding changes in volume produced. Appropriate time must be allowed between measurements, for equilibration of the lung, when all gas movement has ceased.

Dynamic compliance

To measure dynamic compliance a pressure–volume curve is plotted during spontaneous breathing or mechanical ventilation. In this case the changes in volume and pressure are recorded continuously with no pause between measurements. Under these circumstances the value for dynamic compliance is usually lower than the static compliance because:

- Airflow may not have ceased completely within the lung in response to pressure changes, particularly in diseased lungs. Further volume increases can follow gas movement from less distensible areas of the lung to more distensible areas ('pendelluft').
- Relaxation of tissues occurs with applied pressures that are sustained. This is due to the so called 'viscoelastic' nature of tissues. This property of tissues, which mimics the action of hydraulic dampers in mechanical systems, means that when stretching forces are applied to real tissues they do not respond instantaneously, but stretch gradually in a viscous manner.
- The intrapulmonary pressure will be less than the applied airway pressure, because of airway resistance and inertia of the respiratory system. This causes an underestimation of the compliance.

The resultant effect of making dynamic measurements is that airway pressures in the dynamic case will be greater than those in the static case at any given lung volume. This means that the value for dynamic compliance will always be less than the static compliance.

Factor	Change in CR
FRC	
Normal	Maximum
High	Decreased
Low	Decreased
Posture	
Standing	Maximum
Supine	Decreased
Age	
Infant	Decreased
Elderly	Decreased
Pregnancy	Decreased
Disease	
ARDS	Decreased ($\downarrow C_L$)
Pulmonary oedema	Decreased ($\downarrow C_L$)
Ankylosing spondylitis	Decreased ($\downarrow C_L$ and $\downarrow C_W$)

Figure RR9 Factors decreasing respiratory system compliance (C_R)

Factors decreasing respiratory system compliance

Respiratory system compliance is usually maximum or optimal at FRC, and is decreased by both physiological factors and disease. Disease may affect both lung compliance (C_L) and chest wall compliance (C_W). Some examples of these factors are shown in Figure RR9.

Pressure–volume loop for the respiratory system

If a pressure–volume curve for the respiratory system is plotted through a cycle of inspiration and expiration a 'loop' is obtained, as the inspiratory and expiratory limbs of the curve do not exactly coincide (Figure RR10). This 'loop' effect is known as hysteresis, the area of the loop representing the energy expended or 'wasted' as heat in moving through the inspiratory–expiratory cycle. This wasted energy is a result of viscous losses during the stretching and recoil of the tissues, and also the frictional losses due to airway resistance. A factor that reduces this wasted energy and hence improves the efficiency of the breathing cycle is the lining of surfactant in the alveoli.

Surfactant

Surfactant is a phospholipid-based substance secreted by the alveolar type II cells, which lines the alveoli and acts by markedly reducing surface tension. This action has the following effects:

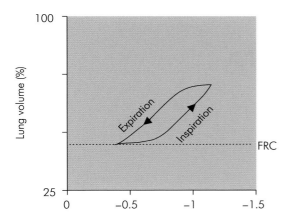

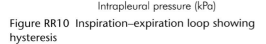

Figure RR10 Inspiration–expiration loop showing hysteresis

- Reduction of surface tension, which helps to even out the distribution of compliance and hence ventilation. Without surfactant, alveoli with low resting volumes are significantly more difficult to expand than those with larger resting volumes. This effect is important in neonates, in whom deficiency of surfactant is associated with infant respiratory distress syndrome.
- Stabilisation of small alveoli. In a bubble wall, surface tension acts to shrink or collapse the bubble. A similar effect is seen in an alveolus. The smaller the alveolus the greater the tendency to collapse. Because of this, small alveoli tend to collapse by forcing their gas into larger communicating alveoli. The reduction of surface tension by surfactant decreases this effect.
- Reduction of the energy expended as heat during each inspiratory-expiratory cycle, i.e. the hysteresis area of the pressure–volume loop is decreased.
- Surfactant also keeps the alveoli dry by reducing the 'suction' effect created by surface tension as it tries to collapse alveoli. Surface tension creates negative interstitial pressures as it tries to shrink alveoli, thus drawing fluid from capillaries into the air spaces.

Distribution of ventilation

When inspiration occurs the fresh gas entering the lung is not evenly distributed. Traditional teaching has upheld for decades that ventilation is distributed unevenly, with the majority of fresh ventilation passing to the more dependent regions of the lung. This model is based on the assumption of gravitationally determined distribution of lung perfusion, which indirectly determines local lung compliance and leads to ventilation inequalities. Thus both ventilation ($\dot{V}$) and perfusion ($\dot{Q}$) become gravitationally determined, ensuring optimum ventilation–perfusion ($\dot{V}/\dot{Q}$) matching.

More recent work, however, challenges this simple model of ventilation distribution by demonstrating significant variations in distribution in sections at the same vertical level, i.e. in areas subject to the same gravitational effect. In addition, the dependence of perfusion on gravitational effects is also challenged. This leads to a different concept of ventilation and perfusion distribution and matching that is based on the structural heterogeneity of the lung.

Gravitational model for distribution of ventilation and perfusion

The mechanism determining the preferential distribution of ventilation to the most dependent regions of the lung during spontaneous breathing depends on the basic assumption of a gravitationally defined distribution of perfusion throughout the lung. Effectively the lung behaves as a continuous volume of fluid with a hydrostatic pressure gradient increasing from apex to base in the upright position. In the upright adult the intrapleural pressure at the base of the lung is approximately 0.7 kPa greater than the pressure at the apex. This variation in intrapleural pressure means that the alveoli will also vary in degree of distension, and correspondingly the alveoli will vary their position on the pressure–volume curve for the lung (Figure RR11). The

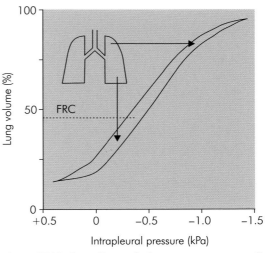

Figure RR11 Compliance during spontaneous ventilation

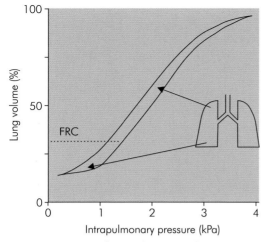

Figure RR12 Compliance during mechanical ventilation

more dependent alveoli will be less distended, and located on the linear part of the pressure–volume curve, compared with the apical alveoli, which are over-distended and situated on the top part of the pressure–volume curve. Thus at the base of the lung the alveolar compliance (gradient of the pressure–volume curve) is greater than that at the apex. Consequently, during inspiration, greater expansion of alveoli in the lower parts of the lung occurs, and ventilation is preferentially directed to the base. The end result is to direct ventilation to the areas of the lung with the most perfusion. In addition to the effects of gravity, airway resistance also plays a part in directing ventilation preferentially to the bases, since airway resistance is lower to the dependent areas of the lung.

This distribution of ventilation during spontaneous breathing contrasts with the situation when a patient is undergoing artificial ventilation. Under these circumstances the FRC is reduced, and this causes a reversal of the distribution of alveolar compliances, producing preferential ventilation of non-dependent areas (Figure RR12).

Structural model for distribution of ventilation and perfusion

The traditional model for distribution of ventilation, as described above, is based on gravity being the most important determinant of local perfusion and hence indirectly regional ventilation. The use of enhanced CT scanning techniques suggests that regional variation of ventilation follows a more centripetal pattern rather than the vertical gravitationally determined distribution described above. Similarly, studies under variable and zero gravity conditions refute the predominant effect of gravity in determining local perfusion and ventilation, and offer the following observations:

- Significant heterogeneity of ventilation and perfusion occurs at the same vertical level (iso-height), i.e. where gravitational effects are excluded.
- The variability in perfusion and ventilation at iso-height level may be much greater than that observed over a vertical (gravitational) gradient.
- Heterogeneity of perfusion and ventilation occurs under zero gravity conditions.
- Postural changes fail to produce predicted changes in ventilation and perfusion, e.g. total lung perfusion in the dependent lung when in the left lateral position is less than in the non-dependent lung.

A more recent concept suggests that the main determinant of regional perfusion differences is regional vascular resistance, which will be largely influenced by changes in lung volume. Ventilation and perfusion remain matched in the lungs by virtue of their development as a twinned system of branching airways and pulmonary vessels. In this way, although regional variations in perfusion may occur independently of gravity, the distribution of ventilation will tend to vary in parallel since the main determinant of regional ventilation will be local airways resistance. The variability of perfusion and ventilation throughout the lung is attributed mainly to the asymmetrical branching nature of the airways and vascular trees, rather than to the gravitational gradient of the traditional model.

Gas flow in the airways

The movement of gas in and out of the lungs is produced by the transpulmonary pressure and is conducted through the airways. The ease with which gas moves through the airways depends on:

- Airway resistance
- Pattern of gas flow

Airway resistance

The gas flow (F, in ml s^{-1} or l min^{-1}) through an airway is determined by the pressure difference between the ends of the airway (ΔP), and the resistance of the airway to gas flow (R). This is loosely analogous to the flow of electrical current through a conductor with electrical resistance. The case of laminar gas flow in an airway can be approximated to fluid (i.e. gas or liquid) flow in a tube, in which

$$F = \frac{\Delta P}{R}$$

This is modified in the Hagen–Poiseuille law, which substitutes factors for the resistance R. These factors include radius, viscosity and length. R is inversely proportional to $(radius)^4$, but dependent on the viscosity of the gas and the length of the tube.

Pattern of gas flow

Gas flow through an airway can occur in a smooth fashion, behaving as if in circumferential layers sliding across each other in the direction of flow. This is laminar flow, which occurs with a 'cone'-shaped gas velocity profile across the airway cross section, the velocity being faster in the centre than at the periphery (cf. Section 2, Chapter 6: Figure CR6).

Alternatively gas flow can be disorderly, with random eddies and whirls occurring across the overall direction of flow. This is turbulent flow, which moves with a relatively flat velocity profile in the direction of flow. Both laminar and turbulent flow exist within the respiratory tract, usually in mixed patterns.

Turbulent flow

In a given airway with a known gas and flow velocity, the likelihood of turbulent flow can be predicted from an index known as Reynolds number (Re), which is calculated from

$$Re = \frac{2rv\rho}{\eta}$$

where

r = airway radius
v = average velocity of gas flow
ρ = gas density
η = viscosity of the gas

Re < 1000 is associated with laminar flow, while Re > 2000 results in turbulent flow.

The pressure–flow relationship for turbulent flow is different because the pressure gradient producing the flow is:
- Proportional to $(flow\ velocity)^2$
- Dependent on gas density and independent of viscosity
- Inversely dependent on $(radius)^5$

The resultant effect of turbulence is to increase the effective resistance of an airway compared with laminar flow.

Turbulent flow occurs at the laryngeal opening, the trachea and the large bronchi (generations 1–5) during most of the respiratory cycle. It is usually audible and almost invariably present when high resistance to gas flow is encountered.

Location of airway resistance

The principal sites of resistance to gas flow in the respiratory system are the nose and the major bronchi rather than the small airways. Since the cross-sectional area of the airway increases exponentially as branching occurs, the velocity of the airflow decreases markedly with progression through the airway generations, and laminar flow becomes predominant below the fifth generation of airway.

Factors affecting airway resistance

The factors affecting airway resistance are:
- Lung volume – the main factor affecting airway resistance. Increasing lung volume decreases airway resistance, and thus patients with high airway resistance often increase their FRC by position or pursed-lip breathing.
- Bronchial smooth muscle tone – airway smooth muscle is primarily under parasympathetic (vagal) control. Reflex constriction occurs with stimulation of the larynx, trachea or bronchi. Sympathetic influence is mediated mainly by β receptors in the airway smooth muscle.
- Histamine release – H_1 receptors cause bronchoconstriction, while H_2 receptors cause bronchodilatation. However, the predominant effect of histamine is bronchoconstriction.
- Properties of inspired gas – flow resistance dependent on the density and viscosity of the inspired gas. Use of a helium–oxygen mixture improves ventilation in some cases of severe bronchospasm.
- Lower airway obstruction, which may be due to mucosal oedema, mucous plugging, epithelial desquamation or foreign bodies.
- Upper airway obstruction secondary to decreased conscious level, drugs, position of head, neck or jaw, tonsils or adenoids.
- Anaesthesia – airway resistance doubles during anaesthesia, due mainly to a reduction in FRC but also to increased upper airway resistance in some patients. Inappropriate selection of breathing systems may also contribute to increased total airway resistance. It is often forgotten that the upper airway contributes significantly to total airway resistance.

Measurement of airway resistance

Airway resistance can be measured during spontaneous breathing by simultaneous recording of air flow and the pressure gradient between mouth and alveoli. In practice the alveolar pressure is difficult to obtain since it must be derived using a body plethysmograph. Intrapleural pressure can be used instead, but will include the pressure gradient required to overcome lung tissue resistance and inertial properties. Thus, this technique measures the resistance to air flow, the viscous resistance due to the lung tissue and the inertia of the lung. Under normal circumstances, these factors are negligible, but tissue viscous resistance may become more significant in pulmonary oedema and fibrosis. Inertia of the lung may be of importance during high-frequency ventilation.

In clinical practice airway resistance can be assessed using forced expiratory flow rates such as FEV_1, peak expiratory flow rate (PEFR), and mid-expiratory flow rate. These indices are more easily measured, but they rely upon expiratory muscle activity in addition to airway resistance, and are affected by patient technique.

Work of breathing

Work is normally expended in inspiration, expiration being passive. The work of inspiration can be subdivided into:

- Work required to overcome the elastic forces of the lung (compliance), which is stored as elastic energy
- Work required to overcome airway resistance during the movement of air into the lung
- Work required to overcome the viscosity of the lung and chest wall tissues (tissue resistive work)

During quiet breathing, most of the work performed is elastic. This inflates the lungs but provides a store of elastic energy to be returned during expiration, and is, therefore, useful work done.

The effect of overcoming tissue resistance and airway resistance is dissipated as heat and can be viewed as wasted energy. Figure RR13 shows an idealised pressure–volume loop, with inspiration occurring along the path AGB and expiration along BEA. The following points illustrate the relationship between the wasted work done and the useful work done:

- In an ideal elastic lung, with no tissue or airway losses, the work stored in inspiration would be completely returned in expiration. Inspiration and expiration would then occur along the straight line AFB, with

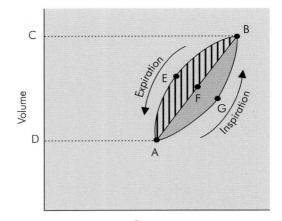

Figure RR13 Work of breathing loop

equal amounts of inspiratory work done and expiratory work, represented by the area AFBCD.
- In the real lung, with tissue and airway losses, inspiration occurs along curve AGB. The inspiratory work done (AGBCD) is thus greater than the ideal case (by the shaded area AGBF). This wasted work is only a fraction of the inspiratory work.
- In the real lung, expiration occurs along BEA. The expiratory work returned (BEADC) is thus less than the ideal case (by hatched area BEAF).
- The total 'wasted' energy due to tissue and airway losses is thus the sum of the shaded and hatched areas, or the area of the loop

In lung diseases all three types of work are increased. Compliance work and tissue resistive work are greatly increased during restrictive diseases such as fibrosis of the lungs, whereas airway resistance work is increased in pulmonary obstructive diseases.

Expiration does not normally entail active work, but this may be necessary in forced breathing or when airway resistance or tissue resistance are increased. In some circumstances, expiratory work may be greater than inspiratory work, for example in asthma.

Gas exchange

The oxygen tension in air (at sea level) is about 20 kPa, falling to 0.5 kPa in the mitochondria, where it is utilised. The transport of oxygen down this concentration gradient is described as the oxygen cascade (Figure RR14). It

Factors influencing oxygen cascade

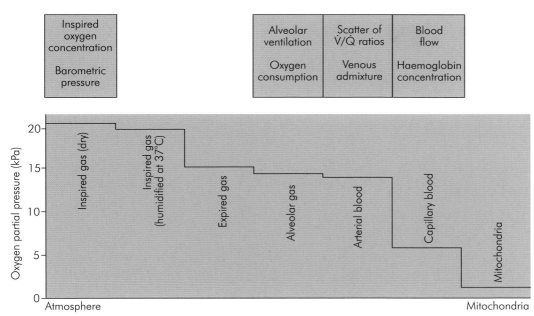

Figure RR14 Oxygen cascade

involves different transport mechanisms, convection, diffusion through gas and liquid media and transport bound to Hb. The same process occurs in the reverse direction for CO_2.

The fractional concentration of oxygen in dry ambient air ($F_{AMB}O_2$) is 0.21, and at sea level with a barometric pressure (P_B) of 101.3 kPa the partial pressure of oxygen ($P_{AMB}O_2$) is given by

$$P_{AMB}O_2 = 0.21 \times 101.3$$
$$= 21.3 \, kPa$$

The addition of saturated water vapour (P_{SVP}) by the upper airway mucosa reduces the tension of inspired gas (P_IO_2) by a small amount:

$$P_IO_2 = (P_B) = P_{SVP} \times F_{AMB}O_2$$
$$= (101.3 - 6.3) \times (0.21) = 20 \, kPa$$

Alveolar oxygen tension

The alveolar oxygen tension (P_AO_2) is less than the inspired oxygen tension (P_IO_2) because some oxygen is absorbed in exchange for CO_2 excreted. Thus, the P_AO_2 is determined by:

- The rate at which oxygen is introduced into the alveoli (dependent on alveolar ventilation and inspired oxygen concentration)
- The rate of removal by absorption into pulmonary capillary blood (oxygen consumption, $\dot{V}O_2$)
- The rate of delivery of CO_2 ($\dot{V}CO_2$) by pulmonary capillary blood

The decrease in oxygen tension caused by oxygen absorption is estimated by using the tension of CO_2 excreted (about P_ACO_2), which must be corrected by the respiratory quotient (because less CO_2 is excreted than O_2 absorbed).

The alveolar gas equation thus becomes

$$P_AO_2 = P_IO_2 - \frac{P_ACO_2}{RQ}$$

where RQ is the respiratory quotient, and

$$RQ = \frac{\dot{V}CO_2}{\dot{V}O_2}$$

which in a normal subject on a mixed diet is about 0.8. For $P_IO_2 = 20 \, kPa$ and $P_ACO_2 = 5 \, kPa$

$$P_AO_2 = 20 - (5 \div 0.8)$$
$$= 13.8 \, kPa$$

(a)

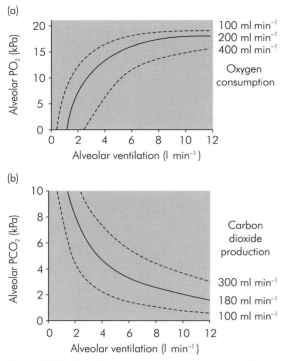

(b)

Figure RR15 Variation of alveolar gas tensions with alveolar ventilation

To summarise: P_AO_2 is intermediate between the inspired oxygen tension (P_IO_2) and the arterial oxygen tension (PaO_2), due to oxygen being absorbed in exchange for CO_2. Its value is given by the alveolar gas equation, which is based on:

$$P_AO_2 = \text{(inspired oxygen tension)}$$
$$- \text{(tension decrease due to oxygen absorbed)}$$

The importance of P_AO_2 in practice is that it determines the partial pressure gradient driving oxygen across the alveolar–capillary membrane. It is not easily measured directly, but an awareness of its value in clinical practice is useful in patient management. The following points should be noted:

- P_AO_2 is most easily increased by increasing inspired oxygen fraction (F_IO_2).
- P_AO_2 will fall with hypoventilation, but it only falls rapidly below alveolar ventilation levels of about 4 litres per minute, assuming normal oxygen consumption (about 250 ml min^{-1}). Figure RR15a

illustrates how varying alveolar ventilation rate affects P_AO_2.

- Hypermetabolic states (sepsis, malignant hyperthermia) will significantly increase the susceptibility to hypoxaemia by increasing oxygen consumption ($\dot{V}O_2$), and by increasing the rate of CO_2 delivery into the alveoli. Thus, both F_IO_2 and alveolar ventilation may need to be increased in such patients.
- P_AO_2 can be decreased iatrogenically by sodium bicarbonate infusion, since this increases body CO_2 levels and hence CO_2 delivery to the alveoli.
- P_AO_2 can be used to calculate the alveolar–arterial PO_2 difference, which is a useful index of gas-exchange efficiency in the lungs.

Alveolar carbon dioxide tension

Alveolar CO_2 tension (P_ACO_2) is determined by the balance between:

- Rate of delivery of CO_2 ($\dot{V}CO_2$) into the alveoli by pulmonary capillary blood
- Rate of removal by alveolar ventilation

P_ACO_2 can be varied by controlling alveolar ventilation. This effect is most noticeable at rates of alveolar ventilation below about 6 litres per minute, given normal rates of CO_2 production (about 200 ml min^{-1}). Hyperventilation above this level produces a more gradual reduction in P_ACO_2. Figure RR15b illustrates the variation of P_ACO_2 (which correlates well with $PaCO_2$ in the normal subject) with alveolar ventilation.

Gas diffusion from alveoli to blood

Gases diffuse between alveoli and pulmonary capillary blood across the blood–gas barrier, which is effectively a membrane with a total surface area about 70 m^2. Over this membrane about 60–140 ml blood is spread as a thin sheet. The rate of gas transfer across this membrane will depend on:

- Properties of the gas (solubility and molecular weight)
- Properties of the membrane (surface area, A, and thickness, D)
- Partial pressure gradient (ΔP) across the membrane

Then according to Fick's Law

$$\text{Rate of gas transfer} \propto \frac{k \times A \times \Delta P}{D}$$

where

$$\text{Diffusion constant, } k \propto \frac{\text{solubility}}{\sqrt{\text{molecular weight}}}$$

The lower molecular weight of oxygen and its greater alveolar-to-capillary partial pressure gradient favour its diffusion compared with CO_2. However, the higher blood/gas solubility coefficient of CO_2 (24 times that of O_2) causes CO_2 to diffuse more readily than oxygen, in spite of a lower partial pressure gradient. Nevertheless, the efficiency of oxygen diffusion across the alveolar–capillary membrane is such that a red cell is fully oxygenated in <50% of the transit time through the pulmonary capillary bed. Any factor that increases the thickness of the membrane, such as pulmonary oedema, interferes with the diffusion of oxygen more than with that of CO_2.

Oxygen transport in the blood

Most of the oxygen (97%) in the blood is transported in combination with haemoglobin (Hb). Once the Hb is saturated, oxygen content can only be marginally increased by dissolved oxygen. Dissolved oxygen is a linear function of P_AO_2 and is 0.023 ml kPa^{-1} per 100 ml plasma. Thus, for a $P_AO_2 = 13$ kPa, only 0.3 ml oxygen (3%) is carried in a dissolved state. Even breathing pure oxygen, where it is possible to increase P_AO_2 to about 80 kPa, the dissolved arterial oxygen content would be only about 2.0 ml per 100 ml blood.

Haemoglobin

Oxygen is transported and delivered to the tissues by haemoglobin. Hb is a conjugated protein with a molecular weight of 66 700 daltons, and is composed of four haem subunits. Each subunit has a central ferrous (Fe^{2+}) atom and is conjugated to a polypeptide chain. The four polypeptide chains collectively form the globin moiety. Different forms of Hb exist, identified by their polypeptide chains. Normal adult Hb consists of HbA_1 (98%) containing 2α and 2β polypeptide chains, and HbA_2 (2%) containing 2α and 2δ chains.

Fetal erythrocytes contain HbF with 2α and 2γ chains. HbF is also modified by having a lower affinity for binding 2,3-diphosphoglycerate (2,3-DPG) than adult forms of Hb. 2,3-DPG is a highly anionic intermediate of glycolysis. It binds to the deoxygenated form of Hb, significantly reducing the affinity of Hb for oxygen. This facilitates the 'unloading' of oxygen in tissues with low oxygen tensions. HbF thus has an increased affinity for oxygen, which adapts its transport and delivery characteristics to the lower oxygen tensions in the placento-fetal circulation. After birth the production of β chains starts, and HbA replaces HbF during the first year of life.

Oxygenation of haemoglobin

Each molecule of Hb can bind four molecules of oxygen. This is not a chemical reaction as in oxidation, but is a readily reversible bond. The following are characteristics of Hb oxygen binding:

- It is determined primarily by local oxygen tension (P_AO_2).
- It is affected by local tissue conditions (e.g. pH, temperature) and local concentrations of substances (e.g. 2,3-DPG, CO_2).
- It produces an allosteric change in the structure of Hb to a 'Relaxed' form, while deoxygenated Hb has a 'Tense' form. This switching between R and T forms underlies the oxygenation and delivery mechanisms.
- It is 'cooperative', meaning that binding O_2 at each site promotes binding at the remaining sites due to allosteric changes. This increases the amount of O_2 delivered under physiological conditions, compared with a carrier having independent binding sites.
- Deoxygenation of Hb increases the affinity of several proton-binding sites on its molecule. This enhances its ability to transport CO_2 from the tissues to the lungs (Haldane effect) and underlies the role of Hb as a major buffer in acid–base regulation.

Oxyhaemoglobin dissociation curve

The percentage of Hb saturation with oxygen (SO_2) at different partial pressures of oxygen in blood is described by the oxyhaemoglobin dissociation curve (ODC). This is a sigmoid curve whose shape is determined by the cooperativity of the oxygen binding process (Figure RR16). The position of the curve is best described by the P_{50}, which is the PO_2 at which Hb is 50% saturated (normally 3.56 kPa). Various factors can 'shift' the ODC to the left or right, altering the characteristics of oxygen uptake and delivery.

'Left shift' of the ODC

This represents an increase in the affinity of Hb for oxygen in the pulmonary capillaries but requires lower tissue capillary PO_2 to achieve adequate oxygen delivery. P_{50} is reduced by factors causing a left shift, which include:

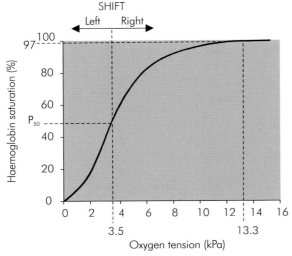

Figure RR16 Oxyhaemoglobin dissociation curve

- Alkalosis
- Decreased PCO_2
- Decreased concentration of 2,3-DPG
- Decreased temperature
- Presence of HbF rather than adult forms of Hb

'Right shift' of the ODC

This represents an increase in the affinity of Hb for oxygen. In this situation P_{50} is increased, requiring higher pulmonary capillary saturations to saturate the Hb, but enhancing delivery at the tissues. Factors causing a right shift of the ODC include:

- Acidosis
- Increased PCO_2
- Increased concentration of 2,3-DPG
- Increased temperature

Bohr effect

The shift in position of the ODC caused by CO_2 entering or leaving blood is known as the Bohr effect. It enhances the 'unloading' of oxygen in the tissues, where PCO_2 levels are high compared with the pulmonary capillaries. In the tissues CO_2 enters the red cells, combining with water and dissociating into H^+ and HCO_3^-. The increased $[H^+]$ shifts the ODC to the right, facilitating the release of oxygen from Hb. The HCO_3^- diffuses out of the cells and is matched by an inward movement of chloride. The reverse change occurs in the lungs, enhancing the uptake of oxygen.

Oxygen content of blood

The theoretical maximum oxygen-carrying capacity is 1.39 ml O_2 g^{-1} Hb, but direct measurement gives a capacity of 1.34 ml O_2 g^{-1} Hb.

The oxygen content of blood is the volume of oxygen carried in each 100 ml blood. It is calculated by

$(O_2$ carried by Hb$) + (O_2$ in solution$)$
$$= (SO_2 \times 1.34 \times Hb \times 0.01) + (0.023 \times PO_2)$$

where

SO_2 = percentage saturation of Hb with oxygen
Hb = Hb concentration in grams per 100 ml (g dl^{-1}) blood
PO_2 = partial pressure of oxygen

For a normal male adult the oxygen content of arterial blood can be calculated.

Given arterial oxygen saturation (SaO_2) = 100%, Hb = 15 g dl^{-1}, and arterial partial pressure of oxygen (PaO_2) = 13.3 kPa, then oxygen content of arterial blood (CaO_2):

$$CaO_2 = 20.1 + 0.3 = 20.4 \text{ ml per 100 ml}$$

Similarly, the oxygen content of mixed venous blood can be calculated. Given normal values of mixed venous oxygen saturation ($S\bar{v}O_2$) = 75%, and venous partial pressure of oxygen ($P\bar{v}O2$) = 6 kPa:

$$C\bar{v}O_2 = 15.1 + 0.1 = 15.2 \text{ ml per 100 ml}$$

Oxygen delivery ($\dot{D}O_2$) and oxygen uptake ($\dot{V}O_2$)

Oxygen delivery is the amount of oxygen delivered to the peripheral tissues, and is obtained by multiplying the arterial oxygen content (CaO_2) by the cardiac output ($\dot{Q}$). For CaO_2 = 20.1 ml per 100 ml and $\dot{Q}$ = 5.0 litres per minute

$$\text{oxygen delivery}(\dot{D}O_2) = 1005 \text{ ml min}^{-1}$$

Oxygen uptake is the amount of oxygen taken up by the tissues, and it can be calculated from the difference between oxygen delivery and the oxygen returned to the lungs in the mixed venous blood. The oxygen return is given by the product of mixed venous oxygen content ($C\bar{v}O_2$) and cardiac output. For $C\bar{v}O_2$ = 15.2 ml per 100 ml and $\dot{Q}$ = 5 litres per minute

$$\text{oxygen return} = 760 \text{ ml min}^{-1}$$

Thus

$$\text{oxygen uptake } (\dot{V}O_2) = (\text{oxygen delivery})$$
$$- (\text{oxygen return})$$
$$= 1005 - 760 = 245\,\text{ml min}^{-1}$$

To summarise: The primary goal of the cardiorespiratory system is to deliver adequate oxygen to the tissues to meet their metabolic requirements, a balance between $\dot{V}O_2$ and $\dot{D}O_2$.

The balance between oxygen uptake by the body tissues and oxygen delivery to them is assessed by:

- The oxygen content of mixed venous blood $C\bar{v}O_2$, which is normally about 15 ml per 100 ml
- The oxygen extraction ratio, which is the ratio of $\dot{V}O_2$ to $\dot{D}O_2$ expressed as a percentage. Normally the extraction ratio is about 25%, but it can double to 50% if tissue demand increases.

Both of the above indices are dependent on mixed venous saturation ($S\bar{v}O_2$) and cardiac output.

Increased tissue demand due to exercise or disease is normally compensated for by increased oxygen delivery. This has to be mediated by increasing cardiac output, since the ability to increase SaO_2 and Hb is limited. However, under extreme conditions (severe exercise, sepsis, malignant hyperthermia) tissue demand can increase 12-fold (requiring a $\dot{V}O_2$ of up to 3000 ml O_2 min^{-1}). Cardiac output can usually be increased by a maximum of up to seven times, and thus under extreme conditions tissue demand can outstrip the body's capacity to increase delivery. In such a case $S\bar{v}O_2$ falls, extraction ratios increase and tissue hypoxia ensues. This susceptibility towards tissue hypoxia will be greatly increased in conditions where cardiac output is limited or compromised.

Carbon dioxide transport

CO_2 diffuses passively down its concentration gradient from the mitochondria to the capillaries. Although partial pressure gradients are low between tissues and blood, transfer is rapid due to the high solubility of CO_2. Partial pressures of CO_2 (PCO_2) in the tissues equilibrate with capillary blood to produce a venoarterial PCO_2 difference of about 0.7 kPa. This corresponds to a CO_2 content difference of about 4 ml per 100 ml blood, depending upon RQ.

The 4 ml CO_2 that is added to each 100 ml arterial blood as it passes through the tissues consists of (Figure RR17):

- 2.8 ml (70%) that enters erythrocytes to form carbonic acid (H_2CO_3). This reaction is catalysed by carbonic anhydrase, which, if inhibited, produces a marked increase in the alveolar–capillary PCO_2 gradient. The H_2CO_3 formed dissociates to give H^+ and HCO_3^-. As noted above, deoxygenation of Hb activates H^+ acceptor sites, increasing its buffering capacity. This encourages the dissociation of H_2CO_3 and as a result enhances the 'loading' of CO_2 in the tissues. The HCO_3^- formed diffuses out of the erythrocytes in exchange for chloride (Cl^-), which enters the red cells to maintain electroneutrality (the 'chloride shift'). The increase in osmotically active ions HCO_3^- and Cl^- in venous red blood cells leads to an increase in their size. This is probably the reason for the venous haematocrit being about 3% greater than that of arterial blood.
- 0.9 ml (22%) carried as carbamino compounds, which are formed by reactions of CO_2 with terminal and side chain amino groups of proteins. Haemoglobin provides most of the amino groups, reduced Hb having at least three times more active sites than oxyhaemoglobin.
- 0.3 ml (8%) carried in solution.

Haldane effect

In the tissues deoxygenation of Hb enhances carriage of CO_2, by activating proton binding and carbamino formation sites. Correspondingly, oxygenation of Hb causes the reverse effect, displacing H^+ and CO_2, thus facilitating the 'unloading' of CO_2 in the lungs. This dependency of CO_2 carrying capacity on the oxygenation state of Hb is known as the Haldane effect.

Body stores of oxygen and CO_2

The oxygen stores of the body are relatively small in comparison to the consumption (around 250 ml min^{-1} for an adult). Total body oxygen is about 1.5 litres, which is held as:

- 50% in combination with Hb
- 30% in the lungs
- 20% in combination with myoglobin

Not all stored oxygen is available for use since severe hypoxaemia occurs before even half of the oxygen stored in combination with Hb and myoglobin is released. These available stores will last only for 3–4 minutes of apnoea, assuming air breathing and normal oxygen consumption. Breathing 100% O_2 increases the oxygen stores to about 4.25 litres, mainly by increasing the O_2 contained in the lungs.

In contrast, total body stores of CO_2 are about 120 litres. During apnoea, $PaCO_2$ increases by about 1 kPa in the first

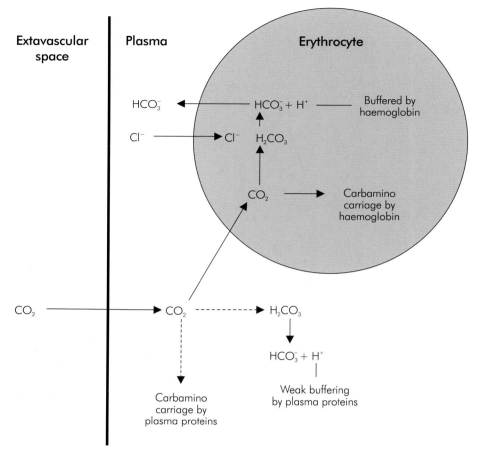

Figure RR17 CO_2 transport in blood

minute. This initial rise in $PaCO_2$ then decreases to a rate of 0.4 kPa min^{-1}, as alveolar PCO_2 levels build up and CO_2 elimination by diffusion through the airways increases.

Pulmonary circulation

The pulmonary circulation is a low-pressure, low-resistance system in series with the right ventricle. The cardiac output from the right ventricle passes through the lungs into the left atrium. The cardiac output from the right ventricle is almost the same as that from the left ventricle.

Blood passes through pulmonary capillaries in about 0.5–1.0 seconds, depending on the cardiac output, during which time it is oxygenated and excess CO_2 is removed. The distribution of blood flow and ventilation throughout the lungs are generally very well matched, but this may vary markedly during anaesthesia or disease.

The pulmonary artery is a thin-walled structure which arises from the right ventricle and divides immediately into left and right branches and then divides successively, following a similar pattern to the conducting airways down to the terminal bronchioles. These small branches give rise to a dense capillary network, which may be viewed as a sheet of blood broken up by 'pillars' of connective tissue that maintain the stability of the alveoli. The oxygenated blood is collected by venules that run between the lobules and then unite to form the four pulmonary veins that drain into the left atrium.

The innervation of the pulmonary vasculature is supplied by the sympathetic nervous system, with α-adrenergic fibres producing vasoconstriction and β-adrenergic fibres vasodilatation. The vagus supplies parasympathetic fibres that produce vasodilatation.

Bronchial arteries from the thoracic aorta supply oxygenated blood to the supporting tissue of the lung, including connective tissue, septa and bronchi, and drain into the pulmonary veins, contributing to the anatomical shunt. An average of 1–2% of the total cardiac output passes through the bronchial arteries, thus making the left ventricular output slightly greater than the right.

Pressures in the pulmonary circulation are about 20% of those in the systemic circulation. Normal pulmonary arterial pressure has a systolic value of 25 mmHg, a diastolic value of 8 mmHg, and a mean of 15 mmHg. The mean pulmonary capillary pressure is 10 mmHg, with a pulmonary venous pressure of 4 mmHg at heart level. Pulmonary arterial and right ventricular pressures are not greatly influenced by increases in cardiac output in normal subjects, demonstrating the distensibility of the pulmonary vasculature.

Pulmonary vascular resistance

Pulmonary vascular resistance (PVR) is influenced by the following factors:

- Autonomic innervation – vasomotor tone is minimal in the normal resting state and pulmonary vessels are maximally dilated. The autonomic system exerts a relatively weak influence on PVR, increases in sympathetic tone giving rise to vasoconstriction.
- Nitric oxide (NO) – an important mediator of pulmonary vascular tone causing vasodilatation (it is also active in systemic vessels). Nitric oxide has been identified as endothelium-derived relaxing factor, which also mediates other processes by the relaxation of smooth muscle. It is derived from L-arginine and increases intracellular concentrations of cGMP. Its actions as a potent vasodilator have led to its use in severe acute lung disease, where inhaled concentrations of 5–80 ppm can improve oxygenation.
- Prostacyclin (prostaglandin I_2) – an arachidonate, which is a potent vasodilator also of endothelial origin.
- Endothelins – potent vasoconstrictor peptides released by the pulmonary endothelial cells.
- Vascular transmural pressure – important in the pulmonary circulation because the thinner vessel walls make them more prone to collapse when alveolar pressure exceeds intravascular pressure. During controlled ventilation, high positive alveolar pressures can cause increased PVR and decrease perfusion in some areas of the lung.
- Lung volume – which also determines the calibre of the vessels embedded in the lung parenchyma. PVR is least at FRC. As the lung increases in volume, the vessels become narrowed and elongated and, as it decreases in volume, the vessels become tortuous.
- Lung disease – both acute and chronic lung disease can result in significant increases in PVR. Long-term increases in PVR due to chronic disease can lead to right-sided heart failure.
- Hypoxic vasoconstriction – a powerful physiological reflex which diverts perfusion away from hypoxic areas of the lung.

Hypoxic pulmonary vasoconstriction

Hypoxic pulmonary vasoconstriction (HPV) is an important mechanism that improves the match between perfusion and ventilation by diverting blood from poorly ventilated areas to better ventilated areas. HPV maintains this balance of ventilation to perfusion on a breath-to-breath basis. The predominant site of HPV lies in the small pulmonary arteries (30–50 μm), with the remaining resistance arising from the capillary bed and venous system.

HPV may also affect the pulmonary vessels in general rather than on a regional basis. Low P_AO_2 levels are responsible for generalised HPV in the fetus, reducing blood flow through the pulmonary vascular bed to about 10–15% of the fetal cardiac output. This generalised response also causes a significant increase in PVR at high altitude.

The exact mechanism of HPV is unknown. It is potentiated by acidosis and modified by various drugs (Figure RR18).

Pulmonary hypertension

Increased pulmonary arterial pressures can be caused by various pathological mechanisms. These are listed in Figure RR19, together with examples of associated clinical conditions.

Drugs	Effect on HPV
Volatile anaesthetic agents	
Nitrates	
Nitroprusside	Attenuate HPV
Calcium channel blockers	
Bronchodilators	
Cyclo-oxygenase inhibitors	
Propranolol	Potentiate HPV
Almitrine	

Figure RR18 Drugs modifying the HPV reflex

Mechanism	Clinical condition
Intracardiac shunt	Atrial septal defect Ventricular septal defect
↑ left ventricular end-diastolic pressure	Mitral stenosis Constrictive pericarditis
Obliteration	Pulmonary fibrosis
Obstruction	Pulmonary embolism
Vasoconstriction	Sleep apnoea syndrome High altitude
Idiopathic	Primary pulmonary Hypertension

Figure RR19 Causes of pulmonary hypertension

Distribution of perfusion

As outlined above, the pulmonary vascular resistance (PVR) is influenced by various factors. Although PVR determines the overall blood flow through the lungs, this blood flow is not evenly distributed throughout each lung. Two contrasting models exist for the distribution of perfusion within the lung, a traditional model based on a gravitational gradient from apex to base (see *Gravitational model for distribution of ventilation and perfusion*, page 367), and a more recent structural model (see *Structural model for distribution of ventilation and perfusion*, page 368).

Functional zones of the lung

The gravitational model for the distribution of ventilation and perfusion has led to a lung model based on 'functional zones' defined by the pressure difference across the walls (transmural pressure) of the pulmonary blood vessels (arteries, capillaries and postcapillary veins). When the extravascular pressure is greater than the hydrostatic pressure in the vessel, the vessel collapses, obstructing flow. If the transmural pressure is reversed (intravascular greater than extravascular pressure) the vessel remains patent.

In the lung, gravity gives rise to an intravascular hydrostatic pressure gradient that increases from the top of the lung to the base. Thus the arterial (Pa) and venous (Pv) pressures in the base are greater than those in the apex by about 23 mmHg. In contrast, extravascular pressure is effectively equal to alveolar pressure (PA), which is approximately atmospheric pressure and is the same throughout the lung.

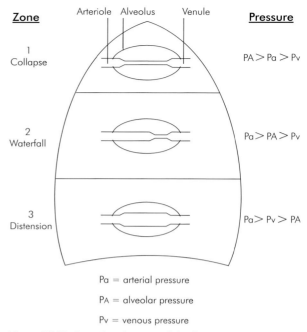

Pa = arterial pressure

PA = alveolar pressure

Pv = venous pressure

Figure RR20 Functional zones of the lung

The relative magnitudes of PA, Pa and Pv define the following functional zones in the lung (Figure RR20).

Zone 1

In zone 1 alveolar pressure (PA) is greater than the arteriolar pressure (Pa) and venular pressure (Pv). Both arterioles and venules will collapse, obstructing blood flow completely. In this case

PA > Pa > Pv

Arterial pressures (Pa) are minimal in the lung apex, and are just adequate to provide perfusion to these areas. In practice, Pa in the apical areas, although low, is not normally less than alveolar pressure (PA), and zone 1 does not exist. Usually this can only occur under conditions of reduced pulmonary arterial pressure (e.g. hypovolaemia, decreased cardiac output) or increased alveolar pressure (e.g. controlled ventilation of the lungs, positive end-expiratory pressure). In such a case, perfusion to this part of the lung is zero and alveolar dead space increases significantly.

Zone 2

In zone 2 alveolar pressure is greater than the venous pressure but less than the arterial pressure. The veins collapse but the arteries remain patent, and blood flow will be partially obstructed. In this case

Pa > PA > Pv

Below the apical regions of the lung, alveolar pressure is less than arterial pressure, but greater than the venous pressure. In these areas the postcapillary veins are collapsed, offering high resistance to flow. The collapsed vessels can open up during systole or if pulmonary arterial pressure increases. This model of a collapsible tube with variable flow resistance due to downstream occlusion by external pressure is sometimes referred to as the Starling resistor or 'waterfall' effect.

Zone 3

Alveolar pressure is less than venous pressure in zone 3, and both arteries and veins will remain patent and blood flow will be unobstructed. In this case

Pa > Pv > PA

In the more dependent regions of the lung arteries, capillaries and veins are patent and pulmonary blood flow is continuous. This zone extends from about 7–10 cm above the heart to the lowermost portions of the lung. There is some increase in perfusion moving down the zone, as pulmonary arterial pressure increases due to the gravitational pressure gradient. This increase in blood flow is achieved by:

- Recruitment of closed pulmonary vessels
- The perfusion of open but not perfused vessels
- Dilatation of vessels already perfused

These mechanisms enable zone 3 blood flow to increase in response to increases in pulmonary arterial pressure. Their overall result is a decrease in pulmonary vascular resistance.

Delineation of the functional zones is variable and affected by different conditions, which alter the relationship between Pa, Pv and PA. In the supine position, nearly all portions of the lung become zone 3, with pulmonary blood flow being more evenly distributed. During exercise, pulmonary artery pressures increase and recruit previously under-perfused capillaries, thus converting most of the lung to a zone 3 pattern of pulmonary blood flow.

A zone 4 is sometimes described for regions in the most dependent parts of the lung where intravascular pressures are highest but blood flow is reduced.

Ventilation: perfusion ratio

Efficient gas exchange in the lung requires the gas flow in and out of each functional unit to be matched by the blood flow through it, i.e. ventilation ($\dot{V}$) must match perfusion ($\dot{Q}$). At rest the overall ratio of total alveolar ventilation (about 5250 ml min^{-1}) to total pulmonary blood flow (about 5000 ml min^{-1}) is about 1. Thus, it is normally assumed that the optimum ventilation:perfusion ($\dot{V}/\dot{Q}$) ratio for any unit of lung tissue is also 1.

When a unit of lung tissue is inadequately ventilated ($\dot{V}/\dot{Q} < 1$), some of the pulmonary capillary blood perfusing it effectively bypasses the lungs, since there is too much perfusion for the blood gases to equilibrate adequately with alveolar gas. This increases the 'shunt' effect in the lungs (see below).

When a lung unit is under-perfused ($\dot{V}/\dot{Q} > 1$), the expired gas from the unit contains a lower than normal concentration of CO_2, since excess fresh gas is supplied which does not exchange gases with pulmonary capillary blood. This increases the 'alveolar dead space' effect in the lungs.

To summarise: Ventilation: perfusion ($\dot{V}/\dot{Q}$) ratio for any area of lung tissue is an index that reflects the efficiency of gas exchange in that region. It has an optimum value of 1.

In an area of lung tissue:
- If $\dot{V}/\dot{Q} < 1$, it increases the 'physiological shunt'
- If $\dot{V}/\dot{Q} > 1$, it increases the 'alveolar dead space'

Distribution of $\dot{V}/\dot{Q}$ ratios in the lung

In the normal lung, although ventilation and perfusion are both distributed to favour the dependent areas, the $\dot{V}/\dot{Q}$ ratios are not uniform and vary from the lung apices to the bases. At the top of the lung $\dot{V}/\dot{Q}$ ratios have been estimated to be about 3.3, and this value decreases passing down the lung to the bottom, where the $\dot{V}/\dot{Q}$ ratios are about 0.6. $\dot{V}/\dot{Q}$ ratios vary in three dimensions, so that a distribution of values will be found across a horizontal section of the lung as well as from apex to base.

In diseased lungs $\dot{V}/\dot{Q}$ ratios vary over a wider range as there is greater non-homogeneity of the lung tissue. The effect on gas exchange of increased $\dot{V}/\dot{Q}$ mismatch is reflected by a deterioration in the following indices from their normal values, so there is:

- An increase in shunt fraction
- An increase in the alveolar–arterial PO_2 difference (PAO_2–PaO_2)

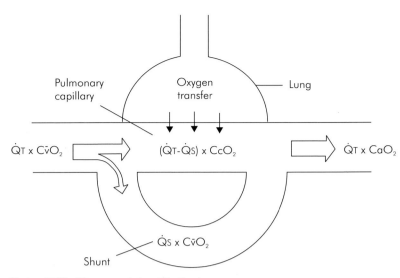

CaO_2 = arterial oxygen content

$C\bar{v}O_2$ = mixed venous content

CcO_2 = pulmonary capillary oxygen content

$\dot{Q}T$ = cardiac output

$\dot{Q}S$ = shunt flow

$(\dot{Q}T\text{-}\dot{Q}S)$ = pulmonary capillary blood flow

Figure RR21 Diagram of shunt in the lung

• An increase in alveolar dead space
• A decrease in PaO_2 or an increase in $PaCO_2$

Alveolar–arterial PO_2 difference

In the normal lung there is a small alveolar–arterial partial pressure gradient for oxygen (PAO_2–PaO_2) of 0.5–1.0 kPa. This difference is the sum of the PO_2 gradient across the alveolar–capillary membrane and the effect of admixture of shunted blood. Any increase in the thickness of the diffusion barrier (e.g. pulmonary oedema or fibrosis) or the shunt effect due to $\dot{V}/\dot{Q}$ mismatch in the lungs will, therefore, produce an increase in this value.

Physiological shunt (venous admixture, shunt fraction)

Arterial blood may be less well oxygenated than blood leaving the alveoli for several reasons, for example:
• Venous blood may bypass the lungs entirely (e.g. intracardiac shunts, thebesian veins, bronchial circulation).
• Blood may pass through parts of the lung which are not ventilated adequately, in which case $\dot{V}/\dot{Q} < 1$ (e.g. pneumonia).
• Blood may pass through areas of the lung which are not ventilated at all, in which case $\dot{V}/\dot{Q} = 0$. This is sometimes referred to as 'true' shunt.

Shunt equation

Physiological shunt can be calculated as a fraction of total pulmonary blood flow (cardiac output). Figure RR21 shows the flows and oxygen contents of systemic, pulmonary capillary and shunt circulations.

Thus, if

$$CaO_2 = \text{arterial } O_2 \text{ content}$$
$$C\bar{v}O_2 = \text{mixed venous } O_2 \text{ content}$$
$$CcO_2 = \text{pulmonary capillary } O_2 \text{ content}$$
$$\dot{Q}T = \text{cardiac output}$$
$$\dot{Q}S = \text{shunt flow}$$
$$(\dot{Q}T - \dot{Q}S) = \text{capillary flow}$$

The total O_2 content of blood leaving the lungs is

$$= (\text{cardiac output} \times \text{arterial } O_2 \text{ content})$$
$$= \dot{Q}T \times CaO_2$$

But the total oxygen content is also

$$= (\text{shunt flow} \times \text{mixed venous } O_2 \text{ content})$$
$$\quad + (\text{pulmonary capillary flow}$$
$$\quad \times \text{pulmonary capillary } O_2 \text{ content})$$
$$= (\dot{Q}S \times C\bar{v}O_2) + (\dot{Q}T - \dot{Q}S) \times CcO_2$$

So

$$\dot{Q}T \times CaO_2 = (\dot{Q}S \times CvO_2) + (\dot{Q}T - \dot{Q}S) \times CcO_2$$

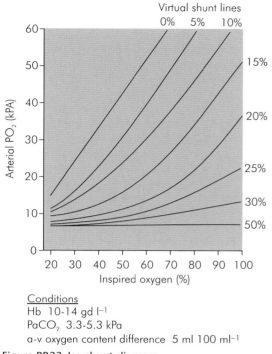

Conditions
Hb 10-14 gd l⁻¹
$PaCO_2$ 3.3-5.3 kPa
a-v oxygen content difference 5 ml 100 ml⁻¹

Figure RR22 Iso-shunt diagram

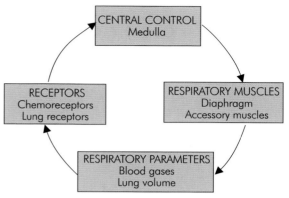

Figure RR23 Central control of ventilation

Control of ventilation

Respiratory control is mediated by neurological and chemical reflexes that involve control centres in the central nervous system, the lungs, respiratory muscles and specialised receptors (Figure RR23).

Neurological ventilatory centres were first localised in the brain stem in 1812 by LeGallois, who demonstrated that breathing did not depend on an intact cerebrum but on a small region of the medulla near the origin of the vagus nerves.

The primary goal of respiratory control is to maintain homeostasis of blood gases. In addition, reflexes also modify the respiratory pattern in order to:

*   Allow speech
*   Enable coughing, sneezing, yawning
*   Protect the airway during eating, drinking and vomiting
*   Minimise the work of breathing

This can be rearranged to give the 'shunt' equation as follows

$$\frac{\dot{Q}s}{\dot{Q}T} = \frac{CcO_2 - CaO_2}{CcO_2 - C\bar{v}O_2}$$

Summarising for physiological shunt: Shunt effectively reduces oxygen content of pulmonary capillary blood by admixture of venous blood bypassing the lungs.

The 'shunt' equation assesses the shunt as a fraction of the total flow, and can be stated as

$$\frac{(shunt\ flow)}{(total\ flow)} = \frac{(reduction\ in\ oxygen\ content\ due\ to\ shunt)}{(total\ oxygen\ content\ added\ by\ lungs)}$$

This fraction is usually quoted as a percentage, and it is a useful clinical index of oxygenation efficiency in critically ill patients. The effect of physiological shunt on arterial blood gases is shown in Figure RR22, which illustrates an 'iso-shunt' diagram. Shunt fractions up to 10% are not considered clinically significant, but when greater than 30% they are associated with poor survival. The iso-shunt diagram is helpful in following clinical progress and in adjusting oxygen therapy.

Central control of ventilation

The respiratory centres in the brain stem have been identified in the past by ablation, electrical stimulation and recording action potentials with microelectrodes. These centres are groups of neurones in the reticular formation rather than defined nuclei, and are described below.

Medullary centres

The medulla contains two pools of ventilatory control neurones, an inspiratory pool and an expiratory pool. These inspiratory and expiratory neurones function by a system of reciprocal innervation. As activity increases in one centre, a rising level of inhibitory activity is relayed from the opposite centre, resulting in a reversal of the ventilatory phase.

- The **inspiratory pool** is located in the dorsal medullary reticular formation and is the source of basic ventilatory rhythm (i.e. it is the pacemaker for the respiratory system). The rhythmic activity persists even when all connections to these neurones are blocked. During inspiration, activity in the inspiratory pool leads to increased output to the muscles of inspiration, principally the diaphragm. At the same time increasing inhibitory activity from the expiratory centre is relayed to the inspiratory neurones, until inspiratory activity ceases and expiration begins.
- The **expiratory pool** is found in the ventral medullary reticular formation. During inspiration, gradually increasing activity is relayed from the expiratory pool, inhibiting the inspiratory pool until expiration begins. At the same time inhibitory activity is relayed to the expiratory neurones from the inspiratory pool, until expiration ceases and inspiration begins.

Pontine centres

There are two respiratory centres in the pons:

- The **pneumotaxic centre** is a region in the upper pons, which 'fine tunes' ventilatory rate and V_T to minimise respiratory work. It controls V_T by switching off the inspiratory centre during the inspiratory phase, which limits V_T. This control of the inspiratory phase also varies the respiratory rate. Even in the absence of the pneumotaxic centre a basic ventilatory rhythm is maintained by the medullary inspiratory group.
- The **apneustic centre** is in the lower pons and is thought to prolong the inspiratory phase by acting on the medullary inspiratory pool of neurones. This also provides some control over the ventilatory rate and pattern. Section immediately above this centre gives rise to 'apneustic' breathing with prolonged inspiration and brief expiratory efforts.

Respiratory control by higher centres

The cerebral cortex also affects breathing pattern, although precise neural pathways are not known. Voluntary hyperventilation and hypoventilation can be performed and maintained to the extent of producing changes in arterial blood gases. The limbic system and hypothalamus can also affect the respiratory pattern, as seen in emotional states.

Reflexes in the control of ventilation

The primary goal of ventilatory control is to maintain homeostasis of PaO_2 and $PaCO_2$. Various reflexes are integrated to produce the responses of the respiratory system to disturbances of arterial blood gases, or to the increased demands of exercise. Other reflexes protect the airway by coordinating breathing with eating, drinking or talking, and enabling coughing and sneezing. An example is the protective reflex that inhibits inspiration momentarily during swallowing, which is usually followed by a single large breath and a brief increase in ventilation. Similarly, it is advantageous to inhibit inspiration during vomiting, because of the risk of aspirating gastric contents.

These reflexes are mediated by specialised receptors that include the following:

- The central chemoreceptors are situated bilaterally 0.2 mm beneath the ventral surface of the medulla and are highly sensitive to changes in hydrogen ion concentration.
- The peripheral chemoreceptors are found in the carotid bodies located bilaterally at the bifurcation of the common carotid artery, and in the aortic bodies located along the arch of the aorta. The afferent nerve fibres of the carotid bodies pass through Hering's nerves to the glossopharyngeal nerves, and those of the aortic bodies pass through the vagi to the dorsal respiratory area. The chemoreceptors have a very high oxygen consumption and respond both to decreases in oxygen content of the arterial blood and to decreases in blood flow. They therefore act as oxygen delivery sensors to the brain, an organ which is particularly vulnerable to hypoxaemia with limited ability to increase oxygen extraction.

The effect of CO_2 and hydrogen ion concentration on the peripheral receptors is much less than the direct effects of both these factors on the respiratory centre itself. However, the peripheral stimulation occurs as much as five times more rapidly than the central effect, so that peripheral receptors will increase the rapidity of the response to CO_2 at the onset of exercise.

Chemical and irritant receptors

These exist in the mucosa of the upper airways and trachea, and help protect the lungs from inhalation of injurious substances, such as gastric acid. These reflexes initiate laryngeal closure, apnoea, hyperpnoea and bronchoconstriction. Similar receptors respond to impending closure of the upper airway during inspiration by increasing pharyngeal dilator activity

Pressure-sensitive receptors

These are located within the smooth muscle of all airways, and help to control the depth of respiration.

'J' receptors

'J' receptors are found in the alveolar walls close to the capillaries. Their stimulation causes rapid, shallow breathing or apnoea. They are thought to be involved in the tachypnoea observed in pulmonary oedema and irritation of the lungs.

Pulmonary stretch receptors

These are believed to lie in the smooth muscle of the airways. These inhibit inspiration in response to lung distension, and slow ventilatory rate by increasing expiratory time. This reflex was first reported by Hering and Breuer in 1868, who noted that lightly anaesthetised, spontaneously breathing animals would cease or decrease ventilatory effort during sustained lung distension. This response is abolished by bilateral vagotomy.

The Hering–Breuer reflex is only weakly present in humans, who can continue to breathe spontaneously with continuous positive airway pressures (CPAP) in excess of 40 cmH$_2$O. This reflex in humans is not activated until $V_T > 1.5$ litres, and it is probably a protective mechanism for preventing excess ventilation, rather than an important component of the normal ventilatory control.

Golgi tendons organs

Golgi tendon organs are particularly plentiful in the intercostal muscles, and are also involved in the pulmonary stretch reflex. When the lungs are distended, the chest wall is stretched and these receptors send signals to the brain stem that inhibit further inspiration.

Muscle spindles

Muscle spindles in the inspiratory muscle and diaphragm contribute to control of depth and effort during inspiration. These receptors are thought to activate when particularly intense respiratory efforts are required, as in airway obstruction. They are also thought to be responsible for the sensation of dyspnoea.

Response of ventilation to carbon dioxide tension

Figure RR24 shows the effect of PaCO$_2$ on alveolar ventilation. Increasing PaCO$_2$ from normal produces an increase

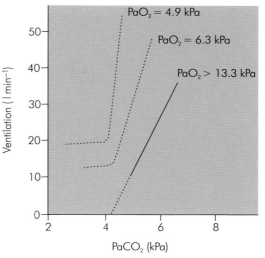

Figure RR24 Ventilatory response to CO$_2$ tension

in alveolar ventilation, which is effectively linear. Alveolar ventilation goes up by 1–2 litres per minute for each 0.1 kPa increase in PaCO$_2$. Decreasing CO$_2$ levels produce a fall in alveolar ventilation, but cease to have effect below a PaCO$_2$ of about 4 kPa. Various factors can displace this line to the left or right, and also alter its gradient. Some examples include:

- Sleep – reduces the gradient of the line and displaces it slightly to the right. These effects represent a decrease in the sensitivity of the ventilatory response to CO$_2$.
- Morphine – also reduces the gradient of the line and displaces it to the right, by central depression of the respiratory centres. Other opioid drugs and barbiturates have a similar effect.
- Work of breathing – increased work of breathing can reduce the response to CO$_2$. This does not appear to depress the respiratory centres, but reduces the peripheral response to central drive. This effect may be noted in some patients with bronchospasm, whose CO$_2$ response may increase with broncodilator therapy.
- Very high levels of CO$_2$ – thought to produce central depression and thus a reduction in CO$_2$ response curve gradient, followed by narcosis and respiratory depression.
- Age, genetics and race.

The effect of increased CO$_2$ levels on ventilation is mediated mainly by the central response to increased $[H^+]$. The central chemoreceptors attempt to maintain the PaCO$_2$

levels within normal range and increase alveolar ventilation. There is some additional response to increased $PaCO_2$ and $[H^+]$ due to peripheral chemoreceptors, but the main effect is central.

The response to CO_2 is maximal over the first few hours and gradually declines to about only 20% of the initial effect over the next 48 hours. This decline is due partly to the renal readjustment of $[H^+]$ back toward normal by reabsorption of bicarbonate ions. More importantly, over a period of time bicarbonate ions slowly diffuse across the blood–brain and blood–CSF barrier, reducing the cerebral $[H^+]$ back to normal.

Response of ventilation to oxygen tension

Changes in oxygen levels mediate their effect on ventilation mainly through the peripheral chemoreceptors. The effect of PaO_2 on ventilation is shown in Figure RR25. These curves are measured with $PaCO_2$ held constant (isocapnic responsiveness). It can be seen that increasing PaO_2 to supranormal levels produces virtually no effect on ventilation. Decreasing oxygen levels from normal also has little effect on ventilation, until PaO_2 is below about 8 kPa. Below this level an exponential increase in ventilation is produced as PaO_2 decreases further. Oxyhaemoglobin saturation and oxygen content start to decrease rapidly at this PaO_2. Thus, the peripheral chemoreceptors play a role in safeguarding cerebral oxygen delivery as well as monitoring PaO_2. At high altitude, hypoxaemia produces a marked increase in ventilatory drive.

Hypoxaemia has virtually no specific effect on central chemoreceptors, but does produce a general depression of cerebral function. Periodic respiration (Cheyne–Stokes breathing) may be induced at moderate levels of hypoxaemia, but the mechanism is unknown.

Simultaneous changes in $PaCO_2$ have a marked effect on the ventilatory response to oxygen levels. Increases in $PaCO_2$ from normal exaggerate the ventilatory response to oxygen levels. Thus, when $PaCO_2$ levels are greater than normal, increasing hypoxaemia produces increased levels of ventilation. In the response to altitude, the hyperventilation due to hypoxaemia is initially blunted by the decrease in $PaCO_2$ produced. With acclimatisation, the $PaCO_2$ returns towards normal and the ventilatory response increases.

The hypoxic ventilatory drive becomes important in some patients suffering from chronic lung disease, who retain higher than normal levels of CO_2. If these patients compensate for their hypercarbia by retaining bicarbonate and producing a normal body pH, they become dependent on hypoxic ventilatory drive to maintain their breathing pattern. Caution is often advised in the administration of high FIO_2 mixtures to such patients for fear of depressing their endogenous drive, but general clinical condition often overrules this effect.

The hypoxic ventilatory drive is reduced or abolished by the same drugs and situations that impair hypercapnic ventilatory drive. The volatile anaesthetic agents are implicated even at sub-anaesthetic concentrations.

Non-respiratory lung functions

Defence mechanisms

The lungs are continuously exposed to particulate matter and infectious material, which demands that they possess well-developed defence mechanisms. These include:

- Filtration – large particles are physically filtered out by the hairs and lining of the nasal passages.
- Sneeze and cough reflexes, which remove foreign bodies or particulate matter physically by the explosive airway pressure and air flow generated.
- Mucociliary clearance – smaller particles that are inhaled become impacted on a thin layer of mucus secreted by goblet cells. This is moved up and out of the respiratory tract by the rhythmic 'beating' of ciliated epithelial cells. The cilia may be paralysed by inhaled toxins or anaesthetic drugs.
- T and B lymphocytes – T cells produce pro-inflammatory peptides (interleukins, interferon γ,

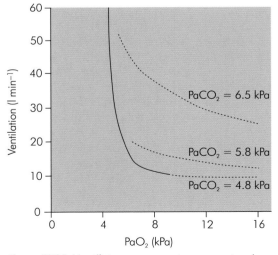

Figure RR25 Ventilatory response to oxygen tension

Type of secretion	Substance secreted
Enzymes	Elastase Plasminogen activator Acid hydrolases
Oxidative radicals	Hydrogen peroxide Superoxide anion Singlet oxygen
Complement components	
Enzyme inhibitors	α_1-antitrypsin
Platelet activating factor	
Leukotrienes	LTB_4, LTC_4, LTD_4, LTE_4
Interferon γ	
Cytokines	Interleukin 1 Tumour necrosis factor

Figure RR26 Secretory products of alveolar macrophages

tumour necrosis factor) that cause multiplication of cytotoxic lymphocytes and recruitment of neutrophils. B lymphocytes secrete IgG and IgA in the airways. IgA promotes clearance of micro-organisms, while IgG opsonises bacteria and fungi for phagocytosis.

• Macrophages and neutrophils, which engulf particles and micro-organisms reaching the terminal airways and alveoli. Macrophages arise from blood monocytes and are capable of secreting a host of substances that are important for lung defence (Figure RR26).

Blood filtration

The pulmonary vasculature acts as a filter in the circulation. Since the diameter of the pulmonary capillaries is about 8 μm, particles greater than this are filtered or slowed during their passage through the lungs.

The lung also filters out small clots, which are then dissolved by the fibrinolytic system. Pulmonary endothelium secretes a plasmin activator converting plasminogen to plasmin, which activates the fibrinolysis. The lung is also a rich source of endogenous heparin and produces a variety of thromboplastins, which play a role in the overall control of coagulation.

Larger clots may obstruct branches of the pulmonary arteries, producing an increase in pulmonary arterial pressure, and tachypnoea. The rise in pulmonary artery pressure is due to reflex vasoconstriction via sympathetic nerve fibres. However, the pulmonary vascular bed has an intrinsic ability to compensate for blocked vessels by opening new channels.

Metabolic functions of the lung

The lung is an important site for the metabolism of both endogenous and exogenous substances. Some of these metabolic functions are shown in Figure RR27.

Function	Substances
Extracellular metabolism by endothelium	Bradykinins Adenine nucleotides
Intracellular metabolism by endothelium	Norepinephrine, serotonin Prostaglandins E and F Atrial natriuretic peptide
Activation	Angiotensin I, enkephalin
Synthesis	Somatostatin, cholecystokinin Opioid peptide, substance P Prostaglandin E and F, prostacyclin Nitric oxide
Systemic release	Prostaglandins, histamine Kallikreins, eosinophil chemotactic factor of anaphylaxis, platelet activating factor
Production of surfactant	
Uptake and metabolism of anaesthetic agents	

Figure RR27 Metabolic functions of the lung

Abnormal metabolic responses of the lungs to drugs, infection or physical injury may lead to lung damage. Among these are:

- Lung injury due to bleomycin, cyclophosphamide and amiodarone. The mechanism suggested is the production of oxidative radicals or the impairment of antioxidant activity.
- Lung injury in acute respiratory distress syndrome is also thought to involve abnormal actions of oxidative radicals and elastases on lung tissue.

Lung function at high altitude

The most important environmental change at high altitude is the decrease in barometric pressure, because this gives a proportional reduction in inspired oxygen tension (P_{IO_2}).

Barometric pressure at an altitude of 5500 m is reduced to about half the value at sea level, i.e. about 50 kPa.

Inspired oxygen tension (P_{IO_2}) at high altitude

P_{IO_2} at an altitude of 5500 m can be calculated by:

- Correcting for humidification, by subtracting saturated vapour pressure of water (about 6.3 kPa)
- Multiplying by the normal fractional oxygen concentration in air (about 0.21)

This gives $P_{IO_2} = 9.2$ kPa instead of the normal value at sea level of about 20 kPa.

Alveolar oxygen tension at high altitude

Applying the alveolar gas equation, the P_{AO_2} at 5500 m can be estimated. The alveolar gas equation is given by

$$P_{AO_2} = P_{IO_2} - \frac{P_{ACO_2}}{RQ}$$

Then for $P_{IO_2} = 9.2$ kPa (see above), assuming a normal value for $P_{ACO_2} = 5.3$ kPa and respiratory quotient (RQ) $= 0.8$

$$P_{AO_2} = 9.2 - 6.6 = 2.6 \text{ kPa}$$

Thus, if P_{ACO_2} levels remain normal at an altitude of 5500 m, the P_{AO_2} would only be 2.6 kPa, which would result in a loss of consciousness in a few minutes. In practice, a marked hyperventilation response occurs at altitude, which increases P_{AO_2}.

Hyperventilation at altitude

Physiological changes occur at high altitude to enable survival. These changes are called acclimatisation. Hyperventilation is one of the most important features of acclimatisation, and is produced by the low P_{AO_2}, which causes a left and upward shift of the ventilation–P_{ACO_2} curve. Under these circumstances, alveolar ventilation can increase by four or five times to give alveolar ventilation rates greater than 20 litres per minute. This can reduce the P_{ACO_2} to levels of about 1 kPa. In such a case the new P_{AO_2} can be found by substituting this value in the aboves equation. Thus, at 5500 m

$$P_{AO_2} = 9.2 - 1.2 = 8.0 \text{ kPa}$$

Although this is less than the normal P_{AO_2} at sea level (about 15 kPa), it is compatible with survival, particularly in combination with the other features of acclimatisation, which help to increase oxygen carriage to the tissues.

The hyperventilation response at high altitude is biphasic. Alveolar ventilation increases rapidly initially, over the first two hours or so, but then a slow steady rise is recorded over the following several days. The initial hyperventilatory phase is the result of a balance between hypoxic stimulation of chemoreceptors and inhibition due to reduced CO_2 levels and respiratory alkalosis. The second more gradual increase occurs because of renal elimination of bicarbonate, bicarbonate shift out of the cerebrospinal fluid compartment and desensitisation of the chemoreceptors.

Acclimatisation

Acclimatisation describes the adaptive physiological changes that occur when a person moves from sea level to high altitude. There are physiological differences between peoples who live their whole lives at high altitude and those who live at sea level, which are referred to as 'adaptation'. The main changes occurring in acclimatisation are:

- Hyperventilation – an immediate and sustained response
- Polycythaemia – Hb levels reach 20 g dl^{-1} or more, increasing the oxygen content of blood to >22 ml O_2 dl^{-1}
- Right shift of the oxyhaemoglobin dissociation curve – due to increased levels of 2,3-DPG
- Increased capillary density – in peripheral tissues, particularly muscle
- Increased mitochondrial density – and increased concentration of respiratory chain enzymes
- Increased pulmonary arterial pressures – due to hypoxic vasoconstriction

- Increased ventilatory capacity – aided by the decreased density of air. Maximum ventilation rates of 200 litres per minute or more may occur
- More even distribution of perfusion

Ventilation–perfusion matching at altitude

The distribution of perfusion is more even throughout the lung due to higher pulmonary arterial pressures and lower alveolar pressures. This has the effect of reducing the transmural pressure of the capillaries and postcapillary venules in perfusion zones 1 and 2. As described above, perfusion in these zones is dependent on the Starling resistor effect of these vessels, which is reduced by the changes at high altitude.

High-altitude disease

Additional physiological changes to those described in acclimatisation may develop. These include:

- Right ventricular hypertrophy
- Muscle atrophy and catabolism
- Antidiuresis and oedema formation
- Increased thyroid activity
- Sleep disturbance and periodic breathing
- Impaired central nervous system performance

These changes may develop into acute and chronic mountain sickness, pulmonary oedema and cerebral oedema.

CHAPTER 9
Physiology of the nervous system

A. K. Gupta and A. M. Sardesai

Structure and function of neurones

The main excitable cell in the nervous system is the neurone. Non-excitable cells or glial cells support neurones and perform various other functions (see Figure NE1). Neurones specialise in processing and transmitting information. The human nervous system contains between 10^{11} and 10^{12} neurones. Functionally, neurones are classified as sensory, motor and interneurone. Structurally, a typical neurone is made up of three parts: a cell body, an axon and terminal buttons (Figure NE2). The cell body consists of intracellular organelles by which the cell maintains its functional and structural integrity. The axon originates from the cell body and divides into terminal branches; each branch terminates in enlarged endings called terminal buttons. The axon is a long projection surrounded by supporting cells (oligodendrocytes or Schwann cells).

When there is a layer of lipid–protein complex deposited within the Schwann cell membrane, the neurone is said to be myelinated, otherwise it is unmyelinated. Myelination allows saltatory conduction with an accompanying increase in speed of propagation of a nerve impulse. Mammalian neurones have varying fibre diameters and speeds of conduction, as summarised in Figure NE3.

The ionic basis of membrane potential
Membrane potential at rest

As in other excitable tissues in the body, the electrical potential of a neurone in the resting state is more negative on the inside of the cell than on the outside. This polarity is maintained by the active transport of Na^+ ions out of the cell, together with the active transport of K^+ ions into the cell. However, there is a tendency for both

Cell	Function
Neurones	Generation, transmission and processing of potentials
Astrocytes	Support neurones and contribute to blood–brain barrier
Oligodendrocytes	Insulate neurones in CNS
Ependymal cells	Line ventricles and spinal canal
Schwann cells	Insulate axons in PNS

Figure NE1 Functions of different cells in the nervous system

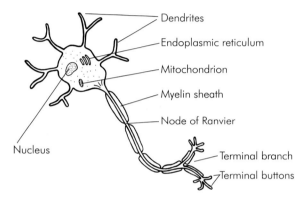

Figure NE2 A typical neurone

ions to diffuse passively down their concentration gradient through leaky ion channels. During its resting state, the membrane is more permeable to K^+ than to Na^+ ions, and therefore more K^+ ions leak out of the neurone than Na^+ ions enter the cell. At the same time, the resting membrane is not permeable to anions. The result is that the interior of the neurone is more electronegative (-70 mV) than the outside. This is the resting membrane potential.

Characteristics of the action potential

Neurones respond to a stimulus by transiently producing changes in ion permeability or conductance in the cell membrane. Ion conductance is defined as the reciprocal of electrical resistance of the membrane to a given ion, and it therefore reflects permeability. When the stimulus is below the threshold potential, the changes produced remain localised. However, when the stimulus reaches the threshold, the membrane becomes depolarised. When this depolarisation is propagated along the axon, it gives rise to an action potential. The latter can be divided into a number of phases (Figure NE4).

At the beginning of an action potential, the rate of depolarisation increases so that the inside of the cell becomes increasingly positive until it rises to a peak, then falls when repolarisation begins. This sharp rise and decline is called the spike potential. The sharp rise is due to an increase in Na^+ conductance, so that Na^+ ions diffuse down their electrical and concentration gradients. However, there are three factors which limit the depolarisation process: first, the Na^+ channels open only very transiently; second, as the inside of the cell becomes increasingly more electropositive, the initial gradients which facilitate Na^+ influx disappear; and finally, K^+ conductance also increases. The rate of repolarisation slows down when the process is about 70% complete; this phase is known as after-depolarisation.

During the final recovery phase, there is a slight but prolonged overshoot after the resting potential is reached. This is due to the slow return of K^+ conductance to normal (Figure NE5). This phase is called the after-hyperpolarisation.

Fibre type	Function	Fibre diameter (m)	Conduction speed (m s^{-1})
Aα	Proprioception, somatic motor	12–20	70–120
Aβ	Touch, pressure	5–12	30–70
Aγ	Muscle spindle motor	3–6	15–30
Aδ	Pain, temperature, touch	2–5	12–30
B	Preganglionic ANS	3	3–15
C dorsal root	Pain, temperature, mechanoreceptors, reflex responses	0.4–1.2	0.5–2
C sympathetic	Postganglionic ANS	0.3–1.3	0.7–2.2

Figure NE3 Classification of mammalian neurones

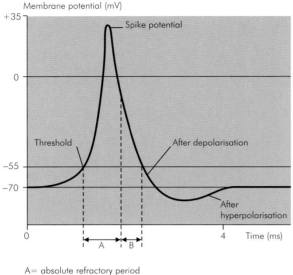

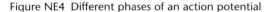

A= absolute refractory period
B= relative refractory period

Figure NE4 Different phases of an action potential

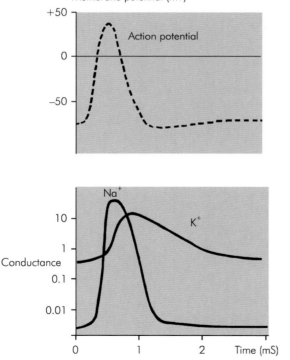

Figure NE5 Changes in Na$^+$ and K$^+$ conductance during the course of an action potential

A neurone is said to be in the absolute refractory period when it is totally unresponsive to any stimulus regardless of its strength. This corresponds to the period between the threshold being reached and when repolarisation is one-third completed. The relative refractory period starts at this point until the beginning of after-depolarisation. During this period, a stronger than normal stimulus may lead to excitation.

Synaptic transmission

Nerve impulses are transmitted from one neurone to another through junctions known as synapses. Synapses are formed between the terminal buttons of a neurone and the cell body or axon of another neurone. The number of terminal buttons forming synapses with a neurone varies from one to several thousand. Synapses almost invariably allow unidirectional impulse conduction, i.e. from the presynaptic to the postsynaptic neurone. This ensures nerve impulses are transmitted in an orderly fashion. Most synaptic transmissions are chemical in nature; others are either electrical or mixed. In electrical synapses, the membranes between the presynaptic and postsynaptic neurones meet to form gap junctions, which contain channels that facilitate diffusion of ions.

Structure of a synapse

Chemical synapses consist of a small gap known as a synaptic cleft. The synaptic cleft measures about 20 nm wide and contains extracellular fluid across which the neurotransmitters diffuse. There are three essential structures that can be found in the cytoplasm of the terminal button: synaptic vesicles, mitochondria and endoplasmic reticulum (Figure NE6). The synaptic vesicles, containing the neurotransmitters, are usually found in large concentrations in the release zone adjacent to the synaptic cleft. The endoplasmic reticulum is responsible for the production of new vesicles, and recycling the used ones. Mitochondria provide the energy required for chemical transmission and the formation of synaptic vesicles by the endoplasmic reticulum.

Synaptic mechanism

When an action potential is transmitted down an axon, the depolarisation opens the voltage-gated calcium channels, allowing an influx of Ca^{2+} ions into the terminal button. In the release zone the Ca^{2+} ions bind with groups of protein molecules in synaptic vesicle membranes. These protein molecules spread apart, allowing fusion between vesicle

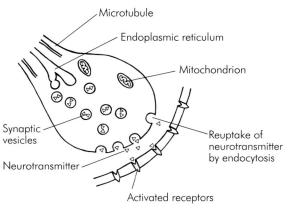

Figure NE6 Structure of a chemical synapse

and terminal button membranes. This releases neurotransmitter into the synaptic cleft. The amount of neurotransmitter released is directly proportional to the Ca^{2+} influx. The postsynaptic receptors are activated by the binding of neurotransmitters which lead to the opening of ion channels, resulting in postsynaptic potentials. Postsynaptic potentials are transient in action because of two mechanisms: first, and predominantly, by transmitter reuptake and, second, by enzymatic deactivation. The terminal buttons at the end of the transmission rapidly and actively take up neurotransmitters. Figure NE7 summarises the different types of neurotransmitter found in the central nervous system (CNS).

The events following the generation of postsynaptic potentials depend mainly on two conditions: first, the amount of neurotransmitter released and, second, the type of ion channel that is being opened. Not all postsynaptic potential changes are propagated as action potentials in the postsynaptic neurone. When an insufficient amount of neurotransmitter becomes bound to the postsynaptic receptor, the change in membrane potential may not reach the firing threshold of the neurone, thus giving rise only to local potential changes. When sodium channels are open, there is a sudden influx of Na^+ ions down its concentration and electrical gradients, producing an excitatory postsynaptic potential (EPSP). However, when K^+ or Cl^- channels are open, K^+ and Cl^- ions move down their concentration gradients, making the inside of the neurone more electronegative with respect to the outside of the neurone, i.e. hyperpolarised, resulting in an inhibitory postsynaptic potential (IPSP) (Figure NE8). When the postsynaptic potential reaches threshold an action potential occurs.

Sensory receptors

Sensory receptors are specialised structures that receive and transmit information from the external and internal environment to the CNS. A sensory receptor may be part of a neurone, such as nerve endings, or a separate structure that is capable of generating and transmitting action potentials to a neurone. They are essentially transducers that respond to different forms of energy, such as mechanical or thermal energy, and convert them into electrical

Neurotransmitter	Location	Function
Acetylcholine	Cerebral cortex, thalamus, limbic system	Likely to be involved in memory, perception, cognition, attention and arousal functions
Norepinephrine	Locus coeruleus	Descending pain pathway
	Cerebellum	Inhibits Purkinje cells
	Hypothalamus	Regulates secretion of anterior pituitary hormones
Epinephrine	Medulla	Functions uncertain
Dopamine	Substantia nigra	Control of motor functions
	Hypothalamus	Regulates prolactin secretion
Serotonin	Neocortex and limbic system	Alters mood and behaviour
	Hypothalamus	Increases prolactin secretion
	Nucleus raphe magnus and spinal cord	Pain modulation

Figure NE7 Locations and functions of different types of neurotransmitter

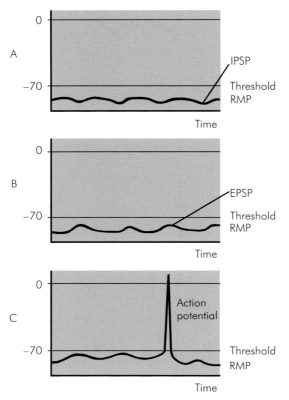

Figure NE8 Synaptic transmission

signals. Special sense organs such as the eye are a collection of sensory receptors supported by highly organised structural and connective tissue.

Sensory receptors may be classified according to whether they perceive visceral or somatic sensory changes:

• Visceral receptors are primarily concerned with perceiving changes in the internal environment; such information does not usually reach consciousness. These include chemoreceptors which are sensitive to changes in glucose level, oxygen tension, osmolality and acidity in the plasma. Stretch receptors in the lungs and pressure receptors in the carotid sinus are other examples of visceral receptors.

• Somatic receptors are sensory receptors that respond to external stimuli such as temperature, light touch, and pressure. Pain is initiated by noxious or potentially damaging stimuli; pain receptors are, therefore, also known as nociceptors. Information from the somatic receptors usually reaches consciousness and is

represented at the cerebral level, giving rise to a variety of sensations. Sensory pathways are multi-synaptic and thus involve a first-order neurone (for example a dorsal root ganglion) which then synapses with a central chain of second-order and third-order neurones, as outlined in Figure NE9.

Functional organisation of the nervous system

The nervous system is divided into two main parts: the central nervous system, consisting of the brain (cerebral cortex, basal ganglia, cerebellum, brain stem) and the spinal cord, and the peripheral nervous system, which includes the cranial and spinal nerves and their ganglia. The autonomic nervous system also forms an important part of the nervous system, and can be subdivided into the sympathetic and parasympathetic nervous system.

Cortex

The cerebral cortex is topographically the highest level of the central nervous system, and always functions in association with the lower centres. The surface of the cerebral cortex is thrown into convolutions called gyri, which are separated by the sulci.

The cortex is divided into various lobes, namely frontal, temporal, parietal and occipital, which have different functions.

• The **frontal lobe** lies in front of the central sulcus and is divided into the precentral area and prefrontal cortex. The precentral area is further divided into anterior and posterior regions. The posterior region is referred to as the primary motor area or Brodmann's area 4, and the anterior region is known as the premotor area. The supplemental motor area is also situated in the frontal lobe. The rest of the frontal lobe, the prefrontal cortex, is divided into superior, middle and inferior frontal gyri. Broca's speech area is situated in the inferior frontal gyrus of the dominant hemisphere. The prefrontal cortex is concerned with personality, initiative and judgement. The frontal cortex controls motor function of the opposite side of the body, insight and control of emotions.

• The **temporal lobe** contains primary and secondary auditory areas. The ability to locate the source of sound is impaired with the destruction of the primary auditory area. Bilateral destruction leads to complete deafness. The secondary auditory area is necessary for the interpretation of sounds. Wernicke's area, which is

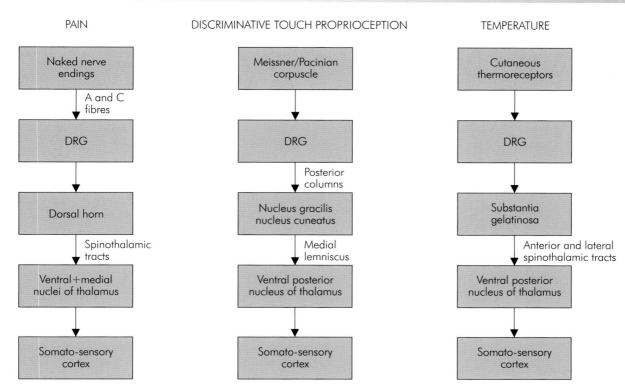

PAIN	DISCRIMINATIVE TOUCH PROPRIOCEPTION	TEMPERATURE

Figure NE9 Somatic sensory perceptions and their afferent pathways to the CNS

the sensory speech area, is located in the categorical (dominant) hemisphere and is associated with comprehension of speech.

- The **parietal lobe** houses the primary sensory area in the postcentral gyrus. The majority of sensations reach the cortex from the contralateral side of the body, although some signals from the oral region go to the same side, and those from the pharynx, larynx, and perineum go to both sides. A secondary sensory area is situated in the wall of the Sylvian fissure. Loss of the primary sensory cortex leads to inability to judge shape or form (astereognosis), degree of pressure or weight of an object. Problems occur with position sense and in localising different sensations occurring in different parts of the body. The secondary sensory area is involved in receiving information and relating it to past experience so that the information can be interpreted.
- The **occipital lobe** contains the primary visual area (area 17) close to the occipital pole. The macula lutea of the retina is represented on the cortex in the

posterior part of area 17 and accounts for a third of the visual cortex. Lesions of the occipital pole produce central scotomas.

Higher functions of the cerebral cortex
Consciousness

There are different levels of consciousness, ranging from alertness to coma. The level of consciousness is determined by activities of both the cerebral cortex and the reticular activating system (RAS). The latter is a diffuse network of neurones situated in the brainstem reticular formation. It receives sensory information from ascending sensory tracts as well as auditory, visual, olfactory and trigeminal tracts. The reticular formation projects to the cerebral cortex directly and indirectly via the thalamic nuclei. RAS activity is closely related to the electrical activity of the cerebral cortex.

Electrical activity of the cerebral cortex can be recorded by scalp electrodes as an electroencephalogram (EEG). Various EEG rhythms can be identified:

- **α rhythm** is seen in an adult human at rest with eyes closed. It is more common in parieto-occipital areas and has a frequency of 8–12 Hz with an amplitude of 50–100 mV.
- **β rhythm** is a lower-amplitude wave with a frequency of 18–30 Hz. It is seen over the frontal region in a normal alert adult.
- **γ rhythm** has a large amplitude with a frequency of 4–7 Hz. It is normally seen in the very old and very young.
- **δ rhythm** consists of large slow waves with a frequency of less than 4 Hz.

Two basic sleep patterns are seen: rapid eye movement sleep (REM) and non-rapid eye movement sleep (NREM).

NREM has four stages. From stage 1 to 4 there is progressive slowing of the EEG with associated increase in EEG amplitude. Stage 1 sleep occurs at the beginning of sleep while stage 4 sleep represents deep sleep. In stage 2 bursts of α-like rhythm known as sleep spindles are seen. In REM sleep the NREM pattern of EEG is replaced by fast low-voltage electrical activity similar to that seen in alert individuals. However, sleep is not disturbed and in fact the threshold for arousal is increased. This kind of sleep is associated with rapid eye movements, hence the name. In REM sleep, large phasic potentials are seen, there is a decrease in muscle tone, and it is also associated with dreaming.

Language

Wernicke's area in the categorical hemisphere receives auditory and visual information and is concerned with comprehension of this information. It communicates via the arcuate fasciculus with Broca's area, which is concerned with output of speech. It processes the information from Wernicke's area to produce appropriate movements of the vocal apparatus.

Memory

Memory is the process of retention and storage of acquired information, and can be divided into **explicit** and **implicit** memory.

Explicit memory involves hippocampus and medial temporal lobes of the brain. It requires conscious retrieval or awareness and can be further divided into **episodic** memory (memory of events) and **semantic** memory, which is memory of words, rules, language and the world around us.

Implicit memory does not require conscious awareness and is not processed in the hippocampus. It is associated with skills required for day-to-day activities and habits. When learning certain tasks, such as driving or cycling, explicit memory is used, but once the tasks are well learned then implicit memory is used to perform them.

Both forms of memory can also be divided into **short-term** and **long-term** memory. Information is processed in the hippocampus as a short-term memory, and then stored as a long-term memory, which lasts for years. Short-term memory lasts from a few seconds to hours, and is easily affected by drugs and trauma.

It is thought that short-term memory is a transient store of limited capacity which permits instantaneous encoding and retrieval, but when the material is no longer the focus of conscious attention, only some of this material may pass on to long-term memory. The latter represents a long-term storage of indefinite capacity that requires effortful encoding and retrieval. The more elaborate and effortful the encoding process, the better the memory of the material.

At the cellular level, it is thought that information is stored in the short-term memory as reverberating electrical activity in the brain, whereas long-term memory is stored in a more robust form. It is thought that memory formation may lead to an alteration in the transmission of electrical signals through parts of the brain. However, it is not clear whether this is the result of facilitation of existing synapses or due to the formation of new synapses. In both situations, however, protein synthesis is thought to be ultimately involved in the formation of long-term memory, and this is brought about through either structural or enzymatic changes in the neurones. The hippocampus is primarily involved in memory storage, since pathological lesions in this area result in both anterograde and retrograde amnesia.

Basal ganglia

The basal ganglia consist of interconnected deep nuclei including the caudate, globus pallidum, substantia nigra and putamen. The basal ganglia are involved in control of posture and movement.

Cerebellum

The cerebellum consists of two cerebellar hemispheres and a central structure. In contrast to the cerebral hemispheres, the cerebellar hemispheres control the structures on the same side of the body. The central cerebral structures control gait and maintain balance, including when seated.

Brain stem

Included in the brain stem are the midbrain, pons and medulla. The brain stem contains the reticular formation, which maintains consciousness, and the nuclei of all the cranial nerves except I and II. It also has ascending and descending tracts from cerebral structures and spinal cord. The corticospinal tract (one of the main descending tracts) and the dorsal columns, which are the ascending tracts, cross over in the medulla. Thus a lesion in the brain stem can produce cranial nerve lesions on the same side but limb signs on the other side.

The brain stem contains control centres for respiration, cardiovascular homeostasis, gastrointestinal function, balance, equilibrium and eye movements. Irreversible brainstem lesions are therefore frequently incompatible with life without artificial support.

Spinal cord

The spinal cord extends from the lower part of the medulla. At birth it ends at the lower border of the third lumbar vertebra, and in the adult between the first and second lumbar vertebral bodies. The spinal cord is an elongated cylinder with cervical and lumbar enlargements corresponding to the origins of the brachial and lumbosacral plexuses. The spinal cord tapers into the conus medullaris.

The spinal cord has three covering membranes, also known as meninges – the dura mater, arachnoid and pia mater. The dura mater, which covers the brain, has two layers – the inner or meningeal layer of the cerebral dura and the outer endosteal layer, which at the foramen magnum merges with the periosteum of the skull. The outer layer of the cerebral dura is represented in the vertebral canal by its periosteum, while the inner layer continues down to cover the spinal cord. The dural sac usually ends at the level of the second sacral vertebra in adults. Dura covering the spinal cord is attached to the edges of the vertebral canal except posteriorly, where it is completely free. The arachnoid mater closely lines the dural sheath, while the pia mater closely covers the brain and the spinal cord. Due to the arrangement of the meninges, the following compartments are formed:

- **Subarachnoid space**. This contains the cerebrospinal fluid, and is traversed by three incomplete trabeculae – a single posterior subarachnoid septum and the ligamentum denticulatum on either side.
- **Subdural space**. This is a potential space only between the arachnoid and the dura mater, and contains a thin film of serous fluid.
- **Extradural space**. A space between the dura and the spinal canal which extends from the foramen magnum downwards as the dura covering the spinal cord fuses with the edges of the foramen magnum. It ends at the sacral hiatus and contains fat, lymphatics, arteries, and veins which are valveless and form the venous plexus of Bateson communicating between the pelvic veins and cerebral veins.

Anterior and posterior spinal roots emerge at the lateral surface of the spinal cord and are covered by the pia and arachnoid mater. They then pierce the dura mater and are subsequently covered by the dura, which fuses with the epineurium of the spinal nerve. Spinal nerves then travel through the epidural space and come out through the intervertebral foramen into the paravertebral space. Paravertebral spaces on either side of the vertebral column are in communication with each other through the epidural space.

Structure of the spinal cord

The spinal cord has an anterior median fissure and a posterior median sulcus which extends as a posterior median septum into the spinal cord. Posterior roots emerge along the posterolateral sulci which are on either side of the posterior median sulcus. Anterior roots emerge as a series of nerve tufts at the front of the cord.

The spinal cord has a central canal, which is the continuation of the fourth ventricle and contains the CSF. An H-shaped zone of grey matter, which contains nerve cells, surrounds the central canal. It has an outer zone of white matter, which contains myelinated nerve cells and forms ascending and descending tracts (Figures NE10, NE11; see also Section 1, Chapter 10, page 185).

Descending tracts

Descending pathways, which start in the cerebral cortex, are usually made of three neurones (Figure NE10). The first-order neurone lies in the cells of the cerebral cortex. The axons of these cells synapse on the second-order neurone situated in the anterior grey column of the spinal cord. The second-order neurone is known as the internuncial neurone, the axon of which is shorter than the axon of the first-order neurone. It synapses with the third-order neurone, known as the lower motor neurone. The lower motor neurone also lies in the anterior grey column of the spinal cord. The axon of this lower motor neurone innervates the skeletal muscle through the anterior root and the

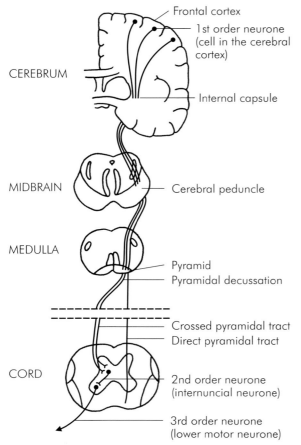

Figure NE10 Descending tract of the spinal cord

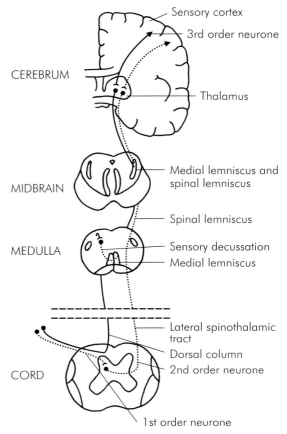

Figure NE11 Ascending tract of the spinal cord

spinal nerve. Figure NE12 gives examples of descending tracts.

Ascending tracts

Like the descending tracts, ascending tracts have three neurones (Figure NE11). The first-order neurone lies in the posterior root ganglia. The peripheral process of this neurone receives the sensory information from the sensory receptor. The central process of this neurone enters the spinal cord via the posterior root and synapses with the second-order neurone. The axon of the second-order neurone crosses the midline and synapses with the third-order neurone in the thalamus. The third-order neurone projects to the sensory cortex. Figure NE13 details important ascending tracts.

Spinal cord transection
Complete transection

In humans, cord transection is followed by a variable period of spinal shock. In this period all spinal reflexes are profoundly depressed or absent. All muscles innervated by spinal nerves below the level of the cord lesion become paralysed. The initial phase of spinal shock is followed by recovery of reflex function but the voluntary control is lost forever. The time of reflex recovery is variable, and can be delayed for up to 6 weeks, although the most frequent interval is about 2 weeks from initial injury. The first reflexes to return are flexor responses to touch and anogenital reflex responses. Reflex responses are hyperactive in the early recovery phase. Tendon reflexes are the slowest to recover. Hyperactivity of tendon reflexes can be accompanied by clonus. In paraplegic patients over time, a mass reflex response develops. This can occur even after a minor

Tract	Detail
Corticospinal tract (pyramidal tract)	First-order neurones originate in the pyramidal cells of the motor cortex. Axons descend, enter the medulla and group to form the pyramid. At the junction of medulla and cord 80% decussate to form the lateral cortocospinal tract, the remainder continuing as the anterior corticospinal tract. The axons synapse in the anterior grey column with internuncial neurones, which in turn synapse with lower motor neurones that innervate skeletal muscle.
Reticulospinal tract	Originates in the reticular formation, pons and medulla. Fibres synapse in the anterior grey column and influence α and γ motor neurones. The reticulospinal tract also carries descending autonomic fibres.
Tectospinal tract	Arises in the superior colliculus of the midbrain. Axons decussate and end in the anterior grey column in the cervical cord. Mediates reflex postural movement secondary to visual stimuli.
Rubrospinal tract	Originates in the red nucleus of the midbrain and decussates. Affects α and γ motor neurones in the anterior grey columns of the cord to facilitate flexor groups of muscles and inhibit extensors.
Vestibulospinal tract	Associated with posture and balance, having a facilitation of extensor muscle groups and inhibition of flexors.
Olivospinal tract	Originates in the olivary nucleus in the pons.
Descending autonomic fibres	Minor significance only.

Figure NE12 Detail of descending tracts of the spinal cord

Tract	Detail
Spinothalamic tract	Originates from free nerve endings in the skin carrying pain and temperature sensation. First-order neurones are Aδ and C fibres which enter the cord and synapse with second-order neurones in the posterior grey columns. Second-order neurones cross to the opposite side within one segment and ascend as the lateral spinothalamic tract. Fibres synapse with third-order neurones in the ventral posterolateral nucleus of the thalamus. Termination is the sensory area of the postcentral gyrus.
Gracile and cuneate tracts	Fibres from receptors for touch, vibration and joint proprioceptors enter the cord via the posterior root ganglia and travel in the posterior white columns of the ipsilateral side. Descending branches affect intersegmental reflexes. Ascending fibres synapse with cells in the posterior grey horn, internuncial neurones and anterior horn cells before travelling up as the gracile and cuneate tracts. Fibres synapse with second-order neurones in the gracile and cuneate nuclei of the medulla, which then decussate to travel as the medial lemniscus. The third-order neurones lie in the ventral posterolateral nucleus of the thalamus and terminate in the postcentral gyrus of the sensory cortex.
Anterior and posterior spinocerebellar tracts	Relay information from muscle and joints to the cerebellum.
Spinotectal tract	Transmits pain, temperature and touch sensation to the superior colliculus of the midbrain. Facilitates spinovisual reflexes.
Spinoreticular tract	Relays various information to the reticular formation. Affects consciousness.
Spino-olivary tract	Minor afferent path to cerebellum.

Figure NE13 Detail of ascending tracts of the spinal cord

noxious stimulus is applied to the skin. This results in evacuation of bladder and bowel, along with signs of autonomic hyperactivity such as sweating, pallor and swings in blood pressure. In complete transection there is total loss of sensation in the dermatomes supplied by the cord below the level of injury.

Hemisection of the spinal cord (Brown–Séquard syndrome)

This affects the pyramidal tracts and posterior columns of the ipsilateral side while the spinothalamic tracts which have crossed over from the opposite side are also affected. Thus there is paralysis of muscles on the same side along with loss of touch, pressure, joint and vibration sense. The pain and temperature fibres coming from the opposite side are also affected.

Blood supply of the spinal cord

Blood supply of the spinal cord arises from a single anterior spinal artery and two small posterior spinal arteries.

The anterior spinal artery is formed by the union of a branch from each vertebral artery and runs along the midline of the cord, supplying the anterior two-thirds of the spinal cord. Thrombosis of this artery can cause anterior spinal artery syndrome, in which there is paralysis due to ischaemia of the pyramidal tract, although there is sparing of the posterior columns so that sensation conveyed by these columns remains intact.

The two smaller posterior spinal arteries lie on each side of the cord posteriorly. They are derived from posterior inferior cerebellar arteries and supply the posterior third of the spinal cord. Blood vessels known as vasa coronae communicate between the anterior and posterior spinal arteries. Various radicular arteries (which arise from deep cervical, intercostal and lumbar arteries) supply the anterior and posterior spinal arteries along the spinal canal. The arteria radicularis magna (major anterior radicular artery) is the principal arterial blood supply of the lower two-thirds of the spinal cord (usually found between T11 and L3). In case of occlusion of the anterior spinal artery the blood supply of the lower two-thirds of the spinal cord may be compromised.

Anterior and posterior spinal arteries do not anastomose with each other except within the spinal cord itself.

The reflex arc

Stimulation of the reflex arc by a specific sensory stimulus produces a repetitive, specific response. The reflex arc begins with a sense organ (e.g. muscle spindle), which transmits information via the afferent neurone to the spinal cord, entering via the dorsal root or cranial nerve. The ganglia of these neurones act as a central coordinating station. The efferent nerve leaves the central station via the ventral roots or a motor cranial nerve and innervates an effector organ such as a voluntary muscle. The activity in this reflex arc is influenced by the central nervous system.

The reflex arc can be monosynaptic, i.e. a single synapse between the afferent and efferent neurone (Figure NE14), or polysynaptic, where two or more synapses occur between afferent and efferent neurones (Figure NE15). The stretch reflex is an example of a monosynaptic reflex. The sense organ for this reflex is the muscle spindle. Skeletal muscle consists of two types of muscle fibres, namely the extrafusal and intrafusal fibres. Contraction of the extrafusal fibres is controlled by motor neurones located in the anterior horn of the spinal cord. These contractions result in contraction of a muscle. The number of muscle fibres controlled by a single motor neurone varies according to the precision of the movement involved. The finer the movement the smaller the number of extrafusal fibres: in the case of muscles controlling finger movement a neurone controls fewer than 10 fibres, whereas for lower limb muscle there may be several hundred extrafusal fibres per neurone.

Structure of muscle spindles

The intrafusal fibres form specialised sensory organs called muscle spindles, which are arranged in parallel with the extrafusal fibres. These spindles respond to the change in length of surrounding extrafusal fibres and form part of the control system for maintaining posture and limb position. Each spindle consists of up to a dozen intrafusal fibres whose ends are attached to the extrafusal fibres. Each intrafusal fibre consists of two portions: the central non-contractile region and a contractile muscle fibre portion at either end. The efferent control of these contractile portions is supplied by the γ motor neurones. The central portion of the intrafusal fibres can take two forms, either a nuclear bag or a nuclear chain. The former consists of an expanded central portion containing a collection of nuclei whereas the latter consist of nuclei arranged in a chain. Two types of sensory nerve fibres innervate the central portion of the intrafusal fibres: type Ia (or annulospiral) and type II fibres. Type Ia fibres innervate both the nuclear bag fibres and nuclear chain fibres, but

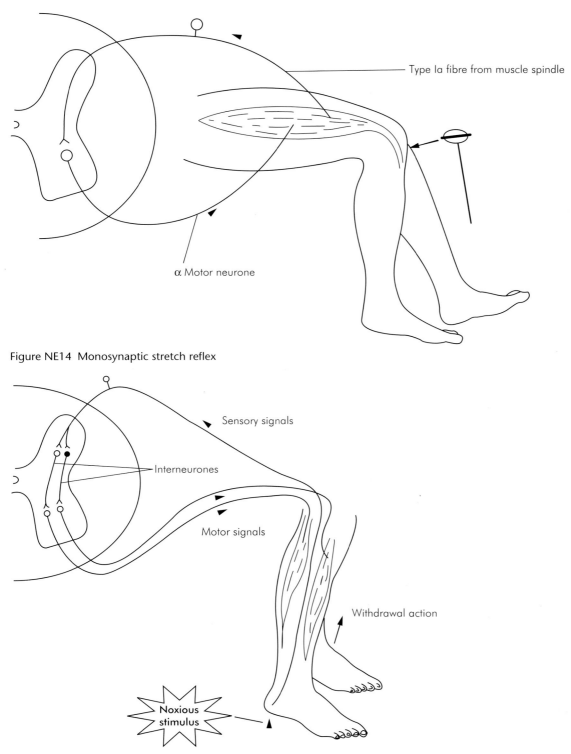

Type Ia fibre from muscle spindle

α Motor neurone

Figure NE14 Monosyntaptic stretch reflex

Sensory signals

Interneurones

Motor signals

Withdrawal action

Noxious
stimulus

Figure NE15 Polysynaptic withdrawal reflex

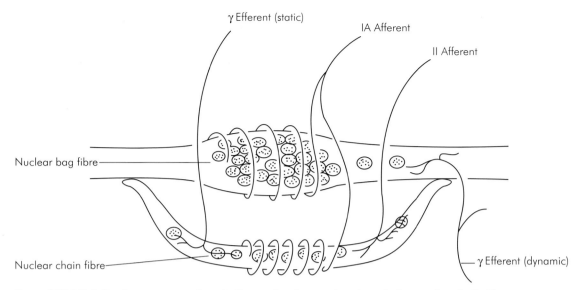

γ Efferent (static)

IA Afferent

II Afferent

Nuclear bag fibre

Nuclear chain fibre

γ Efferent (dynamic)

Figure NE16 Details of nerve connections to the nuclear bag and nuclear chain muscle spindle fibres

the type II fibres only innervate the nuclear chain fibres (Figure NE16).

Function of muscle spindles

The central portion of the muscle spindle detects the change in length of the muscle. When the whole muscle contracts, the muscle spindle relaxes, and firing in its afferent axon stops. However, the opposite occurs when the muscle relaxes or is stretched passively. In other words, the muscle spindle acts as a muscle length detector. This should not be confused with the Golgi tendon organ, which is a stretch receptor within a tendon and responds to tension, not length, within muscle.

One of the most basic functions of the muscle spindle, therefore, is to maintain muscle length. Furthermore, the sensitivity of the muscle spindle is adjustable. When the muscle spindles are relaxed, they are relatively insensitive to stretch. However, when the motor neurones are active, they become shorter and become much more sensitive to changes in muscle length. Therefore by establishing a rate of firing in the motor system, the higher centres control the length of the muscle spindles and indirectly the length of the entire muscle.

During normal movements, both the α and γ motor neurones are activated at the same time. If little resistance is encountered, both the extrafusal and intrafusal muscle fibres will contract at approximately the same rate, and as a result the central portion of the muscle spindle retains its original length before the contraction and little change in activity will be detected in the afferent axons of the spindle. If, however, the limb meets with resistance, the intrafusal muscle fibres will shorten more than the extrafusal muscle fibres, the centre of the muscle spindle becomes stretched, and the rate of firing in the afferent axons increases. This will stimulate the motor neurone and thereby increase contraction of the motor unit.

The inverse stretch reflex implies that the harder a muscle is stretched, the stronger is the reflex contraction. If the muscle tension increases excessively, the Golgi tendon organs, which are attached in series with the muscle, inhibit the activity of the motor neurone, providing an inhibitory feedback mechanism to prevent muscle damage. The relaxation in response to strong stretch is called the inverse stretch reflex. Thus, the muscle spindles and the Golgi tendon organs work hand in hand to make sure that length and tension in a muscle are appropriate to perform a particular task.

The resistance of a muscle to stretch is known as tone. When a motor nerve is cut, the muscle it supplies becomes flaccid. The muscle is hypotonic if the rate of efferent discharge is low and hypertonic when it is high. Another phenomenon seen in the hypertonic state is clonus. This occurs when a sustained and sudden force is applied to a muscle, resulting in regular rhythmic contractions of the stretched muscle.

The withdrawal reflex is a polysynaptic reflex. Contraction of flexor muscles and relaxation of the extensors in response to a painful stimulus results in withdrawal of the stimulated part. When a noxious stimulus is applied to a limb, the signal is first transmitted via sensory fibres to the interneurone(s) in the spinal cord and then on to the motor neurones (Figure NE15). The neuronal circuitry involves not only activation of muscle(s), which carry out the withdrawal, but also the inhibition of the antagonist muscles. Other muscle groups may also be stimulated or inhibited so that the withdrawal of the limb and movement of the rest of the body are coordinated to move safely away from the noxious stimulus.

Motor function

The structures involved in the control of movement are the cerebral cortex, cerebellum and basal ganglia.

Cerebral cortex

The motor cortex is situated in the frontal lobe. It is divided into three parts:

- The **primary motor cortex** is situated in the precentral gyrus. Different areas of the body are represented in the primary cortex. Parts of the body performing the finer functions have the largest representation. The facial area is represented bilaterally.
- The **premotor area** lies anterior to the primary motor cortex immediately superior to the Sylvian fissure. It is concerned with postural adjustment at the beginning of a voluntary movement.
- The **supplemental motor area** is concerned with planning of complex movements.

Motor signals are transmitted directly from the cortex to the spinal cord through the corticospinal tract and indirectly through multiple accessory pathways that involve the basal ganglia, the cerebellum, and the various nuclei of the brain stem.

Cerebellum

The cerebellum is situated in the posterior fossa and has two lateral lobes that are joined in the centre by the vermis. It is functionally divided into three parts:

- The **vestibulocerebellum** has connections with the vestibule of the middle ear and maintains the body's equilibrium during motion.

- The **spinocerebellum** is mainly concerned with proprioception. It receives information from the whole body as well as the motor cortex. Voluntary movements are coordinated here, depending on the sensory information received. The central portion of the cerebellum is concerned with axial and proximal limb muscles while the lobes control the distal musculature.
- The **neocerebellum** is involved in planned execution of voluntary movements. Fast coordinated activity is affected in cerebellar disease. Dysdiadochokinesia (the inability to perform rapid alternating movements) is a feature of cerebellar dysfunction. Other signs of cerebellar dysfunction include ataxia, scanning speech and intention tremor.

Basal ganglia

The term basal ganglia refers to the following structures: caudate nucleus, putamen, globus pallidus, subthalamic nucleus and substantia nigra.

The caudate nucleus and putamen are together called the striatum. The basal ganglia form a loop with the cortex (Figure NE17). The cortex projects to the striatum via the corticostriate projections, the striatum sends efferents to the globus pallidus, and this in turn sends efferents to the thalamus. The thalamus then communicates with the primary motor cortex via accessory motor areas.

Command for voluntary action originates in the cortical association area. It is further planned in the cortex, basal ganglia and lateral portion of the cerebellar cortex. The efferents to muscle travel in the corticospinal tract (pyramidal system) and bring about the voluntary action. The cerebellum and basal ganglia both influence voluntary action. The cerebellum enhances the stretch reflex, fine-tuning of rapid movements preventing oscillations, and the basal ganglia help by carrying out various subconscious movements which are required to carry out a voluntary activity.

Control of posture

Posture-regulating mechanisms involve structures in the spinal cord, the brain stem and the cerebral cortex.

A voluntary action requires smooth coordinated activity in different muscle groups so that posture is maintained. The postural reflexes involved are coordinated at the level of the spinal cord and are influenced by higher centres.

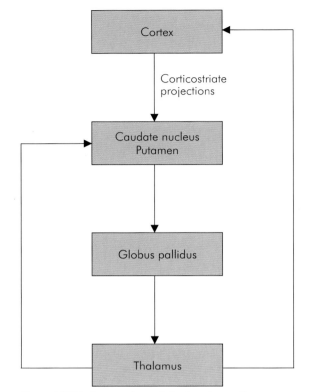

Figure NE17 Connections of the basal ganglia

When the influence of these higher centres is experimentally removed at different levels it is possible to understand the postural reflexes involved.

Spinal cord components

The stretch reflex has already been described in detail earlier. Additionally, proprioceptors in opposing flexor and extensor muscles contribute to the maintenance of an upright stance. Placing a foot on the ground stiffens the leg so that the body can be supported. This is the positive supporting reaction. The disappearance of this is known as negative supporting reaction.

Brain-stem components

These components can be studied by transection of the brain stem at the superior border of the pons. This is known as decerebration, and it causes increased rigidity. In the brain stem there are areas that facilitate and inhibit stretch reflexes. After decerebration the influence of the inhibitory area is reduced whilst that of the facilitatory area is increased, resulting in increased efferent discharge. This facilitates the stretch reflex and causes rigidity. Spasticity produced by decerebration is most marked in the extensor group of muscles as these are the antigravity muscles helping the animal to maintain its posture. In humans decerebrate rigidity causes extension in all four limbs.

The scale of rigidity of the limbs in a decerebrate animal is position-related. In the prone position the rigidity is minimal, while if the animal is on its back the rigidity is maximal. This is known as the tonic labyrinthine reflex. The receptors for this reflex are in the otolithic organs.

When the head of the decerebrate animal is turned to one side, the limbs on that side become more rigidly extended and the limbs on the opposite side become less rigid. Flexion of the neck causes flexion of the forelimbs and hindlimbs. The reverse happens with the extension of the head. This is known as the tonic neck reflex, and it is initiated by the stretch receptors in the neck.

Midbrain components

Midbrain components can be studied by interrupting the neural pathways at the superior border of the midbrain. In the midbrain animal, the phasic postural reflexes are intact so that the animal can stand, walk and correct its position. Rigidity is seen only when the animal is at rest, as it is due to static postural reflexes.

The righting reflexes, such as the labyrinthine righting reflex, body on head righting reflex, neck righting reflex, and body on body righting reflex, are essential for maintaining the normal position of the animal. These reflexes are coordinated by the nuclei in the midbrain.

Cortical components

Removal of the cerebral cortex is called decortication. In the decorticate animal there is loss of the cortical area that inhibits γ-efferent discharge. The increased (γ) efferent discharge causes facilitation of the stretch reflex, leading to rigidity. This is only seen at rest, due to the presence of phasic postural reflexes. Postural reactions like hopping and placing reaction are seriously affected by decortication.

Cerebrospinal fluid (CSF)

Cerebrospinal fluid (CSF) is present in the cerebral ventricles and the subarachnoid space. The total volume of CSF is about 150 ml. Approximately 550 ml of CSF is produced per day in an adult. Most (50–70%) of the CSF is produced in the choroid plexuses of the lateral, third and fourth ventricles, which are highly vascular invaginations of pia mater, covered by single-layered ependymal epithelium. It is formed by secretion and filtration of plasma. Formation of CSF is not affected by intracranial pressure, but removal of CSF increases with increasing pressure. CSF from the lateral ventricles drains into the third ventricle via the foramina of Monro. From the third ventricle it travels to the fourth ventricle via the aqueduct of Sylvius. It enters the cerebral subarachnoid space through the median foramen of Magendie and lateral foramina of Luschka. CSF is absorbed into the venous sinuses by the arachnoid villi. Arachnoid villi are projections of arachnoid into the venous sinuses which are covered by a single-layered endothelium of the venous sinuses. The composition and circulation of the CSF is covered in more detail in Section 2, Chapter 2 (pages 230–1).

Larger molecular weight substances do not pass from blood into the CSF or the interstitial spaces of the brain due to the presence of 'tight junctions' between the endothelium of cerebral capillaries. This blood–brain barrier is highly permeable to water, carbon dioxide, oxygen and most lipid-soluble substances such as volatile anaesthetic agents. The barrier is impermeable to plasma proteins and large molecular weight substances.

Intracranial pressure (ICP)

Intracranial pressure (ICP) is the pressure inside the cranial vault relative to atmospheric pressure. Normal intracranial pressure ranges between 5 and 15 mmHg, although this varies with arterial pulsation, breathing, coughing and straining. The intracranial contents can be divided into four compartments: solid material ($\approx$ 10%), tissue water ($\approx$ 75%), CSF (150 ml, $\approx$ 10%), blood (50–75 ml, $\approx$ 5%).

These compartments are all contained within the rigid cranial vault, and a change in volume of one compartment is accompanied by a reciprocal change in another compartment (The Monro–Kellie doctrine).

Control of ICP

Raised ICP causes brain damage by reducing cerebral perfusion pressure (CPP) or by focal compression of brain tissue due to distortion and herniation of intracranial contents. Control of ICP depends on compensatory mechanisms involving the four compartments described above.

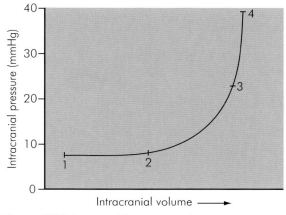

Figure NE18 Intracranial pressure–volume curve

Volume buffering is illustrated in Figure NE18. With an increase in intracranial volume, compensatory mechanisms maintain ICP within the normal range (between point 1 and point 2 on the figure). At point 2, further increases in volume cause a slight rise in ICP. As volume increases, there is a steady decline in compliance, which increases the ICP even more (point 3) until a small rise in volume is associated with a marked rise in ICP, causing a fall in the perfusion pressure and ultimately cerebral ischaemia (between points 3 and 4).

The CSF plays a major part in compensating for an increase in intracranial volume. As a space-occupying lesion expands, it will cause progressive reduction of the CSF space (reduced size of the ventricles and basal cisterns). CSF outflow into the spinal canal increases, and its absorption into the venous system is also increased. Rapid rises in intracranial volume (e.g. acute intracranial haematoma) exhaust spatial compensation quickly, resulting in a rapid rise of ICP.

Another important compensatory mechanism is provided by changes in cerebral blood volume (CBV). Most of the intracranial blood volume is contained in venous sinuses and the pial veins, and only a small change in CBV can have a profound effect on ICP. A rise in ICP decreases cerebral perfusion pressure (CPP). CPP is related to ICP by the formula:

CPP = mean arterial pressure $-$ (ICP $=$ JVP)

Thus a reduction in CPP triggers pressure autoregulation, which causes vasodilatation to maintain a constant cerebral blood flow (CBF). This results in a rise in CBV and consequently a rise in ICP in a non-compliant or swollen

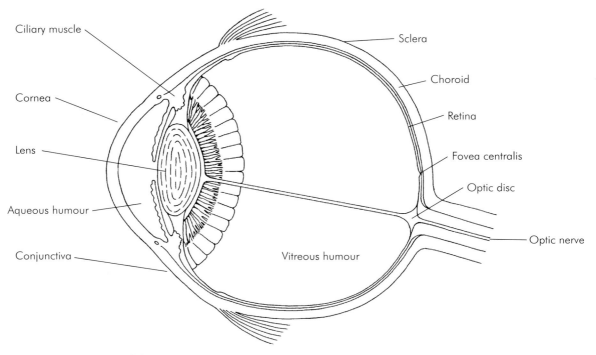

Figure NE19 Structure of the eye

brain. Conversely, a rise in mean arterial pressure will within autoregulatory limits cause cerebral vasoconstriction, resulting in a reduction in CBV and ICP.

Arterial blood gas values also have a major contribution to CBF and CBV. Both CBF and CBV increase with raised $PaCO_2$, but the CBV response curve is flatter than the CBF curve. A reduction in $PaCO_2$ from 5.3 to 2.7 kPa results in a 65% reduction in CBF but only a 28% reduction in CBV. This small decrease in intracranial volume will cause a significant reduction in ICP in the presence of intracranial hypertension, because the system operates on the steep part of the pressure–volume curve. A reduction in arterial oxygen tension causes cerebral vasodilatation, resulting in a rise in CBV.

Increased metabolic demand increases CBF, CBV and ICP due to flow metabolism coupling. Reduction in cerebral metabolism (using intravenous anaesthetic agents, for example) will reduce CBV, and this is a useful therapeutic intervention in patients with raised ICP.

A rise in cerebral venous blood volume will also increase CBV and ICP. Venous distension is a common cause of increased cerebral venous volume and can occur

from jugular venous obstruction, increased intrathoracic pressure, raised central venous pressure, head-down tilt etc. For details see Section 2, Chapter 6 (Figure CR35).

Special senses

Vision

Structure of the eye

Before reaching the photoreceptors on the retina, light must pass through the optical apparatus that is made up of the cornea, aqueous humour, lens and vitreous humour (Figure NE19). The globe is protected by the sclera, which becomes transparent in the anterior part of the eye known as the cornea. Aqueous humour is produced by the ciliary processes and catalysed by the action of carbonic anhydrase; it passes from the posterior chamber through the pupil into the anterior chamber of the eye. It is then drained into a vein via the canal of Schlemm (located at the angle of the anterior chamber).

Pupillary size is determined by the activities of the smooth muscle fibres in the iris: the circular fibres constrict (miosis) while the radial fibres dilate (mydriasis) the

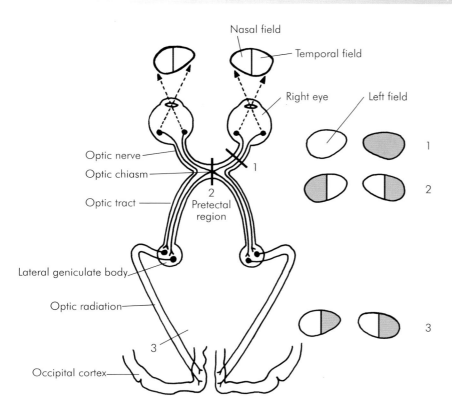

Figure NE20 Visual pathway, and the effect of three different lesions on the visual field

pupil. The interior surface of the globe is lined by the retina, except where the optic nerve leaves the eye and where the ciliary muscle begins. The ciliary muscle changes the tension of the suspensory ligaments, which alters the convexity of the lens and thereby achieves accommodation.

The retina

The retina is made up of photoreceptors – rods and cones. These are located along the outer surface of the retina adjacent to the pigment epithelium. The blood supply of the photoreceptors is derived from the choroid and not from blood vessels on the inner retinal surface. There are about 120 million rods and only 7 million cones in each eye. Rods are uniformly distributed throughout the retina and are responsible for night and monochromatic vision. They contain the pigment rhodopsin. Cones, however, are concentrated in the fovea and are responsible for bright and colour vision. Cones contain opsins that are sensitive to red, green and blue.

The visual pathway

Electrical potential is generated when light reaches the photoreceptors on the retina. This potential is then transmitted to the ganglion cells via the bipolar and/or the horizontal and amacrine cells. Axons from the ganglion cells converge at the blind spot of the optic disc to form the optic nerve. The axons coming from the nasal half of the retina decussate at the optic chiasm, while those situated on the temporal half remain on the ipsilateral side (Figure NE19). These then synapse in the lateral geniculate nuclei. From here, synaptic connections are made via the optic radiation to the primary visual cortex, giving rise to a topographical projection of the visual field around the calcarine fissure. Some fibres of the optic tracts relay to the superior colliculi, which are involved in the control of eye movements or posture. Lesions in the visual pathway will give visual field defects according to their position. Thus, as shown in Figure NE20, the following lesions will give rise to their corresponding defects:

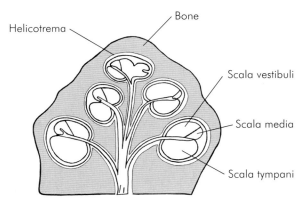

Figure NE21 Cochlea in cross section

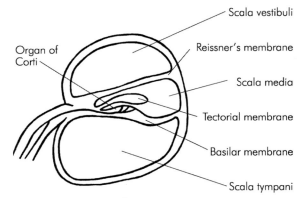

Figure NE22 Organ of Corti

- Lesion 1 – right-eye blindness
- Lesion 2 – bitemporal hemianopia
- Lesion 3 – right homonymous hemianopia

Hearing
Structure of the ear
The ear is divided into external, middle and internal compartments. The external compartment consists of the pinna, which directs sound waves via the external auditory meatus to the tympanic membrane. Vibrations of the tympanic membrane transmit sound energy to the middle ear, which consists of the ossicles: malleus, incus and stapes. The latter stimulates the inner ear through the oval window. The middle ear is air-filled and is connected to the pharynx via the Eustachian tube, which allows equilibration of pressure to occur between the middle ear and the environment. The inner ear consists of the cochlea, which is a bony coiled tube divided lengthwise into three canals by two membranes: the scala vestibuli and scala media (or cochlear duct) are separated by Reissner's membrane, while the scala media and scala tympani are separated by the basilar membrane (Figure NE21). The scala tympani communicates with the middle ear via the round window. The inner ear is fluid-filled: the scala media is filled with endolymph, while the scala vestibuli and tympani, being joined at the helicotrema, are filled with perilymph. The sound receptors are found in the organ of Corti (Figure NE22), which is located on the basilar membrane within the cochlear duct. The organ of Corti is made up of an epithelium of hair cells and supporting cells. Each hair cell is anchored on the basilar membrane and has a bundle of hairs projecting from its tip into the scala media. Directly opposite to these hair cells is the tectorial membrane. The hair cells synapse with dendrites of the ganglion cells, which in turn synapse with fibres from the cochlear nerve. The latter traverses the subarachnoid space and enters the brain stem at the pontomedullary junction.

Mechanism of hearing
Sound waves produce vibrations of the tympanic membrane that lead to movements of the ossicles. Movements of the footplate of the stapes in the oval window are converted to pressure waves in the scala vestibuli. These pressure waves are then transmitted in the endolymphatic canal to reach the basilar membrane. Such oscillations cause displacements of the tectorial membrane with respect to the basilar membrane. The hair cells situated on the latter are thus stimulated and become depolarised. The resulting receptor potential is then transmitted via the underlying ganglion cells to the cochlear nerve. All the cochlear nerve fibres terminate at the cochlear nucleus in the brain stem. From here, second-order fibres project mainly to the contralateral (and to a lesser extent to the ipsilateral) inferior colliculus via the lateral lemniscus. From the inferior colliculus, connections are projected, via the medial geniculate body, to the primary auditory cortex in the temporal lobe.

Taste and olfaction
Taste
Taste buds are made up of specialised epithelial cells (taste cells) and supporting cells, which are located on the surface of the tongue, soft palate and oropharynx.

Most taste buds are found on protuberances called papillae at the back of the tongue. Taste cells have a half-life of about 2 weeks and are constantly being replenished by division of the underlying basal cells. There are four basic tastes: sweet, sour, salty and bitter. All complex tastes are thought to be composed of different combinations of the basic tastes. Nearly all tastes are the combined result of taste and smell. The transduction process of taste is poorly understood: it is thought that chemicals in food interact with chemoreceptors on the surface membrane of taste cells to induce a change in membrane permeability to Na^+ ions. This leads to depolarisation of taste cells, which then leads to the production of generator potentials in the afferent nerve fibres. Taste buds are innervated by the chorda tympani (anterior two-thirds of the tongue), glossopharyngeal (posterior third of the tongue), vagus (epiglottis), and greater petrosal (soft palate) nerves. These then relay in the tractus solitarius in the medulla before projecting to the thalamus and cortex.

Olfaction

Olfactory cells are specialised bipolar neurones found in the olfactory epithelium in the roof of the nasal cavity. The olfactory epithelium also contains basal and supporting cells. Olfactory cells are the only neurones in the body known to be replaced continually by division of the underlying basal cells. Situated at the apical region of these cells are long cilia embedded in a layer of mucus, produced by the supporting cells. Odoriferous compounds reach the olfactory epithelium by diffusion, which is facilitated by sniffing to increase the airflow. These compounds must first dissolve in the mucus; the chemical interactions between odoriferous chemicals and the chemoreceptors on the cilia trigger changes in ion conductance in the olfactory cell, resulting in the generation of action potentials in the olfactory neurones. The axons of the olfactory nerve pass through the cribriform plate and enter the olfactory bulb. Here there is complex signal processing in that there is marked convergence of afferent inputs and also the presence of interneurones. From here second-order neurones project to the olfactory cortex and also to other regions such as the thalamus and the limbic system.

Autonomic nervous system

The autonomic nervous system (ANS) is that part of the nervous system which controls the visceral activities of the body. This control is involuntary and enables the body to adjust to varying physiological demands. For example, one cannot consciously increase cardiac output, but when physical threat is detected, the ANS will initiate changes in various systems of the body which enable the individual to deal with the physical demand. The ANS is controlled mainly by centres in the brain stem and hypothalamus. Sensory inputs are relayed to these areas and reflex responses are effected in the visceral organs. Acting in concert with the hypothalamus and the endocrine system, the ANS is largely responsible for the control of the internal environment of the body.

There are two subdivisions, the sympathetic and the parasympathetic nervous system. In general, the two systems are antagonistic to each other. It is not always predictable whether sympathetic or parasympathetic stimulation will produce inhibition or excitation in a particular organ, but most organs are predominantly controlled by one or the other system. This background activity is known as the sympathetic or parasympathetic tone. For example, arteriolar smooth muscle has a predominant sympathetic tone, whereas the basal tone in the gut is mainly parasympathetic.

Sympathetic nervous system

Neurones of the sympathetic nervous system originate in the thoracic and lumbar segments (from T1 to L2) of the spinal cord, the so-called thoracolumbar outflow (Figure NE23). These synapse in a paired chain of ganglia, the sympathetic ganglia, situated on either side of the vertebral column. The nerve fibres which run from the spinal cord to the sympathetic ganglia are known as preganglionic fibres, while those which leave the ganglia to reach their effector organs are known as postganglionic fibres. A few of the preganglionic fibres pass through the sympathetic chain without forming synapses until they arrive at a more peripheral location in the coeliac and mesenteric ganglia or the adrenal medulla. The adrenal medulla is unique in that it is innervated by sympathetic preganglionic fibres but has no postganglionic nerve fibres.

Parasympathetic nervous system

The parasympathetic nervous system leaves the central nervous system via cranial nerves (III, VII, IX and X) and sacral nerves (S2,3,4). This is called the craniosacral outflow. Approximately three-quarters of all parasympathetic fibres are located in the two vagus (X) nerves. Like the sympathetic pathway, the parasympathetic system has both preganglionic and postganglionic neurones. However, the cell bodies of the parasympathetic ganglia are located within the effector organs themselves, and so the preganglionic fibres travel long distances from the spinal cord and the postganglionic fibres are therefore relatively short.

Parasympathetic system　　　　　　　　**Sympathetic system**

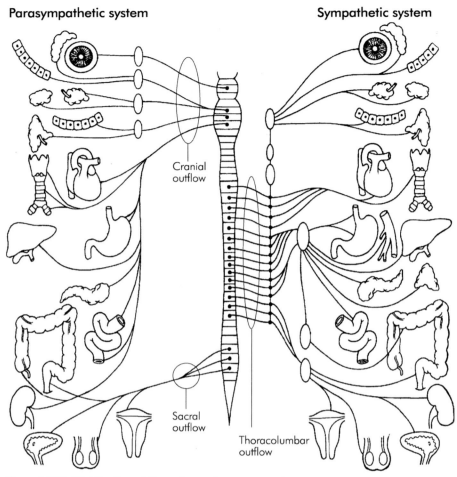

Cranial
outflow

Sacral
outflow

Thoracolumbar
outflow

Figure NE23 Distribution of the autonomic nervous system

Neurotransmitters and receptors in the autonomic nervous system

The sympathetic and parasympathetic nerve fibres release either acetylcholine or norepinephrine in the nerve endings. All preganglionic fibres are cholinergic in both the sympathetic and parasympathetic ganglia. Nearly all the postganglionic neurones of the parasympathetic system are also cholinergic but a few may release vasoactive intestinal polypeptide (VIP). Most of the postganglionic sympathetic fibres are noradrenergic, except in sweat glands, piloerector muscles and a few blood vessels, where they are cholinergic.

Sympathetic stimulation to the adrenal medulla releases epinephrine and norepinephrine into the circulation. In general, about 80% of the secretion is epinephrine and 20% is norepinephrine, but this proportion may change considerably depending on physiological conditions. There are two major types of adrenoceptors: α and β receptors. Norepinephrine acts predominantly on α receptors, whereas epinephrine acts on both α and β adrenoceptors. Alpha receptors can also be divided into two types: α_1 and α_2, and there are three subtypes of β adrenoceptors.

There are two types of cholinergic receptors: nicotinic and muscarinic. Nicotinic receptors are found in both the sympathetic and parasympathetic ganglia. On the other hand, muscarinic receptors are located in the postganglionic parasympathetic synapses. Although five distinct

- Tachycardia
- Raised arterial pressure
- Sweating
- Pupillary dilatation
- Increase in blood glucose concentration
- Increase in glycolysis and gluconeogenesis
- Redistribution of blood flow from splanchnic to cerebral and coronary circulation
- Increase in cellular metabolism throughout the body
- Increase in mental alertness

Figure NE24 'Stress' responses due to sympathetic mass discharge

subclasses of muscarinic receptors have been identified by gene cloning, functionally there are three subtypes: M_1 receptors are found mainly in the CNS; M_2 receptors are located in the heart; M_3 receptors are found in exocrine glands and vascular endothelium.

Consequences of autonomic stimulation

In life-threatening situations, the sympathetic nervous system discharges almost as a complete unit, a phenomenon known as mass discharge. This may occur when the hypothalamus is activated by fear, noxious stimulus or severe pain. There is stimulation of different systems and organs simultaneously to prepare the individual for survival. The resulting sympathetic 'stress' response is summarised in Figure NE24.

The parasympathetic nervous system, on the contrary, is more organ-specific. For example, stimulation of the heart by the parasympathetic system is quite separate from that of gastric secretion. Nevertheless, there is some association between closely related functions; for example, although salivary secretion can occur separately from gastric secretion, they are often coordinated and occur together.

Limbic system

The limbic system is made up of a number of cortical and subcortical structures situated around the basal regions of the cerebrum. It is principally involved in the control of instinctive and learned behaviour, emotions, sexual and motivational drives. The limbic system has extensive neuronal connections with the frontal and temporal cortex. The most important components of the limbic system consist of the hypothalamus, amygdala and hippocampus (Figure NE25).

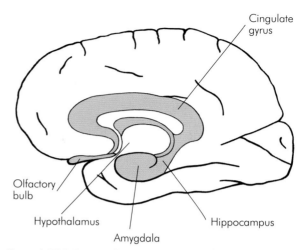

Figure NE25 Paramedian sagittal section of the brain showing different components of the limbic system

Hippocampus and amygdala

As with other structures within the limbic system, stimulation of different areas of the hippocampus also leads to behavioural and emotional changes such as increased sex drive, rage and placidity. In addition, when the hippocampi have been surgically excised, the end result is anterograde amnesia and some degree of retrograde amnesia. It is therefore suggested that the hippocampus may be involved in both short- and long-term memory processes. Due to the extensive neuronal connections between it and various areas of the brain, stimulation of the amygdala not only causes effects similar to that of the hypothalamus, but also widespread behavioural patterns. It is thought that the amygdala projects into the limbic system the current behavioural status in relation to both the surroundings and the thoughts of the individual. It is believed to help pattern the behavioural response of the individual so that it is appropriate for each occasion.

Hypothalamus

The hypothalamus is situated just rostral to the brain stem in the basal region of the brain. Inferior to it is the pituitary gland. It has extensive neuronal connections to the brain stem, pituitary gland and cerebrum. Together with other limbic structures and the endocrine system, the hypothalamus controls the vegetative and endocrine functions of the body as well as many aspects of emotional behaviour. The hypothalamus maintains homeostatic control of the internal environment, and as such it plays a central role

- Control of body temperature
- Regulation of water balance
- Control of food intake
- Control over endocrine system via pituitary gland
- Behavioural and emotional influence

Figure NE26 Functions of the hypothalamus

- Adrenocorticotropic hormone-releasing hormone (corticotropin-releasing hormone)
- Thyrotropin-releasing hormone
- Growth hormone-releasing hormone
- Luteinising hormone-releasing hormone
- Follicle-stimulating hormone-releasing hormone
- Prolactin-releasing hormone
- Prolactin-inhibiting hormone

Figure NE27 Hypothalamic releasing and inhibiting hormones

in the control of body temperature, pituitary secretion, osmolality of body fluids and the drive to eat and drink (Figure NE26).

Control of body temperature

The hypothalamus receives and processes information from both the central thermoreceptors, situated in the preoptic (anterior) part of the hypothalamus itself, and the peripheral thermoreceptors found on the skin. Physiological changes are initiated in response to temperature changes so that a nearly constant body temperature is maintained. For example, in response to cold the hypothalamus will initiate peripheral vasoconstriction and shivering. At the same time, behavioural changes also occur so that a lowering of environmental temperature will lead to an increase in muscular activity to generate heat, and extra layers of clothes may be added to conserve heat.

Control of pituitary secretion

Anterior pituitary secretion is controlled by releasing and inhibiting hormones carried in the portal hypophyseal vessels from the hypothalamus to the pituitary gland. These chemical agents are secreted by nerve endings in the median eminence of the hypothalamus. These nerve endings are in close proximity to the capillary loops from which the portal vessels are formed. There are seven hypothalamic releasing and inhibiting hormones, as summarised in Figure NE27.

The posterior pituitary gland secretes the hormones oxytocin and vasopressin. They are synthesised in the neurones in the supraoptic and paraventricular nuclei of the hypothalamus and are transported down the axons to their endings in the posterior pituitary, where they are released into the circulation. Oxytocin is released when the breast is suckled and is responsible for milk ejection. It also causes contraction of the uterine smooth muscle. The release of vasopressin depends on the osmolality of the plasma. Even small changes in osmolality may cause significant changes

in vasopressin release. The main effect of vasopressin is water retention by the kidneys. It increases the permeability of the collecting ducts of the kidney so that more water is reabsorbed.

Water balance

The hypothalamus maintains water balance by controlling both water intake and water loss. Electrical stimulation or injection of hypertonic saline into the anterior hypothalamus leads to the desire to drink. Drinking is regulated by changes in plasma osmolality and extracellular fluid (ECF) volume. Depletion in ECF volume leads to thirst. The thirst sensation is mediated partly by vasopressin release from the hypothalamus and also via the rennin–angiotensin system. When an individual is dehydrated, plasma osmolality increases and the volume of the ECF (therefore plasma volume) decreases. As a consequence, the hypothalamic osmoreceptors and stretch receptors in the large vessels are stimulated and vasopressin is released from the hypothalamus. However, the stimuli for vasopressin release as a result of changes in plasma osmolality and plasma volume may override one another. For instance, during haemorrhage the resulting hypovolaemia increases vasopressin release even when the plasma is hypotonic.

Food intake

Two hypothalamic centres, the feeding centre and the satiety centre, control food intake. Animal studies suggest that the two centres are antagonistic. Electrical stimulation of the feeding centre results in feeding behaviour, while stimulation of the satiety centre stops feeding behaviour. It is also suggested that the feeding centre is constantly active and its activity is only temporarily inhibited by the satiety centre after food intake. The level of blood glucose probably controls the activity of the satiety centre. After a meal, blood glucose rises and the satiety centre is activated, inhibiting the feeding centre.

Behavioural functions

Apart from the functions described above, animal studies suggest that stimulation of or lesions in the hypothalamus lead to significant changes in behaviour. For instance, stimulation in the ventromedial hypothalamus leads to placidity and satiety whereas stimulation in the lateral hypothalamus leads to increased rage, restlessness and fighting behaviours. Stimulation of the extreme anterior and posterior areas of the hypothalamus increases sexual drive. Destructive lesions such as tumours usually lead to the opposite effects.

Physiology of pain

E. S. Lin

Pain has been defined as 'an unpleasant sensory and emotional experience associated with actual or potential tissue damage' by the International Association for the Study of Pain (IASP), which has become the parent organisation for many national pain societies. This definition has arisen from a consideration of some of the features of pain as a multimodal experience. These include:

- Pain has a protective function, and may or may not be associated with tissue damage.
- Pain should not be equated to nociception. Nociception is usually a component of pain symptoms but not necessarily so.
- Intrinsic modulatory mechanisms exist in the body which attenuate the intensity of the pain experience.
- Sensitisation mechanisms exist which intensify pain symptoms, resulting in the phenomenon of hyperalgesia.
- Pain possesses a subjective and affective element as a result of connections between the pain system, the cortical centres and the limbic system.
- Pain levels are also influenced by past experience and anticipation, due to interaction between the pain system and the prefrontal cortex.
- Pain can affect visceral and neuroendocrine function as a result of interconnections with medullary centres and the hypothalamus.

Nociception

Nociception is the sensory modality by which noxious stimuli are detected peripherally, and transmitted centrally to the central nervous system (Figure PP1). Noxious stimuli may or may not be associated with tissue damage. The pathway by which nociception is mediated consists of:

- Nociceptors
- Dorsal root ganglia containing the body of the nociceptor
- The dorsal horn of the spinal cord
- The primary synapse
- Ascending tracts
- The thalamus and higher centres

Nociceptors

The primary afferent neurones for pain are referred to as nociceptors, which possess specialised nerve endings existing in almost all tissues of the body. These primary afferents respond to different types of intense noxious stimuli. Such stimuli are most commonly mechanical, thermal or chemical. Nociceptors are characterised by:

- The type of stimuli they are sensitive to
- The class of nerve fibre serving the receptor
- The receptor response characteristics – slow or fast, short or long latency
- The ion channel proteins expressed on the receptor cell membrane

Fundamentals of Anaesthesia, 3rd edition, ed. Tim Smith, Colin Pinnock and Ted Lin. Published by Cambridge University Press. © Cambridge University Press 2008.

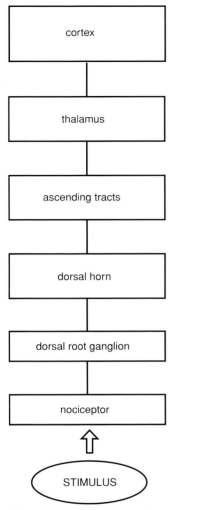

Figure PP1 Nociceptive pathway

Unimodal receptors respond to mechanical distortion, thermal receptors to heat, and polymodal receptors to mechanical distortion, heat, cold or chemical stimuli. The majority of receptors are polymodal, being sensitive to mechano-heat stimuli (MH). Some receptors are sensitive only to mechanical stimuli and are referred to as mechanically sensitive afferents (MSA), while other receptors are insensitive to mechanical stimuli (mechanically insensitive afferents, MIA).

There are two main types of nociceptor fibre which transmit nociceptor signals to the central nervous system, C fibres and Aδ fibres.

C nociceptors

These nociceptors are unmyelinated, with conduction velocities $<2\,\mathrm{m\,s^{-1}}$. They evoke slow-response burning pain and dull aching pain. They are mostly polymodal, responding to heat, mechanical and chemical stimuli. These nociceptors may be referred to using the nomenclature CMH (C mechano-heat nociceptors). Some C-fibre nociceptors are mechanically insensitive, and are referred to as C-fibre MIAs.

Aδ nociceptors

These nociceptors are connected centrally by myelinated fibres, with conduction velocities between $15\,\mathrm{m\,s^{-1}}$ and $55\,\mathrm{m\,s^{-1}}$. Aδ fibres evoke sharp fast-response pains of a burning, stabbing, pricking and aching nature. There are two types of Aδ nociceptor. Type I have higher conduction velocities ($>25\,\mathrm{m\,s^{-1}}$) and are found in hairy and glabrous skin (palms of hands and soles of feet). These Aδ nociceptors may be referred to as AMHs (A mechano-heat nociceptors). Type II are slower, with conduction velocities of around $15\,\mathrm{m\,s^{-1}}$, and are distributed in hairy skin only. An outline of their contrasting responses to stimuli is shown in Figure PP2.

Response	Type I	Type II
Mechanical	Usually sensitive (MSA)	Usually insensitive (MIA)
Heat	Insensitive (high threshold) initially with increasing response to prolonged stimulus (>5 s)	Sensitive (low threshold) initially with decreasing response to prolonged stimulus
	Long latency	Short latency
Chemical	Sensitive	Sensitive

Figure PP2 Responses of type I and type II Aδ nociceptors

Cellular functions of nociceptors

Nociceptors function by:

- Transducing and encoding noxious stimuli to generate afferent action potentials
- Synthesising and releasing neuropeptides such as calcitonin gene-related peptide (CGRP) and substance P, both peripherally and centrally
- Synthesising and releasing neurotrophins such as glial cell line-derived neurotrophic factor (GDNF) and nerve growth factor (NGF), which modulate gene expression in the nociceptor
- Synthesising and releasing neurotransmitters at the primary synapse, e.g. glutamate
- Synthesising and releasing inflammatory mediators which sensitise the nociceptive pathway centrally and peripherally

These functions are initiated by ion channels and receptors in the nociceptor cell membrane. Each nociceptor cell membrane possesses different types of ion channel. They include transient receptor potential (TRP) ion channels, ligand-gated ion channels and voltage-gated ion channels. The nociceptor cell membrane also possesses many different types of receptor. Some receptors control associated ion channels. These are ionotropic receptors. Others, such as tyrosine kinase (trk) receptors, signal intracellular pathway receptors, resulting in the synthesis and release of peptides, neurotransmitters or neurotrophic factors. These are known as metabotropic receptors.

Ion channels

Nociceptors possess families of ion channels in their cell membranes with the following properties:

- They are usually specific for sodium, potassium, calcium or hydrogen ions (acid-sensing ion channels, ASICs). However, non-specific ion channels also exist.
- Some ion channels transduce physical or chemical stimuli into transient changes in membrane potential which initiate action potentials. These are transient receptor potential (TRP) channels which are gated by noxious high-intensity stimuli such as pressure, heat, hydrogen ions (H^+) or chemicals (ligand gating). A spectrum of TRP channels may exist on a nociceptor cell membrane. These may possess different thresholds to temperature, or may be sensitised/inhibited by specific ligands.
- TRP channels can be sensitised or activated by inflammatory mediators released by damaged tissue or by the nociceptors themselves. This results in

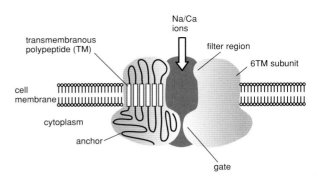

Figure PP3 Transient receptor potential channel (TRP)

hyperalgesia. A prominent TRP channel in hyperalgesic conditions is the TRPV1 (vanilloid 1) channel, which is a calcium/sodium channel. The TRPV1 channel can also be potentiated by heat and H^+, and is inhibited by glycine or intracellular phosphatidylinositol diphosphate (PIP_2) (Figure PP3).

- Voltage-gated channels are opened at different thresholds of membrane potential. Such channels can be triggered by the transient changes in membrane potential produced when TRPV channels are activated. Opening some voltage-gated channels can thus initiate a cascade which leads to the formation of an action potential. In this way a stimulus can be encoded into action potentials with a rate which varies according to the intensity of the stimulus.
- An example of such a channel is the voltage-gated sodium channel. Up to 9 different voltage-gated sodium channels have been identified in a single nociceptor cell membrane. Individual members of such families of ion channels are identified by established nomenclature, e.g. ion channels specific to nociceptors have been identifed as Nav 1.8 and 1.9 (Na, sodium; v, voltage-gated; 1, gene subfamily; 8, isoform).

Nociception and inflammatory mediators

When a noxious stimulus is applied, chemical mediators such as prostaglandins, hydrogen ions and kinins are released by the nociceptor, or as a result of tissue damage. These substances not only initiate nociception but also produce hyperalgesia. In addition to these effects in the pain response, these agents mediate the inflammatory process by inducing the following changes:

- Increases in local blood flow and vascular permeability
- Activation and migration of immune cells

Histamine

Serotonin (5-HT)

Tryptase

Kinins
 Bradykinin
 Kallidin

Eicosanoids
 Prostanoids
 Leukotrienes
  Leukotriene A_4
  Leukotriene B_4
  SRS-A   Leukotriene C_4
      Leukotriene D_4
      Leukotriene E_4

Cytokines
 Interleukins
  IL-1β
  IL-8
 Tumour necrosis factor (TNF)
  TNF-α
  Lymphotoxin (TNF-β)
 Neurotrophic factors
  Nerve growth factor (NGF)
  Brain-derived neurotrophic factor (BDNF)
  Glial cell line-derived neurotrophic factor
   (GDNF)
  Interferon (IFN-α, β and γ)

Figure PP4 Peripheral inflammatory mediators

- Release of growth and trophic factors from surrounding tissues

There are different mechanisms by which inflammatory mediators influence nociceptor function:
- Activation of membrane ion channels, e.g. lipid metabolite activation of TRPV1 channels, proton activation of ASICs, ATP activation of purinergic (P2X) channels.
- Activation of G-protein coupled receptors which increase the activities of second messengers such as cAMP or inositol triphosphate (IP$_3$). These in turn may lead to structural changes in membrane ion channels, or changes in the activity of intracellular enzymes affecting membrane excitability.
- Activation of cytokine receptors by interleukins (IL-1), or tumour necrosis factor α (TNF-α).
- Activation of tyrosine kinase receptors trkA, trkB, by specific neurotrophic factors such as NGF (which

Mediator	Source/origin
Bradykinin	Damaged tissue
Arachidonites	Arachidonic acid
Serotonin	Platelet and mast cells
Histamine	Mast cells
Cytokines (TNF-α, IL-1)	Immune system
Intracellular molecules (ATP, NO)	Damaged tissue
Neurotrophins (NGF, GDNF, BDNF)	Nociceptors

Figure PP5 Some inflammatory mediators and their origins

activates trkA) and brain-derived neurotrophic factor, BDNF (which activates trkB).

A classification of inflammatory mediators is shown in Figure PP4, with examples of the origins of some inflammatory mediators in Figure PP5.

The dorsal root ganglion (DRG)
The dorsal root ganglion contains the cell bodies for all primary afferents, including the nociceptors. The primary afferent fibres are classified according to conduction velocity. Aα and Aβ fibres are the fastest group, with large cell bodies, and form about 40% of the DRG cells. Aδ and C fibres are slower, with small cell bodies, and form about 60% of the DRG population. Nociceptors form the majority of the small cells. They can be further classified into peptidergic if they contain peptides (CGRP, substance P, somatostatin) or non-peptidergic. Approximately 50% of C and 20% of Aδ fibres are peptidergic. Although nociceptors are mainly small-cell-bodied, some nociceptors also exist in the faster larger neurone groups. Specific populations of DRG neurones can be identified by the expression of different neurotrophin receptors on their cell membranes. The DRG is situated in the lateral foramen between neighbouring vertebral bodies and is in close relationship to the sympathetic chain (Figure PP6). This anatomical relationship becomes significant in chronic pain conditions such as complex regional pain syndrome (CRPS), in which abnormal overgrowth of the DRG by fibres from the sympathetic chain is thought to be responsible for the sympathetically maintained symptoms and trophic changes in the affected areas.

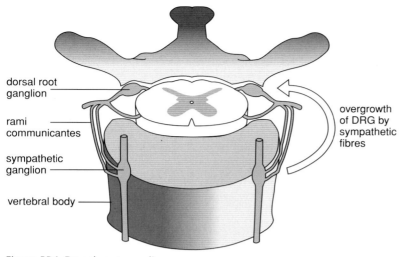

Figure PP6 Dorsal root ganglion

The dorsal horn

Nociceptors terminate almost exclusively in the dorsal horn of the spinal cord. The dorsal horn contains the following neuronal elements which participate in nociception:

- Primary afferent axons and their synapses connecting with secondary neurones or interneurones
- Secondary neurones, which project afferent information to the brain via ascending tracts.
- Interneurones, which form interconnection circuits at one level, or can ascend and descend to interconnect in other segments
- Descending axons from supraspinal centres modulating nociception

The grey matter of the spinal cord was divided into ten laminae (numbered I to X) by Rexed in 1952. The dorsal horn is composed of laminae I to VI (Figure PP7). The majority of nociceptor fibres (Aδ and C) terminate in two areas, laminae I/II (marginal layer and substantia gelatinosa) and lamina V. It should be noted that in addition to Aδ and C fibres, a small fraction of Aβ afferent fibres are nociceptive, with high-threshold mechano-heat characteristics. The nociceptive fibres synapse with second-order neurones or interneurones within the dorsal horn.

The second-order neurones in the dorsal horn may be excited or inhibited by different configurations of the nociceptors and interneurones. Sensitisation of the primary synapse by the descending modulatory system or interneurones can also occur in hyperalgesic states (Figure PP8). Similarly, various configurations of the descending mod-

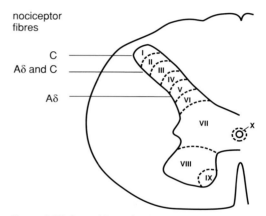

Figure PP7 Dorsal horn laminae in spinal cord

ulatory system and interneurones may occur to inhibit transmission in the primary synapse (Figure PP9).

Interneurones

The great majority of neurones in the dorsal horn are interneurones. Inhibitory and excitatory interneurones exist. Excitatory interneurones release glutamate as the neurotransmitter into the primary synapse. Inhibitory neurones use γ-aminobutyric acid (GABA) and glycine as their neurotransmitters, and may be stimulated by primary afferents, the descending modulatory system or non-nociceptive primary afferents such as Aβ fibres. The interneurones form interconnection circuits that participate in the following aspects of dorsal horn activity:

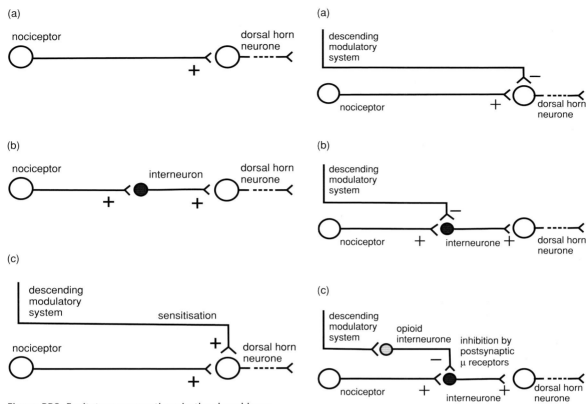

Figure PP8 Excitatory connections in the dorsal horn

- Gating of nociceptive signals
- Sensitisation of the primary synapse
- Presynaptic inhibition of primary afferents
- Relaying primary afferent signals to the appropriate ascending tracts

The primary synapse

Nociceptors are the primary afferent neurones of the pain system and stimulate action potentials in the dorsal horn neurone via the primary synapse. The primary synapse is central to the mechanism by which the pain system controls its sensitivity. The main excitatory neurotransmitter in the primary synapse is glutamate (Figure PP10).

Primary afferents can also inhibit action potentials in dorsal horn neurones by stimulating inhibitory interneurones. The main inhibitory neurotransmitters are GABA and glycine (Figure PP11).

Synaptic transmission is also influenced by a variety of neuromodulators which act through a spectrum of pre-

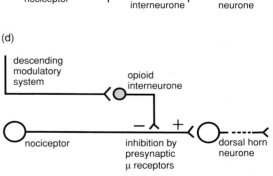

Figure PP9 Inhibitory connections in the dorsal horn

and postsynaptic membrane receptors. These modulators include endogenous opioids, which suppress transmission, but other modulators can enhance transmission. Neuromodulators in the pain system are described further below.

Descending control of the primary synapse is exerted by supraspinal centres, which form the descending modulatory system. This system not only inhibits synaptic transmission but may also facilitate it, leading to sensitisation.

nociceptive afferent

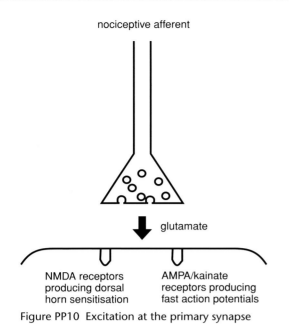

glutamate

NMDA receptors producing dorsal horn sensitisation

AMPA/kainate receptors producing fast action potentials

Figure PP10 Excitation at the primary synapse

non-nociceptive afferent

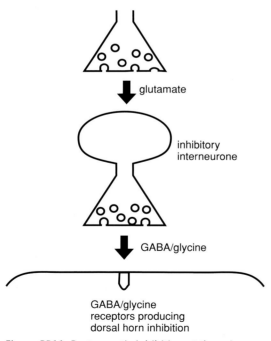

glutamate

inhibitory interneurone

GABA/glycine

GABA/glycine receptors producing dorsal horn inhibition

Figure PP11 Postsynaptic inhibition at the primary synapse

Control of synaptic transmission in the dorsal horn is therefore a result of complex interactions between afferent, descending, ascending and interneurone fibres (Figures PP8, PP9).

Neurotransmitters in the pain system

Many different synapses exist in the pain pathways of the CNS. It is recognised that each synapse operates with multiple transmitters. Some examples of known neurotransmitters in the pain system are presented in Figure PP12.

Receptors in the primary synapse

Primary synapse receptors (Figure PP13) may be classified into metabotropic receptors and ionotropic receptors:

- **Metabotropic receptors** – activate intracellular pathways when triggered by an agonist
- **Ionotropic** receptors – alter conductivity of an associated ion channel

The main excitatory transmitter is glutamate, which activates three different subtypes of ionotropic receptor on the postsynaptic membrane. These are NMDA (N-methyl-D-aspartate), AMPA (α-amino 3-hydroxy 5-methyl 4-isoxazolepropionic acid), and kainate receptors (Figure PP10). The NMDA receptor has a prominent role in chronic pain conditions, while the AMPA receptor mediates the transmission of fast action potentials.

In addition to these ionotropic receptors there are modulatory receptors on the postsynaptic membrane which can facilitate or inhibit action potential formation.

The main inhibitory receptors are GABA and glycine receptors (Figure PP11). Other inhibitory receptors include κ and μ opioid receptors and adenosine receptors, which are G-protein coupled.

The presynaptic nociceptor membrane has a range of receptors, including opioid (δ, κ and μ), nicotinic and muscarinic receptors. These also function to modulate synaptic transmission (Figure PP14).

Ascending tracts

The signals generated by nociception ascend to the brain by sensory-discriminative pathways and affective pathways. The sensory-discriminative pathways enable a nociceptive stimulus to be localised and its different qualities to be distinguished. The affective pathways relay the nociceptive signals with visceral, neuroendocrine and affective centres in the brain to produce the multidimensional nature of the pain response.

Neurotransmitter	Location	Comments
Excitatory neurotransmitters		
Glutamate	Widespread throughout CNS. Primary afferents	Main excitatory transmitter in CNS. >50% of DRG neurones. The main excitatory transmitter in nociception, acting via ionotropic receptors (AMPA, NMDA and kainite receptors)
Substance P	Primary afferents	30% of DRG neurones, mainly small sensory afferents. Small peptide agonist for neurokinin (NK1) receptor. Excitatory role in 'wind up'
Calcitonin gene-related peptide (CGRP)	Dorsal root ganglion cells	50% of DRG neurones, both small and large pain fibres. Released by thermal and mechanical stimuli. Excitatory role in 'wind up'
Inhibitory neurotransmitters		
Gamma-aminobutyric acid (GABA)/glycine	Descending modulation system, dorsal and ventral horn	Potent inhibition of spinal cord neurones. Act through ligand-gated channels
Noradrenaline	Dorsal horn and descending modulation system	Dorsal horn inhibition
Serotonin	Dorsal horn and descending modulation system	Dorsal horn inhibition
Glutamate	Dorsal horn	Inhibitory effects in dorsal horn exerted via metabotropic receptors

Figure PP12 Some examples of neurotransmitters in the pain system

Sensory discriminative pathways

The **spinothalamic** tract (STT) is formed by fibres from dorsal horn neurones which cross the midline and carry touch, pinprick, pain and temperature sensations from below the neck to the thalamus. It is monosynaptic, and phylogenetically the most recent of the nociceptive pathways. It is sometimes referred to as the neospinothalamic pathway.

The STT terminates in the ventral posterior nucleus (VPN) of the thalamus, and is divided into an anterior portion, mainly responsible for touch sensation, and a lateral portion, responsible for pain, temperature and pinprick modes.

The **trigeminothalamic** pathway is responsible for pain, temperature, pinprick and touch sensations in the head and neck, to the thalamus. Fibres from the contralateral spinal trigeminal nucleus form this tract and again terminate in the VPN.

Both pathways tend to lie laterally in the spinal cord and ascend to the contralateral VPN of the thalamus, from which they are projected to the cortex (Figure PP15).

Affective pathways

These pathways are the **spinoreticular** tracts, which are multisynaptic and thought to be phylogenetically the more primitive of the ascending tracts. They are sometimes referred to as palaeospinothalamic projections.

Initially they project to brain-stem areas, including the reticular formation, the parabrachial nuclei, catecholamine cell groups and the periaqueductal grey matter.

Spinoreticular tracts function by integrating incoming pain signals with visceral nuclei (e.g. nucleus tractus solitarius), the limbic system and the descending inhibitory system. They therefore mediate the emotional autonomic responses to pain.

Spinohypothalamic pathways ultimately connect incoming nociceptive signals through to the hypothalamus, and are also relayed to the prefrontal cortex. These hypothalamic connections are reflected by the disturbance

Receptor	Location	Comments
NMDA	Postsynaptic membrane	Important in producing long-lasting sensitisation by allowing calcium influx into the projecting dorsal horn neurones. Normally suppressed by Mg^{2+}, may also be blocked by ketamine
AMPA	Postsynaptic membrane	Produce fast excitatory postsynaptic action potentials. The main receptor responsible for transmission between primary afferents and dorsal horn neurones. Mainly sodium ionophores
Kainate	Postsynaptic membrane	Produce slow postsynaptic potentials associated with activation of high-threshold primary afferents. Sodium and potassium ionophores
NK1		Metabotropic receptors activated by substance P. Activate nociceptive dorsal horn neurones and produce hyperalgesia. Increase intracellular Ca^{++}
CGRP receptors	Postsynaptic membrane	Produce facilitation of the dorsal horn response
Opioid δ, κ and μ	Postsynaptic and presynaptic membranes	Inhibition of dorsal horn neurones
$GABA_A$ and $GABA_B$	Postsynaptic membrane	Inhibition of dorsal horn neurones
		$GABA_A$ increases Cl^- conductance and stabilises postsynaptic membrane potential
		$GABA_B$ decreases Ca^{2+} conductance and causes postsynaptic membrane hyperpolarisation
α_2	Presynaptic membrane	Selective inhibition of nociceptive primary afferents leading to analgesia
Serotonin receptors	Postsynaptic membrane, NMDA receptors	Inhibition of dorsal horn transmission. Some serotonin receptors associated with excitatory action

Figure PP13 Examples of primary synapse receptors

of neuroendocrine function such as ACTH and vasopressin activity, produced by pain. The prefrontal cortex is concerned with the highest cerebral activities such as abstract thought, decision making and anticipation. Such connections enable the prefrontal cortex to influence the response to nociceptive input.

The affective pathways assume a position medial to the spinothalamic tract in the spinal cord (Figure PP16).

The thalamus

The right and left thalami are large oval masses of neurones located deep in the brain, forming the lateral walls of the third ventricle (Figure PP17). Lateral to the thalamus on each side is the internal capsule, and above the thalamus is the floor of the lateral ventricle. The thalamus is a complex collection of nuclei with multiple connections to the cortex and other basal ganglia. No single function can be attributed to the thalamus because of its complexity.

One of its primary functions is the projection of somatosensory signals from the spinothalamic tracts and the trigeminal nuclei, which mediates the localisation and discrimination of painful stimuli. The afferent signals are received by the VPN, which is somatotopically arranged. This 'mapping' of the sensory signals is maintained in the thalamic projection to the cortex, and corresponds to the 'homunculus' representation on the postcentral gyrus (S1 somatosensory area).

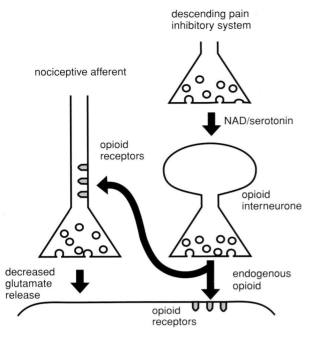

Figure PP14 Presynaptic inhibition at the primary synapse

Spinoreticular projections from the brain stem are received in the reticular, intralaminar and some medial areas of the thalamus. These are thought to exert an inhibitory influence on the VPN via interconnections. Disruption of these interconnections may underlie 'central' or 'thalamic' pain conditions. Part of the thalamic projection also goes to the secondary somatosensory area of the cortex (S2) at the foot of the postcentral gyrus.

Cortical sites of pain projection

Nociception not only activates subcortical structures such as the thalamic and brain-stem nuclei, but also activates a network of cortical sites that is sometimes referred to as the *cortical pain matrix*. Imaging studies have consistently demonstrated activation of the following cortical areas during acute and chronic pain:

- Primary somatosensory cortex (postcentral gyrus, S1)
- Secondary somatosensory cortex (S2)
- Insular cortex (IC)
- Anterior cingulate cortex (ACC)

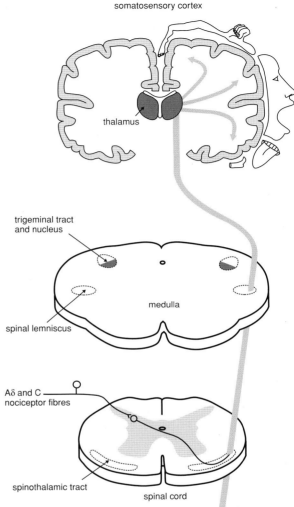

Figure PP15 Somatosensory pain pathway

Activation of the somatosensory areas, S1 and S2, is thought to function in perceiving the location and duration of pain. The ACC, which is part of the limbic system, and the IC, which is close to the limbic system, are thought to be important in the emotional, affective and motivational aspects of pain (Figure PP18).

The prefrontal cortex, which is responsible for higher cortical thought processes such as anticipation, prediction and modelling on past experience, is also activated by noxious stimuli and can exert an enhancing or suppressive

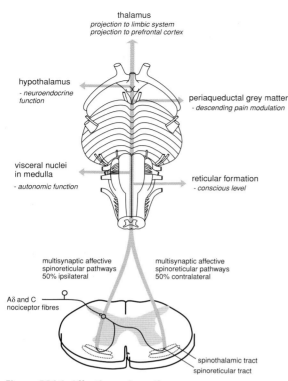

Figure PP16 Affective pain pathway

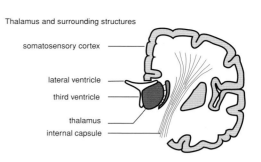

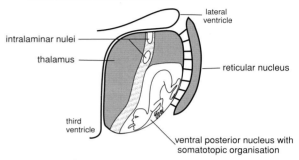

Figure PP17 Thalamus and surrounding structures

effect on the intensity of pain experienced. It is thought to play a part in placebo analgesia.

Sensitisation of the pain system

One of the characteristic features of pain which distinguishes it from other sensory modalities is the ability of the pain pathways to sensitise themselves. This can be regarded as a form of positive feedback control, in contrast to the familiar negative feedback control of homeostatic physiological systems. Sensitisation is recognised as occurring both peripherally at nociceptor level and centrally in the dorsal horn.

Sensitisation is a neurophysiological term used to describe an enhanced response of nociceptors (peripheral sensitisation) or an enhanced efficacy of the primary synapse in the dorsal horn (central sensitisation). It should not be confused with the clinical term *hyperalgesia*, which refers to the overall pain response experienced and may involve supraspinal mechanisms as well as sensitisation. Sensitisation is mediated by chemical factors acting through various cellular mechanisms, outlined below.

Peripheral sensitisation

Nociceptors, like other sensory receptors, are characterised by a response–stimulus curve. These receptors are sensitive to thermal, mechanical and chemical stimuli, but only respond above a certain threshold of stimulus intensity. Peripheral sensitisation usually occurs when tissue damage takes place, and produces a shift of the nociceptor response curve to the left, so that the nociceptor response is enhanced at any given stimulus intensity (Figure PP19). It is dependent on the release of various substances such as inflammatory mediators, prostaglandins and cytokines.

Peripheral sensitisation can also occur in neuropathic pain conditions due to peripheral sympathetic–sensory coupling. Such conditions are referred to as sympathetically maintained pain (SMP). The underlying mechanisms in SMP are thought to be increased adrenergic sensitivity of sensory neurones and proliferation of sympathetic nerve endings. Proliferation of sympathetic nerve endings around the dorsal root ganglion has also been suggested

(a) Lateral aspect of cerebral hemisphere

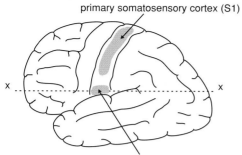

primary somatosensory cortex (S1)

secondary somatosensory cortex (S2)

(b) Horizontal section of brain (xx)   insula

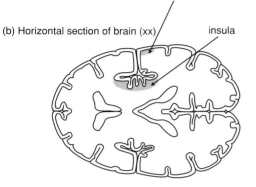

(c) Medial aspect of cerebral hemisphere

anterior cingulate cortex

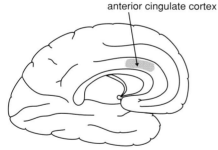

Figure PP18 Cortical matrix for pain

as a site of sympathetic–sensory coupling in chronic pain conditions such as CRPS.

Central sensitisation

A number of mechanisms operate to sensitise nociception centrally, in the dorsal horn:

- **Short-term homosynaptic potentiation** ('wind-up') – Dorsal horn cells can produce progressively increasing outputs in response to prolonged C-fibre nociceptor

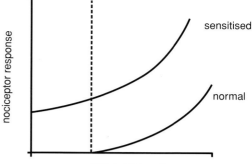

Figure PP19 Nociceptor response-curve shift in hyperalgesia

inputs. When dorsal horn neurones are repetitively stimulated by C fibres at low frequencies, the postsynaptic potentials may steadily increase in amplitude with each stimulus. This type of sensitisation only manifests itself in the primary synapse fed by the stimulated primary afferent (homosynaptic), and only occurs over the duration of the nociceptive stimulus.

- **Long-term homosynaptic potentiation** – This is a prolonged increase in the efficacy of primary synapses which have already been activated by a period of high-intensity nociception. NMDA receptors (Figure PP20) play a key role in a cascade that leads to AMPA receptor sensitisation on the postsynaptic membrane. Other mechanisms include presynaptic sensitisation via tyrosine kinase receptors, which increase the release of glutamate. This type of potentiation may outlast the noxious stimulus by hours or longer.

- **Heterosynaptic sensitisation** – When a nociceptive stimulus is maintained for a period of minutes, synapses outside the directly activated path (heterosynaptic) will also become sensitised. This sensitisation includes non-nociceptive (low-threshold) afferents, such as Aβ fibres serving areas neighbouring the area receiving the noxious stimulus. Heterotopic sensitisation contributes to secondary hyperalgesia and can also be associated with the production of muscular, joint and visceral pains and headache. This form of sensitisation may also outlast the nociceptive stimulus by hours.

- **Transcription-dependent sensitisation** – Intense prolonged nociceptive stimulation, such as that

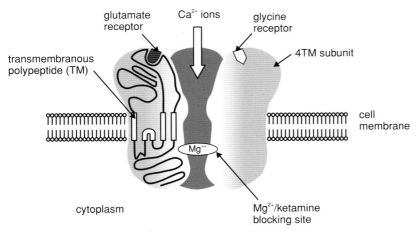

Figure PP20 NMDA channel

produced by inflammation or nerve injury, produces increased levels of factors including substance P and BDNF. These factors activate gene transcription centrally in dorsal horn cells and the primary afferents themselves. This process switches genes in dorsal horn neurones, leading to an increase in levels of receptors such as NK1 and trkB (i.e. the receptors for substance P and BDNF). The gene activation is mediated by an intracellular kinase (extracellular signal-regulated kinase, ERK) which can enter the nucleus and promote transcription. In some chronic inflammatory conditions the promotion of COX-2 transcription contributes to the systemic effects of muscular aches and pains, anorexia and headaches experienced.

- **Loss of inhibition** – As described above, primary afferents not only activate secondary dorsal horn neurones but also inhibit them via inhibitory GABAergic interneurones. Sustained stimulation of Aδ fibres or peripheral nerve injury results in long-term loss of inhibitory activity. In the case of nerve injury this loss of inhibition involves death of the GABAergic inhibitory neurones. GABA mimetics such as gabapentin can thus compensate for this reduction of inhibition in neuropathic pain conditions. Long-term loss of inhibition may also involve resorption of AMPA receptors by dorsal horn neurones. Thus long-term sensitisation occurs via degenerative changes in the dorsal horn in neuropathic pain conditions.

- **Changes in synaptic architecture** – Allodynia following nerve injury is mediated by non-nociceptive Aβ fibres and associated changes in dorsal horn architecture. In particular, low-threshold Aβ afferents sprout and reconnect from their normal position in laminae III and IV to dorsal horn nociceptive neurones in lamina II. This abnormal reorganisation of dorsal horn architecture can be prevented by treatment with neurotrophins (NGF, BDNF).

- **Microglial activity** – There is substantial evidence that activation of microglial tissue follows nerve injury and results in facilitation of glutamate pathways in the dorsal horn.

Modulation of pain

Pain is essential for the survival of an animal. It functions by aiding the animal to avoid harmful external influences and it ensures that an animal takes the appropriate actions to immobilise and protect injured tissue, thus promoting recuperation and healing. Prolongation and sensitisation of the pain response beyond the immediate occurrence of tissue injury or damage is required to fulfil these functions.

However, under certain circumstances survival may be advantaged by transiently suppressing the pain response. This might occur in order to allow escape in the face of threat, to ensure victory in combat, or to protect offspring.

Pain modulation can thus suppress the pain experience or enhance it, and it is thought to occur at cortical, brain-stem and spinal levels. The following mechanisms are discussed in further detail below:

- **Gate control** – This is one of the earliest pain modulation mechanisms proposed.
- **Descending modulatory system** – These pathways originate in the midbrain and medulla and descend to

suppress nociception in the dorsal horn. They not only exert an antinociceptive effect, but can also have a pronociceptive effect, enhancing nociception. Nociceptive sensitivity is therefore a resulting balance of this bidirectional control.

- **Neuromodulators** – These modify neurotransmission both supraspinally and in the dorsal horn. Many modulators have been identified, both enhancing and suppressing neurotransmission. They include endogenous opioids, orphanins and cholecystokinins.

Gate control

The gate control theory was first proposed by Wall and Melzack in 1965. It describes how synaptic transmission between primary nociceptive neurones and secondary nociceptive neurones can be modulated, or 'gated', by internuncial neurones. In particular, inhibitory interneurones in the substantia gelatinosa can exert presynaptic inhibition on primary afferent neurones and postsynaptic inhibition on secondary neurones, thus closing the 'gate' and decreasing the pain response to a nociceptive stimulus (Figure PP21). These inhibitory interneurones may be activated by alternative non-nociceptive primary afferents (e.g. Aβ mechanoreceptor afferents). This enables activated pain fibres to be gated out by other sensations, such as rubbing or pressure, applied to the affected area. Examples of 'gating' at spinal level include:

- Rubbing a sore spot
- Transcutaneous electrical nerve stimulation (TENS)
- Dorsal column electrodes

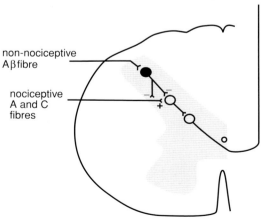

Figure PP21 Gating mechanism

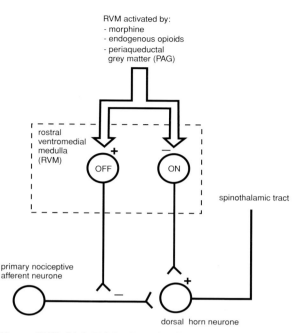

Figure PP22 PAG–RVM axis in the descending modulatory system

Descending modulatory system

Descending modulation of nociception is mediated by a network of pathways. It centres around an axis between the periaqueductal grey (PAG) region of the midbrain and the rostral ventromedial medulla (RVM).

The PAG is believed to be the main descending inhibitory control over nociception. It receives inputs from the hypothalamus, thalamus, limbic system and cortex, and delivers its main projections to the RVM. The RVM is central in a network of medullary nuclei, and exerts bidirectional control over nociceptive transmission in the dorsal horn via *on* and *off* cells (Figure PP22). This medullary network includes the following (Figure PP23):

- Nucleus raphe magnus
- Locus coeruleus
- Dorsolateral pontine tegmentum
- Nucleus reticularis gigantocellularis

Descending modulation therefore results from the integration of multiple inputs enabling diverse cerebral functions such as prediction, anticipation, affect and emotion, as well as the neuroendocrine axes and autonomic function

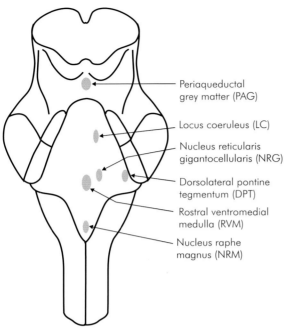

Figure PP23 Components of the descending pain modulatory system

Periaqueductal grey matter (PAG)

Locus coeruleus (LC)

Nucleus reticularis gigantocellularis (NRG)

Dorsolateral pontine tegmentum (DPT)

Rostral ventromedial medulla (RVM)

Nucleus raphe magnus (NRM)

to modulate the intensity of pain. This concept has implications in the management of both acute and chronic pain conditions.

Neuromodulators in the pain system

The neurotransmitters in the pain system are outnumbered by families of neuromodulators, which suppress or enhance synaptic transmission in the pain system. Neuromodulators form the basis for the endogenous control of pain intensity.

- Excitatory and inhibitory modulators operate in the primary synapses and are responsible for producing hyperalgesic states or analgesic states at dorsal horn level.
- Different neuromodulators also act at supraspinal level and ultimately enhance or suppress nociception in the dorsal horn via descending connections.
- Spinal and supraspinal interaction is important in determining the effect of some modulators.
- A modulator released supraspinally may have the opposite effect on nociception if released at spinal level.
- Simultaneous excitation of spinal and supraspinal areas may be essential to produce some analgesic effects.

Thus the clinical effects of neuromodulators depend on their properties and location of action. Properties of some of the recognised neuromodulators in the pain system are summarised in Figure PP24.

Endogenous opioids

Endogenous opioids are peptides that are released supraspinally and spinally. They have a recognised inhibitory effect on the pain response and exert their effects by their selective affinities for a number of receptors. These receptors are the classically described δ, κ and μ receptors, together with the more recently discovered ORL_1 (opioid-receptor-like) type.

The opioid receptors are G-protein coupled receptors with seven transmembrane regions and six extracellular loops (Figure PP25). When activated, they decrease neuronal excitability by inhibiting voltage-dependent sodium channels and activating potassium and calcium channels.

Some properties of endogenous opioids are summarised in Figure PP26.

Clinical aspects of pain

The complex nature of pain conditions has led to the introduction of different methods of characterising pain. Pain has been described by its:

- Temporal variation
- Pathological/physiological mechanism
- Anatomical localisation
- Qualitative descriptors

Pain described according to its temporal variation

The following terms are applied as clinical descriptions of the course of pain symptoms:

- **Phasic pain** – used to describe the short-duration, often high-intensity pain when the immediate impact of trauma or tissue injury is experienced. It is usually accompanied by reflex verbal or non-verbal (facial) expression, withdrawal or protective action.
- **Acute pain** – the pain provoked by tissue damage, consisting of a phasic component of short duration and a tonic component which is of longer variable duration (hours to days). Acute pain occurs in the period initially following trauma or surgery.
- **Chronic pain** – pain persisting beyond the period of time normally expected for healing and recovery from trauma or tissue injury. A chronic pain condition

Neuromodulator	Location	Comments
Excitatory modulators – enhancing nociception		
Cholecystokinin 8	Dorsal horn Supraspinal centres – RVM	Endogenous anti-opioid
Prostaglandins	Dorsal horn	Reduce the inhibitory action of glycine and cause hyperalgesia. Suggest a role for cyclo-oxygenase inhibitors in hyperalgesic conditions
Dynorphin 1–17	Dorsal horn	May be implicated in hyperalgesic and allodynic conditions
Orphanin FQ/nociceptin	Supraspinal inhibition of opioid action	Endogenous agonist for ORL_1 receptor. Reverses opioid analgesia when released at supraspinal sites
Inhibitory modulators – suppressing nociception		
Opioids	Mesencephalon – PAG Basal ganglia – thalamus, amygdala Descending inhibitory pain system – locus coeruleus (LC) Dorsal horn – primary synapse	Some opioids may have excitatory effects producing hyperalgesic conditions. Analgesic effects may depend on synergistic concurrent action at two sites e.g. PAG and LC
Cannabinoids	Wide distribution of cannabinoid receptors (CB1 and CB2) in CNS, including limbic system, descending pain inhibitory system, thalamus and spinal cord	Analgesic effects of cannabinoids probably dependent on complex interaction between supraspinal and spinal sites
Orphanin FQ/nociceptin	Dorsal horn inhibition	Gives analgesia when released at spinal sites
Acetyl choline	Dorsal horn inhibition	Inhibition of nociception mediated by muscarinic and nicotinic receptors in layers I–II of the dorsal horn

Figure PP24 Neuromodulators in the pain system

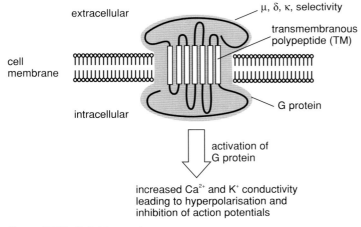

Figure PP25 Opioid receptor

Opioid	Number of amino acids	Receptor affinity
Leu-enkephalin	5	$\delta > \kappa \gg \mu$
Met-enkephalin	5	$\delta > \mu \gg \kappa$
β-endorphin	30	$\delta = \mu \gg \kappa$
Dynorphin	17	κ
Endomorphin 1	4	μ
Endomorphin 2	4	μ
Nociceptin	17	ORL_1

Figure PP26 Summary of endogenous opioid receptor affinities

may therefore exist in the absence of active tissue injury or damage, and can be recognised as early as 6 weeks after trauma. Such conditions, however, are usually diagnosed some months after a precipitating injury, and are frequently associated with depression, social and behavioural dysfunction as well as functional impairment. They may run a progressively deteriorating course over many years. Some commonly recognised chronic pain conditions are outlined in Figure PP27.

Pain described according to its physiological/pathological mechanism

Underlying mechanisms can be used to divide pain into :
- **Physiological (normal) pain** – occurring within the bounds of normal physiological function
- **Pathological (abnormal) pain** – pain outside the bounds of normal physiology

Physiological pain

This term describes pain caused by a noxious stimulus in the absence of actual tissue or nerve damage.

Condition	Signs/symptoms
Complex regional pain syndrome Type I (reflex sympathetic dystrophy) – no nerve injury Type II (causalgia) – nerve injury	Accompanied by abnormal perfusion, localised oedema and abnormal sweating in the affected limb or area. Trophic changes in skin, hair and nails also occur. Impaired limb function is accompanied by muscle wasting and loss of bone density
Trigeminal neuralgia	Unilateral severe shooting/stabbing pains in the territory of one branch of the trigeminal nerve. Background constant burning, gnawing pain may be present
Phantom limb pain	Phantom sensations are felt by virtually all amputees. Severe pain only persists in 5–10%. Stump pain also develops in 5–10%. The role of pre-emptive analgesia is uncertain
Post herpetic neuralgia	This pain syndrome follows shingles (Herpes Zoster infection). Peripheral sensitisation of nociceptors and central sensitisation of the dorsal horn occur. Hyperalgesia, allodynia and spontaneous pain result together with numbness and loss of temperature sensation. Symptoms may persist for years
Low back pain (LBP)	LBP affects a significant proportion of the population, but only 5–10% of these become chronic LBP sufferers. Serious consequences include reduction of individual quality of life, disability and socioeconomic costs. A specific underlying pathology can only be found in 10% of LBP patients
Painful neuropathies	The most common cause of painful neuropathy is diabetes. Other causes include hypothyroidism, alcohol, beriberi and drug toxicity (isoniazid, cytotoxics). Distal symmetrical peripheral neuropathy is present, with associated numbness, paraesthesia, hyperalgesia and burning pain. Symptoms are often most distressing at night

Figure PP27 Common chronic pain conditions

Physiological pain therefore simply warns of impending injury, and can be labelled as *nociceptive*, warning of potential tissue damage (e.g. painful heat sensation without occurrence of burns), or *neuropathic*, warning of possible nerve damage (e.g. nerve compression). In physiological pain no sensitisation of the pain system occurs.

Examples of physiological pain include muscle cramp, tourniquet pain and abdominal colic.

Pathological pain

When tissue or nerve damage occurs, pain becomes pathological. Thus pathological pain may be classified as nociceptive or neuropathic. When tissue or nerve injury occurs, sensitisation of the pain system is mediated through the various mechanisms described above. An *adaptive* function of sensitisation is thought to be the optimisation of conditions for healing. But pain sensitisation may persist, and pain may be experienced long after healing has occurred: this type of sensitisation is *maladaptive*. Sensitisation results in the clinical phenomena of *hyperalgesia* and *allodynia*.

Hyperalgesia and allodynia

Hyperalgesia is an inevitable companion of injury, and in clinical practice the term is used to describe the enhanced pain response resulting from sensitisation, which may be due to both peripheral and central mechanisms.

Primary hyperalgesia is localised in the zone of injury and occurs in response to both mechanical and thermal stimuli. Secondary hyperalgesia is produced in areas neighbouring the primary zone and only occurs in response to mechanical stimuli. It is contributed to by heterotopic sensitisation (see Sensitisation, above).

Two distinct forms of hyperalgesia are recognised, according to the type of mechanical stimulus employed:
- **Punctate hyperalgesia** occurs in response to pressure from a fine probe (e.g. a blunt pin) and is thought to be mediated by small-diameter nociceptive fibres.
- **Allodynia** (stroking hyperalgesia) is a hyperalgesic response to light stroking touch, and is mediated by low-threshold mechanoreceptors.

Hyperalgesia should not be confused with sensitisation, which is a neurophysiological term used to describe an enhanced nociceptor response (peripheral sensitisation) or an enhanced efficacy of the primary synapse in the dorsal horn (central sensitisation).

Neuropathic pain

The concept of pathological pain gives rise to the term *neuropathic pain*. Neuropathic pain is defined by the IASP as 'pain initiated or caused by a primary lesion or dysfunction of the nervous system'.

Neuropathic pain does not necessarily imply physical damage or destruction of nerves, but it may be due to reorganisation or dysfunction of the intact nervous system. Most chronic pain conditions will have a significant neuropathic pain component.

Pain differentiated by anatomical localisation

Somatic pain occurs in structures such as skin, muscle and joints. Visceral pain occurs in internal organs. Consideration of the underlying mechanisms of these pains can be useful in their management.

Joint pain
- Inflammatory changes in the synovium, periosteum and surrounding capsule.
- Stretching and distortion of the periosteum.
- Inflammatory changes in tendon (tendonitis) and their insertions (enthesopathies).

Muscular pain
- Deep, intense, unpleasant sensation associated with ischaemic muscular damage.
- Localised tenderness with referred distribution of pain characteristic of myofascial 'trigger points'.
- Distributed diffuse tenderness and pain associated with chronic conditions such as fibromyalgia.

Visceral pain
- Diffuse and poorly localised due to sparse innervation and spread of spinal input over several segments.
- Convergence of spinal input with somatic afferents, which leads to referred pain in somatic structures such as skin and muscle.
- Viscerovisceral convergence may also occur, leading to referred pain in neighbouring viscera and the diffuse nature of visceral pain.
- Associated with autonomic symptoms because visceral afferents often traverse prevertebral and paravertebral autonomic plexuses, giving rise to dual afferent inputs.
- Stronger emotional and autonomic associations than with somatic pain.

Headache

- Primary neurovascular headaches due to activation of the trigeminocervical complex by changes in intracranial vasculature, e.g. migraine and cluster headaches.
- Associated with head or neck trauma, e.g. whiplash involving myofascial trigger points in neck, cranial and shoulder musculature.
- Headache associated with raised intracranial pressure or intracranial infection involving mechanical or inflammatory meningeal irritation.
- Tension-type headache is the most common type of headache. The underlying mechanism remains uncertain.

Qualitative descriptors of pain

Such descriptors are commonly used by pain patients, and they may be suggestive of underlying mechanisms (Figure PP28).

Psychology of pain

The supraspinal connections of the nociceptive system project via somatosensory and affective pathways to the cortex, limbic system and reticular formation. These projections not only affect the intensity of the pain experienced but also stimulate psychological responses, which include:

- An emotional response
- A cognitive response
- A behavioural response

These psychological processes are inextricably interwoven with the physiological process of nociception. They are important because they play a significant part in determining the intensity of pain perceived and the effect of pain on a patient's life, particularly in the context of chronic pain symptoms. Clinically good management of these psychological responses can not only reduce the intensity of pain symptoms but also help patients to reduce the impact of pain on their lives.

Emotional response

In the context of acute pain, the patient's emotional response can have a significant effect on physiological parameters as well as on analgesic requirements. In chronic pain, the emotional response can often lead to long-term depression and anxiety, which can seriously affect the patient's quality of life. Pain can produce the basic emotions of anxiety, fear, depression, anger and guilt. It is commonly believed that depression and anxiety not only accompany pain symptoms, but also increase their intensity. Such a causal relationship remains controversial, but it is recognised that the treatment of depression and anxiety are an important part of pain management.

Cognitive response

The cognitive response refers to the information-processing functions of the brain, and involves the interaction of variables such as a patient's pain beliefs, pain memories and degree of attention to pain symptoms. Maladaptive cognitive responses include catastrophising and lack of self-efficacy (low self-confidence). Using a patient's cognitive responses to produce coping strategies is a useful part of pain management programmes.

Behavioural response

This refers to the learned patterns of behaviour resulting from the emotional and cognitive responses. Behavioural responses can be adaptive or maladaptive, producing either a beneficial or a detrimental effect on a patient's quality of life. Manipulation of behavioural responses may be useful in managing patients with chronic pain.

Pain management

The management of pain is multidisciplinary, corresponding to the multiple physiological and psychological

Type of pain	Characteristics
Sharp	Localised, sharp sensation transmitted by Aδ fibres. Rapid-response pain
Dull/aching	Diffuse, dull, intense sensation transmitted by C fibres. Slow-onset pain
Burning	Mediated by TRPV receptors on C and Aδ fibres
Pinprick	Mediated by Aδ fibres – mechano-heat sensitive nociceptors
Itching	A nocifensive sensation which provokes a characteristic scratch reflex.
	Subject to peripheral and central sensitisation, as in chronic pain conditions

Figure PP28 Qualitative descriptors of pain

mechanisms that determine the intensity of pain experienced.

In the clinical setting pain management divides into acute pain and chronic pain management. Acute pain usually focuses on postoperative pain, and is increasingly becoming managed outside the recovery room by an acute pain team. Chronic pain on the other hand is managed by the multidisciplinary team of a pain management service, which will operate through pain clinics, day-case procedure lists, specialist nurse-led clinics and a pain management programme.

Acute (postoperative) pain management

The mechanisms underlying acute pain are mainly those of nociception, with a limited degree of sensitisation peripherally and centrally. Supraspinal effects are minimal, with anxiety and fear contributing to the pain experienced to a limited extent. Pain management techniques rely on modifying the nociceptive process, and involve the use of drugs administered by the oral and parenteral routes together with local anaesthetic techniques.

Chronic pain management

In chronic pain conditions, the effect of central sensitisation at dorsal horn level, and of supraspinal mechanisms, is more pronounced. A multidisciplinary team is essential, and pain management may involve multiple inputs in order to achieve a satisfactory result. The approaches used may include:

- Pharmacology
- Local anaesthetic techniques
- Physiotherapy
- Complementary therapies
- Psychological techniques

Pharmacology

The range of drugs used in the pharmacological approach to chronic pain management reflects the diverse physiological factors that determine chronic pain levels. Many exert their effects by multiple actions. They include those listed in Figure PP29.

Local anaesthetic techniques

These methods include spinoaxial blockade, peripheral nerve blocks and sympathetic blockade. In some cases neurolytic blockade may be useful, either with a chemical agent such as phenol or using RF (radiofrequency) lesioning.

Physiotherapy

Physiotherapy remains an essential component of chronic pain management. It reduces pain levels and improves function. In order to reduce pain, physiotherapy employs techniques such as massage and manipulation, injections, acupuncture and acupressure, ultrasound and the application of heat and ice. Active management of rehabilitation is crucial in minimising the impact of injury and pain on a patient's life, and is a major part of the physiotherapist's role.

Complementary techniques

These methods include:

- Osteopathy – a system of medicine based on the principle that many disease conditions can be improved by musculoskeletal manipulation, which reverses dislocations and malalignments in the body's musculoskeletal framework, thus allowing the body to heal itself. This is essentially a holistic approach to the patient.
- Chiropractic – an alternative system of treatment by musculoskeletal manipulation which focuses on treating 'subluxations' and 'malpositioning' of vertebral segments in order to allow the body to heal itself. In common with osteopathy, chiropractic is also a holistic approach to the patient.
- Acupuncture – has been imported from traditional Chinese medicine and is based on restoring the flow of 'chi' (interpreted as 'energy') through a system of 14 meridians in the body by dry needling. The success of acupuncture has led to extensive research into its mechanisms over the past 30 years or more but the picture still remains incomplete, although endorphin release is believed to form an integral part of the process.
- Reflexology – a system of treating patients by stimulating nerves on the feet, hands and ears. Again the practitioners operate on the basis of restoring balance to the flow of 'chi' in the patient's body. It is believed that the body has a topographical representation over the soles of the feet, as well as on the hands and the ears.
- Homeopathy – a holistic system of medicine based on treating 'like with like', using medicines in which the active ingredient has been diluted to virtually undetectable levels. The active ingredient if given in adequate concentrations is thought to reproduce the original patient's symptoms. The dilution process

Type of drug	Examples	Comment
Opioids	Morphine, oxycodone, buporenorphine	Action by opioid receptors
Non-steroidal analgesics	Ibuprofen, diclofenac, celecoxib	COX inhibition
		Selective COX-2 inhibitor
Tricyclic antidepressants	Amitriptyline, imipramine	Inhibit presynaptic uptake of serotonin and noradrenaline in descending inhibitory system
		Block sodium and calcium ion channels
		Block postsynaptic muscarinic and histamine channels
Anticonvulsants	Carbamazepine, phenytoin	Block voltage-dependent sodium channels
		Also serotonergic effects
GABA mimetics	Gabapentin, pregabalin	Modulation of GABA synthesis, release and metabolism
Antispasmodics	Buscopan, baclofen	Relax smooth muscle spasm
		Decreases skeletal muscle tone
Anxiolytics	Diazepam, temazepam	Also relax skeletal muscle spasm
Alpha 2 agonists	Clonidine, tizanidine	Systemic effect in reducing neuropathic pain
		Local effect reducing allodynia
NMDA antagonists	Ketamine	Has been used to treat chronic pain state by infusion
Combination	Tramadol	Opioid action and increases serotonin and noradrenaline activities in the descending inhibitory system

Figure PP29 Some useful drugs in chronic pain management

producing the medicines involves vigorous shaking of the solutions (succussion), which is thought to leave an 'imprint' of the solute molecules in the aqueous solution. Homeopathy is generally accepted as being a safe form of treatment, and it is compatible with other forms of therapy, but mechanisms of action remain unproven.

The underlying mechanisms of complementary therapies remain uncertain, but they may succeed in cases where other therapies fail. Although such complementary therapies are accepted by many workers in chronic pain management, their use remains controversial due to difficulties in evaluating their effects objectively. The possibility of the placebo effect being the primary underlying mechanism is questioned by the successful application of many of these techniques in veterinary practice.

Psychological techniques and pain management programmes

Clinical psychologists are an integral part of the pain management team. As seen from previous sections, pain levels are influenced significantly by the activity of cortical centres and the limbic system. Psychological techniques have long been recognised as playing an important part in helping patients to cope with chronic pain symptoms. This is particularly so in the context of pain management programmes, which provide a structured course of training for patients in psychological and physical methods.

CHAPTER 11

Gastrointestinal physiology

A. Ogilvy

The primary functions of the gastrointestinal (GI) tract are the digestion of ingested food, the absorption of water, nutrients, electrolytes and vitamins, and the excretion of indigestible and waste products. The GI tract should not be thought of as a single organ, but a series of organs each with specialised functions. Each section of the GI tract has characteristic motor and secretory properties to accomplish a particular role in the overall function of the gut.

Gastrointestinal motility

Apart from the proximal part of the oesophagus, the GI tract has a remarkably uniform structure consisting of three layers of smooth muscle. These are arranged as an outer longitudinal layer, a middle circular layer and an inner submucosal layer (muscularis mucosa) (Figure GI1).

The basic contractile unit of the circular and longitudinal muscle layers is the smooth muscle cell. Across each cell membrane a transmembrane potential of between -40 and -70 mV (negative intracellular charge) is maintained by an ATP-dependent Na^+K^+ATPase pump. In most areas of the GI tract, the transmembrane potential of smooth muscle cells rhythmically depolarises and repolarises, which is called basic electrical rhythm, slow-wave activity or electrical control activity (ECA). Gap junctions between individual cells allow transmembrane ionic movements to be conducted from cell to cell. Slow-wave activity is conducted along lengths of bowel in a synchronised pattern due to this electrical continuity between cells. Segments of intestine with similar electrical activity, therefore, behave as a functional syncytium.

Contraction of smooth muscle only occurs when the transmembrane potential activity reaches a threshold voltage during slow-wave activity. Ion channels in the cell membrane open, allowing a rapid influx of sodium and calcium ions with subsequent depolarisation and myocyte contraction. Electrophysiologically, this is recognised as a series of rapid and repeating action potentials known as spike-burst activity (Figure GI2).

The frequency and amplitude of slow-wave activity varies throughout the GI tract and is altered by factors including nervous system control, hormones and pharmacological agents. Inhibition of slow-wave activity hyperpolarises the smooth muscle cell membrane and reduces the likelihood of spike-burst activity occurring. Conversely stimulatory factors increase the transmembrane potential towards zero and make contraction more likely.

The relative density of gap junctions between smooth muscle cells is not constant throughout the intestine. In regions of the gut rich in gap junctions (oesophagus, stomach, upper small bowel) slow-wave activity is easily

Fundamentals of Anaesthesia, 3rd edition, ed. Tim Smith, Colin Pinnock and Ted Lin. Published by Cambridge University Press. © Cambridge University Press 2008.

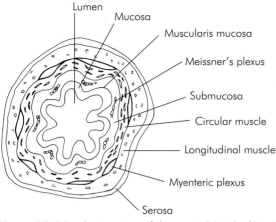

Figure GI1 Muscle structure of the gastrointestinal tract

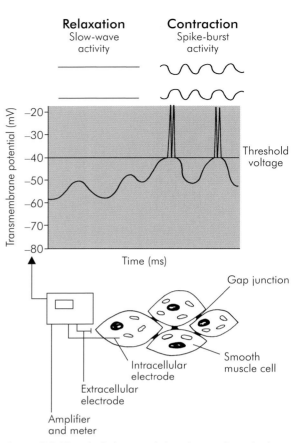

Figure GI2 Electrical characteristics of gastrointestinal smooth muscle

conducted in an orderly coordinated fashion. However, other areas (e.g. colon) have relatively fewer gap junctions, leading to poor intercellular conduction with apparently disorganised and poorly transmitted slow-wave activity.

Gut motility is controlled by the nervous and endocrine systems, which are illustrated in Figure GI3. At any one time, different parts of the gut exhibit different patterns of motility, due to the integration of several different signals from the nervous and endocrine systems.

Nervous control
Neurological control of intestinal motility is modulated by intrinsic and extrinsic nervous systems.

The intrinsic (enteric) nervous system is a complicated latticework of neurones within the bowel wall. It contains nearly as many neurones as the CNS and is organised into a number of plexuses and ganglia, which contain the cell bodies. The most important intrinsic plexus regarding control of bowel motility is the myenteric (Auerbach's) plexus, which lies between the longitudinal and circular muscle layers. Neurones within the myenteric plexus are classified as cholinergic (stimulatory), adrenergic (inhibitory) and non-adrenergic non-cholinergic (NANC) inhibitory neurones. Neurotransmitters in the last group include substance P, vasoactive intestinal polypeptide (VIP) and nitric oxide (NO). The myenteric plexus integrates neural information from the autonomic nervous system and other plexuses within the enteric nervous system to provide the second-by-second control of contractile activity in the gut. Several enteroenteric reflexes rely on the integrity of the myenteric plexus, and will occur even if the gut has no extrinsic nerve supply. The classic example is the peristaltic

reflex, where stretching of a segment of bowel by a bolus of food leads to proximal contraction (cholinergic) and distal relaxation (NANC) causing propulsion of the bolus in a distal direction. It is unlikely that this reflex is important in the normal propulsion of chyme through the bowel, but it neatly demonstrates the circuitry of the enteric nervous system (Figure GI4).

Extrinsic nervous control of intestinal motility is through the somatic (voluntary) and autonomic (involuntary) nervous systems, which includes sympathetic and parasympathetic fibres.

Voluntary control of GI motility only occurs in the pharynx during the initial stages of swallowing and at the anus during defecation.

Parasympathetic innervation of the oesophagus, stomach, small intestine and first half of the colon is by the

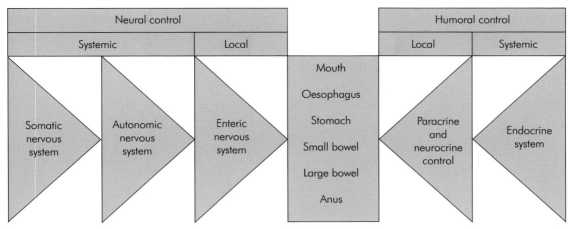

Figure GI3 Control of gastrointestinal motility

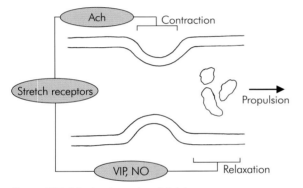

Figure GI4 Mechanism of peristalsis

vagus nerve. The pelvic parasympathetic fibres from the second, third and fourth sacral segments supply the rest of the colon, rectum and anus. These are preganglionic fibres that synapse within the enteric nerve plexuses and have both inhibitory and stimulatory actions within the gut. Sympathetic innervation of the gut arises from the spinal cord between T5 and L3. Preganglionic fibres pass through the paravertebral ganglia without synapsing to form the splanchnic nerves, which then synapse at the superior, middle and inferior pre-vertebral mesenteric plexuses. Postganglionic fibres run with the mesenteric vessels supplying all areas of the gut, and terminate in the enteric nervous system.

Chemical control

Chemical mediators affecting GI motility may be released locally from nerve endings (neurocrine), from endocrine or inflammatory cells within the gut wall (paracrine), or from endocrine glands remote from their site of action (endocrine). Figure GI5 summarises the effects of some of the common mediators on GI motility.

It is somewhat artificial to consider the control mechanisms individually, because in the intact intestine several control systems, both neuronal and chemical, operate simultaneously. In addition, they often have complementary effects on the secretory functions of the intestine which are closely coupled to its contractile state at any one time.

Motility characteristics of specialised regions of the GI tract

Oesophagus

The adult oesophagus is about 30 cm long. Its main functions are to transmit boluses of food and liquid from the mouth to the stomach and to prevent reflux of gastric contents out of the stomach.

The anatomy of the oesophagus is similar to that of the rest of the GI tract except that the upper 6 cm consists of striated skeletal muscle. The rest of the oesophagus is smooth muscle but has no slow-wave activity and therefore has no spontaneous contractile activity.

The oesophagus has two sphincters, upper and lower. The upper oesophageal sphincter (UOS), at the level of the fifth and sixth cervical vertebrae, consists of the cricopharyngeal and pharyngeal constrictor muscles. It is supplied by branches of the vagus nerve and is usually in a state of tonic contraction to prevent entrainment of air during respiration.

Factor	Gastric motility	Gastric emptying	Intestinal motility	Gallbladder emptying
Gastrin	Increased	Decreased	Increased	—
Cholecystokinin (CCK)	Increased	Decreased	Increased	Increased
Secretin (augments CCK)	Increased	Decreased	Decreased	Increased
Gastric inhibitory peptide[a]	Increased	Decreased	—	—
Motilin	Increased	Increased	Increased	—
Somatostatin	Decreased	Decreased	Decreased	Decreased

[a] also called glucose-dependent insulinotropic polypeptide

Figure GI5 Factors affecting GI motility

Increased tone	Decreased tone
Cholinergic stimulation	Cholinergic inhibition
Dopaminergic inhibition	Dopaminergic stimulation
Histamine	Oestrogen
α-adrenergic stimulation	α-adrenergic inhibition
β-adrenergic blockade	β-adrenergic stimulation
Gastrin	Cholecystokinin
Motilin	Secretin
Prostaglandin F_2	Prostaglandin E_1

Figure GI6 Factors affecting lower oesophageal sphincter tone

The lower oesophageal sphincter (LOS) is functionally a zone of increased intraluminal pressure (15–25 mmHg) in the lower 2–4 cm of the oesophagus. Macroscopically this area of smooth muscle is indistinguishable from the rest of the oesophagus. Electrophysiologically, the smooth muscle of the LOS displays continuous spike-burst activity, and therefore the sphincter is usually closed to prevent reflux of gastric contents into the oesophagus. During swallowing the LOS relaxes before a peristaltic wave, but quickly constricts again after a food bolus has entered the stomach. **Barrier pressure** is the pressure difference between that exerted by the LOS and the intragastric pressure. Any decrease in LOS tone or increase in intragastric pressure will reduce barrier pressure and make reflux more likely. Factors affecting LOS tone and hence barrier pressure are listed in Figure GI6. The flutter-valve action of the oesophagus below the diaphragm also helps to prevent reflux whenever the intragastric pressure is increased.

Swallowing

Swallowing is a motor reflex that transmits food from the mouth to the stomach. It is controlled by the deglutination centre in the reticular formation and is divided into voluntary, pharyngeal and oesophageal stages.

In the voluntary stage, masticated food is voluntarily squeezed into the pharynx by upward and backward pressure of the tongue against the hard palate. This initiates a reflex arc that begins with the pharyngeal stage of swallowing.

The soft palate is elevated to close off the nasopharynx and the palatopharyngeal folds are pulled into the midline forming a narrow slit through which boluses of food must pass. The upper airway is protected by the vocal cords closing and by an upward and anterior movement of the hyoid and larynx, which allow the epiglottis to cover the larynx. The upper oesophageal sphincter relaxes and the superior constrictor muscle of the pharynx begins a wave of contraction that passes down through the middle and inferior constrictors and into the oesophagus. The pharyngeal stage lasts about 1–2 seconds, during which time respiration is temporarily halted.

The peristaltic wave started in the pharyngeal stage, known as primary peristalsis, progresses along the oesophagus preceded by a wave of relaxation, aiding the movement of food down the oesophagus. It normally takes 8–10 seconds to complete a single swallow. If primary peristalsis fails, a secondary wave of peristalsis (secondary peristalsis) is generated within the oesophagus by stimulation of stretch receptors.

Nervous control of swallowing

Swallowing is a reflex arc with an afferent and an efferent limb. Once initiated it cannot be interrupted or terminated.

Afferent impulses from the pharynx are transmitted via the trigeminal and vagus nerves to the tractus solitarius. Afferent nerves from the upper middle and lower oesophagus run in the superior laryngeal, recurrent laryngeal and vagus nerves to converge in the tractus solitarius. Efferent motor signals are transmitted by the vagus, trigeminal, facial and spinal accessory nerves.

Gastric motility

Functionally the stomach has a proximal portion, the gastric fundus and upper one-third of the corpus, and a distal portion, which is the lower two-thirds of the corpus and the antrum.

The proximal stomach stores ingested food and controls intragastric pressure, which is important for controlling the rate of gastric emptying for fluids. During a swallow, the fundus relaxes (receptive relaxation) to prevent large increases in intragastric pressure during a meal. The proximal stomach has no phasic contractile activity because there is no slow-wave activity. Instead, muscle activity consists of prolonged tonic contractions lasting between 1 and 6 minutes, which allows stored food in the proximal stomach to be gradually released into the distal stomach for digestion.

The distal portion of the stomach mixes food with gastric juices and grinds it down to a fine paste called chyme. The smooth muscle cells in the distal stomach exhibit slow-wave activity with a resting membrane potential of between -50 and -60 mV. Towards the antrum and pylorus the smooth muscle cells are more polarised with less frequent slow-wave activity. Owing to the abundance of gap junctions between the cells, the corpus acts as the pacemaker region of the stomach whereby slow-wave activity is propagated distally in an orderly fashion.

The contractile status of the stomach alters between the 'fed' and 'fasted' state. For several hours after a meal, rings of peristalsis are generated every 15–20 seconds in the pacemaker centre on the greater curve and sweep down to the pylorus, mixing ingested food with digestive enzymes. The pylorus contracts in concert with the peristaltic waves of the distal stomach to prevent undigested stomach contents entering the duodenum. Food particles are squeezed down the walls of the stomach towards the pylorus and then return in an eddy current to a more proximal region of the stomach. The pylorus does not close completely during a contraction and food particles that are less than 1 mm in diameter can pass through into the duodenum during a contraction. Indigestible particles, such as vegetable fibre, are too large to pass through the pylorus and are removed during the fasted state, when the contractile characteristics of the stomach change.

The fasted state begins when the majority of the stomach contents reach the caecum. During fasting, the stomach and small bowel exhibit a regular and coordinated progressive contraction known as the interdigestive migratory motor complex (MMC). Usually this migratory contraction occurs every 90–120 minutes and starts in the antrum of the stomach. It then progresses down the small bowel at 6–8 cm per minute. This specialised contraction probably acts as a 'housekeeper', periodically sweeping undigested contents, sloughed mucosa, secretions and bacteria along the intestine in a distal direction.

Control of gastric motility and emptying

The rate at which chyme is released from the stomach into the duodenum is carefully controlled, so that the small bowel is presented with partially digested material at the optimum rate to allow further digestive and absorption processes to occur. Several factors affect the tone of the proximal stomach. The activity of the distal stomach and the tone of the pylorus are particularly important in controlling the mixing of gastric contents, and the rate of gastric emptying. The overall integration of these inputs determines the rate of gastric emptying. Although the exact mechanisms that control gastric motility are incompletely understood, it is clear that both neuronal and hormonal factors are important (Figure GI7).

The regulation of the fasting MMC is incompletely understood but motilin, a 22-amino-acid peptide released from the duodenal mucosa, is thought to be an important stimulus. Both stomach and duodenal smooth muscle have receptors for motilin that produce an increase in proximal stomach tone, initiation of the MMC and relaxation of the pylorus.

The 'fed' pattern of gastric motility is triggered by the sight or smell of food, the ingestion of food or gastric distension. The duration of the fed pattern of motility depends on the nutrient content of the stomach and is longer after fatty meals. Liquidised meals induce infrequent low-amplitude antral contractions, whereas solid material produces frequent high-amplitude contractions to aid breakdown into smaller more digestible particles.

The rate of gastric emptying is controlled by central and peripheral mechanisms. Pain, anxiety and stress reduce gastric emptying by activation of the sympathetic nervous system. Peripheral mechanisms include both neuronal and hormonal mechanisms activated in the stomach and small bowel. Distension of the stomach leads to the release of

Hormone	Proximal stomach	Distal stomach	Pylorus	Effect
Gastrin	↓ tone	↑ frequency of pacemaker and amplitude	Constricts	↑ peristalsis and chyme production
Cholecystokinin	↓ tone	↑ frequency of pacemaker and amplitude	Constricts	↑ peristalsis and chyme production
Motilin	↑ tone	MMC activity	Relaxes	↑ gastric emptying in fasted state
Gastric inhibitory peptide	No effect	↓ frequency of pacemaker	Constricts	Decreased emptying

Figure GI7 Effects of hormones on gastric motility

gastrin and stimulation of vagal and local enteric reflexes. The sum effect of these responses is an increase in the secretion of gastric acid and an increase in antral peristaltic activity, thereby increasing the production of chyme.

The composition of chyme entering the duodenum has an important regulatory role in the control of gastric emptying. Receptors within the duodenum are activated by stretch, increasing acidity or osmolarity, and large concentrations of fatty or amino acids (which indicate that stomach emptying is occurring too rapidly). Receptor activation initiates reflex arcs that reduce gastric emptying, and they include vago-vagal and local enteric inhibitory reflexes as well as the release of several inhibitory peptides which act on receptors in the stomach.

If small bowel contents rich in fat reach the ileum, an inhibitory reflex termed the ileal brake occurs whereby gastric emptying, pancreatic secretion and small bowel transit are all reduced to improve further digestion and absorption. This is another hormonally mediated reflex probably involving neurotensin and enteroglucagon.

Small and large bowel motility

The small bowel is about 5 m long in the adult. It has specialised contractile properties to promote the digestion of food, the absorption of nutrients and propulsion of non-digested material along its lumen. Slow-wave activity is present throughout the small bowel but the duodenum acts as the pacemaker. Transit times for intestinal contents are more rapid in the proximal small bowel due to the higher density of gap junctions compared with the distal small bowel. Contractile activity of the small bowel is categorised into several types of contraction (Figure GI8).

On average, transit of intestinal contents through the large bowel takes 33 hours. The colon is important for the absorption of water and electrolytes from the chyme, the fermentation of complex carbohydrates by colonic bacteria and the storage of faeces until a convenient time arises for defecation. The contractile properties of the colon are designed to mix the semi-solid chyme to allow adequate contact with the colonic mucosa, to propel it slowly along the colon, and at certain times to produce mass movements of faeces, e.g. during defecation.

Secretory functions of the gastrointestinal tract

Figure GI9 gives an overview of the composition of fluids secreted into the GI tract.

Salivary glands

The three paired salivary glands produce between 0.5 and 1.5 litres of saliva a day, which consists of water, mucus, digestive enzymes, sodium, potassium, chloride and bicarbonate. The parotid and submandibular glands secrete about 90% of the total volume of saliva.

The electrolyte composition of saliva varies with flow rates. Salivary potassium concentrations are 20 times those of the plasma at low flow rates but decrease at higher rates. Bicarbonate secretion increases at higher flow rates to produce alkaline saliva. Sodium and chloride concentrations are always less than plasma levels but increase at higher flow rates. The functions of saliva are:

- Lubrication to aid swallowing and speech
- Buffering and dilution of irritants
- Antibacterial/antiviral properties due to secretion of lysozyme, lactoferrin and IgA
- Digestion of starch by salivary amylase (optimal pH 7.0, therefore inactivated in the stomach)
- Digestion of fats by salivary lipase (not pH-dependent)

Small bowel

Interdigestive migratory motor complex (MMC)	Similar waveform to gastric MMC, acting as 'housekeeper' to the small bowel. Takes 2 hours to traverse small bowel
Migratory clustered contractions	Highly propulsive contractions over 10–30 cm of bowel. Prominent in terminal ileum to propel viscous contents into caecum
Retrograde giant contractions	Empty upper small bowel contents into stomach prior to vomiting
Giant migrating contractions	Infrequent large-amplitude long-duration contractions in the terminal ileum to return refluxed faecal contents into the ileum. Increased in some disease states

Large bowel

Individual phasic contractions (long and short duration)	Mix and knead faecal contents. Poorly coordinated with little propulsive action. Two to thirteen short-duration and up to two long contractions per minute
Organised groups of contractions	Periodic coordinated peristaltic wave passing along length of colon. Not related to fed or fasted state
Ultrapropulsive contractions	Occur once or twice a day. Responsible for mass movement of faeces in colon and rectum
Defecation	Distension of rectum by faeces produces reflex relaxation of internal anal sphincter (rectosphincteric reflex) followed by reflex contraction of descending and sigmoid colon

Figure GI8 Contractile activity of small and large bowel

The rate of saliva secretion is entirely controlled by the autonomic nervous system, although vasopressin and aldosterone can modify its electrolytic content by decreasing sodium and increasing potassium secretion. Both parasympathetic and sympathetic stimulation produce an increase in salivary gland secretion, although the sympathetic response is less pronounced. Parasympathetic fibres release acetylcholine, which binds to muscarinic receptors with subsequent activation of inositol triphosphate and calcium ion release. Norepinephrine released by sympathetic fibres acts via the cAMP pathway. The common response of the salivary gland is an increase in production and secretion of saliva and local vasodilation.

Gastric secretion

The stomach secretes about 1.2–2.5 litres of gastric juice a day with a pH between 1 and 3.5. The stomach contains principally two types of secretory gland, oxyntic and pyloric. The oxyntic glands are tubular pits of mucosa located all over the gastric mucosa except the lesser curve and are lined by three different types of cell: chief cells, which secrete pepsinogen, mucus cells, which secrete mucus, and oxyntic (parietal) cells, which secrete acid. Pyloric glands are in the pyloric region of the stomach and contain G cells, which secrete the hormone gastrin, and mucus cells.

Hydrochloric acid secretion (parietal cells)

Gastric acid aids protein digestion, activates pepsin, has antibacterial actions and stimulates biliary and pancreatic secretions in the duodenum. A simplified diagram of acid production by parietal cells is given in Figure GI10.

Gastrin, acetyl choline and histamine stimulate gastric acid secretion by binding to specific receptors on the basolateral membrane of the parietal cell, with subsequent activation of intracellular second messenger systems. The final common pathway is an increase in protein phosphorylation and activation of an ATP-dependent H^+K^+ pump, as summarised in Figure GI11.

Pepsinogen secretion (chief cells)

Pepsinogens are secreted mainly by chief cells, and are converted to the active enzyme pepsin by gastric acid. There are eight types of pepsinogen, classified according to the

	pH	Daily volume secreted (ml)	Electrolyte content (low–high secretion rates, mmol l⁻¹)	Enzyme content
Saliva	6.0–7.0	1000–1500	Na^+ 40–140 K^+ 40 HCO_3^- 40–80	Amylase Lipase Mucus Lactoferrin IgA Lysozyme
Gastric secretion	1.0–3.5	1500–2500	Na^+ 100–150 K^+ 10–20 H^+ 20–130 Cl^- 20–160	Pepsin Lipase Mucus Intrinsic factor
Pancreatic secretion	8.0–8.3	1000–1500	Na^+ 150 K^+ 5 HCO_3^- 40–115 Cl^- 110–30	Trypsin Chymotrypsin Elastase Carboxypeptidase A and B lipase Amylase Ribonuclease Deoxyribonuclease Phospholipase A_2
Bile	7–8	700–1200	Na^+ 130–140 K^+ 5–12 HCO_3^- 10–28 Cl^- 25–100 Ca^{2+} 5–23	Bile pigments Bile salts Cholesterol Inorganic salts Fatty acids Lecithin Fat
Small bowel secretion	7–8	1800	(Concentrations from proximal to distal small bowel) Na^+ 140–125 Cl^- 110–60 K^+ 5–9 HCO_3^- 100–74	Mucus Peptidases Lipase Sucrase Maltase Isomaltase Lactase
Large bowel secretion	7–8	200	Na^+ 40 K^+ 90 Cl^- 15 HCO_3^- 40	

Figure GI9 Composition of gastrointestinal secretions

optimal pH for their activation. In normal health, 85% of pepsin secreted is pepsin 3. Pepsinogens are stored in secretory granules within the chief cells, which when stimulated fuse with the apical membrane to release the pepsinogens. In general, stimuli that activate acid secretion also stimulate pepsin secretion.

Mucus secretion

Mucus is secreted throughout the GI tract. It coats and lubricates food particles, protects epithelial surfaces from digestive enzymes and has a small buffering capacity against acid or alkalis. It is also important in the formation of solid faeces by its binding action on faecal particles.

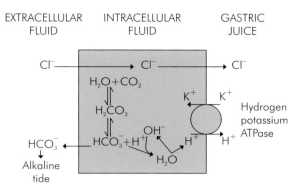

EXTRACELLULAR FLUID   INTRACELLULAR FLUID   GASTRIC JUICE

Figure GI10 Acid production in parietal cells

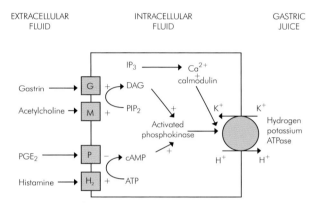

EXTRACELLULAR FLUID   INTRACELLULAR FLUID   GASTRIC JUICE

Figure GI11 Modulators of gastric acid production

In the stomach, mucus is secreted by mucus cells covering the entire mucosa as well as from the pyloric glands in the antrum. Mucus consists of 70% water, electrolytes, sloughed cells and complex glycoproteins called mucins which are important for the viscous and gel-forming properties of mucus. In the normal stomach, the epithelium is covered by a 0.2–0.6 mm layer of viscous mucus that is continually eroded away by the action of pepsins and replaced by newly secreted mucus. Cholinergic stimulation results in an increase in mucus secretion by mobilisation of intracellular calcium. Prostaglandin E_2 stimulates the production of mucus by a cAMP-mediated pathway.

Bicarbonate secretion

Gastric secretion of bicarbonate accounts for about 5–10% of total gastric secretions. Secretion is both an active and a passive process and requires the presence of intraluminal chloride, with which it is exchanged. Bicarbonate alone

would be an ineffectual epithelial defence against intraluminal acid; however, in combination with mucus it provides improves the buffering capacity of mucus. In the stomach this mucus–bicarbonate layer is only effective at pH > 1.5 and is considered as a weak first-line defence. In the duodenum it is a more important mechanism in preventing villous injury.

Intrinsic factor

Intrinsic factor is a mucoprotein essential for the absorption of vitamin B_{12}. It is secreted by parietal cells in the stomach and forms a complex with the vitamin which is actively absorbed in the distal ileum.

Control of gastric secretion

Following a meal there is a rapid increase in gastric secretion, which normally peaks after 30 minutes to 1 hour. Gastric secretion is divided into three stages: cephalic and gastric stages, which are stimulatory, and the intestinal stage, which is inhibitory.

The **cephalic stage** commences even before food enters the stomach. It causes increased gastric secretion in response to the sight, smell, taste or thought of food by vagal stimulation of oxyntic glands. Vagal stimulation of gastrin-producing cells in the pylorus (G cells) leads to an increase in gastrin production, which then stimulates further gastric acid production.

The **gastric stage** begins when food enters the stomach. Gastric distension and an increase in luminal peptides promote the release of gastrin. Secretion of acid ceases when the pH of stomach contents reaches 2.0 to allow the optimum conditions for pepsin activity, but when pH rises above 3.5 acid secretion recommences.

In the **intestinal phase** gastric secretion declines. This usually occurs about one hour after eating, due to a decrease in the stimulatory factors and an increase in the inhibitory factors controlling gastric secretion, which include:
- Distension of the duodenum, or the presence of acid, lipids or carbohydrate in the upper small bowel reducing gastric secretion and stomach emptying by enterogastric reflex.
- Cholecystokinin released from the duodenum in response to an increase in the fat, protein or carbohydrate content will antagonise the effects of gastrin, decrease gastric tone, stimulate gallbladder contraction and pancreatic secretion and augment the effects of the hormone secretin.

- Other hormones may be released in response to nutrients in the small bowel, including gastric inhibitory peptide, secretin, neurotensin and enteroglucagon, all of which reduce gastric secretion.

Pancreatic secretion

The pancreas is a complex alveolar gland similar in structure to salivary glands, with acini (acinar cells) draining into small ductules which then drain into larger ducts and finally the main pancreatic duct. The pancreas has a huge functional reserve, and up to 80% of pancreatic tissue can be removed with no effect on digestion. Normally the pancreas produces about 1.5 litres a day of alkaline fluid (pH 8.0), which consists of digestive enzymes secreted by the acini and bicarbonate produced by the epithelial cells of the ducts.

Pancreatic enzymes are synthesised as inactive proenzymes and stored in secretory granules in the acini. The following enzymatic processes occur:

- Trypsinogen is converted to active trypsin in the duodenum by the presence of enteropeptidase (enterokinase) released from duodenal epithelium, and by the presence of previously activated trypsin. Trypsin is the predominant enzyme produced by the pancreas; it splits ingested proteins into smaller peptide chains and activates most of the pro-enzymes secreted by the pancreas.
- Chymotrypsinogen is converted to chymotrypsin by trypsin in the small bowel, and has a similar action to trypsin,
- Carboxypeptidase cleaves carboxyl groups from peptides to produce free amino acids.
- Ribonuclease and deoxyribonuclease split ribonucleic and deoxyribonucleic acids.
- Fat is digested by pancreatic lipase, which converts it into fatty acids and monoglycerides, cholesterol esterase, which hydrolyses esters, and phospholipase, which cleaves phospholipids into fatty acids.
- Pancreatic amylase hydrolyses starch and other carbohydrates into tri- and disaccharides.
- Bicarbonate and water are secreted entirely by the epithelial cells of the pancreatic ducts.

Other electrolytes secreted by the pancreas include zinc, magnesium and calcium in small amounts, although their functional significance is unknown.

Control of pancreatic secretion

Pancreatic secretion fluctuates throughout the day. Following a meal production of pancreatic fluid increases, and during fasting secretion is dormant except during an interdigestive MMC, when secretion temporarily increases. The dietary content of ingested food determines the magnitude and duration of the pancreatic response to a meal. Intestinal fats and proteins are the main stimuli for pancreatic secretion and produce the biggest response (carbohydrates induce only a weak pancreatic response). Calcium and magnesium are also stimuli for pancreatic secretion, and alcohol may have both inhibitory and stimulatory effects.

Two hormones are responsible for stimulating pancreatic secretion, secretin and cholecystokinin.

- Secretin is released from S cells in the upper small intestine in response to a reduction in duodenal pH < 4.5. Its main effect is stimulation of the ductile systems of the pancreas to produce large volumes of fluid rich in bicarbonate but low in chloride. Bicarbonate neutralises acid in the small bowel, protects intestinal mucosa, and provides the optimal pH for the activation of pancreatic enzymes.
- Cholecystokinin released from duodenal mucosa in response to duodenal amino acids, peptides and fats stimulates the release of pancreatic enzymes from acinar cells. It also augments the actions of secretin on the ductal epithelium.

Several neuronal reflexes are also important in the control of pancreatic secretion. These include a cephalic phase of pancreatic secretion mediated by the vagus nerve. In addition, several enteropancreatic reflexes are probably involved in initiating pancreatic secretion in response to nutrients in the small bowel.

Little is known of the inhibitory control of pancreatic secretion. Glucagon secretion, which increases in the postprandial state, may have an influence, as might somatostatin and vasoactive intestinal polypeptide (VIP). The presence of intraluminal pancreatic enzymes may have a negative feedback effect by reducing the release of cholecystokinin.

Biliary secretion

The liver produces 0.7–1.2 litres of bile a day, of which 30–60 ml can be stored and concentrated in the gallbladder. Bile is a complex mixture of water, bile salts, pigments and other organic and inorganic compounds.

Bile salts are synthesised in the liver by the conversion of cholesterol to the bile acids, cholic and deoxycholic acid.

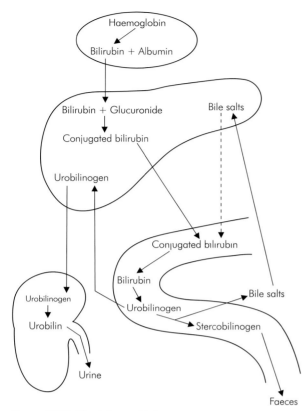

Figure GI12 Physiology of bile

These are then conjugated with glycine and taurine to form bile salts that are secreted in the bile. Over 94% of bile salts secreted by the biliary system are actively reabsorbed in the distal ileum and re-excreted as bile in the liver. This entero-hepatic circulation of bile salts is an important mechanism in maintaining an adequate concentration of bile salts in the upper small intestine necessary for adequate digestion. Approximately 24 g bile salts are required a day for the complete digestion and absorption of fat. As the total body reserves of bile salts are only 6 g and the daily synthesis of bile salts is 0.5 g, the importance of the enterohepatic circulation can be appreciated (Figure GI12).

Bile salts emulsify fatty globules in the small bowel by decreasing their surface tension, thereby breaking them down into smaller particles. They then bind with fats to form micelles that are readily absorbed in the small bowel. The fat-soluble vitamins A, D, E and K indirectly rely on this mechanism for absorption.

The colour of bile is due to the presence of bile pigments (mainly bilirubin) formed from the breakdown products of haemoglobin. Bile pigments have no role in the digestion of fat but are responsible for the normal colour of faeces and urine.

Control of biliary secretion

The secretion of bile into the duodenum varies throughout the day. During fasting, the smooth muscle of the gallbladder and biliary tree exhibits activity similar to the interdigestive MMC seen in the GI tract. Approximately every 2 hours a contraction of the gallbladder expresses about 10 ml bile into the duodenum in the fasted individual.

Gallbladder contraction starts within a few minutes of starting eating, and bile output reaches a maximum at about 1 hour after ingestion of food. Thereafter it reaches a plateau and remains constant until gastric emptying has been completed. The initial rise is due to gallbladder contraction, which empties about two-thirds of the bile stored. Thereafter, during the plateau phase, there is a constant secretion of bile by the liver that bypasses the gallbladder and enters the small bowel through a relaxed sphincter of Oddi. Owing to the enterohepatic circulation, it is estimated that the total pool of bile salts is recirculated two to three times every meal.

The initial gallbladder contraction in response to a meal is vagally mediated. There are also enteric nervous system reflexes that stimulate gallbladder contraction in response to gastric distension. Biliary secretion is affected by the following factors:

- Cholecystokinin is the main hormone controlling biliary secretion. The presence of intraluminal fat in the duodenum stimulates the release of cholecystokinin, which causes relaxation of the sphincter of Oddi and gallbladder contraction.
- Biliary secretion is also stimulated by increasing concentrations of bile salts returning to the liver in the portal circulation, which occurs in the postprandial phase due to the enterohepatic circulation.
- Secretin released in response to acid in the duodenum increases the production of watery alkaline bile and probably augments the action of cholecystokinin.

Digestion and absorption

Digestion is the chemical breakdown of ingested food by GI enzymes into substances that can then be absorbed from the intestines into the systemic circulation. The organ principally responsible for these functions is the small intestine, although some digestion and absorption may occur in the mouth and stomach.

Carbohydrate

The small bowel can only absorb the carbohydrates glucose, fructose and galactose. Therefore, all dietary carbohydrate must be broken down to one of these monosaccharides. Cellulose is a complex polysaccharide with β-glucose linkages, and because humans do not possess enzymes capable of breaking these linkages it is indigestible and forms dietary fibre.

Starch is broken down to oligo- and disaccharides by salivary and pancreatic amylase. Small bowel brush border enzymes cleave larger sugars to monosaccharides, which can then be absorbed. The functional reserve of the enzymes involved in carbohydrate digestion is such that the digestive tract can handle huge carbohydrate loads and still achieve complete hydrolysis by the proximal jejunum. Detail of carbohydrate absorption is shown in Figure GI13.

Protein

Ingested proteins are broken down by digestive enzymes to free amino acids and small di- and tripeptides in the stomach by pepsin, and in the small bowel by pancreatic peptidases. Pancreatic peptidases are either endopeptidases (trypsin, chymotrypsin, elastase), which hydrolyse interior peptide bonds, or exopeptidases (carboxypeptidase), which hydrolyse external peptide bonds. The individual peptidases differ in their ability to cleave peptide bonds containing different classes of amino acid, e.g. neutral or basic, aromatic or aliphatic. The pancreatic peptidases are rapidly inactivated in the duodenum by trypsin. Free amino acids, monopeptides and dipeptides are absorbed by epithelial cells of the small intestine and the remaining larger peptides further hydrolysed by brush border peptidases to smaller peptides, with subsequent absorption. Detail of protein absorption is shown in Figure GI14.

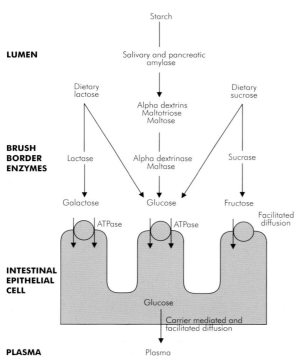

Figure GI13 Carbohydrate digestion and absorption

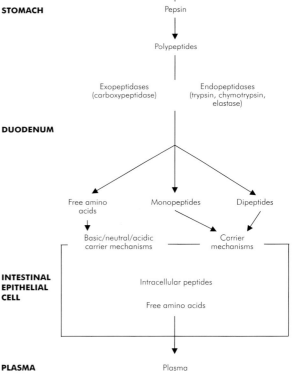

Figure GI14 Protein digestion and absorption

Lipid

Of dietary fat, 90% is triglyceride, with the remainder consisting of phospholipids, cholesterol and cholesterol esters, and fat-soluble vitamins (A, D, E, K). Lingual lipase and pancreatic lipase hydrolyse triglycerides to free fatty acids and monoglycerides.

In combination with bile salts, free fatty acids, glycerides and cholesterol form micelles that fuse with the unstirred layer of the intestinal epithelium to allow the absorption of fats. Phospholipids are metabolised by pancreatic phospholipase A_2 to free fatty acids and lysophospholipids, which are taken up into micelles.

In the intestinal epithelial cell the free fatty acid and monoglycerides are reconstituted back into triglycerides, which are then incorporated into large lipoproteins called chylomicrons. These consist of a hydrophobic core of triglycerides, cholesterol esters and fat-soluble vitamins surrounded by a hydrophilic shell of phospholipid, free cholesterol and protein (synthesised by the rough endoplasmic reticulum as apoprotein). The chylomicrons enter the extracellular fluid by pinocytosis and enter the circulation via the lymphatic system.

The absorption of the fat-soluble vitamins A, D, E and K depends on micelle uptake. With regard to the absorption of water-soluble vitamins:

- Thiamine (B_1) is absorbed in the jejunum by sodium-dependent active transport.
- Vitamin C is absorbed by both active and passive processes in the small bowel.
- Folic acid is actively absorbed from the whole small intestine.
- Vitamin B_{12} requires intrinsic factor for absorption. Initially, the vitamin combines with glycoprotein (R protein) in the stomach. The combination is digested in the duodenum by peptidases to release the free vitamin, which then binds to intrinsic factor. In the terminal ileum the complex is finally absorbed, probably by pinocytosis.

Detail of lipid absorption is shown in Figure GI15.

Sodium and chloride reabsorption

The intestine reabsorbs 25–35 g sodium a day, which accounts for about 15% of the total body sodium. Most of this sodium is from intestinal secretions, with dietary sodium contributing about 5–8 g. Chloride ions are absorbed throughout the intestine, especially the colon.

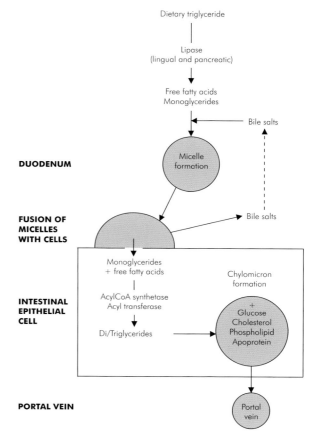

Figure GI15 Lipid digestion and absorption

Water absorption

Dietary fluid and intestinal secretions account for 7.5–10 litres water handled by the intestine per day. Of this, only 200 ml is excreted in the faeces daily, the majority being reabsorbed in the small intestine and about 400 ml in the colon.

Water absorption can be regulated to some extent by the autonomic nervous system by its effects of sodium and chloride absorption. Sympathetic stimulation or cholinergic inhibition leads to an increase in sodium and water absorption. In addition to its renal effects, the mineralocorticoid aldosterone also has effects on sodium and water absorption in the intestine, particularly the colon. Aldosterone increases the number of sodium channels on the epithelium and the number of Na^+K^+ pumps on the basolateral membrane, therefore increasing sodium and water absorption.

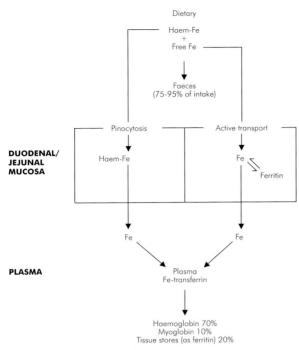

Figure GI16   Iron absorption

Iron absorption

Iron is primarily absorbed in the duodenum and jejunum, either as haem (derived from meat) or as free iron. Absorption is related to the total body iron stores, and normally the amount absorbed is a small fraction of the amount ingested. Haem is absorbed by pinocytosis and broken down to free iron within the enterocyte. Free iron is absorbed using a specific receptor, and once inside the cell it binds with a specific protein, apoferritin, to form ferritin, an intracellular storage complex for iron. Most iron in the form of ferritin is lost in the normal sloughing of epithelial cells. Ferritin-bound iron enters the circulation by cleaving from ferritin and then binding to an intracellular transport protein, which then crosses the basal membrane to release iron into the circulation, where it is bound to a β_1-globulin, transferrin. Iron absorption increases if total body iron is reduced, by increasing the number of iron receptors in the intestine and by increasing the amount of the intra-cellular carrier protein. Iron absorption is summarised in Figure GI16.

Calcium absorption

Calcium absorption occurs mainly in the duodenum, and it is regulated by the hormone 1,25-dihydroxycholecalciferol, synthesised from vitamin D (cholecalciferol) in a series of steps occurring in the skin, liver and kidneys. The action of 1,25-dihydroxycholecalciferol on the intestinal epithelial cells is probably to stimulate the synthesis of a calcium-binding protein which is inserted in the apical membrane of the cells. Intestinal calcium then enters the cell down a concentration gradient through channels gated by the binding protein when it is taken up into intracellular stores to prevent a rise in free intracellular concentrations. Calcium is released from the cell into the circulation by the action of a calcium ATPase pump and by counter-transport with sodium.

Nausea and vomiting

Nausea is an unpleasant but not painful sensation, often relating to the pharynx and abdomen, associated with the desire to vomit. It can be transient or prolonged and often occurs in 'waves'. Vomiting is forceful expulsion of the contents of the upper GI tract out of the mouth. It is an active process, as opposed to regurgitation, which is a passive reflux of stomach contents into the oesophagus. In the animal kingdom, most poisons are ingested orally; therefore, vomiting serves as a protective mechanism in which ingested toxins are detected and expelled from the body. Diarrhoea serves the same purpose except that it clears the lower half of the GI tract. Often in humans the perceived toxin has not been ingested via the oral route, but the basic response is still to purge the GI system. An important example is in postoperative nausea and vomiting.

Mechanisms

Vomiting can be considered as a reflex with a sensory afferent and a motor efferent limb connected by a central integrative centre located in the brain stem. The afferent limb may be activated by a wide range of stimuli using a variety of pathways including fibres from the GI tract, the chemoreceptor trigger zone (CTZ) in the brain stem, the vestibular system and other miscellaneous inputs.

GI tract afferents

Vagal fibres are the main afferent nerve fibres in the GI tract associated with the vomiting reflex. These fibres supply two types of receptor within the GI tract, mechano- and chemoreceptors. Mechanoreceptors are activated by excessive stretching of the gut, such as occurs after overeating or in bowel obstruction. Chemoreceptors detect changes in the intraluminal environment, which may indicate the ingestion of a potential toxin, including excess alkalinity or acidity, certain irritants or bacterial endo- or exotoxins.

Chemoreceptor trigger zone (CTZ)

This is a specialised chemoreceptor region situated in the area postrema in the caudal part of the fourth ventricle. It lies outside both the blood–brain barrier and the cerebrospinal fluid–brain barrier and is ideally situated for the detection of toxins in the plasma and CSF which may have been absorbed from the gut or administered by other routes. Cells of the CTZ contain many types of receptor including muscarinic, histaminic, serotonergic ($5-HT_3$), dopaminergic (D_2), opioid (μ) and α_1 and α_2 adrenoceptors, which may be activated by different chemicals including drugs, or by biochemical and endocrine changes such as in hypoglycaemia or pregnancy.

Vestibular system

Stimulation of the labyrinthine system is a potent stimulus for vomiting (e.g. vertigo), although it is unclear what protective mechanism this has in humans.

Central coordination of the vomiting reflex

The act of vomiting is a highly complex coordinated series of actions involving the GI, respiratory, cardiovascular, somatic and autonomic nervous systems. 'Vomiting centre', which describes the area of the brain stem responsible for the control of vomiting, is a gross oversimplification. In reality, it is probably several discrete areas of the brain stem with complex interconnections that coordinate the reflex. These areas probably include the dorsal and ventral respiratory groups, the dorsal motor vagal nucleus, the nucleus tractus solitarius and the parvicellular reticular formation.

Motor components of vomiting

Vomiting can be divided into two distinct phases: pre-ejection and ejection.

Pre-ejection

The early stages of vomiting usually start with a sensation of nausea, followed by signs of sympathetic activity including peripheral vasoconstriction, hyperventilation, sweating, pupillary dilatation, tachycardia and reduction in gastric secretion. Salivation occurs in response to parasympathetic activity. Vagal impulses arising from the dorsal motor vagal nucleus cause a profound relaxation of the proximal stomach followed by a retrograde giant contraction beginning in the mid-small intestine which propels small-bowel contents proximally back into the stomach in preparation for ejection.

Ejection

Usually, vomiting is preceded by retching, which involves the synchronous contraction of the abdominal wall muscles and diaphragm, producing a rapid rise in intragastric pressure. As the peri-oesophageal portion of the diaphragm contracts during this phase, the oesophagus is tightly compressed, preventing the escape of gastric contents. The exact function of retching is unknown. Vomiting involves exactly the same actions except that the peri-oesophageal area of the diaphragm relaxes, allowing gastric contents to be expelled into the oesophagus and out of the mouth. Respiration temporarily ceases during this phase to protect the airway from aspiration.

Postoperative nausea and vomiting (PONV)

The aetiology of postoperative nausea and vomiting is extremely complicated and almost certainly multifactorial. Various factors are associated with an increased risk of PONV, and they can be broadly categorised into patient, anaesthetic and surgical factors. For details, see anti-emetic pharmacology, Section 3, Chapter 10 (pages 634–9).

CHAPTER 12

Metabolism and temperature regulation

S. Graham and E. S. Lin

Nutrition

Food provides basic energy requirements, and provides the structural building blocks to maintain metabolic integrity. A normal diet consists of carbohydrates, proteins and fats. In addition, small quantities of vitamins and minerals are also required for good health. Nutritional status may be assessed by measurement of skin-fold thickness with callipers (the area overlying the triceps muscle is often used) or by calculation of the body mass index (BMI). BMI is obtained by dividing weight (kg) by the square of the height (m^2). Values between 20 and 24 are normal, with >30 indicating obesity and >40 severe obesity. BMI is also called Quetelet's test after Adolphe Quetelet (1796–1874), a Belgian mathematician who came up with the concept of the 'average' man.

The average calorific requirement for 24 hours in a fit 70 kg man is about 3000 kcal, but this varies greatly with occupation.

Carbohydrates

Dietary carbohydrates may be in the form of simple or complex carbohydrates. Complex carbohydrates, mainly plant starches, are acted upon by salivary amylase, to produce oligosaccharides. The intestinal mucosa secretes maltase, lactase and sucrase to complete the conversion of these oligosaccharides to simple hexoses. The products of carbohydrate digestion are rapidly absorbed in the small intestine. Pentoses are absorbed by diffusion, although glucose utilises a sodium-driven active transport mechanism, with a limit of around 120 g per hour. The average daily requirement of carbohydrate for an adult is between 5 and 10 $g\,kg^{-1}$.

Proteins

Dietary proteins may be classed as grade I (contain all the essential amino acids, usually of animal origin) and grade II (lack one or more of the essential amino acids, almost

Fundamentals of Anaesthesia, 3rd edition, ed. Tim Smith, Colin Pinnock and Ted Lin. Published by Cambridge University Press. © Cambridge University Press 2008.

always of plant origin). Pepsin in the stomach and trypsin and chymotrypsin in the small intestine break down protein into peptides. The peptides are then further degraded to free amino acids by peptidases in the small intestine, where they are absorbed. The average daily requirement of protein is $0.5–1$ g kg^{-1}.

Lipids

Dietary lipids are usually in the form of neutral fats (fatty acids condensed with glycerol to produce an uncharged triglyceride) but may also include phospholipids and cholesterol. Ingested fats are digested by pancreatic lipase to produce free fatty acids, mono- and diglycerides. These are absorbed by simple diffusion, and reconstituted within the mucosal cell. Some lipid crosses the mucosal barrier by uptake as small lipid micelles. Reformed triglycerides, carrier proteins, phospholipids and cholesterol are then combined as chylomicrons. The average intake of fat in the diet is $1–2$ g kg^{-1}, although much lower intakes are well tolerated. A small percentage of the lipid intake must consist of essential fatty acids, which cannot be synthesised by the body. These include linoleic, linolenic and arachidonic acids.

Vitamins and minerals

Vitamins are organic molecules essential for life, but which can no longer be synthesised by higher organisms. Vitamins are only required in small amounts, but fulfil key functions. They are divided loosely into the water-soluble (C, B complex) and fat-soluble vitamins (A, D, E, and K).

Minerals are single elements also essential to life. They include calcium, phosphorus, magnesium, zinc, iron and iodine, all of which have minimal recommended daily intakes for an adult.

In addition, there are also minute quantities of other elements essential to life, such as copper, cobalt, manganese, nickel, molybdenum and chromium, which are known as trace elements.

Deficiencies of vitamins or minerals can produce a wide range of clinical syndromes. Some of these are outlined in Figure MT1.

Energy balance

Energy in the body is obtained by breaking down the larger molecules of digested food or alternatively using stored carbohydrate, fat or protein from body reserves. The degradation of these larger molecules is referred to as catabolism, and it is accompanied by the release of energy as the chemical bonds are broken. The energy released is either used to perform work or appears as heat. Approximately 60% of the energy released during catabolism appears as heat; only 40% produces useful work. The work done may be external work, such as that performed by skeletal muscles. Alternatively, internal work may be done, either mechanically, as in cardiac contraction, or biochemically, in the synthesis of larger molecules and high-energy compounds such as adenosine triphosphate (ATP). Cellular processes such as the active transport of substances across membranes and mucosa also use energy internally.

This energy balance in the body can be summarised as

$$\text{Total energy expenditure} = \text{Heat produced by the body} \\ + \text{External work done} \\ + \text{Energy stored}$$

Metabolic rate

The continuous energy expenditure per unit time in a person is supplied by metabolism, and is known as the metabolic rate. This is measured in kilocalories per hour and is dependent on various factors, which include:

- Age and sex
- Height, body weight and body surface area
- Pregnancy, menstruation and lactation
- Body temperature or environmental temperature
- Muscular activity
- Emotional state
- Circulating levels of hormones, e.g. thyroxine and epinephrine
- Recent ingestion of food
- Conscious level
- Presence of sepsis or other disease

Basal metabolic rate

The basal metabolic rate (BMR) is the metabolic rate of a subject under standardised conditions at mental and physical rest, in a comfortable environmental temperature and fasted for 12 hours. The BMR is not necessarily the minimum metabolic rate, since this may occur with the subject asleep. Under these conditions the BMR can be visualised as the basic metabolic cost of living. For an average young adult the BMR is about 70–100 kcal per hour.

Measurement of BMR

Under the specified steady-state conditions BMR can be measured directly, using a whole-body calorimeter. The subject is placed in the calorimeter chamber and the heat produced per hour is determined by the temperature rise of a steady flow of water through the calorimeter. Since the total energy expenditure of the body ultimately appears as

Substance	Function or coenzyme derivative	Deficiency
Water-soluble vitamins		
Vitamin C (ascorbic acid)	Antioxidant maintaining collagen integrity	Scurvy
Vitamin B_1 (thiamine)	Thiamine pyrophosphate	Beri-beri, congestive heart failure
Vitamin B_2 (riboflavin)	Flavine adenine dinucleotide	Angular stomatitis
Vitamin B_3 (niacin)	Nicotinamide adenine dinucleotide	Pellagra dermatosis, mental disorders
Vitamin B_6 (pyridoxine)	Pyridoxal phosphate	Peripheral neuropathy, convulsions
Panthothenic acid	Coenzyme A	Fatigue, sleep disturbance
Biotin	Carboxylases	Fatigue, depression, dermatitis
Folate	Tetrahydrofolate	Macrocytic anaemia, stomatitis, diarrhoea
Vitamin B_{12} (cyanocobalamin)	Cobamide coenzymes	Macrocytic anaemia, optic neuritis
Fat-soluble vitamins		
Vitamin A	Retinal precursor	Night blindness, xerophthalmia
Vitamin D	Regulation of calcium metabolism	Rickets, osteomalacia
Vitamin E	Antioxidant	Anaemia
Vitamin K	Coagulation cascade	Bleeding diathesis
Minerals and trace elements		
Iron	Component of haemoglobin, myoglobin, cytochromes,	Microcytic, hypochromic anaemia
Zinc	Alcohol dehydrogenase Alkaline phosphatase Carbonic anhydrase Superoxide dismutase	Growth restriction, hypogonadism
Copper	Cytochrome c oxidase Superoxide dismutase	Microcytic, hypochromic anaemia

Figure MT1 Vitamin and mineral deficiencies

heat in the absence of any external work done, the heat produced per hour equals the BMR of the subject.

The BMR can be estimated indirectly by measuring the oxygen consumption of a subject at rest. The oxygen consumption per hour is multiplied by 4.8 kcal of heat produced per litre of oxygen, to give the heat produced per hour. This is an empirical figure representative of heat production regardless of substrate used. The oxygen usage can be measured using a modified spirometer containing oxygen and a carbon dioxide absorber.

Metabolism

This term is used to describe the complex mass of biochemical reactions which break down the absorbed products of digestion to extract chemical energy, synthesise substances for structural maintenance and growth, and synthesise or detoxify waste products.

Organisation

The organisation of metabolism can be visualised as being composed of three sets of interlinked pathways. These deal with the three main types of molecule fed into the system, and are often referred to separately as carbohydrate metabolism, protein metabolism and fat metabolism. The three areas of metabolism are linked by the main energy-producing machinery, which comprises the citric acid cycle and the oxidative phosphorylation cascade (Figure MT2).

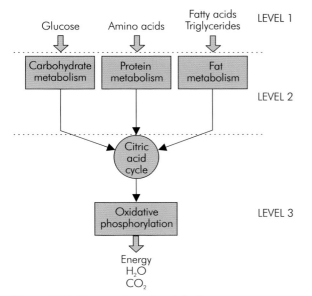

Figure MT2 Organisation of metabolism

The extraction of energy is a primary function of metabolism and provides the driving force that determines the direction taken by the different biochemical pathways. The universal energy currency used to move and supply energy to various pathways is a high-energy compound, adenosine triphosphate (ATP). Figure MT2 also shows how there are three levels of reactions involved in harvesting energy:

- Level 1 – breakdown of carbohydrates, proteins and fats into their simple molecules of glucose and other sugars, amino acids, and fatty acids and glycerol. No energy is produced at this level.
- Level 2 – degradation of these simpler molecules to a common smaller molecule, acetyl-CoA. A small amount of ATP is produced at this stage.
- Level 3 – passage of acetyl-CoA through the citric acid cycle, and an oxidative phosphorylation pathway, which generates >90% of the finally harvested ATP.

The generation and supply of energy for various reactions is the key to maintaining the complex metabolic pathways and keeping them in balance. Most metabolic reactions are potentially reversible, but are directed by the energy released or absorbed during the reaction. The energy exchanged during a reaction is called the free energy of the reaction, (ΔG). All reactions include a free energy component as well as the reagents. Thus, the reaction of reagents A and B to give products C and D can be written as

$$A + B + \Delta G \rightleftharpoons C + D$$

If energy is released, ΔG is negative, and the reaction proceeds spontaneously. If energy is absorbed, ΔG is positive, and the reaction has to be driven by supplying energy.

In general terms, metabolism tends to proceed spontaneously in the direction of catabolism, oxidation and the production of protons. The processes and reactions reversing these trends, i.e. anabolism, reductive reactions and the maintenance of acid–base balance, require energy. Thus, the supply of chemical energy for these reactions is the key to maintaining the life process.

Chemical energy may be supplied in different forms, which are outlined below.

Adenosine triphosphate (ATP)

The majority of reactions and processes requiring chemical energy to drive them use it in the form of ATP. This compound is used in processes such as the myosin–actin interaction in muscle or the active transport of substances across cell membranes, and is sometimes referred to as the common energy currency of metabolism. ATP delivers its energy when it is hydrolysed to adenosine diphosphate (ADP), since its usable energy is carried in a high-energy phosphoryl bond (Figure MT3). The ADP is 'recharged' by various reactions including the citric acid cycle, oxidative phosphorylation and phosphorylation by creatine phosphate. There is a continuous turnover of ATP and at rest an adult can use 40 kg ATP in 24 hours.

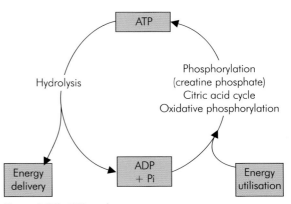

Figure MT3 ATP cycle

Carrier molecule	Group carried
Adenosine triphosphate (ATP)	Phosphoryl
Nicotinamide adenine dinucleotide (NADH)	Electrons
Nicotinamide adenine dinucleotide phosphate (NADPH)	Electrons
Flavine adenine dinucleotide (FADH$_2$)	Electrons
Co-enzyme A	Acyl
Thiamine pyrophosphate (TPP)	Aldehyde
Creatine phosphate	Phosphoryl

Figure MT4 Some activated carriers

Reaction site	Reaction pathway
Cytoplasm	Glycolysis Pyruvate oxidation Glycogenloysis Fatty acid synthesis
Mitochondria	Citric acid cycle Oxidative phosphorylation β oxidation

Figure MT5 Compartmentation of metabolic reactions between cytoplasm and mitochondria

Activated carriers

Although ATP has a universal role in supplying energy to drive reactions, other compounds also have the ability to drive reactions that require energy. The energy in these cases may be carried in the form of a high-potential electron or an activated group. In the case of an electron carrier, donation of an electron to one of the reagents constitutes a chemical reduction, which reverses the spontaneous tendency of the metabolic pathways towards oxidation. ATP can be regenerated with the use of a major electron carrier, nicotinamide adenine dinucleotide (NADH). Figure MT4 shows some of the known activated carriers operating in metabolic pathways.

Control of metabolism

Metabolic reactions are regulated via three basic mechanisms:

- The amounts of enzymes present – enzyme levels are regulated by varying the transcription rate of the genes that encode them. An example of this mechanism is the induction of β-galactosidase by lactose, which can increase enzyme levels by 50 times.
- The availability of substrates. Substrate levels intracellularly can be controlled by hormones that affect the transport of substrates across cell membranes. An example of this mechanism is the action of insulin in promoting glucose entry into cells.
- The activity of the enzymes – enzyme activity is subject to regulation via different biochemical mechanisms. A common mechanism is allosteric modulation, in which the active site of an enzyme is structurally altered by the attachment of a modulator molecule to a separate modulator site (see Section 2,

Chapter 1: Figure PG25). In many synthetic pathways, the final product of the pathway inhibits the first-stage reaction in this way, by reversible allosteric control.

Additional control of metabolism is provided by maintaining separate synthetic and degradative pathways. This may be achieved by physical separation of the pathways, as in intracellular *compartmentation*. In such a case, for example, fatty acid breakdown (β oxidation) occurs in mitochondria while fatty acid synthesis takes place in the cytoplasm (Figure MT5).

Systemic control of metabolic responses is mainly mediated by hormones. Various hormones such as the catecholamines, insulin, cortisol and thyroxine produce their physiological responses through wide-ranging changes in the metabolism of different tissues. Some examples are outlined below, while a summary of endocrine effects on metabolism is given in Section 2, Chapter 13.

Insulin

Insulin secretion is stimulated by glucose and amino acid uptake, and by parasympathetic innervation. Within the liver it increases glycogen synthesis, prevents gluconeogenesis and stimulates the glycolytic production of fatty acid precursors, with resultant increase in fat storage. In the gut it increases the uptake of branched-chain amino acids, and is a stimulant to formation of protein.

Amylin, co-secreted with insulin, may promote lactate transfer back to the liver, and support generation of fat stores.

Glucagon

Released by the pancreas in response to hypoglycaemia, glucagon acts on the liver to inhibit glycogen synthesis and promote gluconeogenesis and glycogen breakdown. In adipose tissue it results in the activation of lipases and fatty acid mobilisation.

Epinephrine and norepinephrine

Secreted as a response to stress or hypoglycaemia, these catecholamines promote glycogenolysis (greater in muscle than in liver) while reducing muscle uptake of glucose. Fatty acids are mobilised from adipose tissue to provide fuel for the increase in muscle activity.

Carbohydrate metabolism

Carbohydrate metabolism is mainly concerned with the generation of energy and the storage of carbohydrate as glycogen. The transportable form of carbohydrate throughout the body is the hexose sugar glucose (six-carbon, termed C6), which can be thought of as a universal fuel for all cells. The circulating levels of this are derived from:

- Dietary intake of carbohydrate
- Breakdown of stored carbohydrate in the form of glycogen, i.e. glycogenolysis
- Synthesis from smaller precursor molecules derived from other pathways, i.e. gluconeogenesis

The energy produced by the metabolism of one mole of glucose can be measured by the number of moles of ATP produced. Under aerobic conditions there is a net gain of 38 moles ATP per mole glucose. Each ATP molecule provides the energy from one activated phosphoryl group (7.6 kcal), which gives a total yield of 288 kcal chemical energy per mole glucose. If 1 mole glucose undergoes complete combustion in a calorimeter, it liberates about 686 kcal heat. The efficiency of carbohydrate metabolism is, therefore, 42%.

The main pathways in carbohydrate metabolism are:

- Glycolysis
- Gluconeogenesis
- Glycogenolysis and glycogenesis
- Hexose monophosphate (HMP) shunt

These pathways and their relationship to each other are illustrated in Figure MT6, and their functions are outlined below.

Glycolysis

Glycolysis (also called the Embden–Meyerhof pathway) breaks down glucose (C6) to the triose, pyruvate (C3). Its main function is to produce pyruvate for oxidation to acetyl-CoA to feed the citric acid cycle. Glucose is activated to glucose 6-phosphate to enter the pathway. This activated form may also be utilised to generate glycogen or for conjugation, but most enters into glycolysis (Figure MT7).

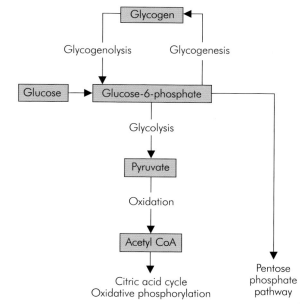

Figure MT6 Overview of carbohydrate metabolism

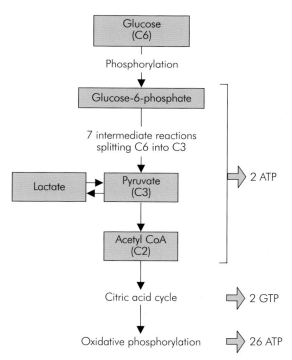

Figure MT7 Glycolysis

This pathway uses up 2 ATP, but generates 4 ATP and 2 NADH per molecule of glucose. Thus overall there is a net gain of 2 ATP and 2 NADH. Under aerobic conditions, the 2 NADH can be oxidised through oxidative phosphorylation to generate further ATP.

Glycolysis can also proceed under anaerobic conditions, but the net energy gain is then only 2 ATP, and lactate accumulates. Anaerobic glycolysis is important to the white muscle fibres of skeletal muscle. These are capable of intense activity disproportionate to their oxygen supply, which incurs an 'oxygen debt' in the form of the accumulated lactate. Lactate itself can be used as a substrate by some tissues. Pyruvate is oxidised to acetyl-CoA, which enters the citric acid cycle (also known as the Krebs cycle, after the biochemist who elucidated it) or can be used in other pathways.

Glycogenolysis

Glycogen is a branched polymer of glucose and is the storage form of carbohydrate in the body. Total body reserves are about 325 g, and these are distributed between skeletal muscle and liver in the ratio of 3 : 1. The pathways for the breakdown of glycogen (glycogenolysis) and its synthesis (glycogenesis) are different, employing different enzymes and controls. They are illustrated in Figure MT6. Glucose is activated by phosphorylation and combination with uridine triphosphate. It is then added to a pre-existing glycogen chain by glycogen synthetase. Branching of the glycogen chains requires a branching enzyme. Glycogenolysis requires a phosphorylase to activate and split off the terminal glucose unit from a glycogen chain. A debranching enzyme is also required to deal with branching points in the glycogen polymer. The enzymes in the glycogenesis and glycolytic pathways are distinct and respond individually to hormonal control. Storage of glucose as glycogen is highly efficient. The energy cost of storage and retrieval is a little over 3% of the total energy available from glucose.

Gluconeogenesis

Gluconeogenesis is the generation of glucose from substrates such as pyruvate and lactate. These in turn may be produced from amino acids by deamination, and consequently muscle mass also serves as a large potential glucose source. This is predominantly a liver function, although it does occur to some extent in the renal cortex. The much smaller mass of the kidney, however, means that the overall renal contribution is small. The purpose of gluconeogenesis is to allow maintenance of

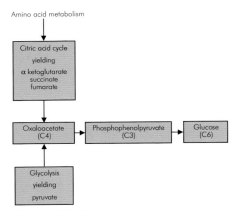

Figure MT8 Gluconeogenesis

plasma glucose for those tissues that preferentially use glucose as an energy source. An outline of the gluconeogenesis pathway is shown in Figure MT8. Gluconeogenesis from pyruvate is not simply a reverse of glycolysis, since the energetics so greatly favour pyruvate formation from the breakdown of glucose. Instead, pyruvate is converted to oxaloacetate at the cost of a single ATP by pyruvate carboxylase, and then phosphorylated and decarboxylated using GTP as an energy source, to give phosphoenolpyruvate. The net cost of glucose synthesis from pyruvate is 6 ATP, whereas only 2 ATP are generated in glycolysis.

Pentose phosphate pathway (PPP) or hexose monophosphate shunt

This is an alternative pathway for the activated form of glucose, glucose 6-phosphate. It is important in tissues that require reductive power for anabolic processes such as cell membrane repair, the synthesis of amino acids, fatty acids and steroids, and the production of nucleic acids.

The PPP is a cyclic pathway that takes in activated glucose units and produces CO_2, ribose 5-phosphate and NADPH (nicotinamide adenine dinucleotide phosphate). The NADPH is important as an activated reducing agent in certain tissues such as the liver, adipose tissue, erythrocytes and the testes.

The cyclic process involves the transfer of a C2 fragment between pentoses (C5), and also provides a source of ribose 5-phosphate, an aldopentose required in the production of nucleic acids (Figure MT9).

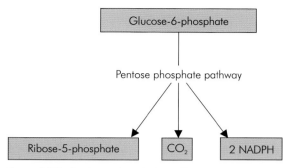

Figure MT9 Pentose phosphate pathway

Oxidation of pyruvate to acetyl-CoA

This step in carbohydrate metabolism occurs inside the mitochondria and is important because it irreversibly funnels pyruvate (C3) into the citric acid cycle. The net reaction is:

$$\text{Pyruvate} + \text{CoA} + \text{NAD}^+ = \text{acetyl-CoA} + CO_2 + \text{NADH}$$

It is a complex reaction requiring pyruvate dehydrogenase (an enzyme complex composed of three different types of enzyme) and several cofactors (including TPP and NAD). This key reaction is subject to feedback control, in which the presence of high levels of energy in the form of NADH, ATP and acetyl-CoA 'switch off' the pyruvate dehydrogenase complex. There is thus a net energy gain in this step of NADH, which can be converted to ATP through oxidative phosphorylation.

Citric acid cycle

The citric acid cycle and the oxidative phosphorylation process both form the core of the energy-producing machinery in metabolism. They take place in the mitochondria and are not exclusive to carbohydrate metabolism, but form a common end pathway for the products of carbohydrate, lipid and protein metabolism. Carbohydrate metabolism and the breakdown of lipids feed acetyl-CoA into the cycle, while protein metabolism can feed into the cycle via several intermediates, including oxaloacetate (C4), α-ketoglutarate (C5) and fumarate (C4).

The main entry to the citric acid cycle is via acetyl-CoA, which is essentially an activated C2 (acetyl) group bound to a carrier (coenzyme A). This C2 fragment is loaded onto a C4 molecule (oxaloacetate) to form citrate (C6), which passes around a cycle of intermediate compounds. Two decarboxylation reactions take place to regenerate the

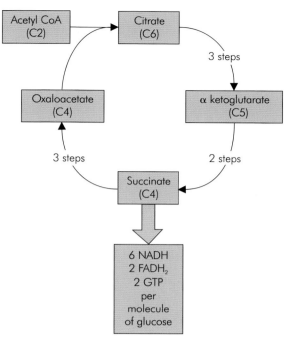

Figure MT10 Citric acid cycle

oxaloacetate (C4). Energy production from each cycle is in the form of:
- Three NADH
- One high-energy phosphoryl bond in guanosine triphosphate (GTP)
- One FADH$_2$

The NADH and FADH$_2$ are high-potential electron carriers, and enter the oxidative phosphorylation process to generate ATP (Figure MT10).

Oxidative phosphorylation

Oxidative phosphorylation is a biochemical process in the mitochondria in which ATP is generated by the high-potential electrons carried by NADH and FADH$_2$. *High potential* refers to the tendency for electrons to be transferred from these activated carriers to a cascade of lower-potential carriers (NADH-Q reductase, cytochrome reductase and cytochrome oxidase) which are located in the inner mitochondrial membrane, and which are sometimes referred to as the *respiratory chain*.

These mitochondrial membrane carriers are basically proton pumps activated by the flow of electrons through them. They pump H$^+$ out of the inner mitochondrion to give an H$^+$ gradient across the inner membrane. This H$^+$

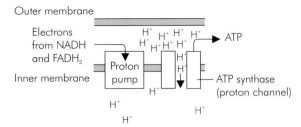

Figure MT11 Oxidative phosphorylation

gradient then generates ATP by driving H^+ back across the inner membrane through channels of ATP synthase. The passage of H^+ through these channels catalyses the synthesis of ATP (Figure MT11).

Defects in carbohydrate metabolism

Inborn errors in the metabolism of carbohydrates can be grouped as follows:

- Intestinal defects
- A deficiency of an enzyme in the intermediary metabolic pathways, with accompanying lactic acidosis
- A deficiency of an enzyme in the intermediary metabolic pathways, without accompanying lactic acidosis
- Glycogen storage disease

Some examples are shown Figure MT12.

Protein metabolism

The basic building block of a protein is the amino acid. Amino acids are characterised by the presence of carboxyl and amine groups on a carbon atom. Also attached is a group R, as shown below:

$$H_2N - \underset{\underset{R}{|}}{\overset{\overset{H}{|}}{C}} - COOH$$

R may be simple, as in glycine, where R = H; or complex, as in glutamic acid, where $R = (CH_2)_2COOH$.

Amino acids can be condensed into chains to form peptides, and these chains can increase in size to form proteins. Protein chains can form a secondary structure by winding and twisting together. Such twisted chains can form more complex molecules by assuming a tertiary structure resulting in sheets or fibres. In a quaternary structured protein, the amalgamation of several tertiary proteins or subunits forms a final complex protein molecule. Examples of such quaternary structures are haemoglobin (formed by four globin subunits connected to a haem core) and apoferritin (20 subunits arranged to form a hollow sphere).

Amino acid pool

Body proteins undergo a continual turnover by being broken down into amino acids and resynthesised from the same amino acids. This creates a metabolic *amino acid pool*, which provides not only precursors for protein synthesis but also many other compounds and pathways, including:

- Purines and pyrimidines
- Hormones
- Neurotransmitters

Disease	Biochemical defect	Clinical features
Intestinal defect		
Lactose intolerance (non familial type)	Gastrointestinal lactase deficiency	Diarrhoea, flatulence, abdominal discomfort
Enzyme deficiency with lactic acidosis		
von Gierke disease	Glucokinase deficiency	Large liver and kidneys, stunted growth, 'doll's face', lactic acidosis
Enzyme deficiency without lactic acidosis		
Galactosaemia	Galactokinase deficiency	Cataracts, hepatomegaly, mental retardation
Glycogen storage disease		
Pompe disease	Lysosomal debranching enzyme deficiency	Infantile cardiomegaly, hepatomegaly, hypotonia

Figure MT12 Examples of defects in carbohydrate metabolism

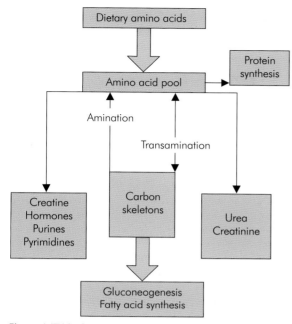

Figure MT13 Overview of protein metabolism

Amino acid	Intermediate
Isoleucine Leucine Tryptophan	Acetyl-CoA (C2)
Alanine Cysteine Glycine Serine	Pyruvate (C3)
Aspartate Phenylalanine Tyrosine	Fumarate (C4)
Methionine Threonine Valine	Succinyl CoA (C4)
Arginine Glutamate Histidine Proline	α-ketoglutarate (C5)

Figure MT14 Conversion of some amino acids to metabolic intermediates

- Creatine
- Gluconeogenesis
- Fatty acid synthesis
- Citric acid cycle

Interconversion of different amino acids, or between amino acids and intermediates of carbohydrate and lipid metabolism, enables specific pathways to link into the amino acid pool. These interconversions occur via transamination, amination or deamination reactions, which are active in many tissues. The metabolic amino acid pool is replenished by the absorbed products of ingested protein.

Excess amino acids from the amino acid pool have their amino groups removed, leaving carbon skeletons. These residues enter other pathways (such as the citric acid cycle), while the excess amino groups are ultimately excreted as urea and creatinine. Figure MT13 gives a simple overview of protein metabolism.

Transamination and deamination

Transamination is the transfer of an NH_2 group to another molecule, usually a keto acid. This common reaction allows excess amino acids to be degraded to intermediates that can be metabolised to give energy. Alternatively these intermediates can be used in gluconeogenesis or the synthesis of fatty acids. An example is the transfer of NH_2 from alanine to α-ketoglutarate, as follows:

$$\text{alanine} + \alpha\text{-ketoglutarate} = \text{pyruvate} + \text{glutamate}$$

Pyruvate can then be oxidised to acetyl-CoA and enter the citric acid cycle.

Deamination is the removal of the amino group from an amino acid to leave a carbon skeleton that can be metabolised. An example of deamination occurs with serine, which can be deaminated to give pyruvate:

$$\text{serine} = \text{pyruvate} + NH_4^+$$

In this way many of the amino acids can be converted to relatively few intermediate molecules (Figure MT14).

Defects in amino acid metabolism

Congenital syndromes are recognised that are due to the disruption of specific amino acid pathways. These are usually rare but illustrate the importance of individual amino acids. Some examples are shown in Figure MT15.

Condition	Biochemical defect	Clinical features
Phenylketonuria	↓ conversion of phenylalanine to tyrosine	1 in 10 000 births Mental retardation
Homocystinuria	↓ levels of cysteine and cystine ↑ levels of homocystine and methionine	Tall, thin body, subluxation of lens, mental retardation
Alkaptonuria	↑ levels of homogentisic acid	Ochronosis (pigmented connective tissues), arthritis

Figure MT15 Examples of defects in amino acid metabolism

Nitrogen balance

Although amino acids are continually recycled from the amino acid pool, a daily loss occurs from the gastrointestinal tract and in the urine. Normally, therefore, protein intake is required to compensate for these losses. The intake and losses of protein may be assessed by their nitrogen content, and these should be balanced in the healthy adult. Normal nitrogen requirements for an adult are a daily intake of about 10 g (approximating to 46 g protein). Dietary intake should be decreased in the presence of hepatic or renal dysfunction since the capacity of the body to produce and excrete urea is compromised. In the case of hypermetabolic and hypercatabolic illness the body requirements are increased.

Negative balance occurs if losses exceed intake, as in illness or starvation. Positive balance, when intake is greater than losses, occurs in growth, convalescence or the use of drugs such as anabolic steroids. Urinary nitrogen losses are mainly contained in the excreted urea, although small amounts of nitrogen are also excreted as creatinine, uric acid and amino acids.

Urea cycle

Excess amino acids are deaminated to release NH_4^+. This reaction occurs mainly in two tissues:

- The kidneys, where the NH_4^+ dissociates into NH_3 and H^+ for excretion into the urine.
- The liver, where the NH_4^+ is converted to carbamyl phosphate, which then contributes to the formation of urea.

The formation of urea is a cyclic process that takes place in the mitochondria. In a normal adult, about 30 g urea is produced daily. In hepatic failure, this conversion is less likely to occur, and an accumulation of ammonia occurs. The formation of urea is illustrated in Figure MT16, which shows how urea, which has two nitrogen atoms, obtains one from carbamyl phosphate and the other by

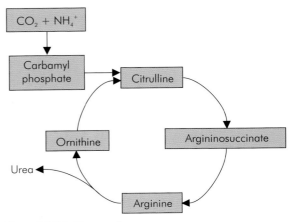

Figure MT16 Urea cycle

transamination from aspartate. The synthesis of one molecule of urea requires the energy from 3 ATP. This process is sometimes referred to as the *ornithine cycle*.

Creatine and creatinine

Creatine is present in muscle, brain and blood. It is particularly important in its phosphorylated form as an immediate store of high-energy phosphoryl bonds for the generation of ATP from ADP. The chemical energy for the first few seconds of muscle contraction is supplied by ATP generated from this source. Creatine is phosphorylated by creatine kinase. The serum levels of this enzyme are used as a marker of muscle damage following trauma or myocardial infarction – although creatine kinase activity may also be raised simply as a result of violent exercise.

Creatinine is the anhydride of creatine and is formed as a metabolite for excretion in the urine. The 24-hour urinary excretion of creatinine is relatively constant for any given individual, while renal tubular reabsorption is small. This means that the value for creatinine clearance can be used as an approximation to glomerular filtration rate.

Purines and pyrimidines

These substances are ring-based structures that occur widely throughout the body. They form the base components in the ribonucleotides and deoxyribonucleotides, i.e. the 'alphabet' triplets that code RNA and DNA strands. Purines and pyrimidines occur throughout the tissues as carriers of high-energy phosphoryl bonds, e.g. adenosine triphosphate (ATP), guanosine triphosphate (GTP) and uridine triphosphate (UTP). These molecules are also ubiquitous as the functional parts of many cofactors.

Purines

Purines are double-ringed molecules with six- and five-membered nitrogenated rings, commonly occurring examples being adenine and guanine. When metabolised, purines ultimately give rise to uric acid, which is excreted in the urine. The average excretion rate for an adult is between 400 and 600 mg over 24 hours. Uric acid and sodium urate are found in the plasma and urine. They have relatively limited solubility at body pH and urine pH, and it requires only a moderate increase in uric acid levels to precipitate the deposition of urate crystals in the tissues or in the kidneys. The clinical syndrome of gout is associated with hyperuricaemia and deposition of urate in soft tissues and joints. The underlying defect is usually a combination of overproduction and increased breakdown of purines, but the cause may range from an enzyme deficiency to a hypercatabolic state.

Pyrimidines

Pyrimidines are based on a six-membered nitrogenated ring. Common pyrimidines in the body are cytosine, thymine and uracil. Breakdown of pyrimidines occurs in the liver and results in highly soluble products, β-alanine and β-aminoisobutyric acid.

Lipid metabolism

The lipids occurring in the body can be classified into the following groups:

- Fatty acids – chains of saturated or unsaturated carbon atoms with a terminal carboxyl group. These form the body's main energy store, and are also components of many structural molecules.
- Triglycerides – storage form for fatty acid chains, in which three chains are attached to a glycerol (C3) mole by ester linkages. Triglycerides are not free in the plasma but are transported as lipoproteins in chylomicra.
- Plasma lipoproteins – 95% of plasma lipids are transported in combination with protein to make them soluble. These lipoproteins have different roles and are targeted to specific tissues.
- Phospholipids and glycolipids – form building blocks for membranes and tissues.
- Cholesterol – precursor of steroid hormones and a component of membranes.

Fatty acids

Fatty acids have the following important functions:
- Fuel molecules
- Components of phospholipids and glycolipids
- Components of hormones and intracellular messengers

Free fatty acids (FFA) only form about 5% of the lipids in the plasma, but this group of lipids is the most active metabolically. They are stored as triglycerides and metabolised to yield energy by β oxidation in the mitochondria. The energy yield from fatty acid oxidation is about 9 kcal g^{-1}, compared with 4 kcal g^{-1} for carbohydrates and protein. In addition, because triglycerides are hydrophobic they are effectively anhydrous compared to glycogen, which binds twice its weight in water. This means weight for weight triglycerides contain more than six times the energy of carbohydrates. A 70 kg man possesses about 11 kg triglycerides, representing a reserve of 100 000 kcal stored energy, compared with 25 000 kcal stored as protein and only 600 kcal stored as carbohydrate. The synthesis of fatty acids takes place in the cytoplasm by using acetyl-CoA to elongate fatty acid chains in C2 steps. An overview of lipid metabolism is shown in Figure MT17.

Beta oxidation of fatty acids

The breakdown of fatty acid chains to give energy is a cyclic process called β oxidation, which takes place in the mitochondrial matrix. Free fatty acids in the cytoplasm are first activated by esterification with acetyl-CoA. The activated fatty acid is then loaded onto a carrier protein called carnitine at the outer mitochondrial membrane. This complex is transported across the inner mitochondrial membrane into the mitochondrial matrix, where it is unloaded by recombination with acetyl-CoA. This is performed by an inner membrane protein called carnitine acyltransferase. Carnitine is then returned to the outer membrane, where it is available to pick up more activated fatty acid. This cyclic process is sometimes known as the *carnitine shuttle*. In the matrix C2 fragments are split off

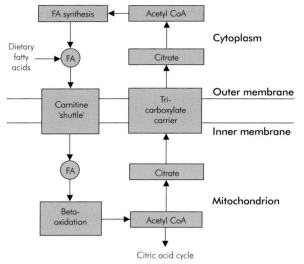

Figure MT17 Overview of lipid metabolism

passes back into the mitochondria, where it is re-converted back to citrate.

Reducing power in the form of NADPH is required for fatty acid synthesis. Some of this is generated by the citrate–pyruvate carrier cycle, while the pentose phosphate pathway provides the rest.

Fatty acid synthesis is regulated by a key enzyme, acetyl-CoA carboxylase, to ensure that synthesis and degradation occur appropriately for the body's needs. This control responds to biochemical feedback as well as hormones such as insulin and the catecholamines.

Plasma lipoproteins

Plasma triglycerides and cholesterol combine with proteins to form a range of lipoprotein particles, the largest being chylomicrons (100–1000 nm diameter), while the smallest are the high-density lipoproteins (7.5–20 nm diameter). These macromolecular aggregates have different lipid contents and are metabolised by specific tissues. Their basic structure consists of a lipid core coated with protein and phospholipid to solubilise them. Specific apoproteins in the particle coatings act as cellular signals for target tissues. The lipoproteins are classified according to density and have different metabolic functions (Figure MT18).

Cholesterol

Cholesterol is a component of all cell membranes and produces membrane fluidity by its interaction with membrane phospholipids. It possesses a steroid-based structure and is also a precursor of the steroid hormones. Cholesterol is, therefore, essential for the growth and viability of the tissues. Tissues outside the liver obtain cholesterol from the plasma low-density lipoprotein (LDL) particles, using membrane LDL receptors to mediate uptake. Normal plasma levels of cholesterol are 2.5–3.5 mmol l^{-1}, and are

from the fatty acid in repeated steps, each C2 fragment producing acetyl-CoA to feed into the citric acid cycle. In this way a molecule of a C16 fatty acid (palmitoyl) can produce 106 molecules of ATP.

Fatty acid synthesis

Fatty acid synthesis takes place in the cytoplasm, in contrast to β oxidation, which is mitochondrial. This is also a cyclic process that builds up fatty acid chains by the addition of activated C2 fragments (acetyl-CoA). These C2 fragments are obtained from the mitochondria and are transferred out to the cytoplasm by a citrate carrier. The acetyl-CoA is removed from the citrate in the cytoplasm, leaving the citrate, which is then converted to pyruvate. The pyruvate

Lipoprotein	Major core lipid	Function
Chylomicrons	Dietary triglyceride	Carries dietary triglycerides to tissues for fuel (e.g. muscle)
Chylomicron remnants	Dietary cholesterol	Taken up by liver for metabolism
Very low-density lipoprotein (VLDL)	Endogenous triglyceride	Exported form of excess triglyceride and cholesterol from liver
Low-density lipoprotein (LDL)	Endogenous cholesterol	Major carrier of cholesterol to peripheral tissues for metabolism
High-density lipoprotein (HDL)	Endogenous cholesterol	Cholesterol from dying cells and membrane repair, for recycling

Figure MT18 Plasma lipoproteins

(a) Normal metabolism

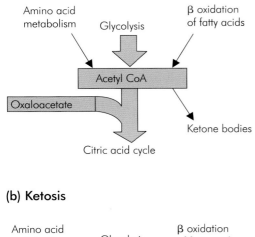

(b) Ketosis

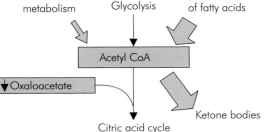

Figure MT19 Ketosis

contributed to by both diet (normal daily intake is about 1 g) and endogenous synthesis. Abnormally high levels of cholesterol result in disease due to deposition of cholesterol in soft tissues and formation of cholesterol-containing plaques in arteries (atherosclerosis).

Eicosanoids

The eicosanoids are C20 unsaturated fatty acids containing a five-carbon ring. They are derived from arachidonic acid, which is synthesised from linoleic acid, one of the essential fatty acids. The eicosanoids include the following compounds:

- Prostaglandins
- Leukotrienes
- Thromboxanes
- Prostacyclin

These substances are local hormones with short-lived and highly localised effects, depending on the tissue in which they are released. Their effects are wide-ranging and include stimulation of the inflammatory response, regulation of local blood flow, control of membrane transport, modulation of synaptic transmission and modulation of platelet adhesion. A key step in the synthesis of prostaglandins is cyclo-oxygenase, which can be inhibited by non-steroidal anti-inflammatory drugs such as aspirin.

Ketones

When excessive levels of acetyl-CoA are present, the acetyl-CoA is diverted to form acetoacetate and γ-hydroxybutyric acid. These compounds are known as ketone bodies, and accumulation of ketone bodies results in the clinical syndrome of ketosis or ketoacidosis (Figure MT19).

Acetyl-CoA represents a crossroads between major metabolic pathways. It can be produced either by glycolysis or by β oxidation. Normally glycolysis is responsible for supplying the acetyl-CoA for the citric acid cycle, but if the glycolytic pathway fails, as in uncontrolled diabetes or starvation, acetyl-CoA is obtained from β oxidation. Under such circumstances excessive levels can result because of:

- Insulin deficiency, leading to increased free fatty acid levels
- Increased glucagon levels, which stimulate β oxidation
- Decreased levels of oxaloacetate, due to increased gluconeogenesis

Starvation

Starvation is a complete absence of dietary intake, and can result in death after about 60 days. This should be differentiated from malnutrition, in which some calorific intake may be present, but which follows a more protracted course accompanied by the effects of chronic lack of protein, fats and essential vitamins and minerals.

In starvation, glucose supplies to the brain are a priority, since it is largely dependent on glucose as an energy substrate. Initially there is an increase in glycogenolysis. However, as glycogen reserves are depleted, blood glucose falls to subnormal levels. Mobilisation of fatty acids occurs to provide energy, and the liver ceases to use glucose as a substrate but uses fatty acids instead. Muscle also adapts to use fatty acids as an energy source.

With the depletion of glycogen, gluconeogenesis increases, using amino acid residues derived from the breakdown of muscle protein. Gluconeogenesis takes place in the liver, which also uses glycerol from lipolysis and oxaloacetate. The use of these substrates leads to the accumulation of acetyl-CoA and hence the formation of ketone bodies. Thus starvation is associated with ketosis. Most tissues, including the brain, can ultimately adapt to the use of ketone bodies as a fuel source. Therefore, protein catabolism is quite rapid in early starvation, but as the body shifts to the use of ketone bodies, the rate of protein breakdown decreases. After three days approximately a third of the brain's energy requirements are derived from ketone bodies, and ultimately this proportion increases to a half. The total reserves of an average adult are sufficient to provide the calorie requirements for about 3 months.

The liver

Structure

The liver weighs 1.5–2 kg and is divided into right and left lobes, the right lobe being much larger than the left (up to six times its size). The functional unit of the liver is the hepatic lobule. These are roughly hexagonal in cross section and possess a central vein from which cords of hepatocytes radiate outwards. In between the lobules are portal spaces through which run a bile duct and branches of the hepatic artery and portal vein. The radial spaces between the hepatocytes are called sinusoids and carry a mixture of arterial and portal blood supplied by the vessels in the portal spaces, towards the centre of the lobule, where it drains into the central vein. The central veins join to form the hepatic vein, which drains into the inferior vena cava.

As the blood flows though the sinusoids it is exposed over a large surface area to the hepatocytes, which are highly active metabolically. The walls of the sinusoids are also lined by macrophages known as Kupffer cells, which are an active part of the reticuloendothelial system.

The cords of hepatocytes are closely apposed to bile canaliculi, which drain centrifugally towards the bile ducts in the portal spaces. These carry the bile secreted by the hepatocytes to the gallbladder and common bile duct (Figure MT20). For detail of bile formation and content see Section 2, Chapter 11 (pages 444–6).

Metabolic functions

The metabolic functions of the liver may be divided into:
- Formation of bile
- Protein metabolism
- Carbohydrate metabolism
- Lipid metabolism
- Detoxification
- Excretion

Protein synthesis

The major proteins synthesised by the liver include albumin, globulins and clotting factors.

Albumin

This is synthesised at about 200 mg kg^{-1} per day in a normal adult. This is about 4% of the total body albumin pool. Plasma albumin correlates well with liver synthetic activity, but with a half-life of about 20 days, it is a poor marker for acute liver injury. Albumin is important in the maintenance of plasma colloid oncotic pressure, and in the transport of drugs, bilirubin and some hormones.

Globulins

These are a range of lipo- and glycoproteins with transport functions (e.g. ferritin, caeruloplasmin). The liver is the principal site for synthesis and recycling of haptoglobin, which serves to bind and conserve free haemoglobin.

Clotting factors

Most clotting factors are synthesised exclusively by the liver. Half-lives vary widely, up to 28 days for prothrombin. Coagulopathies may occur either due to failure of hepatic synthesis directly or because of failure of bile excretion leading to a reduction in the absorption of vitamin K, necessary for the synthesis of factors II, VII, IX and X. Factor VII has one of the shortest half-lives, at about 4 hours.

Protein catabolism

The liver is involved in protein catabolism either directly, in turnover of proteins in the hepatocyte, or indirectly, in handling the products of the absorption of dietary proteins or amino acids from peripheral protein turnover. Amino acids or dipeptides from portal or systemic circulations are absorbed by the liver. They may be used as substrates for new protein synthesis, or used for gluconeogenesis. The conversion of amino acids to carbon skeletons may involve transamination, deamination or modification to primary amines. The by-product from deamination is ammonia, which may be converted by the ornithine cycle to ammonia. In a normal adult, about 30 g of urea is produced daily. In hepatic failure, this conversion is less likely to occur, and an accumulation of ammonia occurs.

Carbohydrate metabolism

The liver's main role in carbohydrate metabolism is in maintaining glucose homeostasis during periods of fasting. It accomplishes this by glycogenesis, storing glycogen and

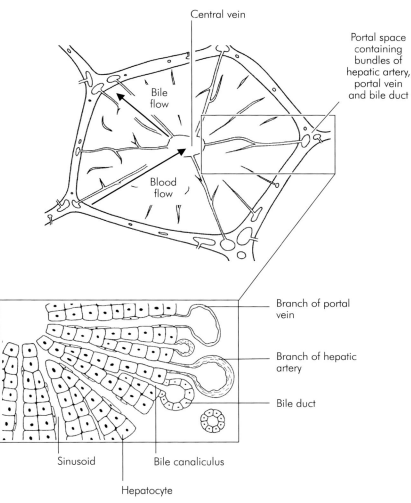

Figure MT20 Structure of the liver

glycogenolysis. When glycogen reserves are depleted it is the site of gluconeogenesis.

Lipid metabolism

The liver synthesises fatty acids and lipoproteins for export. It is also a major site of endogenous cholesterol and prostaglandin synthesis.

Detoxification

The liver has a major function in the detoxification of steroid hormones. The mechanisms for detoxification are also used for the metabolism of exogenous substances, in particular therapeutic drugs.

Drug metabolism

Drug metabolism in the liver is divided into two phases:
- Phase 1 – covers modification of the drug to increase its polar nature and make it hydrophilic. It also provides reactive end groups to act as conjugation sites.
- Phase 2 – involves conjugation of the modified drug with hydrophilic groups to increase its solubility and aid renal excretion.

Phase 1 metabolism is almost entirely oxidative. There is a little reductive metabolism in the gut, and in isolated hepatocytes, as most of the liver is relatively hypoxic, with periportal hepatocytes running at a normal PO_2 of about 3 kPa.

Phase	Reaction
Phase 1	Oxidation
	Hydrolysis
	Hydration
	Dealkylation
	Reduction
	n-oxidation
	Isomerisation
Phase 2	Glucuronidation
	Sulphation
	Acetylation
	Glutathione conjugation

Figure MT21 Hepatic metabolism of drugs

This oxidative activity is carried out by a diverse enzyme superfamily known collectively as cytochrome P_{450}, which occurs in many tissues. A large part of first-pass metabolism may be due to cytochrome activity in the gut mucosa. Similarly, nephrotoxicity after the metabolism of volatile anaesthetic agents may be due to intrarenal metabolism by cytochromes, rather than a consequence of elevated plasma fluoride levels.

Phase 2 metabolism is conjugative. Drugs that have been modified by phase 1 metabolism are usually left with reactive end groups (such as hydroxyl). These groups provide sites for conjugation with more hydrophilic compounds, such as glucuronic acid, acetate, sulphate or glutathione (Figure MT21).

The overall result of phase 1 and 2 metabolism is to produce a modified drug structure that is hydrophilic and rapidly eliminated by the kidneys.

Body temperature and thermoregulation

Body temperature is tightly regulated. Many enzyme and transport systems cannot tolerate excessive temperature changes. Normal body temperature is 37 °C and thermoregulatory mechanisms maintain this temperature with a standard deviation of about 0.2 °C. There are normal variations within this range, such as a circadian variation of up to 0.7 °C. A variation during the menstrual cycle produces a rise in temperature at ovulation. Body temperature may be altered by various factors including exercise, feeding, thyroid disease, infection and drugs.

Physiological mechanisms

The hypothalamus processes temperature information from skin, central tissues and neural tissues. Cold signals travel via A fibres, and warm signals via C fibres in the spinothalamic tracts. This temperature information is integrated and compared to temperature thresholds. Thermoregulation is currently thought to be based on a series of thresholds that activate thermoregulatory responses when crossed by the integrated temperature information. The further the crossed threshold is from the 'normal' temperature, the greater is the response pattern.

If the **warm threshold** is exceeded, heat-loss responses are initiated, which include:
- Behavioural modification, e.g. removal of clothes
- Cutaneous vasodilatation
- Sweating
- Panting

If the **cold threshold** is exceeded, thermogenic activities are initiated. These include:
- Behavioural (turning on heat sources, adding more clothes)
- Exercise
- Cutaneous vasoconstriction
- Shivering
- Non-shivering thermogenesis

Thermoregulatory responses

There are several effective thermoregulatory responses in the normal human. These include:
- Behaviour – in a conscious adult, this is the major regulator of heat loss. The options to move away from heat sources, modify local temperature, or add or remove clothing make this a very powerful mechanism
- Cutaneous blood flow – skin blood flow is a combination of capillary flow and extracapillary shunts. Vasoconstriction minimally reduces capillary flow but has major effects on the shunts, which act as thermoregulator mechanisms. Vasodilatation can increase capillary blood flow up to about 7 litres per minute.
- Shivering – can increase metabolic activity by up to 600% in adults. The effectiveness of this heat source is reduced by the fact that muscle activity also increases blood flow to peripheral tissues, dissipating the heat generated.

- Non-shivering thermogenesis – specialised areas of brown fat are able to increase metabolic output by fat oxidation. This can increase heat production by up to 100% in infants, but is much less effective in adults.
- Sweating – in stressed athletes, sweating can account for the loss of about 2 litres per hour, and increase heat loss by a factor of 10.

Disturbances of thermoregulation
Fever
This is one of the most common manifestations of disease. It is due to the production of endogenous pyrogens, which are most likely to include certain interleukins, interferons and tumour necrosis factor (TNF). These cytokines are thought to act by causing the local release of prostaglandins in the hypothalamus. The antipyretic effect of aspirin and other non-steroidal anti-inflammatory agents is due to the inhibition of cyclo-oxygenase, a key enzyme in prostaglandin synthesis.

Malignant hyperpyrexia
A genetic condition that causes widespread persistent muscle contraction when triggered by stress or specific anaesthetic agents. The result is massive heat production and a rapid uncontrolled rise in body temperature with metabolic acidosis and myoglobinuria. The underlying lesion is a defect in the gene coding for the ryanodine receptors in the sarcoplasmic triads, which leads to excessive Ca^{2+} release.

Hypothermia
Hypothermia is said to be present when body core temperatures are less than 36 °C. It may be associated with:
- Exposure
- Near-drowning
- The elderly
- Hypothyroidism
- Prolonged surgery

Normal metabolic and physiological processes are slowed down, resulting in hypotension, bradycardia, bradypnoea and loss of consciousness. In severe cases, pulmonary oedema and ventricular fibrillation may occur.

Re-warming can be active or passive, and with adequate physiological support humans can be resuscitated from 20–25 °C without permanent sequelae.

Hypothermic effects of anaesthesia and surgery
Anaesthesia has a number of effects on thermoregulation. Behavioural responses are totally abolished. An individual is unable to control his or her environment, clothing levels or level of voluntary muscle activity. Cutaneous vasoconstriction is antagonised by vasodilator anaesthetics. In addition, thresholds are directly affected by anaesthesia, which tends to increase the displacement of the thresholds from normal temperature. The hyperthermic thresholds are increased by about 1 °C, while hypothermic thresholds are markedly reduced, by up to 3–4 °C. This effect also appears to be dose-dependent. Thus, thermoregulatory responses to heat loss are impaired or abolished.

The physical mechanisms during anaesthesia and surgery causing heat loss are:
- Conduction – heat loss due to contact with an object at a lower temperature such as a cold operating table. The rate of heat loss is dependent on the temperature gradient between the body and the table, the surface area of contact, and the thermal conductance of the tissues.
- Convection – heat loss due to the movement of air away from the exposed body surfaces, which will be increased by imposed air-flow currents such as in laminar-flow operating theatres.
- Radiation – heat loss by infrared radiation from exposed portions of the body to neighbouring objects not in contact. This may be reduced by the use of reflective coverings such as a space blanket over the exposed surfaces, or by increasing the ambient temperature.
- Evaporation of sweat from skin or body fluids from mucosal or tissue surfaces – heat loss is due to the latent heat of evaporation lost when fluid changes phase from liquid to vapour. The rate of heat loss is dependent on the mass of fluid evaporated per unit time, since the latent heat of evaporation is a constant.

CHAPTER 13
Endocrinology

J. M. James

Endocrine physiology is the study of hormones, the glands that produce them, and the effects that hormones have on their target organs. Endocrine function is necessary to maintain homeostasis, and is associated with the unconscious and subconscious functions of the body. It is closely linked with areas in the brain and nervous system that control homeostasis, especially the hypothalamus.

The main effects of hormones on the body are control of metabolism, nutrition and growth, sexual and reproductive development, and blood pressure and temperature control.

Traditionally, the gland releases the hormone into the bloodstream, the hormone travels over time to the target organ, and an effect is produced – a relatively slow process. It is now recognised that the physiology is much more complex. Hormones may be produced that act on neighbouring cells (e.g. histamine and prostaglandins), or they may even act on the secreting cell itself. These effects are much more rapid.

Classification of hormones

The more common hormones are listed in Figure EN1.

Polypeptides

Examples – vasopressin, oxytocin, prolactin, insulin, glucagon. These are usually produced as a prohormone which undergoes conversion to its active form. These hormones are stored in granules and secreted by exocytosis and thence into the bloodstream.

Glycoproteins

Examples – TSH, FSH, LH. These are polypeptide hormones linked to carbohydrate residues.

Steroids

Examples – corticosteroids, aldosterone, sex hormones. Steroids are synthesised in the cell mitochondria, from cholesterol. These hormones are not stored in secretory granules, but are produced by the cell as and when required,

Fundamentals of Anaesthesia, 3rd edition, ed. Tim Smith, Colin Pinnock and Ted Lin. Published by Cambridge University Press. © Cambridge University Press 2008.

Polypeptides	Glycoproteins	Steroids	Amines	Fatty acid derivatives
Vasopressin	FSH	Aldosterone	PIH (dopamine)	Prostaglandins
Oxytocin	LH	Corticosteroids	Epinephrine	Vitamin D
ACTH	TSH	Testosterone	Norepinephrine	
FSH-RH		Oestrogen	Thyroxine	
LH-RH		Progesterone	Tri-iodothyronine	
ACTH-RH				
TRH				
PTH				
Calcitonin				
Insulin				
Glucagon				
Somatostatin				

Note that ACTH (adrenocorticotropic hormone) is sometimes still referred to as corticotropin, and ACTH-RH (adrenocorticotropic hormone-releasing hormone) is also frequently called CRH (corticotropin-releasing hormone) or CRF (corticotropin-releasing factor). We have chosen to use the terms ACTH and ACTH-RH in this text.

Figure EN1 Classification of some common hormones

and are bound to protein in the bloodstream en route to the target organ.

Amines
Examples – thyroxine, epinephrine. All the amine hormones are synthesised from the amino acid tyrosine. They are stored in follicles (thyroxine) or granules (catecholamines). Some (e.g. thyroid hormones) may be converted to a more active form nearer to the site of action.

Indole and fatty acid derivatives
Examples – prostaglandins. These produce effects either in the cell or in adjacent cells.

Cellular action of hormones
Hormone receptors
Hormone receptors may be on the cell membrane (or trans membrane) or inside the cell. They increase and decrease in number depending on external stimuli. When there is an excess of hormone the number of receptors decreases (down-regulation); conversely, when there is a deficit of hormone the number of receptors increases (up-regulation). Sometimes down-regulation occurs when the receptors change their chemical structure and become less responsive. The hydrophilic hormones have receptors in the cell membrane, and the lipophilic hormones

(e.g. thyroid and steroid hormones) have receptors within the cell, either cytoplasmic or nuclear.

Some hormones require the presence of small amounts of other hormones in order for their receptors to be fully active. This is known as permissiveness. Small amounts of glucocorticoids, for example, are necessary for catecholamines to produce their lipolytic effects.

Mechanisms of change of cell function
Direct effect on cell membranes
The hormone alters the permeability of the membrane to certain ions, e.g. K^+ and Ca^{2+}, via G proteins. This effect is very rapid.

Effects via second messengers
Hormones bind with receptors in the cell membrane and cause intracellular effects via second messengers.

The second messenger cyclic adenosine monophosphate (cAMP) phosphorylates proteins within the cell. Hormones may increase or decrease levels of cAMP. When a hormone reacts with the receptor within the cell, guanyl nucleotide regulatory proteins are activated within the cell membrane. These may be stimulatory (Gs) or inhibitory (Gi) to the production of cAMP.

Other hormones activate different second messengers, such as IP_3 and DAG. The hormone receptor complex

Affecting permeability	Via G proteins increasing cAMP	Via G proteins decreasing cAMP	Via PIP$_2$,IP$_3$ and DAG	Via mRNA
GH	Oxytocin	Somatostatin	Epinephrine (α_1)	Thyroxine
Prolactin	Vasopressin	Epinephrine (α_2)	Vasopressin	Tri-iodothyronine
Insulin	LH			Steroid hormones
	FSH			
	TSH			
	ACTH			
	Epinephrine (β receptors)			
	PTH			
	Glucagon			

Figure EN2 Common hormones and their mechanism of action

activates an enzyme which breaks down a membrane phospholipid, phosphatidylinositol diphosphate (PIP$_2$), to inositol triphosphate (IP$_3$) and diacylglycerol (DAG). IP$_3$ releases Ca^{2+}; DAG activates protein kinase C, which increases cell division and multiplication. This reaction is enhanced by the released Ca^{2+}.

Protein synthesis

Thyroid and steroid hormones, being very lipophilic, cross the cell membrane rapidly and, once bound with their receptor, cross to the nucleus, where they bind with DNA. This increases mRNA synthesis and via ribosomes leads to an increase in protein production.

Figure EN2 shows the mechanism of action of common hormones.

Control of hormone production

Various mechanisms control hormone secretion. These include levels of inorganic ions (sodium), organic molecules such as glucose and direct physical and chemical stimulation, e.g. gut hormones.

The most important regulator is, however, the negative feedback system. In this system high levels of a substance produced by the hormone reduce the secretion of that hormone, ensuring that the level of the substance itself remains relatively constant.

The negative feedback can be direct or indirect. Direct feedback includes the effect of circulating glucose on insulin production. An example of indirect feedback is shown by the effect that circulating glucocorticoids have on ACTH-RH and thus on levels of ACTH.

Hypertrophy and atrophy

If the level of a specific hormone in the blood remains very low despite maximal production and release, there will be a large increase in the level of the relevant tropic hormone, and the other cells in the producing gland will enlarge and multiply in order to compensate. This is seen as a thyroid goitre in iodine deficiency. Conversely, if there are very high circulating levels of hormone produced by medication (e.g. steroids), the tropic hormones will fall to very low levels and the gland will atrophy. Tropic hormones, therefore, influence both hormone production from the cell and the size of the gland producing the hormone.

Pituitary gland

Anatomy

The pituitary gland is made up of the anterior lobe (adenohypophysis) and posterior lobe (neurohypophysis), which are intimately connected to the hypothalamus.

The anterior and posterior lobes develop quite separately from each other. The anterior lobe develops from Rathke's pouch, an outgrowth from the roof of the mouth. The posterior lobe develops as an extension from the hypothalamus, an evagination of the floor of the third ventricle. The two join together. The part of the anterior lobe which fuses with the posterior lobe is known as the intermediate lobe, which is rudimentary in humans. The remains of Rathke's pouch form the residual cleft (Figure EN3).

The anterior and posterior lobes have independent functions, but both are connected to the hypothalamus by the pituitary stalk. The **anterior lobe** is connected

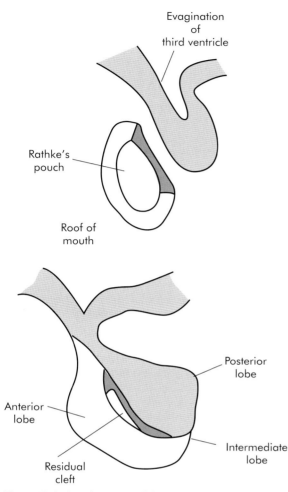

Figure EN3 Development of the pituitary gland

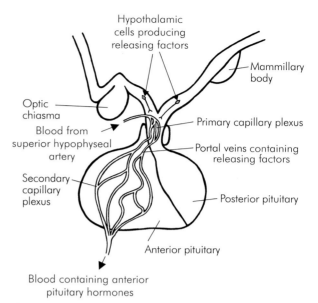

Figure EN4 Portal system of the anterior pituitary gland

- Somatotropes (50%) produce GH
- Lactotropes (10–30%) produce prolactin
- Corticotropes produce ACTH
- Thyrotropes produce TSH
- Gonadotropes produce FSH and LH

Posterior lobe hormones are produced in neurosecretory cells in the hypothalamus. These form granules which pass down the axons through the pituitary stalk and are stored in the posterior lobe, later to be released into the bloodstream when stimulation occurs.

Vasopressin is produced in the supraoptic nucleus of the hypothalamus, and oxytocin from the paraventricular nucleus (Figure EN5).

Pituitary hormones
Anterior lobe
- Thyroid-stimulating hormone (TSH, thyrotropin)
- Adrenocorticotropic hormone (ACTH, corticotropin)
- Growth hormone (GH, somatotropin, STH)
- Prolactin (PRL)
- Follicle-stimulating hormone (FSH)
- Luteinising hormone (LH)

Posterior lobe
- Vasopressin (antidiuretic hormone, ADH)
- Oxytocin

to the hypothalamus by the portal circulation, which transports releasing hormones into the lobe, stimulating the production of tropic hormones into the bloodstream.

The portal circulation is a network of capillaries which arises from the superior hypophyseal artery. The primary capillary plexus, located on the floor of the hypothalamus (known as the median eminence), absorbs releasing factors; the blood then passes via the portal veins in the pituitary stalk to the secondary capillary plexus, where they are released into the anterior lobe. The tropic hormones are then secreted into the plexus and into the bloodstream (Figure EN4).

The anterior lobe hormones are found in five types of secretory cell:

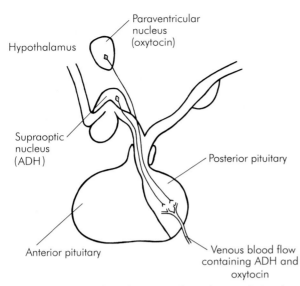

Figure EN5 Secretion of vasopressin and oxytocin by the posterior pituitary

Functions of individual hormones
Thyroid-stimulating hormone (TSH)
Stimulates the production of thyroid hormones from the thyroid gland, and growth of the gland itself.

Adrenocorticotropic hormone (ACTH)
Stimulates the adrenal cortex to produce corticosteroid hormones (mainly cortisol) and also binds to melanotropin receptors in the melanocytes in the skin, which produce melanin and pigmentation.

Growth hormone (GH)
GH causes growth of tissue in the body. It stimulates protein synthesis, lipolysis and a rise in blood glucose. In childhood it is especially active, and it causes an increase in length of the long bones until the epiphyses fuse.

Not all its effects are direct. Some of the effects on target tissues are mediated through polypeptide substances produced by the liver and other tissues called somatomedins. These are closely related to insulin. Insulin-like growth factor I (IGF-I) is involved with skeletal and cartilage growth. IGF-II also exists and is thought to be involved in fetal growth.

Lack of GH in childhood leads to dwarfism, and excess to gigantism – the patient is either very small or very tall but in proportion. Excess in the adult leads to acromegaly. As this occurs after the epiphyses have fused there is little

increase in height, but there is overgrowth of the skull, facial bones and hands and feet. Reduced glucose tolerance is common.

Prolactin
Stimulates milk production post partum, and suppresses ovulation. Excess production can cause lactation and infertility.

Follicle-stimulating hormone (FSH)
Stimulates ovulation in females and spermatogenesis in males.

Luteinising hormone (LH)
Stimulates ovulation and luteinisation of ovarian follicles in females, and testosterone secretion in males.

Vasopressin (ADH)
Vasopressin causes water retention by increasing water absorption from the distal tubules and collecting ducts of the kidney. It is stimulated by a rise in osmotic pressure in the plasma via osmoreceptors in the anterior hypothalamus, by a reduced extracellular volume, a rise in angiotensin II, and by pain, stress and exercise. It is reduced by a decrease in plasma osmotic pressure, and by an increase in extracellular volume and alcohol.

There are several types of receptors, V_{1a}, V_{1b} and V_2, which are all G-protein coupled. The antidiuretic effects are mediated through V_2 receptors, which open aquaporin 2 water channels in collecting ducts of the kidneys. Vasopressin also has a powerful vasoconstrictor effect in vitro on vascular smooth muscle, although this is small in vivo. This is mediated through receptors found in the area postrema in the brain, and the mechanism is very sensitive to haemorrhage. Vasopressin receptors are also found in the liver, where they stimulate glycogenolysis, and in the brain. Figure EN6 shows how these are arranged. V_3 is an alternative classification for V_{1b}.

Type	Location	Function
V_{1a}	Smooth muscle and heart	Vasoconstrictor effect
V_{1b}/V_3	CNS	Mediate release of ACTH-RH
V_{1a}	Collecting ducts	Permit water reabsorption

Figure EN6 Classification of vasopressin receptors

Deficiency of vasopressin leads to diabetes insipidus, where there is polyuria and polydipsia due to water loss. It can be primary, due to disease of the gland, or secondary, where the kidneys are unable to respond to vasopressin.

Excess of vasopressin (inappropriate secretion) leads to fluid retention with low plasma osmolarity and hyponatraemia. Vasopressin-secreting malignant lung tumours are one such cause.

Oxytocin

Oxytocin causes milk ejection from glands in the breast, stimulated by suckling and via touch receptors. It also causes uterine contraction during labour and in the immediate postpartum period.

Pituitary deficiency and excess

Deficiency can be caused by tumours and cysts which press on the pituitary gland. It may also occur in women who have experienced severe hypovolaemia during childbirth leading to necrosis (Sheehan's syndrome). The changes which develop depend on the location of the damage to the gland.

Excess can be produced either by secreting tumours arising from the gland itself or from other sites in the body.

Control of pituitary hormones

The hypothalamus is intimately connected to the pituitary gland, and is responsible for a number of so-called releasing hormones. These polypeptides are produced in the median eminence of the hypothalamus and pass into the portal system to the anterior lobe, where they stimulate or inhibit production of the tropic hormones.

Hypothalamic releasing factors include:
- Thyrotropin-releasing hormone (TRH)
- Adrenocorticotropic hormone-releasing hormone (ACTH-RH)
- Growth hormone releasing and inhibiting hormones (GH-RH and GH-IH) (GH-IH is somatostatin, also produced in pancreatic islet cells)
- Prolactin releasing and inhibiting hormones (PRH and PIF – dopamine)
- Gonadotropic releasing hormone (Gn-RH) – stimulates production of FSH and LH

Some releasing factors have an effect on other hormones. TRH stimulates prolactin production, and GRH inhibits TSH, for example.

The hypothalamus has many inputs which are concerned with vegetative regulation, and it is also connected to other parts of the central nervous system, and its output is affected by stress, diurnal rhythm and emotional factors.

The function of the anterior lobe is under negative feedback control. When the levels of hormones which are produced in the target organs increase, the production of both the tropic hormones and the releasing factors is reduced. Conversely, when the target-organ hormone levels decrease there is increased production of both the tropic hormones and the releasing factors. This keeps the hormone levels relatively constant (Figure EN7).

When steroids are given as medication over a period of time, the anterior pituitary and the hypothalamus produce minimal stimulation of endogenous cortical adrenal steroids, and the adrenal gland atrophies. This can have

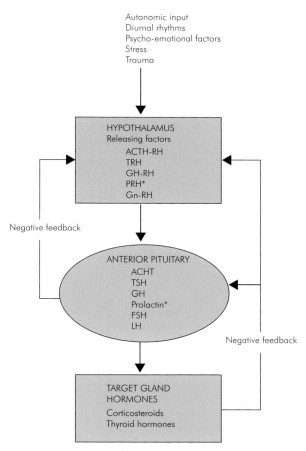

*Main control of prolactin is by PIH

Figure EN7 Feedback control of pituitary hormones

Part of pituitary	Hormone	Main stimulus and control	Action
Anterior lobe	TSH	+ve TRH, −ve thyroid hormones	Thyroid gland to produce thyroid hormones
	ACTH	+ve ACTH-RH, −ve corticosteroid hormones	Adrenal gland to produce corticosteroid hormones
	GH	+ve GH-RH, −ve GH-IH	Increase growth of body tissue especially bone
	Prolactin	+ve PRF, −ve PIF	Milk production, suppression of ovulation
	FSH	+ve Gn-RH	Breast development, milk secretion, spermatogenesis
	LH	+ve Gn-RH	Stimulation of ovulation, testosterone secretion
Posterior lobe	Vasopressin	+ve osmolarity, thirst, pain, haemorrhage	Water reabsorption from distal tubules
	Oxytocin	+ve touch receptors in breast and genitalia	Ejection of milk from breast, uterine contraction

Figure EN8 Pituitary hormones: their production, control and action

serious consequences if the steroids are suddenly stopped, especially if the patient is undergoing a stressful procedure such as surgery.

The pituitary hormones are summarised in Figure EN8.

Thyroid gland

The thyroid gland affects the basal metabolic rate to enable the body to function optimally. It does this via the thyroid hormones, which affect carbohydrate, lipid and protein metabolism, also affecting growth and maturation, and body temperature.

Anatomy

The thyroid gland originates from the floor of the pharynx. The thyroglossal duct marks the path of the gland from the tongue to its final site, and sometimes this persists in adults. The gland is situated in the neck at the level of the second and third tracheal rings. It comprises two lobes on either side of the trachea, joined by the thyroid isthmus. Each lobe has an upper and lower pole. Sometimes there is a third lobe, the pyramidal lobe, which arises anteriorly from the thyroid isthmus. The gland is highly vascular, its arterial supply coming from the superior and inferior thyroid arteries, and its venous drainage via the superior, middle and inferior thyroid veins. The parathyroid glands are located within the thyroid gland.

The gland itself comprises many follicles (acini). The follicles are lined by the thyroid epithelial cells, and within the follicle itself is a variable amount of colloid, which mainly contains thyroglobulin and iodine. There are also parafollicular (C or clear) cells which secrete calcitonin. The thyroid cells rest on a basal membrane, which separates them from the capillaries.

When the gland is inactive the follicles are large and contain substantial amounts of colloid. The cells are small and flattened. When the gland is active, the follicles reduce in size; there is little colloid, and the cells become enlarged and columnar or cuboid. The edge of the colloid develops a scalloped appearance due to reabsorption lacunae at the tips of the cells (Figure EN9).

Thyroid hormones

The most important hormones secreted by the thyroid gland are tri-iodothyronine (T_3) and tetra-iodothyronine (T_4). Both are produced from tyrosine found in thyroglobulin, which combines with iodine in the colloid, and is then secreted by the thyroid cells into the bloodstream.

Iodine is required for synthesis of thyroid hormones. Iodine is ingested from dietary sources. It is converted to iodide (I^-) in the gut and passes into the bloodstream. It is taken up principally by the thyroid gland, but also by the kidney, which excretes it.

Resting state

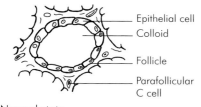

- Epithelial cell
- Colloid

- Follicle

- Parafollicular
  C cell

Normal state

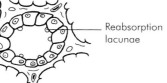

- Reabsorption
  lacunae

Highly active state

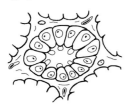

Figure EN9 Follicular structure of the thyroid gland

The thyroid cell membranes which lie next to the capillaries absorb iodide via a sodium and iodide pump which concentrates iodide levels in the cell 20–40-fold. Energy for this is supplied by $Na^+K^+ATPase$. The iodide is secreted into the colloid and oxidised back to iodine.

Synthesis of thyroid hormones

Thyroglobulin is a large glycoprotein, containing about 10% carbohydrate. It is produced by the thyroid cells and secreted onto the colloid by exocytosis. It contains 123 tyrosine residues. In the colloid, iodine combines with 4–8 of these residues to form mono-iodothyronine (MIT) and di-iodothyronine (DIT). MIT combines with DIT to form tri-iodothyronine (T_3) and DIT combines with DIT to form tetra-iodothyronine (T_4) (Figure EN10). MIT and DIT also combine to form isomeric reverse tri-iodothyronine (rT_3), which is inactive.

Alanine is produced in all these coupling reactions as the side chain making up the outer ring of the molecule is eliminated. These reactions are catalysed by the enzyme thyroid peroxidase, which also oxidises iodide to iodine in the colloid (Figure EN11).

FIRST STAGE

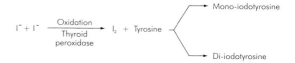

AFTER COMBINATION IN COLLOID

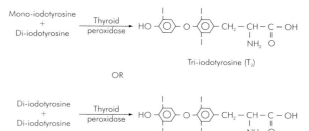

Figure EN10 Thyroid hormone synthesis

The hormones are held bound to thyroglobulin until they are secreted. They then pass into the thyroid cell by endocytosis, and are secreted by the cells into the bloodstream. The removal of the hormones from the colloid adjacent to the cells creates the reabsorption lacunae seen in active cells.

The thyroid cell has therefore three main functions:
- Absorption and concentration of iodide, and secretion into the colloid
- Production of thyroglobulin and thyroxine peroxidase and secretion into the colloid
- Absorption of thyroid hormones from the colloid and secretion into the bloodstream

Secretion, transport and metabolism of thyroid hormones

Secretion is controlled by circulating levels of thyroid-stimulating hormone (TSH). Normal plasma levels for the unbound (free) hormone are about 5 pmol l^{-1} for T_3, and 15 pmol l^{-1} for T_4. Ninety per cent of total secretion per day is of T_4, the remainder being T_3 and a small amount of rT_3, which is inactive. T_3 is, however, up to five times as potent as T_4, which is considered to be a prohormone of T_3. Thirty-three per cent of T_4 is converted to T_3, and much of the remainder to rT_3. The difference in activity is due to differing binding to the intracellular receptors.

Thyroid hormones are transported in the blood by a variety of proteins, including albumin, thyroxine-binding

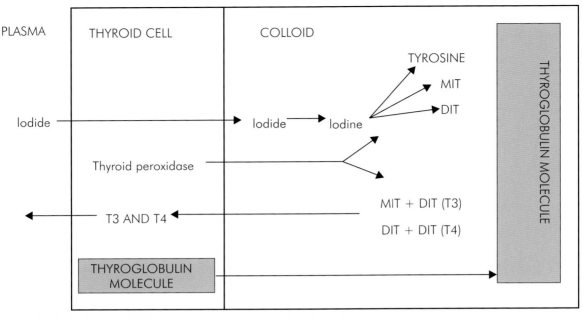

Figure EN11 Outline of thyroid hormone formation in cell and colloid

prealbumin (TBPA or transthyretin) and thyroxine-binding globulin (TBG). Albumin has the greatest capacity, but TBG the greatest affinity, such that most of the hormone is bound to TBG. Less than 1% of the hormones remain unbound. If there is a fall or rise in the total level of the binding proteins the level of the free unbound hormone will remain the same. It is the level of unbound hormone which stimulates or reduces the plasma levels of TSH.

The hormones are deiodinated in the kidney, liver and other tissues, and 33% of T_4 is converted to T_3. Both hormones are also partly broken down to DIT, and also conjugated in the liver to form sulphates and glucuronides, which are excreted in the bile.

Control of thyroid hormone secretion

The main control is the negative feedback system operating via TSH from the anterior pituitary gland, and releasing factor (TRH) from the hypothalamus.

TSH increases secretion of T_3 and T_4 by releasing the hormones from thyroglobulin, from where they are secreted into the thyroid cells and thence into the blood. TSH also increases the size and number of the cells in the thyroid gland itself, which when excessive may lead to goitre. There is also an increase in iodide binding, an increase in T_3 and T_4, release of thyroglobulin into the colloid, and increased endocytosis of colloid by the cells.

Other factors which affect hormone production are trauma, stress and warmth, which decrease it, and cold, which increases it.

Mechanism of action of thyroid hormones

T_3 and T_4 both enter cells and bind with receptors in the nuclei, T_3 more avidly. The hormone receptor complex then binds with DNA, leading to new mRNA and protein synthesis. The number of mitochondria increases, and there is an increase in metabolic rate, with increased oxygen utilisation, energy production and heat.

There is a catabolic effect, with a stimulation of lipolysis and increased protein breakdown. Absorption of carbohydrate from the gut is increased.

Within the cardiovascular system, there is an increase in the number of β-adrenergic receptors in the heart, which also becomes more sensitive to the effect of catecholamines. This leads to a rise in the pulse rate, a decrease in peripheral resistance and an increase in contractility of the heart muscle.

Thyroid hormones are also necessary for normal skeletal and nervous system development. The effects of thyroid hormones are summarised in Figure EN12.

Effect	Mechanism
Catabolic	Increased protein breakdown in muscle
	Increased lipolysis in adipose tissue
Metabolic	Increased absorption of carbohydrate from gut
Developmental	Normal skeletal growth
	Normal brain development
Cardiovascular system	Increase β-adrenoceptors in heart
	Increased sensitivity to catecholamines
	Inotropic and chronotropic effects, reduced peripheral resistance
Heat production	Increased metabolic rate in active tissues

Figure EN12 Summary of main effects of thyroid hormones

Deficiency and excess of thyroid hormones

Deficiency (hypothyroidism)

This may be caused by pituitary or hypothalamic failure, disease of the thyroid gland itself, or iodine deficiency.

In adults this may lead to myxoedema. Symptoms and signs include lethargy, slow mental processes and sometimes severe mental symptoms (myxoedema madness). Metabolism is slow; there may be weight gain and intolerance to cold. The voice becomes husky, and the skin and subcutaneous tissues become thickened and stiff, due to reduced breakdown of proteins which accumulate in those sites. In iodine deficiency there may be goitre due to the increased levels of TSH stimulating gland growth.

Children with hypothyroidism develop cretinism. They are mentally retarded, and have the characteristic signs of dwarfism, pot bellies and large protruding tongues.

Excess (hyperthyroidism)

This may be caused by excess production of TSH, for instance from a pituitary tumour, or due to disease of the thyroid gland itself. Solitary adenomas, toxic multinodular goitres and thyroiditis may all lead to excess hormone production.

Graves' disease is an autoimmune disorder in which there are antibodies to the TSH receptors that stimulate the receptors themselves. In 50% of patients there is also deposition of tissue behind the eyeball, giving the characteristic appearance of exophthalmos. There is also a goitre. The condition is more common in women.

Symptoms and signs of hyperthyroidism include nervousness, tremor, weight loss, sweating and heat intolerance. There may be a tachycardia and a widened pulse pressure.

Parathyroid glands

The parathyroid glands are essential for maintaining normal levels of serum calcium, which are necessary to maintain normal cell function, where Ca^{2+} acts as a second messenger. It is needed for coagulation of blood, transmission of nervous impulses and muscular contraction. Calcium is provided by various dietary sources, and plasma levels are altered by varying absorption in the gut, mobilisation from bone and excretion by the kidney.

Anatomy

There are four disc-like parathyroid glands, two embedded in the upper poles of the thyroid gland, and two in the lower, though their siting and number can be variable.

The cells within the gland are of two types. The so-called chief cells have abundant Golgi apparatus and endoplasmic reticulum, and contain secretory granules that produce parathyroid hormone (PTH). The oxyphil cells are fewer but larger and their function is unknown.

Parathyroid hormone

PTH is a polypeptide produced in the chief cells. It is converted from a preprohormone to a prohormone and thence to PTH, which is stored in the secretory granules before release into the bloodstream.

Action and regulation

PTH has three main actions:

- Mobilisation of Ca^{2+} from bone, raising the plasma Ca^{2+} level.
- Increased reabsorption of Ca^{2+} in the distal tubules, raising the plasma level of Ca^{2+}, and decreased reabsorption of phosphate in the proximal tubules, increasing phosphate excretion.
- Increased production of 1,25-dihydroxycholecalciferol, which increases Ca^{2+} absorption from the intestine.

There are at least three types of PTH receptors. The main mechanism of action appears to be activation of adenyl cyclase via G proteins, increasing cAMP levels.

PTH levels are regulated via a negative feedback linked to Ca^{2+} levels. Low levels of Ca^{2+} stimulate PTH secretion and raise Ca^{2+}; high levels of Ca^{2+} reduce PTH production and lower Ca^{2+}, thus maintaining homeostasis. Magnesium is also necessary for the proper function of the parathyroid glands.

Other hormones affecting calcium levels

Two other hormones have a direct effect on calcium levels. These are vitamin D and calcitonin.

Vitamin D

Vitamin D refers to a group of sterol compounds which are closely related. Cholecalciferol (vitamin D_3) is synthesised in the skin by the action of ultraviolet light on ingested 7-dehydroxycholesterol. This is converted in the liver to 25-cholecalciferol (calcidiol), which passes to the kidney and is converted to the much more active 1,25-dihydroxycholecalciferol (calcitriol). Less than 10% of ingested vitamin-D-related sterols are converted directly to 25-cholecalciferol in the liver, bypassing conversion in the skin (Figure EN13).

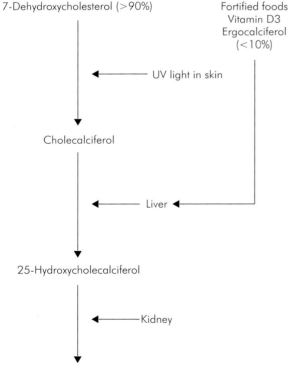

Figure EN13 Formation of 1,25-dihydroxycholecalciferol

Hormone	Ca²⁺	Phosphate
PTH	Increase	Decrease
1,25-dihydroxy-cholecalciferol	Increase	Increase
Calcitonin	Decrease	Decrease
Glucocorticoids	Decrease	Decrease
Thyroid hormones	Variable	Variable
Growth hormone	Increase	Increase

Figure EN14 Summary of main effects of hormones on calcium and phosphate levels

Like other steroid hormones, 1,25-dihydroxycholecalciferol acts by binding to the cell nucleus receptor, exposing DNA binding sites and altering transcription of mRNA. It raises Ca^{2+} and phosphate levels by increasing absorption from the gut, and increases Ca^{2+} absorption in the kidneys. It increases the activity of osteoblasts, laying down Ca^{2+} into the bone matrix.

Calcitonin

Calcitonin is produced by the parafollicular cells (C cells) of the thyroid gland. It reduces Ca^{2+} and phosphate levels in the plasma by reducing bone reabsorption, and is stimulated by high levels of calcium.

The function in humans is unclear. Low levels of calcitonin, which occur following thyroidectomy, do not appear to cause any deficiency syndromes. It may be involved with skeletal development and control of Ca^{2+} levels after meals.

Glucocorticoids lower Ca^{2+} by inhibiting bone breakdown by osteoclasts, but may cause osteoporosis in the long term. Thyroid hormones cause a rise in plasma calcium but also increase excretion in the kidney. Growth hormone increases absorption of calcium from the gut and has a lesser effect on the kidney, causing increased excretion.

The effects of hormones on calcium and phosphate levels are summarised in Figure EN14.

Deficiency and excess of parathyroid hormones

Deficiency

Deficiency of PTH, which may occur following thyroid surgery, can cause hypocalcaemia and hyperphosphataemia, leading to increasing neuromuscular excitability and possible tetany.

In pseudohypoparathyroidism, the levels of PTH are normal, but there is a receptor abnormality leading to a similar picture.

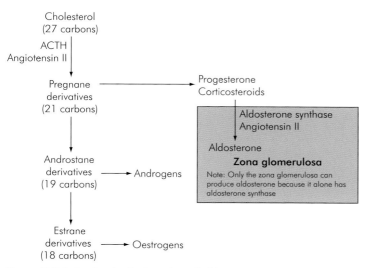

Figure EN15 Synthesis of adrenal cortical hormones

Lack of vitamin D can lead to rickets in children and osteomalacia in adults.

Excess

Excess PTH may be produced by a secreting parathyroid adenoma. There is hypercalcaemia and hypophosphataemia, but the patient is often asymptomatic. There may be associated kidney stones or mental symptoms.

In chronic renal failure the kidney cannot form 1,25-dihydroxycholecalciferol. This leads to a chronically low Ca^{2+}. The parathyroid glands hypertrophy in response to the low Ca^{2+}, leading to secondary hyperparathyroidism.

Excess consumption of vitamin D leads to a rise in both Ca^{2+} and phosphate in the blood.

Adrenal glands

The adrenal glands are found on the upper poles of both kidneys. They comprise two functionally distinct parts, the adrenal cortex and the adrenal medulla.

The cortex is divided into three parts or zones:

- The zona glomerulosa (15% of the gland) secretes mineralocorticoids, which maintain sodium balance and ECF volume
- The zona fasciculata (50%) secretes glucocorticoids, which have widespread effects on metabolism
- The zona reticularis (7%) secretes androgenic hormones

The adrenal medulla (28%) secretes catecholamines, which are produced in 'fight or flight' situations. Both the zona glomerulosa and the zona reticularis are necessary to sustain life. The other parts of the adrenal gland are not.

Adrenal cortex

The zona glomerulosa is situated on the outside layer of cortex, the zona fasciculata in the middle, and the zona reticularis in the inside, next to the adrenal medulla.

All the cortical cells contain large amounts of endoplasmic reticulum, and large amounts of lipid. There is some overlap of hormone production between the three zones, although mineralocorticoids are only produced in the zona glomerulosa. The latter zone is also able to generate new cells for the other zones should they be damaged or removed.

All the cortical hormones are synthesised from cholesterol, and therefore they all have similar chemical structures based around a steroid nucleus. Aldosterone can only be produced in the zona glomerulosa because the enzyme which converts corticosteroids to aldosterone, aldosterone synthase, is only found in that zone.

As with all steroid hormones, they bind with a receptor within the cytoplasm, and the complex so formed moves to the nucleus. There is increased DNA transcription, with increased mRNA synthesis, leading to formation of proteins and enzymes (Figures EN15, EN16).

Mineralocorticoids

The most important of these is aldosterone, which has 95% of the total mineralocorticoids effect, the rest being provided by glucocorticoids. Its production is essential for

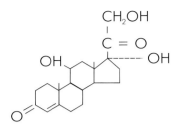

Cortisol

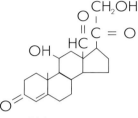

Aldosterone

Figure EN16 Chemical structures of cortisol and aldosterone

water is also absorbed and K^+ and H^+ are excreted into the urine.

Aldosterone is produced in very small amounts, is only slightly protein-bound, and has a very short half-life of about 20 minutes.

Control of aldosterone secretion is influenced by:
- ACTH (very little effect in vivo)
- Plasma potassium levels, with a negative feedback system
- Angiotensin II

The most important is angiotensin II. Low Na^+ levels or reduced perfusion at the juxtaglomerular apparatus cause the production of renin, and via the renin–angiotensin system produce angiotensin II.

Glucocorticoids

The main hormone produced is cortisol (hydrocortisone). Less important ones include corticosterone and cortisone.

Cortisol is bound in the plasma to an α-globulin, transcortin, and to albumin to a lesser extent. The half-life in plasma is about 100 minutes, but the effects of the hormone last much longer.

The level of free unbound hormone activates the feedback control linked to ACTH. If the amount of binding globulin rises, more hormone is bound, which reduces plasma levels. ACTH production is stimulated and more unbound fraction is formed until a new equilibrium is reached.

Glucocorticoids have far-reaching effects on the body and are essential to sustain life. Their effects are summarised in Figure EN17.

Control of cortisol secretion is via the negative feedback system linked with ACTH from the anterior

the maintenance of sodium levels and ECF volume. Its production is stimulated by:
- Increased plasma Na^+
- Decreased plasma K^+
- Reduced ECF volume
- Trauma, stress, surgery, anxiety

The hormone increases reabsorption of sodium from the kidneys, stomach, sweat, saliva and intestine. In the kidneys

Metabolism	Catabolic	↑ Protein breakdown ↑ Gluconeogenesis ↑ Lipolysis Anti-insulin effect (not in brain or heart)
Water		Allows body to excrete a water load (mechanism not understood)
Vascular reactivity and blood pressure control		Allows vascular smooth muscle to respond to circulating catecholamines Facilitates conversion of norepinephrine to epinephrine in adrenal medulla
Blood cells		↑ Red cells, platelets, neutrophils ↓ Neutrophils, basophils, eosinophils
Mineralocorticoid effect		↑ Na^+ ↓ K^+ ↓ H^+ (effect normally small)
Anti-inflammatory		Only at high levels

Figure EN17 Summary of main effects of glucocorticoid hormones

pituitary gland. ACTH is itself controlled by a negative feedback system by ACTH-RH, secreted from the hypothalamus.

Circadian rhythms in the body cause a fluctuation in cortisol levels because of the effects of these on the hypothalamus and ACTH-RH production. Cortisol levels tend to be higher in the morning. Likewise stress and trauma will stimulate ACTH-RH via the hypothalamus, stimulating ACTH and increasing cortisol production.

Adrenocortical androgenic hormones

The main hormones secreted are dehydroepiandrosterone (DHEA) and androstenedione. The latter is converted to testosterone and oestrogens in peripheral tissues and fat. The androgenic effects of the cortical hormones are small unless they are secreted in excess. There is a sensitive negative feedback system linked with ACTH.

Adrenal medulla

The adrenal medulla resembles a large sympathetic ganglion which has lost its postganglionic fibres and become purely secretory. About 90% of the cells secrete epinephrine and 10% secrete norepinephrine. Small amounts of dopamine and opioid peptides are also produced.

Catecholamines are produced in the cells from tyrosine by hydroxylation and decarboxylation (Figure EN18). Norepinephrine is converted to epinephrine by the enzyme N-methyl transferase (more specifically called phenylethanolamine N-methyl transferase, PNMT), which has to be induced by adequate levels of glucocorticoids.

The catecholamines are metabolised by monoamine oxidase (MAO) and catechol-O-methyl transferase (COMT).

The effects of epinephrine and norepinephrine are mediated through two classes of G-protein-coupled receptor, alpha and beta, which are subdivided into α_1 and α_2 receptors, and β_1, β_2 and β_3 receptors. The effects are summarised in Figure EN19.

Figure EN18 Synthesis of epinephrine and norepinephrine

Stimulus and control of medullary hormones

Secretion of medullary hormones is very low during basal states, but is stimulated via the sympathetic nervous system when preparing the individual for 'fight or flight'. Situations which may stimulate secretion include hypoglycaemia, myocardial infarction, heavy exercise, trauma and surgery.

Secretion by the adrenal medulla may be important in the control of blood pressure when changing from a lying to a standing position.

Glucocorticoids are necessary for the secretion of the hormones, as they activate the enzyme which converts norepinephrine to epinephrine.

Metabolic effects	Glycogenolysis in liver and muscle Mobilisation of free fatty acids Stimulation of metabolic rate, increased heat production	
Nervous system	Stimulation	
Cardiovascular system	*Epinephrine*	*Norepinephrine*
Heart rate	raised	lowered
Cardiac output	raised	↓ low dose, ↑ high dose
Peripheral resistance	↓ low levels	raised
Mean arterial pressure	↑ low levels	raised

Figure EN19 Summary of effects of epinephrine and norepinephrine

Abnormalities of adrenal gland function

These manifest themselves in different ways, depending on which part of the adrenal gland is affected.

Adrenal insufficiency

Congenital deficiency in steroid hormone production may give way to adrenogenital syndrome. The pituitary gland produces large amounts of ACTH, which stimulates growth of the adrenal gland and produces a relative excess of androgens. This can cause virilisation in the female and precocious puberty in the male. Basal production of glucocorticoids and mineralocorticoids is enough to sustain life.

Adrenal insufficiency may be due to disease of the adrenal gland itself or to deficiency of ACTH production, and this gives rise to Addison's disease. Lack of mineralocorticoids and glucocorticoids results in:

- Loss of Na^+ and water, and retention of K^+ and H^+
- Hypotension and weakness, hypoglycaemia, weight loss, loss of resistance to infection and trauma
- Inability to excrete a water load, with water retention
- In severe cases, collapse and coma (Addisonian crisis)

In the primary disease there is increased production of ACTH. This can cause increased pigmentation due to its stimulating effect on melanocytes in the skin. The primary disease is usually more serious than the secondary form.

Adrenal excess

This can affect mineralocorticoid or glucocorticoid hormones, and can be primary or secondary.

In primary aldosteronism, which may be due to an adenoma of the zona glomerulosa, excess secretion of mineralocorticoids leads to retention of Na^+ and depletion of K^+, with hypertension, tetany and hypokalaemic alkalosis (Conn's syndrome). The secondary form is due to high renin production, found in cirrhosis, heart failure and some forms of renal disease.

Excess glucocorticoid production gives rise to Cushing's syndrome, where the following occur:

- Muscle wasting, thin hair, poor skin and subcutaneous tissue, and bruising, due to protein catabolism
- Redistribution of body fat to face ('moon face'), abdominal wall and upper back ('buffalo hump'), with numerous striae in the skin
- Hyperglycaemia, which may lead to insulin-resistant diabetes mellitus
- Hyperlipidaemia
- Sodium and water retention due to the mineralocorticoid effects of the glucocorticoids, with accompanying hypertension
- Osteoporosis due to decreased bone formation and increased bone reabsorption
- Mental effects, including increased appetite, insomnia, euphoria and toxic psychosis
- If due to excess production of ACTH there may be hyperpigmentation

Excess catecholamine production from a tumour of the chromaffin cells of the adrenal medulla gives rise to a phaeochromocytoma. These produce varying quantities of epinephrine and norepinephrine. Some tumours arise from extra-adrenal sites. Patients may present with severe hypertension, headaches, sweating and cardiac pathology including arrhythmias and myocardial infarcts.

Pancreas

The pancreas is a gland that has both exocrine and endocrine functions. The pancreas is divided by connective tissue septa into lobules, each of which contains a secretory unit termed the acinus. Lying between the acini and ducts related to the release of digestive enzymes are groups of cells known as the *islets of Langerhans*, which are associated with endocrine function.

The islets of Langerhans

The islets of Langerhans make up about 2% of the pancreas, and produce hormones which regulate the intermediary metabolism of glucose, fat and protein. The hormones are:

- Insulin, produced by the B cells of the islets (60–75%), which is anabolic, increasing storage of glucose, protein and fat
- Glucagon, produced by the A cells (20%), which is catabolic, opposing the effects of insulin
- Somatostatin, produced by the D cells, which helps regulate islet function
- Pancreatic polypeptide, produced by the F cells, the function of which is little understood

It is perhaps worth noting that B, A and D cells are still often referred to as α, β and δ.

Insulin

Insulin is a polypeptide hormone made of two chains of amino acids, the A and B chains, linked by two pairs of disulphide bridges. It is produced in the endoplasmic reticulum and then transported to the Golgi apparatus, where it is stored in granules, and secreted by exocytosis into the capillaries.

It is synthesised from a preprohormone, preproinsulin, which is a much bigger molecule. When this enters the endoplasmic reticulum part of it splits off, and the remaining molecule folds in two and is joined by the disulphide bonds to form proinsulin. The C-peptide part of the molecule, which facilitates the folding, is then removed, leaving insulin.

There is very little difference between insulin produced by different species, which has allowed bovine and porcine preparations to be given in the past, with little antibody production. It is more common nowadays, however, to give human insulin produced by recombinant DNA technology.

Insulin has far-ranging effects on cells throughout the body, the most obvious one being the effect on uptake of glucose.

There is a specific receptor for insulin on certain cells. This is a tetramer of 340 000 daltons which has two α and two β subunits. The α units occupy an extracellular position and directly bind insulin. The β units are membrane-spanning, and their intracellular portion activates a second messenger system via tyrosine kinase.

Glucose enters most cells by facilitated diffusion (although in the intestine and kidney the process is by secondary active transport with sodium), utilising a group of seven distinct glucose transporter proteins. When insulin binds to a receptor on an insulin-sensitive cell a pool of intracellular transporter-containing vesicles moves to the cell membrane and fuses with it, thus actually inserting transporters into the cell membrane. This process is mediated by phosphoinositol 3-kinase. After the action of insulin ceases, the portions of the membrane containing the transporters are endocytosed, in preparation for the process to begin again.

Although insulin is known to facilitate the entry of potassium ions into the cell, it is not known exactly how this occurs. It may be an effect that increases the activity of the Na^+K^+ ATPase pump in a relatively non-specific manner.

The principal anabolic effects of insulin are summarised in Figure EN20.

Glucagon

Glucagon is a polypeptide hormone produced by the A cells of the islets, firstly as a preprohormone, preproglucagon, which undergoes processing to glucagon and a number of other peptides, some with glucagon-like activities. In a similar fashion to insulin, it is stored in secretory granules and secreted by exocytosis.

Glucagon is a catabolic hormone, and most of its effects are therefore opposite to those of insulin. Glucagon receptors lie in the cell wall. They are G-protein-coupled and therefore exert their effect by activation of adenyl cyclase and increased intracellular cAMP.

The main effect of glucagon is to raise blood glucose. It does this by:

- Glycogenolysis in the liver (not muscle)
- Gluconeogenesis
- Lipolysis and ketogenesis

Somatostatin

This hormone is produced by the D cells of the islets. Two forms are secreted, SS14 and SS28, but the latter is more active. It is the same hormone as that produced by the hypothalamus which is termed growth-hormone inhibiting factor (GH-IH). The effects of somatostatin are:

- Inhibition of insulin
- Inhibition of glucagon
- Inhibition of pancreatic polypeptide

The release of somatostatin is stimulated by a rise in plasma glucose, and it generally slows down propulsive movement in the gastrointestinal tract.

	Muscle	Adipose tissue	Liver
Glucose	↑ Glucose entry ↑ Glycogenesis	↑ Glucose entry	↑ Glycogenesis
Protein	↑ Amino acid uptake ↑ Protein synthesis ↓ Protein catabolism ↑ Retention of gluconeogenic amino acids	↑ Protein synthesis	
Fat		↑ Fatty acid synthesis ↑ Activation of lipoprotein lipase	↑ Lipid synthesis
Other	↑ K+ uptake ↑ Ketone uptake Increased cell growth	↑ K+ uptake	↓ Ketogenesis

Figure EN20 Main actions of insulin on muscle, adipose tissue, and liver

Pancreatic polypeptide

This polypeptide hormone is produced in the F cells of the islets. Its function is uncertain, but it may act to smooth out blood levels of glucose and amino acids after a meal. Its effects can be summarised as follows:

- It is stimulated by a protein meal, and by fasting, exercise and hypoglycaemia.
- It is suppressed by somatostatin and hyperglycaemia.
- It slows absorption of food from the intestine.

Role of the pancreatic hormones in metabolism

The role of the separate hormones has been described. The hormones work together to achieve the following:

- Storage of absorbed nutrients (mainly mediated by insulin)
- Mobilisation of energy reserves during times of stress and hunger (mainly mediated by glucagon)
- Maintenance of a steady level of blood glucose (mediated via both insulin and glucagon, with a smoothing effect of somatostatin and possibly pancreatic polypeptide)
- Promotion of growth (insulin)

The stimulating and inhibiting factors acting on insulin and glucagon are summarised in Figure EN21.

Role of other hormones in carbohydrate metabolism

- Epinephrine causes glycogenolysis followed by a rise in hepatic glycogen production. It also decreases peripheral glucose utilisation.

	Stimulating	Inhibiting
Insulin	↑ Glucose (main) Glucagon Selective β-receptor agonists Acetyl choline Sulphonylureas	Epinephrine Somatostatin β-blockers α-agonists Thiazides
Glucagon	↓ Glucose Hunger, stress, trauma, exercise, infection Selective β-agonists	↑ Glucose Somatostatin Insulin Ketones Free fatty acids Selective α-agonists

Figure EN21 Main factors affecting release of insulin and glucagon

- Thyroid hormones tend to cause hyperglycaemia due to increased absorption from the intestine. They also cause increased glycogenolysis in the liver, and possibly increased degradation of insulin.
- Adrenal glucocorticoids cause hyperglycaemia, and in excess can produce a diabetic picture (see above). They are needed for glucagon to produce its gluconeogenic effect during fasting; a deficit can lead to hypoglycaemia and collapse.
- Growth hormone causes hyperglycaemia by decreasing glucose uptake in cells, increased glycogenolysis and decreasing binding of insulin. The rise in blood glucose produced when the hormone is produced in excess may stimulate insulin production and exhaust the B islet cells.

Deficiency and excess
Deficiency of insulin

This results classically in diabetes mellitus.

Type 1, insulin-dependent diabetes (IDDM) commonly develops in childhood and is thought to be an autoimmune disease affecting B cells only. Patients tend to be thin and have a high incidence of ketosis and acidosis. There may be B-cell antibodies, but it is thought the disease may be mediated via T lymphocytes.

Type 2, non-insulin-dependent diabetes (NIDDM) usually develops in older, often obese patients. There is normal or high insulin production but increased insulin resistance. As the B cells become exhausted the insulin levels may fall. Ketosis and acidosis are rare.

Secondary diabetes may occur when there is overproduction of glucocorticoids or growth hormone, or when there is disease of the pancreas.

The effects of diabetes mellitus are summarised below:

- Glucose – hyperglycaemia leads to an osmotic diuresis with loss of water, Na^+ and K^+. This may lead to severe dehydration. There is reduced uptake of glucose into cells, which may lead to hunger. Glycogen stores are reduced.
- Protein – increased protein catabolism leads to a rise in amino acids in the blood and loss of nitrogen in the urine. This can lead to muscle wasting and reduced resistance to infection.
- Fat – increased catabolism of fat leads to an increase in free fatty acids. Metabolism of these fatty acids produces acidosis, ketosis and ketonuria.
- In the severe acute form of the disease the dehydration may lead to coma and death.
- Over a period of time diabetic patients may develop secondary changes in other organs. Microvascular changes can occur in the eye and kidney. Macrovascular changes can lead to strokes and ischaemic heart disease. Peripheral and autonomic neuropathy can also occur. The neuropathy, in combination with the atherosclerosis, can lead to chronic ulceration and gangrene, especially in the feet.

An overview of the effects of insulin deficiency is shown in Figure EN22.

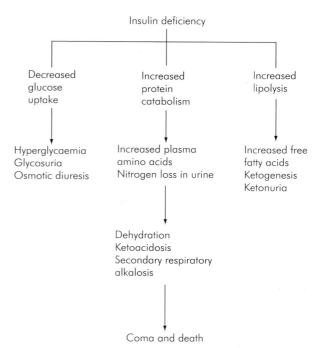

Figure EN22 Effects of insulin deficiency

Excess of insulin

This can occur with overtreatment of diabetes with insulin or with sulphonylureas and biguanides. Rarely, a tumour of the islet cells, known as an insulinoma, can produce insulin excess.

The manifestations of insulin excess are those that occur due to the effect in the central nervous system, which uses glucose primarily as its source of energy. In milder forms there may be anxiety, palpitations and sweating. As the glucose level falls there may be confusion, fits, coma and death.

References and further reading

Mitchell SLM, Hunter JM. Vasopressin and its antagonists: what are their roles in acute medical care? *Br J Anaes* 2007; **99**: 154–8.

CHAPTER 14

Physiology of pregnancy

M. C. Mushambi

Pregnancy

Normal pregnancy involves major physiological and anatomical adaptations by maternal organs. It is important that anaesthetists involved in the care of the pregnant woman understand these changes, to provide safe maternal anaesthetic care which is compatible with safe delivery of the baby.

Cardiovascular system

There are multiple changes in the cardiovascular system, many of which are compensatory changes designed to cope with the growing fetus, uterus and placenta. These are summarised in Figure PN1. Although the majority of changes occur during pregnancy, significant changes also occur during labour and immediately following delivery of the baby.

Cardiac output

Patient posture has been found to influence cardiac output measurements significantly during pregnancy (Figure PN2). Measurements performed in the lateral position, to avoid aortocaval compression, demonstrate an increase in cardiac output by 5 weeks gestation. Cardiac output continues to increase from this time, resulting in a rise of 35–40% by the end of the first trimester, increasing to 50% by the end of the second trimester (Figure PN3). Cardiac output then remains at 50% above non-pregnant levels throughout the third trimester.

A further transient rise in cardiac output occurs at delivery, as a result of labour and uteroplacental transfusion into the maternal intravascular volume.

Heart rate and stroke volume

The increase in cardiac output in pregnancy is produced by a combination of increased heart rate, reduced systemic vascular resistance (SVR) and increased stroke volume. Heart rate is increased above non-pregnant values by 15% at the end of the first trimester. This increases to 25% by the end of the second trimester, but there is no further change in the third trimester.

Stroke volume is increased by about 20% at 8 weeks and up to 30% by the end of the second trimester, then remaining level until term (Figure PN3)

Systemic vascular resistance

SVR is reduced during pregnancy. The average SVR in pregnancy is about 980 compared with about 1150 dynes.s cm^{-5} in non-pregnant women. The decrease in the SVR results from the development of a low-resistance vascular bed (the intervillous space) and vasodilatory effects of oestrogens, prostacyclin and progesterone.

Distribution of the cardiac output during pregnancy is different from that of the non-pregnant state, with increased blood flow to the uterus, kidneys and skin. Uterine blood flow varies from 500 to 700 ml min^{-1} (about 10–12% of the cardiac output) at term, of which >80% perfuses the placenta. The flow to the kidneys is increased, as is the flow to the skin due to peripheral vasodilatation. Flow to the liver and brain remains unchanged.

Blood pressure

Blood pressure falls during pregnancy. Systolic blood pressure is minimally affected, with a maximum decline of

Fundamentals of Anaesthesia, 3rd edition, ed. Tim Smith, Colin Pinnock and Ted Lin. Published by Cambridge University Press. © Cambridge University Press 2008.

	Parameter	Change
Heart	Cardiac output	↑ by 50%
	Stroke volume	↑ by 30%
	Heart rate	↑ by 25%
	Ejection fraction	↑ by 20%
	Left ventricle mass	↑ by 50%
	Left ventricular end-diastolic volume	↑ by 10%
Systemic circulation	Systemic vascular resistance	↓ by 20%
	Pulmonary vascular resistance	↓ by 34%
	Systolic blood pressure	↓ by 6–8%
	Diastolic blood pressure	↓ by 20–25%

Figure PN1 Changes in haemodynamic parameters during pregnancy

Position	Change in cardiac output
Supine	Baseline
Left lateral	↑ by 13.5%
Lithotomy	↓ by 17%
Steep Trendelenberg	↓ by 18%

Figure PN2 The effect of position on cardiac output during pregnancy

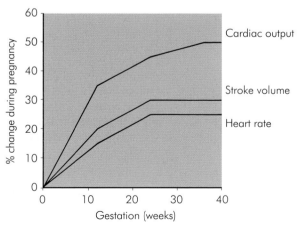
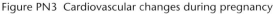

Figure PN3 Cardiovascular changes during pregnancy

8% during early and mid-gestation, returning to non-pregnant levels at term. Diastolic blood pressure falls to a greater extent, with early and mid-gestational decreases of 20–25%, and returns to normal at term. In the supine position, 70% of mothers have a fall in blood pressure of at least 10%, and 8% have decreases of 30–50%.

Aortocaval compression

Compression of the inferior vena cava (IVC) and aorta by the gravid uterus occurs during pregnancy and reduces cardiac output. The severity of this effect is dependent on:
- Patient position
- Gestation
- Systemic blood pressure
- Presence of sympathetic block

In the supine position during pregnancy, IVC obstruction occurs and venous blood bypasses this obstruction primarily via vertebral venous plexuses which empty into the azygos vein. IVC compression develops as early as 13 weeks gestation, causing a 50% increase in femoral venous pressures. This effect becomes maximal between 36 and 38 weeks, after which it may decline as the fetal head descends into the pelvis. Moving from a supine to a lateral position reduces the femoral and IVC pressures, but these are still elevated above those of the non-pregnant woman, indicating that the compression of the IVC is not completely relieved by lateral positioning. In the supine position, 5–8% of pregnant women experience a substantial drop in blood pressure (supine hypotension syndrome), and the patients develop systemic signs of shock, i.e. pallor, sweating, nausea, vomiting and syncope.

Obstruction of the aorta in the supine position has been demonstrated angiographically, but the higher pressures in the aorta prevent total obstruction. This does not cause maternal hypotension but causes arterial hypotension in the lower extremities and in the uterine arteries, which can lead to inadequate uterine blood flow resulting in fetal asphyxia and bradycardia.

Electrocardiogram (ECG) and echocardiogram

The ECG in pregnancy may show the following changes:
- Sinus tachycardia
- Rotation of the electrical axis of the heart to the left
- ST segment depression
- T-wave flattening

However, these changes are thought to be of no clinical significance.

Echocardiographic studies during pregnancy have shown:

- Left ventricular hypertrophy by 12 weeks gestation
- A 50% increase in left ventricular mass at term
- A 12–14% increase in aortic, pulmonary and mitral valve sizes

Heart sounds

The apical impulse moves to the fourth intercostal space and mid-clavicular line. Most pregnant women develop a loud and sometimes split first heart sound. A third heart sound is common, and 16% of women have a fourth heart sound. A grade I–II early to mid-systolic heart murmur is commonly heard at the left sternal edge. This may be due to tricuspid regurgitation resulting from dilatation of the tricuspid valve.

Venous pressure

In the absence of IVC compression by the uterus, central venous pressure (CVP) and pressure in the upper limbs is normal. However, during late pregnancy when in the supine position, IVC compression occurs and CVP may decrease dramatically. IVC compression can also cause increased venous pressure in the lower limbs.

During labour various factors can cause an increase in CVP, including:

- Contractions – can increase CVP by about 5 cmH$_2$O
- Expulsive efforts of the second stage – can create a major rise in CVP by up to 50 cmH$_2$O
- IV ergometrine 0.25 mg after delivery of the baby can produce a rise in CVP of 8 cmH$_2$O, which can last up to 60 minutes

There are no observed changes in pulmonary capillary wedge and pulmonary artery pressures during pregnancy. Recent non-invasive studies have demonstrated a high incidence of asymptomatic pericardial effusion during normal pregnancy.

Haematology

The haematological changes associated with pregnancy are summarised in Figure PN5.

Blood volume

Plasma volume, total blood volume and red blood cell (RBC) volume all increase during pregnancy (Figure PN4). Plasma volume rises by 15% during the first trimester and can reach 50% above non-pregnant values by 32 weeks; it then remains at this level unchanged. Plasma volume

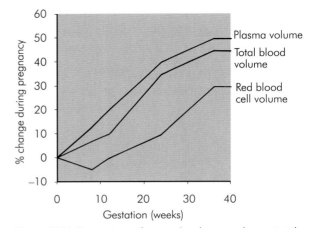

Figure PN4 Percentage changes in plasma volume, total blood volume and red blood cell volume during pregnancy

returns to non-pregnant levels by 6 days post delivery. There is often a sharp rise of up to 1 litre in plasma volume 24 hours after delivery. This is of significant importance in patients with cardiac disease, such as those with fixed cardiac output. Such patients may develop pulmonary oedema during this period.

RBC volume falls during the first 8 weeks of pregnancy, increasing back to non-pregnant levels by 16 weeks and then rising to 30% above non-pregnant levels by term. This increase in RBC volume is due to raised erythropoietin levels that occur from 12 weeks gestation. The lesser increase in RBC volume relative to the increase in plasma volume results in overall reductions of about 15% in haemoglobin (Hb) and haematocrit.

The above changes combine to give total blood volume increases of 10, 30 and 45% at the end of the first, second and third trimester respectively (Figure PN4). Oestrogens and progesterone appear responsible for the increase in plasma volume through their effect on the renin–angiotensin–aldosterone systems.

White cell count (WCC)

The blood WCC rises progressively during pregnancy from non-pregnant levels to 9–11 $\times$ 10^9 l^{-1}. This is predominantly an increase in polymorphonuclear cells. There is a further leucocytosis to about 15 $\times$ 10^9 l^{-1} during labour. White cell count returns to normal by 6 days post delivery.

	Parameter	Change
Blood volumes	Total blood volume	↑ by 45%
	Plasma volume	↑ by 50%
Blood cells	Red blood cell volume	↑ by 30%
	White cell count	↑
	Haematocrit	↓ by 15%
	Haemoglobin	↓ by 15%
Plasma proteins	Total plasma protein	↓ by 18%
	Albumin	↓ by 14%
	Globulin	↓ or ↑
	Plasma cholinesterase	↓ by 20–25%
	Colloid osmotic pressure	↓ by 18%
Coagulation	Platelets	↓ by 0–5%
	Prothrombin time	↓ by 20%
	Bleeding time	↓ by 10%
	Partial thromboplastin time	↓ by 20%
	Antithrombin III	↓ by 10%
	Fibrin degradation products	↑ by 100%
	Plasminogen	↑
	Fibrinolysis	↑
Clotting factors	I	↑ by 100%
	II	↑ or nil
	V	↑ or nil
	VII	↑ by 100%
	VIII	↑ by 150%
	IX	↑ by 100%
	X	↑ by 30%
	XI	↓ by 40–50%
	XII	↑ by 30%
	XIII	↓ by 50%

Figure PN5 Haematological changes during pregnancy

Coagulation

Pregnancy is associated with enhanced platelet turnover, clotting and fibrinolysis (Figure PN5). Thrombocytopenia (platelets $< 100 \times 10^9\,l^{-1}$) occurs in 0.8–0.9% of normal pregnant women, while increases in platelet factor and β-thromboglobulin suggest elevated platelet activation and consumption. Since there is no change in platelet count in the majority of women during pregnancy, there is probably an increase in platelet production to compensate for the increased consumption.

The concentrations of most coagulation factors (I, VII–X and XII) are increased and a few (XI and XIII) are reduced. The levels of factors II and V remain the same during pregnancy. There are increases in fibrin degradation products (FDP) and plasminogen concentrations which indicate increased fibrinolytic activity during pregnancy.

Plasma proteins

The plasma concentration of albumin is reduced to 34–39 g l^{-1}, but globulin and fibrinogen levels are increased. Overall, the total plasma protein concentration falls to 65–70 g l^{-1}. These reductions in plasma proteins are associated with the following changes:

- Total colloid osmotic pressure is reduced by 5 mmHg.
- Drug-binding capacity of the plasma is altered, with consequent changes in pharmacokinetics and dynamics (e.g. a reduction in plasma α-acid glycoprotein concentration reduces the lignocaine binding capacity).
- Plasma concentration of pseudocholinesterase is reduced by 20–25% at term.
- Erythrocyte sedimentation rate (ESR) and blood viscosity are increased.

Fluid compartments

Both extravascular and intravascular water content increases during pregnancy. The increase in extravascular water varies from 1.7 litres in women without oedema to 5 litres in women with oedema.

Respiratory system

Figure PN6 shows a summary of the respiratory system changes associated with pregnancy.

Anatomical changes

Capillary engorgement of the mucosa of nasal cavity, pharynx and larynx begins early in the first trimester. This may explain why many pregnant women complain of difficulty in nasal breathing, have more episodes of epistaxis and experience voice changes. The thoracic cage increases in circumference by 5–7 cm because of the increase in both the anteroposterior and transverse diameters from flaring of the ribs. Flaring of the ribs begins early in pregnancy and is, therefore, not entirely due to pressure from the enlarging uterus. The enlarging uterus displaces the diaphragm upwards in the later weeks of pregnancy, but the internal volume of the thoracic cavity remains unchanged.

Lung mechanics and volumes

Inspiration is mainly as a result of diaphragmatic movement, since flaring of the ribs reduces chest wall movement. Bronchial smooth muscle relaxation decreases airway

	Parameter	Change
Anatomy	Capillary engorgement of URT	↑
	Upper airway	Dilated
	Diaphragm	Elevated
	Thoracic circumference	↑ by 5–7 cm
Lung volumes	Tidal volume	↑ by 45%
	Inspiratory reserve volume	↑ by 5%
	Expiratory reserve volume	↓ by 25%
	Residual volume	↓ by 20%
	Functional reserve capacity	↓ by 30%
	Vital capacity	nil
	Total lung capacity	↓ by 0–5%
	Closing capacity	nil
Ventilation	Minute ventilation	↑ by 50%
	Alveolar ventilation	↑ by 70%
	Respiratory rate	↑ by 0–15%
	Dead space	↑ by 45%
Lung mechanics	Diaphragm movement	↑
	Chest wall movement	↓
	Total pulmonary resistance	↓ by 50%
	Lung compliance	nil
	FEV_1	nil
	FEV_1/VC	nil
	Flow volume loop	nil
Arterial blood gases	$PaCO_2$	↓ to 3.7–4.2 kPa
	PaO_2	↑ to 13.3–14.6 kPa
	pH	↑ to 7.44
	HCO_3^-	↓ to 18–21 mmol l^{-1}
Oxygen consumption		↑ by 30–60%

Figure PN6 Respiratory changes during pregnancy

resistance but lung compliance remains unchanged. Factors contributing to airway dilatation include direct effects of progesterone, cortisone and relaxin.

Forced expiratory volume at 1 second (FEV_1), the ratio of FEV_1 to forced vital capacity (FVC), and the flow volume loop remain unchanged, demonstrating that large airway function is not impaired during pregnancy.

The following changes in lung volumes occur during pregnancy, relative to non-pregnant values:
- Tidal volume increases steadily from the first trimester, by up to 45% at term (Figure PN7).
- Functional residual capacity (FRC) is decreased by 20–30% at term due to reductions of 25% in expiratory reserve volume (ERV) and 15% in residual volume.
- Closing capacity can encroach on FRC, increasing ventilation–perfusion mismatch and leading to the ready occurrence of hypoxia, particularly in supine and Trendelenberg positions.
- Inspiratory capacity increases by 15% at term due to increases in inspiratory reserve and tidal volumes.

Minute ventilation (MV)

MV is increased by up to 50% above non-pregnant values at term. Since respiratory rate remains unaltered, this increase is due to larger tidal volumes. The increased MV levels are stimulated by the high progesterone levels and increased carbon dioxide production occurring during pregnancy.

Dead space is greater by 45% due to dilatation of large airways, but the concomitant increase in tidal volume leaves the ratio of dead space to tidal volume unchanged.

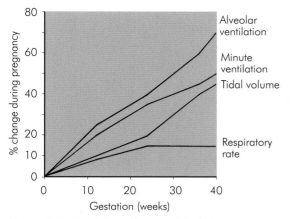

Figure PN7 Respiratory changes (%) during pregnancy

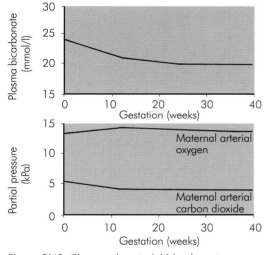

Figure PN8 Changes in arterial bicarbonate, oxygen and carbon dioxide during pregnancy

Diffusing capacity

Diffusing capacity of the lungs for carbon monoxide (DLCO) is increased during the first trimester, but then decreases until 24–27 weeks gestation, after which it remains unchanged until term.

Blood gases

$PaCO_2$ decreases to 3.7–4.2 kPa by the end of the first trimester and remains at this level until term (Figure PN8). This is due to alveolar hyperventilation and gives rise to various compensatory mechanisms in an attempt to maintain normal pH. Metabolic compensation for the respiratory alkalosis reduces the serum bicarbonate concentration to about 18–21 mmol l^{-1}, the base excess (BE) by 2–3 mmol l^{-1} and the total buffer base by about 5 mmol l^{-1}. Metabolic compensation is not complete, which explains the elevation of maternal blood pH by 0.04 units.

PaO_2 in upright pregnant women is in the region of 14.0 kPa, higher than that in non-pregnant women (Figure PN7). This is due to lower $PaCO_2$ levels, a reduced arteriovenous oxygen difference and a reduction in physiological shunt. The small progressive decline in the PaO_2 during the second and third trimesters is due to an increase in arteriovenous oxygen difference.

When PaO_2 is determined in the supine position, the values after mid-gestation are often <13.3 kPa. This occurs because:

- FRC is less than the closing volume in up to 50% of supine pregnant patients.
- Aortocaval compression reduces cardiac output, which increases arteriovenous oxygen difference and reduces mixed venous oxygen content.

Dyspnoea during pregnancy

About 60% of normal pregnant women with no history of cardiorespiratory disease experience dyspnoea. Dyspnoea during pregnancy is, therefore, not always an indication of organic disease. It commonly occurs in the first and second trimesters, and it is probably a result of lowered $PaCO_2$ levels.

Pulmonary circulation

Pulmonary vascular resistance is reduced from 119 dynes.s cm^{-5} in the non-pregnant woman to 78 dynes.s cm^{-5} in the pregnant woman at term. Pulmonary blood flow is increased in pregnancy due to increased cardiac output, and pulmonary blood volume is also greater, as demonstrated by increased vascular markings on chest x ray. The normal woman can cope with these changes, and the pressures in the right ventricle, pulmonary artery and pulmonary capillaries are not raised.

Oxygen consumption

Oxygen consumption is increased in pregnancy by 30–60% because of the metabolic demands of the fetus, uterus and placenta. The decreased FRC and increased metabolic rate predispose the mother to the rapid onset of hypoxia during induction of anaesthesia or airway obstruction.

Human placental lactogen (HPL) and cortisol increase the tendency to hyperglycaemia and ketosis, which may unmask or exacerbate pre-existing diabetes mellitus. The

Parameter	Value (non-pregnant value in brackets)
LOS pressure	15.7 cmH$_2$O (15.2)
Gastric pressure (supine)	11.1 cmH$_2$O (5.7)
Barrier pressure	4.6 cmH$_2$O (9.5)
Heartburn	↑
Gastric acid secretion	↓
Gastric emptying	no change or ↓

Figure PN9 Gastrointestinal tract changes during pregnancy

pregnant woman adapts rapidly to starvation. When feeding is withheld, there is early activation of fat metabolism. Fatty acids are utilised and glucose is saved for the fetus.

Gastrointestinal system

Pregnant women have been regarded for many years as being at higher risk of acid aspiration because of the reduction in barrier pressure, increased gastric secretion, reduced gastric pH and delayed gastric emptying.

Barrier pressure

Barrier pressure (lower oesophageal sphincter [LOS] pressure minus gastric pressure) is reduced significantly during pregnancy compared with the non-pregnant state, due to increased intragastric pressure and reduced LOS pressure (Figure PN9). LOS pressure appears to return to normal by 48 hours post delivery.

Heartburn occurs in 55–80% of pregnant women and may occur at <20 weeks gestation. This is thought to be due to gastro-oesophageal reflux that occurs when barrier pressure is reduced. Lowered barrier pressure can be asymptomatic.

Causes of reduced barrier pressure include:
- The altered position of the stomach, which displaces the intra-abdominal part of the oesophagus into the thorax and lowers LOS pressure
- The relaxant effect of progesterone
- Elevation of intragastric pressure in the last trimester in both standing and supine positions
- Intragastric pressure is raised in the lithotomy position (increased by 5.6 cmH$_2$O) and the Trendelenberg position (increased by 8.8 cmH$_2$O)

Gastric secretion

The total acid content of the stomach and pepsin secretion are reduced during pregnancy. This may be due to decreased plasma gastrin levels. Commonly used criteria assess the risk of acid aspiration as high when gastric pH is <2.5 and gastric volume is >25 ml. During early gestation (<15 weeks), 37% of women have been found to fulfil these criteria, but this percentage was comparable with that in non-pregnant controls. In patients at term undergoing elective Caesarean section, 49% are at risk of acid aspiration, compared with 42% of controls. Approximately 50% of women in labour have gastric pH < 2.5.

Gastric emptying

Gastric emptying is not delayed during pregnancy but becomes delayed during labour, particularly if opioids are administered. When labour is conducted with epidural or no analgesia, gastric emptying is only slightly reduced. The use of epidural opioids as a bolus appears to reduce gastric emptying compared with patients with no epidural opioids, but the effect of low-dose opioid infusions is less clear. Provided that opioids have not been used during labour, gastric emptying returns to normal within 24–48 hours post delivery.

Central nervous system

There are substantial pressure and volume changes in the epidural and subarachnoid spaces, which have important effects upon the spread of solutions within these compartments (Figure PN10).

Parameter	Change
MAC of volatile anaesthetic agents	↓
β-endorphins	↑
Epidural space volume	↓
Epidural space pressure	↑
Cerebrospinal fluid pressure	↑
Cerebrospinal fluid volume	↓
Cerebrospinal fluid composition	nil
Cerebrospinal fluid pH	↑
Sensitivity to local anaesthetics	↑
Local anaesthetic dose requirements	↓

Figure PN10 CNS changes during pregnancy

Epidural space

Compression of the IVC by the gravid uterus results in increased venous pressure below the level of the obstruction. Venous blood is then diverted through vertebral plexuses within the epidural space, and this causes epidural veins to become engorged. Consequently, the epidural volume is reduced and any solutions injected into the lumbar epidural space will spread more extensively.

Pressure in the epidural space of non-pregnant patients is usually negative (-1 cmH$_2$O), but in the pregnant woman it is slightly positive. During contractions, the epidural pressure rises by 2–8 cmH$_2$O, while during expulsion it ranges between 20 and 60 cmH$_2$O.

Subarachnoid space

There are no changes in the constituents or the specific gravity of cerebral spinal fluid (CSF) during pregnancy. CSF pressure is increased by aorto caval compression and by uterine contractions during labour. Baseline pressure in labour in between contractions is 28 cmH$_2$O. It is 22 cmH$_2$O when the uterus is displaced laterally to relieve aorto caval compression. During painful contractions, the pressure is increased and it may reach 70 cmH$_2$O in the second stage.

Sympathetic nervous system

There is increased sympathetic nervous system activity throughout pregnancy, and it is maximal at term. The effect is primarily on the venous capacitance system of the lower extremities, which counteracts the adverse effects of uterine compression of the IVC. Hence, sympathetic block due to either epidural or spinal anaesthesia can result in marked decrease in blood pressure in pregnant women compared with non-pregnant patients.

Drugs and the nervous system

There are reduced requirements for local anaesthetics when administering spinal or epidural anaesthesia during pregnancy. This may be due to decreased volumes of the epidural and subarachnoid spaces, or increased nerve-fibre sensitivity to local anaesthetics.

The minimal alveolar concentration (MAC) of inhalational anaesthetic agents is reduced by 40%, which may be related to gestational increase in progesterone levels. Beta-endorphin levels in the mother are increased during gestation, labour and delivery.

Endocrine system

Thyroid gland

The thyroid gland increases in size during pregnancy. A goitre may develop as a result of increased blood flow and follicular hyperplasia. Iodine uptake by the thyroid gland increases. Thyroxine-binding globulin levels double, but free plasma tri-iodothyronine and thyroxine remain at the non-pregnant level or fall, so that the mother remains euthyroid.

Adrenal gland

The maternal adrenal gland remains the same size but the width and secretion of the zona fasciculata are increased. Plasma cortisol and other corticosteroids increase to 3–5 times the non-pregnant level by term. The half-life of cortisol is prolonged.

Pituitary gland

The pituitary gland increases in weight, making the anterior pituitary very sensitive to haemorrhage and hypotension because its blood supply does not come directly from arterial vessels, but from a portal system whose pressure is below that of the systemic arteries.

Pancreas

The islets of Langerhans and the number of B cells increase during pregnancy, as does the number of receptor sites for insulin. However, there is a resistance to the action of insulin, possibly due to the presence of human placental lactogen, prolactin and other pregnancy hormones. The upper limit of normal blood glucose in the glucose tolerance test is 7.5 mmol l^{-1} in the second trimester, rising to 9.6 mmol l^{-1} in the third trimester.

Renal function

Renal function changes from early pregnancy (Figure PN11). Renal plasma flow increases to 30–50% above the non-pregnant level by 30 weeks, then declines gradually. The glomerular filtration rate (GFR) increases to about 150 ml per minute in the second trimester and falls towards term. As a result the plasma concentrations of urea and creatinine decrease.

The tubules are presented with more urine volume due to the increase in GFR, and they lose some of their reabsorptive capacity. Glucose, uric acid and amino acids are not completely reabsorbed, and there is an increased loss of protein of up to 300 mg a day.

Parameter	Change
Renal plasma flow	↑
Glomerular filtration rate	↑
Urine volume	↑
Renal tubular reabsorption	↓
Glycosuria	↑
Proteinuria	↑
Creatinine clearance	↑
Plasma urea concentration	↓
Plasma creatinine concentration	↓

Figure PN11 Renal changes during pregnancy

Renal sodium retention and therefore water retention are increased in pregnancy. Progesterone helps to conserve potassium during pregnancy.

Musculoskeletal system

Placental production of the hormone relaxin stimulates generalised ligamentous relaxation. This results in widening of the pubic symphysis, increased mobility of the sacroiliac, sacrococcygeal and pubic joints. As the uterus enlarges, lumbar lordosis is enhanced to maintain the woman's centre of gravity over the lower extremity. As a result, most pregnant women experience low back pain.

Hyperpigmentation of the face, neck and abdominal midline (linea nigra) are due to the effects of increased levels of melanocyte-stimulating hormone (MSH).

Weight gain

Weight increases by 10–12 kg due to increases in maternal body water and fat, the fetus, placenta, amniotic fluid and the uterus. At term, 40% of the weight gained is often in the fetus, amniotic fluid, placenta and uterus. Breast enlargement is typical in normal pregnancy, due to human placental lactogen secretion. Enlarged breasts may be a cause of difficult intubation and the use of a short-handle laryngoscope or polio blade may help to overcome this problem.

The placenta

Although the placenta appears as a physical barrier between maternal and fetal tissues, it brings the maternal and fetal circulation into close apposition for physiological exchange across a large area. Fetal wellbeing depends on good placental function for the supply of nutrients and the removal of waste products.

Embryology and anatomy

The ovum is fertilised in the Fallopian tube and enters the uterine cavity, where it rapidly converts to a blastocyst with an inner and outer cell mass. The outer cell layer of the blastocyst then proliferates to form the trophoblastic cell mass. At implantation, the trophoblast erodes into the surrounding decidua of the endometrium and its associated capillaries until the blastocyst is surrounded by circulating maternal blood (trophoblastic lacunae).

The placental tissue develops from the chorion, which consists of the trophoblast and mesoderm of the developing blastocyst. The trophoblast differentiates into two layers, the thick outer syncytiotrophoblast and the thin inner cytotrophoblast. In the second week of development, the (inner) cytotrophoblast layer begins to proliferate and extend cellular fingers into the (outer) syncytiotrophoblast (Figure PN12). The cytotrophoblast cell columns and their covering syncytiotrophoblast extend as villous stems into the lacunae of maternal blood within the decidua. A mesodermal core appears within the villous stems. These villous stems form the framework from which the villous tree will later develop. Cellular differentiation of the villous mesoderm results in the formation of blood cells and blood vessels and forms the villous vascular network. With development, the villi branch out extensively into the lacunae (intervillous spaces), forming the villous tree and thereby increasing their surface area (Figure PN13).

Cytotrophoblastic cells grow into the lumens of the maternal spiral vessels within the decidua, where they replace the endothelial cells, invading and destroying the musculoelastic medial tissue. As a result of the destruction of the smooth muscle, the walls of the spiral vessels in the decidua become thin and their vasoconstrictor activity is reduced. This wave of trophoblastic invasion starts at 10 weeks and is complete by 16 weeks. A second wave of vascular trophoblastic invasion occurs from 16 to 22 weeks and extends more deeply into the myometrial portions of the spiral arteries. These vessels are easily dilated as maternal flow to the placenta increases. Failure of this physiological change is found in pre-eclampsia and intrauterine growth retardation. This means that these vessels still respond to vasoconstrictor stimulation, and there is reduced flow to the intervillous space. Further maturation of the villi results in a marked reduction in the cytotrophoblast component and decreases the diffusional distance between the fetal villi and maternal intervillous blood. At term in humans, only a single layer of fetal chorionic tissue (syncytiotrophoblast) separates maternal blood and fetal capillary endothelium.

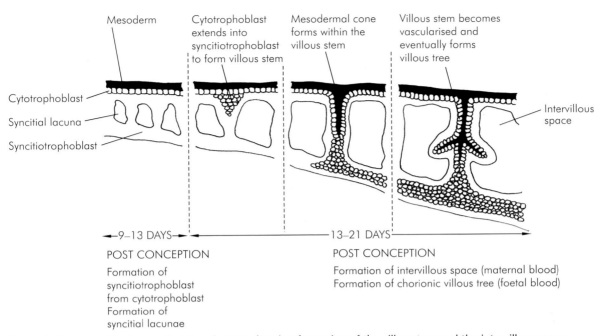

Figure PN12 Early development of the placenta showing formation of the villous tree and the intervillous space

Hence, the human placenta is classified as a haemomonochorial villous placenta.

The placenta is connected to the developing embryo by a connecting stalk that subsequently becomes the umbilical cord containing the umbilical vessels. The placenta is supplied with maternal blood from the uterine blood vessels. Blood enters the intervillous space from the open ends of the uterine spiral arteries (Figure PN13). The intervillous space is a large cavernous expanse into which the villous trees reach. Blood enters the intervillous spaces and flows into loosely packed areas, then into densely packed intermediate and terminal villi. It then empties into collecting veins. However, the relative direction of the blood flow is haphazard and behaves like a concurrent system, though with maternal blood flow exceeding fetal blood flow. The area of densely packed terminal villi is where placental exchange occurs. Maternal placental blood flow is a low-pressure system; the pressure in the intervillous space is on average 10 mmHg. The increasing demands of the growing fetus require 100–150 spiral arteries to feed directly to the placenta. The maternal circulation through the intervillous space is fully developed by 20 weeks. Blood flow will increase from 50 ml min^{-1} at 10 weeks to between 500 and 800 ml min^{-1} at term.

Two umbilical arteries arising from the fetal internal iliac arteries carry deoxygenated fetal blood via the umbilical cord to the placenta, and a single umbilical vein returns oxygenated blood to the fetus. The umbilical arteries divide into chorionic arteries, which feed the multiple placental lobules, and these in turn subdivide into the villous trees, which end as capillaries in the terminal villi (Figure PN13). Fetal sinusoids formed within the terminal villi provide a large endothelial surface area and make it the ideal region for maternal–fetal exchange. Each villous tree drains into a large vein that perforates the chorionic plate to become chorionic veins. Each of the venous tributaries courses towards the umbilical cord attachment site, where they empty into one umbilical vein.

The placenta grows dramatically from the third month of gestation until term. There is direct correlation between growth of the fetus and that of the placenta. By term, the mature placenta is oval and flat with an average weight of 500 g, average diameter of 20 cm and thickness of 3 cm.

Uterine blood flow

Uterine blood flow is influenced by intrinsic and extrinsic factors. Chronic regulation of uterine blood flow

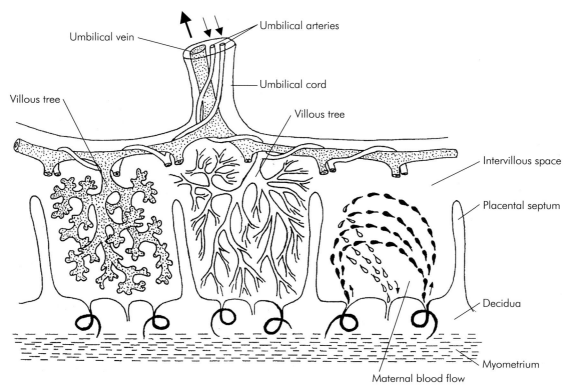

Figure PN13 Placental circulation, showing the villous tree (fetal placental circulation), spiral arteries and intervillous space (maternal placental circulation)

occurs mainly through intrinsic factors. These include prostaglandins (prostacyclin), nitric oxide and oestrogens. Extrinsic factors are more involved in the acute changes of uterine perfusion.

In general, uterine blood flow (UBF) is related to perfusion pressure and vascular resistance according to the following formula:

$$UBF = \frac{\text{Uterine arterial pressure} - \text{Uterine venous pressure}}{\text{Uterine vascular resistance}}$$

Any factors that alter uterine perfusion will affect placental perfusion. Uterine arterial pressure is reduced by systemic hypotension. Uterine venous pressure is increased by IVC compression, uterine contractions and Valsava manoeuvre (i.e. pushing in the second stage of labour).

Uterine vascular resistance is affected by endogenous and exogenous vasoconstrictors. Endogenous vasoconstrictors such as catecholamines are increased by stress and pain during labour.

Functions of the placenta

The placenta is a fetal organ with the following functions:
- Placental transfer of products between maternal and fetal blood
- Transfer of immunity by transfer of immunoglobins from the mother
- Endocrine function
- Detoxification of drugs and substances transferred from the mother

Placental transport

Mechanisms of placental transport

Cellular membrane transport mechanisms are discussed in detail in Section 2, Chapter 1 (pages 208–11). In the case of the placenta these include:
- Simple diffusion
- Facilitated transport
- Secondary active transport
- Active transport

Location	PO$_2$ (kPa)	PCO$_2$ (kPa)
Maternal artery	13.3	3.9
Fetal umbilical artery	2.0	5.9
Fetal umbilical vein	3.9	4.7

Figure PN14 Blood gas tensions in materno-fetal transfer

- Pinocytosis
- Bulk transport

Placental transport of substances

The placenta acts as a barrier between maternal and fetal tissues. However, it is an imperfect barrier, and most substances will cross the placenta as detailed below.

Oxygen

Oxygen crosses the placenta by simple diffusion, depending mainly on the difference between the oxygen tension of the maternal blood in the intervillous space and the fetal blood in the umbilical artery. The PO$_2$ of blood in the intervillous space varies greatly but will be dependent on maternal arterial PO$_2$ (Figure PN14).

Other factors affecting oxygen transfer include the shape of the fetal oxyhaemoglobin dissociation curve and the Bohr effect. The fetal oxyhaemoglobin dissociation curve (P$_{50}$ = 2.5–2.8 kPa) lies to the left of the maternal curve (P$_{50}$ = 3.6 kPa). This favours the transfer of oxygen from the mother to the fetus. A rise or fall in CO$_2$ tension (with corresponding fall or rise in pH) leads to right or left shift response in the dissociation curve and also affects oxygen transfer (the Bohr effect). At the gas exchange interface, fetal blood gives up carbon dioxide, becomes more alkaline (left shift) and develops a greater affinity for oxygen. The maternal blood on the other hand takes up carbon dioxide, becomes more acidic (right shift) and promotes release of oxygen. This is referred to as the double Bohr effect, and it accounts for 2–8% of the transplacental transfer of oxygen. Factors determining oxygen transfer across the placenta are summarised in Figure PN15.

The placenta is a metabolically active organ, using 30% of the total oxygen delivered to it.

Carbon dioxide

CO$_2$ crosses the placenta by simple diffusion. It is present as dissolved CO$_2$ (8%), bicarbonate ion (62%), and carbamino haemoglobin (30%), with very small quantities as carbonic acid (H$_2$CO$_3$) and carbonate ion (CO$_3^{2-}$). Dissolved CO$_2$ is the form that crosses the placenta. The

- High materno-fetal oxygen concentration gradient
- Double Bohr effect
- The shape of the fetal oxyhaemoglobin dissociation curve
- High fetal hemoglobin concentration
- Functional status of the placenta
- Uterine blood flow and placental perfusion

Figure PN15 Factors determining transport of oxygen from the mother to the fetus

placental membrane is highly permeable to CO$_2$, which is 20 times more diffusible than oxygen.

A rise or fall in oxygen tension leads to a reduced or increased affinity for CO$_2$ (Haldane effect) and this affects the transport of CO$_2$. The materno-fetal transfer of oxygen produces de-oxyhaemoglobin in the maternal blood that has a greater affinity for CO$_2$ than oxyhaemoglobin. As the fetal blood takes up oxygen, it enhances CO$_2$ release. This is known as the double Haldane effect and it may account for as much as 46% of the transplacental transfer of CO$_2$. HCO$_3^-$ is not a major contributor to this process because of its ionised form, but it does act as a source of CO$_2$ through the carbonic anhydrase reaction that keeps CO$_2$ and HCO$_3^-$ in equilibrium.

Glucose

Glucose crosses the placenta by facilitated transport, which is stereospecific for the D-isomer. The placenta uses most of the glucose absorbed from the maternal surface.

Amino acids

Amino acids cross the placenta by means of secondary active transport. Much of the transplacental transfer of amino acids occurs by way of linked carriers for both amino acids and sodium. The transport of sodium down its concentration gradient drags amino acids into the cells. The process is stereospecific.

Fatty acids

Fatty acids probably cross the placenta by simple diffusion.

Electrolytes and water

Sodium and water cross the placenta by simple diffusion and bulk transport. Iron, iodine, calcium and phosphate require active transport.

Proteins

The placenta is relatively impermeable to plasma proteins. However, some immunoglobulins, particularly IgG, cross the placenta by pinocytosis.

Hormone secretion

The placenta produces the following hormones:
- Human chorionic gonadotropin (HCG)
- Human placental lactogen (HPL)
- Hypothalamic-releasing factors
- Hypothalamic inhibitory factors
- Oestrogens
- Progesterone
- Thyroid-stimulating hormone (TSH)
- Prostaglandins

A rapid rise in HCG production in early pregnancy stimulates the corpus luteum to secrete progesterone, which is required to maintain the viability of the pregnancy. The role of HCG in late pregnancy is not clear. The presence of HCG in urine forms the basis of the routine urine test for pregnancy.

Until the end of the eighth week, the corpus luteum continues to secrete progesterone. The placenta gradually takes over this role and becomes responsible for the secretion of progesterone which reaches a peak just before labour.

It is likely that the interaction between these placental peptides is important in the control of growth and development of the fetus.

Placental transfer of drugs

Measurement of placental drug transfer

Feto-maternal (F/M) concentration ratios of drugs are frequently used as an index of placental transfer of drugs, but they are influenced by several factors, such as:
- Site of fetal sampling
- Time interval between drug administration and sampling
- Whether drug is given as bolus or infusion

Factors affecting placental drug transfer

Most drugs, given enough time, will cross the placenta. The rate of transfer is dependent on:
- Lipid solubility
- Degree of ionisation
- pH of maternal blood
- Protein binding
- Molecular weight of drug

- Materno-fetal concentration gradient
- Placental blood flow

Lipid solubility

Lipophilic molecules diffuse readily across lipid membranes, of which the placenta is one.

Degree of ionisation

Only the non-ionised fraction of a partly ionised drug crosses the placental membrane. Most drugs used in anaesthesia, analgesia and sedation are poorly ionised in the blood and their placental transfer is almost unrestricted. Muscle relaxants are highly ionised, and therefore their transfer is almost negligible.

pH of maternal blood

The pH of maternal blood can alter the degree of ionisation of a drug. This effect is dependent on the pKa of the drug. If the pKa is near the pH of blood, then small changes (such as may occur during labour) in blood pH produce large changes in drug ionisation.

Protein binding

The diffusibility of a protein-bound drug is negligible compared with that of free drug. Protein binding is influenced by blood pH and concentration of plasma proteins. Acidosis reduces the protein binding of local anaesthetic, and low serum albumin in pre-eclampsia will cause a higher proportion of unbound drug and therefore promote transfer of drugs across the placenta.

Molecular weight of drug

Drugs with molecular weight of 600 daltons or less readily diffuse across the placenta. Most drugs used in anaesthetic practice have molecular weights <600, and therefore diffuse readily.

Materno-fetal concentration gradient

When a drug is transferred by simple diffusion, its rate of transfer is determined by Fick's law of diffusion, which states that:

$$\dot{Q} = kA\frac{(C_m - C_f)}{D}$$

where

$\dot{Q}$ = rate of diffusion per unit time
k = diffusion constant
A = surface area available for exchange
C_m = maternal concentration of free drug

	Half-life (hours)	
	Pethidine	**Norpethidine**
Mother	4	21
Neonate	19	62

Figure PN16 Half-lives for pethidine and norpethidine for mother and neonate

C_f = fetal concentration of free drug
D = thickness of diffusion membrane

The diffusion constant depends on physicochemical properties of the substance such as molecular size, lipid solubility and degree of ionisation.

Placental blood flow

With poorly diffusible drugs, the concentration in maternal and fetal blood changes little during placental transit, and hence blood flow has little impact on transplacental gradient. With highly diffusible drugs, concentration gradient falls significantly as a result of transfer, and hence blood flow has a marked effect on gradient.

Placental transfer of individual drugs
Opioids

All opioids cross the placenta in significant amounts. Pethidine is commonly used during labour. It is about 50% plasma protein-bound and has almost unrestricted placental transfer. Maximum uptake by fetal tissue occurs 2–3 hours after a maternal IM dose, which is when neonatal respiratory depression is most likely to occur. Longer half-lives for pethidine and its active metabolite norpethidine in the neonate, compared with the mother, mean that there is a risk from cumulative side effects in the neonate (Figure PN16).

Morphine is poorly lipid-soluble and weakly plasma protein-bound, but readily crosses the placenta. Fentanyl is highly lipid-soluble, crossing the placental membrane rapidly, but is largely albumin-bound (74%). Alfentanil is less lipophilic than fentanyl but is more highly bound to plasma protein.

Local anaesthetic agents

Local anaesthetic agents cross the placenta by simple diffusion. Commonly used local anaesthetics have molecular weights ranging from 234 daltons (lidocaine) to 288 (bupivacaine). They are weak bases and have relatively low degrees of ionisation and high lipid solubility at normal pH. Local anaesthetic accumulation in the fetus can occur if the fetus is acidotic, due to 'ion trapping'. This occurs when reduced pH in the fetus produces increased ionisation of the local anaesthetic and resultant lower diffusibility.

Drugs that are highly plasma protein-bound (bupivacaine, etidocaine) will have reduced placental transfer and lower F/M ratios compared with those with lower plasma protein binding (lidocaine, mepivicaine).

Transfer to the fetus is also affected by other factors, which include dose, site of administration and effects of adjuvants such as epinephrine. Higher doses result generally in higher maternal and fetal blood concentrations. The vascularity of the site of injection will determine the rate of absorption of the drug. For example, absorption from the paracervical injection is greater than from epidural injection. Addition of epinephrine to local anaesthetic solutions affects the rate of absorption from the site of injection, but the true effect of epinephrine on the various local anaesthetics is still unclear. The addition of epinephrine is thought to reduce absorption of lidocaine but not of bupivacaine.

Inhalational agents

The high lipid-solubility and low molecular weight of these agents facilitate rapid transfer across the placenta. Halothane rapidly crosses the placenta (F/M ratio = 0.87) and can be detected in umbilical venous and arterial blood within 1 minute. Enflurane and nitrous oxide also cross rapidly (F/M ratio = 0.6 and 0.83 respectively), but there is limited information on isoflurane. Diffusion hypoxia may occur in a neonate exposed to nitrous oxide immediately before delivery. It is therefore advisable to administer supplementary oxygen to these neonates.

Induction agents

Sodium thiopental is a highly lipophilic weak acid and it is 75% bound to plasma albumin. It rapidly crosses the placenta (F/M ratio = 0.4–1.1), and so do methohexitone and ketamine. However, the pharmacokinetics of propofol are yet to be investigated fully. Feto-maternal concentration ratios of 0.65–0.85 have been reported.

Muscle relaxants

These drugs are fully ionised and poorly lipid-soluble, and therefore do not readily cross the placenta.

Anticholinergics

The placental transfer rates of anticholinergic drugs correlate directly with their ability to cross the blood–brain barrier. Atropine is detected in umbilical circulation within

1–2 minutes of maternal IV injection. In contrast, glyco-pyrrolate is poorly transferred.

Vasopressors

Vasopressors are often used to treat hypotension secondary to regional anaesthesia. Ephedrine appears to cross the placenta easily.

Benzodiazepines

Diazepam readily crosses the placenta. It is highly non-ionised and very lipophilic. The F/M ratio reaches 1 within minutes of injection and reaches 2 an hour after injection. Midazolam has an F/M ratio of 0.76 but it has a short half-life.

CHAPTER 15

Fetal and newborn physiology

A. R. Wolf

FETAL CIRCULATION
The heart

PULMONARY FUNCTION

RENAL FUNCTION

HEPATIC FUNCTION

THERMOREGULATION

NOCICEPTION

As the fetus develops from a single dependent cell into a fully formed neonate capable of sustained life outside the womb, the physiology of individual organs and the integrated systems of the body undergo substantial developmental changes. Although physiology in the early stages may be crude, and significantly different from that observed in maturity, it usually reflects functional differences that allow the fetus to cope with the challenges of the intrauterine environment, and also with the sudden, extreme changes needed for adaptation to extrauterine life. For example, the presence of fetal haemoglobin in utero allows oxygen to be extracted from the placenta in a very low-oxygen environment compared to after birth. In considering developmental physiology (ontogeny) it is necessary to see fetus, preterm newborn, neonate, infant, child and adolescent as stages of development that merge into each other.

Fetal circulation

The fetus and placenta encompass a unit in which the placenta enables the fetus to eliminate carbon dioxide and metabolic waste products in exchange for oxygen and nutrients from the maternal circulation (Figure FP1). Blood leaves the placenta in the single umbilical vein with an oxygen saturation of approximately 80%. The ductus venosus shunts half of the oxygenated umbilical venous blood through the liver to enter the inferior vena cava (IVC). This mixed IVC blood, with a saturation of 65%, enters the right atrium, but only one-third passes into the right ventricle. The majority is directed through the foramen ovale to the left atrium and left ventricle to supply the heart, brain and upper body with relatively oxygenated blood. Venous blood from the superior vena cava, with low saturation (25%), is directed preferentially to the right

ventricle and pulmonary artery. In the fetus, pulmonary vascular resistance is high, and less than 10% of cardiac output passes through the lungs. This is achieved by intense vasoconstriction in the pulmonary arterioles and patency of the ductus arteriosus, which allows the majority of blood passing into the pulmonary artery to join the aorta. This mixed aortic and ductal blood flow supplies the lower body with blood with a saturation of approximately 55%. Blood returns to the placenta via two umbilical arteries arising from the internal iliac arteries. Placental blood flow is large, comprising 60% of the fetal cardiac output.

At birth, with onset of spontaneous ventilation in the lungs and loss of the placenta, the circulation changes dramatically. The first breath generates a negative pressure of approximately 50 cmH$_2$O, drawing in about 80 ml of air and expanding the functional residual capacity. Pulmonary vascular resistance falls rapidly, allowing blood to flow from the right ventricle through the lungs. As placental flow ceases with clamping of the umbilical cord, systemic vascular resistance rises. The result is a reversal of right to left flow through the ductus arteriosus. Exposure to oxygenated blood and reduced prostaglandin-E$_2$ production stimulates ductal constriction, with functional closure in the majority of newborns by 24 hours. A shunt murmur may be audible prior to closure. Histological obliteration occurs by 3 weeks in most normal term infants. Preterm babies have a higher incidence of patent ductus arteriosus, and may require medical treatment with indomethacin, or surgical ligation. The ductus venosus closes passively, due to absent blood flow.

After the first breath, pulmonary venous blood returns to the left atrium, causing pressure in the left atrium to exceed that in the right. This effect on raised left atrial pressure is enhanced by the sudden rise in systemic vascular

Fundamentals of Anaesthesia, 3rd edition, ed. Tim Smith, Colin Pinnock and Ted Lin. Published by Cambridge University Press. © Cambridge University Press 2008.

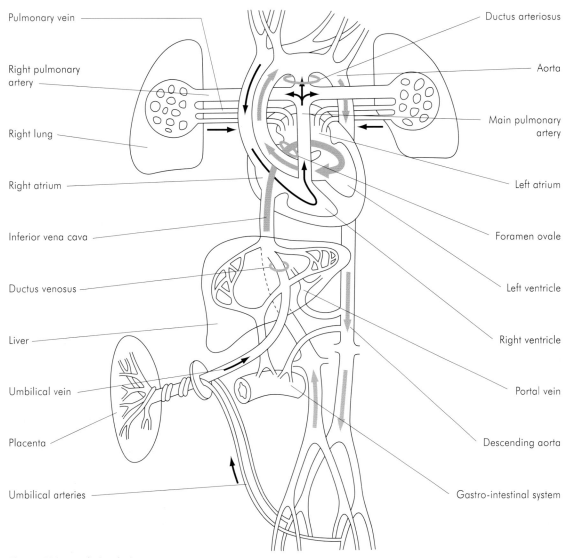

Figure FP1 Fetal circulation

resistance from loss of the placental blood flow. The valve-like foramen ovale closes, thus preventing deoxygenated blood from the right atrium crossing to the left.

Although the pulmonary vascular resistance is reduced after birth, it continues to fall for several days after birth and the pulmonary arteriolar medial walls remain very muscular. This muscle layer reduces considerably over the first few months and becomes thin-walled and elastic with little muscle by 6 months. However, immediately after birth, resistance in the pulmonary circuit is higher than in adults and the pulmonary arterioles remain very reactive. If the neonate becomes hypoxic, hypercapnic or acidotic, pulmonary vasoconstriction can lead to raised right-sided pressures and significant shunting through the foramen ovale, and reversion to a fetal-type circulation. This condition is called persistent pulmonary hypertension of the newborn (PPHN). Oxygen, hyperventilation or nitric oxide may be needed to reverse the condition, and

Age	Systolic BP (mmHg)	Diastolic BP (mmHg)	Heart rate (beats min^{-1})
Preterm 750 g[a]	45	25	>120
Birth	60	35	>120
Neonate	70–80	40–50	120–150
3–6 months	80–90	50–60	120–140
1 year	90–100	60–80	110–130
5 years	95–100	50–80	90–100
12 years	110–120	60–70	80–100

[a] Mean arterial BP ≤ gestational age in weeks is a good rule of thumb for preterm infants.

Figure FP2 Normal cardiovascular values in childhood

extracorporeal membrane oxygenation (ECMO) has been successfully used in severe and persistent cases.

The heart

The newborn heart consists of cardiac myofibrils that are poorly organised and lack the structured architecture of the mature heart. The increased ratio of connective tissue to contractile tissue compared to adults results in limitation in myocyte contractility and ventricular compliance. In addition, calcium metabolism is immature in neonatal myocytes. Consequently there is a relatively flat Starling curve, and while inadequate preload is poorly tolerated, overloading results in early cardiac failure. The stroke volume is relatively fixed, and increases in cardiac output are achieved largely by increases in heart rate. Ventricular end-diastolic volume increases from 40 ml m^{-2} body surface area at birth to 70 ml m^{-2} in children over 2 years of age. Normal heart rate at birth ranges from 100 to 170 beats per minute, decreasing with age and reaching adult values by puberty (Figure FP2). The preterm neonate has significantly lower blood pressure than the term infant, and adult levels are not reached until adolescence.

Autonomic innervation of the heart and blood vessels is incomplete in the newborn, with a relative lack of sympathetic supply. This is highlighted by the relatively small falls in blood pressure associated with high spinal blockade when using regional anaesthesia. Moreover, neonates are also less sensitive to the effects of catecholamines, needing much larger doses than older children or adults to achieve an increase in blood pressure and heart rate. Note the following facts:

- Both ventricles weigh the same at birth, although the right ventricle is the dominant ventricle in fetal life, possessing a thicker wall at the time of delivery.

- In the fetus, the two ventricles are effectively in parallel, with the dominant right ventricle pumping approximately two-thirds of the combined ventricular output via the pulmonary artery, through the ductus arteriosus and into the aorta.
- The left ventricle enlarges rapidly after birth, and by age 6 months reflects the adult ratio. This is mirrored in the ECG, which shows right axis deviation at birth, with an axis of up to +180 degrees, changing to +90 degrees by 6 months.

Pulmonary function

The fetal lung is filled with fluid essential for lung maturation and development. Irregular breathing movements are made in utero, which helps development of respiratory muscles, including the diaphragm and intercostal muscles. As full term approaches, catecholamines and tri-iodothyronine (T$_3$) stimulate the reabsorption of pulmonary fluid by reversal of the chloride pump mechanism. Final reabsorption is stimulated by the physical passage through the birth canal. This stage is less effective in babies born by Caesarean section, and can lead to a condition called transient tachypnoea of the newborn (TTN). Type II pneumocytes produce surfactant under hormonal stimulation (cortisol) from 26 weeks gestation. Surfactant stabilises alveoli by reducing surface tension, and artificial surfactant administration may be needed in preterm infants to prevent them developing respiratory distress syndrome (RDS). Term babies may also be surfactant-deficient if they suffer severe acidosis or hypoxia, or if they are born to mothers with diabetes mellitus.

The bronchial tree is fully developed at birth, in contrast to the alveoli, which continue to expand in both size and number, thus increasing the surface area of the lung by up to 25 times. Newborn infants have extremely compliant chest walls with compressible, horizontally aligned ribs. The diaphragm is the major muscle of ventilation in infancy, but can fatigue more easily in the neonate. In the first year of life, the percentage of type I, slow-twitch muscle fibres, which fatigue more slowly, increases from 10% to 25% (the adult level).

Newborn infants show ventilatory responses to changes in PaO_2 and $PaCO_2$, but these are less responsive and affected by other factors such as gestational and postnatal age, temperature, wake–sleep cycles and drugs. Neonates react to hypoxia with a brief period of hyperpnoea followed by centrally mediated respiratory depression. In the weeks that follow, as chemoreceptors mature, the infant develops a predominantly hyperpnoeic response to hypoxia. In sleeping infants the arousal response to hypoxia (normal in adults) is much diminished, and often completely absent during rapid eye movement (REM) sleep. Intercostal muscle activity is inhibited during REM sleep, and can lead to inefficient ventilation as the chest wall recesses on inspiration. Periodic respiration, where rapid shallow breathing alternates with apnoeas of up to 10 seconds, is normal in many infants.

Renal function

In the developing embryo, the first nephrons form during week 5, are functional from week 8 and have reached their full complement by week 36. After this there is merely growth in size and number of cells in existing nephrons rather than new nephron formation. Renal blood flow comprises 5% of cardiac output at birth, but with reduced renal vascular resistance this increases to 20% by 1 month of age, with increasing flow to cortical areas. The glomerular filtration rate (GFR) is correspondingly low at birth ($30 \ ml \ min^{-1}$), and is even lower in preterm infants ($3 \ ml \ min^{-1}$). By 2 years GFR has increased to near adult levels ($110 \ ml \ min^{-1}$). Low GFR and immature tubular function limits the neonate's ability to deal with water and solute loads, notably sodium and glucose, and they are unable to effectively excrete hydrogen ions or retain bicarbonate as a compensation for acidosis.

Hepatic function

During intrauterine life, the fetus excretes fat-soluble unconjugated bilirubin via the placenta and maternal liver. There is a physiological rise in bilirubin soon after birth, due to both an increased bilirubin load and immaturity of neonatal hepatic enzymes. The peak occurs on day 3–4 of postnatal life, due to immature oxidation-reduction reactions (phase I), with levels dropping in the second week of life as conjugating enzymes needed for glucuronidation mature (phase II). This drop takes longer in preterm babies, and the risk of kernicterus (damage to basal ganglia and auditory pathways) from unconjugated bilirubin entering the brain via an immature blood–brain barrier is significant. Infants handle hepatically excreted drugs differently to older children and adults. Immature enzyme systems play a role, but so does the difference in blood supply to the liver. Infants receive a higher proportion of their hepatic blood supply via the portal vein than via the hepatic artery. Any increase in intra-abdominal pressure, e.g. after abdominal surgery, reduces clearance of hepatically excreted drugs such as fentanyl.

Thermoregulation

Neonates lose heat readily because of their higher ratio of surface area to body weight, and relative paucity of subcutaneous fat. Preterm infants have particularly thin skins, needing higher ambient temperatures and humidity. Heat loss occurs by evaporation, radiation, convection and to a lesser extent conduction, as well as by insensible losses such as through respiration. Infants are seldom able to increase heat production enough to compensate for heat loss, and newborns need to be nursed in a thermoneutral environment (at an ambient temperature that minimises oxygen consumption and heat loss).

Unlike older children and adults, who generate heat involuntarily by shivering, newborns rely on non-shivering thermogenesis to increase their basal metabolic rate and thereby retain heat. This is a function of their unique brown fat, present in the first few weeks of life as an adaptive, protective entity. These specialised adipose cells are situated around the kidneys and adrenals, in the mediastinum and around the scapulae. They are abundant in mitochondria and have a rich blood and autonomic nerve supply. Norepinephrine in sympathetic nerve endings stimulates the hydrolysis of triglycerides to fatty acids and glycerol, resulting in oxygen consumption and heat production.

Nociception

Circumstantially, even the most preterm neonates respond to painful stimuli similarly to an adult, in terms of cardiovascular, stress and behavioural responses, but the presence or absence of pain as a conscious event can never be proven. Little can be inferred about the actual experience of pain in the neonate, or the attendant emotions, if any, relating to it. Much depends on the nature of self aware-ness, consciousness and the development of 'self' in fetal life. Given the impossible task of making judgements on the nature of pain perception in the fetus and neonate, the term nociception is more appropriate.

Nociceptive pathways develop early in gestation, and even in early development and they can produce complex protective responses to painful stimuli. Dorsal horn cells in the spinal cord have formed synapses with develop-ing sensory neurones by 6 weeks gestation, and peripheral nerves migrate to the skin of the limbs by 11 weeks, achiev-ing a density of nociceptive nerve endings similar to that of the adult by birth. The first appearance of transmitter vesicles is seen at 13 weeks gestation, and further synaptic connections and organisation of the dorsal horn structure continues up to 30 weeks.

The fetal neocortex has a full complement of cells by 20 weeks, and thalamocortical tracts can be shown to synapse with dendritic processes of the cells in the neocor-tex by 24 weeks gestation. Myelination of some ascending nociceptive tracts is seen by 30 weeks, but thalamocorti-cal radiations are not myelinated until 37 weeks and some nociceptive tracts are myelinated much later. However, lack of myelination does not imply lack of function: transmis-sion of nerve impulses within the central nervous system still takes place in unmyelinated nerves, albeit at a reduced velocity. Noxious stimuli can produce both haemodynamic and stress responses in a human fetus as young as 18 weeks gestation, and these responses can be reduced by pretreatment with analgesic drugs. Visual and auditory evoked potentials are present by 30 weeks gestation, by which time a complex EEG reactive to external influences has developed.

Overall, even the very preterm infant has complex interneuronal connections capable of integrated responses to tactile or nociceptive input. These infants show inconsis-tent responses to external stimuli, which may reflect the late functional connections of sensory afferents (particularly C fibres) within the spinal cord. However, the combination of larger receptive fields, recruitment of non-nociceptive afferents and reduced inhibitory controls results in 'under-damped' responses (long-lasting, exaggerated and poorly localised) once afferent stimuli have achieved central acti-vation above a threshold level. Inconsistency of response to more complex noxious stimuli may also reflect the profound effects that conscious state and other external responses have on behaviour.

Although newborn infants often have short-lived behavioural and stress responses to noxious stimuli, there is evidence in this age group that surgical trauma or injury can have long-term consequences for sensory and pain behaviour in infancy. It is clear that in neonates repeated noxious stimuli produce hypersensitivity to further stimu-lation, and that poor operative analgesia can be associated with long-lasting hyperalgesia and behavioural changes such as irritability, reduced attentiveness and poor orienta-tion, which may continue long after the expected duration of pain.

CHAPTER 1
Physical chemistry

T. C. Smith

INTERMOLECULAR AND INTERATOMIC BONDS
Atomic structure
Valency
Ionic bonds
Covalent bonds
Dative bonds
Van der Waals forces
Hydrogen bonds
Hydrophobic bonds
Strength of intermolecular bonds

OXIDATION AND REDUCTION

DIFFUSION
Simple diffusion
Non-ionic diffusion

SOLUBILITY AND PARTITION COEFFICIENTS

OSMOSIS
Pharmacological aspects of osmosis

DRUG ISOMERISM
Structural isomerism
Dynamic isomerism
Stereoisomerism

PROTEIN BINDING
Plasma protein binding

Intermolecular and interatomic bonds

The two main types of intermolecular bond are ionic and covalent, although weaker bonds, essential for intermolecular interactions, also exist. The structure of the component atoms determines the type of bonds within the molecule.

Atomic structure

When considering atomic structure, certain definitions aid understanding:

- Atom – the smallest part of an element that can take part in chemical reactions
- Element – a group of atoms all having the same atomic number
- Molecule – a combination of atoms which is the smallest unit of a chemical substance that can exist while still retaining the properties of the original substance
- Atomic number – the number of protons in each atom of an element

Knowledge of the basic structure of atoms is important in understanding the types of intermolecular bond and their functions. A schematic view of atomic structure is shown in Figure PC1.

An atom consists of a nucleus (central core) of neutrons and protons, surrounded by a cloud of negatively charged electrons. Figure PC2 shows the properties of these components. The charge of an atom is the number of protons minus the number of electrons. It is clear that almost all the mass of an atom is in the nucleus. The number of protons (atomic number) defines the element, and the atomic mass is close to the combined masses of protons and neutrons in the atom. Elements may exist with different numbers of neutrons in the nucleus while having the same atomic number. These are called isotopes, and those that release particles (radioactive) are called radioisotopes. Carbon provides an example: it has atomic number 6, and therefore six protons, though ^{12}C (carbon 12) has six protons and six neutrons, while ^{14}C (carbon 14) has six protons and eight neutrons (radioactive). Conventionally, the mass number is shown as a prefix superscript and the atomic number is shown as a prefix subscript, for example $^{12}_{6}C$ for carbon and $^{23}_{11}Na$ for sodium.

Electrons are arranged in orbital shells around the nucleus, from the innermost K shell outwards to L, M,

Fundamentals of Anaesthesia, 3rd edition, ed. Tim Smith, Colin Pinnock and Ted Lin. Published by Cambridge University Press. © Cambridge University Press 2008.

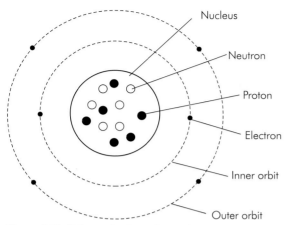

Figure PC1 Schematic view of atomic structure

	Nucleus		
	Proton	Neutron	Electron
Mass number	1	1	1/1836
Charge	+1	0	−1

Figure PC2 Properties of atomic particles

Shell	Maximum number of electrons
K	2
L	8
M	18
N	32

Figure PC3 Capacity of electron shells

N, O, P and Q shells (Figure PC3). These are not precise concentric rings, but the conceptual model helps to predict molecular behaviour. Shells are filled in their alphabetical order. Complete electron shells, pairs and octets of electrons confer stability. Each orbital shell has a maximum number of electrons, and some stability is conferred when this is achieved.

Valency

Valency may be defined as 'the number of atoms of hydrogen that one atom of an element can combine with or replace'.

Each element has at least one valency state, and the valency is used to establish possible intermolecular bonds.

Element	Protons	Neutrons	Electrons in shell					Valency
			K	L	M	N	O	
Hydrogen	1	0	1					1
Helium	2	2	2					0
Carbon	6	6	2	4				4
Nitrogen	7	7	2	5				3
Oxygen	8	8	2	6				2
Sodium	11	12	2	8	1			1
Magnesium	12	12	2	8	2			2
Chlorine	17	18	2	8	7			1
Argon	18	18	2	8	8			0
Potassium	19	20	2	8	8	1		1
Calcium	20	20	2	8	8	2		2
Xenon	54	77	2	8	18	18	8	0

Figure PC4 Electron properties of elements

Each group in the periodic table has a characteristic valency. For example, Group IA elements have a valency of +1. The valency can be predicted from the electron shell configuration, as shown in Figure PC4. Atoms of a particular element lose or gain electrons to achieve the stability described above. This loss or gain of electrons may be complete (in ionic bond) or by sharing with other atoms (in covalent bond). In this way, they adopt the electron configuration of the closest (by atomic number) rare or inert gas (for example helium, neon, argon). The inert gases are already at their most stable and do not gain or lose electrons. Consequently, they have minimal interaction with other atoms and exist as gases. Carbon is the single most important element in organic chemistry because it is chemically versatile – it can either lose or gain electrons to achieve electron stability.

Ionic bonds

The ionic bond (also termed electrostatic) relies on the fact that certain elements (termed electrovalent) have a tendency to lose or gain electrons to form charged atoms or molecules called ions. Like charges repel, but opposite charges attract, and therefore create a bond. This is illustrated by the formation of sodium chloride in Figure PC5.

With respect to the process shown in Figure PC5, the movement of an electron from the sodium atom to the chlorine atom results in both ions having stable

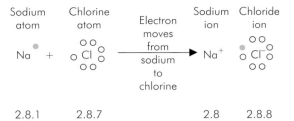

2.8.1   2.8.7   2.8   2.8.8
Electron orbital configuration

Figure PC5 Ionic bonding illustrated by the formation of sodium chloride. In Figures PC5, PC6, PC7 and PC9 the shading of electrons enables identification of any one electron's origin when considering the end result.

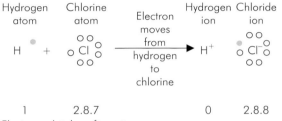

1   2.8.7   0   2.8.8
Electron orbital configuration

Figure PC6 Ionic bonding illustrated by the formation of hydrochloric acid

outermost shells. The sodium ion now has the electron configuration of neon, and chloride that of argon. The resultant change in charge causes a strong attraction between the sodium and chloride ions (the ionic bond) which is sufficient to maintain the precise crystalline structure of solid sodium chloride. Figure PC6 shows another example of ionic bonding with the relevant electron configurations.

Covalent bonds

Covalent bonds have similarities with ionic bonds in that they depend on forming stable electron shells. In contrast with ionic bonding, the atoms share electrons rather than donate them completely. Carbon, nitrogen, hydrogen and oxygen frequently behave in this way. The electron configuration of carbon is 2.4. Stability is achieved either by losing four electrons or by gaining four electrons, resulting in a pair or an octet of electrons in the outer shells, respectively. Covalent bonds may be single, double or triple, depending on the number of electron pairs that are shared. Methane (Figure PC7) is an example of covalent bonding having four single covalent bonds. The carbon atom of methane adopts the electron configuration of neon (2.8) while hydrogen

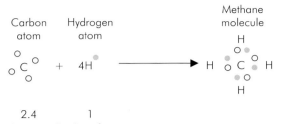

2.4   1
Electron orbital configuration

Figure PC7 Covalent bonding illustrated by the formation of methane

Ionic	Covalent
No sharing of electrons, therefore non-directional bond, therefore no particular shape	Electrons shared, therefore directional bond, therefore definite shape, so isomerism and stereoisomerism possible
Usually solid (crystalline)	Usually highly volatile liquids or gases
Not easily vaporised	Easily vaporised
Fused state	
Melt form is a conductor	Poor conductor
Readily dissolves in water	Not readily soluble in water
Forms electrolyte in water	

Figure PC8 A comparison of the properties of ionic and covalent bonds

adopts the configuration of helium, both being inert gases with stable atomic configurations.

A comparison of the properties of ionic and covalent bonds is given in Figure PC8.

Dative bonds

The dative bond is a type of covalent bond in which both electrons of the shared pair are from the same atom. This bond is a feature of atoms that have complete pairs of electrons in their outer shells in the non combined state. Typical examples are oxygen, nitrogen, phosphorus and sulphur. The formation of ammonium chloride from ammonia and hydrogen chloride (Figure PC9) illustrates this bond, as well as ionic and covalent bonds.

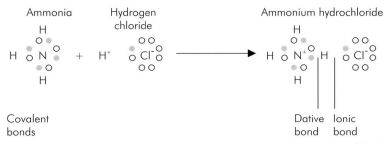

Ammonia Hydrogen chloride Ammonium hydrochloride

Covalent bonds   Dative bond Ionic bond

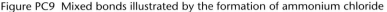

Figure PC9 Mixed bonds illustrated by the formation of ammonium chloride

Van der Waals forces

Because electrons are not rigidly fixed relative to the nucleus, but move in characteristic orbitals, the resulting electron cloud has a characteristic shape. Highly electronegative atoms such as oxygen attract electrons so that the distribution of the electron cloud of the molecule is uneven. This produces dipoles where component atoms of a molecule are not electrostatically neutral. The value of these charges is much less than the +1 or −1 of ions, and the molecule may have a polarity. Van der Waals forces are the attraction and repulsion of these weakly charged areas to similar areas in neighbouring molecules. Graphite is an example of sheets of covalently bonded carbon in which the layers are held together by van der Waals forces, and they are also essential in receptor and enzyme bonding.

Hydrogen bonds

A hydrogen bond is a weak electrostatic bond between the positive nucleus of a covalently bonded hydrogen atom in one molecule and the unshared pair of electrons of a highly electronegative atom of another molecule. Oxygen, sulphur and nitrogen are highly electronegative atoms, and water provides an example of hydrogen bonding (Figure PC10). The hydrogen bonding in water is responsible for the relatively high boiling point (compared with non-polar liquids) and the structure of ice crystals.

Hydrophobic bonds

In water, individual molecules are attracted to each other by hydrogen bonds. Any molecules added to the water will disrupt this loosely held 'structure'. If the electron distribution of the additive is not uniform (it has polarity) or if it is readily ionised, then it too will form bonds with the water molecules. This will allow it to spread readily and evenly throughout the containing vessel. If, however, the electron distribution is even, then the energy required to break the hydrogen bonds of water will be greater than

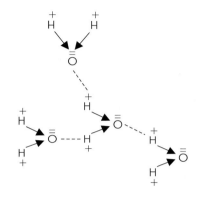

----- = attraction

→ = electron shift within covalent bond

+/− = dipolar non uniformity of electrostatic charge

Figure PC10 Hydrogen bonding in water. Dotted lines represent hydrogen bonds and arrows represent covalent bonds, with the arrow head showing direction of electron donation

that released by the formation of the new bonds. In this case, the most stable arrangement exists when the additive collects together, leaving as much of the water together as possible. This is easily seen when oil is added to water, and is a feature of lipids. Its density relative to water determines where the oil subsequently distributes. Vigorous mixing will provide the energy to break the hydrogen bonds and disperse the fat molecules, temporarily. This is the basis of the hydrophobic bond, which is very important physiologically, occurring at a local level around proteins and other molecules. Areas of membranes and proteins that do not have polarity do not attract water molecules. The water molecules therefore tend to maintain bonds with other water molecules, leaving these hydrophobic

Bond	Bond energy (kcal mol^{-1})
Covalent	50–150
Ionic	5–10
Hydrogen	2–5
van der Waals	0.5

Figure PC11 The strength of intermolecular bonds

areas vacant. This promotes the movement of non-polar hydrophobic molecules to these sites. Looking at this situation in overview gives the impression that the hydrophobic areas and molecules are attracted to each other, but in fact there is little or no attraction at all between the two. It is, in effect, the result of displacement of the hydrophobic molecules by the attraction of water and other hydrophilic molecules.

Strength of intermolecular bonds

The strengths of the main intermolecular bonds are shown in Figure PC11. The stronger the bond the higher the energy required to break it. Covalent bonds are thus very difficult to break without a catalyst or enzyme to facilitate. In physiological and pharmacological systems, therefore, covalent bonds are effectively irreversible. They are 'reversed' by metabolism of the receptor–agonist or enzyme–substrate complex and replacement of the enzyme or receptor. Examples of pharmacological covalent bonding include phenoxybenzamine to α-adrenoceptors, organophosphates to acetyl cholinesterase and monoamine oxidase inhibitors to monoamine oxidase.

The strength of ionic and other bonds decreases with the distance between the molecules such that the force of attraction is given by the following formulae:

Ionic bonds: $\text{force} \propto \dfrac{1}{\text{distance}^2}$

van der Waals forces: $\text{force} \propto \dfrac{1}{\text{distance}^7}$

In the latter, neighbouring groups of electrons cause repulsion once the distance decreases below a critical level.

Oxidation and reduction

Chemically, the loss of electrons is referred to as oxidation, and it involves the use of an electron acceptor (such as oxygen) which is correspondingly reduced. Oxidation can therefore include the binding of oxygen molecules to a molecule, as in the conversion of acetaldehyde to acetic acid:

$$2CH_3CHO + O_2 \rightarrow CH_3COOH$$

In the formation of the new molecule the oxygen accepts an electron from the acetaldehyde in order to complete the formation of a new covalent bond.

Serial oxidations and reductions occur in the mitochondrial release of energy in the cytochrome oxidase electron chain. Anaerobic dehydrogenases facilitate the removal of hydrogen.

In pharmacology, local anaesthetic agent ionisation by the acceptance of a proton (H^+) also constitutes oxidation.

Diffusion

Simple diffusion

Diffusion is a property of gas mixtures and solutions. Molecules of gases can move freely and tend to distribute themselves equally within the limits of the containing vessel (Figure PC12). In a similar way, molecules and ions in solution move freely throughout the solvent, so that the distribution (and therefore the concentration) becomes uniform throughout the solution. Ions and molecules, therefore, move down the concentration gradient and any electrical gradient until those gradients disappear. The result is an even distribution of all the ions and molecules in the container, so that any selected volume, regardless of shape, size or location, will have identical composition.

Graham's law describes gaseous diffusion as follows:

$$\text{Rate} \propto \frac{1}{\sqrt{\text{density}}}$$

The rate of diffusion of a gas at a given temperature and pressure is inversely proportional to the square root of its density. Thus the rate of diffusion increases with rising temperature as the speed of molecular movement increases.

Non-ionic diffusion

Of drugs, the majority is categorised as weak acids or weak bases, which implies that they are encountered in a partly ionised form. A higher degree of ionisation confers water solubility and, thus, is desirable for admixture, for example. In contrast, the unionised form of a drug is required for lipid membrane penetration and, hence, delivery to the target. The proportion of a drug present in ionised form is dependent on environmental pH. A drug that is a weak acid will dissociate in the following way:

$$HA \rightleftharpoons H^+ + A^-$$

Solute added to solvent

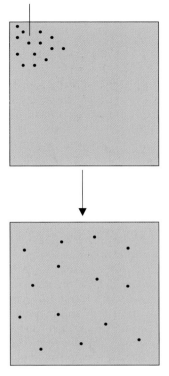

Solute redistributes evenly through solvent, resulting in uniform concentration throughout

Figure PC12 Effect of diffusion on gas molecule distribution

The relationship between dissociation and pH can be obtained by applying the Henderson–Hasselbalch equation:

$$pH = pK_a + \log_{10} \frac{[A^-]}{[HA]}$$

pK_a is the negative logarithm of the dissociation constant and is the pH at which the drug is 50% ionised. As a practical application of this concept consider thiopental (pK_a 7.8), which is deliberately made up in an alkaline solution, pH about 11, to render it more ionised and therefore water-soluble. After injection parenterally, into an environment of pH 7.4, the proportion of un-ionised drug form will become greater, enabling membrane penetration of the CNS.

Solubility and partition coefficients

The partition coefficient of a substance can be defined as a numerical constant that is the ratio at equilibrium of the concentrations of that substance in two adjacent compartments separated by an interface through which that substance readily passes.

When two or more compartments exist together then there will be movement of particles through the interface (permeable) between the compartments. The interface may be a physical boundary such as a cell membrane, or a liquid–gas interface. Unlike simple diffusion, the two compartments in a physiological system are likely to have different affinities for the particles. The resulting equilibrium will therefore have different concentrations of particles in the compartments. Solubility and partition coefficients can be determined for a pair of compartments for a given diffusing molecule. The coefficient is a dimensionless ratio describing the relative concentrations at equilibrium.

Partition coefficients are routinely used to describe the properties affecting distribution of volatile anaesthetic agents. The Ostwald partition coefficients used are specified for a given agent at body temperature (37 °C). Gases and vapours travel down their partial pressure gradient until the partial pressures are equal. The concentration for a given partial pressure in a particular compartment is determined by the affinity of the constituents of the compartment for the specified molecule. The total amount of the molecule in any compartment will also depend on the volume of the compartment. At equilibrium, the partial pressures will be equal but the concentrations will not. Figure PC13 shows these features using sevoflurane

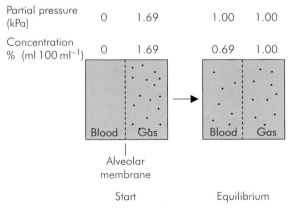

Figure PC13 Distribution of sevoflurane between blood and gas

as an example. Sevoflurane has a blood/gas partition coefficient $= 0.69$. This means that at equilibrium the ratio of sevoflurane concentration in the two compartments is 0.69 in the blood for every 1.00 in the gas phase. Solubility coefficients may also be between different solvents, such as oil and water. A highly oil-soluble molecule such as halothane will have a high oil/water solubility coefficient (220). A highly water-soluble molecule such as sodium chloride will have a low oil/water solubility coefficient. In general, ions are more soluble in water while isoelectric and non-polar molecules are more soluble in oils.

Osmosis

Osmosis is the passage of a solvent through a semipermeable membrane that separates two compartments having different concentrations of a solute (or solutes) to which the membrane is impermeable. A pure semipermeable membrane is one that is freely permeable to the solvent but impermeable to the solute. The glomerular membrane is an example of a functional semipermeable membrane: it is freely permeable to water and smaller molecules but impermeable to larger molecules (molecular weight >69 000 daltons).

In osmosis, an imbalance in the concentration of non-permeable molecules on two sides of a semipermeable membrane causes movement of the freely permeable solute towards the side of higher concentration. The solute tends to move, equalising concentration gradients. The osmotic pressure or potential is the pressure required to prevent this passage of solvent. Figure PC14 shows the effect of osmosis on fluid distribution. Osmotic activity continues until the hydrostatic pressure balances the osmotic potential. All solutions have an osmotic potential for a given semipermeable membrane and concentration. The solvent (e.g. water) moves towards the compartment with the highest concentration of solute and the pressure is, by definition, negative.

Osmotic potential may be the result of a single solute, but is usually due to many different molecules. Osmotically active particles in a solution are those to which the membrane is impermeable. Cell membranes are semipermeable, although ionic transport systems make this picture rather complex.

The difference between osmolarity and osmolality is:
- **Osmolarity** – concentration by volume of solution (in mOsm l^{-1})
- **Osmolality** – concentration by mass of solvent (in mOsm kg^{-1} H_2O)

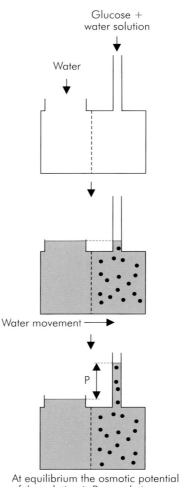

Figure PC14 Osmosis

Pharmacological aspects of osmosis

Drugs affecting the distribution of solutes between compartments will have an osmotic effect. Diuretics interfere with membrane transport of ions and other solutes through the renal cells and in the renal lumen and renal circulation. This manipulates the ionic concentrations in the medulla, and therefore water follows ionic concentrations in the tubules and urine output is increased. Mannitol is a drug used specifically for its osmotic effects. It is a high molecular weight alcohol that remains extracellular, and this produces a negative osmotic potential in the extracellular space that pulls water out of the intracellular space. It is also an osmotic diuretic because it

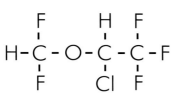

Enflurane

Isoflurane

Figure PC15 Isomerism of enflurane and isoflurane

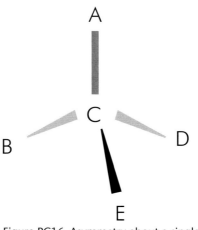

Figure PC16 Asymmetry about a single carbon atom

passes readily through the glomerular membrane but is not reabsorbed.

Drug isomerism

Isomers are chemical compounds that have the same empirical molecular formula (and so the same molecular weight) but differing physical or chemical properties.

Structural isomerism

Structural (or constitutional) isomerism is the presence of different structures with the same empirical molecular formula.

Chain isomerism

In chain isomerism the carbon skeleton varies between isomers whilst retaining the same functional group. Example: butane $CH_3CH_2CH_2CH_3$ and isobutane (2-methyl butane) $CH_3CH(CH_3)CH_3$.

Position isomerism

In position isomerism the component atoms or functional group are in different positions on an identical carbon skeleton. Example: enflurane and isoflurane (Figure PC15).

Functional group isomerism

In this form of isomerism the functional group changes. For example the movement of the oxygen of an alcohol into the carbon chain produces an ether. Example: propanol $CH_3CH_2CH_2OH$ and methyl ethyl ether $CH_3OCH_2CH_3$.

Dynamic isomerism

Dynamic isomerism (tautomerism) is a variant of functional group isomerism in which two isomers exist in dynamic equilibrium obeying the law of mass action. The barbiturates thiopental and methohexital exist in two forms (keto and enol), and the $= S/-SH$ and $= O/-OH$ groups in thiopental and methohexital respectively are in a dynamic equilibrium, the relative proportions of each being determined by the pH of the solution (see also Section 3, Chapter 6, Figure HY4). Nitrous oxide is another tautomer.

Stereoisomerism

Stereoisomerism (spatial isomerism) is another form of molecular rearrangement. Stereoisomers have the same molecular formula, carbon skeleton and structure but have a different spatial arrangement. Each atom in the molecule bonds to the same atoms as in the other stereoisomers. There are two types, optical and *cis–trans*.

Optical isomerism

Optical stereoisomerism requires atoms which are at least tetravalent (having the potential for four bonds), with different groups of molecules on each bond. Carbon is the most important tetravalent atom, and has four hybridised covalent links with neighbouring molecules. Figure PC16 shows the principles of optical stereoisomerism. The carbon atom in the chiral centre has four different groups attached to it. It can be seen that if two of these groups are interchanged then the resulting arrangement is a non-superimposable mirror image of the original. These are

	Traditional term (typically used in physiology)		Contemporary term (typically used in pharmacology)	
	Right	Left	Right	Left
Handedness	D	L	R	S
Rotational effect (on polarised light)	*d*	*l*	+	−

Figure PC17 Classification of stereoisomers

called enantiomers. Enantiomers often have different crystalline structures. Characteristically, they rotate polarised light in opposite directions. The amount of rotation is a feature of the molecular structure. Molecules with multiple chiral centres will not form simple superimposable mirror images unless every chiral centre is mirrored concurrently. Non-superimposable stereoisomers are called diastereomers, and these include isomers with multiple chiral centres and *cis–trans* isomers.

Classification

Several methods exist for classifying optical isomers, and it can seem confusing. Simply put, isomers may be described according to the actual molecular configuration about the chiral centre(s), and also by the direction in which polarised light is rotated (Figure PC17).

The molecular arrangement is described as either right- or left-handed, based on prioritising the groups attached to the chiral atom by atomic number of the attached atoms and molecules. The details of this are beyond the scope of *Fundamentals*. Right-handed isomers are classified as D (from the Latin *dexter*) or R (from the Latin *rectus*), both terms referring to the right. Left-handed isomers are classified as L (from the Latin *laevus*) or S (from the Latin *sinister*), both terms referring to the left.

The optical rotation may be clockwise (to the right) or anticlockwise (to the left). Clockwise rotation is said to be dextrorotatory and is represented by (+) or *d*. Anticlockwise rotation is said to be levorotatory and is represented by (−) or *l*.

Chiral molecules are variously classified in texts, using a mixture of the above terms. It is sufficient to use either handedness or optical rotation to define the enantiomer, but for completeness both terms are often used, especially with drugs. *d* and *l* have largely been superseded by (+) and (−). D and L are still used for physiological components, but R and S are usually used for drugs.

Physiological stereoisomers

Glucose exists naturally as D(+)glucose (which is why it is also referred to as **dextr**ose). Its right-handedness is by comparing carbon-5 with the configuration of D-glyceraldehyde. The mirror image is L(−)glucose, which is a mirror image of all the chiral carbons of glucose. Most naturally occurring carbohydrates are right-handed. Alterations in the chirality about carbon atoms (2, 3, 4) within the carbohydrate ring (interchanging hydrogen and hydroxyl group) result in epimers. Examples include D-galactose and D-mannose. D(−)fructose has the same configuration but in fructose this rotates light to the left, as denoted by the (−). The hexoses are further complicated by their dynamic isomerism into cyclic forms, with variation about carbon-1 leading to α and β forms of D-glucose.

Conversely, the amino acids in proteins (except glycine, which has no chiral atom) all have an absolute configuration similar to that of L-glyceraldehyde. They rotate light in different directions (for example L(+)alanine and L(−)leucine). Some D-amino acids do occur naturally, for example in bacterial cell walls.

Pharmacological considerations

Different enantiomers often have different potencies (stereoselectivity), and may be responsible for different side effects. The manufacture of most stereoisomeric drugs results in equal amounts of each stereoisomer. This is called a racemic mixture, and the rotational effects on light cancel out. Where multiple chiral atoms exist, the number of stereoisomers increases greatly.

The naturally occurring receptors are often stereospecific and will interact mainly or entirely with one racemate (e.g. R(+)etomidate). The rest of the drug may be redundant. As the chemical properties are usually identical, the measurement of drug levels will not distinguish between the species. This affects pharmacokinetic calculations. The elimination of the drug may also be different for each racemate, as will be the activity of any metabolites, so each racemate will have a different pharmacokinetic profile.

H − C − COOH

‖

H − C − COOH

cis form (maleic acid)

H − C − COOH

‖

COOH − C − H

trans form (fumaric acid)

Figure PC18 An example of *cis–trans* isomerism

Unfortunately the 'redundant' stereoisomer (e.g. R-bupivacaine) may be responsible for unwanted effects, and may preclude the drug's use and further development unless the desired stereoisomer can be isolated. This requires special techniques that are costly. Specific manufacture of stereoisomers is advantageous.

Cis–trans *(geometric) isomerism*

Cis–trans (or geometric) isomerism refers to the possible atomic orientational variants about a double bond. Figure PC18 shows an example of this. These stereoisomers are a type of diastereomer (have a non-superimposable mirror image) and are also referred to as *E–Z* isomers. The main parts of each half are in the same plane in the *cis* (Latin: same side) or (*E*) isomers and in opposite planes in *trans* (Latin: other side) or (*Z*) isomers.

Mivacurium contains two such bonds, and the resultant isomers (*cis–cis*, *cis–trans* and *trans–trans*) have different pharmacokinetic profiles (see Section 3, Chapter 8, page 619). *Cis*-atracurium is now available, to minimise the undesirable effects such as histamine release thought to be caused by the *trans* isomers.

Protein binding

Protein binding depends on the structure of the protein. A protein may have up to four levels of structure:

- Primary structure – the chemical formula of the protein, which is usually simplified by using the component amino acids to describe it. It concerns the covalent bonds excluding cross-linking disulphide and hydrogen bonds.
- Secondary structure – the relative spatial positions of neighbouring covalently bonded molecules to each other. Free rotation occurs about single covalent bonds (but not double bonds). This rotation allows the molecule to settle into its most stable orientation, resulting in a specific coiled protein layout held in place by disulphide bridges. This basic coil is often an alpha-helix.
- Tertiary structure – the shape in which the alpha-helix is subsequently arranged, which may be long and straight but usually curls around itself.
- Quaternary structure – the interrelationship between individual protein molecule subunits when more than one subunit constitutes the protein. Subunits are held together by weak bonds such as hydrogen bonds and van der Waals forces.

Proteins are highly complex molecules and potentially have multiple areas or sites with individual properties. These sites vary in size, shape, electrostatic charge and their relationship to other sites. They have the potential to attract molecules of a suitable size, shape and charge in a similar manner to a three-dimensional jigsaw or key. Plasma proteins act in this way to transport poorly soluble molecules to other locations in the body. The bound molecules are generally in equilibrium with their unbound molecules, and are released as the free concentration falls.

Enzymes are specific proteins that bind molecules and then facilitate the formation or destruction of covalent bonds within molecules, allowing synthesis of new molecules and destruction of other molecules. Receptors are usually proteins or glycoproteins that bind or receive specific molecules (agonists and antagonists) producing a conformational change in the receptor that is responsible for the effect. The effect of the agonist–receptor complex may be to open an ion channel in a membrane, for example.

Drugs may interact with binding sites in the following ways:

- Agonist drugs have a similar structure to the intended molecule, bind to the receptor site and mimic the endogenous agonist.
- Antagonist drugs have a similar structure to the intended molecule, bind to the receptor site without causing any change but prevent the endogenous agonist binding to the receptor.

- Drugs may bind to another part of the protein and cause a configuration change that prevents the receptor site from binding to the agonist.
- Drugs may bind to another part of the protein and prevent the configuration change necessary for the physiological effect.
- Drugs may bind to the protein and prevent ions reaching the opened channel.

Plasma protein binding

The degree of drug binding to plasma proteins is relevant to the transport of poorly soluble drugs, and also in determining dose requirements.

Features of plasma proteins

The main plasma proteins involved in drug transport are albumin and globulin. Other molecules, such as α_1-acid glycoprotein, which binds basic drugs, and specific carriers for cortisol and thyroxine, contribute to the transport system. These molecules are large (albumin has a molecular weight of 69 000 daltons) and have multiple, relatively non-specific binding sites. As with all binding sites, the shape and charge of the site are important. The bonds are a combination of any of the relatively weak bonds (hydrogen bonds, hydrophilic bonds and van der Waals forces), which allows rapid dissociation of drugs (determined by concentration) at the site of action and for elimination. A drug will bind to a protein binding site to produce a complex in the following manner:

Drug + protein binding site $\rightleftharpoons$ Drug–protein complex.

According to the law of mass action, as the concentration of free drug falls due to diffusion at locations with a low drug concentration, so the balance of the equation will shift to the left. Figure PC19 shows the different protein binding affinities of some important drugs.

Factors affecting binding

Changes in drug or protein nature alter the amount of protein binding. The amount of protein in the plasma will alter the number of available binding sites, as will abnormalities in the protein structure. Surgery and other trauma, myocardial infarction, carcinoma and rheumatoid arthritis increase the concentration of α_1-acid glycoprotein. Changes in pH may alter the ionisation of some groups on the protein and drug, resulting in either increased or decreased attraction between the molecules as well as the activity of the drug. The presence of other drugs having an affinity for the same binding sites on the protein creates

	Predominantly bound to	
Basic	Albumin	Globulin
	Bilirubin	Chlorpromazine
	Fatty acids	Lidocaine
	Tryptophan	Bupivacaine
		Propranolol
		Opioids
Acidic or neutral	Salicylates	
	Warfarin	

Figure PC19 Drug affinity for plasma proteins

competition and displacement so that less of each drug will be bound. This is particularly relevant when a new drug is added after a patient has been stabilised on the first drug, and can cause toxicity from excessive plasma levels of the first drug.

Effects of changes in binding

Changes in binding alter the amount of free drug. There is considerable interpatient variation in the degree of protein binding for a given drug. Only the unbound drug is available to diffuse and attach to a site of action for pharmacological effect, and the bound portion is effectively inactive. If protein binding for a particular drug is low then the majority of the drug is free to have its effect. Any change in protein binding will need to be large before any significant change in plasma levels of free drug is seen. If, however, the proportion of bound drug is high then even small changes in the proportion of drug bound will have a pronounced effect. Depending on the direction of the effect, these changes can reduce or enhance the therapeutic effect but, more importantly, may permit toxic effects of overdose to develop. Protein binding might appear from this to be a disadvantage. In fact, it is particularly important for the transport of lipophilic drugs, which may not dissolve in aqueous media in sufficient concentration to provide an effective concentration at the target site. There is also a degree of 'buffering' of the administered dose.

Protein binding affects the pharmacokinetic properties of a drug. The greater the degree of binding, the less drug there is available for diffusion into other tissues, and more remains in the plasma. This shows as a low volume of distribution. A low volume of distribution results in higher elimination of the drug.

CHAPTER 2

Pharmacodynamics

T. C. Smith

CONCENTRATION–EFFECT RELATIONSHIPS
Drug–receptor kinetics
Important equations and their derivation

EFFICACY AND DRUG–RECEPTOR INTERACTIONS
Agonists
Partial agonists
Reversible competitive antagonists
Irreversible competitive antagonists
Lineweaver–Burk plot

VARIATIONS FROM PREDICTIONS
Occupancy–response inconsistencies
Hysteresis
General variation
Pharmacogenetics

ENZYMES

Pharmacodynamics is the study of the quantitative effects of drug concentration on the activity and response at specific receptor sites. In simple terms, this is often expressed by the phrase 'what the drug does to the body'.

Both endogenous ligands and exogenously administered drugs interact with receptor sites to produce an effect. Drugs can act in a number of different ways, depending on their characteristics (Figure PD1).

The important equations concerning drug receptor interactions are explained below, aided by graphical representations of these interactions. Although 'drug' is often used to describe the receptor interaction, **endogenous** agonists of the receptor act in exactly the same way.

Agonism – drug binds to the receptor and can produce a maximal response
Partial agonism – drug binds to the receptor and causes a similar but less than maximal response
Antagonism – drug may prevent binding by the agonist or interfere with the response outcome

Figure PD1 Drug properties

Concentration–effect relationships
Drug–receptor kinetics
Key equations in pharmacodynamics describe drug–receptor interactions. The basic equations are the fundamental relationships from which the key equations are built. The following explains the mathematical features of the equations and introduces new terms sequentially. The key equations are displayed graphically to illustrate important comparisons between various drug–receptor interactions.

Important equations and their derivation
The following conventions will be used:

$\Rightarrow$ implies that
$\propto$ proportional to

Consider the basic chemical interaction of an agonist drug with a receptor to form a drug–receptor complex. This interaction is reversible (and note that endogenous agonists act in exactly the same way).

The receptor can be considered to have two states, active and inactive. When unoccupied by an agonist the receptor is predominantly in the inactive state, but when occupied it is predominantly in the active state. The active state tends to increase the strength of the drug–receptor intermolecular bonds. So, in general, the receptor can be considered to be either unoccupied and inactive, or occupied and active.

Derivation of key equation 1
Key equation 1 is built from basic equations 1 and 2, which are detailed below. Terms used are defined as follows:

[D] – concentration of free drug
[R] – concentration of unoccupied receptors
[DR] – concentration of drug-occupied receptors

Fundamentals of Anaesthesia, 3rd edition, ed. Tim Smith, Colin Pinnock and Ted Lin. Published by Cambridge University Press. © Cambridge University Press 2008.

k_1 – constant that defines the rate of the association (forward) reaction

k_2 – constant that defines the rate of the dissociation (backward) reaction

K_D – constant (the dissociation constant) that defines the equilibrium point of the whole interaction

Basic equation 1

Drug + Receptor $\rightleftharpoons$ Drug-Receptor complex

$$D + R \underset{k_2}{\overset{k_1}{\rightleftharpoons}} DR$$

The law of mass action states that the velocity of a chemical interaction is proportional to the molecular concentrations of the reacting components. Therefore:

Forward (association) reaction $\propto [D]$
and also $\propto [R]$, so
Forward (association) reaction $\propto [D] \times [R]$, and
Backward (dissociation) reaction $\propto [DR]$

For clarity the multiplication sign is usually omitted, and $[D] \times [R]$ is written as $[D][R]$.

The next step is to insert the constants to convert '$\propto$' to '$=$', which results in the two terms:

Forward reaction $= k_1 [D][R]$
Backward reaction $= k_2 [DR]$

At equilibrium, there is no net change in the balance of concentrations and the rate of association reaction equals the rate of the dissociation reaction, so generating basic equation 2.

Basic equation 2

$k_1[D][R] = k_2[DR]$

This can also be expressed as:

$$\frac{k_2}{k_1} = \frac{[D][R]}{[DR]}$$

In any equation, constants can be combined as a single constant. In this case, the ratio of the two constants k_1 and k_2 is called the equilibrium or dissociation constant, which is termed K_D.

The final step is to substitute one constant for two, which leads to key equation 1.

Key equation 1

$$K_D = \frac{[D][R]}{[DR]}$$

K_D is a constant for a particular drug–receptor interaction. The dissociation constant is a useful value in pharmacodynamics as it permits quantitative comparisons of the equilibrium points of different drug–receptor combinations. The reciprocal of the dissociation constant represents the affinity of the drug for the receptor. In other words:

$$\text{Affinity} = \frac{1}{K_D}$$

Derivation of key equation 2

Key equation 2 is built from basic equations 3–5. The following definitions are used:

r – receptor occupancy
R_T – total number of receptors

To provide useful information it is necessary to relate receptor occupancy (r) to agonist concentration [D]. To derive key equation 2 the receptor term not featuring in occupancy, [R], must be substituted in key equation 1.

Occupancy is the proportion of receptors occupied by the agonist, and this is described by basic equation 3.

Basic equation 3

$$r = \frac{[DR]}{[R_T]}$$

In other words, the total number of receptors is the sum of free and drug-bound receptors as given in basic equation 4.

Basic equation 4

$[R_T] = [R] = [DR]$

This can also be expressed as $[R] = [R_T] - [DR]$.

Substituting [R] from basic equation 4 in key equation 1 gives

$$K_D = \frac{[D]([R_T] - [DR])}{[DR]}$$

$\Downarrow$ Rearrange

$$\frac{K_D[DR]}{[D]} = [R_T] - [DR]$$

$\Downarrow$ Divide both sides by

$$\frac{K_D[DR]}{[D][DR]} = \frac{[R_T] - [DR]}{[DR]}$$

$\Downarrow$ Simplify

$$\frac{K_D}{[D]} = \frac{[R_r]}{[DR]} - 1$$

Finally, rearrange to produce basic equation 5.

Basic equation 5

$$\frac{K_D}{[D]} + 1 = \frac{[R_r]}{[DR]} = \frac{K_D + [D]}{[D]}$$

When basic equation 3 is substituted in basic equation 5 as follows:

$$\frac{1}{r} = \frac{K_D + [D]}{[D]}$$

and this is shown as a reciprocal, key equation 2 is obtained.

Key equation 2

$$r = \frac{[D]}{K_D + [D]}$$

Key equation 2 shows that when the drug concentration is equal to the dissociation constant the occupancy is 0.5. Therefore, the dissociation or equilibrium constant for a reversible drug–receptor interaction is the concentration of that agent that results in half the receptors being occupied.

Derivation of key equation 3

Derivation of key equation 3 requires basic equation 6. The following definitions are used:

R – response (not the same as [R] in earlier equations)
E – efficacy (a constant for a drug–receptor complex)

The receptor response produced by an agonist binding with the receptor is a function of the occupancy and the effect (efficacy) of the agonist on that receptor. For the purpose of this derivation, response is proportional both to occupancy and to the efficacy of the drug–receptor complex (basic equation 6).

Basic equation 6

R = E r

Substituting r from key equation 2 into basic equation 6 creates key equation 3.

Key equation 3

$$R = \frac{E[D]}{K_D + [D]}$$

This equation shows that when the drug concentration is equal to the dissociation constant then the response is 0.5 times the maximum, as determined by the efficacy. In other words, the dissociation constant is the concentration of drug producing a half-maximal response.

Agonist
Partial agonist
Antagonist
   Competitive – reversible or irreversible
   Non-competitive

Figure PD2 Drug–receptor interactions

Response can be determined from any of the subsequent equations describing occupancy by multiplying by E. Deviations from this model are discussed later.

Efficacy and drug–receptor interactions

Graphical plots based on key equation 3 are used to demonstrate and explain the features of the drug–receptor interactions. These are classified in Figure PD2. In this section the following terms are used:

[B] = concentration of antagonist
[BR] = concentration of receptors occupied by the antagonist
$[D_A]$ = concentration of agonist
$[D_B]$ = concentration of antagonist
r_A = occupancy of receptor by agonist
r_B = occupancy of receptor by antagonist
K_A = equilibrium constant for defining the agonist/ receptor interaction
K_B = equilibrium constant for defining the antagonist/ receptor interaction

Do not confuse the terms K_A and K_B with the terms K_a and K_b used in acid–base calculations.

Figure PD3 lists the values used in the graphical examples that follow. Note that the values for equilibrium constants are not actual ones but represent concentrations for the purposes of illustration.

Agonists

An agonist is an agent that reversibly binds to a receptor site to produce a conformational change in the receptor, which mediates a response. A pure agonist produces the maximum response that the receptor is capable of mediating, and is therefore said to have an efficacy of 1 (E = 1).

Figure PD4 plots receptor occupancy (r) against drug concentration and demonstrates the characteristic rectangular hyperbola. This shows that as the drug concentration increases so the initially high increase in occupancy reduces progressively as more receptors become occupied.

Ligand	Abbreviation	Dissociation constant	Efficacy
Agonist 1	A_1	50	1
Agonist 2	A_2	25	1
Agonist 3	A_3	100	1
Partial agonist 1	P_1	50	0.75
Partial agonist 2	P_2	500	0.75
Reversible competitive antagonist	B	450	0
Irreversible competitive antagonist	I		0

Figure PD3 Values used for the various ligands in the ensuing graphs

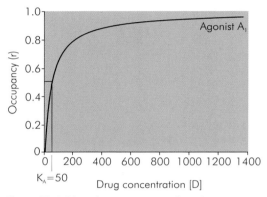

Figure PD4 Plot of occupancy against drug concentration

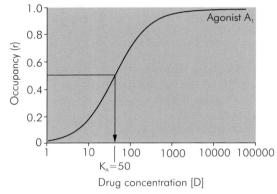

Figure PD5 Semilogarithmic plot of occupancy against drug concentration

The most rapid increase in occupancy occurs when the concentration is low and the number of unoccupied receptors is at its highest. The rate of increase in occupancy rapidly falls off as the agonist concentration rises and unoccupied receptors fall in number. A working model of the mechanics of this may be thought of as a decrease in opportunity for binding as fewer free receptors are left. However, it is important to remember that drug–receptor bonds are constantly being made and broken. The important points to identify on the graph are:

- Zero occupancy with zero agonist concentration
- Maximal occupancy (always 1 with competitive binding)
- Concentration at 0.5 (50%) occupancy (this is K_A)

For a pure agonist (efficacy = 1) the y-axis can also be labelled as response. At this point maximal occupancy and response are by definition both 1, but antagonists and partial agonists alter this finding, and thus identifying the maximal response becomes important.

The shape of the plot makes it difficult to identify the maximum or the equilibrium constant accurately using a single plot even if a relatively small concentration range is used. The plot is useful to demonstrate the pharmacodynamic basis of the drug–receptor interaction but does not lend itself easily to comparisons and predictions with other agonists and antagonists or their interactions.

To address these problems the semilogarithmic plot is used. This plots occupancy on a linear scale against drug concentration on a logarithmic scale. This is the basis of Figures PD5–PD10. Figure PD5 uses the same agonist profile (A_1) as Figure PD4 and shows the characteristic sigmoid shape. The occupancy is plotted as a proportion of full receptor occupancy, and for a pure agonist this equates with response. The 0.5 occupancy point that determines the concentration value for K_A ($K_A = [D]$) is on the 'straight' part of the plot where the direction of curvature changes from upwards to downwards.

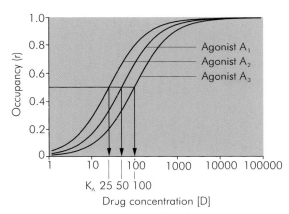

Figure PD6 Semilogarithmic plot of occupancy against drug concentration, showing the effect of changes in equilibrium constant

Figure PD6 shows two more full agonists (A_2 and A_3) with K_A half and double that of the original example ($K_A = 50$). Changing K_A has the following effects:
• Parallel shift to right or left
• No change in maximal occupancy

K_A defines the affinity of the ligand for the receptor (= 1/affinity), so the lower the affinity the higher the equilibrium constant. When the affinity is doubled the K_A is halved, and vice versa. The occupancy profiles for pure agonists, partial agonists and reversible competitive antagonists with identical K_A are identical, but variations in efficacy alter the responses proportionally.

Molecular binding of drugs

Consider 'n' to represent the number of molecules that must bind to each receptor to mediate a response. Frequently each receptor has one binding site for a particular molecule, but this is not always so. The nicotinic acetylcholine receptor has two binding sites for acetylcholine, one on each α subunit. For a response, both sites must be simultaneously occupied by the agonist. Key equation 4 shows this relationship.

Derivation of key equation 4

Key equation 4 is derived using basic equation 1.

$$nD + R \rightleftharpoons D_nR$$

From this modification of basic equation 1 it follows that the forward reaction $\propto [D]^n \times [R]$, and therefore

$$K_D = \frac{[D]^n[R]}{[D_nR]}$$

This may be rearranged to produce an expression for $[D]^n$ as follows:

$$[D]^n = \frac{[D_nR]}{[R]}K_A$$

If top and bottom of the resulting fraction are divided by the total number of receptors, key equation 4 is obtained.

Key equation 4

$$[D]^n = \frac{r}{1-r}K_A$$

If the logarithm of the whole equation is taken the formula below results:

$$n \log [D] = \log \left(\frac{A}{1-r}\right) + \log K_A$$

This formula provides a means of determining 'n'.

Partial agonists

A partial agonist is an agent that reversibly binds to a receptor site to produce a conformational change in the receptor that mediates a response which is less than the maximum possible. It is, therefore, said to have an efficacy of between 0 and 1.

Figure PD7 shows a comparison of the drug–response profile of partial agonists (P_1 and P_2) with that of the standard agonist (A_1). A partial agonist is one that does not elucidate a maximal response regardless of concentration, and it therefore has an efficacy (E) of <1 but >0. A partial agonist with the same affinity for the receptor (P_1) has the same K_A as the agonist (A_1). Characteristically, however, partial agonists also have a lower affinity for the receptor (K_D higher), as demonstrated by P_2.

The following features are apparent:
• Sigmoid-shaped curve
• Response curve shifts downwards
• Shift not parallel
• Maximal response < 1
• Response maximum = efficacy (E)

A partial agonist has the same occupancy profile for a given K_A as a full agonist. The K_A of the partial agonist is a feature of **occupancy** and not response. It is calculated by appreciating that the point of half-maximal occupancy is achieved at half-maximal response. In Figure PD7 the maximal response of each partial agonist is 0.75 of that of the pure agonist, so the K_A concentration is read off at a response (R) of 0.375, as indicated by the line labelled X.

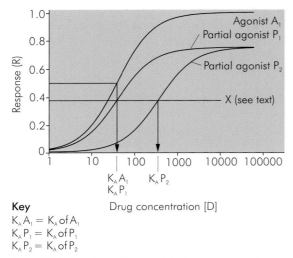

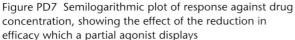

Key
$K_A A_1 = K_A$ of A_1
$K_A P_1 = K_A$ of P_1
$K_A P_2 = K_A$ of P_2

Figure PD7 Semilogarithmic plot of response against drug concentration, showing the effect of the reduction in efficacy which a partial agonist displays

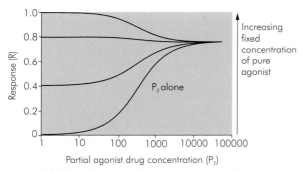

Figure PD8 Semilogarithmic plot of combined response against partial agonist drug concentration. Each line represents the response in the presence of a fixed concentration of pure agonist

Figure PD8 shows the effect on response of the addition of a partial agonist in the presence of various constant concentrations of agonist. For a given concentration of a pure agonist, addition of increasing amounts of partial agonist will eventually result in the observed effect approaching that of the partial agonist alone. At receptor level, competition ensures that the partial agonist displaces the pure agonist from an increasing proportion of the receptor pool until it occupies (almost) all receptors.

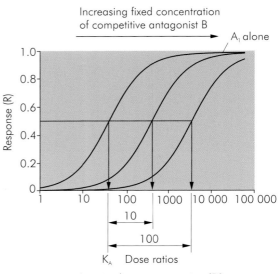

Figure PD9 Semilogarithmic plot of response against drug concentration, showing the effect of introducing increasing doses of competitive antagonist possessing no intrinsic activity

Reversible competitive antagonists

A reversible competitive antagonist is an agent that reversibly binds to a receptor site without mediating a response. A pure antagonist, therefore, has an efficacy = 0. These agents act by preventing the bonding of an agonist with the receptor, and therefore preventing any subsequent response. The occupancy profile of a reversible competitive antagonist is the same as that for an agonist or partial agonist for a given dissociation constant. However, as E = 0 for the antagonist, response will be zero **irrespective of drug concentration**.

Figure PD9 shows the effect of adding fixed concentrations of a reversible competitive antagonist on the agonist dose–response plot. Occupancy is similarly affected. The important features are:
- A parallel shift to the right
- Antagonist overcome by increasing agonist concentration
- No change in maximal response

The effect of the reversible competitive antagonist can always be overcome by increasing the concentration of the agonist. K_A does not change, but the effect is similar to that of a change in agonist affinity. The dose ratio is the quantitative measure of this effect. This is the ratio of the concentration of agonist in the presence of the antagonist at a given level of response (usually 0.5) to the concentration of agonist alone that produces the same response. In other words, the dose ratio is the factor by which the agonist concentration must be increased to achieve the same effect as in the absence of the antagonist. Using Figure PD9 as an example, $K_A = 50$ and the concentration with drug B is 500, producing a dose ratio of 10.

The dose ratio is dependent on antagonist concentration and antagonist receptor affinity, but independent of agonist affinity. The antagonist binds with the receptor in a similar manner to the agonists, and the equations for occupancy derived above apply. Thus for a competitive antagonist:

Antagonist + Receptor $\rightleftharpoons$ Antagonist–Receptor complex
[B] + [R] $\rightleftharpoons$ [BR]

In a similar manner to the agonist binding, this produces the following definition of antagonist affinity for the receptor:

$$\text{Antagonist affinity} = \frac{1}{(K_B)}$$

The antagonist is only effective in the presence of the agonist with which it competes for the binding sites.

Derivation of key equation 5
Key equation 5 is a simple modification of key equation 1 in which the concentrations are represented by their ratio to the equilibrium constant (K_A). A similar ratio for the antagonist, relative to its own equilibrium constant with the receptor (K_B), may be added. This will have the same effect as increasing K_A, because of its mathematical position in the equation. Dividing the terms of key equation 1 by K_A gives

$$r_A = \frac{[D_A]/K_A}{[D_A]/K_A + K_A/K_A} = \frac{[D_A]/K_A}{[D_A]/K_A + 1}$$

and adding the ratio for the antagonist B gives key equation 5.

Key equation 5
$$r_A = \frac{[D_A]/K_A}{[D_A]/K_A + [D_B]/K_B + 1}$$

This predicts that the addition of antagonist B necessitates an increase in the concentration of drug A to achieve the

same receptor occupancy with drug A as in the absence of the antagonist. Taking the term that has replaced K_A/K_A in the equation provides a ratio relative to this which describes the effect of the antagonist on the agonist–receptor interaction. This is the dose ratio:

$$\text{Dose ratio} = [D_B]/K_B + 1$$

This is not constant but is proportional to antagonist concentration and increases linearly. The affinity of the antagonist is defined by the K_B, and the potency pA_2 is derived from this. In a similar way to pH, pA_2 is the negative logarithm of the concentration of reversible competitive antagonist that has a dose ratio of 2. pA_2 is constant for a particular antagonist–receptor interaction. Substituting 2 for dose ratio enables calculation of pA_2, thus:

$$2 = [D_B]/K_B + 1$$
$$\Downarrow \text{Rearrange}$$
$$1 = [D_B]/K_B$$
$$\Downarrow \text{Take logarithms}$$
$$\log 1 = 0 = \log[D_B] - \log K_B$$
$$\Downarrow \text{Rearrange}$$
$$-\log D_B = -\log K_B = pA_2 \text{(as dose ratio is 2)}$$

Therefore, potency as an antagonist is defined by receptor affinity (K_B). Competitive antagonism involves direct competition for the receptor in exactly the same way as the pure agonist and partial agonists.

The competition exists between agonist and antagonist or partial agonist, and there is only space for one drug molecule at each receptor binding site at any time. The balance of this competition is determined by the relative affinities of the competing molecules.

Irreversible competitive antagonists
The irreversible competitive antagonist competes with the agonist for receptor sites but once attached it dissociates only very slowly or not at all because of the strength of the bond, which is usually covalent. There is no change in agonist affinity, and the equilibrium constant for the agonist in the presence of antagonist is unchanged, so the concept of pA_2 is inappropriate.

Figure PD10 shows the effect of adding fixed concentrations of an irreversible competitive antagonist with zero

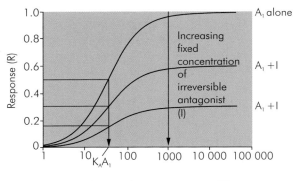

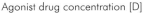

KEY

$K_A A_1 = K_A$ of A_1

Figure PD10 Semilogarithmic plot of response against drug concentration, showing the effect of introducing increasing doses of an irreversible competitive antagonist possessing no intrinsic activity

efficacy on the dose–response plot. Occupancy is similarly affected. The important features are:

- A downward shift
- Antagonism is not overcome by increasing agonist concentration
- Reduced maximal response

The maximal response is reduced in proportion to the reduction in receptors not occupied by the antagonist represented by r_B. A simple modification to key equation 1 to produce basic equation 7 is all that is required to illustrate this point.

Basic equation 7

$$r_A = \frac{D_A}{D_A + K_A}(1 - r_B)$$

Key equation 2 states that the maximum occupancy (and response) cannot be > 1. Basic equation 7 predicts the maximum occupancy, and therefore the maximum response, to be $1 - r_B$. In receptor terms the concentration–effect relationship is based on the interaction of the agonist with the remaining unoccupied receptors. At any given concentration, therefore, the effect will be a constant proportion of the maximal response with that level of antagonist. The equation predicts that the overall effect is similar to that of a partial agonist alone.

Lineweaver–Burk plot

The double reciprocal plot in Figure PD11 is a form of concentration–effect graph to convert a sigmoid curve into a straight line. It is used to determine the type of drug–receptor interaction and the equilibrium constants. The intersection with the y-axis (1/R) gives the reciprocal of efficacy. The intersection with the x-axis gives the negative reciprocal K_A for a single drug.

Variations from predictions

Occupancy–response inconsistencies

Receptor occupancy produces a response at the receptor (R = E r). However, the response is not necessarily identical to the occupancy, even for a pure agonist, because many receptor systems have silent receptors. Silent receptors represent a proportion of the total receptor pool that must be occupied before there is any response at all. This is a conceptual model, and the silent receptors are not a discrete subgroup. Interactions between receptors can also alter the shape of the plots from the theoretical.

Hysteresis

Hysteresis is a feature of changes in a dynamic system in which the response to a stimulus in one direction does not follow the same path when in the opposing direction. The binding of a drug to a receptor confers a degree of stability, and energy must be supplied to break this bond. A rise in drug concentration results in diffusion of drug towards receptors, which facilitates binding. During decreases in drug concentration, there is a lag phase before drug–receptor bonds will break, and thus the system demonstrates hysteresis.

General variation

Within biological systems there is variation between individuals, which usually has a normal distribution. A single individual may also exhibit temporal variation. There are a number of pharmacological terms that use a representative sample of the total population to describe the response. For example:

- ED_{50} – dose causing the specified effect in 50% of the sample population
- LD_{50} – dose causing a lethal effect in 50% of the sample population
- Ratio of $ED_{50} : LD_{50}$ – therapeutic index

Some of these variations originate from identifiable physiological differences such as age, gender and race, but most are the result of pharmacokinetic differences.

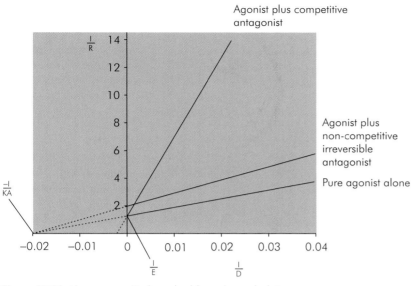

Figure PD11 Lineweaver–Burk or double reciprocal plot

Pharmacogenetics

Genetic variation can alter drug metabolism. For example, the metabolism of warfarin and phenylbutazone varies much less between identical twins than in the rest of the population. Specifically, the drug suxamethonium is metabolised by plasma cholinesterase. Abnormal and deficient plasma cholinesterase result from abnormalities in the gene responsible for transcription of this enzyme, leading to the inherited deficiencies described in more detail in Section 1, Chapter 4 (pages 63-4).

Fast and slow acetylators exist for the metabolism of such drugs as hydralazine, procainamide and isoniazid. Slow acetylators may show a higher incidence of unwanted effects for a given dose. Slow acetylators receiving hydralazine are more likely to develop SLE syndrome, for example.

Enzymes

Enzymes are closely related to receptors in their structure and related functional properties. Many receptors have enzymatic actions (e.g. $Na^+K^+ATPase$ in the cell membrane). They possess binding sites that bind substrates with low-energy bonds. Enzymes are proteins, sometimes linked with coenzymes such as vitamins or ions. They provide a low-energy pathway that facilitates a reaction so that equilibrium is reached more rapidly. Enzymes do not alter the final product, nor do they alter the position of the equilibrium. The effects of an enzyme are similar to those that might result from energy provided in another way, such as thermal energy, but avoid the obvious tissue damage that this would entail. Enzymic processes may be synthetic or destructive. Enzyme kinetics bear a strong resemblance to receptor kinetics, as outlined below.

For a synthetic reaction:

$$xA + yB \rightleftharpoons A_xB_y$$

The law of mass action indicates that the reaction rate in each direction is proportional to the product of the concentrations on each side. x and y represent numbers of substrate molecules A and B; A_xB_y is the product of the reaction. The relative concentrations at equilibrium are defined by the equilibrium constant (K_{eq}):

$$K_{eq} = \frac{A_xB_y}{[A]^x[B]^y}$$

The equilibrium constant is a feature of the reaction itself, regardless of whether or not an enzyme is present. Therefore, an additional concept is required to compare enzymatic function. This is the initial velocity of the enzyme-catalysed reaction, the velocity of the reaction when negligible substrate has reacted.

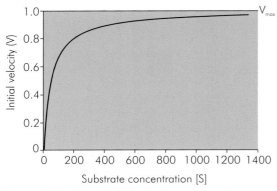

Figure PD12 Plot of initial velocity against substrate concentration

The equation for initial velocity is based on the reaction

Substrate (S) + Enzyme $\rightleftharpoons$ Product (P) − Enzyme

which may be expressed as follows:

$$V = \frac{V_{max}[S]}{K_m} = [S]$$

where

V = initial velocity

V_{max} = maximum initial velocity

K_m = concentration at which the initial velocity is half the maximum initial velocity

Note that this is identical in structure to key equation 3 describing receptor interactions, and therefore describes a rectangular hyperbola (Figure PD12).

Some caution should be exercised when alluding to the similarities. While drug and substrate concentrations are comparable terms, and V_{max} and the initial velocity of the substrate–enzyme interaction might be compared with the efficacy and response of the drug–receptor interaction, K_m is not an equilibrium constant. With this in mind, the equations and plots used in the drug–receptor interactions described above can be used to understand the inhibition of enzyme reactions and their plots. Semilogarithmic plots could be used in exactly the same way as with the receptor interactions, and similar features would be apparent, but by convention the double reciprocal (Lineweaver–Burk) plot is favoured.

Enzyme inhibition may be competitive (reversible) or non-competitive, which may be reversible or irreversible. Neostigmine provides an example of a competitive enzyme inhibitor. Ecothiopate and monoamine oxidase inhibitors are non-reversible enzyme inhibitors.

False substrates compete for the binding site and in addition have a product, so they are reversible and competitive. Methyldopa is a false substrate for the enzyme dopamine decarboxylase. Inhibition of the enzyme will be the result of more prolonged binding to the enzyme during the reaction. Although neostigmine is a competitive inhibitor of acetyl cholinesterase and is hydrolysed by plasma cholinesterase, of which it is a substrate, it is also slowly hydrolysed by the acetylcholinesterase and is therefore a false substrate for this enzyme.

CHAPTER 3
Pharmacokinetics

T. C. Smith

DRUG ADMINISTRATION
Absorption
Enteral administration
Parenteral administration

DISTRIBUTION
Blood flow to tissues
Drug uptake by tissue
Active transport
Protein binding
Placental transfer

ELIMINATION
Enterohepatic circulation
Biotransformation
Extraction ratio
Excretion

PHARMACOKINETIC MODELS
Compartment models
Volume of distribution
Elimination kinetics
Effective levels

Pharmacokinetics is the study of the movement of a drug through the compartments of the body and the transformations (activation and metabolism) that affect it. Pharmacokinetics is often referred to as 'what the body does to the drug'. Figure PK1 shows an overview of these processes.

Drug administration

Drugs are administered by many different routes. The aim of drug administration is to achieve therapeutic levels of the drug at its site (or sites) of action. In general, this is achieved using the vascular compartment as the transport mechanism for redistribution. Drug administration is, therefore, designed to produce suitable drug levels within the blood. The choice of route for a particular drug takes into account physical properties, target site of action, consideration of possible toxic effects and the practicalities of administration. The routes are summarised in Figure PK2 in a practical classification. The enteral and topical routes are most easily accessible, but require absorption across a barrier or membrane to establish their effect.

Absorption

Absorption is the process of taking the drug from the site of administration to the blood. This is necessary for all enteral and parenteral routes except for IV administration. Systemic absorption may occur from topically administered drugs, but this is not the intended route. Absorption involves the crossing of barriers between administration site and vascular compartment with subsequent movement across the physical distance between the two.

The distance within any local compartment is traversed by simple passive diffusion down the concentration gradient. Most barriers are made up of cells closely linked by tight junctions. The cell thus acts as both a filter and a device for active uptake, so the drug must pass into and then out of the cell to cross the barrier. The main principles affecting absorption include:
- Simple passive diffusion
- Facilitated diffusion
- Active uptake
- Pinocytosis

The rate of diffusion is shown by the following formula:

$$\text{Rate of diffusion} \propto \frac{CAP}{T}$$

where

C = concentration difference either side of membrane
A = area of membrane
P = membrane permeability
T = membrane thickness

The ability of a drug (or any molecule) to pass through a membrane is influenced by:
- Solubility in the membrane (lipid solubility)
- Degree of ionisation
- pH
- Size of molecule
- Carrier processes
- Pinocytosis
- Partition coefficient across the membrane

Fundamentals of Anaesthesia, 3rd edition, ed. Tim Smith, Colin Pinnock and Ted Lin. Published by Cambridge University Press. © Cambridge University Press 2008.

INPUT   Gastrointestinal tract

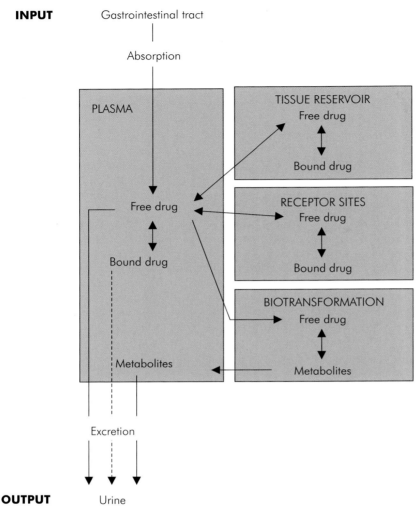

Figure PK1 Overview of pharmacokinetic processes

Enteral administration

Enteral administration encompasses any route that requires the gastrointestinal tract (GIT). Where a patient is incapacitated, access to the stomach and small intestine can still be achieved using a nasogastric tube or an endoscopically sited nasoduodenal small-bore feeding tube. Most enterally administered drugs have sites of action distant from the GIT and therefore require absorption first. This exposes them to the first-pass effect, which is elimination during passage through the liver via the hepatic portal vein. The hepatic portal vein receives blood from the GIT from oesophagus to upper rectum. Oral and nasogastric administrations imply that the drug enters the stomach, but absorption may occur throughout the length of the GIT. Buccal administration, and to a degree rectal administration, bypass the liver and so avoid the first-pass effect. Enterally administered drugs may also be subjected to other effects before absorption, including neutralisation of alkaline drugs by gastric acid and enzymatic action in the intestinal lumen or wall. The

Enteral	Oral
	Buccal
	Rectal
Parenteral	Intravenous
	Intramuscular
	Subcutaneous
	Intradermal
	Transdermal
	Inhalational
	Transtracheal
Topical	Skin
	Eyes
	Ears
	Intranasal
	Vaginal
	Urethral

Figure PK2 Routes of drug administration

advantages and disadvantages of enteral administration are as follows:

Advantages
- Easy to give
- Special equipment not required
- Patient can self-administer

Disadvantages
- May not be appropriate route
- Patient may be unable to swallow
- Drug may be destroyed in the GIT lumen
- May have excessively high first-pass effect
- Drug may be irritant to GIT
- First-pass effect and bioavailability variable
- Effective dose unpredictable

Most drugs administered enterally require absorption followed by distribution via the blood to the effector sites. It is difficult to measure effector levels of drug, but blood levels can be used as a predictor of achievement of an effective level. Absorption is therefore the mechanism for achieving an effective plasma level, and absorption and uptake are essential to this aim. For IV administration, however, this stage is bypassed. IV administration involves administration of a bolus of drug that rapidly becomes distributed throughout the whole circulating volume.

First-pass effect
Enterally administered drugs absorbed from the stomach, small intestine or colon enter the hepatic portal vein. The whole of the absorbed drug dose passes through the liver and is therefore potentially subjected to hepatic metabolism and extraction (elimination) before entering the systemic circulation. This is termed the first-pass effect.

Bioavailability
Bioavailability is the amount of drug administered by a given route that reaches the systemic circulation. IV administration therefore achieves 100% bioavailability. Bioavailability is usually taken to refer to oral administration (oral bioavailability), but other routes also have a bioavailability. Bioavailability is reduced by destruction in the lumen, poor absorption and metabolism. Oral bioavailability is greatly influenced by the first-pass effect, so that a high first-pass effect produces a low bioavailability.

Parenteral administration
By definition, parenteral administration uses routes other than the GIT. Following absorption, the drug is transported in the blood. This may be in the plasma or the red blood cells or both, and may involve protein binding. The absorption process is generally simpler than enteral absorption but still entails some degree of variability between patients, sites and drugs. The advantages and disadvantages of parenteral administration are as follows:

Advantages
- Unaffected by first-pass metabolism
- Plasma levels may be more predictable
- Does not require functioning GIT
- Does not require patient assistance

Disadvantages
- Administration requires training
- Not usually self-administered
- Administration usually requires injection
- Requires special equipment

IM injection is one of the commonest methods of parenterally administering drugs, avoiding the need to cannulate a vein and slowing the onset of the effect, which may confer a safety advantage. The absorption profile means that the drug will be absorbed slowly over a period and will last longer than the same drug administered intravenously.

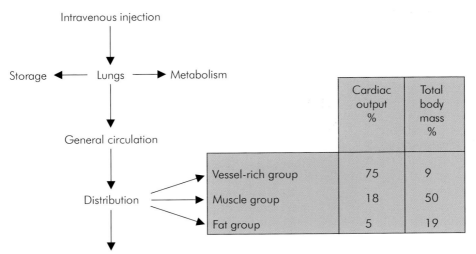

	Cardiac output %	Total body mass %
Vessel-rich group	75	9
Muscle group	18	50
Fat group	5	19

Figure PK3 Overview of drug distribution

The factors affecting absorption from an IM injection are:
- Drug solubility in blood
- Tissue binding
- Protein binding
- Blood flow to site

Transdermal

Fentanyl and glyceryl trinitrate (GTN) are examples of drugs that may be administered transdermally. The method avoids the first-pass effect, and provides a slow absorption and therefore a prolonged effect without significant peaks and troughs in plasma levels. Transiderm-nitro® 5 comprises a reservoir of 25 mg GTN with a contact surface area of 10 cm^2, which achieves an average 24-hour absorption of 5 mg. A plateau in the plasma level of glyceryl trinitrate is achieved within 2 hours of application. This plateau level is directly proportional to the surface area of the permeable membrane of the patch. It is important, therefore, that the patch makes good contact with the skin. Transiderm-nitro® 10 achieves double the transfer (10 mg per 24 hours) by doubling the contact surface area to 20 cm^2.

Inhaled

Inhaled anaesthetic agents are covered elsewhere (Section 3, Chapter 5). Their effect is dependent on achieving sufficient brain concentration of agent (which is produced from an alveolar concentration) secondary to an inhaled dose at the nose or mouth.

Inhaled bronchodilators act in a topical manner, but systemic absorption also occurs.

Distribution

Once a drug is absorbed into the circulation it undergoes distribution. An overview of mass drug movement is shown in Figure PK3.

The distribution to individual tissues depends on the solubility of the drug in those tissues and its delivery to them. The factors determining the uptake of the drug and speed of distribution to an individual tissue are:
- Plasma protein binding
- Blood flow to tissue
- Mass of tissue to which distributed
- Tissue/blood partition coefficient
- Tissue protein binding
- Facilitated transport
- Drug ionisation
- Drug molecular size

Blood flow to tissues

Blood flow determines the speed of distribution and amount of drug reaching the tissue capillaries and, therefore, the amount available for uptake into that tissue.

Three compartments are generally used to explain pharmacokinetic principles: the vessel-rich group (VRG), the muscle group (MG) and the fat group (FG). The vascularity of these tissue groups varies, and the proportion of cardiac output received by them is shown in Figure PK3.

Drug uptake by tissue

Uptake depends on the drug concentration in tissue and blood, and the partition coefficient. The blood concentration will change as it flows through the capillaries provided that tissue and blood are not at equilibrium. The drug will pass into (or out of) the tissue towards equilibrium. The commonest mode of transit is diffusion, but carrier-facilitated diffusion and active transport systems also occur. The partition coefficient indicates the ratio of drug concentration in neighbouring tissue compartments at equilibrium, and drug movement will occur towards this equilibrium point. As blood concentration falls due to redistribution and elimination, then the balance will be restored by movement out of the tissue back into the blood. The speed of transfer to and from compartments depends on the degree of deviation from the equilibrium partition coefficient and the ease of molecular movement. The mass of tissue involved will alter the rate at which equilibrium is reached and so in turn will alter the rate of uptake. For a given partition coefficient, a large volume of tissue will increase both total uptake and rate of uptake of the drug, but will reduce the speed of achievement of equilibrium.

The ease of transfer between compartments is influenced by:
- Ionisation (determined by pH and pK_a)
- Membrane components
- Molecular size

Figure PK4 shows the temporal relationship of drug distribution within various compartments following an IV bolus administration of a typical IV induction agent.

Drug distribution causes the blood concentration to fall. The VRG then has more drug than plasma, so movement is reversed and the drug moves from the tissue back into the blood. At this early stage, the blood concentration is higher than that in either the muscle group or the fat group. There is a net redistribution from VRG to MG and FG. Later the same effect will occur from MG to FG, and much later the drug in FG will return to the blood and be eliminated. All redistribution processes require the blood as an intermediary phase.

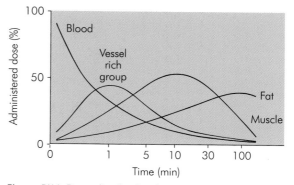

Figure PK4 Drug distribution in various tissues against time following IV bolus administration of thiopental

Active transport

Penicillin is a drug that is actively transported. This is a unidirectional process regardless of the concentration gradient. Probenecid blocks active transport in the liver, kidney and choroid plexus, which increases the proportion in the blood, and so the apparent volume of distribution is reduced.

Protein binding

Protein binding alters the concentration of free drug as a proportion of the total. Different proteins have different affinities for drugs. Albumin mostly binds acidic drugs such as aspirin, whereas α_1-glycoprotein is more important for basic drugs. The amount of drug bound is influenced by plasma pH (which alters the ionisation of the drug), age and certain disease states. Hypoalbuminaemia is a common finding in chronic disease, and in hepatic (reduced synthesis) and renal (increased loss) failure in particular. Such conditions reduce the amount of albumin available for drug binding, and therefore increase the amount of free drug. Note that α_1-glycoprotein is increased in:
- Obesity
- Trauma
- Burns
- Postoperative period
- Myocardial infarction
- Carcinoma
- Inflammatory diseases

Placental transfer

Most drugs cross the placenta to some degree. Transfer is favoured by high lipid solubility and a high un-ionised proportion. Placental blood flow and metabolism also influence transfer. The ratio of concentrations in fetal and

Induction agents	Propofol	0.65–0.85
	Thiopental	0.4–1.1
Volatile agents	Isoflurane	0.7–0.91
	Nitrous oxide	0.83
Opioids	Alfentanil	0.3
	Fentanyl	0.1–1
	Morphine	0.92
	Pethidine	1
Muscle relaxants	Suxamethonium	0.04
	Atracurium	0.05–0.2
	Vecuronium	0.11–0.12
Local anaesthetic agents	Bupivacaine	0.2–0.4
	Lidocaine	0.5–0.7
	Ropivacaine	0.2

Figure PK5 Examples of feto-maternal (F/M) concentration ratios

maternal placental blood is called the feto-maternal concentration ratio (Figure PK5).

Elimination

Elimination is the removal of active drug from the body, and it has two components, biotransformation and excretion. It may thus occur simply as excretion of the unchanged active form of the drug, or after inactivation. Many drugs require biotransformation to enable excretion. Alternatively, an irreversibly inactivated enzyme or receptor (e.g. inhibited monoamine oxidase) may need to be replaced by fresh, unaffected protein.

Enterohepatic circulation

Hepatocytes possess active transport systems that concentrate certain drugs (e.g. digoxin) and conjugates (e.g. morphine) within the bile. In the gut, the glucuronide becomes hydrolysed and active drug is reabsorbed into the hepatic portal vein. Enterohepatic circulation prolongs the half-life of a drug.

Biotransformation

There are two basic phases of biotransformation, I and II.

- Phase I reactions are simple chemical reactions such as oxidation, reduction and hydrolysis, and they tend to be destructive. Oxidation and reduction are mainly hepatic functions in which cytochrome P_{450} is particularly important. Hydrolysis is widespread and

may take place in the plasma by free enzymes such as plasma cholinesterase.

- Phase II reactions are important for the removal of substances that are not readily water-soluble. They are more complex synthetic reactions that add molecular groups (such as acetylation or glucuronide conjugation), and biotransformation often involves several of these reactions before final products are excreted.

Biotransformation predominantly occurs in the liver, but other sites in the body such as lungs, plasma and kidney are also involved.

Extraction ratio

The extraction ratio (ER) is a measure of the effectiveness with which a substance is removed or processed by an organ. Hepatic extraction is the most useful to consider, this being the proportion of drug delivered to the liver which is extracted and does not appear in the hepatic vein. Note that this is a dimensionless ratio, which may be expressed as:

$$ER = \frac{C_a - C_v}{C_a}$$

where

C_a = arterial concentration of a substance
C_v = venous concentration of a substance

The extraction of a drug depends on:

- ER
- Enzyme activity
- Drug–protein binding
- Red blood cell partitioning
- Perfusion

Clearance represents a volume of blood completely cleared of drug in unit time (see Section 2, Chapter 7, pages 331–2). For example, in the case of hepatic clearance

Hepatic clearance = $\dot{Q}_{hep} \times ER$

where

$\dot{Q}_{hep}$ = hepatic blood blow

Hepatic clearance of a drug with a high ER is highly dependent on liver blood flow because most of the delivered drug is extracted. Enzyme activity, protein binding and red cell partitioning, therefore, have less influence on hepatic extraction. Conversely, clearance of a drug with a low ER is relatively unaffected by blood flow but highly dependent on the other factors.

Excretion

Excretion involves the removal of active drug and its metabolites from the body. The main routes of excretion are in urine and bile, but the lungs, faeces and sweat represent other routes. Excretion of a substance relies on it being soluble in the solvent being excreted (usually water). Biotransformation to a water-soluble form is therefore essential for the excretion of highly lipid-soluble drugs. Excretion via the lungs primarily applies to inhaled volatile anaesthetic agents. However, substances administered by other routes, such as ethanol, are also eliminated partially in expired gases.

Molecules presented to the glomerulus in the renal plasma will cross the basement membrane into the renal tubules, but there is a 'cutoff' at a molecular weight of about 69 000 daltons, dependent on shape and charge. In effect, this applies mainly to water-soluble compounds, because highly lipid-soluble substances will only be present free in the plasma in very low concentrations. Similarly, protein binding will reduce the amount of free drug available to cross the glomerulus. If the drug in the filtrate is not reabsorbed as much as the water in the kidney tubule then the concentration of the drug will increase by the time it reaches the renal pelvis. However, it is the amount of drug excreted that is important in elimination and not the concentration, although the two are interdependent. Tubular reabsorption occurs to a limited extent, and this is affected by ionic charge, which is in turn altered by pH. A high filtration rate will facilitate elimination, so good renal blood flow is desirable, but the absolute volume of urine produced is less important.

Active transport systems exist for some drugs (such as penicillin), which are actively secreted into the tubules. Probenecid may be used to block this penicillin transport and thus prolong the half-life of the drug.

Pharmacokinetic models

Measurement of drug levels in blood and other fluids is relatively easy when compared with the measurement of tissue drug levels. Models are created to help to describe, understand and predict the pharmacokinetic behaviour of drugs, and mathematical relationships are used to describe these interrelationships.

Compartment models

Compartment models are based on the body behaving as if it is divided into a number of hypothetical inter-linked spaces or compartments. Each compartment has specific properties of volume and transfer rates for a particular drug. One-, two- and three-compartment models are routinely used, but note that these compartments do not correspond precisely to anatomical structures. Consistent solubilities are assumed throughout, so the volumes are calculated based on partition coefficients $= 1$. The models are used mathematically to describe the changes in plasma concentration with time, and so predict and compare pharmacokinetic profiles. Figures PK6–PK8 illustrate one-, two- and three-compartment models.

One-compartment model

The simplest model is a one-compartment model. In this, all tissues are represented as a composite, single compartment (1). A drug of dose D is administered to the compartment and is considered evenly distributed throughout. The plasma concentration (C) of the drug is measured to calculate the volume (V) of this hypothetical compartment, the plasma being the 'window' through which the compartment can be 'viewed'. By definition:

$$C = \frac{D}{V}$$

The elimination rate constant (k_{el}) defines the overall rate of removal of drug from this single compartment, and is a combination of all the modes of elimination for that drug.

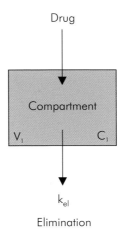

Figure PK6 A one-compartment model

Two-compartment model

The one-compartment model is too simple to describe accurately the behaviour of most drugs, and the single compartment is therefore divided into central (1) and peripheral (2) compartments. Again the plasma is the 'window' to the compartments and is not necessarily equivalent to the central compartment. The central compartment is the intermediary compartment through which the peripheral compartment is accessed. Many drugs, including thiopental, show a good approximation to this model.

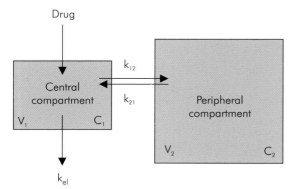

Figure PK7 A two-compartment model

Three-compartment model

Some drugs, such as propofol, require further compartments to be added to allow accurate pharmacokinetic predictions. In this model, a third, deep peripheral compartment is added, and this communicates with the central compartment, but at a much slower rate.

Any model is an approximation, but by increasing the number of compartments, the correlation with the real situation can be improved. However, the size of the improvements diminishes as the number of compartments increases.

Water analogue model

Mapleson described a model for the pharmacokinetic behaviour of inhaled anaesthetic agents using a series of interconnected cylinders of water (Figure PK9). In this model, the height of the water determines the pressure and is analogous to the agent partial pressure. The cross-sectional area of each cylinder is analogous to the solubility of the agent in that tissue, and the amount of agent in the tissue is represented by the volume of water in the cylinder. The resistance of the connecting pipes represents the transfer characteristics, a small-bore (high-resistance) tube representing a slow transfer. The model will proceed towards the equilibrium state in which all the cylinders will have an equal volume of water.

Volume of distribution

Volume of distribution may be explained using the models above. These model compartments are defined as having a consistent concentration throughout. Therefore, if the amount of drug in the compartment is known, measuring the concentration of the drug will enable calculation of the apparent volume through which the drug is distributed. The model works on the basis that the drug is equally distributed throughout that calculated volume.

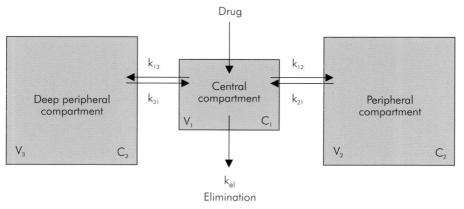

Figure PK8 A three-compartment model

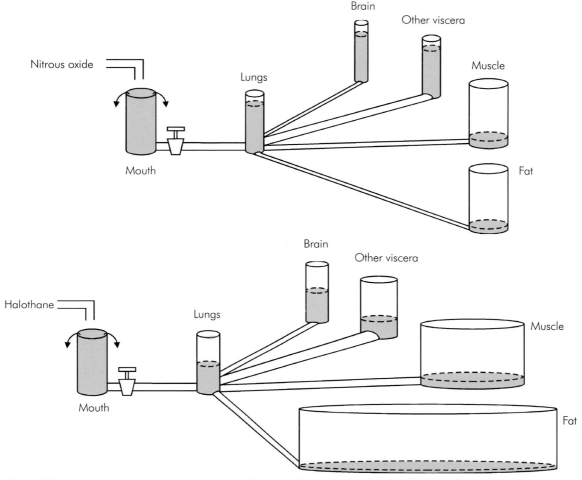

Figure PK9 Mapleson's water analogue models. The levels illustrate the situation in the early part of maintenance

Reproduced with permission from Mapleson WW. Pharmacokinetics of inhaled anaesthetics. In: Prys-Roberts C, Hug CC Jr (eds) *Pharmacokinetics of Anaesthesia*. Oxford: Blackwell, 1984, pp 89–111.

Usually, the drug dose given is known and the plasma concentration that would exist if distribution occurred without elimination can be calculated. The apparent volume of distribution does not exist as an identifiable anatomical entity but rather is a mathematical concept representing the composite result of multiple volumes with differing solubilities for a given drug.

The apparent volume of distribution is thus used as a tool to describe the way in which drugs are distributed. Drugs that are mainly confined to plasma have low volumes of distribution, while drugs that are highly tissue-bound have a high volume of distribution. The volume of distribution may easily exceed the total volume of the body. High tissue binding results in a low plasma concentration. This low concentration spread evenly throughout the calculated volume for a given dose results in a very large value for volume of distribution.

Elimination kinetics
Zero- and first-order kinetics are used to describe the elimination characteristics of a drug. Most drugs are eliminated with first-order kinetics.

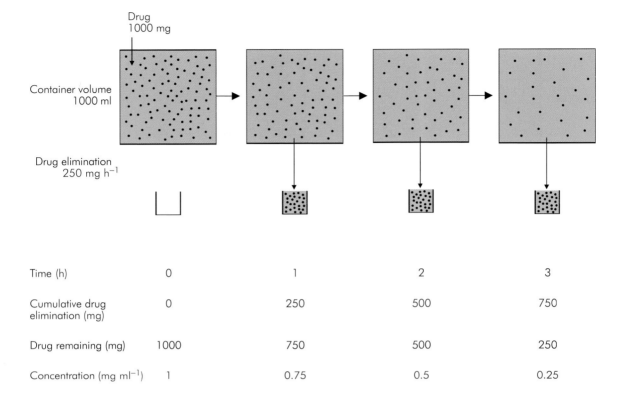

Time (h)	0	1	2	3
Cumulative drug elimination (mg)	0	250	500	750
Drug remaining (mg)	1000	750	500	250
Concentration (mg ml^{-1})	1	0.75	0.5	0.25

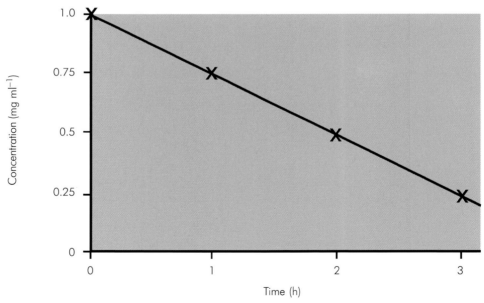

Figure PK10 Effect of zero-order elimination on drug concentration

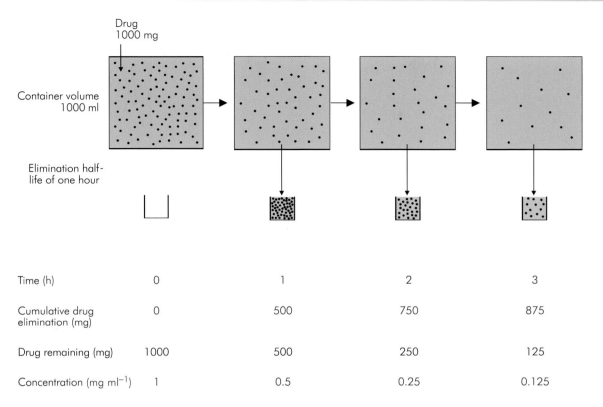

Time (h)	0	1	2	3
Cumulative drug elimination (mg)	0	500	750	875
Drug remaining (mg)	1000	500	250	125
Concentration (mg ml^{-1})	1	0.5	0.25	0.125

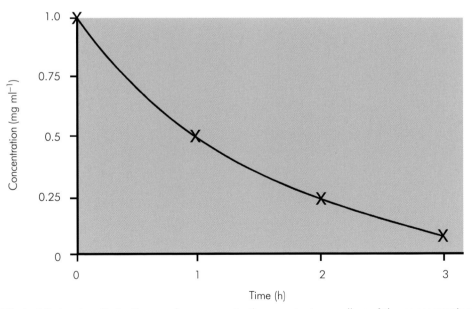

Figure PK11 Effect of first-order elimination on drug concentration constant regardless of the concentration

Zero-order kinetics

In zero-order kinetics the elimination system is saturated at clinical levels, and elimination is therefore constant and unrelated to drug concentration. A fixed mass of drug is eliminated in unit time irrespective of the blood concentration, and the concentration therefore declines at a constant rate. This is demonstrated in Figure PK10, in which a constant amount of drug is removed in each time interval resulting in a similar linear decline in drug concentration.

Ethanol provides an example of zero-order elimination, and high levels of phenytoin, thiopental and salicylates also show zero-order features. As the concentration falls so the elimination pathways may no longer be saturated, and first-order kinetics takes over. Phenytoin exhibits first-order kinetics at low levels and zero-order at higher levels. Kinetics may also be affected by saturation of other components such as protein binding, carrier-mediated active transport mechanisms and enzyme systems.

First-order kinetics

In the first-order model, the rate of drug elimination is proportional to the plasma drug concentration such that:

Elimination $= dC/dt \propto C$

where

dC = a small change in concentration
dt = a small change in time
C = concentration

The elimination pathways are not saturated, but are gradually recruited as the concentration of drug increases, and vice versa. The rate of change of drug concentration is therefore also proportional to the drug concentration. The change in concentration is a lowering of concentration and so the formula has a minus sign. Thus, for first-order kinetics:

$$\frac{dC}{dt} = -kC$$

This can be calculated from the following derived formula, called **key equation 1**:

$C = C_0\, e^{-k_{el}t}$

where:

k_{el} = elimination rate constant
C_0 = concentration (C) at time (t) $= 0$

Figure PK11 demonstrates this process, in which a constant volume is cleared of drug in each time interval, resulting in an ever-declining rate of fall in drug and drug concentration. Although the drug concentration decreases with time, it approaches but never actually reaches zero drug concentration. The rate of that decrease (the gradient of the slope) also falls with time. This is an exponential decay.

Half-lives and time constants

An important feature of the exponential function shown in first-order kinetics is the time taken for the concentration to halve (Figure PK12). This is the half-life ($t_{1/2}$). Half-lives are hybrid constants that are dependent on primary constants. The time constant, another such feature, is based on the rate of change of concentration (the gradient of the plot). The time constant is the time that it would take for the drug concentration to reach zero if elimination continued at the rate of the chosen starting point. Time constants (τ) also apply to exponential functions of the form $y = 1 - e^{-x}$. Figure PK13 shows the proportion of the initial concentration that exists after a given number of time constants. The initial concentration in this sense may be any point on the plot from which timing is started. As the time constant and half-life are constants for a given exponential function, they must have a constant relationship, which is described by the formula:

$$t_{1/2} = \tau \log_e 2 \quad \text{and} \quad \tau = \frac{1}{k_{el}}$$

Derivation of key equation 2

Using key equation 1, an expression relating the half-life and the elimination rate constant can be derived.

Key equation 1

$C = C_0\, e^{-k_{el}t}$

By definition, at one half-life from time zero the concentration will be half that of the concentration at time zero (time zero can be chosen arbitrarily for this calculation).

$\frac{1}{2}\, C_0 = C_0\, e^{-k_{el}\,t_{1/2}}$

$\Downarrow$ Divide both sides by the common factor (C_0)

$\frac{1}{2} = e^{-k_{el}\,t_{1/2}}$

$\Downarrow$ Take natural logarithm of both sides

$\log_e \frac{1}{2} = -k_{el}\,t_{1/2}$

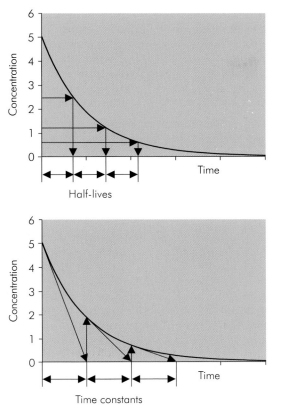

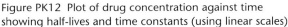

Figure PK12 Plot of drug concentration against time showing half-lives and time constants (using linear scales)

Number of time constants	Proportion of starting concentration remaining
N	e^{-N} (%)
0	100
1	37
2	13.5
3	5.0
4	1.8

Figure PK13 Time constants and the concentration remaining

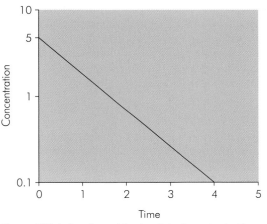

Figure PK14 Semilogarithmic plot of concentration against time

⇓ Rearrange

$$t_{1/2} = -\frac{\log_e {}^1\!/_2}{k_{el}}$$

as $-\log_e {}^1\!/_2$ equals $\log_e 2$, substitute to create key equation 2.

Key equation 2

$$t_{1/2} = \frac{\log_e 2}{k_{el}} = \frac{0.693}{k_{el}}$$

The natural logarithm 'log$_e$' may also be written 'ln'. The concentration and rate of decline of concentration in Figure PK12 fall exponentially with time. Mathematically and graphically, it is easier to work with linear relationships. Using a logarithmic scale for the concentration (or the natural logarithm of the concentration) against time on the original linear scale (Figure PK12) produces a straight line (Figure PK14).

The straight line can now be extrapolated to the y-axis (t = 0) to obtain a theoretical (or apparent) value for concentration at the time of injection (C_0). This is the predicted concentration if there was instantaneous uniform distribution of the drug of dose D throughout the compartment at the time of injection, before any elimination has occurred. This single-compartment model can then be used to calculate the volume of distribution (V_d) as follows:

$$C_0 = \frac{D}{V_d}$$

In practice, this simple exponential decline is masked in the clinical situation by the combined affects of absorption, distribution, redistribution and elimination. Most clinical data sets of plasma (or blood) levels of an intravenously injected drug have a pattern similar to Figure PK15.

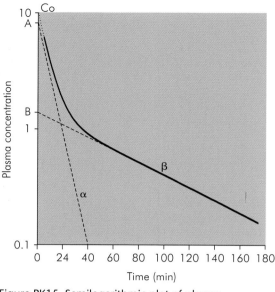

Figure PK15 Semilogarithmic plot of plasma concentration against time

This two-compartment model can be seen to have two linear (graphical) components, which can be separated. The initial rapid decline is the result of rapid redistribution throughout the central compartment being predominant. Later, redistribution to the peripheral compartments is predominant. Clearance is constant throughout, but elimination is proportional to concentration and is greatest earlier in the process. Each component has a half-life and volume of distribution. Elimination half-life ($t_{1/2\beta}$) is the usual value quoted. To calculate elimination half-life using the graph, the following steps may be followed.

Step 1
Extrapolate the straight line of the distribution phase to the y-axis (t = 0). Call this 'C_0' as before.

Step 2
The elimination phase has a slope of β. Extrapolate the straight line of the elimination phase to the y-axis (t = 0). Call this 'B'. This is the initial concentration that would have existed if there was instantaneous distribution to equilibrium on IV injection. This can be used to calculate a value for the volume of distribution following equilibration with the tissues. This is also an approximation of the volume of distribution at steady state (V_{dSS}). However, this is calculated and defined as the volume of distribution when

giving an infusion of a drug at exactly the same rate as total clearance of the drug.

Step 3
Subtract B from C_0 to create concentration A.

Step 4
Subtract the β slope from the concentration plot to create a new straight line of slope α (the distribution element of the graph). Although it may seem unusual that a curve appears as the result of the addition of two straight lines in part of the graph, this is because of the logarithmic scale used for concentration. Observation of this scale shows that it does not reach zero at the x-axis.

Step 5
Use these values mathematically to calculate the following variables:

$$\alpha = \log_e 2/t_{1/2\alpha}$$
$$\beta = \log_e 2/t_{1/2\beta}$$
$$V_{dI} = \text{dose}/C_0$$

Area under the curve (AUC) $= A/\alpha + B/\beta$

Clearance
Clearance (Cl) represents the volume of blood completely cleared of drug in unit time. The amount of drug eliminated is therefore dependent upon the drug concentration, which is a first-order process. Typical units for clearance are 'ml of blood per kg body weight per minute' (ml kg^{-1} min^{-1}). Total clearance is the sum of all the individual clearances, such as hepatic (Cl_H), renal (Cl_R) and others (Cl_X). Clearance can be calculated from a graph using AUC:

$$Cl = \text{dose}/AUC = \frac{\text{dose}}{A/\alpha + B/\beta}$$

In other words, clearance = volume of compartment × elimination rate constant.

Referring back to the two-compartment model, the volume of distribution at steady state (V_{dSS}) is the usual volume quoted, as follows:

$$V_{dSS} = V_{dI}(1 + k_{12}/k_{21})$$

where

k_{12}, k_{21} = intercompartment rate constants
V_{dI} = initial volume of distribution

Compartment	$t_{1/2}$ (min)
Central (1)	2–3
Peripheral (2)	30–60
Deep peripheral (3)	180–480
V_{dl} 230 ml kg^{-1}	
V_{dss} 12 l kg^{-1}	

Figure PK16 Pharmacokinetic values for propofol

As the plasma concentration is determined by the addition of the α and β profiles, $C_p = Ae^{-\alpha t} + Be^{-\beta t}$. Note that at $t = 0$, $e^0 = 1$, so $C_0 = A + B$.

This is a 'best fit', and most drugs fit the two-compartment model. However, it should be remembered that this apparent mathematical model is derived from numerous distribution profiles and a range of tissue profiles. Some drugs, such as propofol, best approximate to a three-compartment model, that is a tri-exponential model. Values pertaining to this are shown in Figure PK16.

Effective levels

Effective levels of volatile agents can be monitored by measurement of the end-tidal concentration. Blood levels of IV agents are not readily monitored, but desired concentrations can be targeted using pharmacokinetic models based on patient demographic data, and compared with plasma equivalents of MAC, which are:
- MIR – minimum infusion rate that prevents response to surgical stimulus in 50% of patients
- ED_{50} – a general term to describe the dose that is effective in 50% of subjects
- EBC – effective blood concentration (sometimes called EC)

The strategy of a target concentration is one method of delivering the anaesthetic dose. A target concentration is chosen in a similar way to volatile agent concentration, and a computer-controlled pump calculates bolus and maintenance infusion rate based on patient details. The target concentration is altered according to clinical need and the pump adjusts accordingly. The concept of an effective blood concentration of the agent depends on the following conditions:
- Intensity of drug action (predictable from concentration at the receptor site)
- Concentration at the receptor site proportional to free plasma concentration

In total intravenous anaesthesia (TIVA) using propofol, the aim is to rapidly achieve a blood level of propofol that will induce anaesthesia, and then maintain this state until the procedure is complete. Discontinuing the infusion will then lead to a rapid recovery of consciousness as blood (and brain) concentrations of propofol fall. A constant infusion achieves a plateau level, but this is slow. A loading dose is therefore used, based on the volume of distribution (V_d) and the desired concentration (C_p) in the following way:

$$Loading\ dose = V_d \times C_p$$

This may be followed by a maintenance dose calculated from the total clearance and the desired plasma concentration (this being equal to the amount of drug being eliminated in unit time) in the following manner:

$$Maintenance\ dose = Cl \times C_p$$

Another method of maintaining a therapeutic level over a prolonged period is to administer intermittent doses so that the bolus is given before the plasma level falling below the therapeutic threshold. For maximum interval, the dose used should raise the plasma level to the top of the therapeutic range without reaching toxic levels. Repetitive dosing results in a plateau once elimination (determined by concentration) equals elimination. The dosing interval is usually approximately that of the terminal elimination half-life.

The various half-lives that are given for the decline in concentration of a given drug apply to specific circumstances. An initial redistribution component ($t_{1/2\alpha}$) and a slower terminal half-life ($t_{1/2\beta}$) describing what happens over a longer period of time, mainly due to elimination, are quoted for two-compartment models. In addition, if a drug is infused over a period of time, eventually a steady state occurs in which all tissues are in equilibrium, the plasma concentration is constant and elimination equals infusion rate. Stopping the infusion gives a decline with the longest possible half-life for that drug. However, usually infusions run for much shorter periods of time and so a steady state has yet to be reached. The half-life in this context (the context-sensitive half-life) is less than the half-life at steady state. The shorter the duration of the infusion the closer the half-life becomes to the redistribution half-life. Drugs with a low lipid solubility (such as alfentanil) are less affected by this than those with a high lipid solubility (such as fentanyl).

CHAPTER 4

Mechanisms of drug action

S. A. Hill

PHYSICOCHEMICAL MECHANISMS
Charge neutralisation
Osmotic effects
Adsorption
Chelation and inclusion complexes
Radio-opacity

PHARMACODYNAMIC MECHANISMS
Drug–cell membrane receptor
Intracellular receptors

PHARMACOKINETIC ACTIONS
Drug interactions with enzymes
Drug interaction with transport proteins

MECHANISMS OF GENERAL ANAESTHETIC ACTION
Anatomical sites of action
Molecular theories
Membrane lipids
Protein site(s) of action

ADVERSE EFFECTS
Physicochemical effects
Pharmacodynamic effects
Pharmacokinetic effects
Idiopathic adverse effects
Hypersensitivity reactions
Pharmacogenetic influences

MECHANISMS OF DRUG INTERACTIONS
Physicochemical
Pharmacokinetic
Pharmacodynamic

Drugs exert their observed effects in a multitude of different ways. They may be physicochemical, pharmacodynamic or pharmacokinetic interactions with biochemical and physiological systems of the body.

The main, intended action of a drug may not be the only effect that substance has on the body, and there may be multiple modes of action. For example, many drugs interact with more than one type of receptor and some may alter the pharmacokinetics of co-administered drugs by enzyme induction or inhibition.

Physicochemical mechanisms

These mechanisms are generally non-specific, and depend on the physicochemical properties of a drug including its molecular size and shape, the degree of ionisation and pK_a of its constituent groups and the lipid and water solubility of the drug.

Non-specific physicochemical mechanisms of action include:
- Charge neutralisation (pH effects)
- Osmotic effects
- Adsorption
- Chelation

Charge neutralisation

This mode of action is typified by the action of the antacid drugs. Sodium citrate is the salt of a weak acid, and combination in the stomach with hydrochloric acid, a strong acid, produces sodium chloride and citric acid, a weaker acid, thus reducing intragastric pH. Calcium bicarbonate is also an effective antacid, but the reaction produces carbon dioxide, which can cause abdominal distension and flatulence. To avoid this problem sodium citrate is preferred preoperatively to reduce the risk of aspiration-induced lung damage in high-risk patients requiring general anaesthesia. Sodium citrate should not be used long-term because of the high sodium load; antacid drugs for prolonged use ideally should not be absorbed. Aluminium hydroxide preparations are relatively insoluble and longer-lasting, so come closest to ideal, although care should be taken in renal failure. Another example of charge neutralisation is the use of protamine in reversing the effects of heparin

Fundamentals of Anaesthesia, 3rd edition, ed. Tim Smith, Colin Pinnock and Ted Lin. Published by Cambridge University Press. © Cambridge University Press 2008.

(see Section 3, Chapter 17, page 701). Protamine is a fish spermatozoal protein that is strongly basic due to a high arginine content, hence a high density of positive charge; heparin carries negative charge. The combination of protamine and heparin produces a complex that has no anticoagulant effect.

Osmotic effects

Mannitol is an alcohol derivative of the sugar mannose. It is not metabolised, but exerts an osmotic effect in the plasma, like glucose, which leads to expansion of the extracellular volume, reduction of blood viscosity and a diuretic effect. It is freely filtered and minimally reabsorbed. Care needs to be taken with the dose of mannitol used in order to avoid impaired tubular function as the result of a high plasma osmolality.

Adsorption

Non-specific adsorption of many drugs to activated charcoal allows the latter to be used in the treatment of drug overdose by effectively removing free drug from the stomach. Charcoal is not effective in lithium, cyanide, iron, ethanol, or methanol poisoning.

Chelation and inclusion complexes

Heavy metal ions such as lead, arsenic and copper can effectively be removed by a mechanism that involves one or more chelating agents. These agents have multiple oxygen, sulphur or nitrogen atoms that form coordinate bonds (where the ligand contributes both electrons) with the metal ion. An ideal chelating agent will be water-soluble, not undergo biotransformation, have a low affinity for calcium and form non-toxic metal complexes that can readily be excreted. Edetate calcium disodium (Ca^{2+} Na_2^+ EDTA) and penicillamine are both used in lead poisoning; penicillamine is also of use in copper and mercury poisoning.

Alpha, beta and gamma cyclodextrins are naturally occurring bucket-shaped oligosaccharides produced from starch; α-cyclodextrins have six β- and eight γ-sugar residues. They present a hydrophilic outer surface and an internal hydrophobic cavity that can trap other molecules by forming an inclusion complex. Modified cyclodextrins are used extensively for masking odours as well as for drug delivery systems, particularly for poorly water-soluble drugs. A novel γ-cyclodextrin reversal agent has been developed that selectively forms an inclusion complex with rocuronium, but less effectively with other non-depolarising muscle relaxants. This drug therefore produces an effective reversal of non-depolarising neuromuscular blockade without the unwanted effects of widespread inhibition of acetylcholinesterase.

Radio-opacity

Contrast media rely on the property of absorption of x rays for their function. Ideal contrast media are otherwise inert but may be selected to possess other properties to ensure that they are concentrated in specific areas such as the urinary system.

Pharmacodynamic mechanisms

Many drugs exert their effects due to an interaction with specific and selective sites on receptors. Receptors are large proteins that are associated with cellular structures such as cell membranes, cytoplasm, intracellular membranes or nuclear material. The selectivity arises from the 3D chemical configuration of the drug, which matches a site on the relevant protein and allows binding to take place. The observed effect then results directly or indirectly from this interaction. This type of action is characterised by a lock-and-key mechanism involving different chemical forces that allow the drug first to approach its active site and then to fit into a selective binding area. Initial attraction may be by ionic forces, but stabilisation is due to van der Waals interactions once the drug is in close proximity to its selective binding site.

Interaction mechanisms include:
- Drug–cell membrane receptor
- Drug–voltage-gated ion channel
- Drug–intracellular membrane receptor
- Drug–cytosolic receptor mechanisms

Drug–cell membrane receptor

Many of the drugs we use in our anaesthetic practice act by interfering with the binding of natural neurotransmitters to their receptor sites on cell membranes. The most important are ligand-gated ion channels and G-protein-coupled receptors. Other membrane-dependent transduction mechanisms, such as the tyrosine kinase receptors activated by insulin, may also be important.

Ligand-gated ion channels

It is important to distinguish ion channels that are opened as a result of changes in membrane potential in the vicinity of an ion channel from those that are associated with the binding of neurotransmitters. Ligand-gated ion channels are generally found at synapses, associated with both

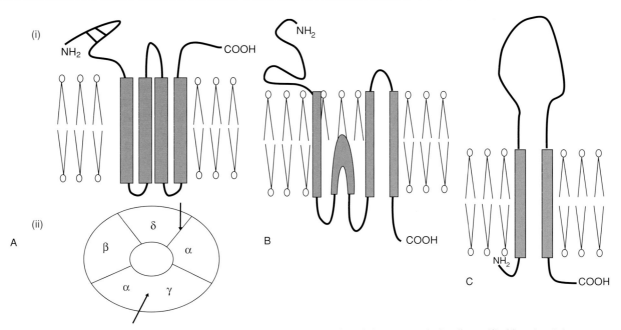

Figure MD1 Schematic illustration of the ionotropic receptor families. (A) Pentameric family typified by nicotinic acetylcholine receptor at the neuromuscular junction; (i) subunit configuration – note four transmembrane domains and two cysteine bridges near the NH$_2$ terminus; (ii) arrangement of subunits as seen from above – arrows show the two acetylcholine binding sites. (B) Ionotropic glutamate family typified by NMDA receptor with three transmembrane domains and one re-entrant loop. (C) Purinergic ionotropic P2X receptors with two transmembrane domains and a large extracellular loop.

pre- and postsynaptic membranes. Although some voltage-gated ion channels are present presynaptically, they are most commonly found in the nerve axon or the non-synaptic regions of membranes of both smooth and skeletal muscle.

Local anaesthetics such as lidocaine and bupivacaine act by blocking voltage-gated sodium channels. They are usually administered in close proximity to peripheral neurones; activity requires access to the cytosolic side of the axon so lipid solubility is important, although the ionised form is active. Some anticonvulsants, such as lamotrigine and carbamazepine, act by blockade of central sodium channels, so reducing neuronal excitability. Voltage-gated calcium-channel blockers such as nifedipine and verapamil act by blocking L-type calcium channels: antihypertensive and antianginal effects are associated with action on vascular smooth muscle, whereas myocardial effects produce their antiarrhythmic action. Central T-type calcium channels are blocked by the anticonvulsant ethosuxamide.

Many of the drugs we use interfere with neurotransmitter-gated ion channels that mediate very

rapid transmission of information through the central and peripheral nervous systems. Activation of ligand-gated channels either depolarises the postsynaptic membrane, allowing forward transmission of electrical signals, or hyperpolarises the membrane, inhibiting such signals. There are three distinct families of ligand-gated receptors, which can be distinguished by their subunit structure: **pentameric**, **ionotropic glutamate** and **ionotropic purinergic** receptors (Figure MD1).

Cys-loop pentameric receptors
Examples – the nicotinic acetylcholine receptor (nAChR), the γ-aminobutyric acid type A receptor (GABA$_A$), inhibitory glycine receptors (GlyR) and the 5-hydroxytryptamine (serotonin) type 3 receptor (5-HT$_3$).

Each subunit of this pentameric family has four helical transmembrane domains (TMDs) – a domain is a part of a protein chain that plays an important role in the function of that protein, often with a specific 3D folded shape – none of which is re-entrant (a term used when a protein chain traverses the membrane and loops back on itself without exiting the opposite side of the membrane). The name *cys-loop* comes from the fact that near the N-terminal extracellularly there are two disulphide cysteine bridges, which force the N-terminal into a looped structure.

The pentameric family provides the most important sites of drug action for neuromuscular blocking agents (nAChR) and, as has been recognised more recently, for many of our general anaesthetic agents (GABA$_A$); the action of general anaesthetic agents is discussed in greater detail below. Subunit composition can vary for the nicotinic acetylcholine receptor. At the neuromuscular junction the composition is $\alpha\epsilon\alpha\beta\delta$, but in the fetus it is $\alpha\gamma\alpha\beta\delta$; acetylcholine binds to the α–ϵ and α–δ subunit interfaces. Cooperative binding of two molecules of acetylcholine is required to produce the required conformational change and open the channel, which is then five times more selective for monovalent cations – Na$^+$ in particular – than for divalent cations such as Ca^{2+}. Depolarising blockers, such as suxamethonium, bind to the same site as the natural transmitter acetylcholine and cause opening of the ion channel by inducing conformational changes similar to those induced by acetylcholine, although channel opening time is increased. However, suxamethonium is not rapidly hydrolysed, as it dissociates from the receptor because it is not a substrate for acetylcholinesterase. As a result the receptor cannot return to the resting conformation, but becomes desensitised and no longer able to respond to agonist. This then produces the observed neuromuscular blockade. Acetylcholine alone can also produce blockade, as is seen when acetylcholinesterase is irreversibly inhibited by organophosphates. In contrast, the non-depolarising muscle relaxants compete for the same binding site as acetylcholine but the conformational change they induce prevents channel opening. Temporarily increasing the concentration of acetylcholine in the synaptic cleft by inhibition of acetylcholinesterase will overcome this blockade.

Nicotinic receptors are found at sites other than the neuromuscular junction (NMJ), in particular at autonomic ganglia and in the central nervous system (CNS). In the CNS the subunit composition is very different from that at the NMJ, $2\alpha3\beta$ or 5β subunits, which accounts for the differing sensitivity of these receptors to cholinergic drugs. In addition, calcium permeability is much greater in CNS nicotinic receptors. As discussed below, these neuronal nicotinic receptors are sensitive to the effects of certain general anaesthetic agents.

The GABA$_A$ and glycine receptors are the major inhibitory signal transducers in the CNS, glycine predominately in spinal cord and hindbrain, GABA supraspinally.

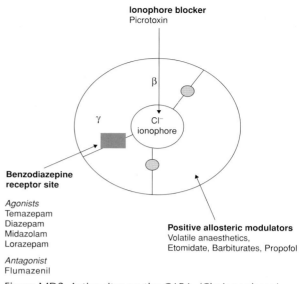

Ionophore blocker
Picrotoxin

Benzodiazepine receptor site

Agonists
Temazepam
Diazepam
Midazolam
Lorazepam

Antagonist
Flumazenil

Positive allosteric modulators
Volatile anaesthetics,
Etomidate, Barbiturates, Propofol

Figure MD2 Active sites on the GABA$_A$/Cl$^-$ ionophore/ benzodiazepine receptor complex, looking from above. The grey circles show the two agonist sites for GABA, which are competitively inhibited by gabazine and bicuculline.

The GABA$_A$ channel, unlike the nACh channel, is an anionic channel favouring chloride passage through the synaptic membrane, resulting in hyperpolarisation and inhibition of forward signalling. Subunit stoichiometry depends on anatomical location but $1\alpha{:}2\beta{:}2\gamma$ and $2\alpha{:}2\beta{:}1\gamma$ are commonly found. The benzodiazepine receptor site is associated with the GABA$_A$ receptor, and is responsible for sedative and anticonvulsant effects due to positive allosteric modulation of the hyperpolarising signal associated with GABA transmission. The benzodiazepine binding site requires both α and γ subunits to be present for positive allosteric modulation whereas etomidate binds with higher affinity to receptors with a β_2 or β_3 subunit. Important sites for drug binding on the GABA$_A$ receptor complex are shown in Figure MD2.

Ondansetron inhibits 5-hydroxytryptamine type 3 (5-HT$_3$) ionotropic channels. Like nACh channels, 5-HT$_3$ receptors are cation channels favouring monovalent over divalent cations. There are several types of serotoninergic receptors, but only subtype 3 are ionotropic; the others are all G-protein-coupled receptors. The centrally mediated anti-emetic action is associated with vagolytic effects, as these receptors are also found on vagal afferents from the gastrointestinal tract (GIT). Ondansetron therefore has both central and peripheral effects.

Ionotropic glutamate receptors

There are three ionotropic glutamate receptor types, NMDA, AMPA and kainite. Other glutamate receptors are metabotropic G-protein-coupled receptors. NMDA receptors require co-activation by glycine and glutamate. They are comprised of two subunits, one pore-forming (NR1) and one regulatory, which binds glycine (NR2 A–D types). In vivo it is thought that the receptors dimerise, forming a complex with four subunits. Each NR1 subunit has three membrane-spanning helices, two of which are separated by a re-entrant pore-forming loop that enters and exits the membrane at its cytoplasmic surface. The C-terminus is cytoplasmic, the N-terminus extracellular. All glutamate receptors are equally permeable to Na^+ and K^+ but have a particularly high permeability to the divalent cation, Ca^{2+}, unlike the pentameric excitatory channels discussed above. NMDA receptors are of great interest to anaesthetists because they are the site of action of ketamine, nitrous oxide and xenon, all of which are non-competitive inhibitors of glutamate. There is a high density of NMDA receptors in the hippocampus and associated regions, all of which are important in the formation and recall of memories. Some evidence points to the novel anticonvulsant topiramate acting by inhibiting kainate receptors, although it can also reduce sodium channel conductance.

Ionotropic purinergic receptors: P2X subtypes

This family of receptors has two TMDs and no pore-forming loops. They form cation channels that are equally permeable to Na^+ and K^+ but also to Ca^{2+}. These receptors are readily inactivated at higher membrane potentials, somewhat like voltage-gated Na^+ channels in nerve membranes. They are activated by ATP and its metabolites and are widely distributed in both central and peripheral neurones. The analgesic property of pentobarbital is thought to be due to inhibition of P2X receptors in the dorsal root ganglia. These ionotropic purinergic receptors are not to be confused with G-protein-coupled receptor forms of purinergic receptors: all P1 (adenosine receptors) and P2Y subtypes.

G-protein-coupled receptors (GPCRs)

Almost 1000 genes for GPCRs have been identified; many have yet to be characterised. Each GPCR has seven helical TMDs that span the cell membrane, starting with the extracellular N-terminus and ending with the intracellular C-terminus. The quaternary structure is such that these helices cluster together, held in the correct alignment by interactions with extracellular/intracellular domains. When a ligand binds, these helices are thought to twist in relation to each other, so inducing a large conformational change that is transmitted to the cytoplasmic elements associated with G-protein coupling. The third transmembrane domain is specific for a given GPCR and does not show a high level of sequence homology between receptor families, unlike the other TMDs. This correlates with the ligand binding site, being associated with the second and third extracellular loops. The second and third intracellular loops are associated with G-protein binding. Seven distinct families of GPCRs have been identified; they differ particularly in terms of the relative proximity of the ligand binding site to the helical domains within the membrane. Compared with other GPCRs, metabotropic glutamate receptors have an extremely large extracellular component.

All adrenoceptors, muscarinic, cholinergic and opioid receptors work through a GPCR mechanism. G proteins are associated with the inner leaflet of the cell membrane and are not normally closely associated with receptors. On binding of the ligand, a conformational change increases the likelihood of the receptor becoming associated with its particular subtype of G protein. The kinetics of GPCR–G-protein interactions requires complex models to explain observed responses. Essentially the receptor can exist in a number of states, which differ in their affinity for agonist, antagonist or inverse agonist; each of these may or may not be associated with G-protein coupling. Response is greatest when a full agonist is bound to the appropriate G protein. Once the GPCR–G-protein association takes place, there is a conformational change in the G-protein α subunit that allows dissociation of bound GDP in exchange for GTP. This in turn allows dissociation of the α subunit from the $\beta\gamma$ dimer. The GTP-bound α subunit now has sufficient energy to interact with intracellular enzymes or cell-membrane-bound ion channels and either activate or inhibit these secondary mechanisms. The GTP-ase activity of the α subunit limits the duration of this activity and, once GTP is hydrolysed to GDP, further interaction is energetically unfavourable and the α subunit then re-associates with the $\beta\gamma$ dimer, which has dissociated from the GPCR. In some situations the $\beta\gamma$ dimer can also act as an activator of secondary mechanisms.

There are many different types of G protein, with subfamilies classified according to their α-subunit activity. There are Gs, Gi, Gq and G_{12} subfamilies: Gs and Gi

Natural ligand/receptor type	G-protein α-subunit type	Agonist/antagonist drugs
Acetylcholine M_1, M_3 and M_5	Gq	Atropine, glycopyrrolate are antagonists
Acetylcholine M_2 and M_4	Gi	Atropine, ipratropium, glycopyrrolate antagonists
Noradrenaline α_1	Gq	Phenylephrine agonist; phentolamine antagonist
Noradrenaline α_2	Gi	Clonidine agonist; yohimbine antagonist
Noradrenaline β_1 and β_2	Gs	Isoprenaline, salbutamol agonist (β2); atenolol, propranolol, labetolol antagonist
Opioid receptors (all types)	Gi	Morphine, fentanyl, alfentanil, remifentanil (μ); pentazocine (κ)
$GABA_B$ receptors	Gi	Baclofen agonist
P1 adenosine receptors	Gi	Adenosine agonist
$P2Y_1$ and $P2Y_2$ receptors	Gi	ADP agonist; clopidogrel irreversible antagonist
Histamine H_1 receptors	Gq	Cetirizine antagonist
Histamine H_2 receptors	Gs	Ranitidine antagonist
Dopamine D_1 and D_5 receptors (postsynaptic)	Gs	Dopamine and dobutamine in kidney agonist
Dopamine D_2, D_3 and D_4 receptors (presynaptic)	Gi	Bromocriptine agonist; haloperidol, risperidone, chlorpromazine and clozapine (D_4 selective) antagonists
Serotonin $5-HT_{1A}$ receptors	Gi	Buspirone antagonist
Serotonin $5-HT_2$ receptors	Gs	Ketanserin antagonist
Angiotensin II AT_1 receptors	Gq	Losartan, valsartan antagonist

Figure MD3 Some important GPCRs and their agonists and antagonists

proteins activate and inhibit adenylyl cyclase, respectively; Gq causes phospholipase C to hydrolyse phosphatidyl-inositol, a phospholipid component of cell membranes, to produce diacyl glyceride (DAG) and inositol triphosphate (IP_3) – both secondary messengers; G_{12} proteins are associated with GPCRs that alter K^+ channel opening in the cell membrane. All catecholamine action is mediated through GPCRs, although different adrenoceptor subtypes are associated with different subfamilies of G protein. Figure MD3 lists some GPCRs and their G-protein associations that are of importance to the anaesthetist.

Tyrosine kinase (trk) receptors
Unlike GPCRs, trk receptors do not rely on an intermediary protein for activity but incorporate the enzyme site on the transmembrane protein itself; the cytoplasmic portion of the receptor is a kinase that is activated by ligand binding to the extracellular portion of the receptor. Insulin receptors

are of the trk type, and it is thought that two receptors must act together (dimerise) in order to elicit a response.

Intracellular receptors
Receptors within the cell can be associated either with the cytosol or with any of the specialised intracellular membranes; of particular importance are receptors associated with the sarcoplasmic reticulum that regulate calcium release.

Cytoplasmic hormone receptors
Lipid-soluble hormones interact with intracellular cytoplasmic receptors. There is a superfamily of such receptors, including those for sex hormones, corticosteroids, thyroxine and vitamin D_3. These receptors act as ligand-regulated transcription factors that bind to DNA and influence the pattern of RNA production by either increasing or inhibiting specific protein production. In the

cytoplasm these receptors are inactive, due to association with inhibitory proteins. Ligand binding produces a conformational change that activates the receptor and initiates translation to the nucleus and association with specific DNA promoter sequences. Gene transcription is influenced by the recruitment of additional proteins that act as co-activators or co-repressors to remodel the quaternary structure of DNA. Chromatin structure may be loosened, so encouraging transcription, or chromatin condensation may be favoured, so inhibiting transcription. The oestrogen-receptor modulator tamoxifen inhibits transcription associated with tumour cells in certain cancers. In addition to hormone receptors, other nuclear receptors can also influence protein production: the new antidiabetic drug rosiglitazone is a peroxisome proliferator-activated receptor type γ (PPAR-γ) agonist that stimulates protein transcription, leading to insulin sensitising activity within adipose tissue.

Adrenal steroid hormones

There are two types of corticosteroid receptor: MR (or type 1) is the mineralocorticoid receptor and GR (or type 2) the glucocorticoid receptor. MR and GR receptors are each composed of four distinct protein regions, including an N-terminal region associated with activation of transcription, a DNA-binding domain, a nuclear localisation signal and a C-terminal hormone-binding region. Glucocorticoid binding displaces the inhibitory heat-shock proteins and triggers a conformational change that facilitates translocation and binding to specific regions on DNA. The GR receptor is widespread in cells, whereas MR is restricted to epithelial tissue such as renal collecting tubules. Cortisol and aldosterone are equipotent at MR receptors: aldosterone-triggered activation is permitted by the presence of 11β-hydroxysteroid dehydrogenase in epithelial cells, which metabolises cortisol to a compound that is inactive at the MR receptor.

Intracellular membrane-bound receptors

Intracellular membranes have GPCRs in addition to receptors that respond to secondary messengers produced by ligand–GPCR coupling at the cell membrane. Of particular importance is the control of intracellular calcium; in endoplasmic reticulum the IP$_3$ (inositol triphosphate) receptor is important. In sarcoplasmic reticulum (SR) the ryanodine receptor in close association with L-type calcium channels, with calmodulin and calcium as modulators, triggers calcium release for excitation–contraction coupling. Dantrolene acts at the ryanodine receptor to inhibit calcium release from the SR. Several families with malignant hyperthermia have genetic abnormalities associated with the ryanodine receptor.

Pharmacokinetic actions

Drugs may exert their effects by interfering with the absorption, distribution and metabolism of endogenous substances involved in biochemical and physiological systems. In this section we consider drug–enzyme and drug–transporter mechanisms.

Drug interactions with enzymes

Enzymes of relevance to anaesthetists are those that metabolise neurotransmitters and those that inhibit non-neuronal homeostatic systems such as elements of the immune or coagulation cascades.

Interaction with neurotransmitter metabolism
Acetylcholine: acetylcholinesterase

All clinically useful muscle relaxants interfere with acetylcholine transmission at the NMJ. The duration of acetylcholine activity is restricted by acetylcholinesterase, a metabolic enzyme associated with the clefts of the synaptic membrane. Several enzyme molecules associate to form an oligomer that is anchored to the synaptic membrane but has the enzymatic sites facing into the cleft. The non-depolarising muscle relaxants, such as vecuronium and atracurium, competitively inhibit the association of acetylcholine with the nACh receptor; this inhibition can be overcome by the use of acetylcholinesterase inhibitors such as neostigmine, resulting in an increase in acetylcholine concentration in the synaptic cleft. The log-dose–response curve for acetylcholine is shifted to the right by the presence of vecuronium; in the presence of neostigmine the acetylcholine concentration increases, so producing a return of muscle contraction (Figure MD4). It is important that some activity is present before neostigmine is given, or the relative increase in acetylcholine concentration is not sufficient to overcome the blockade completely.

There are two binding sites on acetylcholinesterase, the anionic and the esteratic sites. The anionic site attracts the positively charged quaternary nitrogen of acetylcholine, allowing the substrate to approach the esteratic site. This latter site contains a serine residue that is crucial for bond breakage and which is transiently acetylated. Neostigmine binds to both anionic and esteratic sites; it is a substrate for the enzyme but instead of metabolism resulting in acetylation of the enzyme, carbamylation occurs. Although the carbamoyl group can dissociate from the esteratic

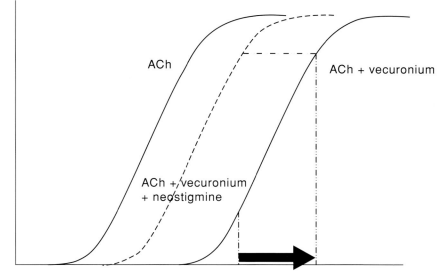

Figure MD4 Addition of vecuronium shifts the log-dose–response curve to the right. Addition of neostigmine has the *apparent* effect of shifting the response back to the left (shown by the dashed arrow), since the concentration of acetylcholine is increased (by an amount indicated by the solid arrow) in the presence of an acetylcholinesterase inhibitor.

site, the rate at which this occurs is very much slower than for an acetyl group; the enzyme remains inhibited sufficiently long for the synaptic concentration of neuromuscular blocking drug to fall to an insignificant level.

Catecholamine neurotransmission

Drugs such as methyl DOPA are substrates for the natural synthetic pathway, and can be packaged into synaptic vesicles in the same way as the endogenous transmitter. Being less active than noradrenaline, autonomic control of blood pressure is impaired.

Endogenous catecholamines are metabolised by monoamine oxidase (MAO) and catechol-O-methyltransferase; inhibition of MAO is associated with antidepressant action. MAO is widespread, but is particularly associated with mitochondrial membranes in the synaptic terminal and hepatocytes. There are two forms of MAO, MAO-A and MAO-B. Non-selective MAO inhibitors (MAOIs) such as tranylcypromine and phenelzine are long-acting. Selective MAO-A inhibitors (e.g. moclobemide) are now available, and are shorter-acting; the MAO-B inhibitor, selegiline, is used in the treatment of Parkinson's disease. The use of pethidine and indirectly

acting synthetic catecholamines, such as ephedrine, is contraindicated in the presence of MAOIs. It is suggested that MAOIs are stopped for 2 weeks before surgery.

GABA metabolism

Enhancement of GABA transmission is a target for development of anticonvulsant drugs. Sodium valproate and vigabatrin both inhibit GABA-transaminase, which is responsible for breakdown of GABA.

Immunomodulatory action

NSAIDs and paracetamol exert their effects by inhibiting cyclo-oxygenase, the enzyme responsible for the production of a variety of prostaglandins and related autocoids. These are derived from arachidonic acid, which is produced by activation of membrane-associated phospholipase C in response to inflammatory mediators. There are two genetically determined forms of cyclo-oxygenase: cyclo-oxygenase 1 (COX-1), which is constitutively active, and cyclo-oxygenase 2 (COX-2), which is inducible. It is this latter form that is produced in response to an inflammatory insult and is associated with the pain of inflammation. Aspirin and non-selective NSAIDs act by inhibiting both forms of the enzyme; reducing the action of the constitutive form is thought to be responsible for many of the unwanted actions of this group of drugs. The selective NSAIDs, such as etoricoxib, have a much higher affinity for the inducible form, COX-2, with an associated reduction in many unwanted effects such as gastric erosions and ulceration. Recent evidence has suggested that a third type of cyclo-oxygenase exists, COX-3, which is found in higher concentrations in the brain, including the hypothalamus. This represents a post-transcriptional modification of the COX-2 gene product, which is not so widely distributed as COX-2 itself. Paracetamol is now thought to inhibit COX-3 as part of its mechanism of action. This aspect provides a unified mechanism of action for all minor analgesics.

Drug interaction with transport proteins

The duration of action of many neurotransmitters is limited by reuptake into neurones, followed either by repackaging into vesicles or by metabolism. The transport proteins associated with the presynaptic membrane responsible for this effect will increase neurotransmitter availability at the postsynaptic membrane. Of particular interest are the selective serotonin reuptake inhibitors (SSRIs), such as paroxetine, which are effective antidepressants with fewer unwanted effects than less selective drugs, such as imipramine.

In the renal tubule furosemide inhibits the $Na^+/K^+/2Cl^-$ symport mechanism in the thick ascending limb of the loop of Henle to produce its diuretic effect. Thiazide diuretics inhibit the Na^+/Cl^- symport in the distal tubule, a weak effect, since electrolyte concentrations in distal tubular fluid are relatively low.

Another transport mechanism of importance is the proton pump in the stomach, responsible for the secretion of hydrogen ions and maintenance of gastric pH. The $H^+K^+ATPase$ enzyme system at the secretory surface of gastric parietal cells is the target for proton pump inhibitors such as omeprazole.

The anticonvulsant tiagabine is an inhibitor of the GABA transport mechanism that is responsible for glial cell uptake of GABA from adjacent synapses.

Mechanisms of general anaesthetic action

Of the mechanisms of drug action described earlier in this chapter, those of particular relevance to anaesthesia predominantly involve neurotransmitter function. Figure MD5 summarises ways in which neuronal traffic can be altered by drugs.

One of the most elusive mechanisms of drug action is that of general anaesthetics themselves. For many years this was thought to involve a non-specific, physicochemical action, but now it is thought more likely that a specific receptor-based mechanism is responsible.

One of the main problems with investigating the mechanism underlying anaesthetic action is the lack of a clear definition of what constitutes general anaesthesia. The definition must include certain clinical observations: loss of conscious awareness, loss of response to noxious stimuli (antinociceptive effect). Importantly, the effect must be reversible. Animal models of anaesthesia can address antinociception and reversibility, but cannot measure conscious awareness.

It is likely that different general anaesthetic agents have differing profiles of pre- and postsynaptic activity at ligand-gated channels within the CNS. All these effects result in depression of signals reaching the hippocampus and cortex so that explicit memory traces are not laid down, information processing is interrupted and unconsciousness ensues. The sedative effects seem to be mediated, at least in part, through the tuberomammillary nucleus, and immobility may be brought about more through spinal than supraspinal mechanisms. The molecular sites of anaesthetic action are likely to be lipophilic sites on mainly ligand-gated ionic channels, although we cannot entirely exclude effects on voltage-gated channels. As a result, an allosteric conformational change in the ion channel either enhances inhibitory or inhibits excitatory currents. At present, the best evidence is for enhancing the inhibitory effect of GABA at $GABA_A$ receptors and/or inhibition of excitatory currents at the NMDA receptor. The contribution made by action on glycine and neuronal nicotinic receptors has yet to be established. Whatever the effects of the anaesthetic agents, clinical anaesthesia is achieved by a balanced combination of agents contributing to the overall effect.

Anatomical sites of action

The anatomical sites of action of general anaesthetics are regions of the brain and spinal cord. Such sites must be involved both in physiological responses to nociception and in consciousness; certainly explicit but possibly also implicit memory mechanisms should be inhibited. Memory is associated with the limbic system, and the degree of awareness is related to depth of anaesthesia. Cortical

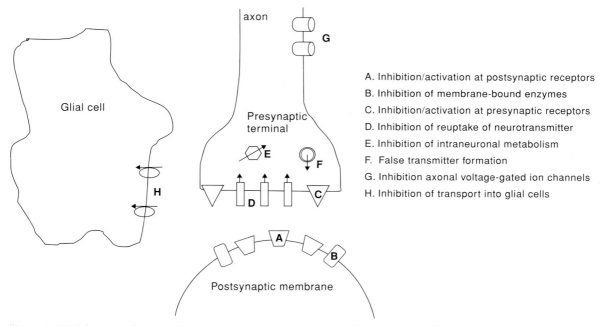

A. Inhibition/activation at postsynaptic receptors
B. Inhibition of membrane-bound enzymes
C. Inhibition/activation at presynaptic receptors
D. Inhibition of reuptake of neurotransmitter
E. Inhibition of intraneuronal metabolism
F. False transmitter formation
G. Inhibition axonal voltage-gated ion channels
H. Inhibition of transport into glial cells

Figure MD5 Schematic diagram showing how drugs can interfere with neuronal traffic

afferent input and motor efferents must also be interrupted. It is likely that both spinal and supraspinal sites are involved.

Auditory and sensory evoked potential data support an anatomical site of action for volatile anaesthetic agents somewhere between brain stem and cortex, with the thalamus the most likely primary target. This fits with the integrative functions of the thalamus, but does not exclude the limbic system or certain cortical areas. Evidence suggests that several brain areas are affected by anaesthetics, each mediating different components of anaesthetic activity. The sedative effect of anaesthetics appears to be associated with the tuberomammillary nucleus. Inhibition of GABA receptors in this region, using the GABA antagonist gabazine, markedly reduces the sedative effects of propofol and pentobarbital, but not those of ketamine.

Molecular theories

At the beginning of the nineteenth century, when the anaesthetic effects of a number of agents were being investigated in animal models, Overton and Meyer independently described the linear correlation between the lipid (in particular olive oil) solubility of anaesthetic agents and their potency (Figure MD6). This correlation was so impressive, given the great variation in structure of these agents, that it suggested a non-specific mechanism of action based on this physicochemical property. Later interpretation pointed out that any highly lipophilic area was a potential site of action, with cell membranes being the most likely contender, given the high concentration of lipids. Not all lipids give as good a correlation between solubility and potency. The best correlation occurs with lecithin, a constituent of cell membranes. However, there are problems with a unified theory based on lipid interactions: some general anaesthetics, such as ketamine, are extreme outliers. The stereoisomeric pair of steroidal agents alphaxalone and betaxalone have identical lipid solubility, but only alphaxalone has anaesthetic properties (perhaps explained by its $GABA_A$ agonism). Thus lipid solubility is likely to be relevant, but it does not in itself explain anaesthesia.

Membrane lipids

The physicochemical correlation between lipid solubility and potency for anaesthetic agents with markedly differing structures is very impressive. To some degree the rejection of prospective agents with low lipid solubility was self-fulfilling, and diverted attention away from seeking out

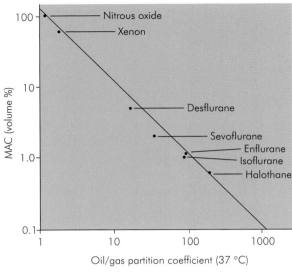

Figure MD6 Meyer–Overton plot

specific receptor sites. There are several potential lipophilic sites in cell membranes, including the lipid bilayer itself and the annular lipids surrounding ionic channels.

Lipophilic anaesthetic agents can penetrate the bilayer and alter the molecular arrangement of the phospholipids in a manner described as 'fluidising' the membrane. The expansion of the membrane was thought to disrupt the function of membrane-spanning ionic channels. This theory explained why general anaesthetic agents could affect a number of ionic currents, as there was a generalised, non-specific change in membrane structure. Calculations identifying the volume of anaesthetic agent required to expand membranes led to a 'critical volume hypothesis'. This suggested that anaesthesia was induced when a certain volume of an anaesthetic agent partitioned into the membrane. Against such a theory, a 1 °C rise in temperature increases membrane thickness to a similar extent as that seen with volatile agents, yet increased temperature lessens anaesthesia. The only lasting reason why such a theory holds any attraction lies with pressure reversal of anaesthesia. In animal models the effects of a volatile anaesthetic can be overcome by pressurising the environment. This is one observation that has yet to be fully explained in our current view of general anaesthetic action.

However, many highly lipid-soluble molecules that can induce changes in lipid bilayers are not anaesthetic. Several halogenated hydrocarbons, including some with multiple

fluorine substitutions, fail to elicit anaesthesia, and some actually induce seizures.

Since the physicochemical theory does not favour any specific lipid environment, it was proposed that deviation from the Overton–Meyer line could be explained by identifying specific lipid site(s) at which anaesthetic agents exerted their action. Discrepancies might then be explained by steric differences. It is known that the composition of phospholipids in the immediate vicinity of ion channels is different from that of the general lipid bilayer, being specific for a given channel. It was therefore proposed that disruption of these so-called annular lipids could account for alteration in specific ion-channel function and therefore account for anaesthesia – the perturbation theory.

Rapid advances in receptor protein identification within the central nervous system, together with the observation that anaesthetic agents can alter enzyme function, led to newer theories based on interactions with specific proteins. It now seems likely that the correlation between potency and lipid solubility reflects the lipophilic nature of specific protein-based binding site(s).

Protein site(s) of action
The evidence for a protein site of action

- General anaesthetic agents, at concentrations close to those producing anaesthesia, inhibit the firefly enzyme luciferase. The order of effective inhibition is the same as the order of potency for those anaesthetic agents.
- Saturable binding of halothane to rat brain synaptosomes suggested a limited number of binding sites. This would not be the case for a non-specific interaction.
- The enantiomers of certain general anaesthetic agents show stereoselective differences in the extent to which they alter ionic currents.

If a specific, saturable, binding site is present it is very likely that stereoisomers of an agent will display different binding and therefore response characteristics. Demonstrating such a difference is good evidence for the existence of specific binding sites, particularly those associated with proteins.

Anaesthetics may prevent afferent signals reaching the brain either by increasing inhibitory or by reducing excitatory pathways, or possibly by a combination of these two actions. Experimental work has therefore looked at both excitatory and inhibitory ionic channel function, including

	Inhibitory transmitters		Excitatory transmitters	
	GABA$_A$	Glycine	NMDA	Neuronal nicotinic cholinergic
R-Etomidate	↑↑↑	–	–	–
S-Etomidate	–	–	–	–
Propofol	↑↑↑	↑	–	↓↓
Ketamine	–	–	↓↓↓	–

Figure MD7 Effect of intravenous anaesthetic agents at ligand-gated ion channels

voltage-gated and ligand-gated channels, in the presence of anaesthetic agents.

We know that anaesthetic agents alter the conductance of voltage-gated sodium and calcium channels, although the concentrations at which such effects can be elicited are generally a little higher than found in vivo. The log-dose–response curve for anaesthesia shows a much steeper, left-shifted curve than that for depression of voltage-gated sodium channels. This suggests not only that anaesthesia occurs at a lower drug concentration, but probably that a different mechanism is responsible.

Several ligand-gated ionic channels are more sensitive to the action of general anaesthetics than are voltage-gated channels. The interactions at inhibitory (GABA$_A$ and glycine) and excitatory (neuronal nicotinic and NMDA) channels have all been studied. Figure MD7 summarises the relative activity of a number of agents at these receptors.

GABA$_A$ receptor

The GABA$_A$ receptor has modulatory sites on the β subunit for benzodiazepines, barbiturates, propofol and volatile agents. In vitro investigation of the stereospecificity of the action of barbiturates and isoflurane support the notion of a specific binding site for each agent.

- Etomidate is clinically presented as an enantiopure preparation of the R(+) isomer; the S(−) form is inactive clinically. At the GABA$_A$ receptor there is a 30-fold difference in activity.
- Stereoisomers of the barbiturates pentobarbital and thiopental show a twofold difference in enhancing GABA activity at the GABA$_A$ receptor. There are no human studies with barbiturate stereoisomers, but animal studies suggest a two-fold difference in potency, with S-barbiturates more potent than R-barbiturates.
- Stereoisomers of isoflurane have a 1.5-fold difference in efficacy at the GABA$_A$ receptor, although there is no clinical evidence for any difference in potency.

Anaesthetics increase channel opening time, so allowing for increased chloride entry resulting in hyperpolarisation. The effect is seen for etomidate, propofol, barbiturates, alphaxalone as well as volatiles. Other pentameric receptors are influenced by some of these agents, but etomidate seems selective for the GABA$_A$ receptor. In contrast, propofol will also increase glycine channel opening time and is inhibitory at neuronal nicotinic and 5-HT$_3$ receptors. Mutation studies suggest each agent occupies a separate site, although all appear to be associated with the β subunit and are distinct from the benzodiazepine receptor site. There are at least 30 types of GABA$_A$ receptor, each with different stoichiometry of subunit composition. Different forms are likely to have varying sensitivities to anaesthetic agents. In vitro it has been shown that the β$_2$ and β$_3$ subunits are more sensitive to the effects of etomidate than is the β$_1$ subunit. A single amino acid substitution on the β$_2$ subunit can reduce the effect of etomidate on chloride conductance. However, animal experiments with genetically modified mice showed only a faster recovery from anaesthesia; EEG changes and loss of the righting reflex were the same as in wild-type mice. A mutation of β$_3$ subunits has been shown to prevent etomidate-induced suppression of hind-limb withdrawal and righting reflex. Animal models thus provide evidence for the importance of GABA$_A$ receptors in producing the state we call anaesthesia.

Glycine receptor

The major inhibitory transmitter in the spinal cord and brain stem is glycine. The glycine receptor is associated with a chloride channel similar to the GABA$_A$ receptor. Electrophysiological evidence suggests that although the spinal cord is not a major anatomical site for signal attenuation by intravenous anaesthetics, the volatile anaesthetics all markedly potentiate the action of glycine, although there is no evidence of stereoselectivity. It has been suggested that the spinal cord is an important site of action for volatile rather than intravenous anaesthetic agents. Efficacy here correlates more with immobility than with awareness.

NMDA receptor

Neuronal signalling may also be reduced by inhibition of excitatory pathways. The excitatory amino acid glutamate has received a lot of attention, but interest has focused on the NMDA receptor as it is involved in long-term signal potentiation associated with learning and memory.

The NMDA receptor is activated by glutamate, modulated by magnesium, and is inhibited in a non-competitive manner by ketamine, nitrous oxide and xenon. It is therefore likely that this glutamate-mediated mechanism represents an additional pathway for the onset of the anaesthetic state. Some other anaesthetic agents, such as barbiturates, can reduce the effectiveness of glutamate but at a lower potency than for inhibition of $GABA_A$ receptor function. Any theory of anaesthesia must therefore include both NMDA- and $GABA_A$-mediated pathways.

Adverse effects

Adverse effects of drugs may be either predictable or idiosyncratic, minor or life-threatening. Genetic factors may influence susceptibility. Predictable adverse effects are usually dose-dependent, and can potentially occur in anyone exposed to the drug in question. The higher the dose of drug, the more likely there will be associated adverse consequences. However, pharmacogenetic and environmental factors contribute to a wide inter-individual variability in occurrence of such unwanted effects.

Physicochemical effects

Many drugs have a complex heterocyclic structure; some, such as sulphonamides, can be photoactivated to produce skin discoloration and dermatitis. This photosensitivity-induced dermatitis is seen in an extreme form in the porphyrias.

The chemical activity of certain drugs can alter the valency of metal ions that play an essential part in enzyme activity. Nitrous oxide is able to induce a change in cobalt from the monovalent to the inactive bivalent form in cyanocobalamin (vitamin B_{12}), which is a co-activator for methionine synthase. Prolonged exposure to nitrous oxide results in megaloblastic anaemia.

Pharmacodynamic effects

Pharmacodynamic effects usually arise from drug action at sites other than those responsible for the required effect. This may involve activity at the same target protein (enzyme or receptor) but at a different anatomical location, activity at a different subtype of the target, or because the drug can interact with more than one target. Such effects are dose-dependent and predictable but there is a wide range of inter-individual variation depending on patient factors such as age, pathophysiology and genetic disposition.

The respiratory depressant effect of morphine typifies the first of these mechanisms: analgesia and respiratory depression are both associated with the μ opioid receptor, but at different central locations. Convulsions arising from toxic levels of local anaesthetic agents such as lidocaine or bupivacaine are due to central inhibition of neuronal voltage-gated sodium channels: clearly a dose-dependent phenomenon occurring at a different anatomic location.

The gastrointestinal effects of aspirin are secondary to its inhibition of the constitutive form of cyclo-oxygenase, COX-1, whereas its anti-inflammatory effect is due to acetylation of the inducible form, COX-2, so this characterises the second type of pharmacodynamic adverse effect. Another example is asthma triggered by the anti-hypertensive agent propranolol, which is due to actions at β_2-adrenoceptors, whereas the blood-pressure-lowering effect is a β_1-mediated action.

The third mechanism is demonstrated by the dry mouth and tachycardia associated with use of intravenous cyclizine, an H_1 antihistamine used as an anti-emetic, which are a consequence of antimuscarinic effects at acetylcholine receptors.

Drugs used by infusion in the intensive care unit (ICU) often induce unwanted effects as duration of infusion increases. One is tachyphylaxis (the reduction in responsiveness of physiological systems to drugs due to continuous exposure), which requires escalating dose and eventually lost responsiveness. This is particularly evident with agonists and is related to receptor down-regulation. Conversely, receptor up-regulation can result in increased responsiveness that can produce adverse effects, such as exposure to suxamethonium several days after denervation injury. Receptor regulation is discussed further below. Other unwanted effects in the ICU are seen with non-depolarising muscle relaxants, which if given continuously can induce myelopathy, and with sodium nitroprusside, where excessive infusion rates can produce cyanide toxicity due to uncoupling of oxidative phosphorylation leading to tissue hypoxia.

Regulation of receptor activity

Some molecular mechanisms of receptor regulation for both GPCRs and ionotropic receptors are now understood.

Interaction of a GPCR with an agonist increases the likelihood of receptor down-regulation and internalisation. The extent to which internalisation occurs depends upon the system in question. Agonist binding may activate GPCR-kinases (GRKs), which phosphorylate both the C-terminal and the domain associated with G-protein binding. Phosphorylation of the C-terminal then increases the affinity of the GPCR for β-arrestin, a protein that triggers receptor internalisation. This down-regulation of receptor activity is seen with β_1-adrenoceptor agonists such as dobutamine. There are families of protein kinases that regulate receptor activity – some of which are being targeted as sites for potential therapeutic intervention.

Up- and down-regulation is also seen in ionotropic receptor populations. Of particular importance are the changes seen at the motor endplate following denervation injury, such as that seen following spinal injury. Under circumstances when acetylcholine is not available for activating postsynaptic receptors the homeostatic response is to manufacture more receptors. Large numbers of these receptors are inserted at extrajunctional sites; most importantly they conform to the fetal subunit configuration ($\alpha\gamma\alpha\beta\delta$) rather than the adult. These fetal-type receptors have a longer channel opening time, allowing a greater efflux of potassium, which may be sufficient to increase plasma potassium levels and trigger arrhythmias. Similar effects are seen in burn injury and acute degenerative disorders. It takes time for a large number of new receptors to be made; suxamethonium can be used safely shortly after injury but is best avoided after 48–72 hours.

Pharmacokinetic effects

Adverse effects resulting from pharmacokinetic mechanisms can be due to alteration in distribution, metabolism or elimination of endogenous bioagents, or they may arise from effects of biotransformation of the drug itself.

The bradycardia associated with neostigmine administration is because of increased acetylcholine concentrations at autonomic sites, particularly cardiac muscarinic M_2 receptors, as well as the intended neuromuscular junction. In anaesthetic practice we anticipate this effect and co-administer an antimuscarinic agent, such as glycopyrrolate.

Drug metabolites can produce unwanted actions. Paracetamol is mostly converted to inactive compounds by conjugation with sulphate and glucuronide, but a small portion is metabolised via the cytochrome P_{450} enzyme system. This is responsible for oxidation of paracetamol to a highly reactive intermediary metabolite, N-acetyl-p-benzo-quinone imine (NAPQI). Under normal conditions,

NAPQI is detoxified by conjugation with glutathione. In overdose the conjugation pathways become saturated, and NAPQI production increases. When hepatocellular supplies of glutathione are reduced by more than 70% NAPQI is free to react with elements of cellular membranes, resulting in acute hepatic necrosis and death.

Idiopathic adverse effects

These adverse effects are generally unrelated to dose, and are often unpredictable. Some involve well-understood hypersensitivity reactions that range from mild skin rashes to anaphylactic shock. Both pharmacogenetic and environmental factors may contribute to an individual's response. Other idiosyncratic effects may result from inherited abnormalities.

Hypersensitivity reactions

These range from mild rashes through angioneurotic oedema to full-blown anaphylaxis. The mechanisms involve immune elements activated either with (anaphylactic) or without (anaphylactoid) previous exposure, and they are described in Section 1, Chapter 2 (pages 27–9). In anaesthetic practice, muscle relaxants account for about 80% of such hypersensitivity reactions; the main culprits are suxamethonium and vecuronium. An immune-mediated mechanism is thought to underlie halothane hepatitis, where the oxidative metabolism of halothane produces a reactive intermediate, trifluoroacetylchloride, which leads to production of trifluoracetylated cellular proteins that act as haptens for immune-mediated fulminant hepatic necrosis on a second exposure. Fatality is high (50%) although the incidence is relatively low, about 1 in 10 000 exposures.

Pharmacogenetic influences

Pharmacogenetic abnormalities can account for several serious adverse effects with anaesthetic agents. Malignant hyperthermia can be triggered by suxamethonium and the halogenated volatile agents. The underlying defect in about 50% of families appears to be associated with an abnormal ryanodine receptor, which is intimately involved in the control of calcium release from sarcoplasmic reticulum in skeletal muscle. Inheritance is autosomal dominant and may also be associated with certain congenital myopathies.

Suxamethonium apnoea is an autosomal co-dominant response to abnormal plasma cholinesterase (pseudocholinesterase) (see Section 1, Chapter 4, page 63). Homozygotes show the most profound prolongation of neuromuscular blockade after suxamethonium use, but supportive ventilation is all that is required. In affected families, avoiding suxamethonium and mivacurium will prevent any problem.

Pharmacogenetics of other drug-metabolising enzymes, including the cytochrome P_{450} system, can profoundly affect extent and duration of response. Although strictly not an adverse action, presence of an abnormal CYP2D6 isozyme can prevent conversion of codeine to morphine, with the unwanted consequence of inadequate analgesia. Slow acetylators will have prolonged effects on drugs such as hydralazine, particularly if they are used intravenously for a short-duration antihypertensive effect.

Mechanisms of drug interactions

We can describe the mechanism of interaction between drugs as physicochemical, pharmacokinetic or pharmacodynamic. The physicochemical interactions influence drug pharmacokinetics, which in turn can affect response. Some of these interactions (e.g. penicillin and probenecid) can be exploited for therapeutic benefit.

Clinically significant drug interactions commonly involve anticoagulants, antiarrhythmics, anticonvulsants and hypoglycaemic agents, where small changes in plasma concentration may produce unwanted effects, i.e. there is a narrow therapeutic index. Furthermore, polypharmacy increases the risk of a significant drug interaction: patients on more than six drugs have an 80% chance of a drug interaction. Since the elderly are more likely to be on multiple therapies, and are often more sensitive to drug effects, they are more likely to experience such adverse interactions.

Physicochemical

The chemical interaction of two drugs may produce an insoluble or non-absorbable product. Of importance is the interaction between an acidic drug such as thiopental and a base such as sodium bicarbonate – when they are given intravenously through the same line an insoluble salt precipitates out. A similar problem occurs with thiopental (acidic) and suxamethonium (basic), as might be used in rapid sequence induction – a saline flush should be used before giving the muscle relaxant. For orally administered drugs, two drugs may interact in the stomach, reducing absorption and causing sub-therapeutic plasma levels of one or both. Antacids are notorious at reducing the absorption of antibiotics from the GIT, particularly ciprofloxacin, rifampicin and tetracyclines. Ketoconazole is administered orally as a poorly soluble base

that has to be changed to the more soluble hydrochloride salt by gastric acid. H_2-antagonists (such as ranitidine) and proton pump inhibitors (such as omeprazole) raise gastric pH, thus reducing the absorption of ketoconazole.

Pharmacokinetic

Drugs that alter the absorption, distribution, metabolism and excretion of other drugs are said to interact pharmacokinetically. Absorption is often affected through physicochemical interactions, and delayed absorption may occur with drugs that produce stasis of the GIT, such as opioids, but in general delayed absorption does not prevent drug entering the plasma, though it may reduce peak concentrations.

Distribution of drugs can be influenced by competition for plasma protein binding sites. This leads to an increased plasma level of free drug that could, theoretically, reach toxic levels. Although many drugs are plasma-protein-bound, changes in the extent of protein binding due to drug displacement are rarely significant. An increase in the free fraction may occur transiently, but increased elimination soon counteracts this effect. Significant interactions involving competition for binding sites occurs only for drugs that are very highly protein-bound (in excess of 95%), and when the displaced drug is eliminated only in a dose-independent manner, i.e. zero-order kinetics (see Section 3, Chapter 3, page 538). In addition, most important interactions of this kind are also associated with alterations in metabolism of the displaced drug. For example, amiodarone and warfarin are highly protein-bound to albumin (99%); the increase in INR when they are used together was thought to be due to displacement of warfarin, but amiodarone also inhibits S-warfarin metabolism. Small changes in free drug may also be of importance where the two drugs act on the same effector system but through different mechanisms. NSAIDs displace warfarin, but one affects blood clotting by reducing platelet adhesion while the other interferes with the coagulation cascade, and the combination results in an increased risk of bleeding.

The majority of clinically significant drug interactions due to pharmacokinetic factors involve induction or inhibition of metabolism. Many drugs are metabolised by the cytochrome P_{450} system of enzymes. These enzymes are subject to induction or inhibition by a wide range of agents, including tobacco, drugs and fruit juices (especially cranberry and grapefruit). Enzyme induction by one drug can increase the clearance of another, so

Drug combination	Drug affected	Result	Mechanism
Cimetidine + theophylline	Theophylline	CNS agitation, arrhythmias, nausea	Inhibition of CYP1A2
Tricyclic antidepressants (TCAs) + paroxetene	TCAs	Serotonin toxicity; agitation, hyperreflexia, arrhythmias	Inhibition of CYP2D6
Amiodarone + S-warfarin	S-warfarin	Increased INR; risk of bleeding	Inhibition of CYP2C9
Fluoxetine + phenytoin	Phenytoin	Phenytoin toxicity: ataxia, nystagmus, slurred speech, nausea & vomiting	Inhibition of CYP2C19
Clarithromycin + terfenidine	Terfenidine	Ventricular arrhythmias	Inhibition of CYP3A4
Carbamazepine + vecuronium	Vecuronium	Reduced duration neuromuscular blockade	Induction of CYP3A4
Rifampicin + S-warfarin	S-warfarin	Reduction in INR; risk of thrombotic events	Induction of CYP2C9
Chlorpropamide + rifampicin	Chlorpropamide	Poor diabetic control; reduced levels	Induction of CYP2C9

Figure MD8 Drug interactions for the cytochrome P_{450} system. CYP2D6 is not inducible, unlike other isoforms. These interactions are considered clinically important according to the *British National Formulary*.

reducing peak concentration and duration of activity. The anticonvulsants phenytoin, phenobarbital and carbamazepine are cytochrome inducers that shorten the duration of aminosteroidal (e.g. vecuronium and rocuronium) non-depolarising neuromuscular blockade; bisbenzylisoquiniliniums are not affected as their metabolism is different. Co-administration of drugs with cytochrome inhibitors such as ranitidine, fluconazole, clarithromycin and amiodarone may lead to toxic levels; the combination of fluconazole and terfenidine in particular leads to a high risk of ventricular arrhythmias (see Figure MD8 for important interactions).

Plasma cholinesterase is responsible for suxamethonium metabolism, and there are several drugs that either inhibit or are substrates for this enzyme. Neostigmine inhibits plasma cholinesterase as well as acetylcholinesterase; suxamethonium-induced neuromuscular blockade is prolonged by neostigmine. Ecothiopate, used in the treatment of glaucoma, is an irreversible inhibitor of plasma cholinesterase.

The interaction between probenecid (a uricosuric used to treat gout) and penicillin is used therapeutically. Both drugs compete for a transport protein for weak acids (such as uric acid) in the renal tubule such that probenecid markedly reduces the rate of penicillin excretion.

Pharmacodynamic

Two drugs that act on a physiological system may either have the same effects (e.g. vecuronium and suxamethonium both produce neuromuscular blockade) or have opposing effects (e.g. phenylephrine vasoconstricts and nifedipine vasodilates). Drugs that have similar physiological effects will, in combination, produce an overall response that is additive, synergistic or antagonistic. Additivity suggests a shared mechanism of action; synergism or antagonism is evidence for differing mechanisms of action. Additivity is seen, for example, when vecuronium and rocuronium or isoflurane and sevoflurane are used together. Both tricyclic antidepressants (TCAs) and selective serotonin reuptake inhibitors (SSRIs) inhibit biogenic amine reuptake at central synapses. The combination of TCA and SSRI is additive, and can produce symptoms of serotonin toxicity such as agitation, hyperreflexia and hyperpyrexia. If a rise in synaptic serotonin concentration is produced by two different mechanisms, synergism can produce the life-threatening serotonin syndrome. The interaction between pethidine and monoamine oxidase inhibitors is now thought to be due to serotonin syndrome, since pethidine is a dose-dependent serotonin reuptake inhibitor.

Synergism is also seen when nifedipine and ACE inhibitors are used together for their antihypertensive effect; doses may need to be adjusted to prevent unwanted hypotension. Similarly, the hypotensive effect of volatile agents is significantly greater in the presence of ACE inhibitors. Synergism in antiplatelet activity is seen with aspirin and clopidogrel, and aspirin and abciximab. Diuretics that increase potassium loss through different mechanisms, such as loop (furosamide) and thiazide (bendroflumethiazide) diuretics, when used together can rapidly precipitate severe hypokalemia with the risk of arrhythmias in susceptible patients. In contrast, a combination of diuretics that have opposing effects on potassium loss can be used together safely, without the need for potassium supplements, such as bendroflumethiazide and amiloride, which is a clinically useful interaction.

Antagonism is seen with the combination of ACE inhibitors and angiotensin II receptor (AT$_1$) antagonists: receptor inhibition minimises the effectiveness of lowering angiotensin II concentration and their combined antihypertensive effect is not as great as would be predicted from their individual activity.

CHAPTER 5

Anaesthetic gases and vapours

T. C. Smith

Administration

Volatile anaesthetic agents are liquids with a low boiling point (BP) and high saturated vapour pressure (SVP) so that they evaporate easily. The physical properties of each agent influence vaporisation. Volatile agents have higher saturated vapour pressures and lower boiling points than water. Most have a characteristic smell, which can also be pleasant.

Volatile agents are administered via inhalation through the lungs and so enter the circulation via the pulmonary alveolar capillaries. Intravenously administered agents are injected into a small part of the venous system and are then diluted by mixing with other sources of the venous blood. The injected agent then passes through the right heart before reaching the pulmonary circulation. Inhaled agents bypass this venous phase and are fairly evenly spread through the ventilated alveoli. However, there is some delay in achieving sufficiently high alveolar concentrations for induction of anaesthesia.

Uptake of inhaled anaesthetic agents

Inhaled anaesthetics are administered so as to achieve levels in central neural tissue sufficient to produce anaesthesia without detrimental effects on other organs. At equilibrium, the partial pressures of the agents will be identical throughout the body, but the concentrations in different tissues will be determined by the partition coefficients. When a difference in partial pressure exists between two compartments, there will be a movement down the pressure gradient until equilibrium is achieved.

Achievement of satisfactory brain levels of anaesthetic agent occurs in three stages:
- Delivery phase
- Pulmonary phase
- Circulatory phase

Delivery phase

The delivery phase involves the introduction of the anaesthetic agents into the gas to be inspired. The fresh gas mixture produced by the anaesthetic machine is passed into the anaesthetic breathing system. This is not usually modified further, but when a circle breathing system is used a vaporiser may be placed within this circuit. While the details of vaporiser and breathing systems are covered elsewhere (Section 4, Chapter 3, pages 840–50), within this chapter it is important to appreciate that the settings dialled up on the anaesthetic machine do not guarantee the same levels in the inspired gas, because anaesthetic agent is lost in several ways:
- Dilution with existing gas in the breathing system
- Uptake by CO_2 absorbers
- Uptake by rubber and plastic components of the circuit

Inspired and expired concentrations of anaesthetic agents should be monitored, whenever possible, at the closest point to the patient.

Fundamentals of Anaesthesia, 3rd edition, ed. Tim Smith, Colin Pinnock and Ted Lin. Published by Cambridge University Press. © Cambridge University Press 2008.

Pulmonary phase

The following factors influence the uptake of anaesthetic agents from inhaled gas to the blood:
- Inhaled concentration
- Alveolar ventilation
- Diffusion
- Blood/gas partition coefficient
- Partial pressure of agent in the pulmonary artery
- Pulmonary blood flow
- Ventilation/perfusion distribution
- Concentration effect
- Second gas effect

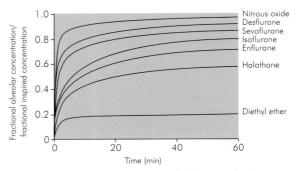

Figure GV1 Wash-in curves for volatile anaesthetic agents

Inhaled concentration

The inhaled concentration directly affects the inhaled partial pressure or tension. The higher the tension the higher the levels achieved in the blood. Levels above the desired maintenance tension for the brain (over-pressure) are often used to speed up arrival at these maintenance levels.

Alveolar ventilation

Ventilation of the lungs carries the volatile agent into the alveoli and the pre-existing gas mixture is gradually replaced. At the same time, vapour is diffusing into the blood, so depleting its concentration in the alveoli. Increasing alveolar minute volume speeds up the approximation of alveolar to inspired levels. Increases in physiological dead space constitute wasted ventilation in terms of supplying vapour to the blood. In general, volatile anaesthetic agents depress respiration, so as anaesthetic depth increases alveolar ventilation falls. This is one reason for a reduction in the rate of uptake of volatile agents as anaesthesia progresses.

Diffusion

The small molecules of volatile agents pass easily through the pulmonary membrane and in health diffusion is not a limiting factor. However, disease processes may reduce the surface area and increase the thickness of the alveolar membrane. For example, emphysema reduces the available area and pulmonary fibrosis increases the thickness of the membrane, so transfer of inhaled agents into the capillary blood may be delayed.

Blood/gas partition coefficient

The blood/gas partition coefficient determines the amount of agent that must be transferred to the blood to achieve equilibrium for a given tension, assuming that the blood volume is known and that there is no transfer to other tissues. This is an important point because it is this tension

that drives the agent into the brain and other tissues. A low blood/gas partition coefficient indicates low solubility in blood, so equilibrium will be reached with relatively small transfers of gas, and therefore equilibrium will be rapid. Conversely, a high coefficient indicates high solubility, and equilibrium will be slow. Nitrous oxide and desflurane, which have low blood/gas solubility coefficients, illustrate this point, and blood levels rapidly approximate to inspired levels. Older agents such as diethyl ether are much more soluble in blood and take considerably longer. Halothane, enflurane and isoflurane lie in the middle, with isoflurane the quickest of these three. In practice, equilibration is affected by distribution to other tissues and the process is slower than the simple model above, and other factors influence the relationship between individual agents. Figure GV1 shows wash-in characteristics for selected volatile agents obtained by plotting the fractional alveolar to inspired concentration as a ratio against time.

Partial pressure of volatile agent in the pulmonary artery

The rate of uptake of volatile agent from each alveolus is dependent on the tension difference between the alveolus and the capillary blood. As the concentration and tension in the blood rises the rate of uptake is reduced and so the rate of tension rise decreases.

Pulmonary blood flow

As blood passes through the pulmonary capillaries the tension of volatile agent in the capillary will increase and so reduce the rate of transfer in the latter part of the capillary. Therefore, increasing the blood flow will increase uptake.

Ventilation/perfusion distribution

Ventilation/perfusion mismatch will reduce perfusion of well-ventilated areas of lung and increase perfusion of alveoli poorly supplied with volatile agent.

Concentration effect

The uptake of volatile agent from the alveolus, during a small part of the respiratory cycle, reduces the amount left in the alveolus for subsequent parts of the cycle. Rate of uptake is proportional to the tension, which is the direct result of the concentration. Assuming that a smaller proportion of the other constituents of alveolar gas (e.g. nitrogen and oxygen) is absorbed, then the concentration of the anaesthetic agent will fall. The degree of fall will be influenced by its concentration, agents in low concentrations suffering a greater proportional loss than those in high concentrations. This means that the uptake of agents inhaled in high concentrations will be better maintained over the respiratory cycle than those administered at lower concentrations.

Second gas effect

The second gas effect embodies the same principles as the concentration effect. However, in this case the administration of a rapidly absorbed gas given in high concentration (typically nitrous oxide), together with a volatile agent of lower solubility, produces an increasing alveolar concentration of the second agent, thus promoting its absorption.

Circulatory phase

The following factors influence the transport of the volatile agent dissolved to the brain:

- Cardiac output
- Cerebral blood flow
- Distribution to other tissues

The distribution of blood to various tissues and compartments is described elsewhere (Section 3, Chapter 3, pages 530–1). While these principles apply to drugs that are intravenously administered, volatile agents behave in a similar fashion, with the driving force of partial pressure (tension) tending toward equilibrium. The uptake of agent by the tissues is proportional to tissue perfusion, solubility and arteriovenous tension difference. The formula is:

$$\text{Uptake} = \text{tissue blood flow} \times \text{tissue/blood solubility} \times \text{arteriovenous tension difference}$$

The formula produces time constants for the exponential function of tissue anaesthetic tension against time. High cardiac output and low tissue solubility produce a low time constant.

Cardiac output

Of cardiac output, 70–80% is distributed to the vessel-rich organs (brain, heart, liver, kidney) that constitute about 9% of body mass. Of the total, 14% goes to the brain (2.2% of body mass). A large proportion of the absorbed anaesthetic is thus directed to the brain. By virtue of their high lipid solubility, the brain has a relatively high affinity for anaesthetic agents.

Cerebral blood flow (CBF)

Factors affecting the proportion of cardiac output going to the brain will influence cerebral uptake of volatile agents. In shock, CBF is relatively well preserved, and therefore more agent will go to the brain and equilibrium will be reached more rapidly. Increasing depth of anaesthesia during spontaneous ventilation increases CO_2 and secondarily CBF. Hyperventilation during induction of anaesthesia will reduce CO_2 and CBF and delay equilibrium.

Distribution to other tissues

Distribution of volatile agent to other tissues (dependent on the factors above) slows the initial rate of uptake by the brain. Later, these depots of anaesthetic agent act to maintain the blood and so brain levels, and they act as a damper to any changes in alveolar and blood levels. This is something of an advantage, but slows recovery as much as it does induction.

Minimum alveolar concentration (MAC)

Minimum alveolar concentration may be defined as the concentration of anaesthetic agent which at equilibrium will prevent a reflex response to skin incision in 50% of subjects. MAC acts as a guide to the concentration required for anaesthesia. Altitude reduces atmospheric pressure, and therefore reduces the concentration of anaesthetic agent for a given percentage, so minimum alveolar pressure might be a more useful concept. It is a form of ED_{50} (effective dose). Other measures of potency include AD_{95} (anaesthetic dose), which is the dose required to prevent response to surgical stimulus in 95% of subjects. Various factors affect MAC for a particular agent, e.g. age, species and concomitant drugs. In clinical practice, it is important to remember that the displayed MAC value on an anaesthetic monitor is calculated from a standard MAC for the identified volatile(s), and does not measure neuronal tissue levels.

The mechanism of action of anaesthetic agents is described in Section 3, Chapter 4.

The ideal volatile agent

Although the ideal volatile agent does not exist, nonetheless it remains a useful concept. The characteristics of an ideal agent are given in Figure GV2. A comparison of the physical properties of the major agents in clinical practice is given in Figure GV3.

Specific pharmacology

The following agents will be considered in more detail: desflurane (D), enflurane (E), halothane (H), isoflurane (I) and sevoflurane (S). Chemical structures are shown in Figure GV4. In the comparative lists for each agent, molecular weight (MW) is given in daltons, boiling point (BP) in °C, MAC in volumes %, and the coefficents are dimensionless.

General features

Physical

Physically, the volatile anaesthetic agents are relatively small, simple molecules, generally denser than water. They rely on physical as well as pharmacological features to achieve their effect. For a particular carbon skeleton, changes in halogenation alter both physical and pharmaco-logical properties. This is best demonstrated by the methyl ethyl ether skeleton common to desflurane, enflurane and isoflurane.

Solubility is reduced with lowering of molecular weight. Fluoride ions are lighter than chloride and bromide ones,

Physical
Liquid at room temperature
Low latent heat of vaporisation
Low specific heat capacity
SVP sufficiently high to allow for easy vaporisation
Stable in light
Stable at room temperature
Non-flammable
Inexpensive
Environmentally safe (locally and globally)

Pharmacological
Pleasant smell
Low blood/gas solubility
Potent enough to provide surgical anaesthesia
    without supplement (low MAC)
High oil/water solubility
Analgesic effect
Non-epileptogenic
No cardiac irritability
No cardiovascular depression
No respiratory depression
Non-irritant to airways
Muscle relaxation
No increase in intracranial pressure (ICP)
Unaffected by renal failure
Unaffected by hepatic failure
Minimal metabolism

Figure GV2 Characteristics of an ideal volatile agent

	MW (daltons)	BP at 1 atm (°C)	SVP at 20 °C (kPa)	MAC (% v/v)	Ostwald solubility coefficients (dimensionless)[a]					
					O/W	Bl/G	W/G	Br/G	O/G	Br/Bl
Desflurane	168	22.8	88.5	6.35	N/A	0.42	N/A	0.54	19	1.3
Enflurane	184.5	56.5	22.9	1.68	120	1.9	0.78	2.6	98	96
Halothane	197	50.2	32.5	0.75	220	2.3	0.8	4.8	224	1.9
Isoflurane	184.5	48.5	31.9	1.15	174	1.43	0.62	21	91	1.6
Sevoflurane	200	58.6	21.3	2.00	N/A	0.69	N/A	1.1	53	1.7
Nitrous oxide	44	− 88	5300	105	3.2	0.47	0.44	1.4	1.0	
Xenon	131.2	−108		71	19	0.12	0.075		1.8	0.17
Ethyl chloride[b]	64.5	13	132							

[a] O/W, oil/water; Bl/G, blood/gas; W/G, water/gas; Br/G, brain/gas; O/G, oil/gas; Br/Bl, brain/blood.
[b] Although no longer used as a volatile agent by inhalation, ethyl chloride remains in practice as a cutaneous analgesic when applied as a spray. It is included here for the sake of completeness.

Figure GV3 Physical properties of volatile agents and anaesthetic gases

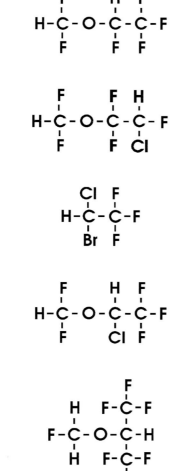

Figure GV4 Chemical structures of volatile agents

	Worst <————> Best			
	0	1	2	3
Induction	D	E/I	H	S
Cardiovascular stability		H	D/E/I	S
Respiratory irritation		D	E/I	H/S
Ease of titration	H	E/I	S	D
Emergence	H	I	E/S	D
Metabolism/toxicity	H	E/S	I	D
Cost (low flow)		S	D/E/I	H

Figure GV5 Ranking of clinical properties of volatile agents

Increasing fluorination of a carbon skeleton increases saturated vapour pressure and stability but reduces boiling point, flammability and toxicity. Methyl ethyl ether is flammable, but desflurane, enflurane and isoflurane are not.

Clinical
The comparative clinical properties of the major volatile agents are summarised in Figures GV5 and GV6.

Central nervous system
Volatile agents cause a dose-dependent depression of cerebral activity on the EEG. Cerebral oxygen consumption reduces in line with this. Epileptiform spikes occur with enflurane. All the volatile agents increase CBF and thus ICP, and should be used with caution where raised ICP may be a problem. Apart from nitrous oxide, analgesia is not a feature of the volatile agents used in current practice.
Relative effects:
- Cerebral blood flow: H, E > D, I, S
- ICP: H, E > D > I, S

Respiratory system
A dose-dependent depression of respiration occurs. This is manifest as reduced tidal volume with increased rate (except sevoflurane, which lowers rate), causing an overall reduction in alveolar minute volume. This is most marked with enflurane. Arterial CO_2 levels rise. The responses to hypercarbia and hypoxia are reduced.

Halothane in particular, but also enflurane and sevoflurane, cause bronchodilatation by reducing bronchial smooth muscle tone.

Desflurane and to a lesser extent isoflurane are irritant and stimulate bronchial and salivary secretion.

and thus desflurane, having fluoride ions in place of chloride, is comparatively less soluble than enflurane or isoflurane. Potency increases with increasing molecular weight, and the lighter desflurane is less potent than either enflurane or isoflurane. This may be related to the strong correlation of oil/water solubility with pharmacological potency (Section 3, Chapter 4, pages 551–2).

	Halothane	Enflurane	Isoflurane	Desflurane	Sevoflurane
Pungency	1	3	3	2	0
Respiratory irritation	0	1	2	3	0
Respiratory depression	2	4	3	4	2
Cardiovascular depression	3	3	2	1	1
Coronary vasodilatation	1	1	2	1	2
Muscle relaxation	2	2	3	3	3
Seizure induction	0	2	0	0	0
Rise in intracranial pressure	4	4	2	3	2

Figure GV6 Grading of clinical properties of volatile agents (0 = least effect, 4 = maximum effect)

Relative effects:
- Respiratory depression: D, E > I > H, S

Cardiovascular system

Cardiovascular depression is usual, with varying effects on contractility, heart rate and vascular resistance. Contractility is reduced by all agents, by interference with calcium ion movement. In clinical practice, contractility is affected by other factors such as preload and sympathetic stimulation. Direct effects, and indirect effects such as hypercarbia from respiratory depression, also influence these factors. Desflurane in particular appears to maintain contractility initially, perhaps as a result of increased sympathetic stimulation. Baroreceptor reflexes are also depressed.

Heart rate is primarily affected by the balance between sympathetic and para-sympathetic nervous systems. In general, heart rate increases in clinical usage. This is more marked with desflurane and isoflurane than with enflurane. However, halothane decreases heart rate, and sinus bradycardia, atrioventricular block, and ventricular premature contractions are not uncommon, especially in the presence of hypercarbia and increased circulating catecholamine levels. Conduction velocity in the atrioventricular node, His–Purkinje system and ventricles is reduced.

Systemic vascular resistance (SVR) is reduced with isoflurane and sevoflurane, and to a lesser extent with enflurane. Desflurane and halothane have little effect.

Blood-pressure changes are the result of the above effects. In general, blood pressure is reduced by a combination of reduced contractility, pre load and after-load.

Coronary vasodilatation alters coronary blood flow and may cause coronary 'steal'. This is more of a problem with isoflurane and sevoflurane than with the other agents.

Sensitisation of the myocardium to catecholamines, both endogenous and exogenous, may result in arrhythmias.

Relative effects:
- Conduction velocity slowing: H > E > I, S
- Catecholamine sensitisation: H > E > D, I, S

Muscle relaxation

There is a dose-dependent depression of neuromuscular function, with potentiation of both depolarising and non-depolarising neuromuscular blocking agents. While this is probably mediated by the neuromuscular junction, there may also be a direct reduction in contractility.

Metabolic rate

A decrease in metabolic rate causes a secondary reduction in oxygen consumption and carbon dioxide production. Inhalation of 2 MAC of a volatile agent reduces basal metabolic rate of oxygen consumption ($BMRO_2$) by 30%.

Toxicity

Increasing fluorination of a carbon skeleton reduces both metabolism and toxicity. While 2.4% of enflurane is metabolised, the corresponding amount for desflurane is 0.02%. Higher levels of metabolism increase the amount of potentially toxic metabolites and so increase toxicity. Fluoride production is greater in the morbidly obese than in non-obese patients when using halothane or enflurane. There is no difference when using sevoflurane.

Soda lime

Formation of carbon monoxide can occur when dry (used) soda lime comes into contact with desflurane, enflurane or isoflurane. Note that this is not a problem with halothane or sevoflurane. To avoid the problem, fresh soda lime should be used and prolonged periods of flushing the soda lime canister with dry oxygen and high gas flows should be avoided. At low flows, humidity will be high and the absorbent will function correctly.

Immune system

Volatile anaesthetic agents reduce the killing function of polymorphonuclear cells by interfering with calcium flux and superoxide generation.

Desflurane

Chemical name – 1,2,2,2-tetrafluoroethyl difluoro-methyl ether (halogenated ether)

Properties

MW	BP	SVP	MAC	O/W	Bl/G	O/G	Br/Bl
168	22.8	88.5	6.35	N/A	0.42	19	1.3

Presentation – pure agent without preservative or stabilisers supplied in brown bottle with self-closing valve, which fits special vaporiser

Storage – at room temperature away from heat

Soda lime – compatible, but avoid exhausted, dry granules

CNS – anaesthesia, no analgesia, not epileptogenic

CVS – dose-dependent depression similar to isoflurane

RS – dose-dependent depression; respiratory irritant; increased secretions

Others – muscle relaxants potentiated; stimulation of salivary secretions

Elimination – predominantly via lungs; 0.02% metabolised in liver

Contraindications – risk of triggering malignant hyperthermia

Desflurane has a boiling point close to ambient temperature with a high saturated vapour pressure. This necessitates the use of a special heated pressurised vaporiser. Superficially, this looks similar to the usual plenum vaporisers, but closer examination reveals a sophisticated microprocessor-controlled unit. The desflurane is heated and the vapour kept under pressure. Pure desflurane is then injected into the incoming fresh gas, which is also heated. The system is very accurate. The vaporiser can be filled without switching off. The unit is mains-operated, and is locked until the operating temperature is reached.

The low blood/gas solubility coefficient is close to nitrous oxide, but desflurane is more potent. This produces a rapid response to changes in inhaled concentration, and rapid recovery. However, to the respiratory tract, it is the most irritant volatile agent and it increases bronchial and salivary secretions. This reduces the rate at which the inspired concentration may be increased during induction and offsets the benefit of its rapid approximation of inhaled and alveolar concentrations. Concentrations of above 6% during induction have a relatively high incidence of coughing, breath-holding and laryngospasm (especially in children under 12 years of age), and it is not recommended for inhalational induction in children.

Desflurane depresses cardiac contractility, but this is less pronounced than with the other agents, perhaps as a result of sympathetic stimulation. During prolonged anaesthesia, this depression is less prominent. Initially SVR does not change, but above 2.2 MAC it falls. As a result, the blood pressure falls and heart rate increases to compensate. Coronary vasodilatation and increased blood flow occur. There is a theoretical risk of coronary 'steal'. Desflurane does not sensitise the heart to catecholamines. There is a dose-dependent depression of the respiratory centre, with reduced tidal volume and increased rate. The response to carbon dioxide is reduced (shifted to the right). Desflurane potentiates the effects of muscle relaxants, benzodiazepines and opioids. As only 0.02% is metabolised, toxicity is likely to be very low.

Enflurane

Chemical name – 2-chloro-1,1,2-trifluoroethyl difluoromethyl ether (halogenated ether)

Properties

MW	BP	SVP	MAC	O/W	Bl/G	O/G	Br/B
184.5	56.5	22.9	1.68	120	1.9	98	96

Colour code – orange

Presentation – colourless liquid in brown glass bottle with keyed filling system collar

Storage – at room temperature away from heat

Soda lime – compatible, but avoid exhausted dry granules

CNS – anaesthesia, minimal analgesia; epileptogenic and excitatory muscular effects

CVS – negative inotrope; vasodilatation with mild reflex tachycardia; coronary vasodilatation; increased rate of phase 4 depolarisation; slight myocardial sensitisation to catecholamines

RS – dose-dependent respiratory depression, predominantly tidal volume, increased or decreased rate; bronchodilator, non-irritant, no increase in secretions

- **Others** – muscle relaxants potentiated; blood pressure-dependent decreased splanchnic circulation; decreased renal blood flow and glomerular filtration rate; decreased uterine tone in pregnancy
- **Elimination** – predominantly via lungs; 2.4% metabolised
- **Contraindications** – epilepsy, risk of triggering malignant hyperthermia

Enflurane is administered using a standard specific plenum vaporiser. It produces anaesthesia without specific analgesia. In concentrations above 3% enflurane causes epileptiform spikes, especially if there is hypocarbia. There is a risk of inducing an epileptic fit in susceptible patients, and enflurane is best avoided in patients with epilepsy. This risk persists for several days after administration.

There is potentiation of neuromuscular blockade, but excitatory muscle twitching may also occur from the centrally mediated activity.

Metabolism of enflurane produces inorganic fluoride ions. These peak within 8 hours of administration and are unlikely to reach renally damaging levels. However, enflurane is best avoided in chronic renal failure.

Halothane

- **Chemical name** – 1-bromo-1-chloro-2,2,2-trifluoro-ethane (halogenated alkane)
- **Properties**

MW	BP	SVP	MAC	O/W	Bl/G	O/G	Br/Bl
197	50.2	32.5	0.75	220	2.3	224	1.9

- **Colour code** – red
- **Presentation** – clear, colourless liquid in brown glass bottle with keyed filling system collar; 0.1% thymol to protect against decomposition by light
- **Storage** – at room temperature away from heat
- **Soda lime** – compatible
- **CNS** – anaesthesia, no analgesia; not epileptogenic
- **CVS** – dose-dependent depression of contractility and heart rate; sensitisation to catecholamines
- **RS** – dose-dependent depression (but may increase rate), reduced tidal and minute volumes; bronchodilatation; non-irritant
- **Other** – postoperative shivering is common; muscle relaxants potentiated
- **Elimination** – 60–80% unchanged via lungs, 20% metabolised in liver (metabolites are excreted in urine for several weeks)
- **Contraindications** – risk of triggering malignant hyperthermia; contraindicated if previous pyrexia or jaundice following prior administration. For

halothane hepatitis see Section 3, Chapter 4 (page 555).

The thymol preservative does not readily evaporate, and therefore builds up in the vaporiser, which requires drainage and cleaning at regular intervals. Halothane may corrode aluminium, tin, lead, magnesium, brass and solder alloys in the presence of water. Halothane is usually administered via a specifically calibrated plenum vaporiser but drawover vaporisers may also be used (e.g. Goldman).

Halothane produces anaesthesia without specific analgesia, and has a low propensity for causing nausea and vomiting. CBF and ICP are increased, and it should be used with caution if ICP is raised.

Halothane reduces myocardial contractility, and decreases heart rate by vagal stimulation. Phase 4 depolarisation and cardiac conduction velocity are slowed. The combination of this and increased irritability may allow ventricular premature beats, bigeminy and other rhythm disturbances to occur. There is no increase in circulating catecholamines, but administered epinephrine increases the risk of cardiac arrhythmias, especially in the presence of hypoxia and hypercarbia. The administration of epinephrine of greater than 1 : 100 000 concentration, more than 100 μg in 10 minutes, and more than 300 μg per hour should be avoided.

SVR is not affected. Blood pressure is reduced and left ventricular end-diastolic pressure is increased, leading to decreased coronary perfusion. This is offset by a reduction in cardiac oxygen utilisation.

Tidal volume is reduced and respiratory rate increased. The ventilatory response curve to carbon dioxide shifts to the right. Minute volume may fall or stay the same. Halothane is non-irritant to the respiratory tract and causes bronchodilatation; anatomical dead space is therefore increased. It reduces salivary and bronchial secretions and is still the agent of choice for inhalational induction where airways obstruction is a significant problem, e.g. epiglottitis.

Halothane reduces gastrointestinal motility and reduces uterine tone. Skeletal muscle tone is reduced and neuromuscular blockade is potentiated, but there may be postoperative shivering.

Increased depth of anaesthesia reduces renal blood flow, glomerular filtration rate and urine output.

The secretion of vasopressin, thyroxine, growth hormone and corticosteroids is increased. Insulin secretion is not affected but insulin sensitivity is increased; glucose levels do not change, however.

Halothane reduces metabolic rate, oxygen consumption and carbon dioxide production. Twenty per cent of halothane is metabolised and it takes 3 weeks to clear completely from the body. The main metabolites are trifluoroacetic acid, chloride and bromide, which appear in the urine. Of patients receiving halothane 50% show a temporary rise in glutathione S-transferase.

Isoflurane

Chemical name – 1-chloro-2,2,2-trifluoroethyl difluoromethyl ether (halogenated ether)

Properties

MW	BP	SVP	MAC	O/W	Bl/G	O/G	Br/Bl
184.5	48.5	31.9	1.15	174	1.43	91	1.6

Colour code – purple

Presentation – colourless liquid in brown glass bottle, with keyed filling system collar, without additive or preservative

Storage – at room temperature away from heat

Soda lime – compatible, but avoid exhausted dry granules

CNS – anaesthesia, no analgesia, not epileptogenic

CVS – decreased blood pressure and systemic vascular resistance; heart rate rises

RS – decreased volume, increased rate, decreased minute volume; moderate respiratory irritant; increases bronchial secretions

Other – muscle relaxants potentiated; stimulation of salivary secretions

Elimination – primarily via lungs; 0.2% metabolised in liver

Contraindications – risk of triggering malignant hyperthermia

Isoflurane is a potent volatile anaesthetic agent, with an average speed of equilibration between inspired and tissue levels. The physical properties of boiling point and saturated vapour pressure are very similar to halothane, so the vaporiser design is also closely related.

Isoflurane causes anaesthesia without specific analgesia. It is not epileptogenic. It causes cerebral vasodilatation and there is a risk of 'steal', where vasodilatation of healthy vessels diverts blood flow away from critically perfused areas supplied by non-compliant vessels, which cannot dilate further. This is compounded by the reduction in blood pressure. Total CBF is increased and ICP may rise.

Isoflurane acts directly on blood vessels, reducing blood pressure by reducing SVR. There is a compensatory increase in heart rate, but cardiac output changes little. Isoflurane has little effect on contractility (excepting at multiples of MAC, when contractility is adversely affected). The baroreceptor reflex is depressed. Myocardial work and oxygen consumption are reduced.

Isoflurane is pungent and causes some respiratory irritation, necessitating slower increases in inspired concentration than with halothane, enflurane or sevoflurane, and making inhalational induction more difficult. Isoflurane reduces tidal and minute volumes with increased respiratory rate. It reduces the responses to hypercarbia and hypoxia and carbon dioxide rises. Bronchial smooth muscle tone is reduced with increasing depth, but during the initial stages of anaesthesia the respiratory irritancy may precipitate coughing and bronchospasm.

Isoflurane facilitates neuromuscular blockade.

Only 0.2% is metabolised, and toxicity from metabolites is therefore very low.

Sevoflurane

Chemical name – fluoromethyl-2,2,2-trifluoro-1-(trifluoromethyl) ethyl ether (halogenated ether)

Properties

MW	BP	SVP	MAC	O/W	Bl/G	O/G	Br/Bl
200	58.6	21.3	2.0	N/A	0.69	53	1.7

Colour code – yellow

Presentation – no preservative; supplied in brown bottle with keyed filling system collar

Storage – at room temperature away from heat

Soda lime – compatible, but may produce Compound A (see below)

CNS – anaesthesia, no analgesia, not epileptogenic

CVS – decreased heart rate, systemic vascular resistance and blood pressure but stable cardiac output; no myocardial sensitisation to catecholamines

RS – dose-dependent depression of respiratory rate and tidal volume; bronchodilatation

Other – muscle relaxants potentiated; uterine relaxation in pregnancy similar to isoflurane

Elimination – predominantly via the lungs; 5% metabolised by cytochrome P_{450}

Contraindications – risk of triggering malignant hyperthermia

Sevoflurane has similar physicochemical characteristics to enflurane and isoflurane, but is a little less volatile. It is administered using a plenum vaporiser. It differs from the other agents in having lower blood/gas and lower oil/gas solubilities. This produces a more rapid response to changes in inhaled concentration, and speedier induction and recovery. The higher MAC (2.0), indicating lower potency, is predictable from the oil/gas coefficient.

Sevoflurane produces anaesthesia without analgesia or epileptogenic spikes in a similar way to desflurane and isoflurane. ICP is raised but this effect is minimal at less than 1 MAC.

Sevoflurane reduces blood pressure primarily by reducing SVR, with little effect on cardiac output until higher doses are used. It lowers heart rate, in contrast with enflurane, isoflurane, and desflurane. There is less coronary vasodilatation than with isoflurane, and coronary blood flow does not change. The reduced heart rate reduces myocardial oxygen consumption so the relationship between supply and demand may be improved.

Sevoflurane reduces tidal volume and respiratory rate. Hypoxic drive is reduced, as is sensitivity to carbon dioxide tension. Sevoflurane reduces bronchial smooth muscle tone and so increases anatomical dead space. It has low respiratory irritancy.

Uterine muscle is relaxed to a similar degree to isoflurane. The potentiation of neuromuscular blockade is similar to other agents. Malignant hyperthermia has occurred with sevoflurane so it should be avoided in at-risk patients.

Most sevoflurane is eliminated via the lungs. Five per cent is metabolised by cytochrome P_{450}, producing hexafluoroisopropanol (CF_3-CHOH-CF_3) and inorganic fluoride ions. A plasma fluoride ion concentration of 50 μmol l^{-1} is quoted as the threshold for renal toxicity. Sevoflurane metabolism can produce levels above this threshold. The potentially hepatotoxic hexafluoroisopropanol is rapidly conjugated before it can cause damage.

Compound A

Sevoflurane is absorbed and degraded by CO_2 absorbers. At temperatures above 65 °C five breakdown products are formed (Compounds A–E). In the lower temperatures encountered clinically, sevoflurane only produces Compound A (CH_2F-O-C(CF_3)=CF_2) and a lesser amount of Compound B (CHF_2-O-CH(CF_2-O-CH_3)-CF_3). The concentrations are higher with baralyme than with soda lime because baralyme attains a higher temperature and the breakdown is temperature-dependent. The concentrations of Compounds A and B are substantially lower than the toxicity threshold in animal studies. A new zeolite-coated soda lime may absorb these compounds. Possible toxicity effects are renal, hepatic and brain.

'Wet' and 'dry' formulations

In 1996 and 1997 specific batches of sevoflurane were found to contain hydrofluoric acid, which reacts with glass and can be toxic. This was because Lewis acids in the presence of some metals such as iron promote the breakdown of sevoflurane. However, the small amounts produced were unlikely to cause serious toxicity. Water inhibits Lewis acids. Two formulations of sevoflurane, 'wet' and 'dry', are now available, the 'wet' having had additional water added at the final stage of production. The 'wet' sevoflurane (330 ppm water) is supplied in a plastic bottle and the 'dry' (130 ppm) in a lacquer-lined aluminium bottle. Clinically there is no difference between the two products, and no convincing evidence of increased risk has yet been found. Stored according to manufacturers' instructions, there should be minimal degradation of either formulation of sevoflurane. Compound A production occurs in the soda lime canister, where water content will be considerably higher.

Nitrous oxide

Structure – resonant hybrid of two forms N=N=O and N≡N–O (anaesthetic gas)

Properties

MW	BP	SVP	MAC	O/W	Bl/G	O/G	Br/Bl
44	−88	5300	105	3.2	0.47	1.4	1.0

Critical temperature – +36.5 °C

Critical pressure – 72.6 bar

Presentation – supplied in cylinders as the pure liquid (no water vapour) under pressure (44 bar at 15 °C); filling ratio 0.75

Colour code – cylinders French blue; rotameter knob blue; pin index 3,5

Storage – at room temperature away from extremes of heat; non-explosive; not flammable but can support combustion because it decomposes to oxygen and nitrogen above 450 °C

Soda lime – compatible

CNS – analgesia, sedation; not epileptogenic

CVS – increased vascular tone, rise in blood pressure

RS – decreased tidal volume, increased rate; non-irritant

Other – increased skeletal muscle activity; emetogenic

Elimination – predominantly via lungs

Contraindications – diffuses into air-filled spaces causing expansion; prolonged use interferes with vitamin B_{12}

Nitrous oxide is a vapour rather than a gas (because it is usually met below its critical temperature). It is manufactured by heating ammonium nitrate (NH_4NO_3) to 240 °C. Toxic impurities (nitric oxide and nitrogen dioxide) and water vapour are removed. The gas is pumped into cylinders and the pressure causes it to liquefy. Any volatile liquid has a specific pressure for any given temperature (the saturated vapour pressure). In use, therefore, the pressure in the nitrous oxide cylinder is maintained until all the liquid nitrous oxide has been used; the pressure then falls rapidly. The pressure does in fact fall slightly during use because conversion of the liquid to vapour uses latent heat of vaporisation, which cools the remaining liquid. The amount of cooling is determined by the specific heat capacity of the liquid nitrous oxide.

As nitrous oxide has a low anaesthetic potency, it is usually administered using a needle control valve and a rotameter marked in litres per minute rather than a vaporiser marked in percentages. It may be administered via a Hudson mask, although scavenging is not then possible.

Rapid equilibration of the brain concentration with the inhaled concentration occurs, but the low anaesthetic potency necessitates the use of adjuncts to provide anaesthesia rather than dissociated sedation. Usually the adjunct is a volatile anaesthetic agent, but intravenous anaesthetic agents are also suitable. The importance of this agent in anaesthetic practice is that it reduces the concentration of volatile agent required so that induction and recovery can be more rapidly achieved than by using the volatile agent alone. This is of limited benefit with the newer agents (desflurane and sevoflurane). But isoflurane, and especially desflurane and sevoflurane, are relatively expensive, and concurrent use of nitrous oxide makes economic sense. The reduced concentration required is also advantageous when the volatile agent is irritant to the respiratory tract.

Nitrous oxide suppresses spinal impulses and may suppress supraspinal pathways in part by activation of inhibitory mechanisms. It has a moderate analgesic effect that may be effected through central nervous system endorphins and enkephalins. The analgesic effects are partly antagonised by naloxone.

Cerebral vasodilatation occurs, with increased CBF and raised ICP.

Myocardial contractility is reduced by a direct effect but this is neutralised by an increased sympathetic tone (alpha and beta stimulation). Vascular tone is increased generally, causing rises in central venous pressure, systemic vascular resistance and peripheral vascular resistance. Blood pressure is usually raised a little, but may decrease if cardiac output is compromised.

Nitrous oxide decreases tidal volume and increases respiratory rate. The overall effect is an increased minute volume. There is little effect on CO_2 tension, but the responses to hypercarbia and hypoxia are impaired. The gas is non-irritant to the respiratory tract but ciliary activity is reduced.

Skeletal muscle activity is increased, probably because of supraspinal excitation. In contrast with the volatile agents, neuromuscular function is not affected and neuromuscular blocking agents are not facilitated. Neutrophil chemotaxis is impaired.

The oxyhaemoglobin dissociation curve (in vitro) is shifted to the left (affinity for oxygen increased).

Nitrous oxide interacts with vitamin B_{12} (cyanocobalamin), converting the monovalent cobalt to the bivalent form. This prevents it functioning as the coenzyme for methionine synthase and methyl malonyl CoA mutase. Methionine synthase catalyses conversion of homocysteine to methionine, and the demethylation of methyltetrahydrate. The latter is an essential step in the synthesis of thymidine for DNA synthesis. Bone-marrow DNA synthesis is impaired, resulting in megaloblastic changes with metabolic precursors appearing in the circulation. Eventually neutropenia and thrombocytopenia also occur. The initial changes are seen with exposure of 6–24 hours duration, but in seriously ill patients as little as 2 hours will show effects. Chronic nitrous oxide abusers develop neurological damage similar to subacute combined degeneration of the cord secondary to a decrease in hepatic S-adenosyl methionine. Nitrous oxide may also have an inhibitory effect on methionine synthesis at very low concentrations (less than 1000 ppm). COSHH regulations specify a time-weighted 8-hour exposure of less than 100 ppm.

Biotransformation occurs in minimal amounts. As nitrous oxide is relatively insoluble, it is excreted predominantly by the lungs. Anaerobic bacteria in the gut can also cause decomposition.

Nitrous oxide is more soluble in blood than nitrogen (34-fold). Nitrous oxide diffuses into air-filled spaces (containing oxygen, nitrogen, carbon dioxide and water vapour) quicker than nitrogen diffuses out, resulting in an increase in volume or an increase in pressure within a fixed volume space.

50% Nitrous oxide in oxygen (Entonox®)

Presentation – supplied in cylinders as a gas under pressure (137 bar); liquefies at −6 °C; filling ratio 0.75

Colour code – cylinder body French blue, shoulder French blue and white quarters; pin index is a specific large single pin offset from centre

Storage – at room temperature away from extremes of heat; may separate if exposed to low temperatures (0 °C), in which case re-warm and invert to restore the mixture

Non-explosive – not flammable but supports combustion

CNS – broadly similar to nitrous oxide

CVS – broadly similar to nitrous oxide

RS – broadly similar to nitrous oxide

Other – mainly used as an inhaled analgesic (e.g. in labour)

Elimination – predominantly via lungs

Contraindications – as for nitrous oxide

Xenon (Xe)

Properties

MW	BP	MAC	O/W	Bl/G	O/G	Br/Bl
131.2	−108	71	19	0.12	1.8	0.17

Soda lime – compatible

CNS – anaesthesia, analgesia

CVS – very cardiostable, no reduction of contractility, increased CBF, no sensitisation to catecholamines

RS – non-irritant, increased tidal volume, reduced rate

Elimination – unchanged, via lungs

Xenon is a possible anaesthetic agent for the future. It is a rare or noble gas (like helium and argon) existing in monovalent form and present in atmospheric air in a concentration of 0.086 ppm (0.0000086%). It is obtained from fractional 'distillation' of liquefied air and is very expensive. Xenon is non-flammable and does not support combustion. As an anaesthetic agent it has a very low Bl/G solubility coefficient, giving rapid induction and emergence. It has a high MAC (low potency). It is highly cardiostable with no sensitisation of the myocardium to catecholamines and no reduction in contractility. It does not trigger malignant hyperthermia or cause respiratory irritation. At concentrations above 60% cerebral blood flow is increased. Xenon inhibits plasma membrane Ca^{2+} pump and inhibits dorsal horn neurones by NMDA inhibition. Problems of expense and availability are the major obstacles to its use, as well as the difficulty of monitoring inspired and expired concentrations. Higher density and (to a lesser extent) higher viscosity than oxygen–nitrous oxide combinations result in the need for higher driving pressures during ventilation.

CHAPTER 6

Hypnotics and intravenous anaesthetic agents

T. C. Smith

General features

Anaesthetic agents are usually administered either by the IV or by the inhalational route, but they may also be given rectally or intramuscularly. The advantages of administering drugs intravenously rather than orally are listed in Figure HY1.

Pharmacokinetics

The pharmacokinetic profiles of most IV anaesthetic agents are similar to that of thiopental, which is shown in Figure PK4 (Section 3, Chapter 3). They result from a rapid transfer of drug from the blood to the brain tissue, followed by a rapid distribution to other tissues. This reduces the plasma level so that the drug diffuses back from the brain into the plasma, from where it is redistributed to other tissues. The result is a brief duration of anaesthesia with

Quick onset as enteral absorption is bypassed
Dose not reduced by the first-pass effect (bioavailability 100%)
Lower total dose required
Quicker recovery with single dose due to redistribution as gut does not act as reservoir
Greater control therefore suitable for infusion

Figure HY1 Advantages of intravenous drug administration, compared with oral administration

a rapid recovery. Elimination of the drugs subsequently occurs more slowly. Thiopental concentrations peak in the vessel-rich group of tissues (including the brain) within 1–2 minutes. Within a further 1 minute the brain level falls again due to redistribution to the muscle group, to reach near equilibrium in about 15–20 minutes. The

Fundamentals of Anaesthesia, 3rd edition, ed. Tim Smith, Colin Pinnock and Ted Lin. Published by Cambridge University Press. © Cambridge University Press 2008.

redistribution to fat tissues is slow, peaking at 3 hours, due to the relatively poor blood supply. However, the capacity of the fat tissues is large. The fat group contributes little to the immediate recovery but accounts for the prolonged elimination.

Adverse reactions

Adverse reactions to IV agents vary from the trivial (muscular movements) to the serious (anaphylactoid or anaphylactic reactions). The incidence of serious adverse reactions to common IV anaesthetic agents is shown in Figure HY2.

Propofol	1 : 50 000–100 000
Thiopental	1 : 14 000–20 000
Etomidate	1 : 450 000

Figure HY2 Incidence of serious adverse reactions to intravenous agents

The ideal agent

No currently available agent fulfils the criteria of an 'ideal' anaesthetic agent. The concept remains useful, nonetheless, as a yardstick for assessing new agents. Properties of an ideal agent are given in Figure HY3.

Barbiturates

Examples – pentobarbital, phenobarbital, thiopental

Chemical structure

Barbiturates are based on barbituric acid, which contains the six-membered pyrimidine nucleus that is a building block of nucleosides. Oxypyrimidines may exist in two structural forms, enol and keto (Figure HY4). Thiobarbiturates have a similar pair of structural forms. Chemically, barbituric acid is a condensation product (formation of the chemical bonds involves the removal of water molecules) of malonic acid and urea. Substitutions on atoms at positions 1, 2 and 5 confer and modulate hypnotic activity.

Structure–activity relationship

Barbituric acid has no hypnotic activity. Clinically active barbiturates are created by the addition of various alkyl groups to C-5. Oxybarbiturates (e.g. phenobarbital) are the basic form of barbiturate. It is thought that the $GABA_A$ receptor has a binding site for these barbiturates, which have a slow onset of action and a long duration. They function well as basal hypnotics and sedatives but are too

Physical
Soluble in aqueous medium
Stable in solution
Stable in air within the container
Stable when diluted
Stable in light
Stable at room temperature
Inexpensive

Pharmacological
Potent enough to provide surgical anaesthesia without supplement
Induction in one arm–brain circulation time
High oil/water solubility
Analgesia
No pain on injection
Non-epileptogenic
No cardiac irritability
No cardiovascular depression
No respiratory depression
Muscle relaxation
No increase in intracranial pressure
Non-cumulative with infusion
Unaffected by renal and hepatic failure
Metabolites inactive and non-toxic
Non-teratogenic

Figure HY3 Properties of an ideal intravenous anaesthetic agent

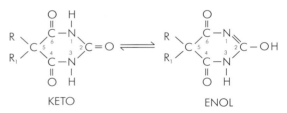

Figure HY4 Basic chemical structure of barbiturates showing enol and keto forms

slow for use as anaesthetic agents. Replacing the oxygen on C-2 with sulphur produces a thiobarbiturate (e.g. thiopental), which has a rapid onset of action and a relatively short duration of action and recovery period. Replacing the hydrogen on N_1 of the basic oxybarbiturate with a methyl group produces a methylbarbiturate (e.g. methohexital). Methylbarbiturates also have a rapid onset and short duration of action plus a short recovery. However, they also produce some excitatory activity that takes the

		Position 2	
		Oxygen	**Sulphur**
Position 1	**Hydrogen**	Oxybarbiturate (phenobarbital)	Thiobarbiturate (thiopental)
	Methyl group	Methylbarbiturate (methohexital)	Methylthiobarbiturate (no clinical use)

Figure HY5 Structural classification of barbiturates

form of sporadic uncoordinated movements during induction of anaesthesia. These may be mild or vigorous, but are usually distinguishable from the repetitive jerking of epileptiform convulsions, or the diffuse muscular shimmering (fasciculation) seen with suxamethonium. Modification of the alkyl groups on C-5 alters the potency of the drug. Oxy-, methyl-, and thio-barbiturates are all clinically useful, but the addition of both sulphur and a methyl group (methylthiobarbiturates) results in excessive excitatory activity precluding its use in the clinical setting.

The structural classification of barbiturates is shown in Figure HY5.

Clinical effects

Phenobarbital and pentobarbital have a slow onset of action, and provide anxiolysis and anticonvulsant activity. The intravenously administered induction agent thiopental is the most relevant to anaesthetic practice: it is a water-soluble barbiturate agent that induces anaesthesia within one arm–brain circulation time of IV injection. It is highly lipophilic, and easily and rapidly crosses the blood–brain barrier to penetrate the brain.

Complications associated with barbiturate usage

Porphyria

The porphyrias are a group of diverse diseases of inborn or acquired errors of metabolism that result in the secretion of excessive amounts of porphyrins and precursors (Figure HY6).

Porphyrins comprise four pyrrole rings linked together to form a larger ring. They are fundamental constituents of haemoglobin, myoglobin, cytochromes and catalases, and all contain iron. Porphyria is very rare in the UK. While still rare, **acute intermittent porphyria** is more common in South Africa, Sweden and Finland, and **variegate porphyria** is more common in Sweden and Finland. These are both inherited by autosomal dominance, and are the most relevant to anaesthesia. They affect the liver, where haem is

Erythropoietic	Congenital erythropoietic porphyria
Hepatic	Acute intermittent porphyria Hereditary coproporphyria Variegate porphyria Porphyria cutanea tarda Toxic porphyria
Erythropoietic and hepatic	Protoporphyria

Figure HY6 Classification of porphyrias

produced as a component of the cytochrome P_{450} enzyme, and therefore affect drug metabolism. Many drugs increase porphyrin production, and administration may result in neurotoxic porphyrin levels. Drugs to avoid include barbiturates, benzodiazepines and steroids, but propofol is thought to be safe.

Subcutaneous extravasation

Extravasation of thiopental, and to a lesser extent methohexital, causes localised pain and tissue damage due to the highly alkaline medium in which it is mixed. It does not usually cause major sequelae, but injection in proximity to a nerve may cause damage. The pain and bruising can be reduced by dilution with a small dose (10 ml) of saline, or 10 ml 1% procaine, which vasodilates as well as diluting the thiopental. The damage is due to the high pH, and is immediate, so any damage limitation measures should be performed as quickly as possible.

Intra-arterial injection

Intra-arterial injection of thiopental is a potentially serious complication, causing endothelial damage. This is related to the change in pH of the solution as it is diluted in the blood, which results in a precipitation of insoluble microcrystals that block the narrowing arterial tree – whereas in veins any such crystals are carried away and diluted so that they dissolve before causing any problems.

The precipitate causes arterial intimal damage, local release of norepinephrine and the release of ATP from damaged red cells and platelets, which initiates vascular thrombosis. Clinically there is pain, with delayed or absent onset of sleep. Blanching or cyanosis of the affected area, loss of the peripheral pulse of the injected limb and gangrene may occur. Arterial thrombosis may gradually develop, progressing for up to 15 days. The treatment is as follows:

- Stop the injection, but leave the needle or cannula in place.
- Dilute immediately by injecting normal saline into the artery.
- Administer local anaesthetic and/or vasodilator directly into the artery.
  - Lidocaine 50 mg (5 ml 1% solution)
  - Procaine hydrochloride 50–100 mg (10–20 ml 0.5% solution)
  - Phenoxybenzamine (α-adrenoceptor antagonist) 0.5 mg or infuse 50–200 μg min^{-1}
- Administer papaverine systemically 40–80 mg (10–20 ml 0.4% solution).
- Consider sympathetic neural blockade (stellate ganglion or brachial plexus block). This produces prolonged vasodilatation to improve circulation and tissue oxygenation while improving clearance of the crystals.
- Start IV heparin.
- Consider intra-arterial injection of hydrocortisone.
- Postpone non-urgent surgery.

Thiopental
Physical
Sodium thiopental is a thiobarbiturate. It is supplied in a rubber-topped bottle, as a pale yellow powder containing 6% anhydrous sodium carbonate (a base). The gaseous environment within the bottle is nitrogen. The sodium carbonate prevents CO_2 in the air from forming free acid that would react with the thiopental. The sodium ion replaces the hydrogen ion that associates with C-1 and C-2 of the base compound, as shown in Figure HY7.

The powder is readily soluble in water, producing a 2.5% (2.5 g 100 ml^{-1}) solution with pH 11. At pH 11, having a pK_a = 7.6, it is almost entirely (99.9%) ionised. However, once in the blood the pH falls towards 7.4 at which 61% of the drug is non-ionised. This non-ionised portion is the more lipid-soluble and readily crosses the blood–brain barrier into the lipid-rich brain tissue. Of the drug,

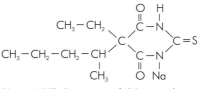

Figure HY7 Structure of thiopental

60–80% is reversibly bound to protein (mainly to albumin) and is therefore non-diffusible and inactive.

Clinical
IV injection of thiopental rarely causes pain, and venous thrombosis occurs in only 3–4% of patients. Characteristically, the subject may be aware of a taste of onions or garlic before the onset of sleep. The redistribution half-life of 4 minutes leads to rapid recovery.

Central nervous system
Thiopental causes cortical depression, with a plasma level of 40 μg ml^{-1} being typical for sleep. Rapid and smooth induction of anaesthesia occurs within one arm–brain circulation time with a low incidence (4%) of minor excitatory movements. Thiopental has no analgesic activity and may be antanalgesic. It is an anticonvulsant agent. During induction, the EEG shows the onset of high-amplitude waves of 10–30 Hz, followed by depression of cortical activity with an iso-electric picture accompanied by occasional bursts of 10 Hz activity.

Cerebral metabolic rate of oxygen consumption ($CMRO_2$) is reduced, which leads to cerebral vasoconstriction with a concomitant fall in cerebral blood flow (CBF) and ICP. The fall in blood pressure that also occurs leads to a fall in CBF, with an opposite effect on cerebral vascular resistance. The reduction in ICP and $CMRO_2$ are useful properties of thiopental for use in cerebral protection for situations such as cardiopulmonary bypass or standstill, and for the prevention of secondary brain damage in trauma.

A single large dose results in the return of wakefulness when the plasma level is higher than if smaller doses are used. This is termed acute tolerance. The technique of injecting a predetermined dose without slowly titrating it to effect allows the use of lower doses while still achieving satisfactory peak concentrations in the cerebral circulation and therefore the brain. A more rapid recovery results from a correspondingly more rapid fall in cerebral plasma thiopental concentration. Late recovery is also improved, as the total dose is lower.

Cardiovascular system

Thiopental causes a dose-dependent reduction in vascular tone with a reduction in SVR, CVP and PCWP. Preload and afterload are therefore both reduced, resulting in a decrease in mean arterial blood pressure and in left and right ventricular work. There is a slight compensatory increase in heart rate. High doses given rapidly can cause severe myocardial depression and hypotension, particularly in hypovolaemic patients or those receiving antihypertensive medication. Extreme caution should be exercised if thiopental is to be used in patients who cannot increase their cardiac output to compensate for a drop in vascular resistance, such as those with valvular stenosis or cardiac tamponade. Gradual administration can produce an iso-electric EEG without any significant effect on blood pressure or heart rate. Cardiac oxygen consumption is increased in normal individuals, but in ischaemic hearts the requirement is reduced.

Respiratory system

Thiopental causes a dose-dependent reduction in both respiratory rate and tidal volume. Manifestations of irritation such as cough and hiccup are uncommon, although it is less effective at depressing the laryngeal reflexes than propofol.

Other effects

Thiopental is not emetic. It has minimal effect on hepatic, renal or adrenal function. Uterine tone is unaffected, but it readily crosses the placenta, also diffusing back into the maternal circulation as plasma levels fall, so this is of little practical significance.

Metabolism

Metabolism occurs in the liver, with an extraction ratio of 0.1 to 0.4. Phase I mechanisms result in oxidation of the C-5 side chains, replacement of the sulphur with oxygen to produce pentobarbital and cleavage of the barbiturate ring into urea and a three-carbon portion. These actions are robust enough to cope with major liver dysfunction, so thiopental may still be suitable in hepatic failure. Clearance is insufficient to deal with repeated doses and cumulation therefore occurs.

Complications

Extravasation causes local damage and intra-arterial injection may cause serious damage distal to injection. Avoid in porphyria.

Steroids

Examples – eltanolone, hydroxydione, minaxolone. At present there are no steroid anaesthetic agents available for clinical use.

Physical

The steroid anaesthetic agents are based on the familiar steroid nucleus. Note that oxy- and hydroxy- substitutions at 3 and 20 appear to be associated with anaesthetic activity.

Clinical
Central nervous system

Most of the steroid agents produce a rapid onset of action (within one arm–brain circulation time) with smooth induction of anaesthesia, and a rapid recovery.

Cardiovascular system

The steroids are less depressant to the cardiovascular system than barbiturates and propofol.

Respiratory system

The steroids are less depressant to tidal volume and respiratory rate than the barbiturates or propofol.

Other effects

Anaesthetic and endocrine activities appear to have no structural relationship. There is a low incidence of postoperative nausea and vomiting. Excitatory phenomena are frequently problematic.

Complications

Toxicity is generally low, with a high therapeutic index. Local irritation is a problem.

Eltanolone (pregnanolone)

Eltanolone produces rapid induction and recovery of anaesthesia. However, this is slower than that of propofol and accumulation occurs. It is insoluble, and a soya bean emulsion is used. It has a terminal half-life of about 50–80 minutes. It has been abandoned because of cutaneous reactions.

Hydroxydione

Hydroxydione is a water-soluble steroid anaesthetic. It has little effect on cardiorespiratory physiology, some neuromuscular blockade with a low incidence of coughing and a very low incidence of nausea and vomiting. However, slow onset of action (several minutes), pain on injection and localised venous irritation have prevented its success.

Minaxolone

Minaxolone is a water-soluble steroid anaesthetic. It has a slower onset of action than althesin, and causes more excitatory activity. Clinical usefulness of minaxolone has been limited by associated convulsions and abnormal liver function tests.

ORG 20599 and ORG 21465

These two water-soluble aminosteroid anaesthetic agents, which have a high therapeutic index (about 13) in animals, have been blighted by excessive excitatory movements and stability problems, which limit human application.

Butyrophenones

Butyrophenones are covered in detail in Section 3, Chapter 10.

Phencyclidine derivatives

Example – ketamine

Physical

Ketamine is a derivative of phencyclidine and cyclohexamine. It is supplied as an aqueous solution in several concentrations, formulated as a weak acid with a pH between 3.5 and 5.5. Ketamine has a single chiral carbon atom. It is supplied as a racemic mixture of the two stereoisomers.

Pharmacodynamics

Ketamine is a non-competitive antagonist of the calcium ion channel operated by the excitatory NMDA glutamate receptor that is likely to be responsible for anaesthesia, analgesia and neurotoxicity. Ketamine also inhibits the NMDA receptor by stereoselectively binding to the phencyclidine (PCP) binding site. Ketamine interacts with the δ, κ and μ opioid receptors. S(+)ketamine provides more potent analgesia than R(−)ketamine. There is stereoselectivity for κ and μ receptors but not δ receptors. Evidence suggests that ketamine may be an antagonist at the μ receptor and that analgesia is not μ-mediated. Ketamine, especially R(−)ketamine, also interacts weakly with the σ receptor (formerly classified as an opioid receptor). The potency of ketamine at the receptors is in the order $\mu > \kappa > \sigma > \delta$.

High doses of ketamine have a local anaesthetic action, and there is supportive evidence of fast sodium channel blockade.

Ketamine also acts stereoselectively at muscarinic acetylcholine receptors. This action is likely to be antagonist, as ketamine produces anticholinergic effects such as bronchodilatation, delirium and a sympathomimetic action. Ketamine anaesthesia is antagonised by anticholinesterases. It is thought that ketamine may also have an effect on voltage-sensitive Ca^{2+} channels.

Clinical

Ketamine has a slow onset of action, taking about 1 minute after IV injection to achieve an effect. Ketamine can be administered intramuscularly, with an onset of sleep in 2–5 minutes and duration of 12–25 minutes. The role of extradurally and intrathecally administered ketamine has yet to be established but, in brief, it causes segmental blockade, and affects the receptors located in the spinal cord as described above.

Central nervous system

Ketamine produces sleep, analgesia and dissociation (a psychological detachment from the surrounding environment). The eyes frequently remain open, and eyelash, corneal and laryngeal reflexes are preserved to a variable extent. Muscle tone is increased and marked involuntary movements are common.

Unlike other typical induction agents, it affects the limbic system rather than the thalamocortical axis. Analgesia is effected by inhibition of the affective, emotional component of pain mediated by the thalamic reticular system rather than the transmission of the nociceptive signals. As well as a slow onset time, the duration of action is much longer than that of the faster induction agents. The recovery may be associated with hallucinations, diplopia or temporary blindness. These effects are a particular problem with short procedures but those lasting beyond an hour when anaesthesia has been maintained with other agents are less of a problem.

Dissociative side effects are less in males and children, and can be reduced by the concomitant use of opioids, benzodiazepine, droperidol or thiopental. There is no retrograde amnesia.

A significant rise (80%) in CBF, ICP, intraocular pressure (IOP) and $CMRO_2$ may persist for 30 minutes. The onset of effect is associated with a loss of α waves followed by a dominant θ wave on the EEG.

The (+) isomer is more potent than the (−) isomer for hypnosis, analgesia and dissociative effects, supporting the hypothesis that ketamine acts via receptor interaction.

Cardiovascular system

Ketamine increases heart rate, blood pressure and catecholamine levels by a generalised increase in CNS activity.

These changes are marked, with 30–100% increases. Direct myocardial depression counteracts the increased sympathetic activity and may leave stroke volume unaffected. Arrhythmias are not common.

Respiratory system

Ketamine has the advantage that, in the absence of opioid, it does not depress respiration greatly. It is a bronchodilator, and protective reflexes are preserved to some extent. Preserved airway maintenance is particularly useful, but reflex protection of the airway from aspiration cannot be guaranteed. Because of the sparing of these reflexes and an increase in secretions, coughing, hiccup and laryngospasm are more prevalent than with thiopental.

Other effects

In both parturient and non-parturient patients, uterine tone is increased. This is a particular problem in the presence of placental abruption or umbilical cord prolapse.

Metabolism

The pharmacokinetic profiles of both stereoisomers are identical. Ketamine is metabolised in the liver by N-desmethylation to norketamine. Norketamine has a half to a third of the potency of ketamine and is subsequently hydroxylated. Hydroxylation of the ketamine ring plays a minor role in its metabolism.

Most appears in the bile, with 20% as metabolites in the urine, but some appears unchanged in urine and faeces.

Imidazoles

Example – etomidate

Physical

Etomidate is a carboxylated imidazole. It is soluble in water but is unstable so it is formulated either in a mixture of water and propylene glycol (pH 8.1) or in a lipid emulsion. Etomidate has two stereoisomers, with R(+)etomidate being the predominant enhancer of GABA binding to the $GABA_A$ receptor. Figure HY8 shows the chiral carbon atom, and the ester linkage which is hydrolysed in its metabolism.

Clinical

Etomidate is a rapidly acting induction agent. It sometimes causes pain on injection, which is considerably less using the lipid emulsion.

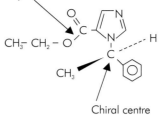

Figure HY8 Chemical structure of etomidate

Central nervous system

There is rapid induction of anaesthesia within one arm–brain circulation time. Excitatory muscle movements are much more frequent than with thiopental or methohexital. The EEG frequently shows epileptiform activity. Cerebral blood flow, ICP, $CMRO_2$ and IOP are reduced.

Cardiovascular system

Etomidate causes less cardiovascular depression than the barbiturates and is indicated when the cardiovascular status is delicate. It has relatively minor effects resulting in a fall in SVR, blood pressure and heart rate. There is a slight increase in contractility and cardiac output but oxygen delivery and utilisation are preserved.

Respiratory system

Etomidate reduces both tidal volume and rate. Depression is much less than that of the barbiturates.

Other effects

Histamine release is minimal. Etomidate has been used by infusion for ICU sedation. Unfortunately, it inhibits 11-β-hydroxylase and cholesterol cleavage, which results in inhibition of corticosteroid and mineralocorticoid synthesis. The suppression of steroid synthesis (part of the stress response to surgery) lasts for 3–6 hours after a single dose, but it is only of clinical significance when infused. It is no longer licensed for use by infusion.

Metabolism

Etomidate is metabolised by esterases in the plasma and liver to produce inactive metabolites that are excreted in the urine and bile. A small amount is excreted unchanged.

Phenols

Example – propofol

Physical

Propofol is an alkyl phenol (2,6-di-isopropyl phenol), having minimal solubility in water. It is formulated as an isotonic 1% emulsion in a mixture of soya bean oil, purified egg phosphatide, glycerol and sodium hydroxide. This has pH 6–8.5. It has a pK_a in water of 11 so at this pH it is almost entirely (>99%) non-ionised. Of the drug, 98% is protein-bound.

Propofol may be diluted using 5% dextrose to a lower limit of 2 mg ml^{-1} (0.2%) for infusion. To reduce the incidence of injection pain, 1 ml of 0.5% or 1% preservative-free lidocaine may be added to 20 ml propofol.

Clinical

Propofol provides a rapid and smooth induction of anaesthesia (within one arm–brain circulation time) and attenuates laryngeal reflexes better than the barbiturates.

Central nervous system

Propofol causes dose-dependent cortical depression. The EEG shows the development of α waves followed by slower δ waves as anaesthesia deepens. There is no epileptiform activity, although, in common with methohexital, excitatory movements are seen particularly with larger doses. Propofol is an anticonvulsant, and reports of epileptic fits following prolonged propofol infusion are now thought to be due to the rapid clearance of the anticonvulsant propofol from the body with a rebound excitation. Arguably it may not be the first choice for electroconvulsive therapy (ECT), as recovery is no better than with other agents and it reduces convulsion duration (although the efficacy may be unaffected). However, with the loss of methohexital from general availability it is becoming the prevalent option. It may have some limited anti-emetic activity.

The incidence of excitation, cough and hiccup are similar to those of thiopental. At equi-anaesthetic doses, laryngeal reflexes are attenuated more than with barbiturates, thus facilitating laryngeal mask insertion.

Cardiovascular system

Propofol causes a dose-dependent reduction in vascular tone that reduces systemic vascular resistance and central venous pressure. The reduction in preload, together with a fall in contractility, contributes to the fall in cardiac output and subsequent hypotension. Heart rate remains relatively unchanged. The reductions in systemic vascular resistance, blood pressure and cardiac output are more pronounced than with methohexital or thiopental. Propofol produces a variable but mild effect on heart rate.

Respiratory system

There is a fall in tidal volume with an increase in rate. The response to CO_2 is attenuated. Propofol is more depressant than thiopental. The response to intubation is suppressed more by propofol than by thiopental.

Other effects

The fat emulsion of propofol can produce hyperlipidaemia. The association of hepatomegaly, metabolic acidosis and mortality with propofol sedation in intensive care has led to the Commission on Human Medicines advice that the use of propofol by infusion is contraindicated in children of 16 years and below. In adults, it is widely used by infusion without apparent problem.

Metabolism

Propofol is conjugated in the liver by glucuronidation to make it water-soluble, with 88% appearing in the urine and 2% in the faeces. Renal and hepatic failure have little effect on propofol metabolism.

Complications

Complications include excitation, and pain on injection, the incidence of which is affected by:
- Site of injection
- Speed of injection
- Concentration of propofol in the aqueous phase
- Buffering effect of blood
- Speed of IV carrier fluid
- Temperature of the propofol
- Concomitant use of adjunct drugs

Immediate pain is probably due to a direct irritant effect, while delayed pain occurring 10–20 seconds after the start of injection is probably the result of activation of the kinin system.

Pain on injection can be reduced by the following measures:
- Using large veins
- Slow administration so that dilution of the injectate occurs
- 1 ml of 0.5% or 1% preservative-free lidocaine added to 20 ml propofol
- Administration of 2 ml lidocaine 1% into the vein prior to propofol injection
- Using different lipid formulations

Extravasation causes no major damage. Intra-arterial injection results in some pain, loss of the pulse and some blanching, but long-term there is no damage. The solvent is non-irritant and there is a low incidence of hypersensitivity, but note that the solvent is a good bacterial culture medium.

Propofol occasionally results in green urine.

Benzodiazepines

Examples – diazepam, lorazepam, midazolam, temazepam

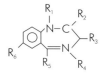

Benzene   Diazepine
ring   ring

Figure HY9 General structure of the benzodiazepine skeleton

Chemical

The benzodiazepine skeleton is a set of two rings (benzene and diazepine: Figure HY9), but most benzodiazepines also have a third ring at the R_5 position.

Structure–activity relationships are not clear, but modifications to the basic structure primarily affect the pharmacokinetic profile of the drug. Benzodiazepines may be classified as in Figure HY10.

Structure	Examples
1,4-Benzodiazepine	Diazepam Temazepam Lorazepam
Substituted 1,4-benzodiazepine	Triazolam
1,5-Benzodiazepine	Clobazepam
Imidazobenzodiazepine	Midazolam Flumazenil

Figure HY10 Structural classification of benzodiazepines

Pharmacokinetics

The benzodiazepines act on specific receptors, which are mainly in the grey matter of the CNS where the majority of synapses are located. The greatest number of receptors is in the cerebral cortex, followed by the cerebellar cortex, thalamus, hypothalamus and limbic system, with the lowest numbers in the brain stem and spinal cord. There are three subtypes of benzodiazepine receptor represented by the abbreviation BDZ or ω. The properties of these are shown in Figure HY11.

The clinical effects appear to be due to agonism at BDZ receptors attached to the $GABA_A$ receptor complex on the postsynaptic membrane. This facilitates the action of GABA, which opens the inhibitory chloride channel and hyperpolarises the membrane. Therefore, benzodiazepines do not act directly on the chloride channels, so the maximum effect is determined by the prevailing levels of GABA, which should ensure a high therapeutic index.

The search for endogenous ligands of the benzodiazepine receptors has not been conclusive. There are agonists at the benzodiazepine receptors (β-carbolines) which have the opposite effect by preventing the binding of GABA to its receptor site. This is called inverse agonism. It is different from antagonism as, rather than acting by preventing the binding of benzodiazepines with no intrinsic activity of its own, the inverse agonist causes a conformational change that is the opposite to that of the agonist. Efficacy is, in effect, negative.

All the benzodiazepines are highly lipid-soluble and cross the blood–brain barrier readily. Used intravenously, the onset of effect usually takes longer than one arm–brain circulation time. Brain levels follow plasma levels closely. Orally administered benzodiazepines are readily absorbed as a result of the lipid solubility.

Drugs with a low lipophilicity have a lower transfer to brain and more drug is distributed peripherally (to vessel-rich tissues). This results in increased persistence of some drugs (although the elimination half-life is shorter) with a prolongation of recovery. For example, lorazepam has a short half-life but is less lipophilic compared with diazepam, so the effects may last less with the latter.

Receptor		Location	On GABA receptor	Postulated clinical effect
BDZ_1	ω_1	Central	yes	Sedation and hypnosis
BDZ_2	ω_2	Central	yes	Anticonvulsant
BDZ_3	ω_3	Central and peripheral	no	Not known

Figure HY11 Properties of benzodiazepine receptors

In rank order of lipid solubility: midazolam > diazepam > temazepam > lorazepam, but onset of action is much the same. The benzodiazepines are bound to albumin in the plasma.

Clinical
Central nervous system
The benzodiazepine family shares the following central effects:

- Anxiolysis
- Sedation
- Hypnosis
- Anterograde amnesia
- Anticonvulsant activity
- Skeletal muscle relaxation

Benzodiazepines reduce both rapid eye movement (REM) and slow-wave sleep, which in the short term may result in a deficit of REM sleep during treatment. Chronic administration results in tolerance, and withdrawal may result in rebound. The benzodiazepines are slow-acting induction agents with a prolonged recovery.

Cardiovascular system
Benzodiazepines administered intravenously have only minor depressant effects on the cardiovascular system in general. There is a slight reduction in SVR, preload, cardiac output and blood pressure. However, elderly and hypovolaemic patients may be particularly sensitive to IV midazolam, and this should be used with caution.

Respiratory system
Oral benzodiazepines have minimal effects on respiration. However, IV benzodiazepines have a very variable although usually slight effect on breathing. Airway maintenance is impaired, and tidal volume is reduced, with reduced sensitivity to CO_2. Respiratory rate usually increases slightly. Depression is especially likely with the concomitant use of opioids and other central depressants.

Other effects
Benzodiazepines reduce skeletal muscle tone via an effect on the dorsal horn of the spinal cord.

Metabolism
A number of benzodiazepines have active metabolites, resulting in prolonged duration of action (Figure HY12). These may have longer half-lives than the parent compound.

Drug	Extraction ratio	Metabolism
Diazepam	Low	Oxidation
Lorazepam	Low	Conjugation
Midazolam	High	Oxidation
Nitrazepam	Low	Nitro-reduction
Temazepam	Low	Conjugation

Figure HY12 Metabolism of benzodiazepines

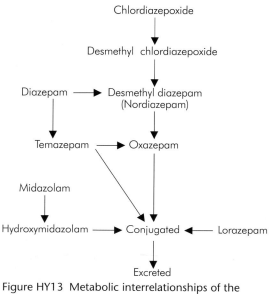

Figure HY13 Metabolic interrelationships of the benzodiazepine family

The metabolism of benzodiazepines produces metabolites that are also administered in their own right. Figure HY 13 shows the important inter-relationships.

Diazepam
Diazepam is a 1,4-benzodiazepine that is insoluble in water. For IV administration, it is therefore solubilised either in buffered propylene glycol and ethanol to a pH of 6.4–6.9 or in a soya bean lipid emulsion, to avoid causing thrombophlebitis and subsequent thrombosis.

It may be administered orally or intravenously. Diazepam is metabolised to N-desmethyldiazepam.

Midazolam
Midazolam is an imidazobenzodiazepine. This results in the ability of a water molecule to open the diazepine ring (Figure HY14), thus encouraging aqueous solubility.

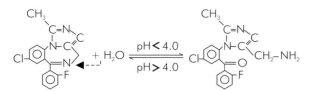

Figure HY14 Structural equilibrium of midazolam

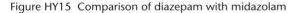

	Diazepam	Midazolam
Physical	No imidazole ring Insoluble in water Lipid emulsion	Imidazole ring Soluble in water Aqueous
Chemical	Consistent structure High FM ratio	Structural change Low FM ratio
Clinical	Anti-epileptic Longer duration	Anti-epileptic Shorter duration

Figure HY15 Comparison of diazepam with midazolam

The equilibrium between the two forms of midazolam is determined by pH. The change from the one form to the other is relatively slow, having a half-life of 10 minutes. The pH in the ampoule containing midazolam hydrochloride is 3.0 and so the ring is open and it is soluble. Once subjected to body pH 7.4, the diazepine ring closes and the midazolam becomes lipid-soluble, allowing it readily to cross the blood–brain barrier. In the plasma most of the midazolam (95%) is protein-bound. Midazolam is redistributed more rapidly than diazepam and so its duration of action is much shorter than that of diazepam.

Midazolam is hydroxylated in the liver to 4-hydroxymidazolam, which has minimal clinical activity. In the elderly, the lower hepatic blood flow and metabolic activity result in a significantly higher elimination half-life.

Diazepam and midazolam are compared in Figure HY15.

Lorazepam

Lorazepam is a 1,4-benzodiazepine used in the alleviation of anxiety and for sedation. It is used as a premedicant. It is available for oral, sublingual, IM and IV administration. The oral dose is 2–4 mg, and IV is 50 μg kg^{-1}. Oral bioavailability is 90%, with 90% protein-bound and a volume of distribution of 1 l kg^{-1}. It is predominantly eliminated by glucuronide conjugation followed by urinary excretion, with an elimination half-life of 10–20 hours.

Temazepam

Temazepam is an orally administered 1,4-benzodiazepine used in the alleviation of anxiety and for sedation. It is used as a premedicant, typically in doses of 10–40 mg (1 mg kg^{-1}, up to 30 mg syrup in children). Bioavailability is high, 76% is protein-bound and the volume of distribution is 0.8 l kg^{-1}. It is predominantly eliminated by glucuronide conjugation followed by urinary excretion, with an elimination half-life of 8 hours.

Flumazenil

Flumazenil is an imidazobenzodiazepine and a competitive benzodiazepine receptor antagonist, bearing the closest resemblance to the structure of midazolam. It is administered intravenously to antagonise the clinical effects of agonist benzodiazepines. It also antagonises inverse benzodiazepine receptor agonists.

Flumazenil is 40–50% protein-bound to albumin and rapidly redistributed, with a volume of distribution of 0.9 l kg^{-1}. Flumazenil has a high hepatic extraction ratio, with a total clearance of 15 ml kg^{-1} min^{-1}. Elimination half-life is about 50 minutes. Flumazenil is metabolised to a carboxylic acid derivative and a glucuronide, which are both inactive.

Cautions

Flumazenil has a short duration of action. It is important to realise that its effects may wear off before the benzodiazepine agonist has been cleared, with a re-emergence of the agonist effects. In addition, rapid antagonism of benzodiazepine sedation in a head-injured patient may precipitate an excessive rise in ICP. After chronic administration of benzodiazepines, flumazenil may provoke abrupt withdrawal effects.

Anaesthetic agents of historic interest
Examples – althesin, methohexital, propanidid

Althesin is a mixture of two steroid induction agents, alphaxolone and alphadolone, solubilised in Cremophor EL. It provides a rapid onset of action and rapid recovery. It was withdrawn because of a strong suspicion of adverse reactions, probably to the Cremophor EL, a derivative of castor oil. It was never reformulated with an alternative solubilising agent.

Propanidid is a eugenol derived from oil of cloves also solubilised in Cremophor EL. It produces a rapid onset of action with a very short duration of action and rapid recovery (6 minutes). It is metabolised by plasma cholinesterase. A possible connection with sudden death led to its withdrawal from use.

Methohexital is a methyl barbiturate which used to be supplied as α isomers only, to minimise the excitatory effects. It enjoyed popularity in ECT, where the excitatory effects were (incorrectly) viewed as contributory to the effectiveness of the treatment. Manufacture ceased in 1998 for commercial reasons.

Other hypnotic agents

Examples – buspirone, chloral hydrate, meprobamate, zolpidem, zopiclone

Buspirone

Buspirone is an azaspirodecanedione used for anxiolysis. It does not appear to act on benzodiazepine receptors, and the most likely mode of action is antagonism at $5HT_{1A}$ receptors. It may also reduce acetylcholine activity and increase catecholamine activity. There is marked first-pass metabolism, with peak levels after 60 minutes. It is 95% protein-bound in the plasma. Buspirone is metabolised in the liver and has a half-life of 2–11 hours.

Chloral and related drugs

Chloral, chloral hydrate, triclofos and dichloraphenazone are interrelated metabolically. These drugs are administered orally as either tablets or elixir. Triclofos is said to cause less gastric irritation than chloral hydrate. Chloral hydrate is useful for premedication of small children. A dose of 50 mg kg^{-1} (up to 1 g) acts within 45 minutes. Doses from 6 mg kg^{-1} in adults will produce sedation.

Clinical effects

Central nervous system

The chloral derivatives cause central depression with a mild anticonvulsant activity. There is little interference with EEG sleep patterns. They have no analgesic activity.

Cardiovascular system

In normal dosage, there is minimal cardiovascular depression, but overdose causes profound depression, with supraventricular tachycardia a feature.

Respiratory system

In normal dosage, there is minimal respiratory depression, but overdose causes profound depression.

Metabolism

Alcohol dehydrogenase, present in the liver, red blood cells and other sites, plays a major role in the inactivation of these drugs. Trichlorethanol is conjugated with glucuronide.

Cautions

Problems include gastric irritation, hepatic enzyme induction or inhibition, and the displacement of drugs such as warfarin from plasma proteins.

Meprobamate

Meprobamate is a carbamate tranquiliser having anxiolytic, anticonvulsant and muscle-relaxant properties. It acts by inhibiting adenosine uptake. It is less effective than benzodiazepines and has a lower therapeutic index. Rapid absorption follows oral administration. Ninety per cent is excreted in the urine (mainly as the hydroxy metabolite and its glucuronide conjugate). It may precipitate convulsions in susceptible patients, particularly following withdrawal of the drug. Meprobamate is contraindicated in acute intermittent porphyria.

Zolpidem

Zolpidem is an imidazopyrine that acts at the benzodiazepine receptor complex of the $GABA_A$ receptor, to produce anxiolysis and sedation. It is selective for ω_1 receptor subtype, producing hypnosis without the ataxia or other ω_2 effects. The effects are reversed by flumazenil. Zolpidem is rapidly absorbed, with a bioavailability of 70%. Concentrations peak at about 1–3 hours, and it is 93% protein-bound. Zolpidem is metabolised to inactive metabolites in the liver, with a half-life of 2.4 hours.

Zopiclone

Zopiclone is a cyclopyrrolone with anxiolytic and sedative properties. It acts at the GABA – benzodiazepine receptor complex but appears to act at a different site from that affected by benzodiazepines. The overall effect is to enhance the action of GABA in promoting opening of the chloride channel. It does not reduce the amount of REM sleep. Zopiclone is well absorbed following oral administration and has a short elimination half-life of 5 hours.

Specific pharmacology

Here, molecular weight (MW) is given in daltons, volume of distribution (V_d) in litres, clearance (Cl) in ml kg^{-1} min^{-1} and half-lives ($t_{1/2}$) in minutes (unless stated otherwise).

Diazepam

Structure – 1,4-benzodiazepine

Presentation

Oral – 2, 5, 10 mg tablets; 2 mg in 5 ml solution

IV – 5 mg ml^{-1} clear yellow solution of diazepam (osmolality 7775 mOsm kg^{-1}) in a mixture of solvents (propylene glycol (40%), ethanol (10%), benzoic acid/sodium benzoate (5%), benzyl alcohol (1.5%), pH 6.2–6.9); or white opaque oil-in-water emulsion (osmolality 349 mOsm kg^{-1}) using soya bean oil similar to intralipid (pH 6.0)

May also be administered rectally and intramuscularly

Storage – room temperature

Dose – IV bolus 0.1–0.3 mg kg^{-1}

Pharmacokinetics

MW	285
bioavailability	oral 86–100%
pH	6.2–6.9
protein binding	99%
V_d	1.2
Cl	0.4
$t_{1/2\alpha}$	70
$t_{1/2\beta}$	30 h

CNS – anxiolysis, hypnosis, sedation, anterograde amnesia; anticonvulsant; CBF, ICP and CMRO$_2$ reduced

CVS – blood pressure, cardiac output decreased; coronary vasodilatation increases coronary blood flow; myocardial oxygen consumption decreased

RS – respiratory depression; hypoxic drive reduced more than response to CO$_2$

Other – clearance reduced by concomitant cimetidine treatment

Elimination – hepatic metabolism to desmethyldiazepam (active $t_{1/2\alpha}$ at least 100 h), oxazepam and temazepam; oxidised and glucuronide derivatives excreted in urine; <1% unchanged

Etomidate

Structure – imidazole

Presentation – clear colourless solution of 20 mg etomidate in 10 ml 35% propylene glycol in water or 20 mg in 10 ml lipid emulsion

Storage – room temperature

Dose – IV bolus 0.15–0.30 mg kg^{-1} (maximum 60 mg)

Pharmacokinetics

MW	342
pH	8.1
protein binding	76%
V_d	3.5
Cl	11.7
$t_{1/2\alpha 1}$	2.6
$t_{1/2\alpha 2}$	27
$t_{1/2\beta}$	75

CNS – rapid induction of anaesthesia (one arm–brain circulation time); excitatory phenomena common, reduced by opioids; recovery is dose-related; IOP, ICP, CBF and brain oxygen consumption (CMRO$_2$) reduced; epileptiform EEG features

CVS – systemic vascular resistance, mean arterial blood pressure fall; cardiac index and heart rate decrease slightly; atrial muscle function or contraction, ventricular dp/dt$_{max}$, mean aortic pressure, coronary blood flow are unchanged; myocardial oxygen delivery and consumption are preserved

RS – dose-dependent depression of tidal volume and rate; at a given CO$_2$ level ventilation is greater than with methohexital; cough and hiccup common

Other – relatively high emesis rate (2–14%); pain on injection; venous thrombosis. There is no effect on renal or hepatic function. Steroid synthesis is inhibited, so infusions should not be used

Elimination – ester hydrolysis in plasma and liver, inactive metabolites; 87% in urine, 3% unchanged, rest in bile

Toxicity – adrenocortical suppression when infused over a long period; suppression direct and via ACTH

Contraindications – porphyria

Flumazenil

Structure – imidazobenzodiazepine, BDZ receptor antagonist

Presentation – clear colourless solution of 500 µg flumazenil in 5 ml

Dose

IV bolus – 100 µg increments up to 2 mg

IV infusion – 100–400 µg per hour

Pharmacokinetics

protein binding	50%
V_d	0.9
Cl	15
$t_{1/2\alpha}$	7
$t_{1/2\beta}$	60

Clinical – antagonises the effects of central benzodiazepines; benzodiazepine withdrawal effects may occur

Elimination – almost entirely metabolised in the liver to the inactive carboxylate, which is excreted in the urine

Ketamine hydrochloride

Structure – phencyclidine derivative

Presentation – white crystalline powder for dilution with water, forming clear, colourless, aqueous solutions of 10, 50 and 100 mg ml^{-1}; 10 mg ml^{-1} isotonic with normal saline; 50 and 100 mg ml^{-1} contain 1 : 10 000 benzethonium chloride as preservative

Dose

IV – 1–4.5 mg kg^{-1}
IM – 4–13 mg kg^{-1}

Pharmacokinetics

MW	237.5
pH	3.5–5.5
protein binding	20–50%
V_d	3
Cl	17
$t_{1/2}\alpha$	10
$t_{1/2}\beta$	120–180

CNS – slow onset of dissociative anaesthesia, light sleep, analgesia, amnesia; the EEG shows θ activity; ICP, CBF and IOP are increased; analgesia is good for burns and fractures but poor for visceral pain

CVS – increases sympathetic tone leading to increases in heart rate, cardiac output, blood pressure, central venous pressure; baroreceptor function is maintained; few arrhythmias

RS – protective respiratory reflexes are usually preserved, but cannot be relied upon; bronchodilatation

Other – nausea and vomiting are common; salivation is increased; uterine tone is increased; levels of epinephrine and norepinephrine are increased

Elimination – N-demethylation and hydroxylation to produce metabolites with reduced activity; metabolites then conjugated and excreted in the urine

Toxicity – rashes 15%; emergence delirium, hallucinations; pain on injection particularly with IM injection

Midazolam hydrochloride

Structure – imidazobenzodiazepine

Presentation – 10 mg midazolam in both 2 and 5 ml; colourless aqueous solution of midazolam hydrochloride. Stable in water by virtue of opening of diazepine ring

Dose

IV – 0.03–0.3 mg kg^{-1} depending on effect (sedation/anaesthesia) required; elderly are particularly sensitive
IM – 0.07–0.1 mg kg^{-1} for premedication

Pharmacokinetics

MW	326
bioavailability	oral 44%; IM 80–100%
pH	3
protein binding	96%
V_d	1.1
Cl	7
$t_{1/2}\beta$	5 h

CNS – slow onset of action; anxiolysis, sedation, hypnosis, anterograde amnesia; anticonvulsant; CBF and $CMRO_2$ reduced

CVS – heart rate, systemic vascular resistance and blood pressure reduced

RS – tidal volume and minute volume reduced; rate increased but may cause apnoea; response to CO_2 impaired

Other – catecholamine levels reduced; renin, angiotensin and corticosteroid levels unaffected; skeletal muscle tone reduced; renal and hepatic blood flow reduced

Elimination – hydroxylated and conjugated with glucuronide in the liver, and is then excreted in urine

Toxicity – occasional pain on injection

Propofol

Structure – alkyl phenol derivative, 2,6-di-isopropyl phenol

Presentation – white, isotonic, neutral aqueous emulsion 10 mg ml^{-1}; 10% soya bean oil, 1.2% purified egg phosphatide, 2.25% glycerol, sodium hydroxide, water

Dose

Anaesthesia – IV bolus 2–2.5 mg kg^{-1}
Anaesthesia – IV infusion 4–12 mg kg^{-1} hour^{-1}
Sedation – IV infusion 0.3–4 mg kg^{-1}

Pharmacokinetics

MW	178
pH	6–8.5
pK_a	11
protein binding	98%
V_d	15
Cl	20
$t_{1/2}\alpha 1$	2.5
$t_{1/2}\alpha 2$	45
$t_{1/2}\beta$	3–8 h

CNS – rapid onset of anaesthesia (one arm–brain circulation); excitatory movements common; ICP, cerebral perfusion pressure and $CMRO_2$ reduced; anticonvulsant

CVS – systemic vascular resistance, cardiac output and blood pressure reduced; variable effect on heart rate, usually a slight increase

RS – tidal volume reduced, rate increased; response to CO_2 reduced; greater suppression of laryngeal reflexes than thiopental

Others – possible anti-emetic effect; pain on injection; excitatory movements; renal and hepatic function unaffected

Elimination – liver and extrahepatic, unaffected by renal or hepatic disease; excreted in urine, 0.3% unchanged; non-cumulative when infused

Toxicity – a small risk of convulsions in epileptic patients; may cause bradycardia or asystole, possibly due to emulsion. Not licensed for use in pregnancy

Sodium thiopental

Structure – thiobarbiturate

Presentation – hygroscopic yellow powder of sodium thiopental with 6% sodium carbonate; reconstituted with water to 2.5% solution. Reconstituted solution must not be used after 24 hours

Dose – IV bolus 4–6 mg kg^{-1}

Pharmacokinetics

MW	264
pH	10.8
pK_a	7.6
protein binding	75%
V_d	1.96
Cl	3.4
$t_{1/2\alpha 1}$	2–6
$t_{1/2\alpha 2}$	30–60
$t_{1/2\beta}$	5–10 h

CNS – smooth, rapid induction of anaesthesia (one arm–brain circulation); CBF, ICP, IOP, $CMRO_2$ reduced; anticonvulsant, antanalgesic

CVS – negative inotropy; cardiac output, systemic vascular resistance and blood pressure reduced

RS – dose-dependent respiratory depression; response to CO_2 reduced; may cause laryngeal spasm or bronchoconstriction

Other – splanchnic vasoconstriction; no effect on pregnant uterus

Renal – vasopressin, renal plasma flow, urine output reduced

Hepatic – no effect, used in hepatic encephalopathy

Elimination – metabolised in the liver at 15% per hour; 30% remains by 24 hours; excreted in urine, 0.5% unchanged

Toxicity – tissue damage with extravasation; arterial constriction and thrombosis with intra-arterial injection

Contraindications – porphyria

CHAPTER 7
Analgesic drugs

I. Power and M. Paleologos

Opioids

The term *opioid* is defined as a natural, semisynthetic or synthetic compound that acts at opioid receptors. *Opiate* is a specific term to describe drugs derived from the opium poppy (*Papaver somniferum*).

Classification

Opioids may be classified in a number of ways according to chemical structure, production, receptor activity and specific receptor subtype affinity. A classification of opioids by origin and structure is shown in Figure AN1.

Naturally occurring opioids fall into two structural categories: those with a phenanthrene nucleus (morphine, codeine and thebaine) and benzylisoquinolines (papaverine and noscopine). Thebaine, despite being a relatively inactive opium derivative, is used as a precursor for the development of many semisynthetic opioid agonists and

antagonists (buprenorphine, naloxone and oxycodone). Semisynthetic opioids are produced from chemical modification of naturally occurring opioids. Synthetic opioids may be further subdivided into four classes: morphinans, diphenylpropylamines, phenylpiperidines and benzomorphans.

Opioids may also be classified by their activity, affinity and efficacy at opioid receptors (Figure AN2).

Partial agonists and mixed agonist–antagonists produce analgesia in opioid-naive patients, but may precipitate withdrawal in individuals who are dependent on full opioid agonists. They usually produce inadequate analgesia for treatment of severe pain, having a ceiling effect at less than the maximal effect of a full agonist. Hence they also produce less respiratory depression, constipation and urinary side effects, and have a lower addiction potential. Mixed agonist–antagonists are associated with a

Fundamentals of Anaesthesia, 3rd edition, ed. Tim Smith, Colin Pinnock and Ted Lin. Published by Cambridge University Press. © Cambridge University Press 2008.

Classification	Structure	Example
Naturally occurring	Morphine analogues	Morphine, Codeine
Semisynthetic	Morphine analogues	Diamorphine
		Dihydrocodeine
		Naloxone
	Thebaine derivatives	Buprenorphine
		Oxycodone
Synthetic	Phenylpiperidines	Pethidine
	Anilinopiperidines	Phenoperidine
		Fentanyl
		Alfentanil
		Sufentanil
		Remifentanil
	Diphenylheptanes	Methadone
		Dextropropoxyphene

Figure AN1 Structural classification of opioid drugs

Classification	Example	Affinity	Efficacy
Pure agonists	Morphine	High	100%
Partial agonists	Buprenorphine	Medium	60–70%
Mixed agonist–antagonists	Pentazocine	Medium	Predominantly agonist
	Nalbuphine	Medium	Predominantly agonist
	Nalorphine	Medium	Predominantly antagonist
Pure antagonists	Naloxone	High	Zero
	Naltrexone	High	Zero

Figure AN2 Functional classification of opioid drugs

much lower incidence of euphoria, but the production of psychotomimetic effects (hallucinations, depersonalisation) limits their clinical use.

Structure–activity relationships

Most opioids demonstrate optical activity, with the majority of the pharmacological effect being produced by one of the stereoisomers – usually the levorotatory (S) isomer. Naturally occurring opioids are produced by stereospecific enzymes and are isolated as a single isomer, while synthetic opioids possessing a chiral carbon can only be synthesised as racemic mixtures. Some opioids require both stereoisomers for maximal efficacy (tramadol).

Phenylalanine and tyrosine are important structural elements of all opioid compounds, including the endogenous opioid peptides. Morphine is synthesised in the opium poppy from two molecules of tyrosine. All opioids have a tertiary positively charged (basic) nitrogen separated by an ethylene chain from a quaternary carbon, which is also attached to a phenyl group (Figure AN3).

The presence of the tertiary nitrogen and its distance from the aromatic ring (4.55 Å for morphine and the related semisynthetic compounds) is considered to be essential for activity. The rigid pentacyclic (phenanthrene) frame of the morphine molecule has a three-dimensional structure in which rings A and B are coplanar and rings C and E are perpendicular to the AB plane. This configuration is common to many compounds with opioid activity. The flat benzene ring (A) lies against the flat part of the receptor, while the piperidine ring (E) fits

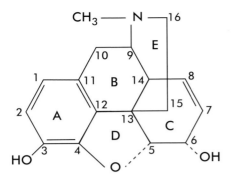

Figure AN3 Chemical structure of opioids

into a groove in the receptor, to which it is attracted by virtue of its positively charged nitrogen atom.

Substitutions of functional groups on the rings or the core morphine molecule produce opioids with different pharmacological properties.

On the tertiary amine N-17, a short-chain alkyl substitution results in mixed agonist–antagonists such as buprenorphine and nalorphine. Hydroxylation of the C-14 in addition to this converts these into full antagonists. Naloxone is such an antagonist, produced by hydroxylation of nalorphine and modification of the C-6 hydroxyl group to double-bond oxygen. Removal of the methyl group (on the tertiary amine N-17) or replacing it with certain alkyl groups markedly reduces opioid agonist activity.

The phenolic group at C-3 probably interacts with the receptor, since the presence of a hydroxyl group maximises potency, whilst substituting it with a methyl to make codeine decreases potency 10 times. Longer alkyl side-chain substitutions produce even weaker agonists. Similar alkyl substitutions on C-1 also reduce potency.

C-6 substitutions with lipophilic groups increase activity. Oxidation of C-6 increases potency and the double acetyl substitution at C-3 and C-6 to produce diamorphine increases potency by increasing lipophilicity, despite the competing effects of the dual substitution.

Alterations to the pentacyclic structure of morphine produce the synthetic opioids. Removal of the oxide bridge between rings A and C produces the morphinans, which are generally more potent. Removal of the C-ring from the morphinans creates the benzomorphan group. Removal of the methylene bridge from the benzomorphans produces the phenylpiperidine structure of which pethidine is the prototype. The molecule unfolds such that the tertiary nitrogen is now further from the aromatic ring. The phenylpiperidines are all developed from modifications to

the structure of pethidine, with sufentanil being a thienyl derivative of fentanyl.

Opioid receptors

Opioid receptors are G-protein-coupled transmembrane receptors. These exist throughout the CNS, with particularly high concentrations in the periaqueductal grey area and the substantia gelatinosa of the spinal cord. They are also present outside the CNS, and this may account for some of the other opioid effects (gastrointestinal) and their postulated value in some peripheral anaesthetic techniques (such as intra-articular injection).

Classification

There have been a number of schemes used to define the various opioid receptor groups. These have in the main been merely new names for the same groups. Three main groups have been classified, to which a fourth (the nociceptin/orphanin receptor) has been added. The grouping has been defined by their response to different *prototype agonists*. The various classifications are shown in Figure AN4. The current International Union of Pharmacology nomenclature for the opioid receptors is MOP (μ, OP_3), KOP (κ, OP_2), DOP (δ, OP_1) and NOP (OP_4). The OP_x type classification can lead to confusion once the receptors are subdivided. Separate genes for each class of opioid receptor have now been identified.

MOP

MOP receptors open potassium ion channels, causing hyperpolarisation and reduced neuronal firing. At the nerve terminal the action potential plateau shortens, thus reducing calcium ion influx and neurotransmitter release. MOP are located in the:

- Primary afferent neurones (pre- and postsynaptic)
- Peripheral sensory neurones
- Periaqueductal grey matter
- Nucleus raphe magnus
- Rostral ventral medulla
- Thalamus
- Cerebral cortex

DOP

DOP receptors also open potassium ion channels, causing hyperpolarisation and reduced neuronal firing. At the nerve terminal the action potential plateau shortens, thus reducing calcium ion influx and neurotransmitter release. DOP are located in the:

- Olfactory bulb
- Cerebral cortex

Classifications	Receptors			
	MOP	**DOP**	**KOP**	**NOP**
	μ	δ	κ	
	OP_3	OP_1	OP_2	OP_4
Subtypes	$μ_1$, $μ_2$	$δ_1$, $δ_2$	$κ_1$, $κ_2$, $κ_3$	
Prototype agonist	morphine	Ala-leu-enkephalin	ketocyclazocine	
Endogenous ligand	Leu-enkephalin	Leu-enkephalin	dynorphin	nociceptin
	Met-enkephalin	Met-enkephalin	β-endorphin	orphanin FQ peptide
	β-endorphin	β-endorphin		

Figure AN4 Opioid receptor classification

- Primary afferent neurones (presynaptic)
- Motor integration areas
- Nociception areas

KOP

KOP receptors, in contrast, directly close calcium channels, so that the end result is reduced neurotransmitter release. KOP are found in the:
- Hypothalamus
- Nociception areas

NOP

NOP receptors directly close calcium channels, so that they too result in reduced neurotransmitter release. NOP are located in the:
- Nucleus raphe magnus
- Primary afferent neurones

Sigma receptor

Following the original discovery of μ, δ and κ subtypes, a fourth variant, σ, was originally classified as an opioid receptor. The selective agonist N-allyl-normetazocine (SKF 10047) had been shown to produce mydriasis, tachypnoea, tachycardia and delirium after occupancy of this receptor. The σ receptor is no longer classified as an opioid receptor as it does not meet the full criteria, notably:
- It has a high-affinity binding for phencyclidine and related compounds.
- The σ-mediated effects are not reversed by naloxone.
- σ receptors are stereospecific for dextrorotatory isomers.

The σ receptor is not affected by opioids but is bound to by phencyclidine and haloperidol.

Pharmacodynamics

All opioid agonists share a similar pharmacodynamic profile, and demonstrate a sigmoidal dose–effect relationship. In addition to the variety of exogenous opioid agonists, there are a number of endogenous agonist ligands which act on opioid receptors. Many of these agonists lack specificity for a particular subtype of receptor, while the mixed agonist–antagonists exhibit agonist, partial agonist and antagonist actions on the various receptor subtypes (Figure AN5).

Each of the opioid receptors arises from a separate gene. Opioid receptors belong to the superfamily of serpentine receptors, which contain seven membrane-spanning domains, with an extracellular N-terminus and an intracellular C-terminus. The transmembrane helices are arranged anticlockwise, forming a tight helical bundle. Importantly, the N-terminal and C-terminal tails, and the second and third extracellular loops, are responsible for ligand binding specificity, and for the differential regulation of, and variation in coupling to effector systems. The four classes of opioid receptors all produce primary inhibitory effects following activation, via receptor-coupling to inhibitory G proteins. This results in inhibition of adenylyl cyclase with reduced formation of cAMP, closure of voltage-sensitive calcium channels, stimulation of inwardly rectifying K^+ channel opening causing membrane hyperpolarisation, and stimulation of phospholipase Cβ. Any excitatory or facilitatory effects of opioids can be explained by the inhibition of inhibitory pathways. Figure AN6 summarises opioid receptor classification and molecular coupling mechanisms.

Stimulation of the NOP receptor may produce either a pro-nociceptive anti-analgesic effect (supraspinal and spinal) or an anti-nociceptive effect (spinal – at high concentrations). The function of this receptor is thought to

Actions	Receptors		
	MOP	DOP	KOP
	OP$_3$ (mu)	OP$_1$ (delta)	OP$_2$ (kappa)
Analgesia: supraspinal	++	++	++
Analgesia: spinal	++	++	++
Respiratory depression	++	++	+
Miosis	++	++	++
Gastrointestinal motility decreased	++	++	0
Smooth muscle	++	++	0
Behaviour	Euphoria	Euphoria	Dysphoria
Sedation	++	++	+
Physical dependence	++	++	+
Other			Diuresis

Figure AN5 Effects of opioid receptor activation

be in setting pain thresholds and in the formation of tolerance to opioid therapy, although tolerance also develops to its antiopioid effects. Importantly, NOP receptor antagonists produce analgesia, prevent the development of tolerance to opioid analgesia, and may be useful for reducing some of the side effects associated with opioid therapy.

Clinical effects

Opioid agonists cause a range of mainly depressant and some stimulant actions on the CNS via specific receptors. Unlike anaesthetic agents, which produce generalised CNS effects, they have little capacity to produce amnesia, have no intrinsic anticonvulsant activity and do not alter seizure threshold. The lack of amnesic properties makes them unsuitable as the sole agents for anaesthesia.

The primary goals of opioid use are for the production of analgesia, and maintaining haemodynamic stability during anaesthesia. Systemically administered opioids produce analgesia through actions at two anatomically distinct regions: supraspinal and spinal sites. Opioids reduce the intensity of pain and reduce the associated fear. They achieve this by raising the pain threshold, altering the reaction to pain, and inducing sleep and hypercapnia. Their efficacy is greater for continuous dull pain rather than sharp intermittent pain, and they tend to be less effective for the treatment of neuropathic pain.

CNS effects

Figure AN7 lists the various effects of opioids on the CNS. Opioids cause a reduction in level of consciousness and eventually produce sleep, with the loss of responsiveness to verbal command. They produce a dose-related decrease in the MAC for volatile anaesthetics, with a ceiling of 60–70% reduction in MAC. They also increase cerebral vasoconstriction in the presence of vasodilating agents such as volatile anaesthetics. They do not cause a loss of cerebral autoregulation or reactivity to CO_2. A ceiling effect is reached on the EEG, with a slowing of EEG frequency and the production of high-voltage (δ) waves.

Cardiovascular effects

Opioids preserve cardiovascular stability to a greater extent than most other anaesthetic drugs. In normovolaemic patients they produce little perturbation in haemodynamic parameters, with minimal cardiac depression, no baroreceptor inhibition and a modest reduction in preload or afterload. Haemodynamic compromise may, however, be observed in individuals whose cardiovascular integrity is dependent on a high level of sympathetic tone, because opioids reduce central sympathetic outflow. In such settings even small doses can cause hypotension or cardiovascular collapse. Morphine has the greatest effect on the vascular system due to its propensity to cause histamine release and subsequent indirect effects on catecholamine release. This may result in a tachycardia with a reduction in the

Receptor	Subtypes	Location	Endogenous ligand	Clinical effect
MOP (μ)	μ_1, μ_2	Pre- and postsynaptic on primary afferent neurones and peripheral sensory neurones Periaqueductal gray matter Nucleus raphe magnus Rostral ventral medulla Thalamus Cortex	β-endorphin Leu-enkephalin Met-enkephalin Dynorphin	Supraspinal analgesia (μ_1) Sedation (μ_1) Spinal analgesia (μ_2) Respiratory depression (μ_2) Bradycardia (μ_2) Hypothermia (μ_2) Miosis (μ_2) Euphoria (μ_2) Pruritis (μ_2) Nausea and vomiting (μ_2) Constipation (μ_2) Urinary retention (μ_2) Physical dependence
DOP (δ)	δ_1, δ_2	Olfactory bulb Cerebral cortex Pre-synaptic on primary afferent neurones, motor integration areas and nociception areas	Leu-enkephalin Met-enkephalin	Supraspinal analgesia (δ_1) Spinal analgesia (δ_1) Respiratory depression Constipation Physical dependence
KOP (κ)	κ_1, κ_2, κ_3	Hypothalamus Nociception areas	Dynorphin	Supraspinal analgesia (κ_3) Sedation Spinal analgesia (κ_1) Dysphoria Psychotomimetic effects ↓ vasopressin + diuresis
NOP		Nucleus raphe magnus Primary afferent neurones	Nociceptin/orphanin FQ peptide	Supraspinal anti-analgesia Spinal anti-analgesia and analgesia Urinary retention

Figure AN6 Opioid receptor molecular pharmacology

SVR and MAP. The risk is increased by increasing the dose and speed of administration, and can be attenuated by pre-treatment with histamine receptor antagonists and volume loading.

Pethidine is unique among the opioids. Opioids generally produce a negative chronotropic effect via central vagal excitation. Pethidine, however, has a homology with atropine and can produce a tachycardia, and it is the only opioid to produce significant direct myocardial depression when used at high doses. Myocardial depression is not observed unless extraordinarily high doses of morphine or the fentanyl congeners are administered. Morphine has indirect positive inotropic effects at doses of 1–2 mg kg^{-1}, and blocks neurally and hormonally mediated venoconstriction to reduce preload,

making it useful in the treatment of acute congestive heart failure.

Effects on other organ systems
The effects of opioids on the cardiovascular system and other organ systems are summarised in Figure AN8.

Opioids are the most efficacious of all anaesthetic drugs for attenuating the stress response associated with pain, laryngoscopy and airway manipulation. The plasma concentrations of stress hormones (catecholamines, cortisol, vasopressin, aldosterone and growth hormone) increase during anaesthesia and surgery in proportion to the degree of operative trauma. This contributes to increased myocardial work, tissue catabolism, and hyperglycaemia – responses associated with increased perioperative

System		Effect
Musculoskeletal	Gait	↓ Physical performance, Ataxia, ↓ Spinal cord reflexes
	Rigidity	Rigidity occurs 60–90 s post-injection and abates spontaneously after 10–20 minutes. Mainly thoracoabdominal and upper limb musculature, ↑ with ↑ age, ↑ speed of injection, ↑ dose, use of N_2O Mediated via nucleus raphe magnus
	Multifocal myoclonus	Non-seizure related, ↑ with pethidine
CNS	Central	Spectrum from abnormal eye movement, to contraction of extremities, to tonic–clonic movements Euphoria: especially for agents which cross the BBB quickly Dysphoria in some individuals Subjective feelings of body warmth and heavy extremities Apathy ↓ Level of consciousness and eventually sleep ↓ Concentration and capacity for complex reasoning
	EEG	Effects vary between different opioids: slowing of frequency, production of high-voltage δ waves. No capacity to produce EEG silence
Cerebrovascular	SSEPs	No effect on SSEPs
	ICP	No effect
	CBF	No effect, but ↑ vasoconstriction with vasodilators No loss of autoregulation or CO_2 reactivity. $CMRO_2$ reduced by up to 10–25%
Vision	Edinger–Westphal nucleus	Miosis (via a ↓ in inhibition to the nucleus) except pethidine. Reversed by hypoxia and atropine
Thermoregulation	Peripheral effects	Promote hypothermia via ↓ BMR (10–20%), venodilatation, and muscle relaxation
	Response	↓ Thermoregulatory responses (as for volatile agents)

Figure AN7 Opioid effects on the CNS

morbidity and mortality. Opioids reduce nociception, inhibiting the pituitary–adrenal axis, reducing central sympathetic outflow and influencing centrally mediated neuroendocrine responses. Fentanyl and its congeners (particularly sufentanil) are the most efficacious, but no opioid is completely effective.

Side effects

The organ-specific adverse effects of opioids observed in an individual depend on age, extent of disease, presence of organ dysfunction, concurrent administration of certain drugs, prior opioid exposure and the route of drug administration. Not all adverse effects are deleterious. A number of opioid-induced side effects are produced by activation of opioid receptors either centrally or peripherally, or in both areas. Serious allergic reactions to opioids are exceedingly rare, although anaphylaxis has been reported.

At equianalgesic doses all opioids produce equivalent degrees of respiratory depression, with the elderly and neonates being at increased risk. Tolerance develops rapidly to this effect (but less slowly than to analgesic effects), and with chronic opioid exposure the risk of significant respiratory depression is reduced. Apnoea may occur in

System		Effect
Cardiovascular	Heart rate	Usually sinus bradycardia via central vagal excitation Occasionally sinus arrest Exacerbated by concomitant vagal stimuli (e.g. laryngoscopy) and β-blockers
	Mean arterial pressure	Usually no effect or a slight ↓ (unless significant bradycardia) Greater ↓ associated with histamine release
	Vascular tree	No effect on SVR (unless histamine release) Mild venodilatation with a ↓ in preload (due to ↓ central sympathetic outflow
	Myocardium	No effect on contractility (except for pethidine which is a depressant) No effect on metabolic rate Possible ischaemic preconditioning
	Excitability	↓ Myocardial conductivity, ↑ Refractory period, ↑ VF threshold
Respiratory	Mechanics	Equivalent ↓ in rate, tidal volume and minute ventilation at equianalgesic doses ↑ Pauses, irregular breathing and apnoeas
	Control	↑ Apnoeic threshold ↓ CO_2 sensitivity ↓ Carotid body chemoreception and hypoxic drive Voluntary control of respiration remains intact No effect on hypoxic pulmonary vasoconstriction
	Airway reflexes	↓ Airway reflexes with improved tolerance of ETT Antitussive via peripheral and central actions ↓ Mucociliary function Brief cough in up to 50% with bolus phenylpiperidines
Gastrointestinal	Stomach and intestines	↓ Peristalsis and secretions, and ↑ tone causing dry stool and constipation ↓ Gastric acid ↓ Gastric emptying with ↑ antral tone and ↓ LOS tone promoting ↑ aspiration risk ↑ tone of pyloric, ileocaecal, and anal sphincters
	Biliary tree	↑ Bile duct pressure Sphincter of Oddi contraction (little clinical significance overall)
	Chemoreceptor trigger zone	Nausea and vomiting (worse with first dose and ↑ dose interval) Worse postprandial due to concomitant ↑ gastric antral tone
Genitourinary	Kidney	Antidiuresis as a result of ↓ RBF and ↓ GFR (predominates) ↓ vasopressin release in response to osmotic stimuli
	Bladder	↑ Bladder and urethral tone Vesicular sphincter contraction
Immunity	Immune system	↓ Immunoglobulin production (uncertain significance) Reactivation of HSV 2–5 days after neuraxial opioid

Figure AN8 Opioid effects on major organ systems

conscious patients, but is usually associated with other signs of CNS depression, and apnoeic patients can be instructed to breathe as voluntary control of ventilation remains intact. Sleep, or the concomitant use of other CNS depressants (except clonidine), potentiates the risk by further reducing sensitivity to CO_2.

Opioid-induced depression of airway reflexes is usually regarded as an advantageous side effect, although the impairment of mucociliary function is not. All opioids possess antitussive activity at less than analgesic doses, acting via central and peripheral mechanisms (opioids that do not cross the blood–brain barrier also depress coughing, e.g. pholcodine).

The incidence of nausea associated with opioid use is 10–60%, and is markedly increased in pain-free and ambulatory patients (via opioid sensitisation of the vestibular nucleus). The ability to produce nausea and vomiting varies between opioids, and also between patients, and tolerance develops rapidly. Substituting one opioid for another may decrease the incidence, as may switching to oral administration.

Constipation remains the most common side effect of chronic opioid administration, and toxic megacolon may occur in patients with ulcerative colitis. Tolerance to this and other smooth-muscle effects develops very slowly. Loperamide is a synthetic opioid which does not cross the blood–brain barrier, and it is used specifically as an anti-motility agent. All opioids increase bile duct pressure and cause contraction of the sphincter of Oddi in a dose-dependent manner. Pethidine has been incorrectly reported to cause less smooth-muscle spasm than the other full agonists, and is equally spasmogenic at equianalgesic doses. Opioid effects on the biliary tree can be reversed by naloxone (except for pethidine, which produces any smooth-muscle contraction via a direct action), nitroglycerine or glucagon.

Other smooth-muscle effects involve the genitourinary system. Urinary retention and urgency occur frequently, and are more common in the elderly, and when opioids are administered neuraxially. This latter situation reflects a centrally mediated mechanism through receptors located in the sacral spinal cord.

There are a number of other centrally mediated opioid effects. The majority of these are of no clinical benefit and usually unpleasant. Opioids may cause pruritis with a spectrum of severity, and the mechanism and physiological significance are unknown. The pruritis predominantly affects the face and nose, and is independent of any histamine release. Substituting opioids may decrease the incidence, and it may be alleviated by low-dose naloxone

therapy. Muscle rigidity begins at or just after the loss of consciousness, and may manifest as hoarseness in mild cases. Severe episodes can make ventilation almost impossible, even after intubation. It can be minimised by co-administration of induction agents and benzodiazepines, and may be prevented by pretreatment with muscle relaxants. It is aggravated by the use of nitrous oxide. It is seen more commonly with the potent phenylpiperidines than with morphine, the risk is increased with increased opioid dose, and it can be reversed by administration of naloxone.

Opioids decrease thermoregulatory thresholds to a similar degree to the potent volatile agents. Pethidine is unique in its ability to reduce shivering probably via a KOP-mediated action, and has been effectively utilised for hypothermic, post-operative, blood transfusion-related, and epidural-related shivering. Tramadol has also been demonstrated to be efficacious in this regard.

All alkaloids of opium cause a histamine weal when injected intradermally. Histamine release and associated hypotension are variable in incidence and severity, and are reduced by slow IV administration and ameliorated by intravascular fluid loading. The phenylpiperidines (except pethidine) are devoid of this side effect. The histamine release may be localised or generalised, and may cause subjective facial flushing and variable itch.

Opioid-specific effects

A number of important opioid-related therapeutic and adverse effects are specific to the individual opioid being used (e.g. codeine – antitussive and constipation). Pethidine is a unique opioid because of its non-opioid effects. It has a local anaesthetic effect of equivalent potency to cocaine, which gives it advantages when administered neuraxially, and it has a quinidine-like effect on cardiac muscle to reduce cardiac irritability and arrhythmias. Pethidine overdose produces the unique combination of cardiovascular collapse, mydriasis, hyperreflexia and convulsions in addition to respiratory depression.

The phenylpiperidine family (excepting remifentanil) has been associated with postoperative respiratory depression after high-dose administration due to secondary peaks in plasma levels. This has been attributed to a number of possible aetiologies, but most probably results from the release of opioid from body stores, with increases in peripheral perfusion and shivering postoperatively.

Opioid metabolites

Some of the significant adverse effects of opioids relate to the production of toxic metabolites. M3G may be

Drug	Protein binding (%)	pKₐ	Octanol/water partition coefficient	V_d (steady state) l kg⁻¹	$t_{1/2\beta}$ (min)	Cl (ml kg⁻¹ min⁻¹)	HER
Alfentanil	92	6.5	129	0.8	100	6	0.4
Buprenorphine	96	8.6		3.0	330	19	0.8
Codeine	10	8.2	0.6	5.4	180	11	0.4
Fentanyl	85	8.4	813	4.0	100	13	0.9
Morphine	35	7.9	1.4	3.5	180	15	0.8
Naloxone	45	7.9	34	2.0	70	25	0.9
Remifentanil	70	7.1	18	0.35	15	50	N/A
Tramadol	20	9.4	1.4	4.0	360	10	0.3

HER, hepatic extraction ratio; V_d, volume of distribution; $t_{1/2}$, half-life

Figure AN9 Pharmacokinetic data for commonly used opioids

responsible for the neuroexcitatory effects observed with large-dose chronic morphine administration. Moreover, it may be an opioid antagonist and possibly associated with hyperalgesia (paradoxical pain) seen after morphine administration. Norpethidine has half the analgesic potency of pethidine, but 2–3 times the convulsant activity. Because of the long half-life of norpethidine, significant accumulation occurs within 48 hours and steady state is achieved within 3–6 days. Greater amounts of norpethidine are produced with oral administration. Norpethidine accumulation initially manifests as subtle mood alteration with anxiety, culminating in potentially fatal reactions at higher concentrations. Norpropoxyphene also has a weak opioid action, but causes central excitatory effects and cardiac conduction disturbances.

Not all opioid metabolites are inactive or toxic. In fact some are necessary for clinical efficacy. Examples include morphine and M6G, codeine and morphine, tramadol and its M_1 metabolite. The main metabolite of naltrexone, 6-β-naltrexone, is active with a longer half-life than its parent, and is necessary for the efficacy of naltrexone.

Pharmacokinetics

Figure AN9 shows pharmacokinetic data for some commonly used opioids.

Administration

The choice of route of administration depends on the opioid being utilised, pain severity, the need for drug titration and any drug or patient contraindications to a particular route. The mode of administration may influence the onset of peak analgesia and side effects. For example, respiratory depression may occur 7 minutes after an IV dose of morphine, but not until ∼30 minutes after IM or 6–10 hours after intrathecal dosing.

Certain routes confer advantages for specific opioids. Intrathecal administration may provide a greater quality and potentially a longer duration of pain relief, with a lower incidence of supraspinal effects. However, a higher incidence of specific side effects (nausea, urinary retention, pruritis) occurs. Hydrophilic opioids (morphine) and the active metabolites of diamorphine remain in the CSF for longer, where they produce prolonged analgesia. At higher doses they ascend to produce analgesia at higher segmental levels. An unfortunate and hazardous consequence of this migration is a dose-dependent risk of late respiratory depression (peak 6–10 hours after dose). The more lipophilic opioids bind rapidly to local sites, and from there are absorbed intravascularly before they can migrate cephalad.

In respect of epidural opioid pharmacokinetics, dural penetration is related to opioid molecular size and lipophilicity, with sufentanil, fentanyl, and morphine peak CSF concentrations occurring at 6, 20, and 60–240 minutes respectively. Only 3–5% of a morphine dose crosses the dura. Opioid lipophilicity is also important for uptake into peridural fat and epidural veins. Hence, plasma opioid concentrations of lipophilic opioids given epidurally are often equivalent to those levels achieved after IM administration.

No opioid agonist demonstrates dose-dependent pharmacokinetics. First-pass metabolism of orally administered opioids occurs in the liver and the intestinal wall (up to 50%). Opioids given IM or SC have 100% bioavailability, but peak plasma concentrations can vary up to fivefold depending on body temperature, site of administration and haemodynamic status. IV administration results in a much narrower range of plasma concentrations.

The lung exerts a significant first-pass effect on several highly lipid-soluble opioids. Prior administration of other lipophilic amines such as propranolol reduces pulmonary uptake, by saturating binding sites.

Distribution

Opioids undergo variable degrees of protein binding, primarily to α_1-acid glycoprotein, but also to albumin. Fentanyl, sufentanil, and alfentanil also bind to β-globulins, while morphine is bound mainly to albumin. Variability in plasma protein concentration only alters the free fraction for highly protein-bound opioids. Those opioids bound to the acute-phase reactant α_1-acid glycoprotein (especially alfentanil) can achieve variable free concentrations in states of inflammation, infection, malignancy and pregnancy. Dilution or states of low protein concentration increase the free fractions of all highly bound opioids, as does competition for binding sites from other drugs that are basic amines.

Due to their high lipid solubility, most opioids tend to be widely distributed throughout the body, resulting in a large volume of distribution (V_d). Redistribution thus has a significant effect on the decline in opioid plasma concentrations after bolus dosing and short-term infusions of certain opioids. Uptake by muscle, visceral organs and the lung contributes to this redistribution.

Receptor kinetics

The diffusion of an opioid to its site of action (biophase) is dependent on its lipid solubility, the driving concentration gradient and uptake into surrounding tissue. Opioid lipid solubility is usually quantified by a specific oil/water (usually octanol/water) partition coefficient. In addition, all opioids are weak bases that dissolve into solutions of protonated (ionised) and free base fractions. The relative proportions of these fractions are dependent on the pK_a of the specific opioid and the plasma pH. The un-ionised free base form is always more lipid-soluble than the ionised form, and thus the pK_a of any particular agonist is another determinant of its lipid solubility in vivo.

The concentration gradient driving diffusion is dependent on the dose and percentage protein binding. Only the unbound fraction of un-ionised drug constitutes the diffusible fraction, which provides the concentration gradient for diffusion into the biophase.

In the biophase the opioid receptor only recognises the protonated form of the opioid, and ion trapping in the context of an acidic CNS secondary to respiratory acidosis therefore amplifies opioid activity.

Binding to receptor sites depends on receptor affinity and on any non-receptor site binding (e.g. brain lipids). Hydrophilic morphine penetrates the blood–brain barrier slowly, but its low lipid solubility and little non-specific brain binding results in a large mass of drug eventually reaching the effect site, where it binds strongly to the μ receptor. Moreover, morphine gets 'trapped' in the CNS, and this explains its longer duration of action than predicted by its elimination half-life. The onset and duration of action of an individual opioid therefore represents a complex interaction between its pK_a and the pH of plasma and the pH of the biophase, lipid solubility, and both protein and tissue binding.

Elimination

Opioids predominantly undergo liver metabolism (phase I and/or phase II reactions), with renal excretion of the more hydrophilic metabolites. Some of these metabolites also undergo biliary excretion. Small amounts of the more hydrophilic opioids may be excreted unchanged in the urine. Hepatic blood flow (HBF) is the primary determinant of plasma clearance (Cl) for most opioids, because of their high hepatic extraction ratios (HER).

Morphine

The biotransformation of morphine is unique among the opioids. In the liver 60–80% undergoes glucuronidation to morphine-3-glucuronide (M3G) and 10% to morphine-6-glucuronide (M6G). The remainder undergoes sulphation (significant in the neonate, where glucuronidation metabolism is immature), 5% is demethylated to normorphine, and a small amount is converted to codeine, with 10% being excreted unchanged in the urine. In healthy individuals up to 10% of glucuronidation occurs in extrahepatic sites (kidney and GIT). The excretion of the morphine-glucuronides is directly related to creatinine clearance. Ninety per cent of conjugated morphine is eventually excreted in the urine, and the remainder excreted in bile, sweat and breast milk. M6G is 2–4 times more potent than morphine, and has a much longer elimination half-life. Despite being more hydrophilic than morphine, M6G crosses the blood–brain barrier, from where its elimination is significantly slower. There is also some enterohepatic recirculation of morphine and its glucuronides, particularly in the setting of chronic oral therapy.

Diamorphine

Diamorphine is inactive and requires rapid deacetylation in the CSF, liver, and plasma to 6-monoacetylmorphine and morphine. These active metabolites are more hydrophilic and their subsequent metabolism is as for morphine.

Codeine

Codeine is mainly metabolised in the liver to codeine conjugates and norcodeine, with some urinary excretion of free codeine. Up to 10% of a dose is also metabolised to morphine by the hepatic microsomal enzyme CYP2D6. This biotransformation is thought to be the major contributor to the analgesia produced by codeine. Due to genetic polymorphisms, 8% of western Europeans are deficient of this enzyme. These individuals require higher doses, although they may still not obtain effective analgesia.

Pethidine

The majority of pethidine metabolism involves hydrolysis to pethidinic acid, with little free urinary excretion (5%) of the parent drug – although this may be increased to 25% with urinary acidification (pH < 5). One-third of metabolism involves N-demethylation to norpethidine, which is then hydrolysed to norpethidinic acid. Enzyme induction resulting from chronic pethidine use (and carbamazepine therapy) increases the proportion transformed to norpethidine.

Fentanyl and sufentanil

The high lipid solubility of fentanyl and sufentanil contributes to their large volume of distribution, which causes rapid and continued peripheral tissue uptake, limiting initial hepatic metabolism. This results in greater variability in plasma concentrations (13-fold range for fentanyl) during the elimination phase, particularly with fluctuations in muscle blood flow that may contribute to secondary peaks in plasma concentration after large doses. Fentanyl, sufentanil and alfentanil undergo little unchanged renal excretion, being metabolised in the liver via similar pathways. These inactive metabolites are subsequently excreted in the urine. Alfentanil is mainly metabolised by CYP3A3/4 – the most abundantly expressed of the hepatic P_{450} enzyme isoforms. Variations in the activity of this enzyme are thought to explain the variability in the kinetics and dynamics of alfentanil infusions.

Remifentanil

Remifentanil is a structurally unique methyl ester that undergoes widespread and rapid extrahepatic metabolism by blood and tissue non-specific esterases. This process is non-saturable and results in a clearance that is several times hepatic blood flow. The primary metabolic pathway is de-esterification to a carboxylic acid metabolite, with 90% of the drug recovered from the urine in this form. This metabolite is also a full agonist at μ receptors, but has a potency 1/4600 that of the parent compound and is of no clinical significance even in renal failure. The high clearance and low volume of distribution of remifentanil mean that the offset of its effect is due to metabolism rather than redistribution; this explains its very short context-sensitive half-life irrespective of the duration of infusion. Hypothermia can reduce remifentanil clearance by up to 20%.

All highly lipid-soluble drugs are sequestered into fat stores after prolonged infusions. Even after large single boluses or sequential boluses there is likely to be a delayed clinical recovery because the fall in plasma drug concentration by elimination of drug from the central compartment is retarded by the return of opioid from the peripheral compartments. Hence, the time for the plasma drug concentration to fall by 50% after an infusion ceases is influenced by the duration of the infusion, representing the degree to which the peripheral compartment has become saturated – so-called 'context-sensitive'. The context-sensitive half-life for most opioids, except remifentanil, increases with increasing duration of infusion. For example, although fentanyl has an elimination half life of 3–5 hours, in the steady state its context-sensitive half-life is 7–12 hours.

Patient factors influencing opioid pharmacokinetics and pharmacodynamics

The pharmacokinetics and dynamics of opioids may be altered in a number of physiological states (Figure AN10). The pharmacokinetic parameters of opioids are unrelated to absolute body weight except for distribution parameters. Rather, they correspond to lean body weight, and dosages should be on the basis of ideal (estimated lean) body weight. Caution in obese individuals is recommended when giving prolonged infusions of all opioids other than remifentanil, because their larger volume of distribution will prolong the elimination half-life.

Renal failure is only of clinical significance for the use of morphine and pethidine. The elimination half-life of morphine-glucuronides increases from 4 to 14–119 hours in renal failure. Fatal and near-fatal CNS toxicities including convulsions and extreme tachycardia and hypertension have occurred with the use of pethidine from

Physiological state	Effect	Mechanism
Obesity	Overdosage	Central V_d is not reflected by actual body weight ↑ Total V_d prolongs elimination half-life
Elderly	↑ Sensitivity to opioid	↓ Neuronal cell mass ↓ Central V_d
	Prolonged effect of infusion	↓ Lean body mass with ↑ adipose tissue causes increase in total V_d ↓ HBF (by 40–50% by age 75)
Infant	Prolonged effect	↓ Conjugating capacity Immature renal function (both approach adult values by 1–3 months)
Renal failure	Morphine toxicity	Accumulation of M6G Possible hydrolysis of glucuronides back to parent compound Uraemia potentiates CNS depression and ↑ blood–brain barrier permeability
	Pethidine toxicity	Accumulation of norpethidine
Hepatic failure	↑ Sensitivity to opioids (in severe liver failure only)	Synergism if encephalopathic Altered integrity of blood–brain barrier ↑ Elimination half-life for pethidine and tramadol

Figure AN10 Factors influencing opioid pharmacokinetics and pharmacodynamics

norpethidine accumulation in individuals with renal failure. These CNS effects are not mediated by opioid receptors, and not reversible with naloxone. A similar accumulation occurs with norpropoxyphene. The clearance of the fentanyl congeners is not altered appreciably, although the reduction in plasma proteins may potentially alter the free fraction of the opioid.

Surprisingly, the pharmacokinetics of most opioids is unchanged in liver failure, except in the setting of liver transplantation. This demonstrates the substantial metabolic reserve of the liver, particularly in relation to conjugation reactions. Liver disease may be reflected by a variable reduction in metabolic capacity, hepatic blood flow (HBF) and hepatocellular mass. It also causes a reduction in plasma proteins and increases in total body water through the formation of oedema, which may alter distribution kinetics and unbound drug fractions. Synergistic and unpredictable CNS depression may occur in the setting of hepatic encephalopathy. The metabolism of morphine is the least likely to be altered by liver disease, mainly because of the preservation of glucuronidation in all but fulminant liver failure. Also, a significant contribution to metabolism (at least 30%) is by increased extrahepatic (kidney and GIT) activity. Importantly, any reduction in liver clearance will increase the oral bioavailability of morphine. During liver transplantation the offset of the effect of morphine is due to redistribution. The metabolism and clearance of the fentanyl congeners is also relatively preserved in most stages of hepatic failure. Fentanyl and sufentanil disposition may be altered only if given in high doses in severe liver dysfunction. There is no change to the pharmacokinetic profile of remifentanil, even during the anhepatic phase of liver transplantation. Pethidine is the only opioid whose clearance is decreased in liver dysfunction. Similarly, considerable dosage reductions are necessary for tramadol, as the clearance is markedly reduced.

Acid–base changes have complex effects on opioid pharmacokinetics, with unpredictable consequences. Alterations in pH have competing effects on drug ionisation (with ion trapping), plasma protein binding and cerebral blood flow, which result in both respiratory acidosis and respiratory alkalosis prolonging the action of opioids.

The use of opioids is also cautioned in hypothyroid patients and those with adrenocortical insufficiency, because of the potential for significant effects on haemodynamics.

Opioid drug interactions

The opioids have limited but important interactions with other drugs. Predictably they produce synergistic effects on the level of consciousness with other CNS depressants. Benzodiazepines, barbiturates and propofol act synergistically on loss of consciousness, but increase the risk of cardiovascular depression. In anaesthesia the use of opioids allows the concentrations of volatile anaesthetic agents to be reduced by up to 50% whilst ensuring amnesia and immobility, with the preservation of haemodynamic stability at low inhaled concentrations ($\leq$1 MAC).

The use of opioids (particularly pethidine and tramadol) with monoamine oxidase inhibitors (MAOI) may result in serious and potentially fatal sequelae. Morphine has been recommended as the preferred opioid for use in these patients. The interaction of pethidine with MAOI may produce excitatory (type I) or inhibitory (type II) reactions. Excitatory phenomena include agitation, headache, haemodynamic instability, fever, rigidity, convulsions and coma. This is attributed to excessive CNS serotonin activity, since both MAOI and pethidine block serotonin reuptake. The inhibitory syndrome consists of respiratory depression, coma and hypotension, and is the result of MAOI inhibition of hepatic microsomal enzymes with secondary pethidine accumulation. A similar excitatory ('serotonergic') syndrome is seen with the combination of tramadol and the selective serotonin and noradrenaline reuptake inhibitors. The risk is increased in individuals with CYP2D6 polymorphisms, which make them extensive metabolisers of tramadol.

Opioid antagonists

The only opioid antagonists currently used in clinical practice are naloxone and naltrexone.

Naloxone

Naloxone is an N-allyl derivative of oxymorphone. It is a pure opioid antagonist, having no intrinsic pharmacological activity. It has a high affinity for MOP but also blocks other opioid receptors. Naloxone reverses the respiratory depression and analgesia of opioids and precipitates withdrawal in opioid addicts. It may also block the actions of endogenous opioids. Intravenous administration of 200–400 μg of naloxone will reverse the respiratory depressant effects of opioids, but incremental titration (1.5–3 μg kg^{-1}) is preferable in order to minimise the reversal of the analgesic effects of the opioids. Naloxone acts for approximately 30 minutes so further doses or an infusion may be necessary to avoid the return of the respiratory-depressant effects of any agonist that outlasts the effects of naloxone. Naloxone is also effective in alleviating the pruritis and urinary retention of intrathecal and epidural opioids. Naloxone has an oral bioavailability of only 2% because of extensive first-pass metabolism.

Naltrexone

Naltrexone is an analogue of naloxone that has a longer duration of action (elimination half-life of 8 hours). Naltrexone is effective orally because it has a low first-pass effect. It is used as maintenance therapy in the management of dependency because it blocks the euphoria of high doses of opioids in relapsing cases.

Tramadol

Tramadol is a unique drug with a complex mode of action, only part of which is mediated through opioid receptors.

Tramadol is a phenylpiperidine analogue of codeine. Tramadol acts as a weak agonist at all types of opioid receptor, with some selectivity for the μ receptor. It has one-tenth the potency of morphine. Tramadol also blocks the reuptake of noradrenaline and 5-HT (serotonin) and facilitates release of the latter, to modify nociceptive transmission by activation of the descending inhibitory pathways in the CNS. Naloxone therefore only partially reverses the analgesic effects of tramadol. Tramadol is a racemic mixture of (+)tramadol and (−)tramadol and it appears that the two enantiomers have separate effects at opioid and non-opioid sites. (+)tramadol affects μ receptors and 5-HT reuptake and release, while (−)tramadol inhibits noradrenaline release. Effects on α_2-adrenergic, NMDA and benzodiazepine receptors may be due to indirect effects secondary to noradrenergic effects.

Tramadol is used in the treatment of moderate to severe pain. Tramadol is well absorbed orally, with a bioavailability of 68%, and only 20% is protein-bound. Tramadol is extensively metabolised in the liver by N-desmethylation, O-desmethylation and conjugation, with 90% being excreted in the urine. The elimination half-life is 4–6 hours. The metabolite O-desmethyltramadol (half-life 9 hours) has 2–4 times greater analgesic potency than tramadol, and caution should be used in hepatic and renal impairment.

Tramadol exhibits little respiratory depression when compared to equianalgesic doses of morphine. Cardiovascular effects are minimal. Other reported side effects include dizziness, sedation, nausea, dry mouth, sweating and skin rashes. There is a low potential for abuse and physical dependence, although abuse has been reported. At present, it is not subject to controlled-drug restrictions.

Concomitant use of monoamine oxidase inhibitors is contraindicated. Co-administration with carbamazepine may decrease the concentration and effect of tramadol.

Non-steroidal anti-inflammatory drugs (NSAIDs)

The non-steroidal anti-inflammatory agents share several properties with aspirin and may be considered together. Injectable preparations of the 'aspirin-like' NSAIDs ketorolac, diclofenac, ketoprofen and tenoxicam promised perioperative analgesia free from opioid disadvantages of respiratory depression, sedation, nausea and vomiting, gastrointestinal stasis or abuse potential. NSAIDs have analgesic, anti-inflammatory and antipyretic effects, and those used for pain relief produce marked analgesia with less anti-inflammatory action.

NSAID absorption is rapid by all routes of administration, whether by mouth or by injection. The drugs are highly protein-bound, have low volumes of distribution and the unbound fraction is active. Consequently, NSAIDs can potentiate the effects of other highly protein-bound drugs by displacing them from protein binding sites (oral anticoagulants, oral hypoglycaemics, sulphonamides and anticonvulsants).

Mechanism of action

Many NSAID and aspirin effects are mediated by inhibition of prostaglandin synthesis in peripheral tissues, nerves and the central nervous system (Figure AN11). Aspirin acetylates and irreversibly inhibits cyclo-oxygenase, whilst NSAIDs act by competitive inhibition. However, the NSAIDs and aspirin may have other mechanisms of action independent of any effect on prostaglandins, including effects on basic cellular and neuronal processes. Prostaglandins were initially described as locally active substances from the prostate gland that produced smooth-muscle contraction. Many are now recognised, based on a 20-carbon chain molecule, being one family of the *eicosanoids* (from Greek *eicosa*, twenty), oxygenated metabolites of arachidonic acid and other polyunsaturated fatty acids that include leukotrienes. The rate of prostaglandin synthesis is normally low, being regulated by tissue stimuli or trauma, which activates phospholipases to free arachidonic acid, from which prostaglandins are produced by prostaglandin endoperoxide (PGH) synthase, which has both cyclo-oxygenase and hydroperoxidase enzymatic sites. Prostaglandins have many physiological functions including gastric mucosal protection,

maintenance of renal tubular function and renal vasodilatation and bronchodilatation. Endothelial prostacyclin produces vasodilatation and prevents platelet adhesion, and platelet thromboxane produces aggregation and vessel spasm.

Cyclo-oxygenase isoenzymes

Two subtypes of cyclo-oxygenase enzyme (*constitutional* COX-1 and *inducible* COX-2) have been identified. NSAIDs, like aspirin, are *non-selective* cyclo-oxygenase inhibitors that inhibit both COX-1 and COX-2. Non-selective COX-1 and COX-2 inhibition confers both the analgesic and the adverse-effect profile of NSAIDs.

The two isolated COX isoenzymes have 75% amino acid homology, with complete preservation of the catalytic sites for cyclo-oxygenase and peroxidase activity, with almost identical enzyme kinetics.

COX-1

COX-1 is a membrane-bound haemoglycoprotein with a molecular weight of 71 000 daltons found in the endoplasmic reticulum of prostaglandin-producing cells. The enzyme cyclises arachidonic acid and then adds a 15-hydroperoxy group to form the endoperoxide PGG_2, which is then reduced to the hydroxy form of PGH_2 by a peroxidase in the same COX enzyme protein. The COX-1 isoenzyme integrates into only a single leaflet of the lipid bilayer, and this is described as a *monotopic* arrangement. The enzyme has three independent folding units: an epidermal growth-factor-like domain, a membrane binding domain and an enzymatic domain. The helices of the membrane binding domains form a channel entrance to the active site, are inserted into the membrane, and thereby allow arachidonic acid to gain access into the interior of the lipid bilayer. The sites for cyclo-oxygenase and peroxidase activity are spatially distinct but are adjacent to each other. The COX active site is a long hydrophobic channel. NSAIDs block COX-1 halfway down the channel by hydrogen bonding (reversible). Aspirin acetylates serine, irreversibly preventing access for arachidonic acid.

COX-2

COX-2 has a molecular weight of 70 000 daltons, with similar sites to COX-1 for the attachment of arachidonic acid, and a similar three-dimensional structure to COX-1. However, its active site has a greater volume, because it has a larger central channel with a wider entrance and a secondary internal pocket, and therefore COX-2 can accommodate larger drugs than COX-1. A single amino acid difference at position 523 is critical for the COX-1

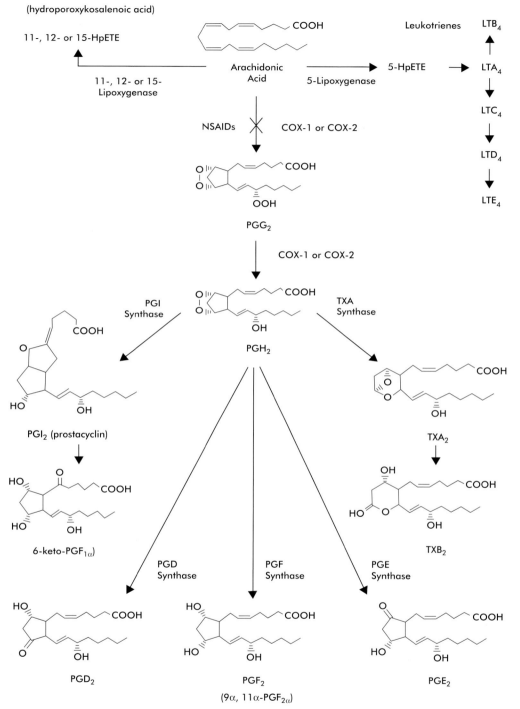

Figure AN11 Prostaglandin synthesis pathways

and COX-2 selectivity of the NSAIDs. In COX-2 a valine molecule replaces the isoleucine molecule present at position 523 in COX-1. This valine molecule is smaller and produces a gap in the wall of the channel, giving access to a side pocket, which is the binding site of the COX-2 selective inhibitors. The larger isoleucine at position 523 in COX-1 blocks access of drug molecules to the side pocket.

The genes for the two isoenzymes are found on different chromosomes. Under physiological conditions COX-1 activity predominates, to produce prostaglandins that regulate rapid physiological responses such as vascular homeostasis, gastric function, platelet activity and renal function. The concentration of the COX-1 isoenzyme is low but this may increase two- to fourfold in response to stimulation by hormones or growth factors. Low concentrations of COX-2 can normally be detected in the brain, kidney and the gravid uterus. COX-2 mRNA expression by monocytes, synovial cells and fibroblasts may be increased 10–80-fold when stimulated by growth factors, cytokines, bacterial lipopolysaccharides or phorbol esters. These factors increase COX-2 production and tissue PGE_2 concentrations resulting in pain and inflammation.

Efficacy of NSAIDs

NSAIDs are effective as postoperative analgesics. The *number needed to treat* (NNT, essentially the number of patients in a study to which the drug must be given to show a benefit) for ketorolac 10 mg is 2.6, diclofenac 50 mg 2.3, and ibuprofen 400 mg 2.4. For comparison the NNT of morphine 10 mg (intramuscularly) is 2.9, and codeine 60 mg (orally) 16.7. When given in combination with opioids, NSAIDs produce better analgesia and reduce opioid consumption by 25–50%. NSAIDs are insufficient for sole use for the relief of very severe pain immediately after major surgery, although they are very useful analgesic adjuncts, improving pain relief whilst reducing opioid requirements.

Adverse effects

Prostaglandins are local tissue hormones regulating function, and interference with their synthesis can produce specific problems. With acute use the main concerns are the potential of producing peptic ulceration, interference with platelets, renal impairment and bronchospasm in individuals who have 'aspirin-induced asthma'. In general, the risk and severity of NSAID-associated side effects increases with age.

The gastric and duodenal epithelia have protective mechanisms against acid and enzyme attack involving prostaglandin production, and chronic NSAID use is associated with peptic ulceration and bleeding. Unfortunately, acute gastroduodenal damage and bleeding can occur even with short-term NSAID use.

Platelet cyclo-oxygenase is essential for the production of the cyclic endoperoxides and thromboxane A_2, which mediate vasoconstriction and platelet aggregation, the primary haemostatic response to vessel injury. Aspirin acetylates cyclo-oxygenase irreversibly, but NSAIDs inhibit platelet cyclo-oxygenase in a reversible fashion. Single doses of NSAIDs such as ketorolac and diclofenac inhibit platelet function (prolong skin bleeding time and inhibit platelet function in vitro), but do not tend to increase surgical blood loss in normal patients. However, the presence of a subclinical bleeding diathesis or administration of anticoagulants may increase the risk of significant surgical blood loss when NSAIDs are given.

Renal prostaglandins have important physiological roles, including the maintenance of blood flow and glomerular filtration, regulation of tubular electrolyte handling and modulation of the actions of renal hormones. The adverse renal effects of chronic NSAID use are well recognised. In certain clinical settings where there are high plasma concentrations of the vasoconstrictors renin, angiotensin, norepinephrine and vasopressin, intrarenal vasodilators including prostacyclin are produced and renal function can then be impaired by NSAID administration. The co-administration of other potential nephrotoxins, such as gentamicin, may increase the renal effect of NSAIDs. Nevertheless, with careful patient selection and monitoring the incidence of NSAID-induced renal impairment is low in the perioperative period.

Precipitation of bronchospasm is a recognised phenomenon in individuals with asthma, chronic rhinitis and nasal polyps. Such 'aspirin-induced asthma' affects 10–15% of asthmatics, can be severe, and features cross-sensitivity with NSAIDs. A history of aspirin-induced asthma is a contraindication to NSAID use after surgery. The mechanism is unclear, but the reaction increases with cyclo-oxygenase inhibitor potency. Cyclo-oxygenase inhibition may increase the arachidonic acid availability for production of inflammatory leukotrienes by lipo-oxygenase pathways. Aspirin-induced asthma is less common in children, and the susceptibility may be precipitated in adult life by viral illness.

Selective cyclo-oxygenase-2 inhibitors

New drugs have been developed that selectively inhibit the inducible cyclo-oxygenase enzyme, COX-2, and spare the constitutive enzyme, COX-1. The COX-2 inhibitors include meloxicam, nimesulide, valdecoxib and parecoxib – the injectable valdecoxib precursor. By sparing physiological-tissue prostaglandin production whilst inhibiting inflammatory prostaglandin release, COX-2 inhibitors offer the potential of effective analgesia but with fewer side effects than the NSAIDs. Unfortunately, associated and unexpected cardiovascular prothrombotic toxicity has minimised their role in clinical practice.

COX-2 inhibitors can produce effective analgesia for moderate to severe acute pain, as after surgery, similar to that of the NSAIDs. Quoted NNTs are comparable to those for conventional NSAIDs: parecoxib 20 mg IV 3.0; parecoxib 40 mg IV 2.2; valdecoxib 20 mg oral 1.7.

COX-2 inhibitors produce less clinically significant peptic ulceration than other NSAIDs. However, peptic ulceration remains a significant adverse effect of the COX-2 inhibitors, and there is continuing debate on the role of COX-2 inhibitors in patients who have other risk factors for complicated ulcer disease: the elderly, those on aspirin or corticosteroids, those with a previous ulcer or *H. pylori* infection.

Platelets do not produce COX-2 (only COX-1), and so COX-2 selective inhibitors do not impair platelet function. Studies have confirmed the lack of an antiplatelet effect of COX-2 inhibitors, and a reduction in surgical blood loss in comparison to NSAIDs. Unfortunately, because they inhibit endothelial prostacyclin production whilst sparing platelet function, it is now apparent that COX-2 inhibitors can produce a tendency to thrombosis, increasing the risk of thrombotic adverse events.

COX-2 is resident (constitutive) in some tissues, including the kidneys, and current opinion holds that COX-2 inhibitors have similar adverse effects on renal function to conventional NSAIDs.

Paracetamol

Paracetamol is the active metabolite of the earlier (more toxic) drugs acetanilide and phenacetin. It can be given orally, rectally or parenterally, has little anti-inflammatory activity, and is an effective analgesic and antipyretic. It is absorbed rapidly from the small intestine after oral administration, and recently parenteral preparations have been introduced into clinical practice, with particular indications for the IV preparation in acute pain. Paracetamol has lower protein binding (hence fewer potential drug interactions than NSAIDs) and a higher volume of distribution than NSAIDs. The recommended dose in adults is 0.5–1 g oral or rectal, every 4–6 hours when necessary, and a maximum of 6 g a day in divided doses for acute use and 4 g a day for chronic use.

The mechanism of action of paracetamol is not well understood, but it may inhibit prostaglandin synthesis in the central nervous system, with little peripheral nervous system effects. Unlike morphine, paracetamol has no apparent binding sites, and unlike NSAIDs it does not inhibit peripheral cyclo-oxygenase activity. There is growing evidence of a central antinociceptive effect of paracetamol. Postulated mechanisms include central COX-2 inhibition, inhibition of a central cyclo-oxygenase, COX-3, that is selectively susceptible to paracetamol, and modulation of descending serotonergic pathways that suppress spinal cord nociceptive transmission. There is also evidence of agonism at the CB_1 cannabinoid receptor. Paracetamol may also inhibit prostaglandin production at the cellular transcriptional level, independent of cyclo-oxygenase activity.

Nitroxyparacetamol (nitroacetaminophen) is a novel potent nitric-oxide-releasing version with anti-inflammatory and analgesic properties that has a described mechanism of action in the spinal cord that differs from paracetamol, and has less hepatotoxicity.

The NNT of paracetamol is 3.8 (compared with morphine 10 mg IM 2.9, ibuprofen 400 mg 2.4, codeine 60 mg 16.7). The combination of paracetamol 1000 mg plus codeine 60 mg has an NNT of 2.2. Paracetamol is therefore an effective analgesic, with potency somewhat less than a standard dose of morphine. Paracetamol is an effective adjunct to opioid analgesia, and regular administration after surgery can reduce opioid requirements by 20–30%; the addition of NSAIDs to paracetamol also improves efficacy. Paracetamol is thus an integral component of multimodal analgesia in combination with NSAIDs and opioids.

Paracetamol has fewer side effects than the NSAIDs, and can be used when the latter are contraindicated (asthma, peptic ulcers, bleeding diathesis). However, paracetamol overdose can produce severe liver damage. A small amount of paracetamol undergoes cytochrome P_{450}-mediated hydroxylation, producing a toxic metabolite that is normally rendered harmless by liver glutathione conjugation. With excessive doses the rate of reactive metabolite formation exceeds that of glutathione conjugation, and the result is centrilobular hepatocellular necrosis. Doses of more than

150 mg kg^{-1} taken within 24 hours may result in severe liver damage, hypoglycaemia and acute tubular necrosis. Individuals taking enzyme-inducing agents are more susceptible. Early signs include nausea and vomiting, with right subcostal pain and tenderness. Damage is maximal 3–4 days after ingestion, and may lead to death. Treatment includes gastric emptying, and administration of methionine or acetylcysteine. Plasma paracetamol concentration versus time from ingestion indicates liver damage risk after overdose (acetylcysteine should be given if the plasma paracetamol concentration is greater than 200 mg l^{-1} at 4 hours and 6.25 mg l^{-1} at 24 hours after ingestion). Nitroxyparacetamol may have less hepatic toxicity than its parent drug.

Other analgesic drugs

Alpha$_2$ agonists

The α_2 agonists clonidine and dexmedetomidine have been shown to provide effective analgesia after a variety of surgical procedures. Attention has concentrated on spinal or epidural administration of clonidine to take advantage of the known attenuating effect of stimulating spinal α_2 receptors on pain perception. In general, α_2 agonists are useful only as adjuncts to conventional opioid analgesics because of the side effects of sedation, hypotension and bradycardia, which can be marked. Epidural administration has been shown to be more effective than the systemic route, supporting the theory that clonidine acts via spinal α_2 receptors. High-dose epidural clonidine has been successfully used as a sole analgesic following major abdominal surgery, but with a significant incidence of sedation and hypotension. There is some evidence that systemic clonidine administration may have some analgesic effect. Clonidine, when given orally as a premedication, reduces both the requirement for postoperative morphine and the incidence of nausea and vomiting. Clonidine is useful in the treatment of neuropathic pain, and can also be used to modify opioid withdrawal states. In addition, spinal infusions of clonidine with opioids and local anaesthetic agents may be of considerable benefit in the treatment of complex regional pain syndromes (CRPS).

Anticonvulsants

Anticonvulsants are useful for the alleviation of neuropathic pain. Drugs used include carbamazepine, phenytoin, sodium valproate and the newer agents gabapentin, pregabalin, lamotrigine and vigabatrin. Suggested mechanisms of action include frequency-dependent block of sodium channels, calcium channel blockade and potentiation of GABA inhibition of spinal nociceptive pathways via increased release or reduced breakdown. Meta-analyses have demonstrated that anticonvulsants are effective for neuropathic pain, but with frequent adverse effects. For example the NNT for carbamazepine for trigeminal neuralgia is 2.6, whilst the *number needed to harm* (NNH) is only 3.4 patients. Therefore the effectiveness of anticonvulsants for neuropathic pain must be balanced against adverse effects, which may be serious. Common side effects include sedation, rashes, nausea, anorexia, dizziness, confusion and ataxia. Serious side effects are blood dyscrasias, subacute hepatic impairment, renal failure and Stevens–Johnson syndrome. Newer agents such as gabapentin (and pregabalin) offer the potential of similar efficacy with an improved safety profile, but gabapentin can produce the significant adverse effects of pancreatitis, altered liver function tests and Stevens–Johnson syndrome.

Antidepressants

The tricyclic antidepressants used to relieve neuropathic pain all have norepinephric activity by inhibition of epinephrine reuptake from nerve endings, probably in descending modulatory inhibitory pain pathways. The antidepressants have similar NNT and NNH to the anticonvulsants and are again effective for the relief of neuropathic pain, but with the cost of common side effects, many related to a vagolytic effect. Some tricyclic side effects are transitory, such as dry mouth and sedation, but others are serious, including postural hypotension, urinary retention, narrow angle glaucoma, paralytic ileus and cardiac arrhythmias. The elderly are particularly susceptible to side effects when given tricyclic antidepressants. Unfortunately newer antidepressants with a better side-effect profile have not been shown to be as effective for the treatment of neuropathic pain.

Cannabinoids

Delta-9-tetrahydrocannabinol (Δ^9-THC) is the main active constituent of the cannabis plant (*Cannabis sativa*). It is used as a recreational drug but is generating interest as an analgesic and anti-emetic in cancer treatment.

Two cannabinoid receptors have been identified, CB$_1$ and CB$_2$. These are both G-protein-coupled receptor complexes. CB$_1$ is the neuronal receptor found in the brain and spinal cord. Relatively few receptors are in the brain stem. CB$_2$ is predominantly found peripherally.

Δ^9-THC is highly lipophilic but has a low potency. Nabilone is a non-selective cannabinoid receptor agonist that is less lipophilic and a more potent agonist. Anandamide, a derivative of phospholipase D, has been identified as an endogenous ligand for CB_1. The breakdown pathway for this is inhibited by NSAIDs. The precise role of this in vivo is yet unclear.

Δ^9-THC causes:

- Anti-emesis
- Analgesia
- Increased pulse rate
- Decreased blood pressure
- Muscle weakness
- Increased appetite
- Euphoria then drowsiness
- Psychological interference

The main use of cannabinoids at present is in anti-emesis. Nabilone is a synthetic dibenzopyran cannabinol that acts on the vomiting centre. It is licensed for use for the antagonism of resistant cytotoxic-induced nausea, but has largely been superseded by ondansetron. Δ^9-THC may have a future role in analgesia, as it appears to cause less dysphoria and drowsiness than nabilone. The route of administration may also affect the spectrum of effects: Δ^9-THC is typically obtained by inhalation in the form of smoke.

Lidocaine

The amide local anaesthetic lidocaine can be a very useful diagnostic test and treatment for neuropathic pain. The dose is 0.5–1.5 mg kg^{-1} h^{-1} by subcutaneous or intravenous infusion, and it may be continued for a number of days to control neuropathic pain quickly before long-term oral therapy is instituted if required.

NMDA antagonists

The activation by excitatory amino acids (glutamate) of spinal cord dorsal horn N-methyl-d-aspartate (NMDA) receptors is essential for the development of central sensitisation after tissue damage. The anaesthetic agent ketamine is a potent NMDA receptor antagonist, and relatively low-dose ketamine given by subcutaneous or intravenous continuous infusion produces significant pain relief. When combined with opioids, ketamine improves analgesia and reduces side effects. Unfortunately the side effects of ketamine, including hallucinations, limit the use of this agent. A notable advantage of ketamine is that it is effective both for nociceptive and for neuropathic pain, which presents as burning stinging pain with allodynia and dysaesthesias. Ketamine can be of particular benefit in

clinical situations where the pain may be of a mixed nociceptive and neuropathic nature (e.g. severe burns or cancer pain with nerve involvement). Dextromethorphan, a component of cough mixtures, is an alternative, although less potent, NMDA receptor antagonist that has been shown to reduce opioid requirements following abdominal surgery.

Steroids

The role of corticosteroids as analgesics is limited to short-term relief of neuropathic pain where nerve compression is a feature.

Future developments

Nicotinic acetylcholine receptor agonists

Epibatidine, from the skin of an Ecuadorian frog (*Epipedobates tricolor*) and used as an arrow poison, has potent analgesic properties, and is an agonist of nicotinic acetylcholine receptors (nAChR). There are two enantiomers of epibatidine, R(+)epibatidine being the naturally occurring agent. Pharmacologically their activity is similar. Nicotinic acetylcholine receptors have five subunits, but it is now known that there is considerable diversity in the amino acid composition of a particular subunit. For example, there are at least nine variants of α and four variants of β subunit, and this may explain the differing affinities for various agonists in different locations. In the CNS, nAChR has a higher affinity for epibatidine than for acetylcholine or nicotine. Currently, however, epibatidine has numerous nicotinic agonist effects that make it unsuitable as a pure analgesic. If drugs with a high affinity for specific central nAChR groups involved in nociception can be developed without the multitude of other effects then this may be a future method of analgesia.

Tachykinins

Tachykinins are a group of neuropeptides including substance P and neurokinins A and B. Substance P and neurokinin A (NKA) are released in the spinal cord in response to peripheral noxious stimuli. Three tachykinin receptors (NK-1, NK-2, NK-3) have been identified. They enhance neurotransmission in the pain pathways. In acute nociception NKA is the main mediator acting on NK-2 receptors. In pathological pain such as inflammatory hyperalgesia NK-1 receptors are more important. Substance P is more active at NK-1, and in addition stimulates the release of peripheral inflammatory mediators such as bradykinin. NK-1 receptor antagonists inhibit pain transmission and appear to reduce inflammatory vasodilatation and plasma protein leakage.

Other centrally mediated contenders

Agonists and antagonists of a number of neurological systems may provide future advances in analgesia:

* Calcitonin gene-related peptide (CGRP) is released in the dorsal horn by afferent fibres in response to noxious stimuli. The neuropeptides somatostatin and galanin cause analgesia, while cholecystokinin inhibits opioid mediated analgesia.
* Galanin is another neuropeptide released from afferent nociceptive neurones. It appears to inhibit nociceptive dorsal horn transmission.
* The amino acid glutamine, released by C fibres, is an agonist at NMDA receptors and may be responsible (in conjunction with substance P) for 'wind-up'. Ketamine blocks the NMDA ion channel and this probably affects analgesia.
* Adenosine acts on A_1 (inhibitory) and A_2 (excitatory) receptors to influence synaptic transmission. Both receptor types are found within the CNS, including the dorsal horn. Intrathecal administration of adenosine analogues produces antinociception.

Specific pharmacology

In this section bioavailability applies to oral administration. Units (unless stated otherwise) are as follows:

Volume of distribution at steady state (V_d): $l\,kg^{-1}$
Clearance (Cl): $ml\,kg^{-1}\,min^{-1}$
Terminal half-life ($t_{1/2}$): minutes

Alfentanil

Structure – anilinopiperidine opioid analogue of fentanyl
Presentation – colourless aqueous solution (500 μg ml^{-1} in 2 and 10 ml ampoules; 5 μg ml^{-1} ampoules also available)
Dose
IV bolus 10–50 μg kg^{-1}
IV infusion 0.5–1 μg $kg^{-1}\,min^{-1}$
Pharmacokinetics

Protein binding	92%
pK_a	6.5
V_d	0.8
Cl	6
$t_{1/2}$	100

Peak effect within 90 s, duration 5–10 min

CNS – potent μ opioid receptor agonist, 10–20 times more potent analgesic than morphine
CVS – bradycardia, hypotension may occur. Obtunds cardiovascular responses to laryngoscopy and intubation in doses of 30–50 μg kg^{-1}
RS – potent respiratory depressant; chest wall rigidity may occur
Other – nausea and vomiting; no histamine release
Elimination – predominantly hepatic metabolism by N-dealkylation to noralfentanil, <1% excreted unchanged via kidneys
Contraindications – concurrent administration with monoamine oxidase inhibitors

Codeine

Structure – a morphine analogue (3-methyl morphine); a principal alkaloid of opium
Presentation
Oral – tablets 15, 30 and 60 mg; syrup 5 μg ml^{-1}
IV – colourless aqueous solution, 60 μg ml^{-1} (1 ml ampoules). Often combined with non-opioid analgesics such as paracetamol as tablets (co-codamol, containing 8 or 30 mg of codeine)
Dose – oral/IM 30–60 mg, 4–6 hourly
Pharmacokinetics

Protein binding	10%
Bioavailability	60–70%
V_d	5.4
Cl	11
$t_{1/2}$	180

CNS – <20% analgesic potency of morphine, low affinity for opioid receptors, low euphoria, rarely addictive, low abuse potential
RS – produces some respiratory depression but not severe even in high doses; antitussive
Other – constipation (used as antidiarrhoeal), mild nausea and vomiting
Elimination – 10% metabolised to morphine in liver by demethylation, remainder metabolised to norcodeine or conjugated to glucuronides. Excretion in urine as free and conjugated codeine, norcodeine and morphine. Less than 17% excreted unchanged

Diclofenac

Structure – phenylacetic acid derivative, NSAID; potent inhibitor of cyclo-oxygenase enzyme (COX-1 and COX-2)

Presentation

Oral – enteric-coated tablets 25, 50 mg; sustained-release tablets 75, 100 mg; dispersible tablets 46.5 mg; suppositories 12.5, 25, 50, 100 mg

IM/IV – aqueous solution in 3 ml ampoules containing 75 mg diclofenac sodium, sodium metabisulphate, benzyl alcohol, propylene glycol and mannitol

Dose

Oral – 75–150 mg day^{-1} in 2–3 divided doses, children 1–3 mg kg^{-1} day^{-1}

Rectal – 100 mg 18-hourly; maximum daily dose 150 mg

Deep IM – 75 mg once or twice daily

IV infusion – 75 mg 6-hourly

Pharmacokinetics

Protein binding	99.5%
Bioavailability	60%
V_d	0.17
Cl	4.2
$t_{1/2}$	90

CNS – analgesic and anti-inflammatory; dizziness; vertigo

RS – bronchospasm in atopic and asthmatic individuals

GIT – gastric irritation, dyspepsia, peptic ulceration; nausea and vomiting; diarrhoea; local irritation from suppositories

Other – renal impairment or failure; decreased renin activity and aldosterone concentrations by 60–70%; platelet aggregation inhibited; pain and local induration with IM injection; rashes and skin eruptions; transaminases raised and hepatic function impaired; blood dyscrasias; increases plasma concentrations of co-administered digoxin, lithium, anticoagulants and sulphonylureas

Elimination – significant first-pass metabolism in liver by hydroxylation then conjugation with glucuronide and sulphate; followed by excretion in the urine (60%) and bile (40%); <1% unchanged in urine

Contraindications – asthma, gastrointestinal ulceration, hepatic and renal insufficiency, bleeding diathesis, haematological abnormalities, pregnancy and porphyria

Fentanyl

Structure – synthetic anilinopiperidine opioid

Presentation – colourless aqueous solution of citrate salt (preservative-free), 50 μg ml^{-1} (2 and 10 ml ampoules)

Dose IV – 0.5–3 μg kg^{-1} for spontaneous ventilation, 1–50 μg kg^{-1} for assisted ventilation. Peak effects in 5 min, duration of 30 min for smaller doses

Epidural – 50–100 μg bolus, infusion 1 μg kg^{-1} h^{-1}

Pharmacokinetics

Protein binding	85%
pK_a	8.4
V_d	4
Cl	13
$t_{1/2}$	180

CNS – potent μ opioid receptor agonist, 60–80 times more potent analgesia than morphine; sedation

CVS – minimal effects even in higher doses, use in cardiac anaesthesia well established. Hypotension and bradycardia may occur particularly in hypovolaemic patients because of reduced sympathetic tone

RS – respiratory depression and reports of delayed respiratory depression probably as a result of enterohepatic circulation; high doses may increase chest and abdominal muscle tone so impairing ventilation

Other – nausea and vomiting, decreased gastrointestinal motility, negligible histamine release

Elimination – predominantly metabolised in liver by dealkylation to norfentanyl, an inactive metabolite; norfentanyl and fentanyl then hydroxylated and excreted in the urine (elimination half-life increased in liver disease and elderly)

Contraindications – concurrent administration with monoamine oxidase inhibitors

Ibuprofen

Structure – propionic acid derivative, NSAID; potent inhibitor of cyclo-oxygenase enzyme (COX-1 and COX-2)

Presentation – coated tablets 200, 400, 600 mg; slow-release tablets 800 mg; capsules 300 mg; syrup 100 mg 5 ml^{-1}; compound preparations with codeine (8 mg codeine/300 mg ibuprofen)

Dose – oral – 1.2–1.8 g day^{-1} in 3–4 divided doses (maximum 2.4 g day^{-1}); children 20 mg kg^{-1} in divided doses (maximum 40 mg kg^{-1} day^{-1}); not recommended in children <7 kg

Pharmacokinetics

Protein binding	99%
Bioavailability	78%
V_d	0.15
Cl	0.75
$t_{1/2}$	120

CNS – mild analgesic and anti-inflammatory properties; malaise; dizziness; vertigo; tinnitus

RS – bronchospasm in asthmatics

GIT – dyspepsia; gastic irritation; nausea and vomiting; diarrhoea

GUS – renal insufficiency and acute reversible renal failure

Other – rashes and hypersensitivity reactions; a few reports of toxic amblyopia

Excretion – metabolised in liver to two inactive metabolites and excreted in urine; <1% excreted unchanged

Contraindications – asthma; history of peptic ulceration; renal insufficiency; haemorrhagic tendencies

Ketorolac

Structure – a pyrroleacetic acid, NSAID; potent inhibitor of cyclo-oxygenase enzyme (COX-1 and COX-2)

Presentation

Tablets – 10 mg ketorolac trometamol

IV/IM – clear, slightly yellow solution, 1 ml ampoules containing 10 and 30 mg ketorolac trometamol

Dose

Oral – 10 mg 4–6-hourly (6–8-hourly in elderly), maximum 40 mg day^{-1} for 2 days

IV/IM – 10–30 mg 4–6-hourly, maximum daily dose 90 mg in non-elderly, 60 mg in elderly, renally impaired and patients <50 kg, for a maximum of 2 days

Pharmacokinetics

Protein binding	99%
Bioavailability	85%
V_d	0.15
Cl	0.35
$t_{\frac{1}{2}}$	300

CNS – dizziness; tinnitus

RS – dyspnoea; asthma; pulmonary oedema

GIT – dyspepsia; gastrointestinal irritation; peptic ulceration; nausea, vomiting and diarrhoea

Other – minimal anti-inflammatory effect at its analgesic dose; renal insufficiency; acute renal failure; hyponatraemia; hyperkalaemia; interstitial nephritis; thrombocytopenia and platelet dysfunction; rashes; pruritis and hypersensitivity reactions; flushing; pain at site of injection; increased risk of renal impairment with ACE inhibitors; reduced clearance of methotrexate and lithium; increased levels of ketorolac with probenecid

Elimination – mainly metabolised to inactive metabolite acyl glucuronide, about 25% metabolised to para-hydroxyketorolac, which has 20% of the anti-inflammatory and 1% of the analgesic activity of the parent drug. Excretion is primarily renal (92%), the remainder in bile (6%), and <1% is unchanged

Contraindications – history of peptic ulcer disease; asthma and atopic tendencies; haemorrhagic diatheses; renal insufficiency; hypovolaemia and dehydration; pregnancy; children <16 years

Morphine

Structure – a phenanthrene; a principal alkaloid of opium

Presentation

Oral – tablets 10, 20 mg; modified release tablets, 5, 10, 15, 30, 60, 100, 200 mg, solution of 10 mg 5 ml^{-1}, 30 mg 5 ml^{-1}; suppositories 10, 15, 20, 30 mg

IV – clear, colourless, aqueous solution of morphine sulphate, 10, 15, 20, 30 mg ml^{-1} (1 and 2 ml ampoules containing preservative 0.1% sodium metabisulphate)

Dose

SC/IM – 0.1–0.3 mg kg^{-1}, peak effect after 30 min, duration 3–4 h

Rectal – 15–30 mg 4-hourly

Intrathecal – 0.2–1 mg

IV – 0.05–0.1 mg kg^{-1}

Epidural – 2.5–10 mg

Pharmacokinetics

Protein binding	35%
Bioavailability	15–50%
pK_a	7.9
V_d	3.5
Cl	15
$t_{\frac{1}{2}}$	180

CNS – potent analgesic, agonist at μ, κ and δ receptors; sedation, drowsiness, euphoria, dysphoria, miosis (stimulation of Edinger–Westphal nucleus); tolerance and dependence

CVS – heart rate, systemic vascular resistance and blood pressure reduced

RS – respiratory rate and volume reduced, response to hypercarbia reduced; bronchoconstriction, antitussive, muscle rigidity

GIT – nausea and vomiting, delayed gastric emptying, constipation, contraction of gall bladder and constriction of sphincter of Oddi causing reflux into pancreatic duct and an increase in serum amylase or lipase

Other – histamine release, itching, urticaria, increased tone of ureters, bladder and sphincter leading to urinary retention, increased vasopressin secretion, transient decrease in adrenal steroid secretion

Elimination – extensive first-pass metabolism: therefore oral dose 50% higher than IM dose. Conjugated in liver to morphine-3-glucuronide (70%) and morphine-6-glucuronide (5–10%), active metabolites more potent than morphine, the remainder demethylated to normorphine. Excreted predominantly in urine as conjugated metabolites; <10% excreted unchanged. Accumulation of morphine-6-glucuronide may occur in renal failure

Naloxone

Structure – N-allyl oxymorphone opioid antagonist

Presentation – clear, colourless, aqueous solution containing 400 μg in 1 ml, or 20 μg in 2 ml naloxone hydrochloride

Dose – IV – increments 1.5–3 μg kg^{-1}, peak effect in 2 min; bolus 0.4–2 mg for suspected overdose repeated up to 10 mg lasts 20 min; may need to follow with infusion. Also administered SC and IM

Pharmacokinetics

Protein binding	45%
V_d	2
Cl	25
$t_{1/2}$	70

Clinical effects – pure opioid receptor antagonist acting at all opioid receptors; effects are related to withdrawal of the effects of any opioids and antagonism of endogenous opioids

Elimination – primarily by hepatic glucuronide conjugation followed by urinary excretion

Paracetamol

Structure – acetaminophen, a hydroxyphenylacetamide

Presentation

Tablets in various forms – 500 mg paracetamol

Suspension – 60 mg 5 ml^{-1}, 120 mg 5 ml^{-1}, 250 mg 5 ml^{-1}

Suppository – 60 mg, 125 mg, 250 mg, 500 mg

IV – clear colourless solution in 100 ml bottles containing 1 g paracetamol in low-pressure atmosphere of argon

Dose

Oral – 500 mg to 1 g, 4–6-hourly, maximum 1 g day^{-1}

IV/IM – over 50 kg: 1 g 4–6-hourly, maximum 1 g day^{-1}; child 10–50 kg: 15 mg kg^{-1} 4–6-hourly, maximum 60 mg kg^{-1} day^{-1}; child < 10 kg: 7.5 mg kg^{-1} 4–6-hourly, maximum 30 mg kg^{-1} day^{-1}; infuse over 15 minutes

Pharmacokinetics

Protein binding	3%
Bioavailability	80%
V_d	1
Cl	5
$t_{1/2}$	150

CNS – analgesia

GUS – potentiation of vasopressin on water retention

Elimination – 80% metabolised by conjugation in the liver to glucuronide or sulphate. 10% hydroxylated by cytochrome P_{450} to the highly reactive and toxic N-acetyl-p-benzo-quinone imine (NAPQI), which is rapidly inactivated by conjugation with glutathione. 4% excreted unchanged in urine

Overdosage – (10 g or 150 mg kg^{-1} in 24 hours) saturates the glutathione leading to free NAPQI, which damages the hepatic cell membrane. Early intervention by providing an alternative source of glutathione (N-acetylcysteine or methionine) can prevent this damage

Caution – Effervescent and soluble paracetamol preparations contain high levels of sodium, a 4 g daily dose typically containing 120–150 mmol of sodium

Remifentanil

Structure – synthetic anilinopiperidine opioid with a methyl ester linkage

Presentation – lyophilised white powder as 1, 2 or 5 mg vials for reconstitution, which forms a clear colourless solution containing 1 mg ml^{-1} remifentanil hydrochloride. Further dilution to a concentration of 50 μg ml^{-1} recommended for general anaesthesia. Reconstituted solution is stable for 24 hours at room temperature

Dose – IV – bolus at induction 1 μg kg^{-1} over not less than 30 s, maintenance infusion 0.05–2 μg kg^{-1} min^{-1} titrated to desired level. For spontaneous ventilation, starting dose 0.04 μg kg^{-1} min^{-1}, with range of 0.025–0.1 mg kg^{-1} min^{-1} titrated to effect

Pharmacokinetics

Protein binding	70%
V_d	0.35
Cl	50
$t_{1/2}$	15

CNS – potent μ opioid receptor agonist; analgesic potency comparable to fentanyl; rapid onset and recovery even after several hours' infusion

CVS – haemodynamically very stable; rarely bradycardia and hypotension

RS – respiratory rate and volume reduced, response to hypercarbia reduced; muscle rigidity, related to dose and rate of administration

Other – nausea and vomiting, no histamine release

Elimination – independent of hepatic and renal function, metabolised by de-esterification by non-specific plasma and tissue esterases to inactive metabolites that are excreted in urine. Unlike suxamethonium it is not a substrate for plasma cholinesterase and clearance is unaffected by cholinesterase deficiency or the administration of anticholinesterases. Not recommended for intrathecal or epidural use

Contraindications – concurrent administration with monoamine oxidase inhibitors

References and further reading

Brown DV, Tuman KJ. Morphine compounds. In: White PF (ed.) *Textbook of Intravenous Anesthesia*. Baltimore: Williams and Wilkins, 1997: 191–211.

Bailey P, Egan T. Fentanyl and congeners. In: White PF (ed.) *Textbook of Intravenous Anesthesia*. Baltimore: Williams and Wilkins, 1997: 213–45.

Cherny NI. Opioid analgesics: comparative features and prescribing guidelines. *Drugs* 1996; **51**: 713–37.

Rang HP, Dale MM, Ritter JM, Flower RJ. *Rang and Dale's Pharmacology*, 6th edn. Edinburgh: Churchill Livingstone, 2007.

CHAPTER 8

Neuromuscular blocking agents

T. C. Smith

Mechanisms of neuromuscular blockade

The transmission of neuronal impulses to skeletal muscle can be prevented in many ways. These are shown in Figure NJ1.

Drugs acting on the postjunctional nicotinic (acetylcholine) receptors of the skeletal muscle neuromuscular junction are generally used in clinical practice. These may be either depolarising or non-depolarising. The features of an ideal neuromuscular blocking agent are shown in Figure NJ2.

Monitoring neuromuscular blockade

Neuromuscular blockade may be assessed both by clinical observation and by response to electrical stimulation. It is important to consider that any assessment will only measure the function of the particular muscle group tested, and that clinical muscle relaxation may vary considerably in different parts of the body.

Clinical assessment

The presence of adequate neuromuscular function at the end of anaesthesia may be crudely determined by grip strength, by the patient (lying supine) being able to lift their head off the pillow for at least 5 seconds, and by the ability to generate a tidal volume between 15 and 20 ml kg^{-1}.

More precise assessment is required for monitoring during anaesthesia, and this may be especially useful in the recovery period.

Electrical stimulation

Most methods of electrical stimulation employ transcutaneous electrical stimulation of a peripheral nerve (most commonly the ulnar nerve at the level of the forearm). It is important to stimulate the nerve rather than neighbouring muscle.

Stimulation can be performed simply using a single pulse lasting 0.2 ms. However, a train of four such pulses produces more information. A train-of-four stimulation is defined as a sequence of four supramaximal, square-wave, electrical pulses each lasting 0.2 ms given at 2 Hz. There must be a gap of at least 10 seconds between each train of four to ensure reliable results. The use of electrical stimulation in the awake person, especially tetanic, is unpleasant and may be painful.

Fundamentals of Anaesthesia, 3rd edition, ed. Tim Smith, Colin Pinnock and Ted Lin. Published by Cambridge University Press. © Cambridge University Press 2008.

Type of blockade

1. Prevention of acetylcholine synthesis
   Hemicholiniums

2. Prevention of acetylcholine release
   Botulinum toxin
   Local anaesthetic agents
   Magnesium ions

3. Depletion of acetylcholine stores
   Tetanus toxin

4. Blockade of the acetylcholine receptor
   (a) Depolarising blockade
       Suxamethonium
       Acetylcholine excess secondary to
         anticholinesterases
       Neostigmine
       Organophosphorus compounds
       Nicotine
   (b) Non-depolarising blockade
       Aminosteroids
       Org 9487
       Pancuronium
       Pipecuronium
       Rocuronium
       Vecuronium
       Benzylisoquinolinium esters
       Atracurium
       Cis-atracurium
       Doxacurium
       Mivacurium

Figure NJ1 Mechanisms of neuromuscular blockade

- Non-depolarising mode of action
- Rapid onset of action
- Short duration of action
- Non-cumulative
- No cardiovascular side effects
- No histamine release
- Spontaneous predictable reversal
- High potency
- Pharmacologically inactive metabolites
- Unaffected by renal or hepatic failure

Figure NJ2 Features of an ideal neuromuscular blocking agent

Measurement of response

Assessment of neuromuscular blockade can be made by the observed or palpated strength of twitch, measuring evoked tension in a certain muscle (e.g. adductor pollicis, which should be preloaded to give an isometric measure).

Alternatively, automated double burst stimulation (DBS) electromyography (e.g. Relaxograph®) can be used, in which case the response from the abductor digiti minimi muscle is recorded following electrical stimulation of the ulnar nerve.

The train of four shows the following correlations:
- At 75% depression of T1, T4 is lost (a count of three twitches).
- At 80% depression of T1, T3 is lost (a count of two twitches).
- At 90% depression of T1, T2 is lost (a count of one twitch).
- When train-of-four ratio (T4/T1) >0.6 the patient is clinically recovered.

Other indices of neuromuscular blockade include tetanic fade and post-tetanic facilitation. Tetanic stimulation is electrical stimulation at 50–100 Hz. The stimulation used to produce post-tetanic facilitation is:
- Single twitch 0.2 ms – measure response
- Delay 5 s
- Tetanic burst 50 Hz for 5 s
- Delay 3 s
- Single twitch 0.2 ms – measure response

During a tetanic stimulation, the presence of a non-depolarising neuromuscular blocking agent is indicated by an exponential decline in muscle response. This is the result of decreasing amounts of acetylcholine being released with subsequent action potentials. In the presence of blockade more acetylcholine is required to achieve a muscle action potential, and the repeated stimulation unmasks this decline in acetylcholine release. Post-tetanic facilitation is the augmentation of muscle response to a single twitch brought about by using a tetanic stimulation in between. This only occurs in the presence of non-depolarising blockade, and is probably the result of stimulation of presynaptic acetylcholine receptors that enhance the subsequent release of acetylcholine from the nerve terminal.

DBS involves administering two short 50 Hz bursts (each containing three stimuli) separated by 750 ms. At a train-of-four ratio of 0.5 the second burst shows a 50% reduction in force.

Depolarising blockade

Examples – decamethonium, suxamethonium

Suxamethonium is the only current therapeutic example of a depolarising blocking drug. However, any agonist of nicotinic acetylcholine receptors can also cause blockade if not rapidly cleared from the neuromuscular junction.

Examples include nicotine and acetylcholine in the presence of excess anticholinesterase.

Mechanism of action

A depolarising block occurs when the agent stimulates the acetylcholine receptor and causes depolarisation. Persistence of the agonist at the receptor prevents repolarisation of the endplate and so it is refractory to further stimulation. As the agent diffuses away from the junctional cleft, repolarisation occurs and muscle action potentials are once more possible. The block is reversible and attachment to the receptors is competitive. The block may be enhanced by a local increase in acetylcholine, as produced by anticholinesterases.

Clinical features

Depolarising blockade is characterised by rapid onset with muscle fasciculation, as groups of muscle fibres are depolarised. This is followed by a prolonged refractory period, which constitutes the blockade.

Neuromuscular test stimulation results in:
- Reduced single-twitch height
- Reduced train of four, all of equal amplitude
- No tetanic fade
- No post-tetanic facilitation

After suxamethonium administration there may be widespread muscular pains, which are worse on movement. They are particularly common in muscular young males after early ambulation. Muscle pains may persist for several days. Pretreatment with benzodiazepines, lidocaine or small doses of non-depolarising agents may help. Dantrolene has also been used with some success.

Plasma cholinesterase abnormalities

Plasma cholinesterase is a lipoprotein enzyme comprising four polypetide chains responsible for hydrolysing esters in many tissues. It is synthesised in the liver and is present in the liver, kidneys, pancreas, brain and plasma but not erythrocytes. The normal range in plasma is 4000–12 000 IU per litre, and a fall of 700 IU per litre or more is significant. Plasma cholinesterase (also known as butyryl or pseudocholinesterase) is responsible for the metabolism of suxamethonium by hydrolysis of the two ester links of choline to succinic acid (Figure NJ8). Suxamethonium is also metabolised, slowly, by acetylcholinesterase.

A reduction in cholinesterase activity may be due either to a deficiency of cholinesterase molecules or to an abnormality of the enzyme. The causes of cholinesterase deficiency are listed in Figure NJ3. Levels fall to 75% of

- Pregnancy, third trimester
- Collagen disorders
- Carcinomatosis
- Myocardial infarction
- Liver disease
- Hypothyroidism
- Blood dyscrasias
- Amethocaine
- Ketamine
- Pancuronium
- Anticholinesterases
- Oral contraceptives
- Propranolol
- Cytotoxic agents
- Ecothiopate eye drops

Figure NJ3 Causes of plasma cholinesterase deficiency

normal during pregnancy and to 67% of normal during the first 7 days post partum. Patients with pre-existing genetic deficiencies are more prone to problems (e.g. suxamethonium apnoea – see Section 1, Chapter 4, pages 63–4) if acquired forms of deficiency coexist.

Plasma cholinesterase synthesis is controlled by a pair of autosomal recessive genes. Figure NJ4 shows possible genetic configurations, their incidence and dibucaine numbers. Assessment of plasma cholinesterase activity includes global plasma cholinesterase activity levels, and dibucaine and fluoride numbers. The dibucaine number quantifies the inhibition, by a 10^{-5} molar solution of dibucaine (a local anaesthetic previously available as cinchocaine), of the activity of plasma cholinesterase in the sample on benzoyl choline. It is expressed as a percentage. The fluoride number is similar but uses 5×10^{-5} molar sodium fluoride.

Plasma cholinesterase may also exist in excess, as a genetic variant or particularly in the presence of obesity or alcoholism. The result is a shortened duration of action of suxamethonium.

Plasma cholinesterase is also responsible for the metabolism of mivacurium, and the concomitant use of these drugs in susceptible patients may exaggerate problems.

Phase I and phase II blockade

Two distinct types of neuromuscular blockade (termed phase I and II blockade respectively) may result after the administration of suxamethonium. Figure NJ5 lists the features of each type.

Type	Genotype		Dibucaine number	Fluoride number	Typical apnoea	Incidence
Normal	$E_1^u E_1^u$	homozygous	80	60	1–5 min	94%
Atypical	$E_1^u E_1^a$	heterozygous	60	50	10 min	1 : 25
Atypical	$E_1^a E_1^a$	homozygous	20	20	2 hours	1 : 3000
Silent	$E_1^u E_1^s$	heterozygous	80	60	10 min	1 : 25
Silent	$E_1^s E_1^s$	homozygous	minimal activity		2 hours	1 : 100 000
Fluoride-resistant	$E_1^u E_1^u$	heterozygous	75	50	10 min	1 : 300 000
Fluoride-resistant	$E_1^f E_1^f$	homozygous	65	40	2 hours	1 : 150 000

Note: u, a, s and f are the four commonest of 25 possible gene variants for plasma cholinesterase

Figure NJ4 Inheritance of abnormal plasma cholinesterase

Phase I blockade
- Well-sustained response to tetanic stimulation
- No post-tetanic facilitation
- Train-of-four ratio > 0.7
- Potentiated by the effect of anticholinesterases

Phase II blockade
- Tetanic fade
- Post-tetanic facilitation
- Train-of-four ratio < 0.3
- Antagonised by the effect of anticholinesterases
- Tachyphylaxis

Figure NJ5 Phase I and II blockade after suxamethonium administration

Non-depolarising blockade

Examples – atracurium, mivacurium, pancuronium, rocuronium, vecuronium

Mechanism of action

Non-depolarising neuromuscular blockade is the result of competitive occupancy of the postjunctional receptors preventing acetylcholine from reaching one or both α subunits of the receptor. This is probably a dynamic process, with both acetylcholine and the blocking agent in equilibrium with the receptors. At least 75% of receptors must be blocked before contraction fails. The process is competitive and reversible. The block can be antagonised by a local increase in acetylcholine, as produced by anticholinesterases. These muscle relaxants have no intrinsic activity at the neuromuscular endplate. Each has one or more quaternary ammonium groups. In the bisquaternary agents, these are usually 140 nm apart.

A graphic illustration of the process by which depolarising and non-depolarising drugs have their effects is shown in Figure NJ6.

Clinical features

The predominant effect of neuromuscular blocking agents is a reversible paralysis of skeletal muscle. This reduction in skeletal muscle activity reduces venous return and therefore reduces cardiac output and blood pressure.

Neuromuscular test stimulation results in:
- Reduced single-twitch height
- Reduced train of four, with twitch amplitude 1 > 2 > 3 > 4
- Tetanic fade
- Post-tetanic facilitation

The neuromuscular blocking agents also have anticholinesterase activity (Figure NJ7).

Aminosteroids

The acetylcholine-type fragment associated with the D ring of the steroid nucleus is probably responsible for most of the neuromuscular antagonism. The acetylcholine-type fragment associated with the A ring is probably responsible for the cardiovascular effects, especially the vagolytic aspects. Histamine release is not expected with the aminosteroid structure. In general, the aminosteroids are more slowly metabolised than the benzylisoquinoliniums.

Benzylisoquinolinium compounds

The chemical structure of benzylisoquinolinium is associated with histamine release. In general, the presence of an ester link promotes rapid degradation and metabolism,

Sequence 1: Normal depolarisation

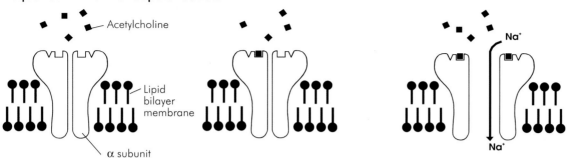

Acetylcholine released into the junctional cleft binds reversibly to receptor sites on the alpha subunits of the sodium ionophore. When the alpha site on each of the two subunits is occupied, the channel opens and allows depolarisation. Rapid metabolism enables rapid dissociation of receptor and agonist and the channel closes.

Sequence 2: Depolarising blockade

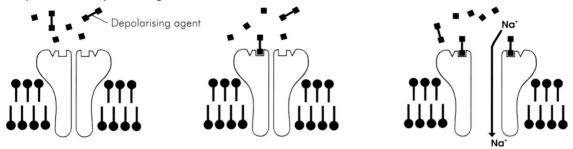

Suxamethonium and the released acetylcholine are both agonists of the receptor. When both receptors are occupied by any combination of these molecules the channel opens. However, the persistence of suxamethonium causes the channel to remain open long after the acetylcholine has been destroyed, maintaining a depolarised refractory endplate.

Sequence 3: Non-depolarising blockade

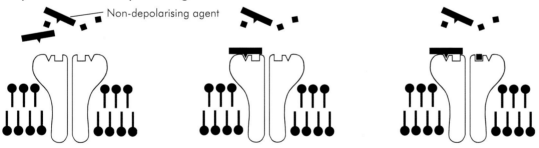

Non-depolarising drugs are antagonists and bind to the receptor without opening the channel. They subsequently prevent acetylcholine from binding and as two acetyl choline molecules are required for depolarisation only one receptor needs to be occupied by the antagonist to be effective.

Figure NJ6 Action of depolarising and non-depolarising muscle relaxants

Drug	Concentration to produce 50% inhibition of enzymatic acetylcholine breakdown (μmol l^{-1}) in the presence of various neuromuscular blocking drugs	
	Acetylcholinesterase	**Plasma cholinesterase**
Suxamethonium	1300	640
Atracurium	340	420
Vecuronium	66	0.62

Figure NJ7 Anticholinesterase activity of neuromuscular blocking agents

leading to a short half-life and rapid transition to complete recovery.

Elimination

The non-depolarising agents are usually metabolised in the liver. Other pathways exist, including spontaneous degradation and enzymatic hydrolysis within the plasma. These pathways are covered under the specific drug details, below.

The non-depolarising blocking agents may be potentiated by suxamethonium, IV and volatile anaesthetic agents, opioids, aminoglycosides, tetracyclines, metronidazole, lincosamides, polymixins, magnesium, verapamil and nifedipine, protamine, diuretics and catecholamine antagonists. The blockade is prolonged by hypothermia.

Anticholinesterases

Mechanism of action

The anticholinesterases inhibit the breakdown of acetylcholine by binding to the acetylcholinesterase enzyme in a competitive manner. This raises the background concentration of acetylcholine near the neuromuscular junction, which in turn overcomes the reduced number of functional nicotinic receptors on the muscle endplate, whether due to a reduced number of receptors (myasthenia gravis) or due to blockade of existing receptors (non-depolarising muscle relaxants). The anticholinesterases can be classified as either reversible anticholinesterases or organophosphorus compounds. While they all act on acetyl and plasma cholinesterase, the specific interaction with the enzyme varies between individual drugs.

Reversible anticholinesterases

Examples – distigmine, edrophonium, neostigmine, pyridostigmine

Acetylcholinesterase has an esteratic site and an anionic site in close proximity. Physiologically, the positively charged quaternary amine of acetylcholine binds to the anionic site. The acetyl ester combines with the esteratic site and the acetylcholine is hydrolysed. The anticholinesterases competitively occupy these sites and prevent acetylcholine access. The anticholinesterases have a quaternary amine group that is attracted to the anionic site and a carbamyl ester that binds covalently to the serine amino acid of the esteratic site. The quaternary amine group is not essential for activity, but when present it conveys enhanced potency and stability. The quaternary group also results in poor absorption following oral administration and a minimal transfer of the drug across the blood–brain barrier. Neostigmine is absorbed poorly from the gut as compared with the IV route. When neostigmine is used orally for the treatment of myasthenia gravis larger doses are, therefore, necessary. Equivalent doses of neostigmine are as follows: IV 0.5 mg; IM 1–1.5 mg; oral 15 mg.

Anticholinesterases also have some direct cholinergic agonist activity.

Physostigmine (no longer available) is an example of an anticholinesterase with several tertiary amine groups rather than the quaternary amine of the others. Consequently it is readily absorbed topically and orally and crosses the blood–brain barrier, but has no cholinergic agonist activity.

Edrophonium is only clinically effective for 5 minutes, and is used in the diagnosis of myasthenia gravis. Longer-acting agents are needed for treatment of the disease. Neostigmine is the only anticholinesterase routinely used to reverse planned neuromuscular blockade in clinical practice. Anticholinesterases have widespread effects subsequent to the stimulation of increased cholinergic muscarinic and nicotinic activity. Heart rate, vasomotor tone and blood pressure are reduced. At high dose levels sympathetic ganglion stimulation may predominate. Excess acetylcholine causes bronchoconstriction and increased bronchial secretion. Increased gastrointestinal tone and secretion occurs. Secretions of saliva, sweat and tears are also stimulated. These problems are prevented by the concomitant use of muscarinic anticholinergic drugs such as atropine or glycopyrrolate. Anticholinesterases can also cause a depolarising neuromuscular blockade when used in excess, or in the absence of non-depolarising blockade.

Neuromuscular blockade is terminated either by endogenous elimination of the drug and diffusion of the blocking agent away from the neuromuscular junction, or, in the case of non-depolarising agents, the effects can be overcome, in part, by inhibiting the metabolism of acetylcholine. If a long-acting muscle relaxant is used, it is possible for the blockade to re-establish if the effects of the anticholinesterase wear off before the neuromuscular blocking agent has left the receptors.

Organophosphorus compounds
Example – ecothiopate

These are primarily used as nerve gases and pesticides, and may feature in cases of poisoning. In general, they have no ionic binding component but bind covalently and irreversibly to the esteratic site of the cholinesterase enzyme by the release of a relatively weakly bound component of the drug. Consequently, the enzyme is not readily reactivated. Organophosphates tend to be highly lipid-soluble and readily cross the blood–brain barrier, causing central nervous system toxicity. Ecothiopate differs from the general features of this group. It is the only organophosphate in clinical use, and is used in the treatment of glaucoma. It too binds covalently to the esteratic site of the enzyme but also has a positively charged quaternary ammonium group that helps binding. This positive charge means that ecothiopate does not readily cross the blood–brain barrier, in contrast with other organophosphorous compounds. Although it is slowly hydrolysed it may nonetheless prolong the action of suxamethonium and mivacurium.

Alternative reversal agents
The development of a selective relaxant binding agent specifically targeting rocuronium has opened the way for a new method of reversal of non-depolarising neuromuscular blockade. Sugammadex (Org 25969) (de Boer *et al.* 2006) is a synthetic γ-cyclodextrin derivative (an oligosaccharide) devoid of intrinsic activity. In effect, it forms a tube into which a single relatively small steroid molecule of rocuronium fits. This binding is specific for rocuronium, effectively encapsulating it to rapidly reduce its unbound plasma concentration and also that at the neuromuscular endplate. Cyclodextrins are highly water-soluble, and sugammadex is excreted rapidly in the urine. The half-life is relatively short and so further administration of rocuronium soon afterwards may be an option. An alternative benzylisoquinolinium non-depolariser could also be used, as these larger molecules will not fit within the cyclodextrin cavity.

In contrast with anticholinesterase reversal, sugammadex:
- Is effective regardless of the state of neuromuscular blockade.
- Is devoid of intrinsic activity.
- Allows subsequent re-paralysis.

Specific pharmacology
Here, units used (unless stated separately) are:
Volume of distribution at steady state (V_d): ml kg^{-1}
Clearance (Cl): ml kg^{-1} min^{-1}
Terminal half-life ($t_{1/2}$): minutes

Pharmacokinetic data for specific non-depolarising drugs are summarised in Figure NJ8, and the chemical structures of atracurium, rocuronium, suxamethonium and neostigmine are shown in Figure NJ9.

Atracurium dibesylate
Structure – bisquaternary benzylisoquinolinium diester. A plant derivative

Presentation – clear, colourless, aqueous solution of pH 3.5 (10 mg ml^{-1}, 2.5, 5, 25 ml ampoules). Storage in fridge at 2–8 °C, protect from light

Dose – IV bolus 0.3–0.6 mg kg^{-1}, infusion 0.3–0.6 mg kg^{-1} h^{-1}. Initial dose lasts 30 min, ED$_{95}$ = 0.2 mg kg^{-1}

Pharmacokinetics

Protein binding	82%
V_d	170
Cl	5.5
$t_{1/2}$	20

CNS – no increase in intraocular pressure (IOP) or intracranial pressure (ICP). Laudanosine, a metabolite and stimulant, crosses the blood–brain barrier and can cause convulsions if plasma concentration >20 pg ml^{-1}

CVS – the small amount of histamine release may lower systemic vascular resistance, central venous pressure and pulmonary capillary wedge pressure

RS – paralysis of respiratory muscles; small risk of bronchospasm due to histamine release

	ED$_{95}$ (mg kg^{-1})	Dose (mg kg^{-1})	V$_d$ (ml kg^{-1})	Clearance (ml kg^{-1} min^{-1})	Elimination t$_{1/2}$ (min)
Atracurium	0.2	0.3–0.6	170	5.5	20
Doxacurium	0.025	0.05	220	2.7	99
Mivacurium	0.08	0.07–0.25			
trans–trans isomer			150–267	51–63	1.9–3.6
cis–trans isomer			290–382	93–106	1.8–2.9
cis–cis isomer			175–340	3.7–4.6	34.7–52.9
Org 9487	1.15[a]	1.5–2.0	293	8.5	74
Pancuronium	0.06	0.05–0.1	200	1.8	115
Pipecuronium	0.049	0.07	309	2.4	137
Rocuronium	0.3	0.6	270	4.0	131
Vecuronium	0.046	0.05–0.1	260	4.6	62

[a] Value quoted for ED$_{90}$

Figure NJ8 Pharmacokinetic data for non-depolarising neuromuscular blocking agents

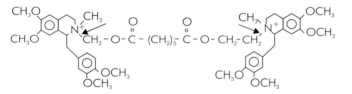

Atracurium

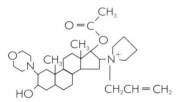

Rocuronium

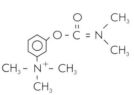

Neostigmine

Suxamethonium

Figure NJ9 Chemical structures of commonly used neuromuscular drugs. The arrows indicate sites of cleavage (Atracurium – Hofmann degradation; Suxamethonium – ester hydrolysis)

Other – no effect on lower oesophageal sphincter pressure; placental transfer insufficient to cause an effect in the fetus

Elimination – non-cumulative. Hofmann elimination is the spontaneous fragmentation of atracurium at the bond between the quaternary nitrogen and the central chain. This occurs at body temperature and pH, producing inactive products – laudanosine ($t_{1/2} = 234$ min) and a quaternary monoacrylate ($t_{1/2} = 39$ min). Atracurium is also metabolised by ester hydrolysis, producing a quaternary alcohol and a quaternary acid. These two mechanisms account for 40% of the elimination of atracurium, the remainder being by a variety of other mechanisms

Metabolites – 55% excreted in the bile within 7 h, 35% excreted in the urine within 7 h

Side effects – histamine release may cause bronchospasm, hypotension, and erythema and weals generally or along the vein of injection

Cis-atracurium dibesylate

Atracurium contains a mixture of ten geometric isomers. One of these, *cis–cis*-atracurium, is marketed as Cis-atracurium. The features are as for atracurium except:

Presentation – clear, colourless, aqueous solution of pH 3.5 (2 mg ml^{-1} in 2.5, 5, 10, 25 ml ampoules, and 5 mg ml^{-1} in 30 ml vial). Store in fridge at 2–8 °C, protect from light

Dose – IV bolus 0.15 mg kg^{-1}; infusion 0.18 mg kg^{-1} h^{-1}

ED$_{95}$ = 0.05 mg kg^{-1}

This single isomer of atracurium avoids the histamine release but is similar to atracurium in other respects.

Doxacurium chloride

Structure – bisquaternary benzylisoquinolinium diester

Presentation – not available in the UK

Dose – IV bolus 0.05 mg kg^{-1}. Initial dose lasts 80–90 min. Can be antagonised within 10 min. ED$_{95}$ = 0.025 mg kg^{-1}

Pharmacokinetics

V_d	220
Cl	2.7
$t_{1/2}$	99

CNS – no effect

CVS – minimal effect, slight decrease in heart rate

RS – paralysis of respiratory muscles

Other – no histamine release

Elimination – doxacurium is non-cumulative. Elimination is mainly renal with some hepatic excretion (unchanged) in the bile. Of it, 31% is excreted unchanged in the urine by 12 h. Doxacurium is also slowly hydrolysed by plasma cholinesterase

Mivacurium chloride

Structure – bisquaternary benzylisoquinolinium diester

Presentation – clear, colourless, aqueous solution of pH 4.5 (2 mg ml^{-1}, 5 and 10 ml ampoules) containing three stereoisomers – *trans–trans* (57%), *cis–trans* (36%), *cis–cis* (6%)

Dose – IV bolus 0.07–0.25 mg kg^{-1}; children 0.1–0.2 mg kg^{-1}; infusion 0.06 mg kg^{-1} h^{-1}. ED$_{95}$ = 0.08 mg kg^{-1} (children 0.1 mg kg^{-1})

Pharmacokinetics

Isomer	V_d	Cl	$t_{1/2}$
trans–trans	150–267	51–63	1.9–3.6
cis–trans	290–382	93–106	1.8–2.9
cis–cis	175–340	3.7–4.6	34.7–52.9

CNS – no effect

CVS – no effect

RS – respiratory muscle paralysis

Other – minimal placental transfer

Elimination – *trans–trans* and *cis–trans* isomers hydrolysed by plasma cholinesterase. The *cis–cis* isomer may be metabolised in part by the liver. Lasts twice as long as suxamethonium (24 min)

Toxicity – block antagonised by neostigmine. Block prolonged by reduced or atypical plasma cholinesterase as with suxamethonium. Block also prolonged if factors interfering with plasma cholinesterase are present. Heterozygotes for atypical plasma cholinesterase show a prolongation of effect of about 10 min

Pancuronium bromide

Structure – bisquaternary aminosteroid

Presentation – clear, colourless, aqueous solution (4 mg in 2 ml)

Dose – IV bolus 0.05–0.1 mg kg^{-1}. Initial dose lasts 45–60 min; ED$_{95}$ = 0.06 mg kg^{-1}

Pharmacokinetics

Protein binding (albumin, γ-globulin)	15–87%
V_d	200
Cl	1.8
$t_{1/2}$	115

CNS – does not cross blood–brain barrier. No increase in IOP and ICP

CVS – increase in heart rate, cardiac output and blood pressure due to vagolytic action. Systemic vascular resistance unchanged

RS – respiratory muscle paralysis; some bronchodilatation

Other – increase in lower oesophageal sphincter pressure; may increase prothrombin time and partial thromboplastin time; small amount of placental transfer but no clinical effect on fetus

Elimination – 50% excreted unchanged, of which 80% appears in the urine. Of it, 40% is deacetylated in the liver to 3-hydroxy, 17-hydroxy and 3,17-dihydroxy derivatives which are eliminated in the bile. The 3-hydroxy compound has some neuromuscular antagonist activity

Note that pancuronium has some prejunctional activity.

Pipecuronium bromide

Structure – bisquaternary aminosteroid

Presentation – not available in the UK

Dose – IV bolus 0.07 mg kg^{-1} for intubation in 3 min (up to a maximum of 0.1 mg kg^{-1}). Initial dose lasts 100 min; ED$_{95}$ = 0.049 mg kg^{-1}

Pharmacokinetics

Protein binding	2%
V_d	309
Cl	2.4
$t_{\frac{1}{2}}$	137

CNS – no effect

CVS – no effect on the cardiovascular system

RS – paralysis of respiratory muscles

Other – does not cause histamine release

Elimination – 40% excreted unchanged in the urine by 24 h, 4% metabolised by the liver to 3-desacetylpipecuronium, 2% excreted in the bile

Rocuronium bromide

Structure – monoquaternary aminosteroid

Presentation – aqueous solution (10 mg ml^{-1}, 5 and 10 ml ampoules)

Storage – in fridge at 2–8 °C; protect from light

Dose – IV bolus 0.6 mg kg^{-1}, infusion 0.3–0.6 mg kg^{-1} h^{-1}, initial dose lasts 38–150 min, ED$_{95}$ = 0.3 mg kg^{-1}. Onset time of 1.5 min using 2 × ED$_{95}$, which may be shortened to 55 s using 4 × ED$_{95}$

Pharmacokinetics

V_d	270
Cl	4.0
$t_{\frac{1}{2}}$	131

CNS – no effect

CVS – increases heart rate, cardiac output and blood pressure slightly due to vagal blockade

RS – respiratory muscle paralysis

Other – no histamine release

Elimination – predominantly hepatic but also some renal elimination. Hepatic or renal failure can cause prolongation of effect

Vecuronium bromide

Structure – monoquaternary aminosteroid, becomes bisquaternary at pH 7.4

Presentation – freeze-dried, buffered, lyophilised cake for reconstitution, containing vecuronium bromide, citric acid monohydrate, disodium hydrogen phosphate dihydrate and mannitol

Storage – avoid light and temperatures in excess of 45 °C. Reconstitution with water for injections produces clear, colourless solution of pH 4.0

Dose – IV bolus 0.05–0.1 mg kg^{-1}, infusion 0.05–0.1 mg kg^{-1} h^{-1}, ED$_{95}$ = 0.046 mg kg^{-1}. Initial dose lasts 30 min

Pharmacokinetics

V_d	260
Cl	4.6
$t_{\frac{1}{2}}$	62

CNS – no increase in ICP

CVS – no effect

RS – respiratory muscle paralysis

Other – no increase in IOP; minimal placental transfer; no histamine release

Elimination – spontaneous deacetylation and hepatic metabolism. Of total dose, 10–25% is excreted in urine; the rest in the bile. Most excreted unchanged. Suitable in patients with absent renal function. Hepatic failure may prolong clinical effect, whereas chronic phenytoin therapy reduces the efficacy of vecuronium. There are three potential metabolites, 3-hydroxy, 17-hydroxy and 3,17-dihydroxy. These have minimal neuromuscular and vagolytic activity; only 3-hydroxy is found in any significant quantity and it has 50% of the neuromuscular blocking potency of vecuronium. Vecuronium is more stable in acidic solutions, and is therefore potentiated by respiratory acidosis

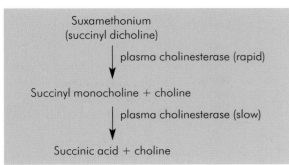

Figure NJ10 Elimination pathway of suxamethonium

Suxamethonium chloride (succinylcholine)

Structure – dicholine ester of acetylcholine

Presentation – clear, colourless, aqueous solution of pH 3.0–5.0 with a shelf life of 2 years (100 mg in 2 ml)

Storage – in fridge at 4 °C; spontaneous hydrolysis occurs in warm or alkaline conditions

Dose – IV bolus 0.3–1.1 mg kg^{-1}; children 1–2 mg kg^{-1}. Infusion 0.1% solution at 2–15 mg min^{-1}. It is effective within 30 s and lasts for several minutes

Pharmacokinetics

$t_{1/2}$ 3.5

Protein binding occurs but the extent is not known because of the transient nature of the drug

CNS – small increase in ICP which may be of relevance in the head-injured patient

CVS – increased blood pressure, bradycardia

RS – paralysis of respiratory muscles

Other – increases IOP and intragastric pressure, and lowers oesophageal sphincter pressure (barrier pressure is increased). Increases gastric secretion and salivary production

Elimination – metabolised by plasma cholinesterase – complete recovery in 10–12 min. 2–20% is unchanged in urine. The elimination pathway is shown in Figure NJ8

Side effects – muscle pains, especially in muscular young males and after early ambulation, malignant hyperthermia trigger. May result in trismus, histamine release and hyperkalaemia – especially if denervation, burns, trauma or renal failure coexist

Contraindications – malignant hyperthermia susceptibility, burns, myotonia

Suxamethonium is a short-acting depolarising neuromuscular blocking agent. It is rapidly acting by virtue of rapid distribution to the neuromuscular junction and its depolarising mode of action. Its effect is terminated by diffusion away from the neuromuscular junction followed by rapid redistribution and hydrolysis. Hydrolysis occurs in two stages each removing choline. 80% is metabolised before reaching the neuromuscular junction.

Neostigmine bromide

Structure – quaternary amine, alkylcarbamic acid ester

Presentation – clear, very pale yellow, aqueous solution in brown ampoule (2.5 mg in 1 ml)

Storage – protect from light

Dose – IV bolus 0.05–0.08 mg kg^{-1}. Peak effect 7–11 min; duration 40 min

Pharmacokinetics

V_d	700
Cl	8
$t_{1/2}$	40

Bioavailability after oral administration < 1%

CNS – central hypotensive effect at high dose; miosis, blurred vision

CVS – causes bradycardia and decreases cardiac output

RS – bronchconstriction and reduces anatomical dead space

Other – increases in all the following: ureteric peristalsis, gastrointestinal peristalsis, sweating, lacrimation, gastric tone and lower oesophageal sphincter pressure

Elimination – hydrolysed by the acetylcholinesterase that it antagonises and by plasma cholinesterase to a quaternary alcohol. Some hepatic metabolism occurs with biliary excretion. 50–67% is excreted in the urine

Side effects – concomitant administration of anticholinergics is essential when used for reversal of neuromuscular blockade. The increased gastrointestinal tone may promote anastomotic breakdown. Neostigmine inhibits the hydrolysis of suxamethonium and mivacurium and other drugs metabolised by plasma cholinesterase. High levels of neostigmine at the neuromuscular junction cause a direct blockade of the acetylcholine receptor, and the raised levels of acetylcholine have a depolarising blocking effect

Reference and further reading

de Boer HD, van Egmond J, van de Pol F, Bom A, Booij LH. Sugammadex, a new reversal agent for neuromuscular block induced by rocuronium in the anaesthetized Rhesus monkey. *Br J Anaesth* 2006; **96**: 473–9.

CHAPTER 9

Local anaesthetic agents

T. C. Smith

Local anaesthetic agents are used directly to block neuronal transmission. They also stabilise other electrically excitable membranes, and some examples, such as lidocaine, have clinically useful antiarrhythmic activity.

Structure

Local anaesthetic agents comprise a hydrophilic tertiary amine group linked to a lipophilic aromatic group. They are divided into esters and amides, based on the linking group. Figure LA1 shows examples of these two types of local anaesthetic agent. Protonation of the highlighted amine nitrogen atom confers activity on the molecule once it is inside the cell.

Local anaesthetic agents exist in two states, acid (protonated) and basic (non-ionised) in equilibrium according to their pK_a and ambient pH, as determined by the Henderson–Hasselbalch equation (Figure LA2).

Local anaesthetic agents are weak bases. At physiological pH, there exists a mixture of non-ionised and ionised drug. This is important, as only the non-ionised drug passes through the membrane, yet it is only the ionised drug that is active. Small changes in pH have marked effects on the proportion of drug that is ionised, and therefore markedly influence the effect.

Mechanism of action

Injectable local anaesthetics must be soluble and stable in water. This is achieved by creating hydrochlorides of the drug. These drugs exist within ampoules in acid solution with a high degree of ionisation, which maintains solubility.

Local anaesthetic agents act by blocking the fast sodium channel in neuronal membranes. To do so the drug must be in the protonated form and the ion channel must be in the open state. The drug enters the ion channel from the intracellular direction, but is administered extracellularly. The process by which local anaesthetic agents reach the sodium channel is illustrated in Figure LA3, using lidocaine as an example. The pK_a of lidocaine is 7.9, so extracellularly (at pH 7.4) 24% is in the non-ionised state and 76% in the ionised state (Figure LA3, stage 1). The non-ionised drug is

Fundamentals of Anaesthesia, 3rd edition, ed. Tim Smith, Colin Pinnock and Ted Lin. Published by Cambridge University Press. © Cambridge University Press 2008.

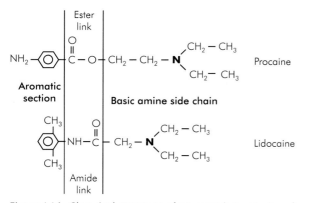

Figure LA1 Chemical structure of an ester (procaine) and an amide (lidocaine)

therefore relatively lipophilic, and it passes passively down the concentration gradient through the membrane into the cell (stage 2). Intracellularly, pH is about 7.1, and this shifts

$$pH = pK_a + \log_{10}\frac{LA\ (base)}{LA - H^+\ (acid)}$$

Figure LA2 Henderson–Hasselbalch equation for local anaesthetic agents (LA)

the balance of ionisation of the intracellular portion of drug towards the ionised state (86%) (stage 3). The ionised drug, attracted by the negative charge of membrane protein, then passes into the open ion channel (stage 4), which remains open but is blocked to further transmission of sodium (stage 5). Blockade by this route is use-dependent, because ionophores are only blocked while open.

Another mechanism of action may contribute to the anaesthetic activity. This involves the passage of non-ionised drug through the membrane directly blocking the sodium channel, an effect that does not rely on the sodium channel being open.

The opening of the fast sodium channels in neuronal membranes and the passage of sodium through them are

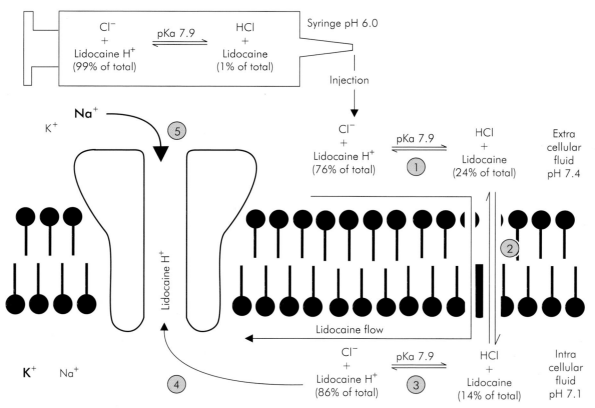

Figure LA3 Mechanism of action of local anaesthetic agents using lidocaine as an example. The stages indicated by circled numbers are described in more detail in the text.

	Molecular weight	pK$_a$ (25°C)	Partition coefficient (heptane buffer)	Protein binding (%)	Onset	Potency (relative to lidocaine)	Duration
Esters							
Amethocaine	264	8.5	4.1	76	Slow	4	Long
Procaine	236	8.9	0.02	6	Slow	$1/2$	Short
Amides							
Bupivacaine	288	8.1	27.5	96	Medium	4	Long
Lidocaine	234	7.9	2.9	64	Rapid	1	Medium
Prilocaine	220	7.9	0.9	55	Rapid	1	Medium
Ropivacaine	274	8.1	6.1	95	Medium	4	Long

Figure LA4 Physicochemical and pharmacokinetic properties of local anaesthetic agents

essential for the development and propagation of the action potential. The sharp upstroke of the action potential is gradually attenuated as more sodium channels become blocked. When the depolarisation is insufficient to generate the currents required to depolarise neighbouring membrane, then action-potential propagation and neuronal transmission cease.

Factors influencing activity
Figure LA4 shows the pharmacological properties of important local anaesthetic agents.

Molecular weight
Molecular weight itself does not affect the pharmacological properties. However, increases in molecular weight tend to be indicative of increased side-chain size and therefore increased lipid solubility.

Lipid solubility
The higher the lipid solubility, the greater the penetration of the nerve membrane by the agent, so that higher lipid solubility results in greater potency. It also results in more toxicity and local irritancy. High lipid solubility also increases the rate of onset and duration of action of local anaesthetic agents.

pK$_a$
The lower the pK$_a$, the lower the degree of ionisation for any given pH and so the more rapid the speed of onset of the block. Increasing pK$_a$ increases the ionised proportion of the drug so that intracellularly a higher proportion is in the active state. However, this also means that less is in the non-ionised, diffusible state, so the onset and offset

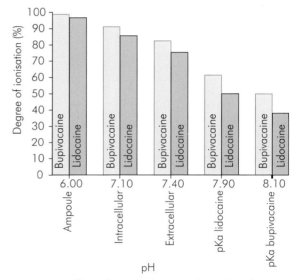
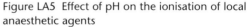

Figure LA5 Effect of pH on the ionisation of local anaesthetic agents

of action are also slower. Figure LA5 shows the effect of differences in pH and pK$_a$ on the proportion of ionised and non-ionised local anaesthetic agents.

pH
Acidosis (low pH) increases the proportion of ionised drug in the interstitium, and therefore reduces the amount of drug able to cross the neuronal membrane. The local anaesthetic is therefore reduced in potency. Manipulation of the pH of the local anaesthetic solution by addition of alkali, buffers or carbonation may be used to alter the proportion of non-ionised drug.

Protein binding

The degree of protein binding reflects the ability of the drug to bind to membrane proteins: the greater the binding, the longer the duration of action. Increased binding to tissue protein correlates with an increase in the duration of action and probably indicates a higher affinity for membrane proteins (for example, the fast sodium ionophore).

Clinical effects and toxicity

Systemic effects

Central nervous system

Central toxicity results from high levels of local anaesthetic agent within the brain. This may be due to direct spread from subarachnoid injection or by excessive systemic absorption. Transfer across the blood–brain barrier is influenced by lipid solubility and ionisation. At a neuronal level, initial inhibitory pathway inhibition results in early excitatory phenomena, superseded by later depressant effects. The toxic CNS effects of local anaesthetic agents are as follows:

- Numbness and paraesthesiae of tongue, mouth and lips
- Metallic taste
- Light-headedness
- Tinnitus
- Slurred speech
- Muscle twitching
- Shivering
- Tremors
- Grand mal convulsions
- Coma
- Apnoea

Apnoea and convulsions result in hypoxia, hypercapnia and metabolic acidosis. The acidosis increases the proportion of ionised local anaesthetic agent. Toxicity results from the presence of ionised drug within the cell blocking the ion channel. Acidosis effectively reduces the proportion of diffusible drug within the cells, and slows clearance.

Cardiovascular system

Most local anaesthetic agents (except cocaine) relax vascular smooth muscle, causing vasodilatation. In addition, centrally administered drugs cause vasodilatation by sympathetic blockade. Direct cardiovascular toxicity is caused by the membrane-stabilising activity of the drugs on myocardial muscle, which is a feature of blockade of voltage-gated fast sodium channels. This reduces the maximum rate of rise of the cardiac action potential and

reduces the duration of the action potential. Conduction of the action potential through the myocardium is slowed. Other voltage-gated and ligand-gated ion channels are also affected. Bupivacaine blocks transient outward potassium flux, interfering with myocardial repolarisation. Calcium ion release from the sarcoplasmic reticulum is impaired. Bupivacaine may bind to the enzyme protein carnitine-acylcarnitine translocase of the mitochondria, preventing entry of the fatty acids which serve as energy substrates to power myocardial contraction.

Cardiac toxicity may result in any of the following effects:

- Prolongation of PR interval
- Supraventricular tachycardia
- Decreased automaticity
- Widening of QRS complex
- Ventricular ectopic beats
- Prolongation of ST interval
- T-wave changes

Note that bupivacaine decreases the baseline cardiac membrane potential.

Respiratory system

The respiratory effects of local anaesthetic agents are due to a combination of peripheral neuronal blockade and systemic toxicity. The following effects may be seen:

- Apnoea with systemic toxicity affecting the respiratory centre
- Bronchodilatation secondary to relaxation of bronchial smooth muscle

Other effects

Local anaesthetic drugs have a weak neuromuscular blocking action. Amides block plasma cholinesterase. A direct antiplatelet effect (probably due to membrane stabilisation) reduces platelet aggregation and blood viscosity. These effects are of minor clinical significance.

Anaphylactoid reactions

Anaphylactoid reactions are very rare with amide local anaesthetics, and some of those reported have been due to preservatives (such as metabisulphite and methylparaben). Effects range from local erythema and swelling to systemic hypotension and bronchospasm. More commonly, the reactions are due to co-administration of epinephrine, intravascular injection or psychological effects (vasovagal episodes). Reactions are relatively common with esters, and cross sensitivity may occur. The metabolism of procaine

	Adult dose (mg)		mg kg^{-1} equivalent	
	Plain	With epinephrine	Plain	With epinephrine
Ester				
Cocaine	100	a	1.5	a
Amides				
Bupivacaine	150	150	2	2
Levobupivacaine	150	150	2	2
Lidocaine	200	500	3	7
Prilocaine	400	600 (felypressin)	6	8.5 (felypressin)
Ropivacaine^b	250	N/A	3.5	N/A

^{a} Unnecessary and contraindicated
^{b} 150 mg (2 mg kg^{-1-1}) for epidural Caesarean section

Figure LA6 Maximum recommended doses (and their mg kg^{-1} equivalents)

produces para-aminobenzoic acid (PABA), which may be allergenic.

Factors affecting toxicity

The toxic effects resulting from systemic absorption of local anaesthetic agent are dependent on:

- Fraction of unbound drug within the plasma
- Peak plasma concentration
- Rate of rise of plasma concentration
- Plasma clearance
- Plasma pH

Following an accidental IV bolus the plasma concentration will fall as redistribution and elimination occur, exactly as with other intravenously administered drugs. Slow absorption from a tissue plane (correctly administered drug) will result in much slower rise and lower peak of plasma concentration. The speed of absorption, and elimination rate, will determine the maximum plasma concentration that occurs. The maximum recommended doses for various local anaesthetic agents are shown in Figure LA6.

Figure LA7 shows how increasing plasma concentrations of lidocaine produce increasing severity of central nervous and cardiovascular toxicity.

The pattern of toxicity is broadly similar for all local anaesthetic agents, but variations exist in the relative severity of the cardiovascular and neurological effects. Bupivacaine has a narrower safety margin between central nervous system and cardiovascular toxicity and is particularly dangerous if cardiac effects do occur, as dissociation from the myocardium is slow, and successful resuscitation following cardiac arrest is unlikely unless prolonged CPR is

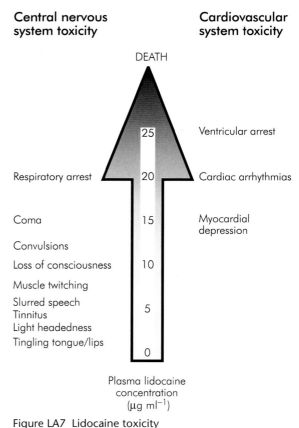

Figure LA7 Lidocaine toxicity

instituted. Bupivacaine should not be used for intravenous regional anaesthesia (Bier's block).

Cardiovascular and central nervous system toxicity depend on the mass of drug reaching the systemic circulation. The transfer of drug (by diffusion) from the circulation to organs is determined by the Fick principle (see Section 2, Chapter 5, page 289). The mass of drug reaching the circulation after peripheral administration is influenced by the following factors:

- Mass of drug administered
- Site of injection
- Tissue protein binding and metabolism
- Vascularity of the injection site

Dose

The volume and concentration of local anaesthetic agents, considered individually, have little influence on systemic spread. Systemically the mass of drug rather than its administered concentration is more important.

Absorption

Absorption from different sites is influenced by the blood flow to the tissue and the uptake of the drug into the vascular compartment, which is a function of solubility. Absorption is in the order of magnitude:

intercostal > epidural > plexus > peripheral

> subcutaneous

Absorption is particularly high when agents are applied topically to mucosa (such as lidocaine spray in the oropharynx). A vasoconstrictor may be added to reduce absorption. Cocaine produces vasoconstriction in its own right and is used on the nasal mucosa to reduce vascularity before some ENT procedures.

Accidental IV injection bypasses the absorption process and subjects the patient to potentially toxic levels of drug. IVRA involves the deliberate introduction of local anaesthetic into the venous system of a limb isolated by tourniquet. The safety of this procedure is dependent on the drug becoming predominantly tissue-bound by the time the tourniquet is released, which should not be for at least 20 minutes. Further improvements in safety can be achieved by using relatively non-cardiotoxic drugs, typically prilocaine.

Distribution

Absorbed drug passes through the lungs, where a large amount of the local anaesthetic agent may become tissue-bound and in some cases metabolised. However, this ability is soon saturated by direct IV injection. After passing through the lungs, local anaesthetic drugs reach vessel-rich tissues which have a high affinity. Some is distributed to muscle and fat, and later gradually released for subsequent metabolism.

Metabolism

Ester local anaesthetics are rapidly metabolised by plasma cholinesterase, and systemic toxicity is rarely a problem. Amide local anaesthetics are metabolised by the liver, but hepatic failure must be very severe before local anaesthetic breakdown is compromised. Lidocaine has a high extraction ratio, and metabolism is therefore dependent on hepatic blood flow, which may be particularly relevant when IV lidocaine is used to stabilise ventricular myocardium in low-cardiac-output states.

Plasma protein binding

α_1-acid glycoprotein and albumin are the main sites for local anaesthetic binding within the plasma. α_1-acid glycoprotein has a high affinity but a low capacity, while albumin has a low affinity but a high capacity for local anaesthetics. Figure LA8 shows the plasma protein binding of drugs at different plasma concentrations.

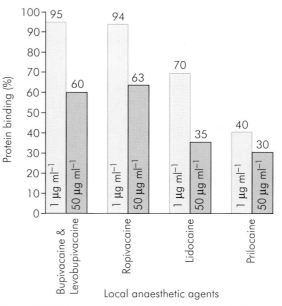

Figure LA8 Plasma protein binding of drugs at different plasma concentrations

Protein binding acts as a buffer to changes in plasma concentration. The chemical bonds are weak and the protein readily releases the local anaesthetic as concentration falls. Toxicity is therefore not directly linked to plasma protein binding, and tissue binding is the more important factor.

Pregnancy

Fetal blood rapidly equilibrates with maternal blood levels of free local anaesthetic agent, but as there is more α_1-acid glycoprotein in fetal blood the overall concentration will be higher. Metabolism is less well developed in the fetus, but the drug rapidly passes back to the mother as maternal levels decline; therefore this does not present a problem. The pH of the fetal fluids is lower than maternal, which acts to increase the proportion of ionised local anaesthetic agent.

Management of local anaesthetic toxicity

Guidelines are available from the Association of Anaesthetists of Great Britain & Ireland (2007).

Prevention

Careful observation of patients having local anaesthetic agents, and a high degree of suspicion both during and after administration, is essential. Make use of the maximum recommended doses as a guide, and combine that with careful technique and an appreciation of the anatomy. If any suspicion of central toxicity arises then stop the injection and re-evaluate.

Treatment

If toxicity does occur, then first stop injecting the local anaesthetic. Call for help. Supportive measures for airway and circulation are the mainstay of successful treatment. Seizures should be controlled with incremental midazolam, thiopental or propofol. Sodium channel blocking agents should not be used, as they will only worsen the situation. If cardiac arrest occurs then inotropes, vasopressors and vagolytics may help. Lidocaine, of course, must be avoided. Bupivacaine is particularly tissue-bound, and cardiac massage of an hour or more may be required.

The use of lipid solutions and the use of insulin/glucose/potassium infusions to improve myocardial energy supply are new developments for the future management of local anaesthetic toxicity.

Insulin/glucose/potassium infusions

Kim *et al.* (2004) induced cardiovascular collapse without arrest in dogs using a bupivacaine infusion. They then stopped the bupivacaine and gave one group a bolus of insulin. Potassium and glucose were then infused. All the dogs in the insulin group gradually improved and survived whilst the entire control group died. It is postulated that the successful resuscitation using insulin was due to a reversal of bupivacaine-induced changes to potassium ion flux, calcium ion transport in the sarcoplasmic reticulum and maybe improved mitochondrial glucose and pyruvate levels too.

Lipid emulsion

The use of lipid emulsion is primarily based on animal studies, although case reports have appeared for bupivacaine, levobupivacaine and ropivacaine. Although the exact mechanism of action is unknown, the following have been postulated:

- Intravascular bupivacaine is absorbed into the lipid (very slow for removing myocardial bupivacaine).
- The lipid delivers a significant concentration of fatty acids to the energy-starved myocardium, allowing replenishment of the ATP as cardiac resuscitation continues.

Picard and Meek (2006) provide a useful discussion of the potential benefits. Uptake into the lipid phase is dependent on the lipid/aqueous plasma partition coefficient, which varies with Intralipid® mixture and species. It is important to appreciate that propofol, whilst useful to treat convulsions, in the volumes that could be given has too little lipid to make any impact on treating toxicity. Intralipid® 20%, by comparison, would be given in a bolus of the order of 100 ml followed by an infusion.

Ester-linked agents

Amethocaine

Amethocaine (tetracaine) is an ester local anaesthetic agent used for topical anaesthesia. It is available as a gel (4%) for local anaesthesia of the skin before intravascular cannulation. Applied to the skin it is effective within 45 minutes. It can then be removed, and remains active for 4–6 hours. The preparation should not be applied to inflamed or damaged skin or highly vascular tissues, as it is rapidly absorbed through mucosal surfaces. More dilute solutions (0.5% and 1%) are available for topical anaesthesia of the conjunctiva. Amethocaine is potent and readily absorbed, but in common with other ester local anaesthetics it may cause hypersensitivity.

Benzocaine

Benzocaine is an unusual ester local anaesthetic agent in that the side chain is an ethyl group with no amine component, and therefore remains un-ionised. Benzocaine has a low potency but it may cause methaemoglobinaemia. It is a component of some throat lozenges, and may be applied directly to painful skin ulcers.

Cocaine

Cocaine is a naturally occurring ester derived from benzoic acid, and extracted from the leaves of *Erythroxylum coca*. It is available in solution and pastes in concentrations ranging from 1% to 10%. It is mainly used for topical anaesthesia and to reduce bleeding during nasal surgery. Cocaine is rapidly taken up into mucous membranes to provide anaesthesia and intense vasoconstriction. This vasoconstriction limits systemic absorption, resulting in a bioavailability by this route of 0.5%. It is well known as a drug of abuse with high addictive potential, and in this role is taken by chewing, inhaling nasally, smoking or intravenously. It causes marked sympathomimetic activity and arrhythmias are a definite risk. Systemic injection must be avoided. Systemically absorbed cocaine has a volume of distribution of $2 \, l \, kg^{-1}$, with 98% being protein-bound. It is eliminated by plasma and liver esterases, having a clearance of $35 \, ml \, kg^{-1} \, min^{-1}$ and a half-life of 45 minutes.

Cocaine shares the same mechanism of action as the other local anaesthetic agents ($pK_a = 8.7$), and also inhibits catecholamine neuronal uptake-1. Synaptic levels of dopamine and norepinephrine increase, resulting in the central stimulation and euphoria, and vasoconstriction. Cocaine initially blocks the inhibitory pathways, resulting in euphoria, hyperthermia, altered vision and hearing, nausea and eventually convulsions. Higher levels of cocaine also block the excitatory pathways, resulting in central nervous depression leading to sedation and unconsciousness, with respiratory depression. Cocaine causes mydriasis and raised intraocular pressure. It is no longer used for local anaesthesia of the eye. The central stimulation increases respiratory rate and volume. A rise in sympathetic tone leads to tachycardia and hypertension, the latter being exacerbated by peripherally mediated vasoconstriction. High doses depress the myocardium. The general excitation also increases metabolic rate, which contributes to the hyperthermia and raises oxygen consumption and CO_2 production. The recommended maximum dose is $1.5 \, mg \, kg^{-1}$. Cocaine should be avoided in porphyria.

Amide-linked agents

Bupivacaine

Bupivacaine is a long-acting local anaesthetic agent with a slow onset of action. Blockade of a large peripheral nerve such as the sciatic nerve may take 60 minutes, depending on the approach, but may last up to 48 hours. Intrathecal injection in contrast produces an acceptable block within a few minutes. Bupivacaine is particularly prone to causing myocardial depression and, once compromised, reversal may be slow and difficult. In part this is due to the relatively high pK_a, but an affinity for cardiac proteins is probably more important. Recommendations to minimise systemic toxicity specific to bupivacaine include:

- Avoid bupivacaine for IVRA
- Avoid 0.75% bupivacaine in obstetric practice
- Limit dose to $2 \, mg \, kg^{-1}$

Bupivacaine is predominantly metabolised by N-dealkylation to pipecolylxylidine (N-desbutylbupivacaine). Hydroxybupivacaine is also produced. The metabolites are excreted in the urine.

Levobupivacaine

Levobupivacaine is the S(−)enantiomer of racemic bupivacaine. It is clinically similar to racemic bupivacaine. The important differences are dose terminology and toxicity. Levobupivacaine is expressed as milligrams of base rather than of hydrochloride salt, so for a given (mg) dose there is 13% more activity. Animal studies demonstrate lower cardiotoxicity but at present the maximum recommended dose remains at $2 \, mg \, kg^{-1}$, and it is contraindicated for IVRA (Bier's block). Lower CNS toxicity is also apparent.

Lidocaine (lignocaine)

Lidocaine is primarily classified as a local anaesthetic agent but is also a Class IB antiarrhythmic. It has a relatively rapid onset of action and intermediate duration. Combination with a longer-acting agent such as bupivacaine may produce a balance of onset and duration between the two component agents alone. The cardiotoxic potential of lidocaine at equivalent levels of central nervous toxicity is about one-ninth that of bupivacaine.

Lidocaine is metabolised in the liver by microsomal oxidases and amidases. N-dealkylation followed by hydrolysis produces ethylglycine, xylidide and other derivatives that are excreted in the urine.

Prilocaine

Prilocaine is closely related to lidocaine in terms of pharmacological activity. It has the same pK_a (7.9) but is less lipid-soluble. Speed of onset and duration are similar. It is less toxic than lidocaine, due to high tissue fixation and rapid metabolism of systemically absorbed drug. Prilocaine is the drug of choice for IVRA.

Prilocaine is metabolised in the liver, lungs and kidney to O-toluidine, and then hydroxytoluidine, leaving less than 1% unchanged. O-toluidine is responsible for methaemoglobinaemia.

Methaemoglobinaemia

Metabolism of prilocaine following significant absorption (e.g. after 600 mg), to O-toluidine results in the oxidation of the ferrous ion (Fe^{2+}) of the haem in haemoglobin to ferric (Fe^{3+}) to produce methaemoglobinaemia. This results in cyanosis, and the abnormal haemoglobin shifts pulse oximeter **readings** towards 85%. Methaemoglobinaemia is not usually clinically detrimental, but when the patient becomes compromised methylene blue (1–2 mg kg^{-1}) may be used as a treatment. Excess methylene blue (>7 mg kg^{-1}) may also cause methaemoglobinaemia, and as the dye has a distinctive spectral absorption it also affects pulse oximeter accuracy.

Children (especially infants) are more susceptible to methaemoglobinaemia, because they have underdeveloped metabolic processes and fetal haemoglobin is more easily oxidised. Methaemoglobinaemia also occurs occasionally after application of EMLA cream.

Ropivacaine

Ropivacaine is closely related to bupivacaine in terms of pharmacological activity, as both drugs are pipecoloxylidides. Ropivacaine is produced as a single enantiomer with an enantiomeric purity of 99.5% for S-ropivacaine. As ropivacaine is less lipid-soluble than bupivacaine and less readily penetrates the neuronal myelin sheaths, C fibres are blocked more readily than A fibres. At high concentrations the blocking effect is similar for both drugs, but at lower concentrations ropivacaine preferentially blocks C fibres over the faster A fibres. Ropivacaine has a potential advantage that motor function can be spared (or show earlier recovery) while still achieving sensory blockade, if a suitable concentration of drug is used. Complete motor and sensory blockade can still be achieved if desired. In summary, ropivacaine provides sensory blockade similar to that of bupivacaine but motor blockade is slower in onset, less pronounced and shorter in duration. Ropivacaine is half as cardiotoxic as bupivacaine. It is mainly bound to α_1-acid glycoprotein in plasma.

EMLA

Eutectic mixture of local anaesthetic (EMLA) is a mixture of 2.5% prilocaine and 2.5% lidocaine used for topical anaesthesia of undamaged skin before intravascular cannulation and minor, superficial dermal and aural surgery. A eutectic mixture is one in which the constituents are in such proportions that the freezing (or melting) point is as low as possible, with the constituents freezing (or melting) simultaneously. The preparation is therefore unusual, as the local anaesthetics are not in aqueous solution, and both agents are in their pure form rather than the hydrochloride preparations used in the solutions. In theory, this means that both drugs are in the non-ionised state in EMLA. Once absorbed into the tissues, ionisation will occur. The commercial preparation (EMLA cream 5%) contains carboxypolymethylene and sodium hydroxide, resulting in an oil–water emulsion.

Additives

Glucose

Standard solutions of local anaesthetic agents are slightly hypobaric at body temperature and pH, and therefore tend to move upwards in the cerebrospinal fluid away from the gravitational pull. Dextrose (glucose) is added to bupivacaine to increase the density of the solution. The specific gravity of hyperbaric (or 'heavy') bupivacaine is 1.026 at 20 °C. The specific gravity of cerebrospinal fluid is 1.005 at 37 °C, so the injected bupivacaine solution will sink due to gravity. Combined with knowledge of the spinal curves and manipulating the position of the patient, this helps to control the distribution of the local anaesthetic. Note that the specific gravity of a substance or solution is the density of that solution relative to the maximum density of water, which occurs at a temperature of 4 °C.

Vasoconstrictors

Epinephrine

Epinephrine is added to local anaesthetic solutions to reduce vascularity of the area by direct vasoconstriction, and in turn to reduce the systemic uptake of the drug. This has the following effects:

- Increased duration of nerve blockade
- Greater margin of safety for systemic toxicity
- Reduced surgical bleeding

Care must be taken to avoid the systemic effects of epinephrine due to systemic uptake. For example, combination with halothane anaesthesia may result in cardiac arrhythmias, especially ventricular excitation and fibrillation. Epinephrine-containing solutions should not be injected in the proximity of end-arteries such as the penile, ophthalmic (central artery of the retina) or digital arteries as there is no collateral circulation to supplement the supply if vasoconstriction is severe. To minimise the risk of serious systemic actions consider the following:

- Avoid hypoxia and hypercarbia
- Use dilute solutions (<1 : 200 000)
- Limit of 100 μg per 10 minutes
- Limit of 300 μg per hour

Felypressin

Felypressin is an octapeptide derived from vasopressin (ADH). In common with vasopressin, felypressin is a powerful direct-acting vasopressor, but it is safe to use with halothane and has no antidiuretic or oxytocic activity. It may, however, cause coronary vasoconstriction.

Hyaluronidase

Hyaluronidase, supplied as a white fluffy powder, is used to facilitate the spread through connective tissues following subcutaneous or intramuscular injection. In addition to promoting the spread of local anaesthetics and other injections, it is also used to promote reabsorption of fluids and blood from extravascular tissues. Its effect is dependent on the temporary depolymerisation of hyaluronic acid. Hyaluronidase is stable in solution for 24 hours at room temperature.

pH manipulation

Alkalination of solutions by addition of bicarbonate increases tissue pH. This results in a higher proportion of non-ionised drug, which diffuses into the neurone more rapidly. Preparation and storage is awkward, and the preparations are not widely available.

Additives with analgesic activity

Other agents developing roles in central and peripheral nerve blockade are shown in Figure LA9. These additives are used to provide a synergistic effect on pain percep-

Drug	Receptor	Uses
Opioids	μ/κ	Central and peripheral
Clonidine	α_2-adrenoceptor	Central and peripheral
Ketamine	NMDA	Central

Figure LA9 Local anaesthetic additives used for receptor-mediated analgesic effect

tion by interaction with specific receptors in the afferent pathways.

Specific pharmacology

n-Heptane/aqueous phosphate buffer partition coefficient indicates lipid solubility. Note that the use of octanol as lipid results in different figures. Units (unless stated otherwise) are:

Volume of distribution at steady state (V_d): $l\,kg^{-1}$
Clearance (Cl): $ml\ kg^{-1}\ min^{-1}$
Terminal half-life $(t_{1/2})$: minutes

Figure LA10 shows the chemical formulae of the commonly used local anaesthetic agents.

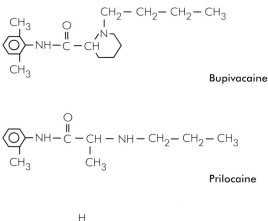

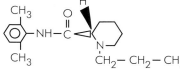

Figure LA10 Structures of common local anaesthetic drugs. The chiral carbon of bupivacaine (levobupivacaine) is shown in bold (C)

Bupivacaine hydrochloride

Structure – amide local anaesthetic agent, pipecoloxy-lidide

Presentation – clear, colourless, aqueous solutions include:

Plain solutions (0.25%, 0.5%)

Solutions with 1:200 000 (5 μg ml^{-1}) epinephrine (0.25%, 0.5%)

'Heavy' 0.5% with 80 mg ml^{-1} dextrose (specific gravity 1.026) for spinal anaesthesia

Recommended maximum dose – 2 mg kg^{-1} (150 mg plus up to 50 mg 2-hourly subsequently). 0.75% is contraindicated in obstetric practice and is no longer available

Pharmacokinetics

MW	288
pK$_a$	8.1
partition coefficient	27.5
protein binding	96%
V$_d$	1
Cl	7
t$_{1/2}$	30

Clinical – intermediate speed of onset, long action, four times as potent as lidocaine; propensity to cardiotoxicity

Elimination – 5% excreted as pipecoloxylidine after dealkylation in the liver, 16% excreted unchanged in urine

Levobupivacaine hydrochloride

As for bupivacaine hydrochloride except:

Structure – Levorotatory enantiomer of racemic bupivacaine

Presentation – Plain solutions (2.5 mg ml^{-1}, 5.0 mg ml^{-1}, 7.5 mg ml^{-1})

Recommended maximum dose – 150 mg (2 mg kg^{-1}), total 400 mg in 24 h. 7.5 mg ml^{-1} contraindicated in obstetric practice

Pharmacokinetics

MW	288
pK$_a$	8.1
partition coefficient	27.5
protein binding	97%
V$_d$	1
Cl	9
t$_{1/2}$	80

Clinical – Levobupivacaine doses are expressed as mg of base compound, whereas racemic bupivacaine is expressed as the hydrochloride salt. Levobupivacaine therefore has 13% more activity than the same dose of racemic bupivacaine. Animal studies indicate lower CNS toxicity than bupivacaine

Elimination – Extensive metabolism with no unchanged levobupivacaine in urine or faeces. The major metabolite is 3-hydroxylevobupivacaine excreted in urine as sulphate and glucuronate conjugates (71% of dose in urine and 24% in faeces by 48 h)

Lidocaine hydrochloride

Structure – amide local anaesthetic agent, derivative of diethylaminoacetic acid

Preparation – clear, aqueous solutions include:

Plain solutions (0.5%, 1%, 2%)

Solutions with 1:200 000 (5 μg ml^{-1}) epinephrine (0.5%, 1%, 2%)

Gel (1%, 2%) with chlorhexidine for urethral instillation

Solutions for surface application to pharynx, larynx and trachea (4%) (coloured pink)

Spray for anaesthesia of the oral cavity and upper respiratory tract (10%)

Dose – topical, infiltration, nerve blocks, epidural and spinal; 0.5–10% available; 100 mg bolus then 1–4 mg min^{-1} for ventricular arrhythmias. Recommended maximum dose 200 mg (3 mg kg^{-1}); with epinephrine 500 mg (7 mg kg^{-1})

Pharmacokinetics

MW	234
pK$_a$	7.9
partition coefficient	2.9
protein binding	64%
V$_d$	1
Cl	9
t$_{1/2}$	100

Clinical – rapid speed of onset, intermediate action; Class IB antiarrhythmic

Elimination – 70% by dealkylation in liver, <10% excreted unchanged in urine

Prilocaine hydrochloride

Structure – amide local anaesthetic agent, secondary amine derived from toluidine

Preparation – clear, colourless, aqueous solutions include:

Plain solutions (1%, 4%)

Solutions with 0.03 unit ml^{-1} felypressin (3%)

Recommended maximum dose – 400 mg (6 mg kg^{-1}); with felypressin 600 mg (8.5 mg kg^{-1})

Pharmacokinetics

MW	220
pK$_a$	7.9
partition coefficient	0.9
protein binding	55%
V$_d$	3.7
Cl	40
t$_{1/2}$	261

Clinical – rapid speed of onset, duration of action intermediate between lidocaine and bupivacaine, potency similar to lidocaine; may result in methaemoglobinaemia

Elimination – rapidly metabolised to O-toluidine by liver, <1% excreted unchanged

Ropivacaine hydrochloride

Structure – amide local anaesthetic agent, pipecoloxylidide

Presentation – clear, colourless, aqueous solutions of S-ropivacaine enantiomer include:

Plain solutions in 10 and 20 ml ampoules (2, 7.5, 10 mg ml^{-1})

Plain solution in 100 and 200 ml bags (2 mg ml^{-1}) for epidural infusion

Recommended maximum dose – 250 mg (150 mg for Caesarean section under epidural); cumulative dose of 675 mg over 24 h according to data so far

Pharmacokinetics

MW	274
pK$_a$	8.1
partition coefficient	6.1
protein binding	94%
V$_d$	0.8
Cl	10
t$_{1/2}$	110

Clinical – intermediate onset, long duration of action between lidocaine and bupivacaine, potency similar to lidocaine; greater separation of sensory and motor blockade, and lower cardiotoxicity than bupivacaine may be advantages

Elimination – aromatic hydroxylation to 3- (and 4-) hydroxy-ropivacaine, and N-dealkylation. 86% (mostly conjugated) excreted in the urine, of which 1% unchanged. 3- and 4-hydroxy-bupivacaine have reduced local anaesthetic activity

Contraindication – IVRA, obstetric paracervical block; not yet recommended in children <12 years of age

References and further reading

Association of Anaesthetists of Great Britain & Ireland. *Guidelines for the Management of Severe Local Anaesthetic Toxicity.* London: AAGBI, 2007.

Kim JT, Jung CW, Lee KH. The effect of insulin on the resuscitation of bupivacaine-induced severe cardiovascular toxicity in dogs. *Anesth Analg* 2004; **99**: 728–33.

Picard J, Meek T. Lipid emulsion to treat overdose of local anaesthetic: the gift of the glob. *Anaesthesia* 2006; **61**: 107–9.

CHAPTER 10
Central nervous system pharmacology

T. C. Smith

ANTI-EMETIC AGENTS
Anticholinergic drugs
Phenothiazines
Butyrophenones
Antihistamines
5-Hydroxytryptamine (5-HT3) receptor antagonists
Cannabinoids
Neurokinin receptor antagonists
Peripherally acting anti-emetic agents

SPECIFIC PHARMACOLOGY
Cyclizine hydrochloride and lactate
Domperidone
Metoclopramide hydrochloride
Ondansetron hydrochloride
Prochlorperazine

ANTICONVULSANT DRUGS
Benzodiazepines
Barbiturates
Phenytoin
Carbamazepine
Gabapentin and pregabalin
Valproate
Lamotrigine
Vigabactrin
Tiagabine
Levetiracetam

ANTIDEPRESSANT AGENTS
Tricyclic antidepressants
Monoamine oxidase inhibitors (MAOIs)
Selective serotonin reuptake inhibitors (SSRIs)
Serotonin–norepinephrine reuptake inhibitors (SNRIs)
Selective norepinephrine reuptake inhibitors
Noradrenergic and specific serotonergic
    antidepressants
Lithium

ANTIPSYCHOTIC DRUGS
Phenothiazines
Thioxanthines
Other antipsychotic drugs

ANTI-PARKINSONIAN DRUGS
Levodopa
Carbidopa
Domperidone
Selegiline
Dopaminergic drugs
Amantadine
Acetylcholine antagonists

Many drugs act on the central nervous system (CNS), with specific aims in mind. While certain categories of drugs are considered elsewhere (anaesthetic gases and vapours in Section 3, Chapter 5, hypnotics and intravenous agents in Chapter 6) other drugs acting on the CNS have been grouped here. Anti-emetic agents are considered in detail, with specific pharmacology of individual agents to reflect their direct relevance to the practice of anaesthesia.

Anti-emetic agents

The causes of nausea and vomiting (NV) are legion, as illustrated by Figure CN1, and anti-emetic therapy is most effective when directed at the likely origin.

Postoperative nausea and vomiting (PONV) is a specific entity. Its treatment is more appropriately directed when other risk factors are considered, and these are summarised in Figure CN2.

Two distinct sites in the CNS, the vomiting centre and the chemoreceptor trigger zone, are implicated in the causes of NV. The chemoreceptor trigger zone lies in the area postrema outside the blood–brain barrier and possesses dopaminergic (D_2) and serotonergic (5-hydroxytryptamine, 5-HT_3) receptors. In contrast, the vomiting centre is a complex entity located in the dorsolateral reticular formation of the brain stem that possesses 5-HT_3, D_2 and muscarinic (M_3) receptors. Histaminic (H_1) and neurokinin (NK_1) receptors are located in the nucleus of the tractus solitarius, which integrates afferent signals associated with emesis. The interaction of various drugs with these sites is shown in Figure CN3.

Fundamentals of Anaesthesia, 3rd edition, ed. Tim Smith, Colin Pinnock and Ted Lin. Published by Cambridge University Press. © Cambridge University Press 2008.

Drug-induced

    Central effect – opioids, nitrous oxide

    Local effect – poisons, copper, sodium chloride

    Systemic effect – cytotoxic drugs

Pregnancy

Radiotherapy

Psychogenic

Vestibular

    Labyrinthitis

    Ménière's disease

    Motion sickness

Stimulation of vagal afferents in the pharynx

Hypotension

Migraine

Abdominal pathology

Raised intracranial pressure

Figure CN1 Causes of nausea and vomiting

Female > male

Children > adults > elderly

Increased if pathology is: gynaecological

                         intractable

                         intraoral

Increased by gastrointestinal stasis

Figure CN2 Factors affecting the incidence of postoperative nausea and vomiting

The major classes of drug used to combat NV possess receptor antagonism at D_2, M_3, H_1 and 5-HT_3 receptors. The more common agents and their receptor specificity are shown in Figure CN4.

Anti-emetic activity is ascribed to the following categories of drug:

- Anticholinergic agents
- Phenothiazines
- Butyrophenones
- Antihistamines
- 5-HT_3 receptor antagonists
- Cannabinoids
- Neurokinin receptor antagonists

Additionally, metoclopramide and domperidone are two peripherally acting anti-emetic agents of importance.

Anticholinergic drugs

Examples – atropine, hyoscine

Atropine and hyoscine cross the blood–brain barrier (unlike glycopyrollate, another commonly used anticholinergic drug) and act on muscarinic cholinergic receptors in the vomiting centre and in the gastrointestinal tract. Anticholinergic agents are antispasmodic, reducing intestinal tone and inhibiting sphincter relaxation. They also reduce salivary and gastric secretions and so reduce gastric distension. These are the drugs of choice for the treatment of motion sickness and opioid-induced nausea. Hyoscine has been popular for premedication in conjunction with opioids for this reason, and because it possesses a sedative effect. The side effects of anticholinergic drugs are predictable from the known effects of muscarinic cholinergic receptors. In particular, dry mouth and blurred vision can be a problem, and drowsiness is not uncommon. Bronchial secretions are rendered more viscid, but a degree of bronchodilatation is seen (increasing anatomical dead space). Pupillary constriction may be abolished, which removes a useful indicator of depth of anaesthesia. Anticholinergic agents that cross the blood–brain barrier are implicated in the development of the central anticholinergic syndrome, which is detailed in Figure CN5.

Treatment of the central anticholinergic syndrome is accomplished by the use of an anticholinesterase that can cross the blood–brain barrier. In practice, this requires a tertiary amine structure, and thus physostigmine is the drug of choice, but is no longer available and at present there is no equivalent drug.

Phenothiazines

Examples – perphenazine, prochlorperazine, promethazine

Phenothiazines have a variety of effects, including anti-emesis. Trifluoperazine is a potent anti-emetic, but its antipsychotic effects preclude its use as a routine anti-emetic. Phenothiazines act on the D_2 receptors in the chemoreceptor trigger zone in the area postrema, and on M_3 receptors in the same way as anticholinergic agents. The major effect of promethazine is antihistaminic, although it has antidopaminergic and antimuscarinic activity that contribute to the anti-emetic effect. Sedation may limit the usefulness of promethazine as an anti-emetic agent. 6 mg

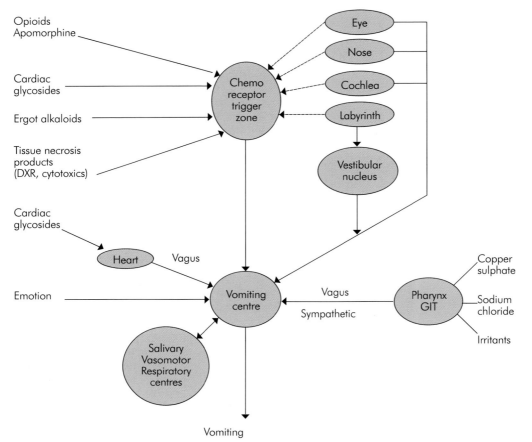

Figure CN3 Causes of NV and sites of drug action

	D_2	M_3	H_1	$5\text{-}HT_3$
Hyoscine	0	++++	+	0
Promethazine	+	++	+++	0
Chlorpromazine	++	+	++	+
Metoclopramide	+	0	+	++
Droperidol	+++	0	+	+
Ondansetron	0	0	0	++++
Prochlorperazine	++++	+	+	0

Figure CN4 Receptor antagonism of anti-emetic agents

of buccal prochlorperazine may be a useful alternative to IM injection.

Butyrophenones
Examples – benperidol, droperidol, haloperidol

Causes
• Muscarinic anticholinergic drugs which cross the blood–brain barrier (typically atropine and hyoscine)

Risk factors
• Elderly patients most at risk

Features
• Excitement
• Drowsiness
• Ataxia
• Coma

Figure CN5 The central anticholinergic syndrome

Droperidol (no longer available in the UK) is an antagonist of D_2 receptors in the chemoreceptor trigger zone. It has potent anti-emetic activity but can cause a dissociative phenomenon even in relatively small doses, when the patient appears outwardly content but experiences an unpleasant feeling of helplessness and vulnerability.

Haloperidol and benperidol are primarily used as antipsychotic agents, but haloperidol possesses substantial anticonvulsant activity. It causes α_1-adrenoreceptor blockade, which may result in postural hypotension.

Butyrophenones are metabolised in the liver. Side effects include extrapyramidal phenomena, neuroleptic malignant syndrome and hyperprolactinaemia with gynaecomastia.

Antihistamines
Examples – buclizine, cinnarizine, cyclizine, diphenhydramine

Several categories of drug may show antihistaminic activity. Figure CN6 lists the main categories.

Antihistamine is a term used for a group of chemically different agents that are antagonists at histaminergic receptors. Despite the discovery of a second type of histamine receptor (H_2 in gastric mucosa), the general term 'antihistamine' is used to describe anti-H_1 drugs alone. These are particularly effective in the treatment and prevention of motion sickness. The anti-emetic action is centrally mediated, but H_1 antagonism may not be the sole mechanism of anti-emesis. The sedative effects of antihistamines contribute to the treatment of nausea.

Ethanolamines (such as diphenhydramine) are potent antihistamines with some anticholinergic activity, which are thought to work at the labyrinth and the neural interface between the labyrinth and the vomiting centre.

Cyclizine is used for motion sickness and for PONV. It has anticholinergic activity, resulting in dry mouth, and can cause tachycardia if given intravenously. Cinnarizine is almost insoluble in water and only available in the tablet form. Buclizine has a long duration of action but is only available in combined formulation with other drugs.

Ethanolamines	Diphenhydramine
	Dimenhydrinate
Piperazines	Cyclizine
	Buclizine
	Cinnarizine
Phenothiazines	Promethazine

Figure CN6 Anti-emetic drugs with antihistamine activity

5-Hydroxytryptamine (5-HT$_3$) receptor antagonists
Examples – granisetron, ondansetron, tropisetron

There are four basic types of serotonergic (5-HT) receptors (5-HT$_{1-4}$). 5-HT$_1$ receptors are subdivided further (5-HT$_{1A}$, etc.). An especially high density of 5-HT$_3$ receptors is found in the area postrema and nucleus tractus solitarius, where they are probably on the vagus nerve terminals. Receptors have also been identified on peripheral sections of the vagus nerve in the gastrointestinal tract, and the emetogenic effect of 5-HT release can also be blocked here.

Cannabinoids
Example – nabilone

Cannabis is derived from the plant *Cannabis sativa*. The active constituents of cannabis are called cannabinoids. Δ-9-tetrahydrocannibol is the major active cannabinoid. A specific cannabinoid receptor has been identified in the CNS, and it is thought that cannabinoids act at the chemoreceptor trigger zone. Naloxone may be used to overcome their effects. Nabilone is a synthetic derivative of the naturally occurring tetrahydrocannibol. It is effective against NV induced by opioids, cytotoxic therapy and radiotherapy. Taken orally it is well absorbed and has a half-life of 120 minutes. Indications for cannabinoid therapy are limited by the side effects of hallucinations, psychosis, dizziness and dry mouth.

Neurokinin receptor antagonists
Example – aprepitant

Selective neurokinin (NK$_1$) receptor antagonists have been shown to have anti-emetic activity via the nucleus of the tractus solitarius and dorsal motor nucleus of the vagus nerve. Aprepitant has a broader spectrum of anti-emetic activity than 5-HT$_3$ antagonists. It has a half-life of 11 hours.

Peripherally acting anti-emetic agents
Examples – domperidone, metoclopramide

Metoclopramide and domperidone are chemically unrelated yet functionally similar. Metoclopramide hydrochloride is a white crystalline salt that is chemically related to procaine. It is readily soluble and stable in water. It has anti-dopaminergic (D$_2$) activity in the chemoreceptor trigger zone and also inhibits the emetic effects of gastric irritants. It also antagonises H_1 and 5-HT_3 receptors and promotes gastric emptying through the pylorus. Extrapyramidal effects (such as oculogyric crisis) are the major potential side effects. Metoclopramide is indicated for PONV, opioid-induced nausea and NV related to cytotoxic drug treatment and radiotherapy.

Domperidone is a benzimidazole derivative that has both centrally and peripherally mediated effects. Peripherally, domperidone promotes gastric emptying and increases lower oesophageal sphincter tone. It crosses the blood–brain barrier (but only slowly) and then acts on dopamine receptors in the chemoreceptor trigger zone. This impaired transit across the blood–brain barrier reduces the incidence of extrapyramidal side effects. Domperidone is indicated for the treatment of PONV and opioid-induced NV but it is limited in its application as it cannot be given parenterally. The major application of the drug is in the treatment of cytotoxic and radiotherapy-induced NV. These agents may also be useful in promoting gastric transit when impaired by diabetic autonomic neuropathy.

Miscellaneous anti-emetics

- Sedatives and anxiolytics often have an anti-emetic effect by reducing the psychological component of the nausea. Propofol appears to reduce PONV.
- Betahistine is a histamine analogue used for the treatment of Ménière's disease and its associated NV.
- High doses of methylprednisolone or dexamethasone (glucocorticoids) are useful against the nausea of cytotoxic agents. Their mode of action is not known.

Specific pharmacology

Here, the units (unless stated) are:
Volume of distribution at steady state (V_d): $l\,kg^{-1}$
Clearance (Cl): $ml\,kg^{-1}\,min^{-1}$
Terminal half-life ($t_{1/2}$): hours

Cyclizine hydrochloride and lactate

Structure – piperazine
Presentation – tablet 50 mg, IV/IM 50 mg in 1 ml, and in combination with morphine
Pharmacokinetics

Bioavailability	80%
$t_{1/2}$	10

Blood–brain barrier – crossed
CNS – anti-emetic, with some sedation

CVS – slight tachycardia
RS – minimal effect
Other – increase in lower oesophageal sphincter pressure
Elimination – N-demethylation to norcyclizine (half-life 20 h, minimal activity), and also some to the oxide
Side effects – anticholinergic; dry mouth, blurred vision, drowsiness

Domperidone

Structure – butyrophenone derivative
Presentation – tablets 10 mg, suppositories 30 mg
Pharmacokinetics

Bioavailability	15%
Protein binding	92%
V_d	5.7
$t_{1/2}$	7.5

Blood–brain barrier – poorly crossed
CNS – anti-emetic, acting predominantly outside the brain, but some antagonism of D_2 receptors in the chemoreceptor trigger zone
CVS – minimal effect
RS – minimal effect
Others – acts on peripheral dopaminergic (D_2) neurones. Increased lower oesophageal sphincter tone, increased gastric emptying, increased prolactin secretion
Elimination – metabolised by hydroxylation and oxidative N-dealkylation (90%); 30% in urine, 60% in faeces
Side effects – galactorrhoea, gynaecomastia

Metoclopramide hydrochloride

Structure – chlorinated procainamide derivative
Presentation – tablets 10 mg, syrup 1 mg ml^{-1}; IV 10 mg in 2 ml
Pharmacokinetics

Protein binding	18%
V_d	2.8
Cl	10
$t_{1/2}$	4

CNS – anti-emetic via chemoreceptor trigger zone, and by decreasing afferent activity from viscera to vomiting centre
CVS – some reports of hypotension, dysrhythmias and cardiac arrest
RS – minimal effects

- **Others** – lower oesophageal sphincter pressure increased, gastric contractility and emptying increased, small intestine transport time accelerated; prolactin and aldosterone secretion increased; may increase ureteric peristalsis
- **Elimination** – 80% in urine within 24 h, of which 20% unchanged, the rest conjugated or as sulphated metabolite
- **Side effects** – drowsiness, dizziness, extrapyramidal effects

Ondansetron hydrochloride
Structure – 5-HT$_3$ receptor antagonist
Presentation – tablets 4 mg; IV 4 mg in 2 ml (protect from light)
Pharmacokinetics

Bioavailability	60%
V_d	1.8
Cl	6
$t_{1/2}$	3

CNS – anti-emetic
CVS – no effect with therapeutic doses
RS – no effect on respiratory regulation
Others – antagonises 5-HT$_3$ receptors on vagal afferents in small intestine, no effect on platelet function or prolactin secretion
Elimination – extensively metabolised in liver, main metabolite 8-hydroxyondansetron; metabolites conjugated; <5% unchanged via urine
Side effects – constipation, headache, flushing

Prochlorperazine
Structure – piperazine phenothiazine
Presentation – tablets 5 or 25 mg, buccal tablets 3 mg, suppositories 5 or 25 mg, IM clear colourless solution 12.5 mg in 1 ml
Pharmacokinetics

V_d	20
$t_{1/2}$	6

Blood–brain barrier – crossed
CNS – anti-emetic with neuroleptic effects, acting via dopaminergic (D$_2$) receptors
CVS – α blockade occasionally causes postural hypotension; QT increased, ST depressed, T and U wave changes on ECG
RS – mild respiratory depressant effect
Other – lower oesophageal sphincter tone increased, anti-adrenergic activity, antihistaminic and anticholinergic effects

Elimination – S-oxidation to a sulphoxide by the liver
Side effects – extrapyramidal effects

Anticonvulsant drugs
Epileptic events are the result of repetitive neuronal discharges in the CNS involving many neurones. Anticonvulsant drugs act by breaking these propagating and recycling currents either by increasing inhibitory neurotransmitter levels or by facilitating their action by modulating the γ-amino butyric acid (GABA) receptor function. There is the potential for new drugs to be developed that would inhibit excitatory neurotransmitters and their receptors (the N-methyl-D-aspartate agonist–receptor interaction is a likely target). The modes of action of anticonvulsants are listed in Figure CN7.

The drug chosen for treatment of epilepsy depends greatly on the type of fits. Figure CN8 shows treatment guidelines for different types of epilepsy.

In pregnancy, most anticonvulsant drugs carry a risk of causing neural tube defects, teratogenicity and coagulation disorders in the newborn. Counselling, antenatal screening, folate supplements and pre-delivery vitamin K should be considered. The greatest risk to mother and baby, however, is that of the re-emergence of convulsions. Fears about the drugs may lead to poor compliance in the complacent patient. In addition, the increase in body water during pregnancy will dilute the concentration of the anticonvulsant agent, thereby reducing its clinical effect.

GABA facilitation	Benzodiazepines
	Barbiturates
GABA agonism	Progabide
GABA transaminase inactivation	Valproate
	Vigabatrin
Fast sodium channel blockade	Phenytoin
Presynaptic sodium channel stabilisation	Lamotrigine Valproate

Figure CN7 Modes of action of anticonvulsants

Benzodiazepines
Examples – clobazam, clonazepam, diazepam

Benzodiazepines act by attaching to a specific area of the GABA–receptor complex. The benzodiazepine has an agonist activity at this site that facilitates the opening of the chloride channel by GABA. Chloride ions then flow down

Status epilepticus	First line	IV diazepam
	Subsequently	Phenytoin or Phenobarbital or Chlormethiazole or Paraldehyde
Prevention	Absences (petit mal)	Ethosuximide or Valproate
	Tonic–clonic	Carbamazepine or Phenytoin or Valproate or Phenobarbital
	Myoclonic	Valproate or Clonazepam or Ethosuximide
	Atypical (usually childhood, especially if any cerebral damage)	Clonazepam or Ethosuximide or Lamotrigine or Phenobarbital or Phenytoin or Valproate

Figure CN8 Types of epilepsy and drug choice

the concentration gradient into the cell, making it hyperpolarised (more negative) and so less excitable.

Diazepam is primarily used for the acute treatment of convulsions. It has the disadvantage of pronounced sedation, long half-life and active metabolite. Other benzodiazepines may be used prophylactically.

Barbiturates

Examples – phenobarbital, primidone

All barbiturates possess anticonvulsant activity, but phenobarbital is less sedative for a given anticonvulsant activity. It binds to the GABA receptor at a site distinct from the benzodiazepine receptor area, and facilitates the chloride channel opening. It is inhibitory at some excitatory synapses. The barbiturate primidone acts by being converted to phenobarbital.

Phenytoin

Phenytoin is a hydantoin that also has local anaesthetic and antiarrhythmic properties. It has structural similarities with the barbiturates. The site of action of phenytoin is the fast sodium channel responsible for depolarisation during an action potential. It binds to the channel when it is refractory following opening, and is therefore most effective when repetitive discharges occur. It may also interfere with calcium entry and with calmodulin protein kinases. Phenytoin can cause hirsutism, gum hyperplasia, megaloblastic anaemia and fetal malformations.

There is the potential for interaction with other drugs, including other anticonvulsants. The high degree of protein binding (85% bound to albumin) results in competition for the binding site with salicylates, phenylbutazone and valproate. Phenytoin metabolism is competitively inhibited by phenobarbital due to enzyme induction in the liver. The same hepatic microsomal enzymes are induced by phenytoin, phenobarbital, steroids, oestrogens and coumarins. As with ethanol, the enzyme system is readily saturated, so that as doses increase the metabolism changes from first-order kinetics (metabolism proportional to concentration) to zero-order kinetics (metabolism constant and maximal), thus 'half-life' increases with dose.

Carbamazepine

Carbamazepine is structurally similar to the tricyclic antidepressants and has pharmacological similarities with phenytoin, but the precise mode of action is not known. With chronic usage, the half-life decreases from 30 to 15 hours due to enzyme induction.

Gabapentin and pregabalin

Gabapentin is an amino acid. The postulated mechanisms of action are listed in Figure CN9. Gabapentin is used as adjunct treatment for partial seizures. It is also used to treat neuropathic pain, trigeminal neuralgia and post-herpetic neuralgia. Pregabalin has the same mechanism of action

- Competes with Leu, Ile, Val, Phe for specific amino acid transmembrane transporter
- Increases concentration and synthesis of brain GABA
- Binds to $\alpha_2\delta$ subunit of voltage-sensitive Ca^{2+} channels
- Reduces release of monoamine transmitter (norepinephrine, dopamine and 5-HT)
- Inhibits voltage-sensitive Na channels
- Increases 5-HT
- Prevents neuronal death by inhibition of glutamate synthesis

Figure CN9 Postulated mechanisms of action for gabapentin

but it is claimed to have more specificity for the target receptors, leading to a higher therapeutic index.

Valproate

Sodium valproate is a monocarboxylic acid that increases brain levels of GABA by inhibiting GABA-transaminase and inactive presynaptic Na^+ channels. It is used for petit mal, myoclonic epilepsy and infantile spasms. It also has a role in the management of chronic pain, especially trigeminal neuralgia. It interferes with platelet numbers and function, and can cause neural tube defects.

Lamotrigine

Lamotrigine stabilises inactive presynaptic sodium channels and so reduces neurotransmitter release. It is used to treat partial seizures, tonic–clonic and myoclonic seizures. Concentrations are increased by carbamazepine and phenytoin (enzyme inducers) and reduced by valproate.

Vigabactrin

Vigabactrin binds to and inhibits GABA transaminase, resulting in increased GABA levels. It is used for partial epilepsy in combination therapy and as a sole agent for the treatment of the brief infantile spasms of West syndrome. Particular concerns are that a third of patients develop visual field defects, and that it may cause behavioural problems.

Tiagabine

Tiagabine is an adjunct antiepileptic used for treating partial seizures. It is a selective inhibitor of the GABA uptake carrier. A recent Cochrane review which found insufficient evidence of benefit in bipolar disorders noted that a significant proportion of patients had episodes of seizure or syncope (Vasudev *et al.* 2006). It is 96% protein-bound. It should be avoided in porphyria.

Levetiracetam

For use alone or as an adjunct for partial seizures and myoclonic seizures. No binding to the usual neurotransmitter agonist sites has yet been found, but it may work at a specific neuronal binding site, resulting in a selective action on epileptogenic neuronal tissue only. Non-epileptic neuronal tissue may therefore be unaffected.

Tricyclic antidepressants	Dibenzazepines Dibenzocycloheptenes
Monoamine oxidase inhibitors	Hydrazines Propargylamines Cyclopropylamines Reversible MAOI (RIMA)
Selective serotonin reuptake inhibitors (SSRI)	
Serotonin–norepinephrine reuptake inhibitor (SNRI)	
Selective norepinephrine reuptake inhibitor (NARI)	
Noradrenergic and specific serotonergic antidepressants (NaSSA)	
Other antidepressants	Lithium

Figure CN10 Classes of antidepressants

Antidepressant agents

There are several different classes of antidepressant agents. The classic groups of tricyclic agents and inhibitors of monoamine oxidase have recently been joined by the serotonin reuptake inhibitors and norepinephrine reuptake inhibitors. The major categories of antidepressant drugs are listed in Figure CN10.

Miscellaneous agents unrelated either structurally or functionally may also show antidepressant activity. Among these are nomifensine, maprotiline, venlafaxine, nefazodone, flupenthixol and L-tryptophan.

Tricyclic antidepressants

Examples – dibenzazepines (clomipramine, imipramine), dibenzocycloheptenes (amitriptyline, nortriptyline)

Tricyclic antidepressants are chemically related to the phenothiazines, but differ in that the central ring has an additional carbon atom. This changes the shape of the molecule from the planar phenothiazine molecule to a three-dimensional skeleton. Tricyclic antidepressants act by preventing reuptake of neurotransmitter (primarily norepinephrine) into the nerve terminal of monoaminergic neurones. This action is stronger at noradrenergic and serotonergic sites than at dopaminergic sites. Some drugs also act on presynaptic α_2 receptors to increase neurotransmitter release. Tricyclic agents also antagonise muscarinic cholinergic (amitriptyline is used in the treatment of nocturnal enuresis), H_1 histaminergic, and α_1-adrenoceptors. In addition to the antidepressant effects, they cause sedation, weakness and fatigue. Cardiac effects include postural hypotension, sinus tachycardia and cardiac arrhythmias. Amitriptyline prolongs the PR and QT intervals on the ECG. In the plasma tricyclic antidepressants are 90–95% bound to albumin, and may become displaced by drugs such as aspirin which compete for the same binding sites.

While reuptake blockade occurs soon after administration, the onset of antidepressant action takes several weeks to develop. It is not clear why this is so, but it may be due to down-regulation of adrenergic and 5-HT receptors.

Tricyclic agents are metabolised by hepatic microsomal enzymes, and are therefore competitively antagonised by some neuroleptic drugs which share the same route of excretion. There are two main methods of metabolism: either N-demethylation, converting the tertiary amine to a secondary amine, or ring hydroxylation.

Monoamine oxidase inhibitors (MAOIs)

Examples – cyclopropylamines (tranylcypromine), hydrazines (iproniazid, phenelzine), propargylamines (pargyline, selegiline)

Two variants of monoamine oxidase have been described (MAO-A and -B). MAO-A is more effective at oxidising norepinephrine and 5-HT than MAO-B, but types A and B are equally effective in the metabolism of dopamine and tyramine. Antidepressant activity is conferred by inhibition of MAO-A. MAOIs act by antagonising the breakdown of monoamine neurotransmitters after uptake into the nerve terminal.

The classical MAOIs are irreversible (although a new class of reversible MAOIs now exists). Pargyline, phenelzine, tranylcypromine and iproniazid nonselectively inhibit both MAO-A and MAO-B, while clorygyline is selective for MAO-A. Selegiline is selective for MAO-B and is therefore not antidepressant but is used in Parkinsonism, acting by inhibition of dopamine oxidation. Reuptake blockade occurs soon after administration, but the onset of antidepressant action takes several weeks to develop. In a similar fashion to the tricyclic antidepressants, this may be due to down-regulation of adrenergic and 5-HT receptors. Patients being treated with MAOI drugs also become compromised in their ability to metabolise exogenously administered amines. The pressor effect of tyramine (which is found in cheese, broad beans, red wine and Marmite) is greatly enhanced. Indirect sympathomimetic drugs such as those found in cough medicines will show enhanced effects. A specific interaction with pethidine may result in profound coma.

Reversible MAOIs

Example – moclobemide

These drugs reversibly inhibit MAO-A (also called RIMA – reversible inhibition of MAO-A). Caution should still be exercised with foods rich in tyramine and sympathomimetic agents, but the problem is likely to be less marked. The advantage of RIMAs is that they can be stopped and another antidepressant started without the need to wait several weeks for MAO enzyme regeneration.

Selective serotonin reuptake inhibitors (SSRIs)

Examples – fluoxetine, paroxetine, sertraline

SSRIs act by increasing the level of 5-HT at the neuronal receptors. The specificity for 5-HT results in fewer antimuscarinic and cardiac side effects than with other antidepressants. Sedation is less marked than with the tricyclic antidepressants. Diarrhoea and NV are more common, and headache, restlessness and anxiety may occur. Withdrawal should be slow, over several weeks, and MAOI therapy should not be started until 2–5 weeks after stopping the SSRI treatment (dependent on which drug was being taken). SSRI should not be started until 2 weeks after stopping MAOI therapy.

Serotonin–norepinephrine reuptake inhibitors (SNRIs)

Example – venlafaxine

Serotonin–norepinephrine reuptake inhibitors inhibit both norepinephrine and serotonin (5-HT) neuronal reuptake. Venlafaxine is a bicyclic phenylethylamine antidepressant that inhibits presynaptic reuptake of 5-HT, norepinephrine and to a much lesser extent dopamine. There is no effect on adrenergic, cholinergic or histaminergic **receptors**. The specificity results in lower adverse effects than with the tricyclic antidepressants.

Selective norepinephrine reuptake inhibitors

Example – reboxetine

Reboxetine is a selective inhibitor of norepinephrine reuptake. Again the specificity results in lower adverse effects than with the tricyclic antidepressants.

Noradrenergic and specific serotonergic antidepressants

Example – mirtazapine

Mirtazapine increases norepinephrine and 5-HT neurotransmission by blockade of α_2-adrenoceptors, and also blocks 5-HT$_2$ and 5-HT$_3$ receptors. The 5-HT$_3$ blockade reduces the incidence of nausea. The specificity results in lower adverse effects than with the tricyclic antidepressants.

Lithium

Lithium is used prophylactically to suppress the manic element of bipolar depression (manic–depressive psychosis). It is unclear how the pharmacological activity of lithium produces the clinical effect. The active component of lithium carbonate is the lithium cation (Li$^+$). Chemically, lithium is the first element in group IA of the periodic table (same group as sodium and potassium). It has the atomic number 3 and a molecular weight of 7. It mimics cations, especially sodium. It passes through the fast sodium channels easily, being smaller, but the Na$^+$K$^+$ATPase pump does not readily extract lithium from the cells, and it therefore tends to accumulate intracellularly, which in turn displaces potassium and reduces the outward leakage of potassium responsible for maintaining the negative intracellular potential. In this way, the transmembrane potential becomes reduced and neuronal depolarisation is facilitated. Lithium also reduces brain levels of norepinephrine and 5-HT acutely, reduces cyclic AMP production, and reduces inositol triphosphate.

Lithium has a low therapeutic index, and plasma levels should therefore be maintained between 0.4 and 1.0 mmol per litre. Toxicity occurs with levels of over 2.0 mmol per litre. The half-life of the extracellular ion is about 12 hours, and lithium should be stopped 2–3 days before using a muscle-relaxant drug. This is particularly important for non-depolarising relaxants that are potentiated. It may also delay the onset and prolong relaxation with suxamethonium. The intracellular lithium takes a further 1–2 weeks to excrete. Lithium inhibits vasopressin activity in the kidney via cyclic AMP and increases aldosterone secretion, which can result in renal tubular damage. Lithium inhibits thyroid hormone release and thyroid hypertrophy, and hypothyroidism may occur. Neurological effects include thirst, tremor, muscle weakness, confusion and seizures. Cardiac arrhythmias may be induced, and all toxic effects are enhanced if dehydration occurs. Close monitoring of clinical state, lithium levels and renal function is essential to minimise toxicity.

Antipsychotic drugs

A wide variety of drugs has antipsychotic activity. These have been variously referred to as neuroleptics, major tranquillisers and anti-schizophrenia drugs. Specific categories of drug that have antipsychotic activity include:

- Phenothiazines
- Butyrophenones
- Thioxanthines
- Benzamide
- Diphenylbutylpiperidine
- Dibenzodiazepines

The mode of action of these drugs in the treatment of psychosis is not precisely known. Various receptor systems have been implicated including dopaminergic, noradrenergic and 5-hydroxytryptaminergic (serotonergic). It is likely that many different receptors are affected, but D$_2$ dopaminergic receptors are currently thought to be the most important. While D$_1$ receptors increase adenylyl cyclase activity generally, D$_2$ receptors are found both pre- and postsynaptically, and blocking potency at these receptors correlates closely with clinical potency. The delay in onset of a therapeutic effect from these drugs may in part be explained by a slow increase in the numbers of D$_2$ receptors over several weeks. Some antipsychotic drugs are formulated so that they may be administered by deep IM injection given at intervals of 1–4 weeks.

As antipsychotic agents affect so many receptors, a wide diversity of adverse effects results. These are listed in Figure CN11.

Phenothiazines

Phenothiazines may be classified chemically by the side chain on the nitrogen atom of the phenothiazine base as follows:

- Aliphatic – chlorpromazine
- Piperazine – fluphenazine
- Piperidine – thioridazine

The side chains alter the potency and specificity for the receptor types and in turn alter the clinical features (Figure CN12).

Antidopaminergic

Anti-emesis

Extrapyramidal features

    Facial grimacing

    Involuntary movements of tongue and limbs

    Oculogyric crises

    Torsion spasms

    Tasikinesia

    Akithisia

    Parkinsonism

    Tardive dyskinesia

    Increased prolactin secretion

Antimuscarinic

    Dry mouth

    Constipation

    Urinary retention

    Blurred vision

    Precipitation of glaucoma

Anti-alpha-adrenergic

    Postural hypotension

Antihistaminergic

    Sedation

Figure CN11 Adverse effects of antipsychotic drugs

Thioxanthines

Examples – flupenthixol, zuclopenthixol

Thioxanthines are similar in structure and function to the aliphatic phenothiazines, and therefore block D_2 receptors more than D_1. Flupenthixol is also employed clinically as an antidepressant agent.

Other antipsychotic drugs

Other miscellaneous antipsychotic drugs include sulpiride, which has a greater affinity for D_2 than D_1 receptors; pimozide, which may prolong QT interval on the ECG; and clozapine, which has been associated with agranulocytosis.

Anti-Parkinsonian drugs

Parkinson's disease is caused by a dysfunction within the basal ganglia. The predominant change is a deficit of dopamine with an increase in dopamine D_2 receptors, but other neurotransmitters are also implicated in the pathology of the disease. Drugs that affect Parkinson's disease may act in any of the following ways:

- Increased dopamine synthesis (levodopa)
- Decreased peripheral conversion of levodopa (carbidopa)
- Decreased dopamine breakdown (selegiline)
- Dopamine receptor antagonists (bromocriptine)
- Dopamine receptor facilitators (amantadine)
- Acetylcholine antagonists (benztropine)

Levodopa

Levodopa is used to increase brain levels of dopamine. Dopamine does not cross the blood–brain barrier, and racemic DOPA produces numerous systemic side effects without being effective. DOPA is well absorbed orally and 95% is converted into dopamine by DOPA-decarboxylase. This is then metabolised by monoamine oxidase and catechol-O-methyl transferase (COMT). About 1% of the drug enters the brain, where it is converted into its active form, dopamine. Levodopa causes an increase in the number of dopamine (D_2) receptors in the brain.

Carbidopa

Used in conjunction with levodopa, carbidopa increases the proportion of the oral dose of levodopa entering the brain by inhibiting its peripheral conversion to dopamine. Carbidopa itself does not cross the blood–brain barrier, and

Chain	Receptor blockade		Clinical effect		
	D_2	α-adrenergic	Muscarinic	Extrapyramidal	Sedation
Aliphatic	+	+++	++	++	+++
Piperidine	++	++	+++	+	++
Piperazine	+++	+	+	+++	+

Figure CN12 Receptor sensitivity of phenothiazines

therefore does not interfere with subsequent conversion in the brain.

Domperidone

Used in conjunction with levodopa, this dopamine antagonist only crosses the blood–brain barrier slowly, and it is used to reduce the peripheral effects of dopamine. It has important anti-emetic activity peripherally and also at the chemoreceptor trigger zone. Domperidone permits the use of larger doses of levodopa than would otherwise be possible without gross unwanted effects.

Selegiline

Selegiline is a selective MAO-B inhibitor. This selectivity reduces the peripheral effects of conventional MAO inhibitors, which are largely due to MAO-A inhibition. There is no effect from tyramine-containing foods and drug interactions are less severe and less common.

Dopaminergic drugs

Examples – bromocriptine, carbergoline, quinagolide

Dopaminergic drugs act by direct stimulation of central dopamine (D_2) receptors. They are reserved for patients in whom levodopa is ineffective. Predictably, these drugs inhibit prolactin secretion. They are sometimes referred to as 'dopamine facilitators'. Carbergoline lasts longer than bromocriptine and has fewer side effects. Bromocriptine and carbergoline are chemically related to the ergot alkaloids and may be associated with retroperitoneal, pulmonary and pericardial fibrosis. Quinagolide is not derived from ergot and may avoid this risk.

Amantadine

The mode of action of amantadine remains obscure. Possibilities include facilitation of dopamine release, inhibition of dopamine metabolism and direct D_2 agonist activity.

Acetylcholine antagonists

Examples – benzhexol, benztropine, orphenadrine, procyclidine

Certain muscarinic antagonists can cross the blood–brain barrier having a preferential action on central muscarinic receptors, thus minimising their peripheral side effects. The central excitatory effects of acetylcholine are inhibited, and this may restore the imbalance between cholinergic and dopaminergic activity that occurs in Parkinson's disease. Cholinergic antagonists also antagonise presynaptic inhibition of dopaminergic neurones, so increasing dopamine release, which may prove therapeutic.

References and further reading

Diemunsch P, Schoeffler P, Bryssine B *et al.* Antiemetic activity of the NK1 receptor antagonist GR205171 in the treatment of postoperative nausea and vomiting after major gynaecological surgery. *Br J Anaesth* 1999; **82**: 274–6.

Taylor CP, Gee NS, Su T *et al.* A summary of mechanistic hypotheses of gabapentin pharmacology. *Epilepsy Res* 1998; **29**: 233–49.

Vasudev A, MacRitchie K, Rao SNK, Geddes JR, Young AH. Tiagabine in the treatment of acute affective episodes in bipolar disorder: efficacy and acceptability. *Cochrane Database Syst Rev* 2006; Issue 3: CD004694.

Williams PI, Smith M. An assessment of prochlorperazine buccal for the prevention of nausea & vomiting during intravenous patient-controlled analgesia with morphine following abdominal hysterectomy. *Eur J Anaesthesiol* 1999; **16**: 638–45.

CHAPTER 11

Autonomic nervous system pharmacology

T. C. Smith

CHOLINERGIC SYSTEM
Muscarinic receptors
Muscarinic agonists
Muscarinic antagonists
Nicotinic receptors
Nicotinic agonists
Nicotinic antagonists
Drugs interfering with synthesis, release and
  metabolism of acetylcholine

ADRENERGIC SYSTEM
Adrenoceptors
Adrenoceptor agonists
α-adrenoceptor antagonists
β-adrenoceptor antagonists
Drugs interfering with synthesis, storage, release
  and metabolism of catecholamines

DIRECT-ACTING VASODILATING AGENTS
Calcium channel antagonists
Organic nitrates, nitrites and related drugs
Potassium channel activators

Endothelin receptor antagonists
Prostacyclins
cGMP phosphodiesterase inhibitor
Other agents of importance

SPECIFIC PHARMACOLOGY
Dobutamine hydrochloride
Dopamine hydrochloride
Dopexamine hydrochloride
Ephedrine
Epinephrine
Isoprenaline
Norepinephrine acid tartrate
Clonidine hydrochloride
Esmolol hydrochloride
Labetalol hydrochloride
Atropine sulphate
Glycopyrrolate
Hyoscine hydrobromide or butylbromide
Glyceryl trinitrate
Sodium nitroprusside

The autonomic nervous system (ANS) comprises the sympathetic and parasympathetic nervous systems. Ganglionic synaptic transmission in the ANS is mediated by the release of acetylcholine from the preganglionic neurone. Both muscarinic and nicotinic receptors are involved in mediation of the postganglionic response, as are inhibitory dopaminergic interneurones. In general, sympathetic postganglionic neurones are noradrenergic, and parasympathetic postganglionic neurones are muscarinic (cholinergic). The two systems tend to have opposite actions. Deliberate pharmacological manipulation of the ANS is therefore aimed at sites where physiological or anatomical differences exist between the two systems.

Cholinergic system

The important structural features of the neurotransmitter acetylcholine are the strongly positive quaternary amine in the choline part of the molecule and the ester component with its partial negative charge. Choline receptor antagonists have either a tertiary or a quaternary amine (or both). Acetylcholine receptors are classified as either muscarinic or nicotinic. Nicotinic receptors are widespread in the body, and are found in both sympathetic and parasympathetic nervous systems. Drug actions at the nicotinic receptors of the neuromuscular junction, which is not part of the ANS, are covered in Section 3, Chapter 8.

Muscarinic receptors

The muscarinic receptors are G-protein-coupled receptors. Five subtypes have been identified (M_{1-5}), but the most important ones are M_1, M_2 and M_3, which are all antagonised by atropine. M_1 receptors are found in the central nervous system (CNS), autonomic ganglia and gastric parietal cells, M_2 receptors are found in the heart and at presynaptic sites, and M_3 receptors are found in smooth muscle, vascular endothelium (causing vasodilatation) and in exocrine glands.

Fundamentals of Anaesthesia, 3rd edition, ed. Tim Smith, Colin Pinnock and Ted Lin. Published by Cambridge University Press. © Cambridge University Press 2008.

Muscarinic agonists
Examples – carbachol, pilocarpine

Pharmacological features
In common with other agonists, these drugs bear a structural relationship to the relevant endogenous agonist (acetylcholine). Pharmacological activity is reduced by changing the nitrogen unit from quaternary to tertiary, by removing the ester and by increasing the length of the aliphatic component on the quaternary nitrogen. Such changes also reduce hydrolysis and increase the half-life. This is essential to enable the drug to be given by conventional intermittent doses.

Carbachol has a quaternary amino group with the acetyl component changed to a carbamyl group so that it produces both nicotinic and muscarinic effects. Pilocarpine has a tertiary amino group and possesses muscarinic effects only.

Clinical effects
Muscarinic agonists are used to constrict the pupil to reduce intraocular pressure in glaucoma, and to improve micturition by increasing detrusor muscle contraction.

The muscarinic agonists are often referred to as parasympathomimetics, because the peripheral muscarinic receptors are predominantly located in the parasympathetic system. Their effects are predictable from this knowledge, and are summarised in Figure AS1.

Muscarinic antagonists
Examples – atropine, glycopyrrolate, hyoscine

Pharmacological features
Muscarinic antagonists compete with acetylcholine in the end effector organs of the parasympathetic system, and in the sweat glands, which are also muscarinic yet innervated by the sympathetic system. Atropine and hyoscine are naturally occurring agents formed from esters of tropic acid and either tropine or scopine. The tertiary amines such as atropine and hyoscine cross the blood–brain barrier, whereas quaternary amines such as glycopyrrolate and ipratropium do not.

Clinical effects
Muscarinic antagonists increase cardiac activity by increasing heart rate (blood pressure often rises as a result). They inhibit most secretions and sweating. In the gastrointestinal and urinary systems there is increased sphincter tone

Cardiovascular system
- Atrial contractility decreased
- Heart rate decreased
- Blood pressure decreased
- Systemic vascular resistance decreased

Respiratory system
- Mucous secretion stimulated
- Bronchoconstriction with increased resistance and decreased deadspace

Gastrointestinal system
- Propulsive activity increased
- Salivary, exocrine pancreatic, gastric and intestinal secretions stimulated

Urogenital system
- Sphincter tone decreased
- Detrusor tone increased

Eye
- Miosis
- Ciliary muscle stimulated (poor focusing on far objects)
- Lacrimation increased

Figure AS1 Clinical effects of muscarinic agonists

and reduced motility. The pupils are dilated and accommodation is blocked, causing blurred vision. The clinical effects of the muscarinic antagonists are the opposite of those of the agonists, and are shown in Figure AS2.

Atropine
Atropine is initially synthesised in the S(−) form by plants but it spontaneously racemes so that the commercial preparation of atropine contains a mixture of both enantiomers, which are frequently referred to as hyoscyamine, in particular the R(+) enantiomer. There is an aromatic group in place of the acetyl group of acetylcholine, and there is a tertiary amino group in place of the quaternary one. The muscarinic effects are mainly due to the L form. Atropine is chemically related to cocaine and consequently it has a weak local anaesthetic effect. Atropine readily crosses the blood–brain barrier and the placenta. Initially the drug causes CNS excitation, followed by depression.

Glycopyrrolate
Glycopyrrolate has a quaternary ammonium group and does not readily cross the blood–brain barrier, and therefore central anticholinergic effects are minimal. It also has

Peripheral

Cardiovascular system
- SA node and atria hypopolarised
- Refractory period of SA node and atria increased
- Refractory period of AV node decreased
- Conduction velocity in SA node, atria and AV node increased
- Atrial contractility increased
- Heart rate increased
- Systemic vascular resistance increased (vascular receptors not innervated)
- Salivary gland arterioles vasoconstricted

Respiratory system
- Mucous secretion inhibited
- Bronchodilatation

Gastrointestinal system
- Sphincter activity increased
- Propulsion reduced
- Biliary tree constricted
- Salivary, exocrine pancreatic, gastric and intestinal secretions inhibited

Urogenital system
- Sphincter tone increased
- Detrusor tone reduced
- Erectile tissue vasoconstricts

Eye
- Mydriasis
- Ciliary muscle relaxed
- Lacrimal secretions reduced

Central
- Sedation
- Anti-emesis
- Anti-Parkinsonian

Figure AS2 Clinical effects of muscarinic antagonists

the advantage that its duration of effect is similar to that of neostigmine, with which it is given concomitantly for the reversal of neuromuscular blockade.

Hyoscine

The muscarinic effects of hyoscine are mainly due to the L form. Hyoscine causes CNS depression and has a useful role as a sedative and anti-emetic in premedication.

Nicotinic receptors

The nicotinic acetylcholine receptors are part of a transmembrane protein ion channel. In the ANS, they are located in the ganglia. The pharmacology of the nicotinic receptors at the neuromuscular junction is discussed in detail in Section 3, Chapter 8.

Nicotinic agonists

Nicotine is the most prevalent exogenous agent active at the nicotinic receptors. It preferentially affects autonomic ganglia rather than the neuromuscular junction, and causes central stimulation. When an excess of acetylcholine occurs, such as when acetylcholinesterase is blocked by an anticholinesterase (for example, neostigmine or an organophosphorus compound), there will be nicotinic stimulation of the ganglia. Stimulation of autonomic ganglia has no clinical application but the following effects will be seen: vasoconstriction, hypertension, sweating and salivation. Gut motility may increase or decrease.

Nicotinic antagonists

Nicotinic antagonists cause blockade of autonomic ganglia. They have been superseded by drugs targeting more specific parts of the autonomic system. The neuromuscular blocking agent D-tubocurarine caused ganglion blockade as a side effect and has also been superseded by drugs with more specificity for the nicotinic receptors of the muscle endplate. This is made possible by the different sub-chain types (specifically the α subunit) and subtypes that make up the pentameric nicotinic receptor (see Section 3, Chapter 4, pages 544–5).

Clinical effects

Drugs causing ganglion blockade reduce blood pressure by a combination of vasodilatation and inhibition of compensatory effects such as tachycardia. The vasodilatation affects both arterioles (afterload) and venules (preload). The effect on the capacitance vessels reduces venous pressure and consequently intraoperative venous oozing. In general use, ganglion blockade causes postural hypotension, as the venous tone does not increase to compensate for the upright position.

Drugs interfering with synthesis, release and metabolism of acetylcholine

Hemicholinium is an example of a drug preventing acetylcholine synthesis. It does so by preventing the uptake of choline into the nerve terminal. It is not taken up and does not produce a false transmitter effect. It is also a nicotinic receptor antagonist causing autonomic ganglion blockade, but it is no longer available.

Magnesium ions and aminoglycosides inhibit calcium entry into the synaptic terminal, and so prevent neurotransmitter release. Botulinum toxin and β-bungarotoxin bind irreversibly to nicotinic nerve terminals and prevent neurotransmitter release (α-bungarotoxin blocks postsynaptic acetylcholine receptors). The main effect of these compounds is that of muscle paralysis. However, if ventilation support is instituted then the excessive parasympathetic blockade is still a serious problem.

Metabolism of acetylcholine is inhibited by anticholinesterases and organophosphorus compounds, resulting in excess levels of acetylcholine. Initially, these cause increasing levels of stimulation of the parasympathetic system, but further rises cause depolarising blockade of the postsynaptic membrane with muscle paralysis.

Adrenergic system

The postganglionic neurones of the sympathetic nervous system provide the adrenergic component of the ANS. The adrenoceptors (adrenergic receptors) are located on the postsynaptic membrane of the end organ. Catecholamines are the agonists at these receptors, which are readily affected by circulating catecholamines and adrenergic drugs. The ubiquity of the sympathetic nervous system results in diverse effects when drugs interfering with adrenergic neurotransmission are used.

Adrenoceptors

The adrenoceptors are structurally similar. They are G-protein-coupled receptors with seven transmembrane α-helical segments (see Section 3, Chapter 4, page 546). Drugs affecting the adrenergic system work either by being structurally similar to the neurotransmitter, or by interfering with storage, release or metabolism. Drugs with a structural similarity take the place of the endogenous agonist and either mimic (agonism) or block (antagonism) the effect on the receptor. The endogenous neurotransmitters and hormones norepinephrine, epinephrine and dopamine are used pharmacologically. The two basic divisions of adrenoceptors (α and β) are affected to different degrees by various drugs. They were originally defined by their responses to norepinephrine, epinephrine and isoprenaline in the following manner:

Agonist responses of adrenoceptors
- α-adrenoceptor:
  norepinephrine ≥ epinephrine > isoprenaline
- β-adrenoceptor:
  isoprenaline ≥ epinephrine ≥ norepinephrine

Receptor	Location	Effect on neurotransmission
α_1	Postsynaptic	Excitatory
α_2	Presynaptic	Inhibitory
β_1	Postsynaptic	Excitatory
β_2	Postsynaptic	Inhibitory
β_3	Postsynaptic	–

Figure AS3 Characteristics of the adrenoceptor subtypes

The subclassifications are now performed using selective antagonists. α and β receptors are further subdivided into α_1 and α_2, and β_1, β_2 and β_3. They may be located at different sites or at the same synapses, and drugs may have specificity for one subtype over another, although this is not usually exclusive. Figure AS3 details the receptor subtypes and their characteristics.

Clinical effects
The clinical effects of the adrenoceptors are as follows:
- α_1 – vasoconstriction, gut smooth muscle relaxation, increased saliva secretion, hepatic glycogenolysis
- α_2 – inhibition of autonomic neurotransmitter (norepinephrine and acetylcholine) release, stimulation of platelet aggregation
- β_1 – increased heart rate, increased myocardial contractility, gut smooth muscle relaxation, lipolysis
- β_2 – vasodilatation, bronchiole dilatation, visceral smooth muscle relaxation, hepatic glycogenolysis, muscle tremor
- β_3 – lipolysis, thermogenesis

Drugs acting on the adrenoceptors may cause agonism, antagonism or partial agonism, and often have a mixture of effects at different receptor types. Figure AS4 shows the relative agonism and antagonism of various drugs on the adrenoceptor subtypes.

Adrenergic drugs will be considered further according to their primary effect in the clinical setting.

Pharmacological features
The structure–activity relationship of adrenergic drugs is marked. The basic catecholamine structure consists of an organic ring and side chain. Increasing the size of the attachment to the amino group of the side chain increases the affinity for β receptors, which increases the effect of both agonists and antagonists, and reduces the effect of

	α_1	α_2	β_1	β_2
Agonists				
Norepinephrine	+++	+++	++	+
Phenylephrine	++	0	0	0
Clonidine	0	+++	0	0
Dopamine	+	0	++	++
Epinephrine	++	++	+++	+++
Dobutamine	0	0	+++	+
Salbutamol	0	0	+	+++
Isoprenaline	0	0	+++	+++
Antagonists				
Phentolamine	– – –	– – –	0	0
Phenoxybenzamine	– – –	– – –	0	0
Prazocin	– – –	–	0	0
Indoramin	– – –	–	0	0
Ergotamine	pa	– –	0	0
Labetalol	– – –	–	– –	– –
Propranolol	0	0	– – –	– – –
Atenolol	0	0	– – –	–

+, agonist activity
–, antagonist activity
pa, partial agonist activity

Figure AS4 Drug–receptor interactions at adrenoceptors

Figure AS5 Catecholamine structures

monoamine oxidase and the uptake 1 mechanism (U1) which removes catecholamines from the synaptic cleft. The β-hydroxy group is important for α-agonist activity and β antagonism, while removal reduces receptor affinity. Substitution or repositioning of the catechol hydroxyl groups results in resistance to catechol-O-methyl transferase (COMT) and uptake 1. Removal of one or both catechol hydroxyl groups reduces or obliterates receptor affinity but leaves uptake 1 intact. The structure of the more common catecholamines is shown in Figure AS5.

Adrenoceptor agonists

Examples – clonidine, dobutamine, dopamine, dopexamine, epinephrine, isoprenaline, norepinephrine

Note that β-adrenoceptor agonists are covered in more detail in Section 3, Chapter 13 (pages 674–5).

Clinical uses

Adrenoceptor agonists are administered systemically for myocardial failure (inotropic), sepsis (vasoconstriction and inotropy), anaphylaxis, nasal congestion and bronchospasm. They may be administered peripherally to cause local vasoconstriction and so prolong the effects of local anaesthetics and reduce bleeding in the operative field. β₂ agonists are effective in the treatment of asthma when inhaled, which reduces systemic effects.

Epinephrine

Epinephrine has both α and β agonist effects and many applications. It is an inotrope and chronotrope but sensitises the myocardium to arrhythmias. The ventricles in particular become hyperexcitable. There is generalised vasoconstriction, but dilatation of skeletal muscle arterioles.

Dobutamine

Dobutamine is a non-selective β agonist and has both chronotropic and inotropic effects. It is usually used for its inotropic effect, but tachycardia may limit the dose. It causes some vasodilatation, and this may require concurrent treatment with an α agonist such as norepinephrine.

Dopamine

Dopamine is an agonist at α₁, β and dopamine receptors. The balance of these effects is dose-related. Initially only dopamine receptors are affected, but with increasing doses β receptors and then α receptors are also affected. Peripheral dopamine receptors are located in the renal arterioles and are responsible for vasodilatation. Dopamine is often used to maintain renal perfusion when this may be compromised. Increasing the dose recruits the β receptors with their positive inotropic effect. This is limited by the onset of a tachycardia. Vasoconstriction (α_1) may become a problem as the drug dose increases.

Dopexamine
Dopexamine is an agonist of β_2 and dopaminergic (D_1 and D_2) receptors in the periphery. It also inhibits neuronal norepinephrine reuptake (uptake 1), so enhancing the β effects. It is a positive inotrope but has the principal effect of peripheral vasodilatation, especially of the splanchnic and renal arterioles. The resulting reduction in afterload improves cardiac output.

Isoprenaline
Isoprenaline is used in the treatment of bronchospasm, bradycardia and heart block. It is used to increase heart rate in complete heart block while electrical pacing is instituted. It is agonist at β_1 and β_2 receptors.

Norepinephrine
Norepinephrine is primarily an α_1 agonist and causes vasoconstriction (although it does have some β-agonist effects). It is particularly useful in patients with septicaemic shock, as they have a pathological reduction in systemic vascular resistance resulting in hypotension and hypoperfusion due to diversion of blood away from essential organs. The inotropic effect, although small, may also help. It may cause a reflex bradycardia if hypotension is overcorrected.

Salbutamol
Salbutamol is an effective bronchodilator, used in both the treatment and prophylaxis of obstructive airway disease. It is a selective β_2 agonist, and this minimises the undesirable effects such as tachycardia, although this β_1 effect does still occur with higher doses. It also has a role as a uterine relaxant for the treatment of premature labour and before delivery during Caesarean section.

Clonidine
Clonidine is an α_2 agonist used as a centrally acting antihypertensive agent that works by reducing norepinephrine release. Its role in preventing migraine is controversial. α_2 receptors are located on the presynaptic membrane of noradrenergic neurones, and have also been found in the spinal cord and at peripheral nerve endings. Clonidine may prolong the effect of epidurally administered local anaesthetic agents, although it is not licensed for this route.

Metaraminol
Metaraminol tartrate has both α and β agonist effects, with the α effect predominating. It increases systemic and pulmonary vascular resistance and causes increased systolic and diastolic blood pressures. Heart rate decreases in response and some inotropy occurs, although overall cardiac output may fall or may not change. Cerebral and renal blood flow are reduced by the vasoconstriction, and during pregnancy uterine tone is increased. β effects increase blood glucose levels.

α-adrenoceptor antagonists
Examples – alfuzosin, doxazocin, phenoxybenzamine, phentolamine, tamsulosin

Uses
α_1-adrenoceptor antagonists are used as antihypertensives and in benign prostatic hyperplasia.

Clinical effects
α blockade causes vasodilatation with reduced systemic vascular resistance and lowered blood pressure. There is a reflex increase in heart rate and cardiac output.

Phenoxybenzamine
Phenoxybenzamine is a haloalkylamine. The N-chloroethyl group binds covalently to part of the receptor. It therefore detaches from the receptor very slowly and behaves like a competitive irreversible antagonist. The recovery half-life is about 24 hours. Phenoxybenzamine is also an antagonist of acetylcholinergic, 5-hydroxytryptaminergic and histaminic receptors. Its primary effect is that of vasodilatation.

Phentolamine
Phentolamine affects both α_1 and α_2. It does not bind covalently and so is reversible.

Labetalol
Labetalol is an antagonist at both α_1 and β receptors. The reflex tachycardia from the α blockade is antagonised by the β blockade. α blockade is more prominent when used intravenously, whereas β blockade is the main effect when used orally.

Tamsulosin and alfuzosin

Tamsulosin and alfuzosin have specificity for the α_{1A}-adrenoceptor, giving targeted treatment of benign prostatic hypertrophy by smooth muscle relaxation.

β-adrenoceptor antagonists

Examples: acebutolol, atenolol, metoprolol, nadolol, oxprenolol, pindolol, propranolol, sotalol

Mode of action

β-adrenoceptors activate adenylyl cyclase. There are two subtypes of β receptor (β_1 and β_2). In general, β_1 receptors tend to be excitatory and β_2 inhibitory. β-adrenoceptor antagonists with a specific affinity for β_1 receptors alone are called selective, and those also affecting β_2 receptors are called non-selective. Even those classified as selective still have some β_2 antagonism. Some β blockers are partial agonists (intrinsic sympathomimetic activity), so that at low dose there is increasing agonism as the dose increases, but a plateau is reached and there is antagonism of circulating catecholamines. They may have an advantage over the others in minimising bradycardia, reducing heart failure and maintaining perfusion to the extremities. The membrane-stabilising effect that some β blockers have is, however, of little clinical importance. Figure AS6 shows the selectivity and partial agonist properties of the β blockers.

	Antagonist	Partial agonist
Selective	Atenolol	Acebutalol
	Betaxolol	Alprenolol
	Bisoprolol	
	Esmolol	
	Metoprolol	
	Nadolol	
Non-selective	Propranolol	Celiprolol
	Sotalol	Oxprenolol
	Timolol	Pindolol

Figure AS6 Partial agonism and selectivity of β blockers

Uses

β blockers are used in the treatment of angina, hypertension, tachyarrhythmias, anxiety, glaucoma, migraine, phaeochromocytoma and thyrotoxicosis.

Clinical effects

The clinical effects are predictable from knowledge of receptor locations. The important effects for clinical use are those of negative inotropy and negative chronotropy,

Peripheral

Cardiovascular system
- Conduction velocity in SA node, atria, AV node and ventricles reduced (β_1)
- Atrial contractility reduced (β_1)
- Heart rate reduced (β_1)
- Blood pressure reduced (β_1)
- Class II antiarrhythmic activity (β_1)
- Skeletal muscle (β_2) and coronary vasomotor tone increased
- Coronary blood flow reduced
- Cardiac oxygen demand reduced

Respiratory system
- Bronchoconstriction with increased resistance and reduced dead space (β_2)

Renal system
- Renin secretion inhibited (β_1)

Metabolic
- Less free fatty acid release (β_1)
- Glycogenolysis reduced (β_2)
- Insulin release reduced (β_2)
- Lipolysis (β_3)
- Thermogenesis (β_3)

Eye
- Reduced production of aqueous humour
- Constriction of ciliary muscle (β_2)

Central
- Reduced sympathetic tone
- Anxiolysis
- Tiredness
- Nightmares
- Sleep disturbance

Figure AS7 Clinical effects of β blockade

which reduce blood pressure and myocardial work. Coronary blood flow is reduced but this effect is less than the reduction in myocardial work. These drugs are particularly effective when sympathetic tone is increased, for example following myocardial infarction, but care must be taken not to block a protective inotropic effect in incipient heart failure. The undesirable effects include bradycardia, bronchoconstriction, sleep disturbance, hypoglycaemia (especially with exercise) and cold extremities.

β blockers (whether selective or not) should be avoided in asthmatic patients. They should be used with caution in diabetes, peripheral vascular disease and heart failure.

Calcium antagonists with negative inotropic effects (verapamil and diltiazem) act synergistically with β blockers to cause hypotension, bradycardia and conduction defects, and they should not be administered contemporaneously.

Atenolol, celiprolol, nadolol and sotalol are very water-soluble and therefore penetrate the brain poorly and are primarily excreted in the urine. In general, the β blockers are well absorbed orally, but the first-pass effect is particularly high with alprenolol, propranolol, metoprolol, oxprenolol and timolol. Bisoprolol and sotalol have a high bioavailability.

Atenolol

Atenolol is a popular selective β blocker for the control of essential hypertension. In the clinical setting, patient compliance with the treatment is often apparent from a relatively slow heart rate. Bioavailability is 50% and protein binding is low. Atenolol is highly water-soluble and is largely excreted unchanged in the urine.

Esmolol

Esmolol hydrochloride is a short-acting β_1-adrenoceptor antagonist, and class II antiarrhythmic. This aryloxypropanolamine is rapidly hydrolysed to a low-activity acid by red cell esterases and has a half-life of only 9 minutes. It is used in the acute management of supraventricular tachycardias, hypertension and myocardial infarction, and is an option for suppression of the hypertensive response to laryngoscopy and intubation.

Propranolol

Propranolol is a non-selective β blocker with no intrinsic sympathomimetic activity. It has been largely superseded by selective antagonists but still has a role in the management of phaeochromocytoma (in conjunction with α blockade), thyrotoxicosis and crisis, acute hypertension and tachyarrhythmias. Propranolol has a high first pass with a bioavailability of only 10–30%. It is lipid-soluble and highly protein-bound (90–95%).

Drugs interfering with synthesis, storage, release and metabolism of catecholamines

Examples – bretylium, carbidopa, guanethidine, methyldopa, reserpine

A few drugs act by interfering with the metabolic elements of the catecholamines rather than with receptor interactions. While not widely used now as they lack specificity, these agents merit brief consideration.

Synthesis

Carbidopa inhibits dopa decarboxylase and so prevents the formation of dopamine, the first catecholamine in the chain of synthesis. Carbidopa does not cross the blood–brain barrier and is therefore used to minimise the peripheral effects of L-dopa used in the treatment of Parkinsonism. The antihypertensive agent methyldopa is a false substrate for dopa decarboxylase and dopamine hydroxylase and results in the synthesis of a false transmitter – methyl norepinephrine. This is ineffective, and as it is not metabolised by monoamine oxidase it accumulates within the nerve terminal and displaces the true neurotransmitter, which becomes depleted.

Storage

Reserpine blocks the uptake and reuptake of norepinephrine, dopamine and 5-hydroxytryptamine in the neuronal terminals. The neurotransmitter accumulates within the cytoplasm where MAO inactivates it and transmitter levels fall. It affects both the sympathetic and CNS but has been superseded by drugs that are more specific.

Release

Guanethidine was originally used as an antihypertensive but is now mainly used in the management of chronic pain. It is transported by the uptake 1 mechanism and accumulates in the nerve terminals. Initially it causes release of norepinephrine from the vesicles and then inhibits release of the diminishing levels of norepinephrine. Bretylium has a similar mode of action. Guanethidine is used to treat reflex sympathetic dystrophy by IV regional sympathetic block (chemical sympathectomy), in which guanethidine is injected intravenously into an isolated limb.

Direct-acting vasodilating agents

Calcium channel antagonists

Examples – amlodipine, felodipine, nicardipine, nifedipine, nimodipine, nisoldipine

The calcium channel antagonists are covered in detail in Section 3, Chapter 12 (pages 666–7). The calcium channel antagonists are a mixed group of drugs having in common the blockade of various calcium ionophores in cell and intracellular membranes. These vasodilators relax vascular smooth muscle preferentially and dilate coronary and other arterial smooth muscle. They can be used in conjunction with β blockers. Amlodipine, felodipine, nicardipine and nifedipine are used to treat both hypertension and angina. Isradipine and lacidipine are only useful in the treatment of hypertension. Nimodipine has a specificity for cerebral arterioles and is used to treat vascular spasm following subarachnoid haemorrhage or neuroradiological instrumentation.

Organic nitrates, nitrites and related drugs

Examples – glyceryl trinitrate, isosorbide di- and mononitrate, nitric oxide, nitroprusside

Uses

These are direct-acting vascular smooth muscle relaxants that are used to control and reduce blood pressure and to alleviate angina.

Mode of action

Both organic nitrates (NO_3^-) and sodium nitroprusside act in a similar way. Having diffused from the vascular lumen through to the smooth muscle they are converted to nitrites (NO_2^-) by reacting with –SH groups (thiols) in the tissues. Hydrogen ions within the cells then react with the nitrite to produce nitric oxide (NO). This in turn reacts with more thiols in the muscle cell to produce nitrosothiols. These stimulate guanylyl cyclase to convert guanosine triphosphate (GTP) to cyclic guanosine monophosphate (cGMP) in a comparable way to adenylyl cyclase. The cGMP then relaxes the smooth muscle. Nitric oxide may be administered by inhalation to selectively dilate pulmonary arterioles. It mimics the physiological mediation by the vascular endothelial cells of a number of circulating autacoids such as bradykinin, which stimulate nitric oxide synthase to convert arginine to citrulline and nitric oxide. This nitric oxide (formerly identified as endothelium-derived relaxing factor, EDRF) diffuses into the muscle cell, where it has its effect.

Clinical effects

The predominant effect is that of vasodilatation affecting the venous system (preload) in particular. The reduction in preload reduces cardiac output, cardiac work and myocardial oxygen demand, and so these drugs are used to treat angina. Higher or more prolonged doses also dilate arterioles including the coronary vessels, and therefore reduce afterload. In the ischaemic heart, these drugs may increase the blood flow to ischaemic myocardium by dilating collaterals that bypass partial vessel occlusions.

Flushing and headaches are common, and a reflex tachycardia develops, putting a practical upper limit on the degree of vasodilatation. All smooth muscle is affected somewhat, but the clinically important effect is confined to the cardiovascular system.

Patients using isosorbide dinitrate and other longer-acting nitrates may develop tolerance, perhaps because of depletion of the tissue thiols. Excessive levels of nitrates convert haemoglobin to methaemoglobin.

Glyceryl trinitrate

Glyceryl trinitrate reduces blood pressure and coronary vascular resistance and increases subendocardial coronary blood flow by decreasing left ventricular end-diastolic pressure. It may be administered by infusion, by transdermal absorption using a skin patch, or by sublingual absorption using a spray or a tablet. Gastric acid rapidly inactivates glyceryl trinitrate, and once the desired effect is achieved it may be swallowed. Within the body it is rapidly hydrolysed in the liver, producing inorganic nitrite. Some is also converted to glyceryl dinitrate and glyceryl trinitrate, which have a small amount of activity and a half-life of 2 hours.

Isosorbide dinitrate

Isosorbide dinitrate is usually given orally by a slow-release preparation, and so its effect is delayed compared with glyceryl trinitrate. It may also be given sublingually for rapid onset, and by infusion for precision control of symptoms or blood pressure. The effects are similar. It is converted to isosorbide mononitrate in the liver with a half-life of 4 hours.

Isosorbide mononitrate

Isosorbide mononitrate, the active metabolite of isosorbide dinitrate, is given orally and is similar to its precursor.

Nitric oxide

Inhaled nitric oxide (in concentrations of about 40 ppm) is used to treat pulmonary hypertension in the intensive care setting. It diffuses through to the pulmonary vascular smooth muscle, where it interacts to cause cGMP-mediated relaxation. Further diffusion to the vascular lumen results in rapid inactivation as it combines with haemoglobin to form methaemoglobin.

Nitroprusside

Sodium nitroprusside is used in the control of hypertension, and for induced hypotension during surgery. It affects both arterial and venous systems to cause a reduction in systemic vascular resistance followed by a compensatory tachycardia. It is administered by infusion in systems protected from light (brown syringes and yellow infusion lines are available). Nitroprusside metabolism produces the highly toxic cyanide ion (CN^-), some of which combines with haemoglobin to produce methaemoglobin, and the rest is converted to thiocyanate by rhodonase in the liver and subsequently excreted in the urine. Thiocyanate levels can be measured to monitor toxicity. A small amount combines with vitamin B_{12} to form cyanocobalamin. In excess the cyanide ion saturates these elimination processes and damages the cytochrome oxidase chain (fundamental for aerobic cellular energy production).

Potassium channel activators
Examples – minoxidil, nicorandil

Potassium channel activators act by opening potassium channels, resulting in hyperpolarisation of the cell membrane with a reduction in electrical activity. ATP has the opposite effect, closing the channels and depolarising the membrane. Nicorandil relaxes arterial smooth muscle and reduces systemic vascular resistance. The nitrate component of the drug causes venous smooth muscle relaxation with a fall in preload. It also has a direct dilating affect on coronary arterioles, to improve perfusion of ischaemic myocardium. The intended role for nocorandil is in the treatment of angina.

Minoxidil is also a potassium channel activator, and is reserved for resistant severe hypertension. The resulting vasodilatation causes a tachycardia and increased cardiac output, and fluid retention is also a problem. Concomitant use of a β blocker and diuretic are essential. It causes hypertrychosis, and has been used as a treatment for baldness.

Endothelin receptor antagonists
Examples – bosentan, sitaxsentan

Endothelin receptors ET_A, ET_{B1} and ET_{B2} are G-protein-coupled receptors located in the endothelium and vascular smooth muscle. The endogenous agonist endothelin causes an increase in free intracellular calcium ions. Bosentan is a competitive antagonist at both ET_A and ET_B receptors, causing vasodilatation. It is licensed for some types of pulmonary hypertension. Sitaxsentan is a sulphonamide that is very selective for ET_A. It is also used as a pulmonary antihypertensive.

Prostacyclins
Examples – epoprostenol, iloprost

Epoprostenol (synthetic prostacyclin, PGI_2) and iloprost (a synthetic analogue of prostacyclin) are both potent vasodilators. Epoprostenol is used for inhibition of platelet aggregation, for example during haemodialysis. Iloprost is presented as a solution for nebulised inhalation, and so targets pulmonary vessels for the treatment of pulmonary hypertension.

cGMP phosphodiesterase inhibitor
Example – sildenafil

Sildenafil inhibits PDE_5 (phosphodiesterase 5) to inhibit the nitric oxide stimulation of guanylyl cyclase to produce cGMP, causing vascular smooth muscle relaxation. Its specificity leads to its use as a pulmonary vasodilator, but it is perhaps better known for its use in treating erectile dysfunction.

Other agents of importance
Diazoxide
Diazoxide is a thiazide, but unlike its diuretic counterparts it causes sodium and water retention. Diazoxide antagonises the effect of ATP on potassium channels. It has a direct effect on arteriolar smooth muscle, and given intravenously causes marked hypotension and a reflex increase in heart rate and cardiac output. The increased sympathetic outflow also increases free fatty acids and blood glucose.

Hydrallazine
Hydrallazine acts both centrally and peripherally. The peripheral effect causes direct vascular smooth muscle relaxation. There is also a mild α blocking action. The drop in blood pressure causes a reflex increase in sympathetic tone. Renal blood flow is increased. Headache, dizziness, nausea and vomiting are common side effects.

Specific pharmacology
Units (unless stated otherwise) are:
  Volume of distribution at steady state (V_d): $l\,kg^{-1}$
  Clearance (Cl): $ml\,kg^{-1}\,min^{-1}$
  Terminal half-life ($t_{1/2}$): minutes

Dobutamine hydrochloride

Structure – catecholamine; β_1 and β_2 (and α_1) agonist

Preparation – 250 mg dobutamine and 4.8 mg sodium metabisulphite in 20 ml for further dilution prior to administration

Dose – infusion 0.5–40 μg kg^{-1} min^{-1}

CNS – stimulant at high dose

CVS – heart rate, stroke volume, cardiac output increased, atrioventricular node conduction enhanced; vasodilatation; systemic vascular resistance and left ventricular end-diastolic pressure (LVEDP) reduced; coronary perfusion may increase

RS – no effect

Other – β_1 effect increases renin output; urine output increases secondary to increased cardiac output

Metabolism – converted to 3-O-methyldobutamine by COMT; this is conjugated and excreted in urine (80%) and faeces (20%)

Contraindications – increasing doses cause tachycardia, hypertension and arrhythmias; angina may occur in susceptible patients; allergic reactions to the metabisulphite preservative have occurred

Dopamine hydrochloride

Structure – catecholamine; β and α agonist

Preparation – 400 mg (1600 μg ml^{-1}) and 800 mg (3200 μg ml^{-1}) in 250 ml 5% dextrose (other mixtures available)

Dose – IV infusion

1–20 μg kg^{-1} min^{-1}

1–5 μg kg^{-1} min^{-1} increases renal blood flow

5–15 μg kg^{-1} min^{-1} inotropic

15–20 μg kg^{-1} min^{-1} vasoconstricts

CVS – contractility, stroke volume increased; little effect on heart rate; systemic vascular resistance, systolic, mean and diastolic blood pressures decreased; coronary blood flow increased

RS – carotid bodies stimulated, leading to reduced respiratory response to hypoxia

Other – splanchnic (including renal) vasodilatation; renal blood flow, glomerular filtrate, urine (volume and sodium content) increased; prolactin secretion inhibited (also known as prolactin-inhibiting hormone (PIH) secreted by the posterior pituitary)

Metabolism – by COMT and MAO to homovanillic acid and 3,4-dihydroxyphenylacetic acid. Predominantly excreted in urine, conjugated and unconjugated; 25% of the dopamine is taken up into adrenergic nerve endings and is converted to norepinephrine

Contraindications – nausea, tachycardia and arrhythmias; caution with MAO inhibitors

Dopexamine hydrochloride

Structure – catecholamine; dopamine (D_1 and D_2) and β_2 agonist

Preparation – colourless aqueous solution adjusted to a pH of 2.5, containing 50 mg dopexamine hydrochloride in 5 ml, and 0.01% disodium edetate; requires dilution prior to use

Dose – IV infusion – 0.5–6 μg kg^{-1} min^{-1} (start at 0.5 and increase by 0.5–1 μg kg^{-1} min^{-1} increments with at least 15-min intervals according to need

CNS – cerebral blood flow increased; dopexamine causes nausea by its action on D_2 receptors in the chemoreceptor trigger zone

CVS – stroke volume, heart rate and cardiac output increased; systolic blood pressure increased; systemic and pulmonary vascular resistance, diastolic blood pressure, LVEDP, pulmonary artery pressure reduced; coronary blood flow increased

RS – bronchodilatation

Other – mesenteric and renal vasodilatation with increased blood flow, diuresis and natriuresis; hyperglycaemia, hypokalaemia; splenic platelet sequestration; 40% of dose is bound to red cells

Metabolism – rapid tissue uptake, methylation and conjugation eliminate the drug

Contraindications – caution with MAO inhibitors

Ephedrine

Structure – sympathomimetic amine; α and β agonist

Preparation

Oral – tablets 15, 30 and 60 mg; elixir 15 mg in 5 ml

IV – clear, colourless, aqueous solution containing 30 mg ephedrine in 1 ml

Dose – IV – 3, 6 or 9 mg increments at minimal interval of 3–4 min. Maximum of 30 mg as tachyphylaxis ensues

CNS – stimulant effect (drug of abuse)

CVS – heart rate, stroke volume, cardiac output, myocardial oxygen consumption increased; SVR, diastolic, systolic and pulmonary pressures increased; coronary blood flow increased; splanchnic and renal vasoconstriction

RS – bronchodilator; respiratory rate and tidal volume increased; irritant to mucous membranes

Other – uterine, bladder and gastrointestinal smooth muscle relaxation; bladder sphincter tone increased;

gluconeogenesis, metabolic rate and oxygen consumption increased; irritant to mucous membranes

Metabolism – up to 99% eliminated in urine unchanged; the rest by oxidation, demethylation, and hydroxylation of the aromatic part plus conjugation

Contraindications – tachyarrhythmias (especially with halothane), nausea and central stimulation

Epinephrine

Structure – catecholamine; α and β agonist

Preparation – IV/subcutaneous – 1 mg in 1 ml (1 : 1000) and 1 mg in 10 ml (1 : 10 000), also added to local anaesthetics 1 : 200 000 (1 mg in 200 ml)

Dose – highly variable, depending upon indication and route

CNS – limited crossing of the blood–brain barrier but does cause excitation. Neuromuscular transmission facilitated

CVS – heart rate increased (may be reflexly reduced); contractility, stroke volume and cardiac oxygen consumption increased; systemic vasoconstriction but vasodilatation in skeletal muscle; mean arterial pressure, systolic and pulse pressure increased, diastolic decreased; coronary blood flow increased

RS – bronchodilatation; respiratory rate and tidal volume increased; secretions more tenacious

Other – gastrointestinal tract tone and secretions decreased, splanchnic blood flow decreased; renal blood flow increased; bladder tone reduced but sphincter tone increased; clotting factor V increased, leading to enhanced platelet aggregation and coagulation; metabolic effects to increase gluconeogenesis and increase metabolic rate

Metabolism – by catechol-O-methyl transferease (COMT) in the liver and monoamine oxidase (MAO) in adrenergic neurones to inactive metabolites 3-methoxy-4-hydroxy phenylethylene and 3-methoxy-4-hydroxy mandelic acid

Contraindications – beware arrhythmias with halothane; caution with MAO inhibitors

Toxicity – there are many adverse effects but the major ones are cardiac; increases cardiac sensitivity and irritability, so arrhythmias including VF and asystole are likely if given too quickly

Isoprenaline

Structure – catecholamine; β agonist

Preparation

Oral – tablets 30 mg

IV – colourless, aqueous solution adjusted to a pH of 2.5–2.8, containing 2 mg isoprenaline hydrochloride in 2 ml, with ascorbic acid and disodium edetate; requires dilution prior to use

Dose – IV infusion – 0.02–0.4 μg kg^{-1} min^{-1}

CNS – stimulant

CVS – heart rate, stroke volume and cardiac output increased; SA node automaticity and AV nodal conduction increased; systemic vascular resistance and diastolic blood pressure reduced; coronary blood flow increased; splanchnic and renal vasoconstriction, but flow may improve if treating low cardiac output

RS – bronchodilatation

Other – uterine and gastrointestinal smooth muscle relaxation; gluconeogenesis increased; antigen-induced histamine release is inhibited

Metabolism – extensive first-pass effect if taken orally. 15–75% unchanged in the urine; the rest by COMT then conjugated

Norepinephrine acid tartrate

Structure – catecholamine; α (and β) agonist

Preparation – clear, colourless, aqueous solution containing 0.2 mg ml^{-1} (in 2, 4 and 20 ml ampoules) or 2 mg ml^{-1} (2 ml ampoule) with sodium metabisulphite and sodium chloride. 1 mg norepinephrine acid tartrate (1 ml) contains 0.5 mg norepinephrine base, so the preparations contain 0.1 and 1 mg norepinephrine base per ml respectively

Dose – IV infusion 0.05–0.2 μg kg^{-1} min^{-1}

CNS – cerebral oxygen consumption reduced

CVS – generalised peripheral vasoconstriction, systolic and diastolic blood pressure increased; a reflex fall in heart rate occurs; cardiac output may fall slightly; coronary vasodilatation causes coronary blood flow to increase; ventricular rhythm disturbances may occur

RS – mild bronchodilatation, minute volume increases

Other – hepatic, renal and splanchnic blood flow reduced; pregnant uterus contractility increased, and this may compromise fetal oxygen supply; insulin secretion reduced; renin secretion increased; mydriasis; plasma water reduced by contraction of vascular space, and this increases haematocrit and plasma protein concentration

Metabolism – by MAO and COMT, which in combination produce 3-methoxy-4-hydroxy mandelic acid (VMA) in the urine. 5% excreted unchanged

Contraindications – caution with MAO inhibitors

Clonidine hydrochloride

Structure – imidazoline-aniline derivative

Preparation

Oral – tablets/capsules 25, 100, 250 and 300 µg

IV – clear, colourless, aqueous solution containing 150 µg in 1 ml

Dose

Oral migraine/flushing – 50–75 µg twice daily

Oral antihypertensive – 50–600 µg 3 times daily

Slow IV – 150–300 µg for control of hypertensive crisis

Pharmacokinetics (IV dose)

onset	10 min
peak	30–60 min
duration	3–7 h
V_d	2
Cl	3
$t_{1/2}$	6–23 h

CNS – analgesia

CVS – transient α_1 effect causes increased systemic vascular resistance and blood pressure; α_2 agonism produces presynaptic inhibition of sympathetic norepinephrine release with reductions in SVR, blood pressure, venous return and heart rate; cardiac contractility and output are preserved; coronary blood flow increased; renal blood flow increased; rebound tachycardia and hypertension can result from sudden withdrawal

RS – no effect

Other – plasma catecholamine and renin reduced; blood glucose increased; reduction of MAC; may cause dizziness, drowsiness, headache, dry mouth and impotence

Metabolism – 65% unchanged in urine, 20% in faeces, 15% inactivated in liver

Esmolol hydrochloride

See Section 3, Chapter 12 (page 672).

Labetalol hydrochloride

Structure – 2-hydroxy-5-[1-hydroxy-2-(1-methyl-3-phenyl-propylamino) ethyl] benzamide hydrochloride; combined α_1, β_1 and β_2-adrenoceptor antagonist

Preparation

Oral – tablets 50, 100, 200, 400 mg

IV – clear, colourless, aqueous solution containing 100 mg in 20 ml

Dose

Oral – 100–1200 mg twice daily

IV – slow bolus of 50 mg at 5-min intervals until blood pressure is controlled (duration 6–18 h, maximum dose 200 mg); IV infusion 15–160 mg h^{-1}

Pharmacokinetics

V_d	10
Cl	23
$t_{1/2}$	6 h

CNS – fatigue, confusion

CVS – heart rate, contractility, stroke volume, cardiac output, systemic vascular resistance, systolic and diastolic blood pressure decreased; coronary and renal blood flow increased

RS – potential risk of bronchoconstriction in asthmatics

Other – with IV use there is a compensatory increase in endogenous catecholamines; renin and angiotensin II reduced; platelet aggregation may be reduced

Metabolism – hepatic

Contraindications – as for other β blockers; may interact with antiarrhythmics of Class I and IV; crosses the placenta and causes clinical effects in the fetus, including bradycardia, hypotension, respiratory depression, hypoglycaemia and hypothermia in the neonate

Atropine sulphate

Structure – tertiary amine; muscarinic, anticholinergic antagonist

Preparation

Oral – tablets 600 µg

IV/IM – clear, colourless, aqueous solution containing a racemic mixture of 600 µg atropine in 1 ml

Dose – 10–20 µg kg^{-1}

Pharmacokinetics

Bioavailability	10–25%
Protein binding	50%
pK_a	9.8
V_d	3
Cl	17
$t_{1/2}$	150

CNS – variable stimulation or depression, anti-emetic, anti-Parkinsonian; competitive antagonism of muscarinic receptors causes blockade of parasympathetic system and sweating

CVS – heart rate, AV nodal transmission and cardiac output increase (initial temporary bradycardia with low doses due to centrally mediated increase in vagal tone); blood pressure may increase; tachyarrhythmias

RS – bronchodilator with increased anatomical dead space; respiratory rate increased; secretions reduced

Other – gastrointestinal motility and secretions reduced; biliary anti-spasmodic effect; lower oesophageal sphincter pressure reduced; urinary tract tone and peristalsis reduced, bladder sphincter tone increased and retention may result; pupillary dilatation, inability to accommodate for near objects (may persist for several days) and raised intraocular pressure occur; metabolic rate increased

Metabolism – atropine ester hydrolysed into its component parts tropine and tropic acid by the liver, 94% of the dose appearing in the urine in 24 hours

Contraindications – beware glaucoma, hyperpyrexia especially in children; central anticholinergic syndrome

Glycopyrrolate

Structure – quaternary amine; muscarinic anticholinergic antagonist

Preparation – IV – clear, colourless, aqueous solution containing 200 µg ml^{-1} in 1 and 3 ml ampoules

Dose

IV – 4–5 µg kg^{-1} (10–15 µg kg^{-1} in conjunction with neostigmine)

Children – 4–8 µg kg^{-1} (10 µg kg^{-1} in conjunction with neostigmine 50 µg kg^{-1})

Pharmacokinetics

Bioavailability	5%
V_d	0.4
Cl	13
$t_{1/2}$	50

CNS – does not cross the blood–brain barrier, so there is no effect on the eye; competitive antagonism of muscarinic receptors causes blockade of parasympathetic system and sweating

CVS – heart rate, AV nodal transmission and cardiac output increase, blood pressure may increase; tachyarrhythmias less common than with atropine

RS – bronchodilatation with increased anatomical dead space; secretions reduced

Other – gastrointestinal motility and secretions reduced; lower oesophageal sphincter pressure reduced; urinary tract tone and peristalsis reduced, bladder sphincter tone increased and retention may result; metabolic rate increased

Metabolism – excreted unchanged in the urine (85%) and faeces (15%)

Contraindications – in high doses the quaternary ammonium has a nicotinic antagonist effect of significance in myasthenia gravis; limited crossing of the placenta but can still cause fetal tachycardia

Hyoscine hydrobromide or butylbromide

Structure – tertiary amine, muscarinic anticholinergic antagonist; S-hyoscine (scopolamine) used

Presentation – hyoscine-N-butylbromide tablets 10 mg; IV – clear colourless solution, 20 mg in 1 ml, hyoscine hydrobromide 20 mg in 5 ml

Pharmacokinetics

Bioavailability	10%
Protein binding	11%
V_d	2
Cl	10
$t_{1/2}$	150

CNS – sedation, anti-emesis, anti-Parkinsonian

CVS – initial tachycardia given IV, but may later cause bradycardia due to central effect

RS – decreases secretions, bronchodilatation, slight ventilatory stimulation

Others – anti-sialagogue, anti-spasmodic for biliary tree and uterus; marked decrease in tear and sweat formation; decreases bladder and ureteric tone

Elimination – metabolised in the liver to scopine and scopic acid; unchanged, urine 2%, bile 5%

Toxicity – potential problem in patients with porphyria

Glyceryl trinitrate

Structure – organic nitrate ester of nitric acid and glycerol (glycerine)

Preparation – sublingual tablets and oral spray, transdermal patches (5 and 10 mg), IV – clear colourless, aqueous solution containing 1 mg glyceryl trinitrate per ml with polyethylene glycol and dextrose; stored in amber ampoules with 5 and 50 ml solution

Dose

SL – 300 µg

TD – 5 or 10 mg per 24 h

IV – 0.2–3 µg kg^{-1} min^{-1}

Pharmacokinetics

V_d 0.04–2.9

Cl   600

$t_{1/2}$ 2

CNS – intracranial pressure increased as a result of vasodilatation and headache ensues if sublingual dose continues beyond desired anti-anginal effect

CVS – venodilator with arterial dilatation as dose increases; SVR, systolic, diastolic, venous and pulmonary artery pressures reduced, myocardial oxygen demand reduced; cardiac output and coronary blood flow little effected; heart rate is unchanged in failure but increased reflexly in normal state

RS – bronchodilatation, and may increase shunt

Other – relaxes other smooth muscle such as biliary and gut

Metabolism – hydrolysis of the ester bonds by red cells and the liver, and 80% of the dose is excreted in the urine

Contraindications – substantial amount of intravenously administered GTN binds to the plastic of giving sets and syringes, therefore reduced availability

Sodium nitroprusside

Structure – inorganic complex

Preparation – red-brown powder containing 50 mg sodium nitroprusside in a brown glass ampoule which is reconstituted in 2 ml 5% dextrose before further dilution. It should be protected from light, and yellow and brown giving sets and syringes are available for this purpose

Dose – IV infusion 0.1–1.5 μg kg^{-1} min^{-1} (maximum of up to 8 μg kg^{-1} min^{-1}). Maximum dose 1.5 mg kg^{-1}; starts to accumulate once rate > 2 μg kg^{-1} min^{-1}

Pharmacokinetics

V_d 0.2

Elimination   1 μg kg^{-1} min^{-1}

nitroprusside $t_{1/2}$ very short

thiocyanate $t_{1/2}$ 2.7 days

CNS – cerebral vasodilatation increases intracranial pressure

CVS – dilates arterioles and venules with reduced blood pressure, reduced LVEDP, reduced myocardial oxygen demand; heart rate increases but contractility is unaffected

RS – hypoxic pulmonary vasoconstriction is impaired and arterial oxygen tension may fall

Other – gastrointestinal motility and lower oesophageal sphincter pressure are reduced; metabolic acidosis may occur

Metabolism – reacts with sulphydryl groups of plasma amino acids; higher concentrations cause non-enzymatic hydrolysis in red blood cells to produce five cyanide ions from each nitroprusside molecule. One of these combines with haemoglobin (iron in ferrous state) to form methaemoglobin (iron in ferric state); most of the rest is converted to thiocyanate by rhodonase in the liver and is then excreted in the urine; small amount of thiocyanate combines with vitamin B_{12} to form cyanocobalamin

Toxicity – cyanide ions inhibit the cytochrome oxidase chain; plasma levels of >80 μg l^{-1} produce tachycardia, sweating, hyperventilation, cardiac arrhythmias and retrosternal pain

CHAPTER 12

Cardiovascular pharmacology

T. C. Smith

Antiarrhythmic agents

Antiarrhythmic agents are usually classified according to their effect on the electrophysiology of cardiac myofibrils. Figure CV1 shows the different sites in the heart on which these drugs act. There are four basic classes of antiarrhythmic agent, with considerable variation in the chemical structure of the drugs within each functional class (Vaughan Williams 1970). Examples of the drugs by class are shown in Figure CV2.

Class I

Class I drugs work in a similar way to local anaesthetic agents (lidocaine is used for both roles). They act by slowing sodium entry into cells through the fast, voltage-gated sodium channels that primarily affect the non-nodal areas characterised by a fast depolarisation action potential. They reduce the maximum rate of rise of phase 0 depolarisation. The rate of phase 4 sinoatrial node depolarisation may also be reduced, and with it spontaneous automaticity.

Fast, voltage-gated sodium channels may exist in three states – resting, open and refractory. In normal myocardium their state switches between resting and open, but ischaemia results in prolonged depolarisation and the channel becomes refractory. The class I antiarrhythmics block open channels so that the more frequent the action potentials the more ionophores become blocked. The first action potential shows a slight reduction in phase 0 depolarisation. Subsequent action potentials show a progressive reduction in the rate of depolarisation as more channels are blocked. The block is therefore use-dependent.

Class I has three subdivisions, based on the effect on the action potential duration. The effect on action potential duration is related to the type of sodium channel affected, as follows:

- Class IA (e.g. quinidine) – action potential duration increased
- Class IB (e.g. lidocaine) – action potential duration decreased

Fundamentals of Anaesthesia, 3rd edition, ed. Tim Smith, Colin Pinnock and Ted Lin. Published by Cambridge University Press. © Cambridge University Press 2008.

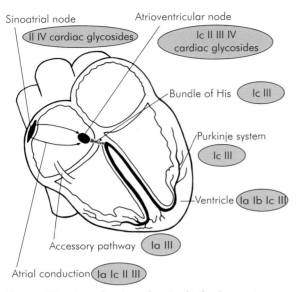

Sinoatrial node

II IV cardiac glycosides

Atrioventricular node

Ic II III IV
cardiac glycosides

Bundle of His — Ic III

Purkinje system

Ic III

Ventricle — Ia Ib Ic III

Accessory pathway — Ia III

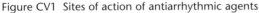

Atrial conduction — Ia Ic II III

Figure CV1 Sites of action of antiarrhythmic agents

- Class IC (e.g. flecainide) – action potential duration unaffected

The key features of the subdivisions of class I antiarrhythmics are listed in Figure CV3, and their ECG effects are shown in Figure CV4.

Class IB antiarrhythmics have a receptor association/dissociation cycle shorter than the cardiac cycle. The initial drug effect causes gradual blockade of the ionophores to develop during the action potential depolarisation. By the time the next action potential occurs, however, the drug will have dissociated from its receptor again. If a premature depolarisation (e.g. a ventricular premature beat) occurs then the myofibril will still be blocked. Class IB antiarrhythmics bind preferentially to refractory channels, and are therefore selective for ischaemic myocardium. Class IB drugs also elevate the fibrillation threshold. Lidocaine is discussed in Section 3, Chapter 9 (page 629). Mexiletine is similar but also has anticonvulsant properties, possibly due to GABA reuptake inhibition.

Class IC drugs have a much slower association/dissociation cycle, lasting longer than the cardiac cycle, so the block is relatively constant from cycle to cycle. The overall effect is a general reduction in excitability, and this is therefore more suitable for re-entrant-type rhythms. There is little selectivity for the refractory channels of ischaemic myocardium.

Class IA drugs have features midway between those of IB and IC.

Class IA drugs are primarily used for supraventricular tachycardias, and Class IB and C for ventricular tachycardias.

Class I
IA
Quinidine
Procainamide
Disopyramide
Cibenzoline
IB
Lidocaine
Phenytoin
Mexiletine
Tocainide
Ethmozine
IC
Flecainide
Lorcainide
Propafenone
Indecainide
Encainide
Class II
Propranolol
Esmolol
Sotalol
Class III
Amiodarone
Bretylium
Sotalol
n-acetyl procainamide
Class IV
Verapamil
Diltiazem

Figure CV2 Antiarrhythmic drugs by class

Class	Example	dV/dt of phase 0	Repolarisation	PR	QRS	QT
IA	Quinidine	Slowed	Prolonged	↑	↑	↑
IB	Lidocaine	Little effect	Shortened	0	0	↓
IC	Flecainide	Marked slowing	Little effect	↑↑	↑↑	0

Figure CV3 Features of the subdivisions of class I antiarrhythmic drugs

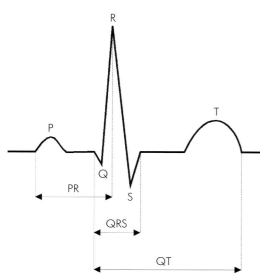

	Anti-arrhythmic group		
	I A	I B	I C
PR Interval	↑	—	↑
QRS Duration	↑	—	↑
QT Interval	↑	↓	—

Figure CV4 ECG effects of antiarrhythmic drugs

Class II

Class II antiarrhythmics (β blockers) competitively block the effects of circulating and neurotransmitter catecholamines, reducing arrhythmogenicity, heart rate and contractility. This slows and so lengthens phase 4 depolarisation, the phase which is shortened by catecholamines. The action potential is shortened and the refractory period of the AV node is prolonged. These GS-coupled effects are mediated by a slow L-type Ca channel influx that may be particularly useful in preventing post-myocardial-infarction ventricular arrhythmias, when catecholamine levels may be high. Some potassium, chloride and even sodium channel modulation may also be involved. β blockers are covered in detail in Section 3, Chapter 11 (pages 652–3).

Class III

Class III drugs (amiodarone, bretilium, sotalol) prolong repolarisation and therefore the action potential, and increase the effective refractory period. Their principal uses are for the following arrhythmias:

- Atrial tachycardia
- Atrial flutter and fibrillation
- Re-entrant junctional tachycardia
- Ventricular tachycardia

Amiodarone is particularly effective for the treatment of atrial tachyarrhythmias when Wolff–Parkinson–White syndrome is also present. At higher doses, the effect may be similar to β blockade and there is a quinidine-like action. Marked hypotension may result from IV administration.

Bretylium tosylate is reserved for use in resuscitation. It is given intravenously or intramuscularly in the treatment of ventricular fibrillation after DC shock and lidocaine have been tried. It accumulates in sympathetic ganglia and reduces norepinephrine release. There is an initial postganglionic discharge. It may cause hypotension, nausea and vomiting, and should be used with caution when a cardiac glycoside has been previously administered.

Sotalol is a β-adrenoceptor antagonist and is classified as both a Class II and a Class III antiarrhythmic. Sotalol causes both β_1 and β_2 antagonism (mainly by the L isomer). Its place amongst the Class III antiarrhythmics is due to K^+ channel inhibition, which is equally attributable to both stereoisomers. It is indicated for the treatment of paroxysmal supraventricular tachycardia, ventricular premature beats and ventricular tachycardia. It is more suitable than lidocaine for the treatment of spontaneous sustained ventricular tachycardia secondary to coronary disease or cardiomyopathy. The usual precautions for β-blocker therapy apply. Use with caution when there is hypokalaemia and when other agents that prolong the QT interval are concurrently administered.

Class IV

There are numerous calcium antagonists (pages 666–7), having different sites of action. Verapamil and diltiazem have antiarrhythmic activity, but nifedipine does not. Slowing of calcium influx reduces the duration of phases 2 and 3 of the action potential. At the atrioventricular node, this action is particularly beneficial in preventing re-entry rhythm problems.

Adenosine

Adenosine is used for rapid conversion of paroxysmal supraventricular tachycardias back to sinus rhythm (including Wolff–Parkinson–White syndrome). It may also be used in the diagnosis of conduction defects. Adenosine is ubiquitous in the body, in combination with phosphate (e.g. cyclic AMP) and has predominantly inhibitory effects. There are four specific types of adenosine receptor, A_1, A_{2A}, A_{2B} and A_3, the effects of which are detailed in Figure CV5.

The effect of adenosine in causing transient slowing of AV nodal conduction allows normal sinus nodal discharge to initiate a normal pattern of electrical depolarisation throughout the heart, and so normal sinus rhythm resumes, before the drug has been eliminated. This appears to be mediated by increasing myocardial K^+ flux. The A_1 purinoceptors are linked by a stimulatory G protein to the same transmembrane K^+ channels that are opened by M_2 muscarinic acetylcholine receptors. It is an unusual drug in that a key to successful use is that its IV injection must be rapid. This is because it is metabolised rapidly, with

A_1
- Inhibition of AV nodal conduction
- Reduced heart rate
- Reduction of atrial contractility
- Decreased cardiac excitability in response to adrenaline
- Antihypertensive
- Inhibition of excitatory amino acid release in CNS and PNS
- Decreased cerebral excitability during hypoxia and epilepsy
- Renal vasoconstriction leading to reduced diuresis
- Bronchoconstriction
- Enhanced response to insulin
- Anti-lipolytic

A_{2A}
- Vasodilatation (increasing coronary and cerebral blood flow)
- Inhibition of platelet aggregation
- Stimulation of nociceptive neurones

A_{2B}
- Anti-inflammatory
- Inhibition of GIT tone

A_3
- Cardioprotection

Figure CV5 Receptor effects of adenosine

a half-life of only 8–10 seconds. Unlike verapamil, it can be used safely in conjunction with β blockers, but is contraindicated in asthma, sick sinus syndrome and second and third degree AV heart block.

Cardiac glycosides

The cardiac glycosides are a group of naturally occurring compounds used to improve myocardial contractility and reduce cardiac conductivity. Cardiac glycosides are found mainly in three botanical species, white foxglove (*Digitalis lanata*), purple foxglove (*D. purpurea*) and climbing oleander (*Strophanthus gratus*).

Chemistry

The cardiac glycosides share the same basic structure:
- Steroid nucleus (cyclopentanophenanthrene)
- Lactone ring (five- or six-membered) – the aglycone
- Carbohydrate (up to four monosaccharide units)

The carbohydrate moiety is responsible for solubility, and the lactone ring confers pharmacological activity. Saturation of the lactone rings reduces potency, and opening of the ring abolishes the pharmacological activity. Only rings A and D of the steroid nucleus are coplanar, whereas in adrenal steroids rings A and C, and B and D are coplanar.

Pharmacological effects

Cardiac glycosides increase myocardial contractility and slow conduction at the atrioventricular node. Isometric and isotonic contraction of both atrial and ventricular muscle is improved. Cardiac glycosides cause directly mediated vasoconstriction.

Clinical uses

Cardiac glycosides are used to improve contractility in hypervolaemic myocardial failure. In chronic atrial fibrillation ventricular rate becomes slower because of a direct reduction in AV nodal conduction and by a secondary reduction in vagal tone.

Mechanisms of action

Sodium–potassium adenosine triphosphatase (Na$^+$K$^+$ATPase)

Cardiac glycosides specifically and reversibly bind to cardiac cell membrane Na$^+$K$^+$ATPase, which alters the electrolyte balance inside the myocardial fibres with more sodium and less potassium intracellularly. This results in a reduction of the transport of sodium into the cell using the Na$^+$Ca^{2+} ion exchange system, and intracellular calcium is better maintained and increased. The increased calcium may be responsible for the positive inotropy. However, at higher doses this interference with an essential membrane pump may be responsible for toxicity.

Interference with neuronal catecholamine reuptake

At low biophase concentrations, there is an increase in local catecholamine levels due to interference with neuronal catecholamine reuptake. This has positive inotropic and chronotropic effects, and may in fact increase overall Na$^+$K$^+$ATPase activity. There is also an increase in local acetylcholine levels, resulting in negative inotropic and chronotropic effects.

Elimination

The glycosides are highly bound to cardiac muscle, and therefore have very high volumes of distribution. This slows

- Heart block
- Cardiac arrhythmias
- Fatigue
- Nausea
- Anorexia
- Xanthopsia
- Confusion
- Neuralgia
- Gynaecomastia

Figure CV6 Side effects of cardiac glycosides

elimination considerably as most are excreted unchanged in the urine, both by simple filtration and also by tubular secretion. Digitoxin is the exception, being primarily metabolised by hepatic microsomal enzymes.

Toxicity

The cardiac glycosides have a very low therapeutic index. Most of the toxic effects are due to potassium loss. It is therefore particularly important to consider potassium-sparing diuretics when diuretics are needed in conjunction with cardiac glycosides. Side effects of the cardiac glycosides are listed in Figure CV6.

Contraindications

Digoxin is contraindicated in hypertrophic cardiomyopathy as it may increase outflow obstruction and cause sudden failure. It is also contraindicated in cardiac amyloid.

Magnesium

Magnesium is the fourth most prevalent cation in the body, and the second intracellularly. Of total body magnesium, 53% is in bone, with 27% in muscle and only 0.3% in plasma. Its physiological roles include incorporation as a cofactor in over 300 enzyme systems, inhibition of IP$_3$-gated calcium channels, muscle contraction, neuronal activity, neurotransmitter release and adenylyl cyclase regulation.

Pharmacologically, magnesium is used as replacement therapy. It is recognised now that magnesium deficiency is not uncommon in hospital patients, and in particular two-thirds of intensive care patients may be magnesium-depleted. There is now good evidence that magnesium is effective in the treatment of eclampsia, and some evidence to support its use in pre-eclampsia and in preventing the hypertensive response to intubation. The treatment of cardiac dysrhythmias is particularly indicated if

- Correction of magnesium deficiency
- Control of eclampsia and pre-eclampsia
- Inhibition of premature labour
- Improvement of cardiac contractility
- Limitation of myocardial infarct size
- Component of cardioplegia (a mixture to arrest the heart during cardiac surgery)
- Correction of cardiac dysrhythmias: emergency treatment of torsades de pointes, digoxin toxicity, life-threatening atrial and ventricular dysrhythmias
- Prevention of hypertensive response to intubation
- Pre-eclampsia
- Reduction of catecholamine release in phaeochromocytoma surgery
- Treatment of asthma

Figure CV7 Possible pharmacological uses of magnesium therapy

hypokalaemia coexists. A list of possible uses is given in Figure CV7.

Calcium antagonists

Calcium is involved not only in muscle contraction but also in neurotransmitter release, hormone secretion, platelet aggregation and enzyme function. There are numerous calcium channels across cell and other membranes. These may be active or passive, triggered by chemical mediators or voltage changes, and may be coupled with other ionic exchange. The term calcium antagonist is generally used to describe those agents with a role in cardiovascular manipulation. These act primarily on the voltage gated (L-type) calcium channels, preventing opening of the ionophore. There are three main groups (papaverines, benzothiazepines, dihydropyridines), each having characteristic actions. However, even within these groups, there is considerable difference between the individual chemical structures of the drugs, and in their calcium-channel specificity. The myocardial depression caused by the volatile anaesthetic agents halothane, enflurane and isoflurane is also the result of an alteration in calcium flux. Figure CV8 shows the relative potencies of the three representative calcium antagonists.

All three groups of calcium antagonist reduce systemic vascular resistance and central venous pressure by vasodilatation. This vasodilatation is more pronounced in the arterial system, and as it is combined with a slight negative inotropic effect blood pressure falls. The reduction in afterload and contractility reduces myocardial workload and oxygen requirement. All calcium antagonists cause coronary vasodilatation, but this is only of clinical relevance in coronary artery spasm.

Calcium antagonists may also interfere with noncardiac calcium channels, affecting, for example, neuromuscular blockade and insulin secretion.

Papaverines

Examples – methoxyverapamil, teapamil, verapamil

Papaverines predominantly act on cardiac muscle, by inhibiting the slow calcium entry during phases 2 and 3 of the cardiac-muscle action potential. This lengthening of the action potential makes them appropriate for tachyarrhythmias, especially re-entry supraventricular tachycardias and others of atrial origin. They also slow AV conduction, giving them a role in the management of atrial flutter and tachycardia. Papaverines have relatively little effect on vasomotor tone, but the reduction in contractility is more marked than with the calcium channel blockers.

	Verapamil (papaverine)	Diltiazem (benzothiazepine)	Nifedipine (dihydropyridine)
Reduction in SVR	++	+	+++
Coronary vasodilatation	++	++	++
Reduction in contractility	++	0	+
Reduction in blood pressure	+	0	++
Reflex increase in sympathetic tone	+	0	++
Slowing of AV nodal conduction	+++	++	0

Figure CV8 Relative clinical effects of calcium antagonists

Benzothiazepines
Example – diltiazem

Diltiazem affects both cardiac and smooth muscle, causing relatively mild reductions in systemic vascular resistance, blood pressure and cardiac output. It is used as an antiarrhythmic agent and for the treatment of angina and hypertension.

Dihydropyridines
Examples – amlodipine, nicardipine, nifedipine, nimodipine

The dihydropyridines predominantly act on smooth muscle. Clinically this mainly affects vascular tone, causing peripheral vasodilatation primarily on the arterial side, and so reduces afterload. This reduces cardiac workload and may improve peripheral perfusion. The resultant drop in blood pressure results in a partial compensatory increase in heart rate and cardiac output. They also cause coronary vasodilatation, but this is not generally of clinical benefit. Dihydropyridines are used to treat hypertension, angina and heart failure. Nimodipine acts preferentially on cerebral arteries and is used to prevent vascular spasm after subarachnoid haemorrhage.

Phosphodiesterase inhibitors
Selective phosphodiesterase inhibitors are used for their inotropic and vasodilator properties. They selectively inhibit the phosphodiesterase III isoenzyme (PDE III) responsible for the breakdown of cAMP in myocardial muscle and vascular smooth muscle. This is in contrast with the methylxanthines such as theophylline (see Section 3, Chapter 13, page 676), which non-specifically inhibit all five phosphodiesterase isoenzymes. There are two chemical types of PDE III inhibitors, bipyridines and imidazolines.

Mode of action
Inhibition of PDE III causes an increase in intracellular cAMP, and to a lesser extent cGMP, in myocardial and vascular smooth muscle cells. The cAMP is responsible for phosphorylation of protein kinases in the cell. In the myocardium, this increases the influx of calcium through the slow calcium channels of the sarcolemma by increasing both the number of channels open and the duration of the open state. The sarcoplasmic reticulum is also affected, facilitating faster calcium release. The net effect is an increase in calcium ion availability in the cell for contraction. The raised level of cAMP is also responsible for improved reuptake of calcium into the sarcoplasmic reticulum, so that active myocardial relaxation is also improved, leading to an overall improvement in myocardial function.

In smooth muscle, the cAMP causes phosphorylation of the myosin light chain kinase which reduces the affinity for the calmodulin complex and dephosphorylates the myosin light chains. This results in relaxation and secondary vasodilatation. The increase in cGMP also mediates smooth muscle relaxation.

Clinical effects
PDE III inhibitors improve contractility in the failing heart without increasing the myocardial oxygen utilisation. The positive inotropic effect is greater than that of the cardiac glycosides and there is little chronotropic activity. Conduction in the atrium and AV node is increased, with little effect on the His–Purkinje system. PDE inhibitors cause vasodilatation, and therefore reduce preload and afterload. Coronary vascular resistance is also reduced, but this does not appear to cause coronary steal. PDE III inhibitors also cause some bronchodilatation, but this is not a major feature. These agents are used in the short-term treatment of severe congestive cardiac failure when other measures have failed. They work synergistically with β-adrenoceptor agonists, and can work when the latter used alone have failed.

Bipyridines
Example – milrinone

Milrinone is supplied as a pale yellow solution of the lactate salt. It is administered as a loading dose followed by infusion. It may potentially cause hypotension because of vasodilatation, necessitating close monitoring. Eighty per cent is eliminated unchanged in the urine, and it is therefore greatly influenced by decreases in renal function. In severe myocardial failure, glomerular filtration rate is often reduced and so half-life is increased from the normal 1 hour to several hours.

Imidazolines
Example – enoximone

Enoximone is supplied as a pale yellow solution in ethanol, propylene glycol and sodium hydroxide and has pH of

12. It is administered as a loading dose followed by infusion. Enoximone reduces the refractoriness of the atrium and AV node and shortens the ventricular refractory period. Ventricular tachycardias and ectopic beats have been observed in some patients who have received enoximone. The propensity to cause hypotension (due to vasodilatation) necessitates monitoring of blood pressure. Enoximone is metabolised in the liver, producing a mixture of active and inactive metabolites, and has a half-life of about 4 hours.

Selective imidazoline receptor agonists (SIRAs)

Example – moxonidine

Selective imidazoline receptor agonists are used for antihypertensive therapy. These drugs act by selective agonism at the imidazoline subtype 1 receptor (I_1) in the rostral-ventrolateral pressor area and ventromedial depressor areas of the medulla oblongata. This area is responsible for sympathetic activity, and an agonist effect at I_1 receptors results in a reduction of general sympathetic nervous system activity which produces the desired effect. SIRAs have a minor effect at the α_2 receptor which might potentially result in sedation, but in practice this is not seen, and the commonest side effect is dry mouth.

An example from this group is moxonidine, a centrally acting antihypertensive agent for mild to moderate hypertension. Moxonidine is also an α_2-adrenoceptor agonist acting similarly to clonidine. Moxonidine improves insulin release in response to glucose in animal studies, which could favour its use in obese or diabetic hypertensives in the future. It may exacerbate cardiac conduction defects and should be withdrawn slowly over a 2-week period. Caution is necessary when administering moxonidine with benzodiazepines, as the sedative effects of the latter become enhanced.

Renin–angiotensin system

Antagonism of the renin–angiotensin system at various levels is used to control hypertension by reducing vasomotor tone and by reducing salt and fluid retention. The first site of interference in this cascade is by antagonism of the β-adrenoceptors responsible for renin secretion. Next in line are the angiotensin-converting enzyme (ACE) inhibitors, then the angiotensin II receptor antagonists.

Angiotensin-converting enzyme inhibitors

Examples – captopril, enalapril, lisinopril, perindropril, ramipril

Mechanism of action

ACE inhibitors block the action of angiotensin-converting enzyme (ACE), a carboxypeptidase in the lungs that converts the inactive angiotensin I (Ang I) into the active angiotensin II (Ang II, an octapeptide). Angiotensin II causes profound vasoconstriction and release of aldosterone, resulting in sodium and water conservation. ACE is relatively non-specific, and it also inactivates bradykinin (a vasodilator) and other kinins. These three activities produce a rise in intravascular volume and vasomotor tone with the resultant increase in blood pressure. ACE inhibitors antagonise these effects. ACE inhibitors may also cause specific renal vasodilatation, and so further enhance sodium and water excretion. The reduced breakdown of bradykinin is responsible for the side effect of dry cough experienced with ACE inhibitors. The effects of ACE inhibitors include a reduction in:
- Sodium and water retention
- Vasomotor tone
- Preload
- Afterload
- Myocardial work

ACE inhibitors are indicated in hypertension, congestive cardiac failure, myocardial infarction and diabetic nephropathy. They are particularly effective when renin levels are raised, such as when sympathetic tone is increased. Myocardial infarction and congestive cardiac failure may show such increases. In antihypertensive therapy the ACE inhibitors may be used alone or in conjunction with other agents using different systems, such as diuretics and calcium antagonists. β blockers reduce renin secretion, so the benefit of adding an ACE inhibitor will be limited.

Angiotensin$_1$ inhibitors

Examples – irbesartan, losartan, valsartan

Mechanism of action

The classification of the AT_1 receptor deserves further clarification. ACE converts Ang I to Ang II. Ang I is inactive and does not have identified receptors, whereas Ang II is highly active. Two receptor subtypes for Ang II (roman numerals) have been identified and numbered (with arabic numerals) AT_1 and AT_2. AT_1 receptors are G-protein-coupled

- Reduced sodium and water retention
- Reduced vasomotor tone
- Reduced preload
- Reduced afterload
- Reduced blood pressure especially if sodium depletion
- Reduced myocardial work
- Variable reduction in aldosterone levels
- Blockade of negative feedback produces a rise in renin, Ang I and Ang II
- Increased insulin sensitivity and reduced catecholamines and atrial natriuretic peptide (ANP)
- Increased plasma potassium concentration

Figure CV9 Clinical effects of AT_1 inhibitors

receptors responsible for vasoconstricton and aldosterone secretion. The role of the AT_2 receptors is less clear, but they are thought to be antiproliferative for endothelial cells and to be involved in smooth muscle proliferation and differentiation.

Uses

The AT_1 inhibitors are used as antihypertensive agents and have clinical effects similar to the ACE inhibitors. Their main advantage is the absence of an effect on kinins, so the persistent dry cough of ACE inhibitors is not seen.

Features

The clinical features of AT_1 inhibitors are very varied. The main effects are shown in Figure CV9.

Diuretics

Diuretics promote the loss of water and sodium via the urine. Interference with sodium reabsorption in the renal tubule causes increased sodium loss, and the sodium takes water with it. Their precise effect is determined by which part of the renal tubule they affect. Other drugs may also indirectly increase renal water loss. The sites of action of the various diuretics are shown in Figure CV10.

Loop diuretics

Example – frusemide

These act on the thick (upper) part of the ascending loop of Henle by reducing sodium and chloride reabsorption. This interferes with the generation of the interstitial hypertonicity which is used by the collecting duct to reabsorb water. A smaller effect is due to the increased delivery of filtrate to the distal tubule. These are the most efficacious diuretics, causing up to 25% of sodium and water in the filtrate to be excreted. Loop diuretics also cause vasodilatation either directly or indirectly. This increases renal blood flow without affecting the glomerular filtration rate. The protein left in the efferent capillaries supplying the remainder of the nephron is therefore more dilute and has a lower oncotic pressure, which reduces reabsorption from the nephron. Subsequently more filtrate enters the loop of Henle, which is the primary site of action of the loop diuretics. In congestive cardiac failure, the venodilatation reduces preload before any diuretic effect is seen.

Loop diuretics work as antihypertensives by reducing both blood volume and vascular tone. The vascular effects may be mediated by interference with prostaglandin E_2 and I_2 degradation.

Loop diuretics present more filtrate to the distal convoluted tubule. The sodium–potassium exchange pump reabsorbs more sodium, and therefore more potassium is excreted. Hydrogen ions are also excreted in exchange for some of the potassium, and bicarbonate concentration increases. Patients on loop diuretics are therefore at risk of hypokalaemia and metabolic alkalosis. Calcium and magnesium loss also occurs. Uric acid secretion is reduced.

Loop diuretics are highly protein-bound, and therefore do not readily pass through the glomerular membrane. They are actively secreted into the proximal convoluted tubule (via the organic acid transport system) and then travel along the tubule to the luminal membrane of the loop of Henle. Excretion occurs via the urine, and they are non-cumulative.

Thiazide diuretics

Example – bendrofluazide

Thiazides act on the luminal membrane pump of the distal convoluted tubule by inhibiting active sodium and chloride reabsorption. They are medium-efficacy diuretics, causing up to 10% of sodium and water in the filtrate to be excreted. More sodium reaches the distal tubules, and this results in high potassium loss in the same way as with the loop diuretics, but because this is the main mode of thiazide action potassium loss is a much greater problem.

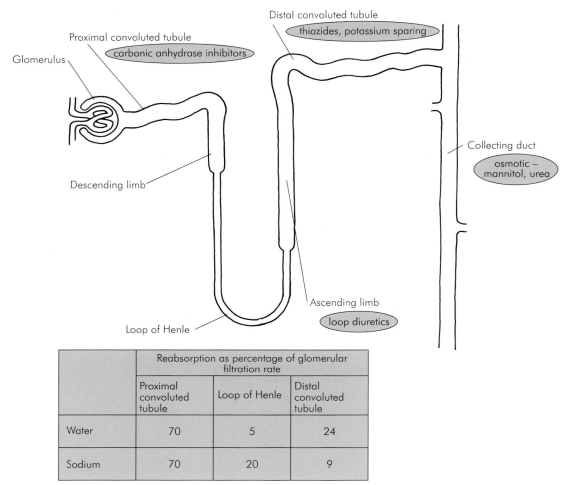

Figure CV10 Sites of action of diuretics

	Reabsorption as percentage of glomerular filtration rate		
	Proximal convoluted tubule	Loop of Henle	Distal convoluted tubule
Water	70	5	24
Sodium	70	20	9

Magnesium excretion is increased, but calcium and uric acid excretion are reduced.

Thiazides also cause direct vasodilatation. Owing to the ability to cause hyperglycaemia they are best avoided in diabetics. Excretion is by glomerular filtration and by tubular secretion using the uric acid secretion mechanism, which reduces uric acid excretion.

Potassium-sparing diuretics
Examples – amiloride, spironolactone

Potassium-sparing diuretics act on the distal convoluted tubule and collecting duct. They are low-efficacy diuretics, causing only 5% of sodium and water in the filtrate to be excreted, but have the advantage that they conserve potassium and are mainly used to minimise potassium loss caused by more effective diuretics. The decrease in potassium secretion increases the hydrogen ion secretion and thus reduces bicarbonate excretion. They also reduce uric acid excretion. Spironolactone inhibits the sodium–potassium exchange pump of the extraluminal membrane of collecting duct cells. Triamterene and amiloride interfere with the sodium channels through which the effects of aldosterone are mediated. Amiloride also inhibits sodium–potassium exchange in the proximal tubule.

Osmotic diuretics

Examples – mannitol, glucose, urea

Osmotic diuretics (such as mannitol and glucose) act by passing freely through the glomerular basement membrane, but being non-reabsorbable once in the tubule. The resultant effect is dependent directly upon the number of molecules, and so a large number of molecules is required to produce a clinical effect. They must usually be given intravenously. Urea is classified as an osmotic diuretic but is actively secreted into the tubule as well.

Carbonic anhydrase inhibitors

Example – acetazolamide

Carbonic anhydrase inhibitors inhibit the enzymatic breakdown of carbonic acid, and so interfere with the reabsorption of sodium in exchange for hydrogen ion secretion, especially in the proximal tubule. Their diuretic effect is mild. Their use is now mainly reserved for treatment of glaucoma and epilepsy. Other examples of carbonic anhydrase inhibitors are methazolamide and dichlorphenamide.

Specific pharmacology

Here, bioavailability applies to oral administration. Units (unless stated otherwise) are:

Volume of distribution at steady state (V_d): $l\,kg^{-1}$
Clearance (Cl): $ml\,kg^{-1}\,min^{-1}$
Terminal half-life $(t_{1/2})$: hours

Adenosine

Structure – a nucleoside comprising adenine (6-amino purine) and D-ribofuranose (pentose sugar)
Presentation – IV – clear aqueous solution of adenosine 6 mg in 2 ml 0.9% sodium chloride
Dose – IV – bolus 3 mg over 2 s, then bolus 6 mg after 1–2 min if necessary, then bolus 12 mg after 1–2 min if necessary; stop if high nodal block develops
Pharmacokinetics

$t_{1/2}$	8–10 s

CNS – rare occurrence of blurred vision, headache, dizziness
CVS – inhibits AV nodal conduction, reduces contractility, vasodilatation; palpitations, flushing, hypotension, severe bradycardia may occur
RS – dyspnoea, bronchospasm may occur
Other effects – nausea

Elimination – rapid cellular uptake, adenosine deaminase, phosphorylation to nucleotide
Contraindications – second and third degree heart block and sick sinus syndrome unless artificial pacemaker functioning; asthma
Interactions – dipyridamole inhibits adenosine uptake (if essential, use 0.5–1 mg dose); xanthines (caffeine, aminophylline) are potent inhibitors of adenosine; drugs slowing AV nodal conduction

Amiodarone hydrochloride

Structure – iodinated benzofuran derivative – class III antiarrhythmic
Presentation – tablets 200 mg, 100 mg; IV – clear, pale yellow solution, 150 mg in 3 ml
Dose – oral loading regimen then 200 mg per day; IV 5 mg kg^{-1} over 20 min to 2 h; onset of action by oral route is 6 days
Pharmacokinetics

Bioavailability	22–86%
Protein binding	97%
$t_{1/2}$	1300

CNS – peripheral neuropathy rare; nightmares, tremor, ataxia; corneal microdeposits (benign and reversible)
CVS – slows heart rate and may cause bradycardia, and AV block
RS – may rarely cause diffuse pulmonary alveolitis and fibrosis
Other effects – metabolite blocks conversion of T_3 to thyroxine and may therefore cause hypo- or hyperthyroidism. Thyroid function should be monitored. It may cause chronic liver disease, and transaminases often rise, especially at start of treatment
Elimination – it is de-iodinated and has a very long half-life because it is highly lipid-soluble and highly tissue-bound, which may result in cumulation; toxic effects may still be present months after treatment stopped

Digoxin

Structure – sterol lactone with sugar moiety – cardiac glycoside
Presentation – tablets 62.5, 125 and 250 μg, elixir; IV, clear, colourless, aqueous solution, 125 μg ml^{-1}
Dose: IV – up to 1 mg loading dose by slow (25 μg min^{-1}) injection; typically 10 μg kg^{-1} once daily oral or IV, monitor levels, plasma concentrations $(nmol\,l^{-1})$ – therapeutic 1.3–1.5; toxic 3.5

Pharmacokinetics

Bioavailability	75%
Protein binding	25%
V_d	8
$t_{1/2}$	35

Clearance $= 0.88 \times$ creatinine clearance $+ 0.33$

CNS – nausea, vomiting, dizziness, anorexia, fatigue, apathy, malaise, visual disturbance, depression and psychosis

CVS – positive inotropy, especially in hypervolaemic failure; negative chronotropy; slowing of AV conduction; in excess may cause complete heart block, and most rhythm disturbances, especially bradycardias

Other effects – mild intrinsic diuretic affect; abdominal pain, diarrhoea; gynaecomastia (steroid-related); intestinal necrosis (oral route); skin rashes; thrombocytopoenia

Elimination – 10% metabolised in the liver by progressive removal of the sugar moieties; 60% excreted unchanged in the urine by glomerular filtration and active tubular secretion

Toxicity increased by low potassium, low magnesium, high sodium, high calcium, acid–base disturbance and hypoxaemia. Poorly removed by dialysis as highly tissue-bound; digoxin-specific antibody fragments available for treatment of poisoning.

Diltiazem

Structure – benzothiapine calcium antagonist – class IV antiarrhythmic

Presentation – tablets 60 mg; slow-release 90, 120, 180, 200, 240 mg

Dose – 60–120 mg, 6–8 hourly

Pharmacokinetics

Bioavailability	35%
Protein binding	80%
V_d	5.3
Cl	15
$t_{1/2}$	5

CNS – no effect

CVS – causes peripheral and coronary arterial vasodilatation; decreases systemic and peripheral resistance; slows AV nodal conduction; exacerbates the negative inotropic effects of volatile agents

RS – antihistamine effect

Other effects – renal artery dilatation increases renal plasma flow; local anaesthetic effect; reduced lower oesophageal sphincter pressure in achalasia; may inhibit platelet aggregation

Elimination –2% is excreted unchanged in the urine; deacetylation and demethylation produce active metabolites which are conjugated with glucuronides and sulphates; renal failure has no effect on elimination

Esmolol hydrochloride

Structure – aryloxypropanolamine – β blocker – class II antiarrhythmic

Presentation – IV – clear aqueous solution 10 ml of 250 mg ml^{-1} for dilution and infusion; 10 ml of 100 mg ml^{-1} for undiluted boluses; 250 ml of 100 mg ml^{-1} for infusion

Dose – 50–200 μg kg^{-1} min^{-1}; a loading dose may be used

Pharmacokinetics

Protein binding	56%
V_d	3.43
Cl	285
$t_{1/2}$	9.2 min

CVS – mainly β$_1$; used for acute SVT, acute control of hypertension and myocardial infarction; negative chronotrope and inotrope, cardiac output falls by 20%

RS – selectivity minimises increases in airway resistance

Elimination – metabolised by red cell esterases producing methanol and a primary acid (70–80% as this in urine) which has weak β antagonism and half-life of 3.5 hours; < 1% is excreted unchanged in the urine. Use with caution in renal failure; hepatic failure has no effect

Nifedipine

Structure – dihydropyridine calcium antagonist – class IV antiarrhythmic

Presentation – tablets 10 and 20 mg and capsules 5 and 10 mg; the yellow, viscous liquid in the capsules has been used sublingually for speedy control of blood pressure; a solution is available for direct intracoronary injection

Dose – oral 10–20 mg 8 hourly, 20–40 mg 12 hourly slow-release formulation

Pharmacokinetics

Bioavailability	65%
Protein binding	95%
V_d	0.8
Cl	10
$t_{1/2}$	5

CNS – marginal increase in cerebral blood flow; headache, flushing, dizziness

CVS – decreases systemic and peripheral vascular resistance, decreases pulmonary artery pressure, reflex increase in heart rate and cardiac output; increases epicardial and coronary blood flow, negative inotrope

RS – no effect

Other effects – increases red cell deformability, decreases platelet aggregation, decreases thromboxane synthesis; reduces lower oesophageal sphincter pressure; increases renin, increases catecholamines; increases hepatic blood flow; oedema of legs; eye pain; gum hyperplasia

Elimination – 85% in urine; 15% in bile; non-cumulative

Verapamil

Structure – synthetic papaverine derivative – class IV antiarrhythmic

Presentation – tablets 40, 80 and 120 mg; IV 5 mg in 2 ml

Dose – oral 40–120 mg 8 hourly; IV 10 mg (0.075–0.20 mg kg^{-1})

Pharmacokinetics

Bioavailability	20%
Protein binding	90%
V_d	4.5
$t_{1/2}$	5

CNS – dizziness, headache

CVS – slows cardiac action potential; slows AV nodal conduction; decreases systemic vascular resistance; decreases blood pressure, heart rate and cardiac output; increases coronary blood flow

RS – no effect

Other effects – local anaesthetic effect; constipation

Elimination – 70% excreted in urine as conjugated metabolites, 5% unchanged; non-cumulative; half-life is increased in hepatic disease

Interactions – avoid concurrent use with β blocker as it may cause asystole or hypotension

References and further reading

Small R. Anti-arrhythmic drugs. *Anaesth Intensive Care Med* 2006; **7**: 294–7.

Vaughan Williams EM. Classification of anti-dysrhythmic drugs. In: Sande E, Flensted-Jensen E, Oleson KH (eds.) *Symposium on Cardiac Dysrhythmias*. Södertälje: Astra, 1970: 449–72.

CHAPTER 13
Respiratory pharmacology

T. C. Smith

ADMINISTRATION AND MODES OF ACTION

CONTROL OF BRONCHIAL CALIBRE
Adrenoceptor agonists
Anticholinergic agents
Methylxanthines
Steroids
Cromoglicate
Leukotriene receptor antagonists

RESPIRATORY CENTRE STIMULANTS

MUCOLYTICS

SURFACTANT

SPECIFIC PHARMACOLOGY
Aminophylline
Beclomethasone
Budesonide
Doxapram
Ipratropium bromide
Salbutamol
Sodium cromoglicate
Zafirlukast

Administration and modes of action

Drugs acting on the airways may be administered systemically or by inhalation. The inhaled mode allows a higher concentration of agent to be delivered directly to the bronchial tree, which minimises absorption and accompanying systemic effects. Some drugs are metabolised in the lungs, resulting in a non-hepatic first-pass effect.

Typically, only 10% of an inhalationally administered bronchodilator reaches the lungs. Most of this is deposited in the upper airways with little benefit, with about 3% reaching the alveoli. Distribution is little affected by the presence of obstructive airways disease, or by particle size.

Bronchial calibre is fundamentally affected by two opposing systems. Factors that cause an increase of intracellular cyclic AMP (such as sympathetic stimulation) result in bronchodilatation. The reverse situation involves factors that raise the intracellular concentration of cyclic GMP (such as parasympathetic stimulation) to cause bronchoconstriction. The physiological and pharmacological influences on bronchial calibre are summarised in Figure RP1.

Leukotrienes are involved in the development of bronchospasm. They are so-named because of their presence in white blood cells (the *leuko* component) and their chemical bonds (a *triene* system of double bonds). They are a group of eicosanoids (bioactive lipid derivatives of arachidonic acid). Leukotrienes are produced by the action of the enzyme 5-lipoxygenase, which is found in white

blood cells (particularly eosinophils) and mast cells, among other tissues. When activated, 5-lipoxygenase binds to the cell membrane and associates with five-lipoxygenase-activating protein (FLAP), the resulting complex causing change in arachidonic acid to produce leukotriene A_4 (LTA_4). This is a precursor of a whole family of leukotrienes, LTA_4 to LTF_4. LTC_4, D_4 and E_4 are spasmogenic, and comprise the substance formerly termed 'SRS-A' (see Section 2, Chapter 10, Figure PP4).

Control of bronchial calibre
Adrenoceptor agonists
β_2-agonists
Examples – bambuterol, formoterol, salbutamol, salmeterol, terbutaline

Selective β_2-adrenoceptor agonists are used in the treatment of bronchospasm and for prophylaxis. This selectivity is not absolute, and high doses of these drugs will cause β_1 effects (tachycardia, tremor, hyperglycaemia, increased insulin secretion and hypokalaemia).

β_2-agonists reverse bronchospasm caused by histamine release, platelet-activating factor and members of the leukotriene family, particularly C_4, D_4 and E_4.

The β_2-agonist salbutamol is the most widely used agent in the treatment of asthma. It is conjugated in the liver and excreted in both conjugated and unchanged forms in urine and faeces. Terbutaline is a similar agent that may

Fundamentals of Anaesthesia, 3rd edition, ed. Tim Smith, Colin Pinnock and Ted Lin. Published by Cambridge University Press. © Cambridge University Press 2008.

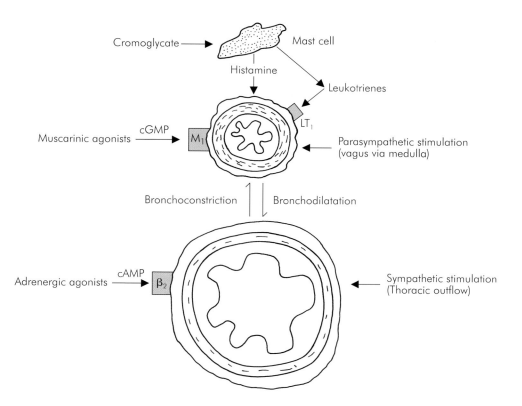

Figure RP1 Causes of changes in bronchial calibre

have advantages in some patients due to fewer sympatho-mimetic side effects. Terbutaline may be used antenatally to stimulate fetal lung surfactant production. Bambuterol is a prodrug of terbutaline.

β_2-agonists (in particular ritodrine, salbutamol and terbutaline) may be used as uterine relaxants for the management of premature labour or excessive contractions, or during Caesarean section to facilitate delivery. Administration for this purpose may be inhalational.

Other adrenoceptor agonists
Examples – ephedrine, epinephrine, isoprenaline, orciprenaline

Ephedrine, isoprenaline, orciprenaline and epinephrine are non-selective sympathetic agonists with bronchodilator (β_2) actions, which are infrequently used. Epinephrine has re-emerged as an effective inhaled agent for the treatment of acute tracheolaryngobronchitis (croup)

and laryngeal oedema. A dose of 0.5 ml kg^{-1} 1 : 1000 epinephrine up to a maximum of 5 ml may be nebulised, and given according to effect.

Anticholinergic agents
Examples – ipratropium and tiotropium bromide

Anticholinergic agents are given inhalationally and, as with other inhaled bronchodilators, only 10% of the dose reaches the lungs. These drugs act at muscarinic acetylcholine receptors and so inhibit bronchoconstriction. Systemically administered anticholinergic drugs also affect these receptors. Anticholinergic agents have the following respiratory effects:
• Bronchodilatation
• Reduced airways resistance
• Increased anatomical dead space
• Increased physiological dead space

Ipratropium bromide (N-isopropylatropine) is a non-selective muscarinic antagonist at M_1, M_2 and M_3. It has a rapid onset of action, but takes 2 hours to peak, lasting for 4–6 hours. Of the orally deposited drug, 70% passes unprocessed into the faeces. A small amount of drug is absorbed systemically from the oral mucosa, and this is metabolised by the liver. Antagonism at the (negative feedback) M_2 receptor increases acetylcholine release, which may limit the effectiveness of its M_1-mediated bronchodilatation. Ipratropium also blocks the M_1 muscarinic acetylcholine receptors on mast cells, limiting degranulation. It is primarily used for prophylaxis of bronchospasm, frequently in combination with other inhaled agents.

Tiotropium has a longer half-life, allowing once-daily administration, and remains preferentially bound to M_1 and M_3 compared with M_2, so improving efficacy.

Methylxanthines
Examples – caffeine, theophylline

The methylxanthines are stimulant bronchodilators derived from plant alkaloids which have both a local effect on the bronchial tree and a general central stimulating effect which increases respiratory drive. They have a multimodal mechanism of action that includes:

- Phosphodiesterase inhibition
- Facilitation of β_2 action
- Enhanced Ca^{2+} release from sarcoplasmic reticulum in striated muscle
- Adenosine receptor antagonism

Inhibition of phosphodiesterase directly and via β_2 effects causes bronchodilatation similar to that of β_2-agonists. The enhanced release of calcium within the sarcoplasmic reticulum improves the function of the respiratory muscles. Methylxanthines are potent inhibitors of adenosine receptors and inhibit smooth muscle contraction by increasing cAMP and by direct interference with calcium entry.

Clinical effects
Respiratory system
Methylxanthines cause bronchodilatation, with increased anatomical dead space. They are effective against bronchospasm due to the release of histamine, platelet-activating factor and leukotrienes. The force of respiratory skeletal-muscle contraction is increased, as is respiratory rate. Respiratory work is increased with relatively less fatigue. Methylxanthines are effective prophylactically, and are also indicated for the treatment of acute attacks of bronchospasm.

Cardiovascular system
Heart rate and cardiac contractility are increased and peripheral vascular resistance is markedly reduced due to smooth muscle relaxation. This combination of effects may be helpful in the treatment of left ventricular failure.

Central nervous system
There is general stimulation, which increases respiratory rate. Although CNS excitation is relatively non-specific, both vasomotor and respiratory centres are markedly affected. Convulsions are a potential hazard.

Other effects
These include the stimulation of gastric acid and pepsin secretion, diuresis (by dilatation of afferent glomerular arterioles) and inhibition of uterine contraction.

The methylxanthines can be considered as a family of agents with theophylline as the parent compound. Although theophylline is well absorbed orally, its rapid elimination in the liver by cytochrome P_{450}, and variable protein binding of about 40%, leads to unpredictable clinical effects. Theophylline levels are measured in the plasma during chronic administration to ensure adequate therapeutic concentrations. Aminophylline, the ethylene diamine salt of theophylline, is more water soluble (but highly alkaline in solution). This improved water-solubility is required for intravenous administration.

Steroids
Examples – beclometasone, budesonide, fluticasone

Inhaled and systemic steroids may be used in the treatment and prevention of bronchospasm secondary to obstructive airways disease. Steroids act directly on intracellular receptor sites, have an anti-inflammatory action that reduces mucosal oedema and swelling, and also interfere with many mediators of airways resistance. Chemical mediators suppressed by steroid treatment include prostaglandins, thromboxanes, prostacyclin, leukotrienes, platelet-activating factor and histamine. There are multiple other effects of steroids, including reductions in inflammation, smooth muscle tone, vascular permeability and pulmonary vascular resistance, all of which are useful in the treatment of bronchospasm.

The effects of inhaled steroids can be summarised as follows:

- Inhibition of arachidonic acid metabolites
- Inhibition of inflammatory response
- Stabilisation of mast cells
- Catecholamine synergism

Although inhaled steroids are used for prophylaxis, acute attacks require systemic steroids – but their action by this route is slow in onset.

Beclometasone is an inhaled steroid given in typical doses of 100–400 μg, 2–4 times a day. Budesonide may have advantages in reaching the bronchioles in a more reliable manner, with less systemic effects.

Cromoglicate

Cromoglicate, an inhaled membrane-stabilising agent, is only effective in the **prevention** of bronchospasm. It inhibits the action of platelet-activating factor on eosinophils, mast cells and platelets, suppresses axonal reflexes caused by irritants and acts as a mild mast-cell stabiliser. This may be mediated by inhibition of calcium entry into the mast cell.

Bioavailability by the inhaled route is 10% (1% orally). Of the drug, 70% is protein-bound and it is excreted unchanged (50% in urine, 50% in bile). It has a half-life of 90 minutes, but its duration of action is several hours.

Leukotriene receptor antagonists
Examples – montelukast, zafirlukast

The release of cysteinyl leukotrienes C_4, D_4, and E_4 from eosinophils, basophils and mast cells is involved in the genesis of asthma. Leukotrienes increase mucus production, cause airway wall oedema, eosinophil migration, airway smooth muscle proliferation, bronchoconstriction and airway hyperresponsiveness. The leukotriene receptor antagonists are highly selective, and competitive. They block the effects of leukotrienes on the LT_1 receptor on bronchial smooth muscle and so antagonise the bronchoconstriction. They also reduce leukotriene production.

Montelukast and zafirlukast are indicated for the **prevention** of mild to moderate asthma as an adjunct to inhaled steroids, cromoglicate and intermittent β_2-agonists, but not in the treatment of acute attacks. Exercise-induced and aspirin-induced asthma may be particularly suitable for treatment. They are administered orally with a bioavailability of 60–80%, although with food this drops substantially. They achieve peak plasma levels at 2–3 hours. Metabolism is hepatic.

Respiratory centre stimulants
Example – doxapram

Respiratory centre stimulants act by increasing respiratory drive. As their site of action is not purely the respiratory centre, increasing doses produce the effects of generalised central nervous system stimulation such as restlessness, anxiety and convulsions. Doxapram is useful in the management of central respiratory depression either as a result of chronic lung disease or from drug therapy, but should not be used in patients with respiratory obstruction in whom the normal central drive is preserved, as this may lead to further exhaustion and precipitation of respiratory collapse.

Doxapram acts via the carotid sinus chemoreceptors (and also centrally causing stimulation of the respiratory centre) to cause increased respiratory rate and tidal volume. Clinical effects last only 5–10 minutes, and further boluses or infusion may be required for longer duration of effect. Doxapram has a higher therapeutic index than the other respiratory stimulants, and because of this it has found a limited niche in the recovery area.

Other general analeptics also cause respiratory centre stimulation, but the more generalised CNS excitation precludes their use as specific respiratory stimulants.

Mucolytics
Examples – carbocisteine, methylcysteine

Carbocisteine and methylcysteine (given orally) may be used to reduce the viscosity of sputum as an aid to expectoration. Dornase alpha is a specific mucolytic agent that is a genetically synthesised enzyme acting by cleavage of extracellular DNA. The specific use of dornase alpha is administration by inhalation in selected cystic fibrosis patients.

Surfactant
Surfactant is a physiologically occurring lipid–protein complex produced in the lung by type II alveolar cells. It lines the alveolar lung surface and has its effect by reducing surface tension, which increases pulmonary compliance. Surfactant mainly comprises dipalmitoylphosphatidylcholine. Synthetic, porcine and bovine forms of surfactant have been used to treat respiratory distress in neonates, the route of administration being by direct instillation into the lungs.

Specific pharmacology

Here, units (unless stated otherwise) are:

Volume of distribution at steady state (V_d): $l\,kg^{-1}$

Clearance (Cl): $ml\,kg^{-1}\,min^{-1}$

Terminal half-life ($t_{1/2}$): hours

Aminophylline

Structure – ethylene diamine salt of the methylxanthine theophylline

Presentation – modified release tablets 225 mg; IV clear solution 25 mg ml^{-1}

Dose

Oral – up to 300 mg three times daily

IV – cautious slow infusion 500 $\mu g\,kg^{-1}\,h^{-1}$ adjusted by serum theophylline concentrations

CNS – direct respiratory stimulant, may cause convulsions

CVS – myocardial contractility and heart rate rise, cardiac output increased; marked peripheral vasodilatation (offset slightly by vasomotor centre stimulation)

RS – bronchodilatation by β_2 action, direct respiratory centre stimulation; rise in respiratory rate

Other – general smooth muscle relaxation; renal blood flow increased

Elimination – demethylation and oxidation in the liver followed by urinary excretion

Caution – rapid IV administration may result in convulsions, tachycardia and collapse

Beclomethasone

Structure – synthetic corticosteroid

Presentation – metered inhaler, 50, 100 or 200 μg per puff

Dose – up to maximum of 800 μg daily (adult)

CNS – steroid psychosis rare but possible in high dosage

CVS – hypertension and fluid retention possible in high dosage

RS – reduction in airway sensitivity, reduction of bronchospasm; risk of *Candida albicans* infection

Other – adrenal suppression possible; osteoporosis is a risk in chronic therapy

Budesonide

Structure – synthetic corticosteroid

Presentation – metered inhaler, 50 or 200 μg per puff

Dose – 200–400 μg twice daily

CNS – steroid psychosis rare but possible in high dosage

CVS – hypertension and fluid retention possible in high dosage

RS – reduction in airway sensitivity, reduction of bronchospasm; risk of *Candida albicans* infection

Other – adrenal suppression possible; osteoporosis a risk in chronic therapy

Doxapram

Structure – monohydrated pyrrolidinone

Presentation – IV, clear colourless solution, 100 mg in 5 ml, or 2 mg ml^{-1} in 500 ml 5% dextrose

Dose – IV, 1–1.5 mg kg^{-1}, onset 30 s, peak 2 min, lasts 10 min

Pharmacokinetics

V_d	1.5
Cl	5
$t_{1/2}$	3

CNS – carotid body chemoreceptors and respiratory centre stimulation; higher doses cause restlessness, dizziness, headache, hallucinations, convulsions

CVS – stroke volume and cardiac output increased; heart rate and blood pressure may increase

RS – tidal volume increased; rate increased with higher doses or if slow; minute volume increased. CO_2 response curve shifted to left

Others – may increase urine output, salivation, and motility of GI and urinary tracts

Elimination – 95% metabolised primarily by liver, 5% unchanged in urine

Side effects – potentiates sympathomimetic amines; increased effect if on MAOI; may cause agitation and increased skeletal muscle activity when concurrent with aminophylline therapy

Caution – if respiratory failure not due to inadequate respiratory drive, will cause agitation and convulsions

Ipratropium bromide

Structure – quaternary derivative of N-isopropyl atropine

Presentation – Aerocap® 40 mg dry powder formulation, metered inhaler 20 μg per puff, nebuliser solution 250 $\mu g\,ml^{-1}$ also available; maximum effect 30 min after administration, duration 6 h

Dose – up to 40 μg three times daily

CNS – no effect

CVS – no effect

RS – bronchodilatation, occasional irritation and cough; paradoxical bronchospasm possible but rare

Other – may produce glaucoma and urinary retention (anticholinergic effects)

Salbutamol

Structure – synthetic amine

Presentation – IV, clear solution 5 mg in 5 ml, tablets 4 and 8 mg, syrup 2 mg in 5 ml, inhalation powder 200 and 400 µg, nebuliser solution 5 mg ml^{-1}

Dose – IV, 250 µg bolus; 3–20 µg min^{-1} by infusion

Pharmacokinetics

Protein binding	8–64%
V_d	2.2
Cl	6.7
$t_{1/2}$	4

CNS – may cause excitation, anxiety, tremor

CVS – β_2 effects cause vasodilatation with decreased blood pressure; higher doses cause β_1 effects with tachycardia

RS – bronchodilator for prophylactic and therapeutic use

Other – crosses placenta and may causes fetal tachycardia

Elimination – 30% unchanged in urine; the rest unchanged in faeces, small amount of conjugated form also appears in urine and faeces

Sodium cromoglicate

Origin – derivative of khellin, found in the oil of a Middle Eastern herb, *Ammi visnaga*

Presentation – metered inhaler, 5 mg per puff, Spincap® 20 mg, nebuliser solution 10 mg ml^{-1} (also available as eye drops)

Dose – up to 20 mg four times daily; duration of single dose 6 h

Pharmacokinetics

Bioavailability	10%
Protein binding	70%
$t_{1/2}$	90 min

CNS – no effect

CVS – no effect

RS – prophylactic against bronchospasm; may produce coughing and throat irritation

Other – used in food allergy and inflammatory eye conditions

Zafirlukast

Structure – a complex cyclopentyl carbamate; a leukotriene receptor antagonist

Presentation – film-coated tablet 20 mg

Dose – 20 mg twice daily, peak 3 h

Pharmacokinetics

Bioavailability	73%
Protein binding	99%
Cl	5
$t_{1/2}$	7

RS – bronchodilator by inhibition of leukotriene-mediated smooth muscle contraction

Elimination – hepatic by cytochrome P_{450}

Side effects – Churge–Strauss syndrome has been reported. Look out for eosinophilia, vasculitis, rhinitis and sinusitis

Caution – it inhibits cytochrome P_{450}, so caution should be exercised with concomitant use of warfarin, phenytoin or phenobarbital

Contraindications – moderate to severe renal or hepatic impairment

CHAPTER 14

Endocrine pharmacology

T. C. Smith

BLOOD SUGAR CONTROL
Insulin receptor
Glucose
Glucagon
Insulin
Oral hypoglycaemic agents

THYROID HORMONES AND ANTI-THYROID DRUGS
Hypothyroidism
Hyperthyroidism

ADRENOCORTICAL STEROIDS

OXYTOCIC DRUGS
Oxytocin
Ergometrine
Carboprost

RENAL HORMONES
Vasopressin and analogues
Vasopressin antagonists
Renin–angiotensin system

SPECIFIC PHARMACOLOGY
Dexamethasone
Ergometrine maleate
Hydrocortisone
Insulin (soluble)
Oxytocin

Blood sugar control

The physiological control of blood glucose is complex. While the major role belongs to insulin, a multitude of other hormonal influences apply. It should also be remembered that insulin has other actions beyond the regulation of blood glucose. Pharmacological control of blood glucose becomes necessary in situations of elevation and depression of blood glucose beyond the homeostatic limits, in other words due to hyperglycaemia or hypoglycaemia. The causes of failure in regulation of blood glucose are given in Figure EP1.

Treatment of hypoglycaemia is directed towards administration of glucose and removal of the root cause. Treatment of hyperglycaemia includes removal of the cause, administration of insulin in the acute phase and at a later stage augmentation of both the secretion and effect of endogenous insulin.

Insulin receptor

The insulin receptor is a complex of four glycoprotein subunits ($\alpha\alpha\beta\beta$) linked by disulphide bridges to form a cylinder. The α units are entirely extracellular and contain the insulin binding site. The β subunit spans the cell membrane, and the intracellular part has tyrosine kinase activity. The α subunit has a repressive effect on this activity that is removed by the conformational change resulting from insulin binding. The tyrosine kinase acts on insulin receptor substrate 1 (IRS-1), triggering a chain of action culminating in the activation of glycogen synthetase, phosphorylase kinase and glycogen phosphorylase. IRS-1 is also a substrate for insulin-like growth factor 1 (IGF-1) receptors. The binding of insulin to the α subunit changes the insulin receptor formation to form a transmembrane tunnel allowing glucose (and other molecules) to pass through the membrane. The activated β subunit autophosphorylates at six or more tyrosine residues and these phosphorylate intracellular proteins, resulting in second messenger effects on fat, protein and glycogen synthesis. Insulin has a very high affinity for the insulin receptor. This may be due to subsequent binding to the second α subunit. The interaction does not conform to the law of mass action. The insulin–receptor complex is internalised and the receptors recycled, while the insulin itself is degraded in lysosomes.

Glucose

Ideally, glucose should be administered by mouth. Its rapid absorption ensures rapid correction of limited hypoglycaemia. In more severe situations, the unconscious patient requires IV administration. Dextrose (5%) has little calorific value ($840 \, J \, l^{-1}$). The treatment of hypoglycaemia

Fundamentals of Anaesthesia, 3rd edition, ed. Tim Smith, Colin Pinnock and Ted Lin. Published by Cambridge University Press. © Cambridge University Press 2008.

Hypoglycaemia
Deficiency of glucose intake and failure of
  compensatory mechanisms
Excess insulin   insulinoma
                      iatrogenic

Hyperglycaemia
Deficiency of insulin
Decreased end organ sensitivity to insulin
Excess administration of glucose solutions

Figure EP1 Failure of glucose control

	Onset (hours)	Peak (hours)	Duration (hours)
Short-acting	0.5–1	2–4	8
Intermediate-acting	1–2	4–12	12–24
Long-acting	2–4	24–40	36

Figure EP2 Temporal characteristics of subcutaneous insulin preparations

usually requires a 20% dextrose solution (3.36 MJ l^{-1}) or alternatively a 50% solution (8.4 MJ l^{-1}). Glucose (20%) requires a large vein but can be administered peripherally, but 50% glucose should always be given via a central venous line. Both 20% and 50% solutions can cause damage to the blood vessels and are viscous. Extravasation of concentrated glucose solutions will cause local necrosis.

Glucagon
Glucagon is a polypeptide (smaller than insulin) formed in the A cells of the pancreas and also in the upper gastrointestinal tract. Glucagon has a large number of roles in the regulation of metabolism, all of which are directed to the raising of blood glucose. Although the majority of effects are physiological, glucagon has been used therapeutically in two main areas, for the rapid restoration of blood glucose in severe hypoglycaemia and in cardiogenic shock, due to its positive inotropic effect.

Insulin
Soluble (otherwise known as unmodified) insulin may be given subcutaneously or intravenously. It is short-acting and has a half-life in the circulation of 5 minutes. Subcutaneous administration results in more gradual absorption. Administration of IV insulin allows rapid control in ketoacidotic hyperglycaemia.

Long-term control of diabetes requires a variety of preparations of insulin with differing absorption characteristics for precise control. Longer-acting insulin may be obtained by the formation of insulin complexes using either zinc or protamine or both. The addition of zinc produces a crystalline insulin of intermediate action. The addition of protamine produces isophane insulin, which also has an intermediate duration of action. These insulin preparations may be mixed with soluble insulin (to make *biphasic* insulins), which will lessen temporal fluctuations in plasma insulin.

Long-acting insulin is produced by combination with both protamine and zinc (protamine zinc insulin). This preparation should not be mixed with soluble insulin because the soluble insulin will combine with any free protamine in the solution. Figure EP2 gives a guide to the time-related effects of the different categories of insulin.

Insulin may be bovine, porcine or human, the animal products being purified by crystallisation. Bovine insulin has three differences from human in its amino acid sequence, and porcine one. These foreign sequences in the insulin or in impurities may be antigenic, leading to insulin resistance and immunoreactivity. To overcome this the insulin is highly purified, but alternatively human insulin may be used. This is the preferred choice in modern therapy. Human insulin is either synthesised by bacteria or created by enzymic modification of porcine insulin.

Insulin is mainly used in the treatment of diabetes mellitus, but it may also be indicated in parenteral feeding to aid glucose utilisation.

Oral hypoglycaemic agents
Sulphonylureas
Examples – chlorpropamide, glibenclamide, gliclazide, glipizide, tolbutamide

Sulphonylurea drugs act by augmenting endogenous insulin secretion from existing B cells within the islets of Langerhans. Sulphonylureas bind to receptors on the pancreatic B cells and increase the sensitivity of the cells to glucose. The potassium permeability of B cells is reduced by blockade of the ATP-dependent potassium channel. The membrane becomes depolarised, leading to calcium influx and subsequent secretion of insulin.

In excess, sulphonylureas have the propensity to cause hypoglycaemia. Most are metabolised in the liver,

Augmented by	Phenylbutazone
	Salicylates
	Alcohol
	Monoamine oxidase inhibitors
Diminished by	Thiazides
	Corticosteroids
	Oestrogens
	Frusemide

Figure EP3 Effect of sulphonylureas

resulting in the formation of active metabolites. The sulphonylureas and metabolites are excreted in the urine. They cross the placenta and can cause hypoglycaemia in the newborn. There is competition for albumin binding sites with sulphonamides, aspirin and other highly protein-bound drugs. Factors affecting the action of the sulphonylurea family are given in Figure EP3.

Chlorpropamide is active for 1–3 days, inactivated in the liver and excreted in the urine. It has vasopressin-mimicking action on renal tubules and a disulfiram-like effect in the presence of alcohol. Glibenclamide has a duration of about 24 hours. Tolbutamide has a short half-life of about 5 hours, and may decrease thyroid iodide uptake. The third-generation sulphonylureas (such as gliclazide) have a biphasic effect and are metabolised in the liver.

Biguanides
Example – metformin

Biguanides decrease hepatic gluconeogenesis and increase insulin-mediated peripheral glucose uptake. They act by increasing the sensitivity of target tissues (skeletal muscle, adipose tissue and hepatocytes) to insulin. They have no effect on insulin secretion and do not require functioning B cells in the islets of Langerhans. Metformin also lowers low density lipoproteins (LDL) and very low density lipoproteins (VLDL) in the plasma.

Metformin does not bind to plasma protein and is excreted unchanged in the urine, with a half-life of 3 hours. All biguanides carry a risk of lactic acidosis, possibly due to inhibition of oxidative phosphorylation, and are gradually falling into disuse.

Thiazolidinediones
Examples – pioglitazone, rosiglitazone

Thiazolidinediones are new agents intended for the treatment of type 2 diabetes mellitus. Like the biguanides, they sensitise target tissues to insulin. The thiazolidinediones activate nuclear peroxisome proliferator-activated receptor γ (PPAR-γ), predominantly in adipose tissue. This increases transcription of genes in adipocyte differentiation and lipid and glucose metabolism, resulting in reduced blood glucose and a corresponding fall in insulin secretion. Thiazolidinediones increase high density lipoprotein cholesterol and may prove to reduce cardiovascular risk. They are to be used in conjunction with sulphonylureas or metformin. Disadvantages include weight gain and possible risks of hepatotoxicity.

Meglitinide analogues
Examples – nateglinide, repaglinide

Nateglinide and repaglinide belong to a class of oral hypoglycaemic agents structurally related to meglitinide (the non-sulphonylurea moiety of glibenclamide). They inhibit ATP-sensitive K^+ channels in pancreatic B cells in the presence of glucose. They bind to a receptor site distinct from that of the sulphonylureas and stimulate prandial insulin release. They act synergistically with metformin and thiazolidinediones by specifically targeting postprandial hyperglycaemia. Nateglinide is a phenylalanine derivative and repaglinide is a carbamoylmethyl benzoate.

Thyroid hormones and anti-thyroid drugs
Hypothyroidism
Deficiency of thyroid hormones is treated with replacement therapy, usually with L-thyroxine (T_4). If a rapid onset of action is required (e.g. hypothyroid coma) then tri-iodothyronine (liothyronine) is used. This is effective within a few hours and lasts up to 48 hours.

Hyperthyroidism
Excess of thyroid secretions may be treated in several ways: surgical reduction of the thyroid gland, inhibition of the peripheral actions (β-adrenoceptor antagonists) or specific targeting of thyroid hormone synthesis and secretion.

Specific anti-thyroid drugs have a variety of effects; the thioureylenes (such as carbimazole) block organification of iodine, potassium iodide inhibits secretion of thyroid hormones, and radio-iodine causes destruction of thyroid follicle cells.

Drug	Glucocorticoid	Mineralocorticoid
Hydrocortisone	1	1
Cortisone	0.8	0.8
Prednisone	4	0.25
Prednisolone	4	0.25
Methylprednisolone	5	minimal
Dexamethasone	25	minimal
Aldosterone	0.3	400
Fludrocortisone	10	300

Figure EP4 Relative potencies of the effects of corticosteroids

Thioureylenes
Examples – carbimazole, propylthiouracil

Thioureylenes may take 3–4 weeks to take effect. Their major action is the inhibition of iodination of thyroglobulin-bound tyrosine by opposing thyroperoxidases. There is also evidence of inhibition of iodinated tyrosine coupling, and suppression of antibody synthesis in Grave's disease. The thiocarbamide group is essential for the therapeutic activity of carbimazole. Carbimazole is rapidly converted to another, active, thioureylene called methimazole. A rare but serious side effect of carbimazole therapy is the development of agranulocytosis.

Iodine/iodide mixtures
These inhibit iodine substitution on the tyrosine moieties, resulting in a decreased output of thyroid hormone by the gland.

Radio-iodine
Radio-iodine (^{131}I radioisotope) emits β rays. These cause cellular destruction but are rapidly attenuated and have an effective penetration of only 2 mm. Iodine-131 also emits γ rays that enable imaging.

Adrenocortical steroids
Examples – betamethasone, cortisone, fludrocortisone, hydrocortisone, prednisolone, prednisone, triamcinolone

Hydrocortisone (cortisol) is naturally occurring whereas the other examples are synthetically derived. Cortisone has minimal activity and must be converted to hydrocortisone in the liver first. Corticosteroids are used as replacement therapy in Addison's disease and similar conditions, and in higher doses for suppression of various inflammatory processes. Steroid choice is determined in part by the relative glucocorticoid and mineralocorticoid effects. Hydrocortisone is suitable for replacement therapy and short-term use. Long-term use causes excessive fluid retention compared with alternatives such as prednisolone. The relative glucocorticoid and mineralocorticoid potencies are given in Figure EP4. The pharmacological effects of steroids are manifold, including:

- Inhibition of inflammation
- Improved transport of cellular oxygen
- Preservation of lysosome membrane integrity
- Inhibition of complement C5 activation
- Inhibition of plasminogen activator
- Negative feedback on hypothalamus, and pituitary and adrenal cortex atrophy
- Inhibition of neutrophil and macrophage recruitment
- Red cell and neutrophil counts selectively increased

Corticosteroids diffuse into cells and act on specific intracellular receptors. The complex subsequently produced then moves to the nucleus and increases synthesis of certain enzymes. Glucocorticoids are lipid-soluble and are transported in the plasma by corticosteroid-binding globulin (CBG) and albumin. CBG is relatively specific for endogenous steroids and does not bind synthetic steroids readily. Because of its low capacity, it may become saturated when therapeutic doses of steroids are used.

The therapeutic effects of steroids are primarily a feature of the glucocorticoid effects. The side effects may be caused by either glucocorticoid or mineralocorticoid components. Mineralocorticoid side effects are seen early and mimic those of hyperaldosteronism – sodium and water

Mineralocorticoid
- Sodium retention
- Potassium loss
- Water retention
- Renal calcium loss
- Hypertension

Glucocorticoid
- Muscle wasting
- Fat deposition
- Liver glycogen deposition
- Thin, friable skin
- Poor wound healing
- Reduced immunity
- Cataracts
- Raised intraocular pressure
- Osteoporosis
- Hyperglycaemia

Figure EP5 Side effects of steroids

retention, and increased renal potassium and calcium excretion. Glomerular filtration rate is increased. In the gut, there is increased calcium absorption but this is insufficient to offset the renal loss. The glucocorticoid side effects tend to be seen with chronic administration and are seen relatively late on, mimicking Cushing's syndrome. The side effects of steroid therapy are listed in Figure EP5.

Oxytocic drugs

Oxytocin

Oxytocin is an octapeptide similar to vasopressin. The pharmacological preparation is synthetic, hence the name 'syntocinon'. It binds to specific sites in the myometrium, causing uterine contraction. This is probably mediated by increases in potassium permeability which reduce the membrane potential, making it more excitable. Uterine sensitivity to oxytocin increases from minimal in the non-pregnant to maximum at term. Oxytocin also causes contraction of breast-duct smooth muscle with milk ejection.

Oxytocin causes direct vasodilatation, and a mild vasopressin-like antidiuretic effect, which may become significant if used for prolonged infusion. There is metabolism by both renal and hepatic routes.

Ergometrine

Ergometrine stimulates uterine contraction (possibly via 5-HT receptors), and also causes vascular smooth muscle contraction although the effect is slight. It has a very mild α-adrenergic blocking action. These effects are mediated via dopaminergic and 5-HT receptors. Ergometrine is a potent emetic, acting on the chemoreceptor trigger zone and vomiting centre (via D_2 receptors). After treatment with ergometrine there may occasionally be a clinical picture of hypertension with headache and blurred vision which lasts several days. Ergometrine acts within 30–60 seconds of IV administration (IM 2–4 minutes, orally 4–8 minutes), and lasts 3–6 hours. The drug is metabolised by the liver and excreted in the bile.

Carboprost

Carboprost tromethamine is a prostaglandin used in the management of severe obstetric haemorrhage secondary to uterine atony that is unresponsive to oxytocin and ergometrine. It may be administered by deep intramuscular injection. Side effects include nausea and vomiting, diarrhoea, flushing and bronchospasm. There have been very rare reports of cardiovascular collapse with prostaglandin use.

Renal hormones

Vasopressin and analogues

Vasopressin

Vasopressin (antidiuretic hormone, ADH) is an octapeptide similar to oxytocin. It may be used pharmacologically but its short half-life (10 minutes) is a disadvantage. Vasopressin acts on the vasopressin 2 (V_2) receptor to permit water reabsorption from the renal collecting duct and is a very potent direct-acting vasoconstrictor (V_{1a} receptor). Vasopressin also increases hepatic glycogenolysis, increases factor VIII activity and encourages platelet aggregation and degranulation. It is also involved in the release of ACTH-RH in the hypothalamus (V_{1b}/V_3). The vasopressin receptors are all G proteins. An IV preparation of vasopressin is available, but synthetic analogues last longer and are more useful.

Desmopressin (1-deamino-8-D-arginine vasopressin or DDAVP)

Desmopressin is used for the diagnosis and treatment of diabetes insipidus. It has an antidiuretic potency about 12 times that of vasopressin, but it has only 0.4% the vasoconstrictor activity. Desmopressin increases factor VIII activity in the same manner as vasopressin and is used to cover minor surgical procedures in mild haemophilia. It may be

Drug	$V_2 : V_{1a}$ relative potency
Conivaptan	30
Lixivaptan	100
Tolvaptan	10

Figure EP6 Relative potency of vasopressin antagonists

given by oral, IV, IM, subcutaneous or nasal administration. Desmopressin is metabolised by proteases and then excreted in the urine. It has a half-life of 75 minutes.

Other vasopressin analogues include felypressin, which has a predominantly vasoconstrictor action and is used as an adjunct for local anaesthetics in place of epinephrine, and lypressin, which is similar but shorter in duration (10 minutes).

The nasal route of administration is used for these agents. Terlipressin, a prodrug for vasopressin, is used to control bleeding from oesophageal varices. Terlipressin requires IV administration.

Vasopressin antagonists
Demeclocycline
Demeclocycline is a tetracycline derivative which opposes the effect of vasopressin. It has been used in cases of inappropriate vasopressin secretion.

Future developments
Specific vasopressin receptor antagonists (tolvaptan, conivaptan and lixivaptan) are being developed. Figure EP6 shows their relative potencies. Tolvaptan is therefore a combined V_{1a}/V_2 receptor antagonist.

These drugs have potential uses in chronic heart failure with high levels of circulating vasopressin, and in hyponatraemia when water loss can be specifically facilitated. The drugs also inhibit cytochrome $P_{450}3A4$, a potential problem with concurrent use of drugs such as clarithromycin and simvastatin.

Renin–angiotensin system
Inhibition of the renin–angiotensin system (see Section 2, Chapter 7, and Section 3, Chapter 12, pages 346 and 668–9) may be effective in the control of hypertension. Renin secretion is increased by catecholamines (β_1 effect) and reduced by β blockers. Angiotensin-converting enzyme (ACE) inhibitors inhibit the conversion of angiotensin I to angiotensin II. Angiotensin II receptor inhibiting drugs inhibit the vascular receptor for this pathway thus preventing vasoconstriction.

Specific pharmacology
Dexamethasone
Structure – glucocorticoid steroid
Presentation – IV, clear colourless solution; 8 mg dexamethasone in 2 ml
Dose – IV, 0.5–20 mg initial bolus, particularly indicated where sodium and water retention are to be avoided
CNS – may cause convulsions and increase ICP (but indicated for treatment of cerebral oedema)
CVS – minimal effect
RS – may be used for asthma and aspiration pneumonitis
Other – mineralocorticoid effects may be present to a limited extent
Elimination – liver metabolised
Side effects – as for hydrocortisone

Ergometrine maleate
Structure – ergot alkaloid
Presentation – IV/IM, colourless solution, 500 μg in 1 ml (available in combination with oxytocin; see above)
Dose – slow IV 125–250 μg; IM 500 μg
CNS – potent emetic, avoid in pre-eclampsia
CVS – direct vasoconstriction, avoid in hypertension
RS – occasional dyspnoea, chest tightness
Side effects – nausea, vomiting, vasoconstriction (potential for stroke, myocardial infarction)
Contraindications – induction of labour, first and second stages of labour; avoid in presence of cardiac or vascular disease, or porphyria

Hydrocortisone
Structure – glucocorticoid steroid
Presentation – IV/IM, white powder as sodium succinate for reconstitution with water for injection (many other preparations are available)
Dose – IV 100–500 mg 6–8 hourly, onset 2–4 h, lasts 8 h
CNS – mood changes
CVS – restores vasomotor tone of small blood vessels, reduces vascular permeability and resultant tissue swelling
RS – reduces bronchial wall swelling caused by asthma or anaphylaxis
Other – anti-inflammatory agent with multiple uses
Elimination – hepatic conversion to tetrahydrocortisone
Side effects – anaphylactoid reactions have occurred

Cautions – congestive cardiac failure, hypertension, peptic ulceration, glaucoma, epilepsy, diabetes mellitus, history of tuberculosis, effect of anticholinesterases antagonised

Insulin (soluble)

Structure – glycopeptide; formed as pro-insulin with a connecting peptide, the C fragment

Presentation – clear colourless solution of human insulin pH 6.6–8.0 (containing glycerol and m-cresol)

Dose – SC/IM/IV, typically up to 8 IU per hour, based on intermittent blood glucose monitoring; used as replacement for low endogenous insulin, may be necessary in total parenteral nutrition to facilitate glucose uptake into cells

Oxytocin

Structure – synthetic octapeptide identical to human oxytocin

Presentation – IV/IM, clear colourless solution, 5 or 10 IU in 1 ml (available in combination with ergometrine 500 μg in 1 ml, as syntometrine)

Dose – IV to augment labour by infusion of variable magnitude; following Caesarean delivery slow bolus of 5 or 10 IU

CNS – no effect

CVS – bolus administration causes transient hypotension with reflex tachycardia. Following term delivery usually offset by placental autotransfusion

RS – no effect

Other – breast duct smooth muscle contraction, promoting milk ejection

Elimination – rapid metabolism by plasma oxytocinase (use separate line if transfusing blood or plasma)

Side effects – uterine spasm or rupture, hypotension, water intoxication (secondary to the vasopressin-like effect)

References and further reading

Mitchell SLM, Hunter JM. Vasopressin and its antagonists: what are their roles in acute medical care? *Br J Anaesth* 2007; **99**: 154–8.

CHAPTER 15

Gastrointestinal pharmacology

T. C. Smith

REDUCTION OF GASTRIC ACIDITY
H_2 receptor antagonists
Proton pump inhibitors
Prostaglandins
Antacids

MUCOPROTECTIVE DRUGS
Chelates and complexes
Carbenoxolone

ANTISPASMODICS
Anticholinergics
Direct-acting smooth muscle relaxants

PROKINETIC AGENTS

LAXATIVES
Bulking agents
Faecal softeners
Osmotic laxatives
Stimulants

SPECIFIC PHARMACOLOGY
Cimetidine
Omeprazole
Ranitidine

Reduction of gastric acidity

Although gastric acidity is extremely variable, in health gastric pH may be as low as 1.0 (hydrogen ion concentration 100 mmol l^{-1}). In anaesthetic practice a pH > 3.5 (hydrogen ion concentration 300 mmol l^{-1}) is sought, to minimise the risk of acid aspiration syndrome. Many drugs may be used to reduce gastric acidity, acting in a variety of ways. The sites at which agents work are detailed in Figure GP1.

Site	Example
H_2 receptor	Ranitidine
Proton pump	Omeprazole
Prostaglandin receptor	Misoprostol
Gastric mucosa	Aluminium hydroxide

Figure GP1 The sites of action of drugs used to reduce gastric acidity

H_2 receptor antagonists

Examples – cimetidine, famotidine, nizatidine, ranitidine

Histamine has two primary effects on the gastrointestinal tract, mediated by H_1 and H_2 receptors. H_1 agonism causes contraction of gut smooth muscle, whereas H_2 agonism causes secretion of gastric acid. The H_2 antagonists typically resemble the imidazole ring end of histamine and are hydrophilic. The H_2 antagonists are competitive reversible antagonists which each feature a five-membered ring similar to the imidazole of histamine, with a specific structure as follows:

- Cimetidine – imidazole ring
- Famotidine – guanidinothiazole ring
- Nizatidine – thiazole ring
- Ranitidine – furan ring

H_2 antagonism inhibits both basal levels and stimulated release of gastric acid. Pepsin secretion is reduced in line with the decrease in gastric volume even though secretion of pepsin is mediated by acetylcholine. As pepsin is usually secreted in excess of requirements, this does not present a problem. H_2 receptors are also present in the uterus, heart, blood vessels, ductus arteriosus and the lower oesophageal sphincter. Clinically, the H_2 antagonists have little effect on these other tissues, and there are no clinical applications related to these sites.

Cimetidine

Cimetidine is an H_2 antagonist with slight anti-androgenic effect that may cause gynaecomastia and impotence. Peak effect is achieved 80 minutes after oral administration, and the terminal half-life is 2 hours. It is given twice daily,

Fundamentals of Anaesthesia, 3rd edition, ed. Tim Smith, Colin Pinnock and Ted Lin. Published by Cambridge University Press. © Cambridge University Press 2008.

is metabolised in the liver and binds to cytochrome P_{450}, causing inhibition. It also reduces hepatic blood flow. Seventy per cent of cimetidine is excreted unchanged in the urine. T lymphocytes have H_2 receptors, and blockade of these may inhibit suppressor T-cell function, resulting in enhanced immune system activity. This effect may be harmful in the presence of autoimmune conditions or after organ transplantation. H_2 receptors in the atria are responsible for atrial rhythmicity, and cimetidine may cause bradyarrhythmias, especially when given intravenously.

Famotidine
Famotidine is an H_2 antagonist that may be intravenously administered twice daily. It reduces acid and pepsin content, reduces gastric volume, and is about 50 times more potent than cimetidine. It is excreted in the urine, having a half-life of 3 hours and a duration of action of 10 hours. Cytochrome P_{450} is unaffected.

Nizatidine
Nizatidine is currently the H_2 antagonist with the shortest half-life (1.3 hours). It may be given orally or intravenously. It does not affect cytochrome P_{450}. In high doses, nizatidine may increase salicylate absorption. Nizatidine also causes non-competitive inhibition of acetylcholinesterase similar to that caused by neostigmine, and so possesses prokinetic activity too.

Ranitidine
Ranitidine is the most widely used H_2 antagonist at present. Peak effect occurs 100 minutes after oral administration and the terminal half-life is 2.5 hours. There is a substantial first-pass effect that is avoided by use of the IV preparation. It is metabolised in the liver and binds to cytochrome P_{450}, causing inhibition, but this effect is only about one-tenth that of cimetidine and thus rarely achieves clinical significance.

Proton pump inhibitors
Examples – esomeprazole, omeprazole, pantoprazole

The proton pump inhibitors directly affect the acid-secreting pump of the gastric parietal cells, and therefore bypass the muscarinic, gastrin and H_2 receptors. Proton pump inhibitors bind to the sulphydryl groups of cysteine amino acid residues in the $H^+K^+ATPase$ pump and prevent hydrogen ion passage. These agents are administered orally in buffered capsules to minimise the effects of gastric acid before arrival at the site of action. This allows slow release and gradual absorption of the dose. They are readily absorbed in the non-ionised form. Exposure to acid conditions (pH 0.8–1.0) in the gastric parietal-cell cytosol causes protonation and therefore ionisation of the drugs, and the ionised form is the active component. The active form accumulates within the parietal canaliculi near the luminal surface and binds to the target enzyme. These inhibitors are therefore very selective. The enzyme is irreversibly inhibited, and reversal of effect relies on the production of replacement $H^+K^+ATPase$. The site of action of proton pump inhibitors is shown in Figure GP2.

Omeprazole
The structure of omeprazole constitutes substituted benzimidazole and pyridine rings joined by a sulphoxide link. It is a prodrug, converted within the parietal cell to sulphenamide, the active form. It has a highly selective effect that increases over several days to a plateau, probably because the reduced gastric acid reduces its degradation and increases bioavailability. Plasma distribution half-life is only 3 minutes, but gradual absorption and accumulation in the parietal cells results in a prolonged therapeutic effect. There is minimal crossing of the blood–brain barrier but free crossing of the placenta. Omeprazole undergoes hepatic metabolism. Untoward effects are limited, although long-term use may result in hypergastrinaemia, thought to be of little consequence. Cytochrome P_{450} is inhibited, leading to a prolonged half-life of benzodiazepines and phenytoin as well as other agents sharing this elimination pathway.

Pantoprazole, a second-generation agent, is similar to omeprazole although it has higher bioavailability (75%). Gradual absorption and accumulation in the parietal cells results in a prolonged therapeutic effect. The drug is conjugated in the liver and excreted in the urine (80%) and faeces.

Prostaglandins
Example – misoprostol

Prostaglandins E_2 and I_2 (PGE_2, PGI_2) inhibit gastric acid secretion and stimulate the production of mucus and bicarbonate, and therefore have a protective effect on the gastric mucosa. Natural prostaglandins are rapidly eliminated, and synthetic analogues have therefore been developed.

Misoprostol is a synthetic prostaglandin E_2 analogue that reduces gastric acid secretion and antagonises the antiprostaglandin effects of the NSAIDs. It is most useful when these are a factor in the causation of ulcer formation, and

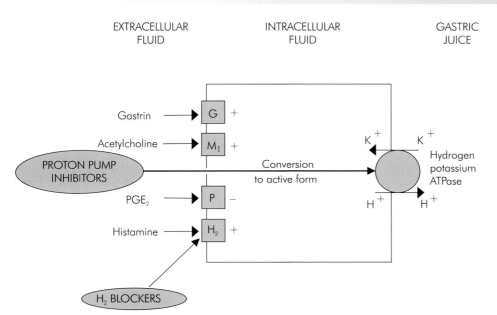

EXTRACELLULAR FLUID   INTRACELLULAR FLUID   GASTRIC JUICE

Figure GP2 Gastric parietal cell and proton pump

it can be used in conjunction with NSAIDs (to prevent further ulceration) when alternatives to NSAIDs are unacceptable. The only untoward effect of note is the occurrence of diarrhoea.

Antacids

Examples – aluminium hydroxide, sodium citrate

Antacids act in a simple chemical manner by neutralising acid in the stomach in the following manner:

$$acid + base \rightarrow salt + water$$

It is important that the by-products of this reaction are not toxic and cause minimal side effects. The commonest problem encountered is the production of CO_2 causing gastric distension with discomfort, nausea and belching. Antacids are given to alleviate symptoms of dyspepsia and reflux oesophagitis, or to neutralise acid preoperatively when a significant risk of acid aspiration exists. In the awake patient laryngeal reflexes protect the lungs from damage. In the anaesthetised patient the antacid may be aspirated and cause damage, a factor which influences antacid choice. Sodium citrate (0.3 molar) is the commonest antacid used in anaesthetic practice, because it is non-particulate.

The simplest antacids are those containing the following bases, either alone or in combination: magnesium carbonate, hydroxide or trisilicate; aluminium hydroxide or glycinate. Sodium bicarbonate may also be used. Calcium and bismuth bases are no longer in general use. Solubility and speed of reaction are important in antacids suitable for clinical use; sodium and potassium hydroxide are very soluble and are therefore very basic. These readily neutralise the acid, but any excess would render the stomach contents alkaline, causing potentially more damage than gastric acid. A solution is to use agents that either dissolve slowly or are less soluble. Magnesium carbonate has a crystalline structure that slows its reaction with the acid even though it is highly soluble, and the hydroxides of aluminium and magnesium have a low solubility but react rapidly. The problems of antacid therapy are summarised in Figure GP3.

A relatively large number of molecules is required for a chemical effect compared with receptor-based pharmacological methods. This can lead to excess salt and water

- Salt and water retention
- Alkalosis
- Belching and regurgitation
- Constipation or laxative effect
- Lung damage from aspiration

Figure GP3 Problems of antacid therapy

absorption, with predictable consequences. Sodium bicarbonate is so readily absorbed that it may cause iatrogenic non-respiratory alkalosis. Bicarbonate and carbonate compounds release CO_2 within the stomach, resulting in belching and the risk of regurgitation. Calcium compounds cause constipation, and magnesium compounds have a laxative effect. Most of the antacids are suspensions and are therefore particulate in nature. Such particles if aspirated may lead to lung damage similar to acid aspiration syndrome.

Mucoprotective drugs

Mucoprotective drugs achieve their principal effects either through cytoprotective activity or by enhancing endogenous defence mechanisms. A mechanically protective barrier against acid damage to the gastric mucosa may be formed, and some agents stimulate endogenous secretion of mucus from the gastric mucosa.

Chelates and complexes

Examples – bismuth chelate, sucralfate

Bismuth chelate

The bismuth chelate tripotassium dicitratobismuthate promotes the healing of peptic ulcers. Its mechanism of action is unclear but may be related to its binding to glycoproteins at the base of the ulcer.

Sucralfate

Sucralfate is a complex of sulphated sucrose and aluminium hydroxide that, although possessing little antacid activity, has a profound cytoprotective effect. It may be used, with caution, in critically ill patients unable to tolerate enteral feeding, to protect the gastric mucosa, and it is also used in ulcer treatment to promote healing in conjunction with acid-lowering drugs. It adheres to damaged gastric mucosa perhaps by virtue of its negatively charged component and forms a protective layer. It also stimulates the production of prostaglandins (particularly E_2), bicarbonate and mucus. Thromboxane release is inhibited, and the production of natural sulphydryl compound is increased. Sucralfate stays in the stomach for many hours, and only small amounts are absorbed. Aspiration of the drug may lead to pneumonitis, and the absorption of digoxin and warfarin is inhibited.

Carbenoxolone

Carbenoxolone is used to promote peptic ulcer healing. It is a synthetic derivative of glycyrrhisinic acid which is found in liquorice. It probably enhances mucous secretion from the gastric mucosa and so provides protection from the hydrochloric acid and pepsin in the stomach. Carbenoxolone has mineralocorticoid effects, and patients may develop sodium and water retention with hypertension, signs of fluid overload and potassium depletion.

Antispasmodics

Antispasmodic agents mostly comprise muscarinic anticholinergic drugs, but include direct-acting smooth muscle relaxants. They are used for irritable bowel syndrome and diverticular disease.

Anticholinergics

Examples – atropine, dicycloverine, hyoscine, propantheline

Muscarinic anticholinergic agents reduce acid secretion and reduce gastrointestinal tone, including lower oesophageal sphincter tone. The dose required usefully to reduce gastric acid secretion causes numerous side effects related to inhibition of other muscarinic receptors. At lower doses they function as antispasmodics and are used in irritable bowel syndrome and diverticular disease. Selectivity is improved by using quaternary amino agents that do not cross the blood–brain barrier (poldine methylsulphate and propantheline bromide) and by using anticholinergics specific for the M_1 receptor (dicyclomine, now renamed dicycloverine). The muscarinic M_1 receptors are present in parasympathetic ganglia supplying parietal gastric cells. The muscarinic receptors affecting the heart, eyes and bladder are primarily M_2 receptors.

Pirenzipine is a tricyclic antimuscarinic agent which inhibits oesophageal motility and reduces gastric volume and acidity. Pirenzipine is a relatively selective antagonist at the M_1 receptor that is found on the postganglionic fibres in the gastric mucosal plexus. In contrast, it is the M_3 receptor subtype that is located on the parietal cell. The reduction of lower oesophageal sphincter pressure caused by pirenzipine renders the drug unsuitable in anaesthetic practice (no longer available).

Direct-acting smooth muscle relaxants

Examples – alverine, mebeverine, peppermint oil

This mixed group of drugs has its effect by direct relaxation of gastric mucosal smooth muscle.

Prokinetic agents
Examples – domperidone, erythromycin, metoclopramide

Prokinetic agents are drugs used to stimulate enteral propulsion. Most are drugs known for other uses. The final common pathway seems to be via acetylcholine, but many other neurotransmitters are involved in the production of activity.

Domperidone and metoclopramide act via peripheral dopaminergic (D_2) antagonism. These are detailed in Section 3, Chapter 10 (pages 637–9).

Erythromycin is an agonist of the motilin receptor. Motilin is a powerful prokinetic acting on the G-protein-coupled motilin receptor in the mucosa. Motilin and erythromycin release nitric oxide. Erythromycin is covered in more detail in Section 3, Chapter 18 (page 711).

The H_2 antagonist nizatidine (see page 688) also has an anticholinesterase effect similar to that of neostigmine and thus has prokinetic properties.

Laxatives
Constipation may result from a variety of causes. Within the hospital population, it is commonly iatrogenic. Drugs that cause constipation are listed in Figure GP4.

- Opioids
- Phenothiazines
- MAOIs
- Antacids
- NSAIDs
- Ganglion blockers

Figure GP4 Drugs causing constipation

There are four main categories of laxative: bulking agents, faecal softeners, osmotic laxatives and stimulants.

Bulking agents
Bulking agents are usually derived from bran, and increase the bulk of stools by absorbing and retaining water. These agents are usually administered as a dietary supplement. The only minor untoward effect is that of a minor reduction in the absorption of some drugs.

Faecal softeners
Faecal softeners are oily compounds that soften the consistency of stools. Liquid paraffin is the most common agent given by mouth. It is unpleasant tasting and potentially dangerous if aspirated. There may be a minor reduction in the absorption of fat-soluble vitamins.

Osmotic laxatives
Osmotic laxatives include magnesium salts (usually sulphate), phosphates and lactulose. These agents act by drawing water into the large bowel by an osmotic effect. Their major use is in the preparation of bowel before surgery.

Stimulants
Stimulants are poorly understood drugs that can have profound effects. It is thought that mucosal permeability is increased, although other effects may be mediated via the prostaglandin system. This group includes danthron derivatives (senna), diphenylmethane derivatives (bisacodyl) and anthraquinones. Absorption may occur, and there is a risk of hepatotoxicity. Some of these agents may be abused by patients.

Specific pharmacology
Here, bioavailability applies to oral administration. Units (unless stated otherwise) are:
Volume of distribution at steady state (V_d): $l\,kg^{-1}$
Clearance (Cl): $ml\,kg^{-1}\,min^{-1}$
Terminal half-life ($t_{1/2}$): hours

Cimetidine
Structure – histamine-related imidazole ring
Presentation – tablets 200, 400, 800 mg, suspension 100 mg in 5 ml
Dose – 400 mg twice daily
Pharmacokinetics
Bioavailability	60%
Protein binding	20%
V_d	1–2
$t_{1/2}$	1–2.5
CNS – headache, dizziness, confusion
CVS – bradycardia, AV block, hypotension
RS – no effect
Other effects – gynaecomastia; impotence; thrombocytopenia; muscle pains; occasionally pancreatitis

Omeprazole
Structure – substituted benzimidazole
Presentation – tablets 10, 20, 40 mg
Dose – 20 mg daily, increasing to 40 mg daily

Pharmacokinetics

Bioavailability	35%
Protein binding	95%
pK_a	3.97
$t_{\frac{1}{2}}$	1

CNS – headache, dizziness

CVS – no effect

RS – no effect

Other effects – rash; pruritus; eosinophilia; gynaecomastia; liver dysfunction

Ranitidine

Structure – furan derivative – five-membered oxygen-containing ring with three tertiary amine groups in the side chains

Presentation – tablets 150 and 300 mg; clear aqueous solution (50 mg in 2 ml) for IV/IM use

Dose – slow IV/IM, bolus 50 mg 6–8 hourly; oral 150 mg twice daily

Pharmacokinetics

Bioavailability	50–60%
Protein binding	15
V_d	1.5
Cl	10
$t_{\frac{1}{2}}$	2

CNS – no effect

CVS – no effect

RS – no effect

Other effects – placenta is readily crossed

Interactions – the increase in gastric pH increases the non-ionised proportion of some drugs (such as benzodiazepines) and so increases their absorption

CHAPTER 16
Intravenous fluids

T. C. Smith

CRYSTALLOIDS
Water
Electrolytes
Solutions

COLLOIDS
Gelatins
Dextrans
Hydroxyethyl starch (HES)
Human albumin solutions (HAS)

HAEMOGLOBIN SOLUTIONS (EXPERIMENTAL)
Stroma-free haemoglobin (SFH)
Microencapsulated haemoglobin

SYNTHETIC OXYGEN CARRIERS
Chelating agents (experimental)
Perfluorocarbons

Intravenous fluids are characterised by being given in relatively large volumes compared with other drugs. This is in part a feature of their non-receptor mode of action, and often there are multiple functional components in the fluid administered. The uses of IV fluids are shown in Figure IV1.

Volume replacement	Total body water
	Extracellular water
	Intravascular (blood) volume
Provision of metabolic substrates	Electrolytes
	Carbohydrate
	Amino acids and protein
	Fatty acids
Manipulation of acid–base balance	Forced acid or alkaline diuresis
Coagulopathy correction	Platelets
	Clotting factors
Improving oxygen carriage	
Diluent for drugs	If caustic
	If low solubility
Osmotic effects	
Manipulation of blood viscosity	

Figure IV1 Uses of IV fluids

Crystalloids

Crystalloids are relatively small molecules that dissociate into ions and form true solutions. In clinical terms, crystalloids pass through the capillary and glomerular membranes easily, but do not readily pass through cell membranes. This situation only applies immediately after administration, as metabolism and membrane pumps soon alter the distribution. The constituents of the commonly used IV fluids are shown in Figure IV2.

Water

Water is the essential solvent of all the IV fluids. A figure of 1.5 ml kg^{-1} h^{-1} is a typical requirement for IV maintenance, which is the primary determinant of the volume given. The solutes determine how widely the water will be distributed in the body.

Electrolytes
Cations

Sodium is primarily an extracellular ion. Typical sodium requirement is 1 mmol kg^{-1} day^{-1}. In contrast, **potassium** is primarily an intracellular ion. In concentrations similar to plasma levels, potassium solutions can be given rapidly, but this will have little effect on total body potassium. Replacement of potassium by the IV route should be done slowly and requires careful monitoring when more concentrated solutions are used, to avoid cardiac arrhythmias and cardiac arrest. The addition of potassium to crystalloid solutions such as Ringer's lactate (Hartmann's) is an attempt to mimic the electrolyte composition of plasma.

Fundamentals of Anaesthesia, 3rd edition, ed. Tim Smith, Colin Pinnock and Ted Lin. Published by Cambridge University Press. © Cambridge University Press 2008.

	Na⁺	K⁺	Ca²⁺	Cl⁻	HCO₃⁻	Osmolality	pH
Sodium chloride 0.9%	150	0	0	150	0	300	5
Dextrose 5%	0	0	0	0	0	280	4
Dextrose 10%	0	0	0	0	0	560	4
Dextrose 4% saline 0.18%	30	0	0	0	30	255	4.5
Hartmann's solution	131	5	2	111	29	278	6
Sodium bicarbonate 8.4%	1000	0	0	0	1000	2000	8

Ionic concentrations in mmol l^{-1}, osmolality in mOsm l^{-1}

Figure IV2 Constituents and physicochemical properties of crystalloids

Calcium may be used to improve myocardial contractility when plasma levels are depleted. It is available as calcium chloride 10% ($CaCl_2$, which contains 0.68 mmol ml^{-1} = 680 mmol l^{-1} calcium ions). Note that using the combined atomic weight of calcium and two chlorine atoms (MW 111) does not provide the actual molarity of calcium. This is because calcium chloride (dihydrate) has two water molecules closely associated with it in the crystalline form in which it is weighed ($CaCl_2.2H_2O$). Calcium is also available as the gluconate 10% (0.22 mmol ml^{-1}). However, this preparation may be negatively inotropic, and can cause coronary vasoconstriction. Calcium may be useful when large amounts of blood and fresh frozen plasma have been rapidly transfused.

Magnesium is important in enzyme systems, and in muscle and neuronal function. Magnesium can be used therapeutically for arrhythmias (especially torsades de pointes), myocardial infarction, eclampsia and pre-eclampsia.

Anions

Chloride is the predominant anion in the body, and is a constituent to maintain the cationic/anionic balance of most IV fluids. **Bicarbonate** may be used to manipulate the pH of IV fluids. As heat sterilisation destroys the ion and thus produces CO_2, these solutions are sterilised by filtration and are relatively expensive. Phosphorus in the form of **phosphate** is the main intracellular anion. It is not routinely required in IV fluids but is important in long-term nutrition. Phosphate buffers are an important constituent of blood cell storage solutions.

Solutions

Sodium chloride 0.9% is the correct generic term for the solution isotonic with body fluids. It is also referred to as *normal saline*. 'Normal' in this sense is used to mean that it has the same tonicity as physiological fluids, and *twice normal saline* refers to sodium chloride 1.8%, which is used in cases of hyponatraemia. Unfortunately, 'normal' is an imprecise term that could also be interpreted in this case as 1 molar sodium chloride.

Hartmann's solution uses lactate (another base present in the body) in place of bicarbonate and is heat-sterilised. Lactate is readily metabolised in the liver.

Sodium bicarbonate 8.4% solution is used for the immediate correction of metabolic acidosis. Its alkalinity and high osmolality can easily cause tissue damage if small veins are used or if extravasation occurs. It contains 1000 mmol of sodium ions per litre and this carries a risk of fluid retention, which may be a particular problem if the acidosis is the result of renal failure.

Bags of IV fluid typically contain more volume than stated on the packaging. A litre bag of Hartmann's solution, for example, may contain 1050 ml. This is to offset the priming volume of the giving set, but this clearly only applies to the first bag.

Colloids

Colloids tend to be larger molecules than crystalloids, and are dispersed throughout the solvent rather than forming true solutions. The component particles tend to arrange as groups of molecules and so do not readily pass through clinical semipermeable membranes. They therefore have an oncotic potential that is usually measured as colloid osmotic pressure (COP). As the number of molecules per volume of solution is usually lower than crystalloid solutions, boiling point and freezing point are less affected for a given mass of solute. Increasing the amount of colloid has little effect on osmotic pressure so electrolytes are used to achieve iso-osmolality with blood. The constituents of common colloids are shown in Figure IV3. The frequency

	Na+	K+	Ca²⁺	Mg²⁺	Cl⁻	Osmolality	pH
Gelofusine	154	0.4	0.4	0.4	125	279	7.4
Haemaccel	145	5.1	6.25	0	145	301	7.3
Dextran 70 (dextrose 5%)	0	0	0	0	0	287	3.5–7
HAS 4.5%	100–160	<2	0	0	100–160	270–300	6.4–7.4
HAS 20%	50–120	<10	0	0	<40	135–138	6.4–7.4

Ionic concentrations in mmol l⁻¹, osmolality in mOsm l⁻¹

Figure IV3 Constituents and physicochemical properties of colloids

Solution	Frequency
Succinylated gelatin	1 : 13 000
Polygeline	1 : 2000
Dextran 70	1 : 4500
Hetastarch	1 : 16 000
Human albumin	1 : 30 000

Figure IV4 Serious adverse reactions following the use of intravenous colloids

of serious adverse reactions varies between solutions, and a comparison is given in Figure IV4.

Gelatins

These are prescribed by their proprietary names, as the generic term gelatin does not indicate the various component differences of the solutions. The two major gelatin solutions in widespread use are Gelofusine and Haemaccel.

Gelofusine® (Braun)

Gelofusine is a 4% solution of succinylated gelatin in saline in which the gelatin is prepared by hydroxylation and succinylation of bovine collagen. Other ions are present in negligible amounts because of the manufacturing process. The calcium present does not warrant line flushing before giving citrated blood.

Characteristics

- Relative viscosity 1.9
- Gel point 0 °C
- t½ 2–4 hours
- COP 35 mmHg

The majority of renal excretion occurs within 24 hours, and the incidence of severe anaphylaxis is about 1 : 13 000 (Figure IV4).

Haemaccel® (Hoechst)

Haemaccel is a 3.5% solution of polygeline in a mixed salt solution. Polygeline is a degraded and modified gelatin with 6.3 g nitrogen equivalent per litre containing traces of phosphate and sulphate. The gelatine is cross-linked with urea, which may be released after hydrolysis, a potential problem in patients with renal failure.

Characteristics

- Relative viscosity 1.7
- Gel point <3 °C
- t½ 6 hours
- COP 28 mmHg

Dextrans

The dextrans are glucose polymers that are available in several different average molecular weight preparations: Dextran 40 (average MW 40 000 daltons) and Dextran 70 (average MW 70 000 daltons). Dextran 110 is no longer available because of an unacceptable incidence of anaphylactoid reactions. Their main application is in the prevention of thromboembolism by blood volume expansion, reduction of blood viscosity and lowering of erythrocyte and platelet aggregation, although they are also used as plasma volume expanders. Dextrans are available in solution with either sodium chloride 0.9% or dextrose 5%.

Hydroxyethyl starch (HES)

These are composed of at least 90% amylopectin that is etherified with hydroxyethyl groups. The degree of etherification is indicated by the prefix, with hetastarch more etherified than pentastarch. The degree of substitution reflects the number of hydroxyethyl groups per glucose unit. The starch solutions have a large range of molecular weights. The polymerised glucose units are primarily joined by 1–4 linkages and the hydroxyethyl groups are attached to the 2 carbon of the glucose moiety, making the resultant polymer similar to glycogen.

Hetastarch

Hespan® (Geistlich) is 6% hetastarch in sodium chloride 0.9% with pH modification by sodium hydroxide. It is almost entirely derived from amylopectin. Molecules with a molecular weight below 50 000 daltons readily pass through the glomerular membrane and 40% is excreted by this route within 24 hours. The hydroxyethyl-glucose bond remains intact and usually <1% of the total dose remains in the body after 2 weeks. Hetastarch has a colloid osmotic pressure of 20 mmHg. Other starch solutions such as hexastarch and pentastarch have comparable characteristics.

Human albumin solutions (HAS)

Derived from human plasma by fractionation (the old term is plasma protein fraction), human albumin is heat-sterilised, and thus the risk of infective transmission is very low. It may be supplied as 4.5% (40–50 g l^{-1}), to reflect normal plasma, or 20% (150–250 g l^{-1}), in which water is removed together with the dissolved salts. It is sometimes called 'salt-poor albumin', as the sodium concentration is also lowered. At least 95% of the protein in HAS is albumin and this has been stabilised using sodium n-octanoate. HAS is used as a colloid especially if high albumin loss has been a problem (burns, for example). The 20% albumin solution will oncotically draw water from tissues and may be useful in the treatment of hypoalbuminaemia. A simple formula for calculating the amount of albumin needed in hypoalbuminaemia is:

$$\text{Albumin required (g)} = [\text{desired total protein (g } l^{-1})$$
$$- \text{actual total protein (g } l^{-1})]$$
$$\times \text{plasma volume(1)} \times 2$$

The use of HAS is still controversial. In addition to its colloid properties, it is involved in plasma molecular carriage, coagulation and membrane integrity. It is also a free radical scavenger. Low serum albumin is associated with poor outcome. Large volume resuscitation depletes albumin probably due to redistribution. Theoretical benefits of albumin replacement are yet to be proven in practice. At present, it is important to refrain from routine use of HAS as colloid and blind replacement, but considered use may be beneficial.

Haemoglobin solutions (experimental)

Stroma-free haemoglobin (SFH)

Stroma-free haemoglobin has shown some promise experimentally as a blood substitute. The advantages and disadvantages of SFH are outlined in Figure IV5.

Advantages
- Effective oxygen carrier
- Passes easily into smallest capillaries
- No need for cross-match
- Infection risk minimal
- Storage and transport at ambient temperature
- Long shelf life

Disadvantages
- Low P_{50}
- Poor intravascular persistence
- Nephrotoxicity
- Immunological effects
- Free radical production
- Increased nitric oxide scavenging

Figure IV5 Stroma-free haemoglobin

Oxygen affinity

The P_{50} of intracellular haemoglobin is 3.6 kPa, but this drops to 1.6 kPa when free in the plasma due to loss of 2,3-DPG from the haemoglobin molecule. This very high affinity for oxygen severely reduces its release to the tissues. In the clinical setting extra-erythrocytic haemoglobin coexists with intra-erythrocytic haemoglobin, and it has been shown that intracellular haemoglobin supplies most oxygen to the tissues until very low haematocrits (<0.2) are reached. Pyridoxylation of haemoglobin reduces the high oxygen affinity.

Intravascular persistence

Free haemoglobin dissociates to monomers and dimers with molecular weights well below the renal threshold (69 000 daltons) and is rapidly excreted. The dimer binds to haptoglobin in plasma but within 4 hours 25–40% of unmodified haemoglobin will have passed into the urine. Polymerisation of the haemoglobin produces a molecule of MW 600 000 daltons ($t_{1/2}$ 38 hours). Other methods include intramolecular cross-linking of haemoglobin, and conjugation of haemoglobin with large molecules (for example dextran).

Nephrotoxicity

Red cell lysis releases haemoglobin and stroma. Minute amounts of stroma can cause renal damage, so the haemoglobin solution must be washed thoroughly following lysis to produce stroma-free haemoglobin. Haemoglobin is not nephrotoxic, but severe hypovolaemia itself can cause clogging of the distal tubule.

Nitric oxide scavenging

This is increased by permeation of haemoglobin into the tissues. It results in vasoconstriction and possible neurotoxicity.

Microencapsulated haemoglobin

The physiological carriage of haemoglobin in erythrocytes avoids the problems of high oncotic pressure, prevents loss in the urine, and provides the most efficient microenvironment for the haemoglobin. Microencapsulated haemoglobin (non-capsule) is like an artificial red blood cell. A membrane of synthetic polymers, cross-linked protein, lipid protein, and lipid polymer is created with a solution of haemoglobin and enzyme inside. The haemoglobin cannot leak out and therefore remains as a tetramer. There is no membrane antigen. Ideally the membrane is permeable to hydrophilic material but does not allow leakage of 2,3-DPG. These artificial cells are about 1 μm in diameter (compare the red cell – diameter 7 μm), which results in rapid clearance from the circulation. A less sophisticated alternative is to use a phospholipid and sterol bilayer liposome to encapsulate the haemoglobin.

Synthetic oxygen carriers

Normally only 4% of the oxygen delivered is carried in solution (0.0225 ml O_2 100 ml^{-1} blood kPa^{-1}), the rest being carried as oxyhaemoglobin. To rely entirely on dissolved oxygen (if this could all be extracted) would require either an increased cardiac output to 13 litres per minute or an inspired oxygen pressure of 2–2.5 bar. The latter is the principle behind the treatment of carbon monoxide poisoning, but it requires hyperbaric equipment and risks oxygen toxicity. Therefore, an oxygen carrier is required that will carry oxygen more efficiently than plasma or plasma substitutes, and that will release it to the tissues. There are two options: perfluorocarbons and chelating agents.

Chelating agents (experimental)

These are synthetic compounds based on porphyrin. They can contain iron or another metal. They need modification to avoid oxidation of the ferrous ion, a function normally carried out by the globulin, after which they may be incorporated into a membrane.

Perfluorocarbons

Perfluorocarbons (PFCs) are based on a carbon skeleton with fluorine atoms, but they may also have oxygen and nitrogen atoms as part of this skeleton. PFCs absorb oxygen without having a specific binding site. This produces a linear increase in oxygen content proportional to the oxygen partial pressure. They also absorb other low-polarity gases (CO_2, carbon monoxide, nitrogen) and volatile anaesthetic agents in proportion to the individual partial pressures. Fluosol-DA is a mixture of F-decalin (FDC) and F-tripropylamine (FTPA) in a ratio of 7 FDC : 3 FTPA. The only clinical use was for distal coronary perfusion during angioplasty, because the maximum concentration possible did not carry sufficient oxygen. Sufficient oxygen transport is only achieved by hyperbaric partial pressures of oxygen. Second-generation PFCs using egg yolk lecithin emulsions allow much higher concentrations of PFC to be used, thus raising the oxygen-carrying capacity to clinically useful levels for whole-body perfusion at atmospheric pressure.

CHAPTER 17

Pharmacology of haemostasis

T. C. Smith

ANTICOAGULANTS
Oral anticoagulants
Heparins
Activated factor X inhibitor
Calcium chelating agents

FIBRINOLYTIC AGENTS
Plasminogen activators
Fibrinolytic inhibitors

ANTIPLATELET DRUGS
Aspirin
Prostacyclin

OTHER HAEMOSTATIC MODIFIERS
Viscosity
Coagulation factors
Platelet action

The ways that haemostatic processes may be altered pharmacologically are classified in Figure CP1, while Figure CP2 shows the effects of the commoner drugs on the coagulation system.

Anticoagulants

Anticoagulants are drugs that interfere with the process of fibrin plug formation, to reduce or prevent coagulation. This effect is used to reduce the risk of thrombus formation within normal vessels and vascular grafts. The injectable anticoagulants are also used to prevent coagulation in extracorporeal circuits and in blood product storage. There are two main types of anticoagulants: oral anticoagulants and injectable anticoagulants (heparins).

Oral anticoagulants

Oral anticoagulants inhibit the reduction of vitamin K. Reduced vitamin K is required as a cofactor in γ-carboxylation of the glutamate residues of the glycoprotein clotting factors II, VII, IX and X, which are synthesised in the liver. During this γ-carboxylation process, vitamin K is oxidised to vitamin K 2,3-epoxide. The oral anticoagulants prevent the reduction of this compound back to vitamin K in the liver, and they do this by virtue of their structural similarity to vitamin K. Their action depends on the depletion of these factors, which decline according to their individual half-lives (Figure CP3).

There are two groups of oral anticoagulants:
- Coumarins (warfarin and nicoumalone)
- Inandiones (phenindione)

Warfarin has the most widespread use. Phenindione is more likely to cause hypersensitivity, but is useful when there is intolerance to warfarin.

Warfarin sodium

Warfarin is administered orally as a racemic mixture. It is rapidly absorbed, reaching a peak plasma concentration within 1 hour with a bioavailability of 100%. However, a clinical effect is not apparent until the clotting factors become depleted after 12–16 hours, reaching a peak at 36–48 hours. Warfarin is 99% protein-bound (to albumin) in the plasma, resulting in a small volume of distribution. Warfarin is metabolised in the liver by oxidation (L-form) and reduction (D-form), followed by glucuronide conjugation, with a half-life of about 40 hours.

Warfarin crosses the placenta and is teratogenic during pregnancy. In the postpartum period it passes into breast milk, which is a particular problem as the gut flora responsible for producing vitamin K_2 and hepatic function in the newborn are not fully developed.

Warfarin has a low therapeutic index and is particularly prone to interactions with other drugs. Interactions increasing the effect of warfarin occur in several ways:
- Competition for protein binding sites
- Increased hepatic binding
- Inhibition of hepatic microsomal enzymes
- Reduced vitamin K synthesis
- Synergistic anti-haemostatic actions

Drugs such as NSAIDs, chloral hydrate, oral hypoglycaemic agents, diuretics and amiodarone displace warfarin from albumin binding sites, resulting in higher free plasma

Fundamentals of Anaesthesia, 3rd edition, ed. Tim Smith, Colin Pinnock and Ted Lin. Published by Cambridge University Press. © Cambridge University Press 2008.

Mechanism	Class	Examples
Coagulation (fibrin clot formation)	Procoagulants	Desmopressin
		Vitamin K
	Anticoagulants	Coumarins
		Inandiones
		Heparin
		Calcium chelating agents
Fibrinolysis	Fibrinolytic drugs	Streptokinase
		Urokinase
	Antifibrinolytics	Aprotinin
		Tranexamic acid
Platelet function	Antiplatelet drugs	Aspirin
		Prostacyclin
	Platelet enhancers	Ethamsylate

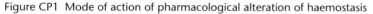

Figure CP1 Mode of action of pharmacological alteration of haemostasis

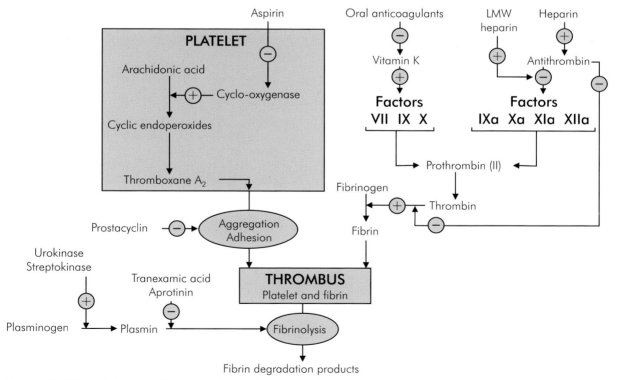

Figure CP2 Effect of drugs on the coagulation pathway

Factor	half-life (hours)
II	60
VII	6
IX	24
X	40

Figure CP3 Half-lives of vitamin-K-dependent clotting factors

levels and greater effect. This effect is made more significant because normally only 1% of warfarin is free and a small change in protein binding has a dramatic effect on free warfarin levels. D-Thyroxine increases the potency of warfarin by increasing hepatic binding. Ethanol ingestion may inhibit liver enzymes responsible for warfarin elimination. The effect of warfarin may also be increased by acute illness, low vitamin K intake and drugs such as cimetidine, aminoglycosides and paracetamol. Broad-spectrum antibiotics reduce the level of gut bacteria responsible for vitamin K_2 synthesis, and may enhance the effect of warfarin where the diet is deficient in vitamin K. Other anticoagulants, and particularly antiplatelet drugs, increase the clinical effects of warfarin.

Interactions decreasing the effect of warfarin can occur in several ways, notably:
- Induction of hepatic microsomal enzymes
- Drugs that increase levels of clotting factors
- Binding of warfarin
- Increased vitamin K intake

The effect of warfarin may be reduced by induction of hepatic enzymes by barbiturates and phenytoin. Oestrogens increase the production of vitamin-K-dependent clotting factors (II, VII, IX, X). Cholestyramine binds warfarin, reducing its effect. Carbamazepine and rifampicin reduce the effect of warfarin, but the mechanism of this effect is not clear.

Heparins

Heparins are injectable anticoagulants that act by binding to antithrombin, resulting in a profound increase in antithrombin activity.

Structure

Heparins are a group of sulphated acid glycosaminoglycans (or mucopolysaccharides) comprising alternate monosaccharide residues of N-acetylglucosamine and glucuronic acid and their derivatives. The glucuronic acid residues are mostly in the iduronic acid form and some are ester-sulphated. The N-acetylglucosamine residues may be de-acylated, N-sulphated and ester-sulphated in a random manner. This results in a chain of 45–50 sugar residues of variable composition based on the above units. The molecules are attached by the sulphated components to a protein skeleton consisting entirely of glycine and serine amino acid residues. The molecular weight of heparin ranges from 3000 to 40 000 daltons, with a mean of 12 000–15 000. Endogenous heparin is located in the lungs, in arterial walls and in mast cells as large polymers of molecular weight 750 000. It is present in the plasma at a concentration of 1.5 mg per litre.

Heparin has a strong negative charge and is a large molecule, so there is minimal absorption following oral administration. It is supplied as heparin sodium and heparin calcium.

Mechanism of action

Heparin has the following effects:
- Inhibition of coagulation by enhancing the action of antithrombin on the serine protease coagulation factors (IIa, Xa, XIIa, XIa and IXa)
- Reduced platelet aggregation
- Increased vascular permeability
- Release of lipoprotein lipases into plasma

The negatively charged heparin binds to the lysine residue in antithrombin, an α_2-globulin, which in turns increases the affinity of the arginine site of antithrombin for the serine site of thrombin (factor II). This increases the inhibitory activity of antithrombin 2300-fold. This reversible bond is the feature of a specific antithrombin binding site comprising five particular residues. This particular pentasaccharide sequence is present randomly in about one-third of the heparin molecules. For full activity of heparin on thrombin (IIa) a heparin molecule must have at least 13 extra sugar residues in addition to the pentasaccharide antithrombin binding site sequence. The covalently bonded thrombin–antithrombin complex is inactive, but once it is formed the heparin is released and the complex is rapidly destroyed by the liver. The active heparin section is then free to act on more antithrombin. Heparin acts in a similar way on the other activated serine protease coagulation factors (XIIa, Xa and IXa). The binding of heparin to both the clotting factor and antithrombin is important in the above enhancement of antithrombin. The activity of heparin on factor Xa is also mediated by increasing the affinity of antithrombin for the clotting factor, but heparin does not bind to factor Xa. Factor Xa inhibition is enhanced with lower levels of heparin than those required for thrombin inhibition. Heparin reduces platelet aggregation secondary to the reduction in thrombin (a potent platelet aggregator). The increase in plasma lipase results in an increase in free fatty acid levels.

Low molecular weight heparins
Examples – dalteparin, enoxaparin, tinzaparin

The low molecular weight (LMW) heparins are fragments of depolymerised heparin purified to contain the antithrombin-specific binding site. Therefore they all inhibit factor Xa. The molecular weight of LMW heparins ranges from 3000 to 8000, with a mean of 4000–6500. They comprise 13–22 sugar residues. The LMW heparins have a full anti-Xa activity but much reduced antithrombin activity, and require the presence of antithrombin for their effect. The reduction in interference with thrombin gives LMW heparins the following advantages:
- Minimal alteration of platelet function
- Better intraoperative haemostasis
- Possible better venous thromboembolic prophylaxis in orthopaedic practice

Administration
Heparin is administered intravenously and subcutaneously. A typical adult dose for thrombosis prophylaxis is 5000 IU subcutaneously 8–12-hourly. For full anticoagulation, as used during cardiopulmonary bypass, a dose of 3 mg kg^{-1} (300 IU kg^{-1}) is used to achieve 3–4 IU heparin ml^{-1} blood. Heparin has an immediate action within the plasma. It has a volume of distribution of 40–100 mg kg^{-1} and is bound to antithrombin, albumin, fibrinogen and proteases. Increase in acute-phase proteins (during acute illness) can significantly alter the clinical effect. Heparin also binds to platelet and endothelial protein, reducing bioavailability and effect. The drug is metabolised in the liver, kidney and reticuloendothelial system by heparinases that desulphate the mucopolysaccharide residues and hydrolyse the links between them. Heparin has a half-life of 40–90 minutes.

LMW heparins are also administered subcutaneously, and have the advantage of once-daily administration. They may be used in extracorporeal dialysis circuits, and have been used in cardiopulmonary bypass. LMW heparins are much less bound to proteins in the plasma, platelets and vascular walls, and bioavailability after subcutaneous administration is at least 90%. The levels of free LMW heparin are therefore much more predictable and require less monitoring. Peak anti-Xa activity is achieved within 3 to 4 hours after subcutaneous injection and activity has halved after 12 hours. Elimination is predominantly renal, and half-life may be raised in renal failure.

Effects on coagulation studies
Heparin increases activated partial thromboplastin time (APTT), thrombin time (TT) and activated clotting time (ACT) but does not affect bleeding time. Heparin therapy is routinely checked using the APTT and, on cardiopulmonary bypass, using ACT.

Heparin relies on the presence of antithrombin for its activity. Prolonged heparin therapy may lead to osteoporosis by an unknown mechanism.

Protamine
Protamines are a group of basic, cationic (positively charged) proteins of relatively low molecular weight. Protamine is used to neutralise the effects of heparin and LMW heparins. This occurs because the negative charge of the heparin is attracted to the positive charges of the protamine. 1 mg of protamine sulphate neutralises 1 mg (100 IU) heparin. Protamine (in excess) has anticoagulant activity, although this effect is not as powerful as that of heparin.

Activated factor X inhibitor
Example – fondaparinux

Fondaparinux is a synthetic pentasaccharide based on a sequence of sugars found in heparin that forms a highly specific binding site for antithrombin III. This binding substantially increases the anticoagulant effect of heparins and is likely to be the mechanism of action of fondaparinux. It may be of particular use when heparin-induced thrombocytopenia is a risk. It is contraindicated in the presence of bacterial endocarditis.

Calcium chelating agents
Calcium is an essential cofactor in the coagulation system. Agents that bind calcium will therefore inhibit coagulation. Citrate is used to bind calcium in stored blood to prevent its coagulation. In vivo, the citrate is metabolised by the liver, reversing this inhibition. However, massive transfusion may temporarily overload the liver's capacity to metabolise citrate, particularly if metabolic rate is reduced by the cooling effect of the transfusion or by deliberate

hypothermia, as used in cardiac surgery. To some extent this may be overcome by administering calcium ions.

Fibrinolytic agents

Fibrinolysis may be **activated** or **inhibited** pharmacologically.

Plasminogen activators

Examples – alteplase, reteplase, streptokinase

The plasminogen activators act by catalysing the conversion of plasminogen to plasmin, the enzyme responsible for the enzymatic degradation of fibrin clot. Plasminogen activators are used to destroy clots in the following situations:

- Venous thrombosis
- Pulmonary embolus
- Retinal thrombosis
- Myocardial infarction

The drugs may also remove clot formed in response to haemorrhage, so bleeding from other sites is a risk. In some cases this can be minimised by administering the activator directly to the desired site of thrombus by catheter. However, this is technically difficult and the delay in doing so may remove any benefit. Some of these agents require heparin and/or aspirin to prevent reformation of thrombus. They may reduce levels of plasminogen, α_2-antiplasmin, α_2-macroglobulin and C_1-esterase inhibitor.

Alteplase (rt-PA) is a synthetic form of tissue-type plasminogen activator (a glycoprotein). Anistreplase is a ready-combined complex of plasminogen and streptokinase that is blocked by an anisoyl group. Once in the body the anisoyl group leaves the complex, which produces plasmin and so activates fibrinolysis. Reteplase is another recombinant plasminogen activator. These three agents act on fibrin-bound plasminogen.

Streptokinase is obtained from group C **haemolytic streptococci** cultures. Streptokinase induces an immune response that produces antibodies to the drug, limiting its useful duration to 6 days. Allergy is common. Patients frequently have antibodies to protein from previous exposure to the *Streptococcus*.

Fibrinolytic inhibitors

Examples – aprotinin, tranexamic acid

The fibrinolytic inhibitors act by inhibiting the enzymatic activity of plasmin on fibrin. They are used to prevent the breakdown of fibrin clot when excessive bleeding during surgery is a risk. Uses include the reduction of blood loss during surgery in haemophiliacs, cardiac surgery and in thrombolytic overdose.

Aprotinin is a polypeptide and inhibitor of proteolytic enzymes in general, but specifically it is used for its action on plasmin and kallikrein. It has also been tried in the treatment of acute pancreatitis. Tranexamic acid inhibits the fibrinolytic activity of both plasmin and pepsin. It is useful in upper gastrointestinal haemorrhage and in surgery in haemophiliacs, and it can be administered orally or intravenously.

Antiplatelet drugs

Aspirin

Aspirin irreversibly inactivates platelet cyclo-oxygenase (COX-2) by acetylation of the terminal serine amino acid. This inhibits endoperoxide and so thromboxane (TXA_2) production within the platelets. More importantly, endothelial cells generate new cyclo-oxygenase, whereas platelets are unable to. As it is an irreversible process, the effect on an individual platelet is permanent for the 4–6-day life span of the platelet. Aspirin is not specific for platelet cyclo-oxygenase, but this is more readily inactivated than endothelial cyclo-oxygenase responsible for prostacyclin production. Aspirin should be stopped 7–10 days before surgery to allow regeneration of normally functioning platelets. It may be restarted 6 hours postoperatively. Prolonged aspirin usage may reduce circulating levels of factors II, VII, IX and X.

Other NSAIDs also inhibit COX, but are generally less potent, and the inhibition is reversible, so that the overall effect on platelet function is small.

Prostacyclin

Synthetic prostacyclin (epoprostenol) inhibits platelet aggregation and dissipates platelet aggregates. It can be used in haemodialysis, but must be given as an infusion because of a short half-life (about 3 minutes). Prostacyclin is also a potent vasodilator, so patients should be observed for hypotension, flushing and headaches.

Other haemostatic modifiers

Viscosity

Dextrans reduce the viscosity of blood and may reduce the incidence of venous thrombus formation by improving the flow characteristics of the relatively slow-flowing venous circulation.

Coagulation factors

Coagulation factors may be administered as extracts (antithrombin III and factors VIIa, VIII, IX and XIII) or as fresh frozen plasma (FFP). Vitamin K may be used to increase levels of factors II, VII and IX when there is a deficiency of vitamin K or excess of oral anticoagulant therapy. Vitamin K_2 is produced by gut bacteria. These are reduced by broad-spectrum antibiotics and are deficient in the newborn (haemorrhagic disease of the newborn). Desmopressin increases levels of Factor VIII. This may be useful to decrease surgical oozing in mild haemophilia, and in cases of massive transfusion, when clotting factors are reduced.

At present, anticoagulants either rely on a reduction in levels of clotting factors (oral anticoagulants) or on the enhancement of antithrombin. Future developments may involve the direct inhibition of specific clotting factors.

Platelet action

Ethamsylate reduces capillary bleeding, probably by correcting abnormal platelet adhesion. Ethamsylate inhibits the antiplatelet action of some NSAIDs, in addition to a weak arteriolar constricting action. It is contraindicated in porphyria.

CHAPTER 18
Antimicrobial therapy

J. Stone

Principles of antimicrobial therapy

The factors that must be assessed before choosing antimicrobial therapy are shown in Figure AB1.

After treatment has commenced, the duration of therapy must be determined and regularly reassessed, together with the need to modify the antibiotic(s) in terms of both type and dose, depending on the clinical condition of the patient and laboratory results, e.g. sensitivity tests, plasma drug levels.

Antimicrobial therapy in renal failure

Most antibiotics or their metabolites are renally excreted. Accumulation of potentially toxic compounds may therefore arise unless careful monitoring and dose adjustments are performed. Some antimicrobials are nephrotoxic while others should be avoided if there is pre-existing renal disease, and different methods of dialysis have differing abilities to clear certain compounds.

Fundamentals of Anaesthesia, 3rd edition, ed. Tim Smith, Colin Pinnock and Ted Lin. Published by Cambridge University Press. © Cambridge University Press 2008.

Patient factors
* Age
* Weight
* Renal function
* Hepatic function
* Antimicrobial allergy
* Immune deficiency or suppression
* Pregnancy
* Significant medical conditions
* Site of infection
* Severity of infection
* Prophylaxis or treatment required

Organism factors
* Virulence
* Predicted microbe population
* Predicted antimicrobial susceptibility

Drug factors
* Spectrum of antimicrobial activity
* Route of administration
* Pharmacokinetics
* Synergy or antagonism with other antimicrobial agents
* Toxicity profile
* Interactions with non-antimicrobial compounds
* Local antibiotic prescribing policies

Figure AB1 Factors influencing antimicrobial therapy

Mechanisms of action

Antimicrobials work by interfering with cellular functions. They target structures and functions specific to the target microbe or those that have an alternative metabolic pathway in human cells. These mechanisms target four groups of microbial sites:
* Cell wall
* Cell membrane
* Protein synthesis
* Nucleic acid synthesis

Cell wall synthesis

Bacteria have a cell wall to prevent swelling and lysis in hypotonic environments. The cell wall comprises N-acetyl glucosamine, acetyl muramic acid and a polypeptide, which form multiple cross-links. This maintains the three-dimensional integrity of the structure. The cell wall can range from several molecular layers thick in Gram-negative bacteria to 100 layers in the Gram-positive organisms. Antimicrobials that inhibit cell wall synthesis cause the cell to burst, and so are bactericidal. Antibacterial drugs targeting the cell wall cannot affect eukaryotic cells by this mechanism.

Cell membrane permeability

Drugs that selectively interfere with cell membrane permeability are active against bacterial and fungal cells. Selectivity is conferred by targeting components of bacterial or fungal cell membranes that are not found in the host. Negatively charged lipids are abundant in the cell membranes of Gram-negative bacteria and are the target of polymyxins such as colistin and polymyxin B. Sterols are present in both fungal and human cell membranes. Imidazoles and triazoles interfere with sterol synthesis, and toxicity occurs with higher doses. Polyenes such as amphotericin and nystatin bind to the fungal sterols and open pores in the membrane, leading to destruction of the molecular composition of the cytoplasm.

Protein synthesis

Where bacterial and human ribosomes differ, they can be targeted by antibiotics. Those agents that reversibly inhibit protein synthesis are bacteriostatic. Those that bind to the 30S subunit of the bacterial ribosome are bactericidal.

Nucleic acid synthesis

Rifampicin inhibits DNA-dependent RNA polymerase. The quinolones inhibit DNA synthesis and disrupt the final coiling of the DNA helix essential for its transcription. Nucleic acid analogues such as acyclovir attach to the active site of the enzymes of DNA synthesis and so block DNA synthesis.

Beta-lactams

This is the single largest group of antimicrobial agents presently available, and includes penicillins, cephalosporins, carbapenems and monobactams.

Mechanism of action

The β-lactam antibiotics target the penicillin-binding proteins (PBPs). These are cell-wall synthesising enzymes located in the cytoplasmic membrane. PBPs are not present in mammalian cells, which accounts for the low toxicity of these drugs. The bacterial cell wall is weakened and osmotic lysis occurs. Penicillins and cephalosporins show synergy with antibiotics acting on targets within the bacterial cell because the cell-wall changes increase the permeability of the cell to other compounds.

Acquired resistance

Bacteria exhibit resistance to β-lactams by four mechanisms:

- Enzymatic destruction of β-lactam
- Bacterial modification of PBP target (MRSA)
- Impermeability of cell membrane to β-lactams
- Active efflux (mainly Gram-negative bacteria) – the bacterium excretes the drug

Penicillins

Examples – amoxicillin, azlocillin, benzylpenicillin, flucloxacillin, mezlocillin, piperacillin

Adverse effects

These are few. Allergy is the most common problem. True anaphylaxis is rare (0.005%) but has a mortality rate of 10%. In very high doses with meningitis and renal impairment it may cause convulsions.

Benzylpenicillin
Spectrum of activity

Benzylpenicillin is active against Gram-positive bacteria, most anaerobes and certain Gram-negative cocci (*Neisseria* spp.). Most strains of *Staphylococcus aureus* produce β-lactamase and are resistant.

Pharmacokinetics

Benzylpenicillin is unstable in acid and must be given parenterally. It is distributed widely, penetrating pleural, pericardial, peritoneal and synovial spaces, but not cerebrospinal fluid in the absence of meningeal inflammation. Low levels are found in saliva. It is excreted mainly by tubular secretion in the kidney with an elimination half-life of 30 minutes. This process is blocked by probenecid. Aspirin and sulphonamides also prolong the half-life.

Amoxicillin

Amoxicillin has a relatively broad spectrum of activity. It is active against bacteria covered by benzylpenicillin and several Gram-negative species, *Haemophilus influenzae* and most fecal streptococci. Resistance is common, due to β-lactamase.

Amoxicillin is stable in gastric acid, and achieves good bioavailability after oral administration. It is otherwise very similar to benzylpenicillin. It has a half-life of 1–1.5 hours. Skin rashes are more common with amoxicillin than with benzylpenicillin.

Amoxicillin is the drug of choice for most acute lower respiratory tract infections acquired in the community, for *Neisseria gonorrhoeae* and for fecal streptococcal infections. It remains effective as prophylaxis for patients at risk of developing endocarditis.

Flucloxacillin

Flucloxacillin and related compounds (methicillin, cloxacillin) are unaffected by staphylococcal β-lactamase but have a narrower spectrum of activity than benzylpenicillin. Resistance to them is conferred by an altered target site (the PBP). These are the methicillin-resistant *Staphylococcus aureus* (MRSA) – methicillin sensitivity being the basis of the laboratory method of typing the bacterial subspecies.

Flucloxacillin is well absorbed orally but high protein binding (95%) limits its diffusion into some compartments, notably cerebrospinal fluid. It has a half-life of 45 minutes. Flucloxacillin remains the drug of choice for staphylococcal infections.

Flucloxacillin may rarely cause cholestatic jaundice and hepatitis, and it must be used with caution in patients with hepatic impairment.

Piperacillin, azlocillin and mezlocillin

These drugs are distinguished from amoxicillin mainly by their activity against *Pseudomonas aeruginosa* and related species. They are destroyed by β-lactamase.

Poor absorption necessitates parenteral administration. These drugs are sodium salts, and the high doses required to treat severe sepsis may cause sodium overload. They are mainly used for known or suspected *Pseudomonas* infections and, in combination with aminoglycosides, for the treatment of febrile neutropenic patients. Most β-lactam antibiotics exhibit antibacterial synergy when given with aminoglycosides, and there is some evidence that they may also be synergistic against Gram-negative bacteria when given with quinolones.

Clavulanic acid

Clavulanic acid is not an antibiotic but is an inhibitor of most β-lactamases. In combination with amoxicillin it improves the spectrum of activity.

Co-amoxiclav (clavulanic acid and amoxicillin combination) has been particularly successful. Pharmacokinetically the combination closely mimics that of amoxicillin alone. In addition to the side effects of amoxicillin, there is a small risk of cholestatic jaundice. Co-amoxiclav is

Group	Generation	Examples	Effect of β-lactamase	Antibacterial activity
1	1st	Cephazolin	Stable	Moderate
2	2nd	Cephalexin Cefaclor	Moderately stable	Moderate
3	2nd	Cefuroxime Cephamandole	Resistance	Moderate
4	3rd	Cefotaxime Ceftriaxone	Stable	Potent: especially Gram-negatives
5	3rd	Cefixime Cefpodoxime	Stable	Potent: especially Gram-negatives
6	3rd	Ceftazidime Cefsulodin	Stable	Potent: especially Gram-negatives and *Pseudomonas*
7	4th	Cefpirome	Stable	Enterobacteriaceae

Figure AB2 A classification of cephalosporins

used in the treatment of soft tissue infections, surgical prophylaxis, lower respiratory infections and urinary tract infections.

May rarely cause cholestatic jaundice and hepatitis and must be used with caution in patients with hepatic impairment.

Cephalosporins

Examples – cefotaxime, ceftazidime, cephalexin, cefuroxime

These compounds are based on cephalosporin C, a fermentation product of *Cephalosporium acremonium* cultivated from a Sardinian sewage outfall in 1948. They may be classified into seven groups (Figure AB2).

Cephalexin

Cephalexin is active against most Gram-positive cocci, except fecal streptococci and MRSA. It is also moderately active against some enterobacteria (including *Escherischia coli*). It has negligible activity against *Haemophilus influenzae*.

Pharmacokinetics

Cephalexin is stable to gastric acid and almost completely absorbed when given by mouth, and 10% is protein-bound. There is reasonable penetration into bone and purulent sputum. It is almost entirely excreted in the urine, with a half-life of 50 minutes.

Adverse effects

Cephalexin occasionally causes hypersensitivity, diarrhoea and abdominal discomfort, and rarely Stevens–Johnson syndrome.

Cefuroxime

Cefuroxime is more active than cephalexin against most of the Enterobacteriaceae, and has useful activity against *Haemophilus influenzae*. It is similar to cephalexin against Gram-positive cocci. It is not absorbed from the intestinal tract and is usually administered intravenously. It is well distributed, but cerebrospinal fluid levels are not sufficient to treat bacterial meningitis. It is excreted unchanged in the urine, one-half being the result of tubular secretion, with a half-life of 80 minutes.

Cefuroxime is used in the treatment of urinary, soft-tissue, bone, intra-abdominal and pulmonary infections and septicaemia. It is ineffective against fecal streptococci and most anaerobes.

Cefotaxime

Cefotaxime is similar to cefuroxime but with greater activity against many Gram-negative bacteria (e.g. coliforms and Gram-negative cocci including β-lactamase-producing strains). It is usually active against penicillin-resistant strains of *Streptococcus pneumoniae*. It has moderate activity against *Listeria monocytogenes* and limited efficacy against anaerobes. It has only slight activity against *Pseudomonas aeruginosa*.

Cefotaxime is administered intravenously. Unlike other cephalosporins, cefotaxime is metabolised in the body to desacetylcefotaxime, and both the parent compound and metabolite are renally excreted. It has an elimination half-life of 80 minutes.

Cefotaxime has a very wide range of indications, including lower respiratory infections, septicaemia, meningitis, intra-abdominal sepsis, osteomyelitis, pyelonephritis, neonatal sepsis and gonorrhoea.

Ceftazidime

Ceftazidime is similar to cefotaxime but much more active against *Pseudomonas aeruginosa*. It is less active against Gram-positive cocci than other cephalosporins.

It is 17% protein-bound. Distribution of the drug around the body is similar to cefotaxime. It is mainly excreted renally, with a half-life of 2 hours.

Carbapenems

Examples – ertapenem, imipenem, meropenem

Carbapenems are bicyclic β-lactam compounds with a carbapenem nucleus. Their mechanism of action is similar to that of other β-lactam antibiotics but they seem to have a greater affinity for penicillin-binding protein 2 (PBP-2). This results in faster bacterial death and less endotoxin release. They are extremely broad-spectrum antibiotics, because they are resistant to β-lactamase.

Pharmacokinetics

Carbapenems are administered intravenously. Excretion is predominantly by glomerular filtration. Carbapenems exhibit a phenomenon known as the *post-antibiotic effect*. This is a prolonged inhibition of bacterial growth for a period of time after the concentration of antibiotic has fallen below the accepted minimum inhibitory concentration (MIC). Therefore 6-, 8- and even 12-hourly dose regimes can be effective.

Adverse effects

Adverse effects are similar to those of other β-lactams. Neutropenia is a rare complication and is reversible on stopping the drug. Neurotoxicity appears to be more of a problem than with other β-lactam antibiotics but is primarily seen in patients with renal insufficiency and on high doses, particularly neonates and the elderly.

Imipenem

Imipenem is chemically unstable in its natural form and is supplied in crystalline form. It is highly active against virtually all Gram-positive and Gram-negative pathogenic bacteria, including anaerobes. Poor intracellular penetration of eukaryotic cells prevents its use against intracellular infections such as *Legionella*. It is rapidly bactericidal against a majority of organisms but is only bacteriostatic against fecal streptococci. MRSA is not susceptible, and *Pseudomonas aeruginosa* can rapidly develop resistance.

Pharmacokinetics

Imipenem is rapidly destroyed by dehydropeptidase 1 in renal tubules. It is administered with cilastatin, a selective competitive inhibitor of this enzyme. Cilastatin has similar pharmacokinetic properties to imipenem, and inhibition of dehydropeptidase has no apparent adverse physiological consequences.

Meropenem

Meropenem is similar to imipenem but is stable to human renal dehydropeptidase, rendering the addition of cilastatin unnecessary. It is more active than imipenem against some Gram-negatives but less active against Gram-positives. The main benefit is that it is less neurotoxic than imipenem.

Monobactams

Example – aztreonam

Monobactams only have a single β-lactam ring, while penicillins, cephalosporins and carbapenems all have two. Note that only Gram-negative aerobic bacteria are sensitive. It is highly active against most of the Enterobacteriaceae, *Haemophilus influenzae* and *Neisseria*, and has some activity against *Pseudomonas aeruginosa*.

Pharmacokinetics

Intestinal absorption is poor, so aztreonam is given by IV or IM injection. Distribution in the body is similar to other β-lactams. Elimination is renal, by a combination of glomerular filtration and tubular secretion. Aztreonam has a half-life of 2 hours.

Adverse effects

Aztreonam is similar to other β-lactams. However, as a monobactam, there appears to be very little cross-hypersensitivity with penicillins or cephalosporins. Aztreonam should still be used with caution in patients with severe penicillin allergy. Aztreonam does not seem to interfere with platelet function, unlike some cephalosporins and penicillins.

Glycopeptides
Examples – teicoplanin, vancomycin

The glycopeptides are a group of complex, high molecular weight compounds that are usually bactericidal and prevent bacterial cell wall synthesis at the substrate level. Glycopeptides are active against most Gram-positive bacteria but they do not penetrate the outer membrane of Gram-negative organisms because they are large polar molecules.

Acquired resistance
Acquired resistance is uncommon. Gene mutations occur, which alter cell-wall precursors. These precursors are called Van-A (which produces resistance to both vancomycin and teicoplanin and is inducible and present on plasmids – allowing transfer between strains), Van-B and Van-C (which produce resistance to vancomycin only and are present on bacterial chromosomes – less easy to transfer to other species). Resistance has been reported principally in various *Enterococcus* species, which have been named vancomycin resistant enterococci (VRE).

The mechanism of resistance is not clear. The presence of mucopolysaccharide slime reduces the susceptibility of coagulase-negative staphylococci. This is often present when there are microcolonies on the surfaces of joint and heart valve prostheses or on IV and peritoneal dialysis cannulae.

Vancomycin
Vancomycin is used to treat difficult Gram-positive bacterial infections including MRSA, staphylococcal or streptococcal infective endocarditis, coagulase-negative staphylococci on indwelling materials and antibiotic-associated colitis (*Clostridium difficile*).

Spectrum of activity
Vancomycin is effective against Gram-positive cocci (including MRSA), coagulase-negative staphylococci (e.g. *Staphylococcus epidermidis*), streptococci, enterococci, bacilli, corynebacteria, *Listeria monocytogenes* (moderate), Gram-positive anaerobes (*Clostridium perfringens* and other *Clostridia* spp.).

Pharmacokinetics
Vancomycin is administered intravenously, because intestinal tract absorption is poor and IM injection causes pain and necrosis. It is widely distributed, reaching most body compartments except the cerebrospinal fluid. It may also be administered into CSF shunts and into the peritoneum, and for antibiotic-associated colitis it is given orally. Vancomycin is 55% protein-bound. It is excreted, unchanged, mainly by glomerular filtration, with a half-life of 6–8 hours. Plasma monitoring is usually required only in those with renal impairment or those on prolonged high-dose regimes. It is not removed effectively by either haemodialysis or haemofiltration.

Adverse effects
Adverse effects include hypersensitivity, nephrotoxicity, ototoxicity and occasionally neutropenia. Chemical thrombophlebitis is relatively common when vancomycin is administered via a peripheral vein. Vancomycin-induced histamine release with rapid infusion produces the 'red man syndrome'. This comprises itching, flushing, angioedema, hypotension and tachycardia. Bronchospasm does not occur. It normally resolves within 1 hour of the infusion stopping. It is prevented by antihistamines. The hypotensive effect may be severe. Nephrotoxicity and ototoxicity may be related to impurities in earlier preparations, and are now rare.

Teicoplanin
Teicoplanin has slightly greater activity against some streptococci and slightly less activity against staphylococci than vancomycin. It is distributed similarly to vancomycin but is more protein-bound (>90%). The serum half-life is considerably longer (47 hours) than vancomycin, partly because of the protein binding. It may be given by rapid IV infusion or intramuscularly.

Aminoglycosides
Examples – amikacin, gentamicin, netilmycin, streptomycin, tobramycin

Aminoglycosides are naturally occurring or semisynthetic polycationic compounds with aminosugars glycosidically linked to aminocyclitols.

Mechanism of action
Aminoglycosides bind to the 30S subunit of the bacterial ribosome, causing inhibition of protein synthesis. It is not known why aminoglycosides are usually rapidly bactericidal, but other inhibitors of protein synthesis are bacteriostatic. They cause cell-membrane leakiness and consequent cell death. In general, aminoglycosides are active against *Staphylococcus aureus*, a majority of the coagulase-negative staphylococci, the Enterobacteriaceae, and most

are effective against *Pseudomonas aeruginosa* and other *Pseudomonas* spp.

Acquired resistance

There are three mechanisms of resistance to aminoglycosides:

- Altered binding site
- Reduced uptake/permeability
- Aminoglycoside-modifying enzymes

Adverse effects

Aminoglycosides are nephrotoxic and ototoxic (vestibular and auditory). Toxicity is directly related to plasma levels, which should be monitored closely, particularly with impaired renal function. Slow IV injection will minimise the risk, but toxicity is principally associated with elevated trough levels. Ototoxicity is usually irreversible, but renal function often recovers.

The ototoxicity is put to use in chemical vestibular labyrinthectomy, with gentamicin delivered to the middle ear to treat Ménière's disease.

Gentamicin

Gentamicin is active against the Enterobacteriaceae, some *Pseudomonas* spp. (e.g. *Ps. aeruginosa*) and staphylococci. It has limited activity against streptococci and *Listeria* spp. Gentamicin is used for serious Gram-negative bacterial infections. It is rapidly bactericidal and has a strong synergistic effect with β-lactams. Poor tissue penetration limits its usefulness in the treatment of deep soft-tissue infections and abscesses. Similarly, typhoid and other intracellular infections are relatively resistant. Selective decontamination of the intestine by oral administration may be useful, but may increase bacterial resistance.

Pharmacokinetics

Gentamicin is administered parenterally because oral bioavailability is low (1%), in a dose of 1–2 mg kg^{-1}, 8-hourly. Tissue and cell penetration is poor but it crosses the placenta. Excretion is renal, mainly by glomerular filtration, with an elimination half-life of 2 hours.

Amikacin

Amikacin has a similar antibacterial spectrum to gentamicin, but is less susceptible to most of the aminoglycoside-modifying enzymes. It is reserved for specific sensitive strains. It is also active against *Mycobacterium tuberculosis*

and other 'atypical' mycobacteria, including strains resistant to streptomycin. Any nephrotoxicity and ototoxicity that occurs is usually reversible.

Streptomycin

Streptomycin is particularly effective against *Mycobacterium tuberculosis*, but is also active against many Gram-negative aerobic bacteria and staphylococci. Resistance can develop as a single-step mutation that changes the structure of the ribosomal target site.

Macrolides

Examples – clarithromycin, erythromycin

Macrolides are naturally occurring antibiotics produced mainly by streptomyces. They comprise a macrocyclic lactone ring with two sugars attached, one being an amino sugar. They are grouped according to the number of atoms in the lactone ring, e.g. 14 for erythromycin and clarithromycin.

Mechanism of action

Macrolides bind to the 50S ribosome of bacteria to inhibit protein synthesis, probably by preventing the first translocation. Macrolides appear to have a therapeutic effect below their in vitro minimum inhibitory concentration. This may be achieved by inhibiting attachment and adherence by bacterial protein adhesions and by suppressing bacterial toxin and coenzyme production. Macrolides are active against most Gram-positive bacteria, Gram-negative organisms, some strains of *Haemophilus*, *Legionella*, *Campylobacter jejuni* and *Helicobacter pylori*. Some anaerobes are sensitive, including most Gram-positive streptococci and some species of *Bacteroides*.

Acquired resistance

Acquired resistance is relatively common. There are three mechanisms of resistance to macrolides:

- Altered binding site (the ribosome)
- Drug inactivation
- Active efflux of the drug from the bacterial cell

Changing the target site results in resistance to all the macrolides and also to lincosamides and streptogramins. The resistance genes can be on either the bacterial chromosome or the plasmid.

Erythromycin
Pharmacokinetics

Erythromycin is bitter, insoluble in water and inactivated by acid. The estolate and ascitrate are the most stable in gastric acid. Enteric and film-coated tablets of the base are available, but incomplete absorption occurs, with considerable inter-patient variation. Erythromycin is distributed widely throughout the body. It tends to be retained longer in liver and spleen. Very low levels are obtained in the cerebrospinal fluid, even in the presence of meningeal inflammation. The normal serum half-life is 1.4 hours, increased to 5 hours in anuric patients, so that only slight dose adjustment is required in renal failure. It accumulates with liver disease. It is eliminated primarily by hepatic inactivation and excretion in the bile, with active intestinal reabsorption. Less than 15% of active drug is excreted in the urine. It is usually given 6-hourly.

Adverse effects

Erythromycin causes gastrointestinal upset, hepatotoxicity, ototoxicity and cardiotoxicity. Erythromycin is a gastric irritant, and stimulant of intestinal motility (prokinetic). Nausea, vomiting and diarrhoea are common. Erythromycin may cause intrahepatic cholestasis, particularly during pregnancy. Ototoxicity is usually due to high-dose erythromycin lactobionate administration in patients with renal or severe liver dysfunction. Cardiotoxicity is very rare but potentially fatal. Allergic reactions are rare (<0.5%). Thrombophlebitis is a major problem with IV administration. Drug interactions include increased serum levels of prednisolone, theophylline, carbamazepine, cyclosporin, warfarin and terfenadine.

Clarithromycin, a derivative of erythromycin, has slightly greater activity and higher tissue levels. It requires only twice-daily administration.

Tetracyclines

Examples – doxycycline, minocycline, tetracycline

Mechanism of action

Tetracyclines bind to the 30S subunit of the bacterial ribosome and prevent the binding of aminoacyl-tRNA. Protein synthesis is prevented, resulting in a bacteriostatic effect. Tetracyclines have a very broad spectrum, including Gram-positive and Gram-negative bacteria, spirochaetes, some mycobacteria, mycoplasmas, *Chlamydia*, *Rickettsia*, *Coxiella* and protozoa. Minocycline even shows some activity against the fungus *Candida albicans*.

Acquired resistance

Acquired resistance is very common. This is plasmid-mediated and so is easily spread between different bacterial species, and is associated with multiple resistance genes. There are four mechanisms of resistance:
- Decreased cell entry
- Increased drug efflux
- Ribosomal protection by the formation of a cytoplasmic protein
- Chemical modification requiring nicotinamide adenine dinucleotide phosphate (NADPH) and oxygen

Tetracycline

Tetracycline is particularly active against *Vibrio cholerae*, *Aeromonas hydrophila* and *Plesiomonas shigelloides*.

Pharmacokinetics

Tetracycline is less protein-bound (24%) and less lipophilic than doxycycline and minocycline. Penetration is quite good into most body tissues, although levels in tears and saliva are low. The serum half-life is about 7 hours. Excretion is mainly renal (by glomerular filtration) and biliary. The bioavailability of tetracycline following oral administration is less than for minocycline and doxycycline and declines proportionally with increasing doses. Absorption is better in the fasting state but impaired by ferrous ions.

Adverse effects

Adverse effects include gastrointestinal (nausea, epigastric pain, vomiting and diarrhoea), superinfections, hyperpigmentation, photosensitivity, dental discolouration in children, hepatotoxicity, nephrotoxicity, haematological (leucopenia and thrombocytopenia) and benign intracranial hypertension.

Bacterial and fungal superinfections are particularly frequent with tetracycline treatment. There are four types of nephrotoxicity:
- Aggravation of pre-existing renal disease
- Association with acute fatty liver
- Interstitial nephritis
- Nephrogenic diabetes insipidus and renal failure

Weak neuromuscular blockade and potentiation of non-depolarising neuromuscular blockade is seen, and this is not reversed by calcium or anticholinesterases. Metronidazole elevates lithium and digoxin levels and interferes with the effectiveness of the contraceptive pill.

Resistance and newer, more effective antibiotics have limited the use of tetracyclines, but they remain the preferred treatment for chlamydial and rickettsial infections, Q-fever, anthrax and plague (*Yersinia pestis*).

Doxycycline

Doxycycline is semisynthetic. It is active against some tetracycline-resistant strains of *S. aureus*. It is more active than most other tetracyclines against *Streptococcus pyogenes* and *Nocardia* spp. It is strongly lipophilic, allowing widespread tissue distribution. 80–90% is protein-bound, the highest of any tetracycline. It has a long half-life of 15–25 hours. Specific uses include chlamydial infection of the eye and genital tract.

Chloramphenicol

Mechanism of action

Chloramphenicol reversibly binds to the 50S subunit of the bacterial ribosome to inhibit bacterial protein synthesis. Chloramphenicol is therefore bacteriostatic against most organisms, but at high concentrations it is bactericidal against *Haemophilus influenzae* and *Neisseria meningitidis* and some streptococci.

Chloramphenicol is a broad-spectrum antibiotic, active against most Gram-positive bacteria, anaerobic streptococci, Gram-negative bacteria, branching bacteria (*Actinomyces israeli*) and some mycobacteria.

Acquired resistance

Resistance is widespread, largely plasmid-mediated, and readily transferred between species.

Pharmacokinetics

Chloramphenicol is well absorbed from the intestinal tract, and IV and topical ophthalmic preparations are available. It is well distributed throughout the body, including the cerebrospinal fluid and the eye. The serum half-life is 1–3 hours. It is inactivated by hepatic glucuronide conjugation, then excreted by glomerular filtration with some active tubular secretion.

Adverse effects

Chloramphenicol causes the following adverse effects:
- Bone marrow suppression
- Grey baby syndrome
- Optic neuritis
- Ototoxicity

Bone marrow suppression is the most important toxic effect of chloramphenicol. There are two types: an idiopathic aplastic anaemia with pancytopenia (incidence 1 in 24 500 to 1 in 40 800) with a high mortality rate, and more commonly a dose-related and reversible marrow depression.

Grey baby syndrome results from reversible myocardial dysfunction causing circulatory collapse. This is seen in premature neonates who have very high serum levels of chloramphenicol. It has a mortality rate of 50%, but survivors recover 24–48 hours after chloramphenicol is stopped.

Chloramphenicol inhibits the activity of several liver enzymes, and concomitant administration may result in elevated levels of tolbutamide and phenytoin.

Fusidanes

Example – fusidic acid

Mechanism of action

Fusidanes are a group of naturally occurring antibiotics that inhibit bacterial cell protein synthesis. They are active against most Gram-positive bacteria (including MRSA) and Gram-negative cocci. Tolerance rapidly develops if used as monotherapy.

Pharmacokinetics

Fusidic acid is well absorbed following oral administration. Ninety-five per cent is protein-bound. It penetrates pus and wound exudates well and achieves high concentrations in brain abscess cavities, although it does not enter the cerebrospinal fluid. Levels in bone and joint are high following either IV or oral administration. It is eliminated by liver metabolism and biliary excretion, with a half-life of 9 hours. Fusidic acid is reserved for severe staphylococcal sepsis, in combination with a second anti-staphylococcal agent.

Adverse effects

Fusidic acid may cause abnormal liver function, jaundice and thrombophlebitis.

Quinolones

Examples – ciprofloxacin, ofloxacin

The quinolones are synthetic antimicrobials having a dual ring structure based on the 4-quinolone nucleus, and are closely related to nalidixic acid.

Mechanism of action

Quinolones inhibit bacterial DNA-gyrase, which promotes the supercoiling of double-stranded DNA. Quinolones are particularly potent against Gram-negative bacteria, including the Enterobacteriaceae (*E. coli*, *Klebsiella aerogenes*, *Salmonella typhimurium* etc.), *Haemophilus influenzae* and *Neisseria* spp. Quinolones are also active against *Pseudomonas aeruginosa* and related species, *Legionella pneumophila* and *Chlamydia* spp.

Acquired resistance

Acquired resistance is uncommon. Three mechanisms are known:

- Altered target site (DNA-gyrase enzyme)
- Reduced permeability of bacterial cell
- Active efflux of the quinolones from the bacterium

Reduced bacterial permeability also reduces susceptibility to β-lactams. Resistance is relatively common in *S. aureus* (including MRSA), *Pseudomonas aeruginosa* and some Enterobacteriaceae.

Ciprofloxacin

Ciprofloxacin is active against the vast majority of Gram-negative aerobic bacteria, including *Pseudomonas* and *Legionella* species. Aerobic Gram-positive bacteria and mycobacteria are generally moderately susceptible. Ciprofloxacin is active against *Chlamydia* spp., *Rickettsia* spp., *Coxiella* spp. and *Plasmodium falciparum*. There is little activity against most spirochaetes.

Pharmacokinetics

Most quinolones have a similar pharmacokinetic profile. Ciprofloxacin is readily absorbed, with a bioavailability of 80%. Tissue penetration is generally good except for cerebrospinal fluid, even with inflamed meninges. Prostatic tissue levels are approximately twice those in the plasma. Ciprofloxacin is inactivated in the liver and excreted in the urine and faeces, but 70% is excreted unchanged. There is active tubular secretion. The elimination half-life is about 4–5 hours. Eleven per cent is also excreted by direct transepithelial elimination into the intestinal tract.

Adverse effects

Adverse effects include gastrointestinal symptoms; headache, dizziness, insomnia; arthralgia, acute interstitial nephritis; leucopenia, eosinophilia, thrombocytosis and thrombocytopenia; and hypersensitivity reactions. Ciprofloxacin inhibits cytochrome P_{450}, resulting in increased serum concentrations of some drugs, including theophylline and caffeine.

Ofloxacin

Ofloxacin has a similar activity to ciprofloxacin but the longer half-life allows once-daily administration. It is mainly excreted in the urine.

Nitroimidazoles

Example – metronidazole

Mechanism of action

Nitroimidazoles are synthetic antimicrobials that act by destroying DNA. They are only active when the nitro group is in the reduced form induced by the very low redox values achieved by anaerobic bacteria and some protozoa. Nitroimidazoles are only active against anaerobes, some micro-aerophilic bacteria (*Helicobacter pylori*) and certain protozoa.

Acquired resistance

Resistance in *Helicobacter pylori* is thought to be due to the redox potential internally not being low enough. Resistance in anaerobic bacteria is very rare.

Metronidazole
Spectrum of activity

Metronidazole is active against anaerobes (*Peptococcus* spp., *Clostridium* spp., *Bacteroides* spp., fusobacteria), micro-aerophilic organisms (*Helicobacter pylori*, *Gardnerella vaginalis*), protozoa (*Entamoeba histolytica*, *Giardia intestinalis*, *Trichomonas vaginalis*) and a few helminths.

Pharmacokinetics

Oral metronidazole is rapidly absorbed, almost completely. Bioavailability is 60–80% when given rectally. Only 20% is protein-bound. It is widely distributed in body tissues, including cerebrospinal fluid, pleural fluid, breast milk, saliva, vaginal secretions, abscess cavities and the prostate. The elimination half-life is 6–10 hours, and 60–80% is excreted in the urine.

Adverse effects

The adverse effects of metronidazole include central nervous (headache, dizziness, confusion, depression, incoordination and peripheral neuropathy); gastrointestinal (nausea, vomiting, abdominal discomfort and diarrhoea); haematological (neutropenia and thrombocytopenia). It has a metallic taste, and may cause intrauterine mutation. Metronidazole gives a disulfiram-type reaction with alcohol, enhances warfarin anticoagulation, and impairs phenytoin and lithium clearance. Concomitant administration of cimetidine increases plasma metronidazole.

Rifamycins
Example – rifampicin

Mechanism of action
Rifamycins specifically inhibit bacterial DNA-dependent RNA polymerase, preventing the transcription of RNA from the DNA template. Eukaryotic RNA polymerase is unaffected. They have indications beyond anti-tuberculous therapy due to their wider spectrum of action than other anti-mycobacterial agents.

Rifamycins are particularly active against Gram-positive bacteria, Gram-negative cocci and mycobacteria. Resistance is rapid so combination therapy is essential.

Pharmacokinetics
Rifampicin is well absorbed following oral administration. Eighty per cent is protein-bound. Rifampicin is distributed throughout the body, including CSF, bone, tears, saliva, abscesses and ascitic fluid. The plasma half-life is 4 hours. Elimination is mainly by liver metabolism, producing an active metabolite. The urine turns an orange-red colour.

Adverse effects
Rifampicin is well tolerated but may cause:
- Hypersensitivity reactions
- Gastrointestinal effects
- Hepatotoxicity
- Thrombocytopenia
- Acute renal failure
- Influenza syndrome

Rifampicin induces liver microsomal enzymes, increasing the rate of metabolism of the contraceptive pill, corticosteroids, anticoagulants, digoxin, quinidine and tolbutamide.

Trimethoprim
Mechanism of action
Trimethoprim inhibits dihydrofolate reductase, the enzyme catalysing the conversion of folinic acid to folic acid. It therefore indirectly inhibits DNA synthesis.

Trimethoprim is active against many Gram-negative bacteria, including most enterobacteria, *Haemophilus influenzae* and *Bordetella*. It has moderate activity against Gram-positives, including MRSA and streptococci. *Enterococcus faecalis* can utilise preformed folinic acid and becomes relatively resistant if the patient receives supplements containing folinic acid. Anaerobes are intrinsically resistant. Trimethoprim is active against some non-bacterial pathogens.

Acquired resistance
Resistance is increasingly common. The mechanisms are:
- Modification of target enzyme
- Altered metabolic pathway
- Reduced cell-membrane permeability

Plasmid-coded synthesis of a mutant enzyme is probably the most important mechanism, and enables easy inter-species transfer.

Pharmacokinetics
Trimethoprim is almost insoluble in water, and is rapidly absorbed from the gastrointestinal tract. Forty-two per cent of the drug is protein-bound. Trimethoprim is extensively distributed in the body, and reaches cerebrospinal fluid and prostatic tissue. Excretion is almost entirely renal, with about 70% excreted in the first 24 hours. Trimethoprim is a weak base, so elimination is facilitated by acidic urine.

Adverse effects
Adverse effects are due to folate deficiency. This can be offset by giving a folate supplement, which the bacterium cannot use.

Sulphonamides
Examples – sulphadiazine, sulphadimidine

Mechanism of action
Sulphonamides inhibit folic acid synthesis (at an earlier stage than trimethoprim). Sulphonamides inhibit the incorporation of para-aminobenzoic acid (PABA) into folinic acid, and therefore indirectly inhibit DNA synthesis. Sulphonamides are broad-spectrum agents, active against Gram-positive and Gram-negative bacteria and some protozoa (*Toxoplasma gondii* and *Plasmodia*).

Acquired resistance

This is very common, with complete cross-resistance between sulphonamides. Of *Neisseria meningitidis* in the UK, 15% is resistant, and most species of Enterobacteriaceae are now resistant.

Pharmacokinetics

Sulphonamides are well absorbed from the intestine and are widely distributed around the body, including cerebrospinal fluid and the eye. Elimination is mainly by hepatic acetylation, but some oxidation and glucuronidation occurs. The parent compound and metabolites are excreted in the urine.

Adverse effects

Sulphonamides cause renal damage, rashes and bone marrow depression, and they interfere with fetal bilirubin transport. Older sulphonamides cause crystalluria. Newer sulphonamides produce a hypersensitivity reaction resulting in tubular necrosis or vasculitis. Rarely, they may cause Stevens–Johnson syndrome, which is often fatal. Sulphonamides cross the placenta, increase free plasma bilirubin and may cause kernicterus. Sulphonamides compete for plasma protein binding sites to affect oral anticoagulants and oral hypoglycaemic agents.

Antimycobacterials

Examples – ethambutol, isoniazid, pyrazinamide

These drugs are used specifically for their antimycobacterial action. Some aminoglycosides, quinolones and macrolides are also active against mycobacteria.

Ethambutol

Ethambutol inhibits the synthesis of arabinogalactan, a cell-wall polysaccharide. It is employed in combination with other agents when resistance is suspected. The most important side effect is optic neuritis, which can be irreversible.

Isoniazid

Isoniazid inhibits mycolic acid synthesis. Resistance is common but toxicity is unusual. The neurological effects can be minimised by using pyridoxine (vitamin B_6). Isoniazid forms part of all standard anti-tuberculous regimes.

Pyrazinamide

Pyrazinamide is bactericidal and resistance is uncommon. It is particularly active against intracellular bacilli. It is usually well tolerated but uric acid excretion may be inhibited, resulting in gout. It is a component of all modern short-course anti-tuberculous regimes.

Antivirals

The main mechanisms of action of antiviral agents are:

- Direct inactivation of virus prior to cell attachment and entry
- Blocking viral attachment to host cell membranes
- Blocking virus uncoating
- Preventing integration of virus into the host cell membrane
- Blocking transcription or translation into viral messenger RNA
- Interfering with glycosylation steps, viral assembly and release

Currently most compounds in clinical use are nucleoside analogues that block nucleic acid metabolism. They include the anti-herpes virus agents (e.g. acyclovir), the broad-spectrum antiviral ribavirin, and the anti-HIV agents zidovudine, stavudine and didanosine.

Two agents that are active against influenza virus are amantadine and rimantadine. They appear to prevent acidification of the virus interior, required to allow fusion of the viral envelope to the endosome, which normally leads to the release of viral RNA.

Human α-interferon is produced by recombinant DNA technology using *E. coli*. It renders cells resistant to infection by a wide range of viruses. Its main clinical use is the treatment of some cases of hepatitis B and hepatitis C.

CHAPTER 19

Clinical trials: design and evaluation

L. A. G. Vries

TYPES OF TRIAL
Phased clinical trials
Crossover studies
Multi-centre trials
Meta-analysis

DESIGN OF A TRIAL
Sample size
Variability
Bias

IMPLEMENTATION OF TRIAL DESIGN
Ethics committee approval
Data collection
Data analysis
Presentation of results

A clinical trial is a study of the efficacy and value of treatments or interventions, and most such trials involve comparing the treatment or intervention under investigation to a control group.

This should be a prospective process (as opposed to a retrospective one), in which participants or subjects are identified at the start of the process and followed forward in time. Investigators implement carefully defined interventions. Data are then gathered, evaluated and analysed and the results may be published. Interventions may include treatments, screening programmes, preventative measures and diagnostic tests.

Types of trial

Phased clinical trials

Phase I trials

In phase I trials, new treatments are administered to small groups of people. Often, useful information on safety and efficacy has been obtained from animal studies before the phase I trial. People who participate in phase I trials are often those who have failed to improve on existing, conventional therapies, or they may be healthy volunteers. One of the main purposes of this type of trial is to ascertain what the maximum safe dose of the study drug is and how it is metabolised. This maximum dose is usually referred to as the maximum tolerated dose (MTD).

Phase II trials

After the safety and maximum tolerated dose have been established, the investigators may proceed to a phase II trial. Typically, small groups of patients are started on different doses and frequencies of administration. Neither a phase I or a phase II trial is randomised. Patients may for example be given a new treatment for a certain type of cancer. If fewer people than expected die of their illness in the treatment group, and side effects or toxic effects are tolerable, then the investigators may proceed to a phase III trial. The results obtained in a phase II trial will be used to design the more comparative phase III trial.

Phase III trials

Phase III trials use the optimum treatment dose and regimen determined by the phase I and II trials to set up a randomised controlled trial (RCT). The main aim of the phase III trial is to determine the effectiveness of the new intervention. In an RCT there is a control group receiving standard treatment, a placebo, or no treatment at all, and one or more treatment groups receiving the intervention(s) of interest. Randomisation means that all participants have the same likelihood of ending up in any of the groups.

Following phase III a drug licence may be granted. The licence is time-limited, and additionally new drugs are kept under heightened surveillance using the yellow card system as denoted by a black triangle in the BNF.

Phase IV trials

Often the effectiveness referred to in phase III trials is only measured over the short term. Phase IV trials are designed to monitor the long-term safety and efficacy of

Fundamentals of Anaesthesia, 3rd edition, ed. Tim Smith, Colin Pinnock and Ted Lin. Published by Cambridge University Press. © Cambridge University Press 2008.

the new intervention. They are also called post-marketing surveillance studies and need not contain a control group.

Crossover studies

Crossover studies are the opposite of parallel design studies, because in the crossover model each participant will receive each of the study interventions. In effect, each participant acts as his/her own control. The main advantage of this type of controlled study is the ability to determine whether a particular patient does better on a specific treatment. The simplest crossover study design contains two periods during which the subject receives two different treatments. It is crucially important that the interventions are of rapid onset and short duration. If not, then the effect of the treatment in period A may interfere with the effect of the treatment in period B. For example, if a particular disease is cured during period A, then clearly the patient will not enter period B in the same pretreatment state as in period A. It follows that chronic, incurable conditions are better suited to a crossover study.

Multi-centre trials

The multi-centre trial has gained recent popularity because it increases the power of the study by recruiting larger patient numbers. The multi-centre effort is used when a single centre cannot provide sufficient patients. The cost of a multi-centre trial is invariably higher than that of a single-centre type, and it takes a lot more organisational effort. A universal study protocol must be devised and followed by all participants. Inter-centre differences in patient management may be difficult to eliminate, as variations in working practices in the contributing sites may not be apparent to the investigators immediately and may be difficult to alter.

The need to perform a multi-centre trial arises when the variable in question occurs infrequently. For example, a study is set up to compare the incidence of neurological damage after a spinal anaesthetic with two different types of spinal needle. A large number of patients will be required to show whether or not there are any statistically significant differences because the incidence of these complications very low. An alternative to a multi-centre trial in this case would be a meta-analysis.

Meta-analysis

A meta-analysis is a statistical combination of a number of independent trials, usually expressed with confidence intervals. These pooled data summarise the effect of the intervention. The main aim of a meta-analysis is to maximise the statistical precision of the effect of a particular intervention.

Suppose a researcher wants to review all the published data on the mortality rate of patients in intensive care units who have been treated with drug A. The usual format would be to express all the studies in terms of odds ratios with 95% confidence intervals (see Section 4, Chapter 4, page 881).

A meta-analysis combines many studies, some of which may lack statistical significance on their own, to generate a larger sample that may in totality answer the research question. The potential problems of combining individual studies, with vast differences in outcomes and outcome measures, must not be underestimated. Other limitations of meta-analyses result from the potential for bias from various sources. Investigators may choose to include or exclude certain trials, and reviewers and editors, both of the source journals and those assessing the meta-analysis, may be more inclined to accept studies showing positive findings, as the criticism of Type II error is less likely (publication bias). Also, meta-analyses use statistical techniques that are still poorly understood by reviewers and readers. At times, a meta-analysis is wrongly seen as a substitute for a large, well-conducted, randomised controlled trial.

Design of a trial

As can be seen from the above, there are a variety of study designs available to investigate the efficacy of a medical intervention or treatment. The strength of the evidence depends on the chosen design, and varies from anecdotal evidence to a randomised, controlled, double-blind trial. It is of pivotal importance that a trial starts with a clearly defined question and an outlined means of assessing the outcome, including statistical methods. Issues which should be addressed from the outset when designing a trial will now be considered further.

Sample size

A power analysis is used to maximise the chance of finding a statistical difference between groups, where a real difference exists. This calculation of the required number of subjects should take place early on in the planning of the trial. The difficulty with this calculation is that it is often based on pilot studies or previous studies with very small numbers. Estimates derived from these small studies are frequently too optimistic. This is often due to the fact that these initial studies are not randomised and have a huge potential for bias. In deriving the required number

Type of bias	Description
Selection bias	Systematic difference in acceptance or rejection for inclusion in trial
	Systematic difference in assignment of treatment
Ascertainment bias	Patient or investigator knows which treatment is administered
Publication bias	Tendency to submit and publish trials with positive findings
Dropout/withdrawal bias	Dropout may be more frequent in one treatment group
Protocol violation bias	Failure to follow protocol (for example on missing data)
Inappropriate crossover design bias	Curable or lethal conditions are inappropriate
Time-lag bias	Studies with positive findings are published much quicker
Potential breakthrough bias	Overemphasis of a positive finding whilst ignoring a previous negative finding

Figure CT1 Examples of bias in clinical trials

of patients, the measured change must also be of **clinical** significance.

The power of a study is the likelihood of the null hypothesis being rejected correctly. This is given as 1 minus β, where β is the type II error, or false negatives. A power of 0.8 or above is generally acceptable, as this equates to an 80% chance of showing a statistical difference, where such a difference truly exists.

Variability

Variability in the interpretation of the outcome measures can reduce the chance of finding a statistically significant difference. Such variability may arise from instrument precision, observer variability, or a combination of the two. Both intra-observer and inter-observer variability are well-recognised sources of error. Ways of reducing variability include the introduction of technology (for example automated rather than manual blood pressure measurement), and repeated and blinded assessments. Repeated assessments take a pooled value for the variable, and this may be a better reflection of the required variable.

Bias
Bias types

The main strength of a randomised controlled trial depends heavily on its potential to minimise selection bias. With the correct application of the appropriate techniques, the study groups can be kept as similar as possible from the outset of the study. This will enable the investigators to establish more reliably the true effect of the intervention studied. Despite attention to detail, the groups sometimes become different during the conduct

of the trial and bias arises. Bias may arise from several sources, not all of them due to the investigators' instigation. Investigators may inadvertently favour particular observations or changes, or they may deliberately introduce bias. One source of inadvertent bias is the ongoing analysis of cumulative data, which may lead to the study terminating once a 'statistically significant' result has been found. Figure CT1 summarises the most common types of bias.

Randomisation

The purpose of randomisation is to ensure that every participant in the study has the same chance of ending up in any of the treatment groups. A logical consequence of this will be that each group will contain subjects with similar characteristics. Simple as it may sound, randomisation is not always easy to achieve. Allocating patients on the basis of year of birth (odd or even), hospital number, day of admission or by alternating allocation to each group leads to imbalance or bias. Acceptable methods include the use of computer-generated random numbers, flipping a coin or rolling dice.

Despite the use of these randomisation methods, groups may become vastly different at some point during the study. There are basically two types of randomisation techniques available to try and minimise these differences:

- The number of patients in each group can be kept as close together as possible by the process of *block* or *restricted randomisation*. The total number of patients to be studied is divided into blocks of equal numbers. In each block the same number of patients will be allocated to each group.

- To minimise the differences in age, sex and other characteristics, *stratified randomisation* may be used. Block randomisation is used for each variable, thus ensuring equal distribution of these characteristics across all groups.

Blinding

Bias frequently results from either the patient or the investigator(s) knowing which type of treatment is being administered. To minimise this potential for distortion, the investigator and the patient should be unaware of the type of treatment assigned. In a single-blind trial, the investigators are aware which group the patient is allocated to. A clinical trial should ideally have a double-blind design, in which neither the patient nor the investigator is aware of the treatment identity.

Although the term double-blind is frequently used in medical literature, it is likely that many such studies are not completely double-blinded. For example, a drug which is being investigated may have a clear therapeutic or side effect. The investigator and even the patient may recognise these effects, and this is then a source of (ascertainment) bias.

Implementation of trial design

Ethics committee approval

The most important function of a local ethics committee is to protect the potential subjects of medical research. They should also ensure that valuable resources are not wasted on research that is unlikely to answer the proposed question. In the United Kingdom, these committees are set up either at county level, or even at hospital trust level, particularly at teaching trusts. Most ethics committees have lay members on them, to represent the views of the public.

Before the recruitment of patients may begin, approval of the local ethics committee should be obtained. A detailed explanation of the proposed study must be enclosed, including a review of previously published papers. The reason for undertaking the study must be explained and potential advantages to medical science or practice demonstrated. A patient information leaflet explaining the purpose of the study and a consent form, which is to be signed by the patient and the investigator, are also necessary before ethics committee approval can be obtained.

Data collection

The data to be collected in a clinical trial may come from various sources. For example, these could be questionnaires, laboratory results, patient interviews or pain scores. To minimise the potential for bias, the method of data collection and interpretation should be determined when the study protocol is drawn up.

Problems in data collection can occur because of incorrect data, missing data or problems arising as a result of variability. Incorrect or missing data is usually linked to human error or the inability to collect all the necessary information. As discussed before, inter- and intra-observer variability can be responsible for failing to detect a real statistical difference.

There are several ways to minimise the potential errors in data collection. Firstly, there should be clear guidelines regarding the variables to be measured. Ideally, the investigators should produce a manual for reference. The data collectors should have adequately detailed knowledge of the study protocol. Secondly, the data collectors should have forms with a brief synopsis of the guidelines on them, to refer to as necessary. Closed questions with yes or no answers or tick-boxes are preferable to open-style essay questions. Thirdly, the people collecting the data should have had sufficient training in the process of data collection. Whenever possible, a test period should precede the start of the clinical trial to highlight any potential pitfalls or flaws in the protocol.

Machines and monitors used in a clinical trial should be checked and calibrated regularly according to the manufacturers' instructions.

Data analysis

As with the collection of data, it is crucially important to determine the analysis technique to be used when the protocol is being drawn up. The statistical tests that will be employed should be appropriate for the type of data. Subsequent exclusion of a number of randomised patients from a clinical trial is a problem that is often difficult to prevent. Patients may have to be excluded from analysis for a variety of reasons. They may develop complications or morbidity that precludes them from further participation in the study. Non-compliance of the patient may lead to exclusion from the trial. The problem of missing or incomplete data can be particularly difficult to prevent. It is essential that the number of patients excluded from the study be mentioned in the publication, as well as the reason for elimination.

Presentation of results

The results obtained from a trial may be discussed at a local level, presented at national or international meetings or published in scientific journals. The investigators must review their data critically and truthfully, and when submitting material to journals, adhere to the guidelines for manuscripts. It is obvious that the article must be submitted to an appropriate journal. The manuscript should provide a detailed account of the methods employed in the trial, so readers can assess the validity of the procedures, including the statistical methods that were used. The authorship of the publication is an important issue. An author is someone who has been involved in the design, the implementation, the data analysis and the drawing of conclusions from that study. The manuscript should include a comparison with other articles published on the same or similar subject, with references supplied. Finally, the clinical implications of the results must be discussed. It may be that the outcome of the trial raises more questions than it has answered. In this case, suggestions for further research could be given. If appropriate, the social and financial implications must be discussed, and whether the patients and circumstances in the trial are in any way comparable and suitable to the general population.

CHAPTER 1

Applied physics

E. S. Lin

Some useful mathematics

Functions

Functions help us to understand how physical materials and systems behave, and to predict what will happen when conditions change. When two variables (x and y) are related, changes in one variable produce a change in the other: e.g. increasing the stretching force to a spring produces an extension in length. A mathematical function expresses this relationship as

$$y = f(x)$$

This means that y is a function of x. Here x is called the independent variable and y is the dependent variable. Functions can be visualised as a graph by plotting x and y on two axes.

Fundamentals of Anaesthesia, 3rd edition, ed. Tim Smith, Colin Pinnock and Ted Lin. Published by Cambridge University Press. © Cambridge University Press 2008.

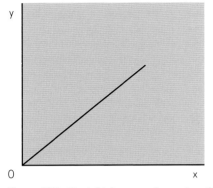

Figure PH1 Straight-line graph passing through origin

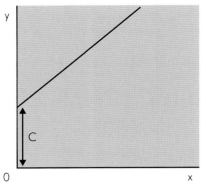

Figure PH2 Straight-line graph with intercept

By convention x, the independent variable, is plotted on the horizontal axis and y, the dependent variable, on the vertical axis.

Linear functions and proportionality
If two variables, x and y, are proportional to each other, fractional changes in x will produce similar changes in the value of y. Thus if x is doubled, y will be doubled, and if x is halved the value of y is also halved. This relationship can be written as the function

$$y = Mx$$

where M is a constant. An example of such a relationship exists when a spring is stretched, where $x =$ the **stretching force** applied to the spring, and $y =$ the **extension** produced. In this case the graph of y against x is a straight line passing through the origin. The gradient or slope of the line is M (Figure PH1).

If we now consider the effect of the force (x) on the **length** (y) of the spring, then the graph of y against x is different. It is still a straight line with a gradient $= M$, but it no longer passes through the origin. It now passes through a point $y = C$, where C is the original length of the spring (Figure PH2). The relationship between y and x then becomes:

$$y = Mx + C$$

C is known as the intercept. Any straight-line graph will be represented by the above function. A function of this form is said to be linear. Other examples of linear functions are:
- The variation of voltage with current in an electrical resistor
- The increase in length of a metal rod with temperature

Relationships between physiological variables are generally non-linear, but some can be approximated to linear functions over limited ranges: e.g. pressure–volume curve for the lung.

Non-linear functions
When the graph of a function does not take the form of a straight line, the function is said to be non-linear. Often non-linear functions contain multiple terms which are higher powers of x (i.e. x^2, x^3 etc). These are called polynomials. A polynomial in which the highest power term is x^2 is called a quadratic function, and has a graph in the shape of a parabola. The simplest quadratic function is

$$y = Ax^2 \text{ (Figure PH3)}$$

A general quadratic function is

$$y = Ax^2 + Bx + C \text{ (Figure PH4)}$$

Quadratic functions commonly occur when considering energy stored or dissipated in a system, for example:
- The energy stored in a stretched spring is proportional to the square of the displacement.
- The energy stored in a gas compressed by a piston is proportional to the square of the displacement of the piston.
- The energy dissipated in a linear electrical circuit is proportional to the square of the applied voltage.

Logarithms and logarithmic curves
Another type of non-linear function occurring in biological systems is the logarithmic function. Logarithms are a method of expressing numbers as a power of a chosen number, or base.

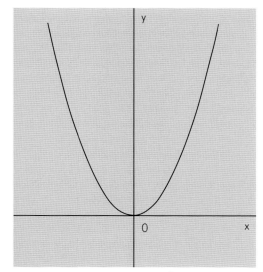

Figure PH3 Parabola for $y = Ax^2$

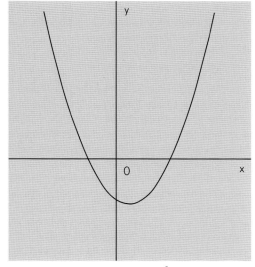

Figure PH4 Parabola for $y = Ax^2 + Bx + C$

For example if a base equal to 2 is chosen, then any number can be expressed as a logarithm to the base 2 as follows:

Express the number 8 as a logarithm to the base 2.

$8 = 2^3$

therefore

$\log_2 8 = 3$

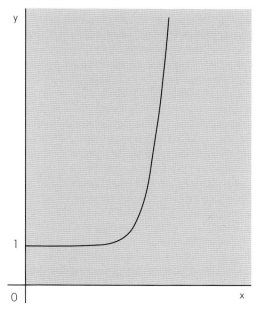

Figure PH5 Graph for $y = e^x$

Express the number 100 as a logarithm to the base 10

$$100 = 10^2$$
$$\log_{10} 100 = 2$$

Common logarithms are calculated to the base 10. **Natural** logarithms are calculated to the base e, where e is a constant equal to 2.718281. Thus if the natural logarithm of a number y is equal to x, this can be written as:

$y = e^x$

or

$\log_e y = x$

(Natural logarithms can also be denoted as ln y.)

If a graph of $y = e^x$ is plotted, the result is a non-linear curve which rises rapidly at an increasing rate, and in which the gradient is equal to the height of the curve (Figure PH5). If $y = e^{-x}$ is plotted, a falling curve is produced in which the gradient is negative but is again proportional to the height of the curve (Figure PH6). These curves are called exponential curves.

Exponential functions of time

Exponential functions occur very commonly when examining the behaviour of physiological systems. The

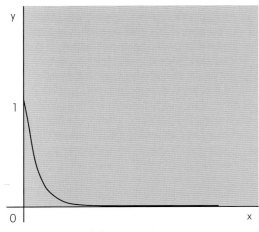

Figure PH6 Graph for $y = e^{-x}$

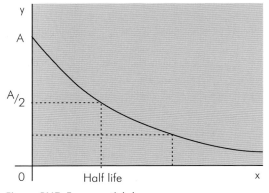

Figure PH7 Exponential decay curve

exponential function is written in two ways:

$$y = A\exp(-kt)$$

or

$$y = Ae^{-kt}$$

This is merely a notational difference between the two forms. The above function is illustrated in Figure PH7, and has an initial amplitude A. This curve is called an exponential decay curve. The time taken for the function value to reduce to half its initial value is the half-life. The rate of decay is determined by the time constant, which is given by

Time constant $= -1/k$

This is related to the half-life by

Half-life $= 0.693 \times$ time constant

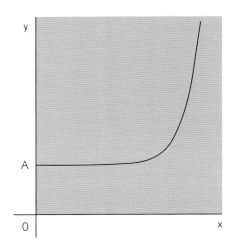

Figure PH8 Exponential growth curve

Exponential decay curves occur when k is negative, and are encountered in:

- Drug washout curves, where the concentration of the drug remaining in the blood stream is proportional to the rate of drug excretion from the body
- Expiration, when lung volume is approximately proportional to the rate of lung emptying

When k is positive, a different curve is produced, as shown in Figure PH8. This is an exponential growth curve and can represent growth of a population, where the rate of population growth is proportional to the population at any given time. In this function, k determines the rate of growth. Exponential growth is seen in:

- The early phase of growth in bacterial and cell cultures. Exponential growth remains until the availability of the food supply becomes the growth-limiting factor.

Trigonometric functions

The three most common trigonometric functions, sine (sin), cosine (cos) and tangent (tan), can be thought of as ratios of lengths in a right-angled triangle. This is illustrated in Figure PH9, which shows a right-angled triangle with a hypotenuse length of c, a side of length a adjacent to the angle α, and a side of length b opposite. Thus:

$$\sin\alpha = \frac{b}{c} \qquad \cos\alpha = \frac{a}{c} \qquad \tan\alpha = \frac{b}{a}$$

The sine and cosine functions are found in many physical situations, because they define a common type of repetitive or cyclical motion called simple harmonic motion. The

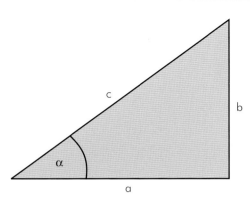

Figure PH9 Right-angle triangle showing sine, cosine and tangent

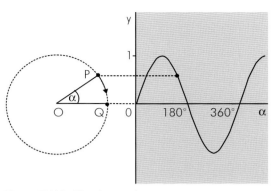

Figure PH11 Circular motion

Another version of the sine function equation is:

$$y = \sin(2\pi f t)$$

Thus the movement of P can be described in two ways, either as a function of angle α or as a function of time. This angle–time equivalence is useful in the analysis of any system subjected to repetitive (or 'periodic') disturbances or displacements. Physiological examples of such systems include:

- Clinical measurement systems processing periodic electrical signals such as arterial pressure waveforms
- The respiratory system making cyclical respiratory movements or being driven by the cyclical pressure from a ventilator
- The arterial system subjected to the periodic outflow of the left ventricle

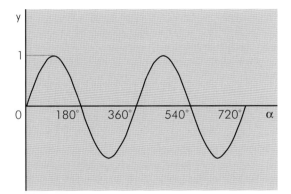

Figure PH10 Sine wave

tangent function in Figure PH9 defines the gradient of side c.

Sine function and circular motion

If the function $y = \sin$ is plotted as a graph (Figure PH10), a 'wave' is produced which is repeated as the angle α passes through each successive 360° (or 2π radians). The sine curve starts at zero, increasing to a maximum value of 1 at 90°, reducing to 0 at 180° and then decreasing to a minimum of -1 to return back to zero at 360°. This graph can also be thought of as describing the circular motion of a point P as it moves round in a circle (Figure PH11), where α is the angle between OP and OQ. The graph plots the value of the vertical height of P above OQ.

Since α (in radians) can also be expressed in terms of the frequency (f) of the circular movement of P and time (t):

$$\alpha = 2\pi f t$$

Phase angles

It can be seen that the equivalence between angle and time in sine functions enables time delays or differences to be expressed as angles. These are usually referred to as phase angles (phase shifts or phase differences). Thus a time delay of a whole cycle is equal to a phase angle of 360° (2π radians). A phase shift equal to half a cycle is 180° (π radians), while a quarter of a cycle is equal to 90° ($\pi/2$ radians). Such time delays measured in seconds would vary depending on the frequency of the sine wave involved: e.g. the duration of one cycle at 50 Hz is 1.2 seconds, while at 100 Hz a cycle is 0.6 seconds.

In many applications of sine waves to a system it is more useful to deal with phase angles rather than absolute times measured in seconds. An electrical example is the behaviour of a capacitor when a voltage is applied across it. In such a case the voltage changes are delayed compared to

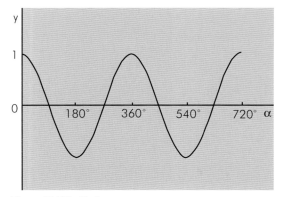

Figure PH12 Cosine wave

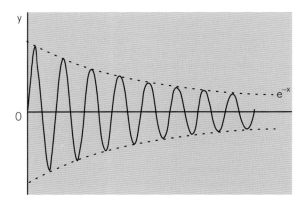

Figure PH13 Damped oscillation of a sine wave

the current changes in the circuit (see below, pages 752–3). The time delay measured in seconds would depend on the frequency of the applied voltage. However, if a sine wave is applied to the capacitor and the delay is measured as a phase angle, it is found to be 90° no matter what the frequency.

Cosine function
The cosine function has a similar graph to the sine wave. However, the cosine curve is shifted sideways relative to the sine function by an angle of 90°, as illustrated in Figure PH12. When the angle equals zero, cos is equal to its maximum value of 1, but as it increases to 90°, cos decreases to 0.

Sine and cosine functions in electrical signals
Sine and cosine waveforms often occur as electrical signals. In this context the signals are plotted as voltages (or currents) in time and are characterised by two parameters – the amplitude (A) and frequency (f).

For the sine wave

$$y = A\sin(2\pi f t)$$

and for the cosine wave

$$y = A\cos(2\pi f t)$$

The amplitude gives the height of the wave, and the frequency shows how many oscillations occur per second.

When oscillation is combined with energy dissipation, the result is known as *damped oscillation* (Figure PH13). This occurs in systems that have some form of energy stor-

age and exchange, but also some energy dissipation. The shape of the resulting function depends on the amount of damping. As the damping increases, the number of oscillations seen before the function dies away is reduced. In the situation known as *critical damping* (see Section 4, Chapter 2, page 792), the damping is high enough that no oscillations occur, and the function then looks similar to an exponential curve. Damped oscillatory motion is seen in mechanical systems which have compliance, inertia and friction. Damping is due to the frictional elements in the system, which tend to dissipate energy. When inertia and compliance dominate, many oscillations are seen, but as damping increases, the number of oscillations seen reduces to the point of critical damping, when the system does not oscillate at all.

Some degree of damping occurs in most oscillatory systems, for example:
- In resonant electrical circuits, due to the resistance of electrical components
- In mechanical systems, due to friction
- In respiratory muscle and lung tissue, due to tissue viscoelasticity
- In the airways, due to viscosity of gases and viscous interaction with the airway walls

Fourier analysis
Many functions occurring in physiology have a repetitive form when plotted as a graph: e.g. ECG waveform, respiratory waveform. These functions are generally referred to as periodic functions. A sine wave is one of the simplest periodic functions. Fourier analysis is a mathematical method of breaking down any periodic function into sine and cosine wave components.

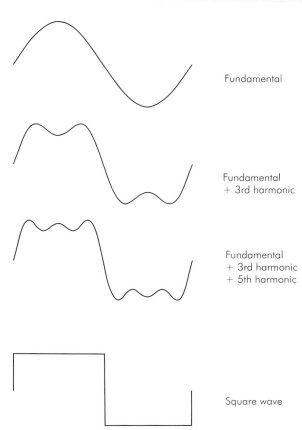

Fundamental

Fundamental
+ 3rd harmonic

Fundamental
+ 3rd harmonic
+ 5th harmonic

Square wave

Figure PH14 Summation of fundamental and harmonics to approximate square wave

The sine and cosine components exist at the fundamental frequency and multiples of the fundamental (harmonics). Figure PH14 shows how a square wave signal can be approximated to by the summation of its fundamental and some harmonics.

Fourier analysis can be used to:
- Determine the frequency spectra of electrophysiological signals (EEG, ECG, EMG)
- Determine the frequency response of electronic or mechanical systems in clinical measurement systems
- Design filters in signal-processing units
- Analyse signals in cerebral function monitors
- Analyse signals in Doppler systems

Calculus
Calculus is based on two mathematical operations, those of **integration** and **differentiation**. These operations are applied to mathematical functions of the form

$$y = f(x)$$

If this function is plotted as a graph, then integration and differentiation can be described in relation to this curve as follows:
- **Integration** is a mathematical operation which results in a second function (or *integral*, denoted $\int f(x)$), which can be used to determine the area under the curve between any two values of x.
- **Differentiation** is a mathematical operation which results in a second function (or *derivative*, denoted dy/dx) which defines the gradient of the curve at any point.

Integration and differentiation are reciprocal mathematical operations. Differentiation of a mathematical function gives a derivative function, which can be integrated to restore the original function. These basic mathematical operations are not simply tools which can calculate areas and gradients in graphs, but they define the dynamic relationship between two variables. In advanced calculus, differential equations are developed whose solutions enable the behaviour of complex systems to be modelled and predicted. This can be applied to physical, chemical and biological systems.

Integration
Integration is best described by considering an application. A useful application is provided by the calculation of volumes from a graph of gas flow against time. Consider the case of a patient blowing through a pneumotachograph (see Section 4, Chapter 2, page 806). The pneumotachograph records the expired gas flow as a function of time. If the flow were constant from the beginning to the end of expiration, the graph would look like Figure PH15. Calculation of the expired volume is then given by

Expired volume = flow rate × time

= area under the flow curve.

In practice, however, expiratory flow is not constant but is continuously variable, and the expiratory flow curve may be as illustrated in Figure PH16. Here the flow rate is not constant, but varies with time and can be written as a function $Q(t)$. In order to find the expired volume, the patient's total expiratory time is first split into small intervals of length δt (see Figure PH17). The flow rate can be considered approximately constant over each time interval, δt.

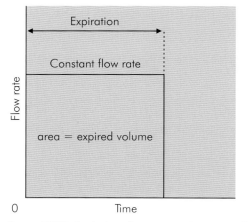

Figure PH15 Expiratory flow curve at constant flow rate

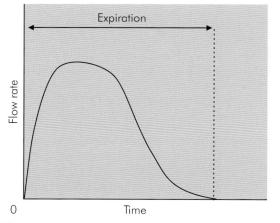

Figure PH16 Expiratory flow curve with varying flow rate

The incremental volume, δV, which flows during each δt is given by

$$\delta V = Q(t) \times \delta t$$

The expired volume is then the sum of (Σ represents 'the sum of') these individual increments in volume:

Expired volume $= \Sigma\, Q(t) \times \delta t$

where $Q(t)$ is the volume flow rate at any instant in time, and is thus the height of the rectangular strips in Figure PH17. Of course, the flow rate is not constant over each increment in time, particularly when the flow rate is changing rapidly during the rise and fall of the curve. However, in the mathematical operation of integration, the width of each rectangular strip is allowed to become

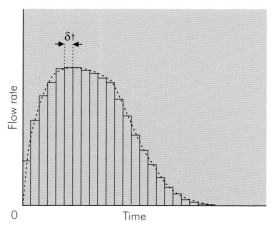

Figure PH17 Expiratory flow curve divided into time intervals of δt

infinitely small. In this case the flow rate becomes effectively constant for this instant in time. The sum of instantaneous flow rates is then written:

$$\text{Expired volume} = \int_{t=t_1}^{t=t_2} Q(t) \times \mathrm{d}t$$

The symbol $\int$ is called the integral sign. It is a stylised S, indicating that we are performing a sum of infinitely narrow strips of $Q(t)$. The numbers t_1 and t_2 at the top and bottom of the integral sign are the times for starting the summing process, and finishing it.

Evaluation of an integral
If a graph can be described by a mathematical function, then the integral of this function can be found, which can be used to determine the area under the curve. Once the integral of a function has been found it is relatively simple to calculate the value of the integral (area under any section of the curve) by substituting numerical values into the integral. Figure PH18 shows some common mathematical functions and their integrals.

For example, a flow-controlled ventilator gives an accelerating inspiratory flow represented by

Flow rate $V(t) = 1.4\mathrm{e}^{-0.8t}$ litres per second

What is the tidal volume if the inspiration phase lasts 4 seconds?

The tidal volume can be written as the integral of flow rate between the start of inspiration ($t = 0$) and the end of

Function f(t)	Integral
1	t
t	$\dfrac{t^2}{2}$
t^2	$\dfrac{t^3}{3}$
e^{at}	$\dfrac{1}{a}e^{at}$
$\sin(at)$	$-\dfrac{1}{a}\cos(at)$
$\cos(at)$	$\dfrac{1}{a}\sin(at)$

Figure PH18 Some examples of common integrals

inspiration ($t = 4$):

$$\text{Tidal volume} = \int_{t=0}^{t=4} = 1.4e^{-0.8t} \times dt$$

So, from the table of integrals in Figure PH18:

$$\text{Tidal volume} = -\frac{1.4}{0.8}e^{-0.8t} \Big|_{t=0}^{t=4}$$

The symbol

$$\Big|_{t=0}^{t=4}$$

means that the expression to the left of the vertical bar is to be evaluated first with $t = 4$ and then with $t = 0$. The difference between these values is then the value of the integral (area under the flow curve) between 0 and 4 seconds.

$$\text{Tidal volume} = 1.75(e^{\circ} - e^{-3.2})$$
$$= 1.68 \text{ litres}$$

In practice, integration calculations can be evaluated using computers with appropriate software, or by microprocessors built into monitoring equipment or ventilators.

Differentiation

Consider the problem of determining gas flow rate using a spirometer, which measures expired volume. The recording from the spirometer is a graph of total expired volume as a function of time. If the average flow is required, a simple ratio of total expired volume over expiratory time is taken:

$$\text{Average flow} = \frac{\text{total expired volume}}{\text{expiratory time}}$$

However, in order to determine the flow rate at each instant in time, the following approach is taken. The expiratory time is again split up into small increments, as in Figure PH17, each of duration δt, during which the change in expired volume is δV. Then, at any given time, the average flow over this small interval δt is given by

$$\text{Average flow} = \frac{\delta V}{\delta t}$$

This also represents the average gradient of the graph over δt.

The mathematical operation of differentiation then allows the time interval, δt, to become infinitely short, so that the above flow becomes an instantaneous flow. This is then written as

$$\text{Instantaneous flow} = \frac{dV}{dt}$$

The letter d is used to show that the intervals in V and t have become infinitely small. This mathematical process is called *differentiation*, and it can be applied to any function. Differentiation of a function produces another function called the *derivative*. This can be written as:

$$\text{Derivative of } f(t) = \frac{df(t)}{dt}$$

The derivative defines the gradient of the function at any point on its curve. Figure PH19 shows some common mathematical functions and their derivatives.

A comparison of the tables in Figures PH18 and PH19 shows that differentiation can be thought of as the inverse of integration. For example, if the function $\sin(t)$ is differentiated, the result is $\cos(t)$. Integration of $\cos(t)$ then gives $\sin(t)$, the original function. This holds true for any function.

Function f(t)	Derivative
t	1
t^2	$2t$
t^3	$3t^2$
$\exp(at)$	$a \cdot \exp(at)$
$\sin(at)$	$a \cdot \cos(at)$
$\cos(at)$	$-a \cdot \sin(at)$

Figure PH19 Some common derivatives

For example, during an expiration that lasts 6 seconds, the volume V (litres) of air expired is described by:

$$V(t) = 2.5 \sin\left(\frac{\pi}{12}t\right)$$

What is volume flow rate after 3 seconds of expiration?

Differentiating the equation above gives:

$$\text{Flow} = \frac{dV(t)}{dt} = 2.5 \times \frac{\pi}{12} \times \cos\left(\frac{\pi}{12}t\right)$$

Therefore, for $t = 3$, flow $= 0.46$ litres per second.

Scalars and vectors

A scalar quantity is defined solely by its magnitude. Scalars include quantities such as temperature and mass.

A vector quantity requires both magnitude and direction to be defined. Vectors include quantities such as force, velocity and displacement (change in position). Simple addition or subtraction of vector quantities cannot be performed without reference to their direction. Consider the sum of a force of 1 newton added to another force of 1 newton. If the forces are in opposite directions the result is zero; if they act in the same direction the result is a force of 2 newtons.

Vector addition

Vector quantities may be added using simple geometrical rules, to give a resultant vector. If a person walks from A to B in Figure PH20, and then from B to C, the same could have been achieved by walking directly from A to C. In other words, the resultant of the two component vectors AB and BC is the vector AC. This can be obtained graphically by simply completing a parallelogram and drawing the diagonal.

Vector resolution

The reverse of vector addition is to resolve it into a number of components. Resolving a vector into two component vectors can be performed graphically by reversing the parallelogram construction shown in Figure PH20. If the two components required are at 90° to each other, i.e. along x and y axes, they can be calculated by simple trigonometry (Figure PH21). The magnitude of the component in the x direction can be found by dropping a perpendicular from the vector to the x axis giving OB (a mathematical statement of this procedure is $OB = OA \cos \theta$). Similarly the magnitude of the y component can be found as

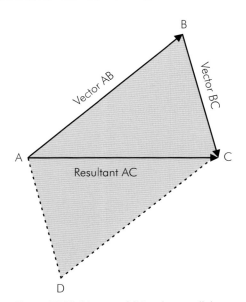

Figure PH20 Vector addition by parallelogram construction

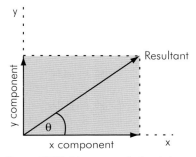

Figure PH21 Vector resolution into x and y components

$OC = OA \sin \theta$. If OB and OC are added they give the original vector OA as their resultant.

The leads of an ECG

A vector can be resolved in any direction by dropping a perpendicular to that axis as described above. In the electrocardiogram (ECG), we are presented with the components of the cardiac vector in various directions. These are the leads of the ECG. Thus lead I in the anterior chest leads of an ECG is the component of the cardiac vector acting at 0°. Similarly, lead II is the cardiac vector component acting at 60°, and lead III the component acting at 120°. Any two of these components can be used to find the direction and magnitude of the cardiac vector, by the following

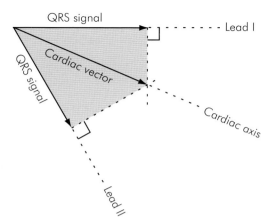

Figure PH22 Cardiac axis and ECG leads

construction. Draw perpendiculars from the tips of the two chosen components and find the point of intersection (Figure PH22). This gives the tip of the cardiac vector. Further discussion of calculation of the cardiac axis from the frontal ECG leads is presented in Section 2, Chapter 5.

Units

Quantifying physical dimensions and properties requires the definition of units of measurement. Many traditional and varied systems of measurement have evolved, but progress towards standardisation of units continues. The system adopted in 1960 was the International System of Units (SI, *Système International d'Unités*). The SI system is a coherent system based on the use of seven fundamental units, two supplementary units and an unlimited number of derived units. 'Coherent' in this context refers to the fact that there is a single unit for each fundamental quantity in the SI system, and all derived units are formed by single multiplication of fundamental units. This means that consistent use of SI units in all equations and calculations produces an answer in the appropriate SI unit automatically without scaling or conversion. Unfortunately in medical sciences traditional units still persist, and it is necessary to be aware of some inter-conversions between units.

Fundamental units

The seven fundamental units and two supplementary units in the SI system are shown in Figure PH23.

Derived units

Some of the units that are derived from the fundamental SI units have no specific names (Figure PH24). Most derived

Quantity	Unit	Symbol
Fundamental		
Length	metre	m
Mass	kilogram	kg
Time	second	s
Electric current	ampere	A
Temperature	kelvin	K
Amount of substance (specify particles, e.g. atoms, molecules, ions)	mole	mol
Light intensity	candela	cd
Supplementary		
Angle	radian	rad
Solid angle	steradian	sr

Figure PH23 Fundamental units and supplementary units in the SI system

Phenomenon	Derived unit	Symbol
Area	square metre	m^2
Volume	cubic metre	m^3
Density	kilogram per cubic metre	$kg \cdot m^{-3}$
Velocity	metre per second	$m \cdot s^{-1}$
Acceleration	metre per second per second	$m \cdot s^{-2}$

Figure PH24 Derived SI units

units, however, are named after the famous scientists who originally investigated those physical laws (Figure PH25).

Unit multiplication factors

Basic or derived units may be prefixed by a letter that denotes a multiplying factor. The more common multiplying factors are shown in Figure PH26. These letters increase or decrease the value of the unit by powers of 10.

Conversion between pressure units

As noted above, many non-SI units are still commonly used in clinical practice, mainly because of tradition or context. This particularly applies to pressure measurements in anaesthesia, where pressures may range from airway pressures (measured in cmH_2O) through to gas cylinder pressures (measured in atmospheres). There are many different units of pressure still used, and it is therefore

Phenomenon	Derived unit	Name (symbol)	Unit description
Force	$kg·m·s^{-2}$	newton (N)	Force required to accelerate a mass of 1 kg at 1 $m·s^{-2}$
Pressure	$kg·m^{-1}·s^{-2}$	pascal (Pa)	Pressure which exerts a force of 1 newton per square metre of surface area
Frequency	$1·s^{-1}$	hertz (Hz)	Number of cycles of a periodic activity per second
Energy	$kg·m^2·s^{-2}$	joule (J)	Energy expended in moving a resistive force of 1 newton a distance of 1 metre
Power	$kg·m^2·s^{-3}$	watt (W)	Rate of energy expenditure of 1 joule per second

Figure PH25 Named derived units

Prefix	Letter	Multiplying factor
exa	E	10^{18}
peta	P	10^{15}
tera	T	10^{12}
giga	G	10^{9}
mega	M	10^{6}
kilo	k	10^{3}
hecto	h	10^{2}
deca	da	10
deci	d	10^{-1}
centi	h	10^{-2}
milli	m	10^{-3}
micro	m	10^{-6}
nano	n	10^{-9}
pico	p	10^{-12}
femto	f	10^{-15}
atto	a	10^{-18}

Figure PH26 Prefixes used to denote unit multiplication factors

Basic unit		Converted equivalent
1.0 kPa	1000	$N·m^{-2}$
	0.01	bar
	0.01013	atmospheres
	104	$dyne·cm^{-2}$
	7.5	mmHg
	10.2	cmH_2O
	0.145	pounds force per square inch
	20.9	pounds force per square foot

Figure PH27 Conversion between pressure units

so dividing both sides of the conversion factor equation by 7.5 gives

$$1.0\,mmHg = 1.0/7.5 = 0.133\,kPa$$

and multiplying both sides by 158 gives

$$158\,mmHg = 158 \times 0.133 = 21\,kPa$$

useful to be familiar with inter-conversion between pressure units (Figure PH27).

When converting physical values between one system of units and another, it is useful to treat the conversion as an equation. In this case each side of the equation must be multiplied or divided by the same factor in order to keep the equation valid.

For example, if the partial pressure of oxygen is 158 mmHg, what is the partial pressure of oxygen in SI units?

$$7.5\,mmHg = 1.0\,kPa\,(Figure\ PH27)$$

Fundamental constants
These are basic constants which have internationally agreed values. An example is the speed of light in a vacuum, which is now given the value of 299 792 458 m s^{-1}. In fact, the fundamental SI unit of length, the metre, is now defined as the length of the path travelled by light in a vacuum during a time interval of 1/299792458 of a second.

Other fundamental constants include the elementary charge of an electron (1.602×10^{-19} coulombs), the Faraday constant (9.648×10^4 coulombs per mole), Avogadro's number and the gas constant (R).

Quantity	Vector or scalar	Description	SI unit
Displacement	Vector	Distance measured in a given direction	m
Velocity	Vector	Change in displacement per second	$m \cdot s^{-1}$
Acceleration	Vector	Change in velocity per second	$m \cdot s^{-2}$
Mass	Scalar	Amount of matter present in an object	kg
Force	Vector	An external 'push' or 'pull' which when applied to an object can change its state or motion	N
Weight	Vector	Gravitational pull acting on an object	N
Pressure	Scalar	Force per unit area	Pa
Energy	Scalar	Capacity to do work (stored work)	J
Work	Scalar	Energy expended when a force moves its point of application	J
Power	Scalar	Work done per second	W

Figure PH28 Some basic quantities in mechanics

Mechanics

Mechanics is the study of how objects around us move or remain at rest. This subject therefore requires an understanding of the quantities shown in Figure PH28.

Dimensional analysis

Three basic dimensions are described in mechanics, mass (M), length (L) and time (T). Any mechanical quantity can be defined in terms of its dimensions. An example is **velocity**, which is displacement per unit time. This will have the dimensions of length divided by time, which can be expressed as

Dimensions of velocity $= [L/T]$

Similarly, **force** is mass times acceleration, and thus

Dimensions of force $= [ML/T^2]$

Dimensional analysis can be applied to test the validity of equations, since both sides of an equation should be dimensionally equivalent.

Mass and weight

Sometimes some confusion can arise between mass and weight. Dimensional analysis can be applied to help distinguish between them. Mass is the amount of matter present and has the dimensions $[M]$. Mass is a property of an object which remains constant no matter where the object is situated.

Weight is the gravitational force acting on an object and is given by the product of mass (m) times the acceleration due to gravity (g):

Weight $= m\,g$

Weight therefore has the dimensions of mass times acceleration, and varies according to the location of the object. The weight of an object will be less on the moon than on earth, and it will be greater at the north pole than at the equator.

Applications of mechanics in anaesthesia

Mechanics can be applied to help in understanding the functioning of various mechanical devices or physiological mechanisms. Some examples include:

- Pressure measurement by a barometer or manometer
- Work done in compressing gases by a ventilator
- Work of breathing done by the body
- Work done by the myocardium in providing the cardiac output

Hydrostatic pressure

Manometers and barometers measure pressure using a column of fluid. This is done by balancing the unknown pressure against the pressure produced by the weight of a column of fluid. The pressure exerted at the base of a column of fluid is effectively the pressure exerted at an equivalent depth in the fluid. In the barometer and sphygmomanometer this fluid is mercury, while the manometer usually uses water. In practice the pressure measured is often expressed simply as the height of the specific fluid column (e.g. cmH_2O or mmHg). Calculating the pressure

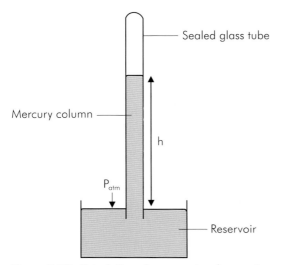

Figure PH29 Calculation of pressure in a barometer

at the base of a column of fluid enables a conversion to be made from the height of the column to SI units (Pa).

Barometric pressure

A barometer balances atmospheric pressure (P_{atm}) acting on the surface of a reservoir (Figure PH29) against the pressure at the base of a column of mercury. The mercury column must therefore be in a sealed glass tube, since if it were open, as in the sphygmomanometer, no difference in mercury levels would exist. Consider the pressure at the base of the mercury column:

$$Pressure = \frac{force}{area}$$
$$= \frac{weight\ of\ mercury\ column}{cross\text{-}sectional\ area}$$
$$= h\rho g$$

where

h = height of column = 0.76 m
ρ = density of mercury = 13.6×10^3 kg m^{-3}
g = acceleration due to gravity = 9.81 m s^{-2}

Therefore the atmospheric pressure measured by a column of mercury 760 mm tall is given by:

$$Atmospheric\ pressure = 0.76 \times 13.6 \times 10^3 \times 9.81$$
$$= 101\ 396\ Pa$$
$$= 101.4\ kPa$$

This can be used to convert between kPa and mmHg, thus:

$$760\ mmHg = 101.4\ kPa$$
$$7.49\ mmHg = 1\ kPa$$

Gauge pressure

When an unknown pressure is measured relative to atmospheric pressure (as is usually the case in clinical practice) the value obtained is referred to as a *gauge pressure*. This is the case in measurements such as blood pressure or airway pressure.

Absolute pressure

An absolute pressure measurement includes the effect of the atmosphere, and is therefore equal to the sum of atmospheric pressure plus the gauge pressure. Clearly barometric pressure is an absolute pressure measurement.

Force required when injecting with a syringe

The relationship between force and pressure is illustrated by the higher resistance experienced when injecting with a large syringe compared to a small syringe. In order for fluid to pass out of the barrel of the syringe the same pressure must be developed in the syringe. Let this pressure equal 4 kPa (30 mmHg). Then the force required to depress the plunger of the syringe will be dependent on the cross-sectional area of the syringe barrel, since

$$Force = pressure \times cross\text{-}sectional\ area$$

Consider a 2 ml syringe with a diameter of 1 cm. The force required is given by

$$Force = 4 \times 10^3 \times \pi \times (0.5 \times 10^{-2})^2$$
$$= 32\ N$$

If this is compared with a 20 ml syringe, the diameter of the larger syringe is approximately double that of the smaller syringe (2 cm). The cross-sectional area will be four times that of the smaller syringe and consequently four times the force is required to depress the plunger (Figure PH30). Thus it is easier to inject with a small syringe than with a larger syringe.

Work, energy and power

Work and energy are closely related, since the expenditure of energy usually results in the performance of useful work, and similarly the performance of work often produces changes in energy levels. Energy is not destroyed but merely converted from one form to another. In a

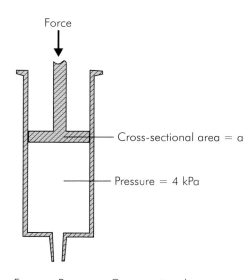

Force = Pressure x Cross-sectional area

Figure PH30 Force required to depress plunger in a syringe

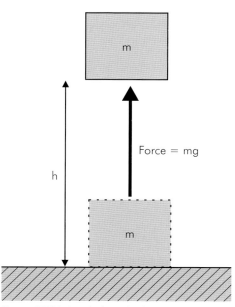

Figure PH31 Work done by force raising a mass

mechanical system, when energy is expended in doing work or converted from one form to another, there is usually an apparent 'loss' due to the inefficiencies of any real system (e.g. friction). This apparent loss of energy often appears as a production of heat.

Power

Power is the rate of doing work or the energy expended per unit time. To calculate the power output of a machine or process, divide the total energy expended by the time taken.

For example: calculate the power output of intermediate metabolism over 24 hours, given a basal metabolic rate of 2400 kcal per day.

$$\text{Total energy expended} = 2400 \times 10^3 \text{ cal}$$
$$= 9.98 \times 10^6 \text{ J}$$
$$\text{Total time taken} = 24 \text{ h}$$
$$= 86\,400 \text{ s}$$
$$\text{Average power output} = 115 \text{ W}$$

Work done by a force

The work done by a force acting on an object can be calculated as the product of the force and the distance moved by the point of application of that force. Consider the work done by a force F raising an object of mass m through a height h (Figure PH31). In order to lift the mass the force must be at least equal to the weight of the object. So:

$$F = m g$$

where g = acceleration due to gravity. So:

$$\text{Work done} = m g h$$

The work done in raising the object has resulted in a gain in potential energy due to its increase in height (energy by virtue of position or state). This potential energy represents a capacity to do work, or may be converted to another form of energy such as kinetic energy, if the object were allowed to fall. As the object falls it loses potential energy but gains kinetic energy (energy by virtue of its velocity).

Use of potential energy in the Manley ventilator

An example of the application of potential energy lies in the action of the bellows weight in a Manley ventilator. When this weight is raised by the driving gas, it gains potential energy. This potential energy is then used by allowing the weight to fall and compress the bellows of a ventilator. The work done in compressing the ventilator bellows is converted into the potential energy gained by the gas as it becomes pressurised.

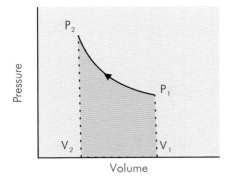

Figure PH32 Pressure–volume curve for ventilator during inspiratory phase

Work done by a ventilator in compressing inspiratory gases

When a volume of gas is compressed, work is done, and potential energy is gained by the gas. This is analogous to the storage of potential energy in a spring when it is compressed. The work done in compressing a volume of gas from volume V_1 to V_2 with a pressure (P) can be found by plotting a pressure–volume curve and finding the area under the curve (Figure PH32).

$$\text{Work} = \int_{V_2}^{V_1} p \, dV$$

In order to estimate the inspiratory work in delivering a breath of 500 ml, a simple example can be taken. Consider a constant inspiratory pressure of 1.0 kPa applied to produce a tidal volume of 500 ml in a patient (Figure PH33). The inspiratory work done per breath would then be $1000 \times 0.5 \times 10^{-3}$ J $= 0.5$ J.

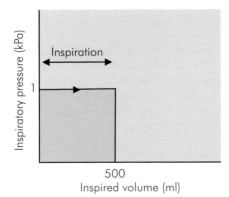

Figure PH33 Pressure–volume curve during inspiration with constant pressure

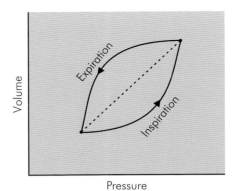

Figure PH34 Pressure–volume loop for a ventilator cycle

When the complete inspiratory–expiratory cycle of a ventilator is plotted, the pressure and volume axes are traditionally shown as in Figure PH34. Note the arrangement of the axes, with pressure on the x axis and volume on the y axis: this is done to give the familiar inspiratory–expiratory loop. Work is performed in compressing the inspired gas and expanding the patient's lungs (inspiratory curve). This stores potential energy as elastic energy in the gases and tissues of the respiratory system, which then performs work in restoring the lungs to their original volume (expiratory curve). In an ideal system with 100% efficiency the inspiratory and expiratory curves would coincide since no energy is wasted in frictional losses. The amount of energy put into the system during inspiration is thus returned in full during expiration. In practice, when this cycle of events is plotted on a pressure–volume curve as in Figure PH34, the inspiratory and expiratory curves do not coincide, and a loop is formed. This phenomenon is known as *hysteresis*, and the area of the loop represents the inspiratory and expiratory work 'wasted' over the complete cycle.

Work of breathing

Under resting conditions the work done in inspiration can be approximated by considering a simple model as described above. At an expenditure of 0.5 J per breath and a resting respiratory rate of 12 per minute:

$$\text{Work done per minute} = 12 \times 0.5$$
$$= 6 \text{ J}$$
$$\text{Power used} = 6/60 \text{ J s}^{-1}$$
$$= 0.1 \text{ W}$$

Allowing for the fact that respiratory muscles are only about 10% efficient, the total expenditure on work of breathing is approximately 1 W, which is equivalent to 1% of basal metabolic requirements. Under stressful or pathological conditions work of breathing may increase tenfold or more and represent a significant energy requirement. The work of breathing during spontaneous respiration is considered in further detail in Section 2, Chapter 8 (page 370).

Work done by the myocardium

The work performed by the myocardium of the ventricle during each cycle of the heart can also be derived from a pressure–volume loop, as described in detail in Section 2, Chapter 5 (pages 283–4). Calculation of the area of this loop gives the work done per cycle by the ventricle, which can then be normalised for body surface area to give left or right ventricular stroke work index (LVSWI or RVSWI). A gross simplification of the loop enables an estimate to be made. Figure PH35 shows an example for the left ventricle. The work done per cycle is then given by:

Stroke work done = (MAP − PCWP) × SV

where

MAP = mean arterial pressure = 90 mmHg (12 kPa)

PCWP = mean pulmonary capillary wedge pressure

= 7.5 mmHg (1 kPa)

SV = stroke volume = 80 ml $(0.080 \times 10^{-3} \, \text{m}^3)$

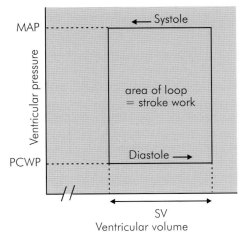

Figure PH35 Pressure–volume loop for left ventricle

So: stroke work done

$$= (12 \times 10^3 - 1 \times 10^3) \times 0.08 \times 10^{-3}$$
$$= 0.88 \, \text{J}$$

for a heart rate of 70 beats per minute.

$$\text{Power output} = \frac{0.88 \times 70}{60}$$
$$= 1 \, \text{W}$$

Assuming a 10% efficiency for the myocardium, the total energy requirements to provide 5.6 litres per minute of cardiac output becomes approximately 10 W (approximately 10% of basal metabolic requirement).

Heat

Heat is a form of energy which can be transferred from hot objects to cooler objects. Temperature is a measure of how hot or cold an object is, in other words a measure of its thermal state. Therefore heat energy will tend to pass across a temperature gradient from high to low temperatures. When heat is transferred to an object its temperature will increase, and the loss of heat energy from an object will be accompanied by a fall in temperature.

Units of heat energy

Heat energy is measured in joules (J), but traditionally has also been measured in calories (cal) or kilocalories (kcal or Cal).

1 calorie is defined as the amount of heat required to raise the temperature of 1 gram of water by 1 °C.

1 cal = 4.16 J

Temperature scales

Temperature scales have been defined in the past by using known fixed temperatures, such as the boiling and freezing points of water at one standard atmosphere pressure. Some temperature scales are compared in Figure PH36 using these points.

Scale	Freezing point H₂O	Boiling point H₂O
Kelvin	273.15 K	373.15 K
Celsius	0 °C	100 °C
Fahrenheit	32 °F	212 °F

Figure PH36 Commonly used temperature scales, showing freezing and boiling points of water

The boiling and freezing points of water, however, vary according to ambient pressure, and nowadays a more invariant point called the *triple point of water* (see below, pages 738–9) is used to define the two most commonly used temperature scales of Kelvin and Celsius. The unit used in the Kelvin scale is the kelvin (K), which has precisely the same magnitude as a one-degree increment (°C) on the Celsius scale. Practical methods of measuring temperature are discussed in Section 4, Chapter 2 (pages 825–6).

Specific heat capacity and heat capacity

In an object the relationship between temperature change and amount of heat energy added or removed depends on the size of the object and the material it is composed of.

Specific heat capacity, c (kJ kg^{-1} K^{-1}) is the amount of heat required to raise the temperature of 1 kg of a substance by 1°C. The specific heat capacity of water is 4.16 kJ/kg/°C. The average specific heat capacity of body tissues is between 3 and 4 kJ kg^{-1} K^{-1}.

Heat capacity (kJ K^{-1}) is the amount of heat required to raise the temperature of an object by 1 °C. Various symbols are used to denote heat capacity, with a capital C being the most prevalent, usually followed by a subscript letter to denote the conditions, as follows:

C_p heat capacity at constant pressure
C_V heat capacity at constant volume
C_m molar heat capacity

If the object has a mass M with a specific heat capacity c then it has a capacity given by

$$C_p = Mc \, (\text{kJ K}^{-1})$$

Thus the heat capacity of a 70 kg adult, assuming a specific heat capacity of 3.5 kJ kg^{-1} K^{-1}, is given by

$$= \frac{70 \times 3.5}{245 \, \text{kJ}} (= 58.9 \, \text{kcal})$$

Gases, liquids and solids

The addition or removal of heat energy to or from a substance will not only cause a variation in its temperature, but can also cause that substance to change its physical state. Any substance can exist in three states (phases) as a solid, a liquid or a gas. The conditions determining which state exists are temperature and pressure. At any given pressure the transition between solid and liquid occurs at a fixed temperature, the *freezing point*, while the transition between liquid and gas occurs at the *boiling point*. However, changes in ambient pressure cause boiling and

freezing points to vary. At sea level water boils at 100 °C, but at 5500 m, where atmospheric pressure is approximately halved, the boiling point of water decreases to 80 °C.

Critical temperature

Both pressure and temperature can change the state of a substance. Thus gases can be liquefied either by cooling or by increasing the pressure. However, there is a temperature above which any gas cannot be liquefied by increasing pressure. This is the critical temperature. The critical temperature for oxygen is -119 °C, and therefore oxygen in a cylinder at room temperature is always gaseous. But the critical temperature for nitrous oxide is 36.5 °C. This means that at normal room temperature a cylinder of nitrous oxide contains a mixture of liquid and gas, unless the ambient temperature exceeds 36.5 °C (as in a tropical country), in which case the nitrous oxide can only exist in gaseous form.

Variation of physical state with pressure and temperature

The way in which temperature and pressure determine the physical state of a substance is illustrated in Figure PH37. This figure shows curves plotting volume against pressure for a given mass of substance. Each curve is plotted at a given temperature and is called an isotherm. The middle curve is plotted at the critical temperature (T_C), while T_H is plotted at a temperature above T_C, and T_L is less than T_C. Note the following:

- T_H – at temperatures higher than the critical temperature, the substance exists only as a gas and the variation of volume with pressure at constant temperature follows a simple hyperbolic curve or inverse relationship, according to Boyle's law.
- T_C – at the critical temperature, the substance exists as a vapour at low pressures (i.e. below critical pressure). But when pressure increases above critical pressure the vapour liquefies, producing an inflexion point in the curve. Further increases in pressure do not then decrease the volume as the liquid state is effectively incompressible.
- T_L – at temperatures less than critical temperature, the substance exists as a liquid at high pressures. As the pressure decreases the volume remains constant until a point is reached when the liquid begins to boil (i.e. at the saturated vapour pressure, SVP) and a mixture of liquid and vapour is produced. The volume of this mixture at SVP varies according to the degree of vaporisation. When complete vaporisation has

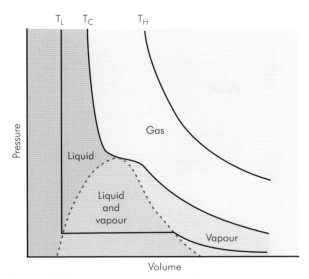

Figure PH37 Isotherms for nitrous oxide

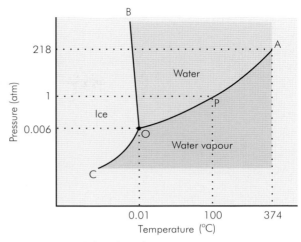

Figure PH38 Triple point of water

occurred, volume again follows an inverse relationship with pressure.

The isotherms (Figure PH37) map out areas which define the physical state of the substance. At temperatures above T_C (lightest shaded area) the substance exists only as a gas. At temperatures below T_C the substance may be in liquid form (darker shaded area); it may exist as a vapour (lighter shaded area); or it may be a mixture of both. This diagram is representative of the behaviour of nitrous oxide, since T_C for nitrous oxide is 36.5 °C.

Critical pressure
This is the minimum pressure at critical temperature required to liquefy a gas.

Critical volume
This is the volume occupied by 1 mole of gas at critical temperature and critical pressure.

Triple point of water
Water can exist in three phases, as water vapour, liquid water and ice. These phases will depend on temperature and pressure as shown in Figure PH38. The transition between water and water vapour is demarcated by the boiling point of water (P), which is 100 °C at 1 atmosphere, but which increases with increasing pressure (OA).

Water vapour and water therefore coexist along OA. Similarly the freezing point of water (0 °C at 1 atmosphere)

separates water and ice, but decreases with increasing pressure (OB). Ice and water thus coexist along OB. Finally OC separates ice and water vapour, and these phases coexist along this line. There is only a single point (O) at which the three phases of water coexist, at a pressure of 0.006 atmospheres and 0.01 °C. This is the triple point of water.

Vapours and gases
The term **gas** is applied to a substance which is normally in its gaseous state at room temperature and atmospheric pressure. Its critical temperature is below room temperature and therefore it cannot exist as a liquid.

The term **vapour** refers to a gaseous substance which is normally in liquid form at room temperature and atmospheric pressure, since its critical temperature is above room temperature. Thus a vapour is a gaseous substance which is below its critical temperature under ambient conditions.

Saturated vapour pressure and its relationship to boiling point
A vapour is formed from a liquid by *evaporation*, or the escape of molecules from the liquid surface. This process also occurs from the surface of solids to small extent by a process known as *sublimation*.

When evaporation takes place from the surface of a liquid the concentration of vapour above the liquid increases. This process continues until a state of equilibrium is reached when no further increase in vapour concentration occurs. At this stage the vapour is said to be saturated,

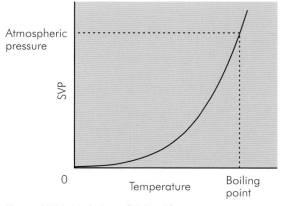

Figure PH39 Variation of SVP with temperature

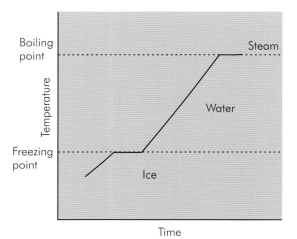

Figure PH40 Variation of temperature of a block of ice being heated

and the vapour pressure is the *saturated vapour pressure* (SVP).

SVP can therefore be defined as the pressure exerted by a vapour when in contact and equilibrium with its liquid phase. The SVP of a liquid increases with temperature (Figure PH39). The temperature at which the SVP becomes equal to atmospheric pressure is the boiling point of the liquid.

Latent heat

When a substance changes phase from liquid to gas or from solid to liquid the molecular separation and bonding change. Water molecules in steam are about 12 times further apart than in liquid water. This increased separation of the molecules represents stored potential energy since the *hydrogen bonds* between water molecules in liquid water are very strong. Work is therefore required to achieve this molecular separation, which is provided by the latent heat absorbed.

If ice is heated from a subzero temperature (Figure PH40), its temperature will rise steadily except when it passes through the two transitions in phase from solid to liquid (freezing point) and from liquid to gas (boiling point). At these transition points the temperature remains constant while latent heat is absorbed to increase molecular separation. The latent heat associated with these changes in state is known as *latent heat of fusion* and *latent heat of vaporisation* respectively.

Liquids also evaporate at temperatures lower than their boiling point, and will also require latent heat of vaporisation to achieve this change in state. However, the cooler the liquid the greater the amount of latent

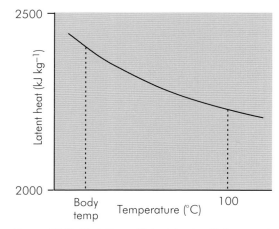

Figure PH41 Variation of latent heat with temperature

heat required to increase the liquid molecular energy levels to those possessed by vapour molecules. Thus specific latent heat of vaporisation increases as temperature decreases (Figure PH41), and is usually quoted at a given temperature.

- **Specific latent heat of fusion** is the energy required to change 1 kg of substance from liquid to solid, without change in temperature. The specific latent heat of fusion for water is 334 kJ kg^{-1}.
- **Specific latent heat of vaporisation** is the energy required to change 1 kg of substance from liquid to vapour, without change in temperature. The specific latent heat of vaporisation of water at 100 °C is

2260 kJ kg^{-1}. At 37 °C, the specific latent heat of water is 2420 kJ kg^{-1}.

Heat loss due to ventilation with cool dry gases

Poor preparation of inspired gases can cause a patient to lose body heat, because:
- The gases are not warmed, and heat is lost in warming the gases to body temperature.
- The gases are not humidified, and heat is lost due to evaporation in order to humidify the gases in the respiratory tract.

Heat loss in warming gases

Consider ventilating with air at 20 °C (body temperature = 37 °C) with a minute volume of 6 l min^{-1}. The specific heat capacity (c) of air is 998 J kg^{-1} K^{-1} and the density of dry air at normal temperature and pressure (NTP) is 1.29 kg m^{-3}.

Mass (M) of air in the minute volume

$$= \text{volume (m}^3) \times \text{density}$$
$$= 0.006 \times 1.29 = 7.74 \times 10^{-3} \text{ kg}$$

Heat required to warm air to body temp

$$= Mc\,(37 - 20)$$
$$= 7.74 \times 10^{-3} \times 998 \times 17$$
$$= 131 \text{ J min}^{-1}$$
$$= 2.2 \text{ W}$$

If basal metabolic requirements are approximately 100 W this represents just over 2% of basal requirements.

Heat loss in humidifying gases

Fully saturated air at 37 °C contains approximately 43 g m^{-3} (0.043 kg m^{-3}) of water. Assume 6 l min^{-1} of ventilation with dry gases which become 100% humidified in the respiratory tract. If the specific latent heat of vaporisation of water at 37 °C is 2420 kJ kg^{-1}, then the amount of water vapour required to humidify the inspired minute volume is given by

Mass of water evaporated per minute

$$= 6 \times 10^{-3} \times 0.043$$
$$= 2.58 \times 10^{-4} \text{ kg}$$

Heat lost by evaporation per minute

$$= 2.58 \times 10^{-4} \times 2420 \times 10^3$$
$$= 624 \text{ J}$$
$$= 10.4 \text{ W}$$

Thus the total heat losses due to using cool unhumidified gases are

$$2.2 + 10.4 = 12.6 \text{ W}$$

Humidity

Humidity is a measurement of the amount of water vapour present in the air. It may be presented in two ways, either as an **absolute humidity** value or as a **relative humidity** value.
- **Absolute humidity** is the mass of water vapour present in a given volume of air. The units of measurement are grams per cubic metre (g m^{-3}) or kilograms per cubic metre (kg m^{-3}). Absolute humidity value will not vary with the temperature of the air.
- **Relative humidity** is the ratio of the mass of water present, in a given volume of air at a given temperature, to the mass of water required to saturate that given volume at the same temperature. Relative humidity is usually expressed as a percentage, and it varies with temperature.

Figure PH42 shows how the relative humidity (RH) of a sample of air which is saturated at 20 °C (RH = 100%) decreases as temperature increases. The amount of water vapour required to saturate air at 20 °C is approximately 17 g m^{-3}. However at 37 °C, approximately 43 g m^{-3} is required for saturation, so the RH of the given sample decreases to 39%. From this example it can be seen that humidifying inspired gases at room temperature results in only 40% RH or so at body temperature.

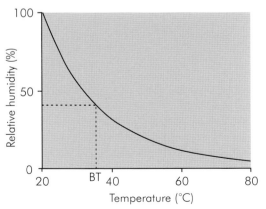

Figure PH42 Variation of relative humidity with temperature

Calculation of RH from water vapour pressure and SVP

Since the partial pressure exerted by a gas is proportional to the mass of gas present, the relative humidity can be determined from the actual water vapour pressure and the saturated water vapour pressure at the given temperature:

$$\text{Relative humidity} = \frac{\text{actual water vapour pressure}}{\text{saturated vapour pressure}}$$

Methods of humidity measurement are discussed in Section 4, Chapter 2.

Heat transfer

Heat energy can be transferred by different mechanisms:

- **Conduction** – When one end of a bar of metal is held in a fire the cool end gradually gets hotter as heat travels along the bar. This form of heat transfer is due to heat conduction. In the metal the atoms maintain a mean fixed position, unlike the case of a liquid or gas. The atoms, however, are free to vibrate about their mean position, the amplitude of this motion being dependent on the temperature of the solid. When this vibration is increased by raising the temperature in one region, the vibration is transmitted to neighbouring atoms, causing their temperature to increase and heat to be transferred. Clearly conduction requires physical continuity or contact. Gross movement of the medium transferring heat does not occur in conduction. Conduction also occurs in liquids and gases, but the transfer of heat in these cases occurs mainly by convection.
- **Convection** – This mechanism describes the transfer of heat in a liquid or gas when one region becomes heated. Increasing the temperature locally in a liquid or gas causes the density locally to decrease. This less dense fluid then rises, to be replaced by cooler denser fluid. This results in a *convection current* or the bulk movement of the fluid, with an accompanying transfer of heat energy. Hot air currents in the atmosphere and the continuous movement of water in a kettle as it boils are examples of convection.
- **Radiation** – Heat energy can also be transferred by electromagnetic radiation in the form of infrared radiation (see Figure PH96, below). This enables heat transfer to occur across a vacuum in the absence of any physical continuity or surrounding medium. Radiation is the mechanism by which heat is transferred from the sun to earth. Any object is capable of both emitting and absorbing infrared radiation, with a resultant loss or gain of heat energy.

The importance of these mechanisms in anaesthesia lies in heat losses suffered by a patient during prolonged periods of anaesthesia or sedation. These mechanisms are considered, together with additional factors such as losses due to evaporation from the respiratory tract and by sweating, in Section 2, Chapter 12.

Gases

Gases, unlike solids and liquids, are compressible and change their volume when different pressures are applied to them. Therefore the physical behaviour of a gas can be described by three parameters, pressure (P), volume (V) and temperature (T). This is summarised by the three **gas laws** for a fixed mass of gas:

(1) The relationship between volume and pressure at constant temperature is described by Boyle's law:

Pressure is inversely proportional to volume

$P \propto 1/V$

or $PV = \text{constant}$

(2) The relationship between volume and temperature at constant pressure is described by Charles's law:

Volume is proportional to temperature (kelvin)

$V \propto T$

or $V/T = \text{constant}$

(3) The relationship between pressure and temperature at constant volume is described by Gay-Lussac's law:

Pressure is proportional to temperature (kelvin)

$P \propto T$

or $P/T = \text{constant}$

The ideal gas equation

The above three laws can be summarised into a single equation, the **ideal gas equation**:

$$\frac{PV}{T} = \text{constant}$$

This equation enables us to convert from one set of conditions to another when a fixed mass of gas undergoes changes in pressure, volume or temperature, since:

$$\frac{P_1 V_1}{T_1} = \frac{P_2 V_2}{T_2}$$

The gas constant (R)

The ideal gas equation may be written as

$$PV = kT$$

where k is a constant dependent on the mass of gas present. If n = number of moles of gas present, the ideal gas equation becomes

$$PV = nRT$$

where R is known as the **universal gas constant**, and can be evaluated by considering 1 mole of gas at 273 K (0 °C) at a pressure of 1 atmosphere. This gives a value of R = 8.32 joules per °C.

Gas contents in a cylinder

From the ideal gas equation, the pressure exerted by any gas is dependent on the number of moles present. Therefore, in a fixed volume such as a gas cylinder, the pressure is a measure of the amount of gas contained. This applies to a gas (e.g. an oxygen cylinder), but not to a vapour (e.g. a full nitrous oxide cylinder, where liquid and gas phases are present), since the pressure then reflects the saturated vapour pressure. However, it should be noted that the critical temperature (T_C) for nitrous oxide is only 36.5 °C, and if ambient temperature rises above this value nitrous oxide cannot exist in its liquid state.

Avogadro's hypothesis

The above gas laws apply to any gas as long as the *given mass* of gas remains the same, since gas behaviour is determined by the number of molecules present rather than the absolute mass present. This idea is based on a hypothesis proposed by Avogadro in 1811 which stated:

Equal volumes of gases, under the same conditions of temperature and pressure, contain equal numbers of molecules.

An important conclusion following from this hypothesis was that gaseous elements exist as molecules (O_2 and N_2) rather than as single atoms. This explained apparent anomalies in behaviour between gaseous elements and gaseous compounds.

Avogadro's number

1 mole of gas or vapour contains the same number of molecules. This is Avogadro's number:

Avogadro's number $= 6.022 \times 10^{23}$

One mole of any gas or vapour occupies 22.4 litres at NTP (0 °C or 273 K, and 1 atmosphere).

Dalton's law of partial pressures

This states that if a mixture of gases is placed in a container then the pressure exerted by each gas (partial pressure) is equal to that which it would exert if it alone occupied the container.

Thus in any mixture of gases (e.g. alveolar gas, fresh inspired gases, air), the partial pressure exerted by each gas is proportional to its fractional concentration.

Consider a mixture of 5% carbon dioxide, 15% oxygen and 80% nitrogen. If the mixture exerts a total pressure of 100 kPa, then the partial pressures exerted by each gas are PCO_2 = 5 kPa, PO_2 = 15 kPa and PN_2 = 80 kPa.

Similarly, if the total pressure exerted by the gas mixture is increased to 200 kPa, then the partial pressures become PCO_2 = 10 kPa, PO_2 = 30 kPa and PN_2 = 160 kPa.

Adiabatic compression or expansion of gases

Adiabatic, when applied to the expansion or compression of a gas, means that heat energy is not added or removed when the changes occur. Thus when compression of a volume of gas occurs, it is accompanied by a temperature rise, and similarly expansion of a volume of gas will produce a temperature fall. Practical consequences of this are that compression of gases will require added cooling to avoid unwanted heating of the system.

Alternatively, expansion of gases in the airway during jet ventilation can produce localised cooling, which in turn can reduce the humidity of injected gases. A practical application of the adiabatic expansion of gases lies in the cryoprobe. Here expansion of gas in the probe is used to produce low temperatures in the tip for cryotherapy.

Hydrodynamics

Gases, liquids and fluid behaviour

Although gases and liquids differ considerably in their physical properties, they display similar behaviour under flow conditions, and can both be described as being *fluid*. The following points are similarities in behaviour between gases and liquids:

- Liquids and gases both fill the shape of their container, and are subject to constraints imposed by gravity. However because of their lower density, gases are less affected by gravity than liquids.
- The flow behaviour of gases and liquids is still largely determined by density and viscosity, although gases have much lower density and viscosity than liquids.
- Flow is produced, in both gases and liquids, by the application of a pressure gradient.

The similarity between gases and liquids in flow behaviour has led to the development of *fluid mechanics*, which is the study of fluids in motion, and applies equally to both gases and liquids.

Viscosity

Viscosity may be thought of as the 'stickiness' of a fluid. This property of a fluid can show itself in many ways. Imagine trying to pour treacle from a bottle compared to pouring water from the same bottle. Viscosity will affect the flow of fluids through a tube: the more viscous the fluid, the slower the flow. Gases are far less viscous than liquids, and viscous effects only become apparent at much higher flow velocities in gases compared to liquids.

The viscosity of a fluid can be quantified by its *coefficient of viscosity*. In order to understand how the coefficient of viscosity for a fluid is obtained, the concepts of *shear stress* and *shear rate* are required.

Shear stress and shear rate

A viscous force, or drag, is felt on any object moving through a fluid, and also when a fluid moves past a stationary object. Figure PH43 shows a thin, flat plate with a fluid flowing past it. Away from the plate the fluid flows faster, but closer to the plate the fluid is slowed down by the presence of the plate until at the surface the fluid is not moving. This happens at any surface because of adhesion between the fluid and the solid surface; it is known as the *no-slip* condition. Near to the surface, the flow pattern is deformed from one of uniform flow velocity to one in which layers of fluid parallel to the direction of flow 'slip' against each other, giving rise to a drag effect or *shearing* action. This shearing action at the surface gives a drag force per unit area of the plate, which is called the *shear stress*. The lengths of the arrows in Figure PH43 represent the velocity of the fluid, which diminishes to zero next to the plate. The velocity of flow thus varies between these fluid layers, i.e. a velocity gradient perpendicular to the direction of flow, or *shear rate*, is produced.

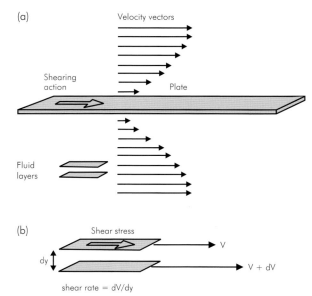

Figure PH43 Shear stress and shear rate

Coefficient of viscosity

The coefficient of viscosity (or simply the 'viscosity') of a fluid can be defined by considering laminar flow in which two parallel layers of fluid are slipping against each other. As described above this produces two effects, a shear stress between the layers, and a velocity gradient at right angles to the direction of flow (shear rate). The coefficient of viscosity (or viscosity) is defined by:

$$\text{Viscosity, } \eta = \frac{\text{shear stress}}{\text{shear rate}}$$

The units of viscosity are *poises*, after Poiseuille, who discovered the laws governing the flow of fluids through tubes. Water has a viscosity of 0.0101 poises at 20 °C, while air has a viscosity of 0.00017 poises at 0 °C.

Viscosity varies with temperature. Liquids generally become less viscous with increasing temperature, while gases become more viscous as temperature rises.

Newtonian fluids are fluids in which viscosity, η, is constant, regardless of the velocity gradients produced during flow. Many fluids, including water, are Newtonian. Some fluids, however, do not behave in this way, such as the shear-thinning fluids, whose viscosity falls as the shear rate between layers increases, and the rheotropic fluids, which become more viscous the longer the shearing persists. Blood is a well-known shear-thinning fluid.

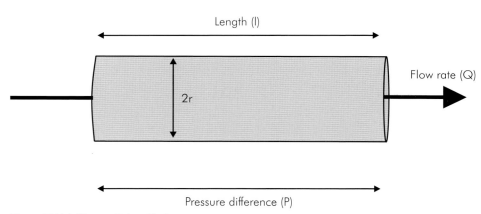

Figure PH44 Hagen–Poiseuille law

Measurement of viscosity

Viscometers are used to obtain a measurement for the coefficient of viscosity. The simplest form of viscometer allows fluid to flow under the influence of gravity down a fine-bore calibrated tube. The rate of fall of the fluid meniscus is detected by photocells from which the viscosity can be calculated.

A more complicated device uses the viscous drag created by spinning a small drum containing a sample of fluid. A pointer is mounted on a float suspended in the sample and is displaced by the torque due to the viscous drag. This records the viscosity measurement on a scale.

Viscosity and the damping of fluid flow

The viscous shearing action in a fluid flow dissipates energy as heat and is analogous to frictional effects between two solid surfaces rubbing against each other. This dissipative effect dampens the motion of fluid in a system, and thus viscous effects form a major component of damping in any hydrodynamic system. As with mechanical or electrical systems, damping is an important factor in determining the behaviour of the system.

Viscous effects can also affect the pattern of flow, since fluid flow can occur with two different basic patterns: **laminar flow** and **turbulent flow**. Laminar flow is smooth and streamlined while turbulent flow is rough, containing eddies of swirling fluid, which disrupt the flow and create greater drag. The characteristics of these flow patterns are discussed in more detail below.

Flow through tubes

When a pressure difference is applied across the ends of a tube, fluid will flow from the high pressure to the low pressure. An analogy can be drawn with an electrical circuit. Fluid flow (electrical current) occurs along the tube (conductor) because of the driving pressure difference (voltage), and energy is dissipated by the viscous drag (shear stress) between the fluid and the tube (electrical resistance).

Hagen–Poiseuille law

Hagen (in 1839) and Poiseuille (in 1840) discovered the laws governing laminar flow through a tube. Consider a pressure P applied across the ends of a tube of length l and radius r (Figure PH44). Then the flow rate, Q, produced is proportional to:

- The pressure gradient (P/l)
- The fourth power of the tube radius (r^4)
- The reciprocal of fluid viscosity $(1/\eta)$

This is often combined as:

$$Q = \frac{\pi P r^4}{8\eta l}$$

and attributed to Poiseuille, a surgeon, who verified this relationship experimentally.

Kinematic viscosity

As noted above, the viscosity of a fluid influences its flow pattern by creating a damping effect. However, the inertial properties of the fluid (dependent on fluid density) also affect the flow pattern. Thus the relative effects of inertial and viscous forces can determine the nature of fluid flow in any given situation. This is taken into account by using the kinematic viscosity (μ), which is defined as the ratio of the viscosity (η) to the density (ρ):

Kinematic viscosity, $\mu = \eta/\rho$

If the kinematic viscosity is high, rapid irregular flow patterns in a fluid will be well damped, but if it is low then disturbances such as swirling eddies may persist for a long time.

Reynolds number

The Reynolds number (Re) is used to determine whether the flow will be laminar or turbulent in any given situation. It includes the kinematic viscosity (μ), and the ratio of the inertial forces to the viscous damping forces in the fluid and is given by

$$Re = vl/\mu$$

where $v =$ the mean flow velocity through a tube, or the velocity a long way from an object, and $l =$ a characteristic length of the system, such as the diameter of a tube.

At low Reynolds numbers, the viscous forces dampen minor irregularities in the flow, resulting in a laminar pattern. A high Reynolds number means that the inertial forces dominate, and any eddies in the flow will be easily created and persist for a long time, creating turbulence. For flow through a tube, a Reynolds number of less than 2000 tends to give laminar flow, while between 2000 and 4000 the flow may be a mixture of laminar and turbulent, depending on the smoothness of the fluid entering the tube. Above 4000, the flow will certainly be turbulent.

Velocity profiles for laminar and turbulent flow in a tube

If we looked at the velocities across a tube (the velocity profile), the shapes would be different for laminar and turbulent flow, as shown in Figure PH45.

- **Laminar flow** – Figure PH45a shows the profile (dotted line) for laminar flow. It is much more pointed than the flat central portion of turbulent flow. The arrows are flow velocity vectors and are all parallel to the axis of the tube. There is a gradual decrease in flow velocity as the walls of the tube are approached. Laminar flow tends to occur when viscous effects predominate, i.e. with viscous fluids, in narrow tubes or at low flow velocities.
- **Turbulent flow** – In turbulent flow (Figure PH45b) the tube contains swirling eddies and the velocity varies continuously in time, and therefore the velocity profile is averaged in time. For the same net flow rate as in the laminar case, the flow velocity at the centre of the tube is flatter across the centre of the tube and has a lower peak value. However the velocity gradient at the walls is steeper because of an increased viscous

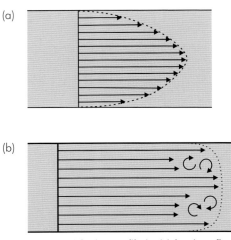

Figure PH45 Velocity profile in (a) laminar flow, (b) turbulent flow

drag associated with the turbulence. Turbulent flow tends to occur when density (inertial) effects predominate, i.e. thin fluids, wide-bore or uneven tubes and high flow velocities.

Transition between laminar flow and turbulence

When flow is slow it remains laminar, and both viscous drag and pressure drop along the tube increase in proportion with flow velocity. As the flow velocity increases, there is an increased tendency for small eddies to disrupt the flow until at higher velocities the flow becomes turbulent. When flow is turbulent there is an abrupt change in the viscous forces, as reflected by an increased pressure drop along the tube. The slope of a graph plotting pressure drop against flow velocity becomes steeper at the laminar–turbulent transition (Figure PH46): at this point the Reynolds number exceeds the threshold of approximately 2000.

A mixture of laminar and turbulent gas flow patterns is found in the airways of the lung during normal breathing. Turbulent flow occurs in the trachea and main bronchi at peak flow rates during quiet breathing, while flow in the small airways remains laminar under virtually all conditions.

Effect of varying cross section on flow velocity

In many situations flow occurs through tubes with a varying cross-sectional area, as illustrated in Figure PH47. The fluid is assumed to be incompressible, an assumption which is clearly valid for liquids, and which under

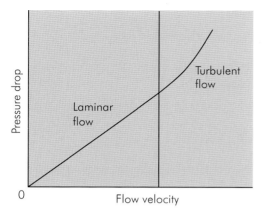

Figure PH46 Velocity–pressure drop curve, showing transition between laminar and turbulent flow

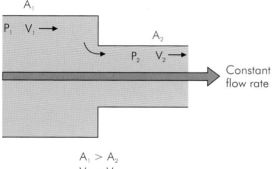

$A_1 > A_2$
$V_1 < V_2$
$P_1 > P_2$

Figure PH47 Constant-volume rate flow through a tube with varying cross section

normal circumstances remains surprisingly valid for gases. The volume flow rate is the product of the area of the tube (A) and the average flow velocity (v), and since no fluid leaves or enters the tube, the volume flow rate must be the same at point 1 as it is at point 2. This statement can be written as

$$A_1 v_1 = A_2 v_2$$

As the fluid moves from a larger cross section (point 1), to a smaller cross section (point 2), the velocity increases (from v_1 to v_2). Similarly, on moving from a smaller cross section to a larger cross section the velocity of flow will decrease.

Pressure and velocity: Bernoulli's equation

The pressure in the fluid can be related to its flow velocity by considering the balance between potential and kinetic energy for the fluid. The fluid has potential energy due to the pressure driving it in the direction of flow, and kinetic energy because it is moving. Since it is moving faster at point 2 than at point 1, its kinetic energy at point 2 is higher. For a gain in kinetic energy to occur, some potential energy must have been lost, i.e. a pressure drop occurs between point 1 and point 2. Thus the increased velocity at point 2 is accompanied by a reduced pressure. The relationship between pressure (P), and velocity (v) at any point in a fluid is given by

$$\frac{1}{2}\rho v^2 \text{(kinetic energy)} + P \text{(potential energy)} = \text{constant}$$

This is Bernoulli's equation for incompressible flow, assuming no change in potential energy due to gravity (i.e. flow does not occur uphill or downhill). This is a good approximation for gases, in which gravitational effects are usually negligible, or liquid flow in horizontal tubes.

Bernoulli's equation shows that as the velocity of a fluid increases, the pressure falls, or alternatively if the pressure of a gas flow falls, it gains velocity. This is illustrated by the example of gas escaping from a cylinder at high pressure through a nozzle to the atmosphere. The gas in the cylinder acquires a high speed as it exits through the nozzle to atmospheric pressure. The potential energy initially contained in the gas due to it being compressed has been converted to kinetic energy as the pressure falls to atmospheric pressure.

Venturi effect

The Venturi effect refers to the low pressure that is produced by a constriction in a duct with fluid flowing through it. As seen from the above discussion, this arises as a result of the Bernoulli principle. The Venturi effect is applied in devices such as the flow-driven nebuliser. The Venturi flow meter (Figure PH48) also uses the Venturi effect to estimate flow velocity from the drop in pressure at a tube constriction. However, the pressure drop is not proportional to the flow velocity, and the device needs careful calibration.

Injection of gas through a jet

The use of gas injected through a narrow jet or cannula occurs in jet ventilation, the Sanders injector and some types of fixed-performance oxygen masks. In these devices high-pressure gas is injected through a small orifice into a duct or airway open to the atmosphere. The injected gas forms a high-velocity stream which drags surrounding air

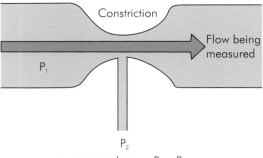

pressure drop $= P_1 - P_2$

Figure PH48 Principle of a Venturi flowmeter

behind it (entrainment) due to the viscosity of the gases. This is often erroneously referred to as a Venturi effect, but it can more accurately be attributed to viscous drag.

Electricity

Basic quantities and units
Electric charge
An electric charge may be positive or negative, and is produced by the accumulation of an excess or deficit of electrons in an object. Charge is measured in coulombs. Like charges tend to repel each other and opposite charges attract each other.

One coulomb is defined from the unit of current (the ampere: see below) as that charge which passes any point in a circuit in a second, when a steady current of 1 ampere is flowing.

A coulomb is equal in magnitude to the electric charge possessed by 6.24×10^{18} electrons.

Electric current
Most electrical effects are produced by the movement of charge. Any movement of electric charge forms an electric current. The current flowing in a conductor can be measured as the number of coulombs passing any given point per second. The unit of current is the ampere (amp – SI symbol A), where

$$1 \text{ ampere (A)} = 1 \text{ coulomb s}^{-1}$$
$$1 \text{ milliampere (mA)} = 1 \times 10^{-3} \text{ A}$$
$$1 \text{ microampere(}\mu\text{A)} = 1 \times 10^{-6} \text{ A}$$

When a current flows through a conductor it produces magnetic lines of force around the conductor (Figure PH49). This effect was discovered by Oersted and later

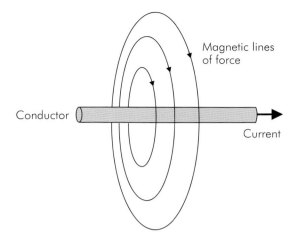

Figure PH49 Magnetic effect of current

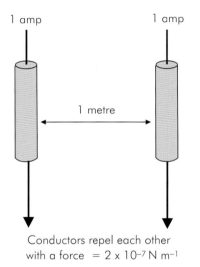

Figure PH50 Definition of the ampere

applied by Michael Faraday to give rise to the development of electric motors and generators.

Definition of the ampere
If two conducting wires are close to each other they will produce a force between them due to their magnetic fields, which depends on the size of the current in the wires. The ampere is defined as the current which, if flowing in two parallel wires of infinite length, placed 1 metre apart in a vacuum, will produce a force on each of the wires of 2×10^{-7} newtons per metre (Figure PH50).

Currents flow easily in *conductors*, which commonly include metals and electrolyte solutions. Materials which do not conduct current are *insulators*. There are some materials with intermediate conducting properties (*semi-conductors*), e.g. silicon, which have revolutionised electronic technology.

Electrical potential

If a positive electrical potential exists at a point, any positive charge at that point will possess potential energy and will tend to move away from it to a point at lower potential. Electrical potential is analogous to height in a gravitational field, where a mass possesses potential energy due to its height, and always tends to move downhill. The electrical potential of the earth is taken as a reference point for zero potential, and is usually referred to simply as *earth*.

Potential is measured in volts (V). Charge will only move between points separated by a potential difference (also measured in volts).

Potential difference (voltage)

When a potential difference (often referred to as voltage, since these terms have become interchangeable) is applied across a conductor it produces an electric current. A current is a flow of positive charge from the higher potential to the lower.

One volt can be defined as a potential difference producing a change in energy of 1 joule when 1 coulomb is moved across it.

Electric circuits

The flow of electric current in circuits is a critical concept. Consider a simple circuit, as in Figure PH51. An electric current flows from positive to negative and lights the lamp. However, as electrons are the only mobile form of charges in a conductor, this current is actually formed by a movement of electrons in the opposite direction.

Ohm's law

Electrical resistance is the electrical property of a conductor which opposes the flow of current through it. Electrical resistance is measured in ohms (Ω).

Ohm's law states that the current flowing through a resistance is proportional to the potential difference across it. In Figure PH52, the potential difference across the resistance $= V$ volts, the current $= I$ amps and the resistance has a value of $R\,\Omega$.

So

$V = IR$ volts

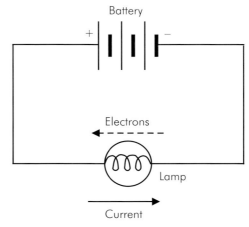

Figure PH51 Simple circuit

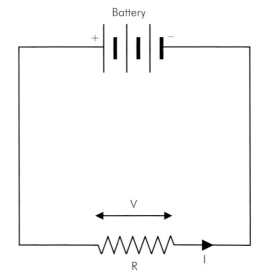

Figure PH52 Ohm's law

The flow of current through the resistance requires the expenditure of energy, which appears as heat. The power, P, dissipated as heat is given by

$P = VI$ watts

Substituting for I or V, this may become

$$P = I^2 R \text{ watts}$$
$$= V^2 / R \text{ watts}$$

For example, find the current flowing when a resistance of 250 Ω is connected across a 12 volt battery:

$$V = IR$$
$$I = V/R$$
$$= 12/250$$
$$= 0.048 \, A$$
$$= 48 \, mA$$

Direct current (DC) and alternating current (AC)

The terms DC and AC are normally used to describe the electricity supply to a circuit or system, and are applied to either voltages or currents.

DC describes current which only flows in one direction (i.e. the polarity always remains the same). Generally DC is supplied by a battery (or power adaptor), and if the current supplied is plotted against time it will give a graph as shown in Figure PH53a.

AC describes a supply in which the current reverses direction cyclically. If the current is plotted against time the sinusoidal curve shown in Figure PH53b is produced. AC is the normal mains supply, and has this form because of the way in which electricity is generated and distributed. An AC voltage is described by its amplitude (peak value) and frequency. The amplitude of mains voltage in the UK is 340 V, and it has a frequency of 50 Hz.

Usually mains voltage is quoted as 240 V, which is the *root mean square* (RMS) value. The RMS value for an AC voltage is the DC voltage or current which would have the same heating effect. This is used to compare AC and DC because the heating and lighting effects (power dissipation) of a current are not dependent on the direction of flow. It is obtained mathematically by squaring the value of the voltage/current, averaging this squared value over time and then taking the square root value.

AC currents and voltages are important because they can be used to carry information. In this case they are usually referred to as signals. The properties of signals measured and generated in the body, *biological potentials*, are discussed in more detail in Section 4, Chapter 2 (pages 794–5). Often electrical currents and signals are a combination of DC and AC (see Figure PH53c).

Impedance and reactance

The response of many circuit elements to DC and AC can be very different. Some devices may have a very low ability to resist the flow of AC but offer a high resistance to DC, or vice versa (see below).

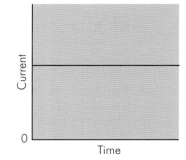

(a) DC

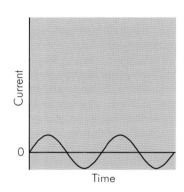

(b) AC

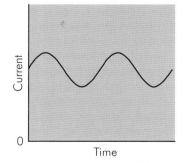

(c) DC and AC combined

Figure PH53 (a) Direct current (DC); (b) alternating current (AC); (c) DC with AC superimposed

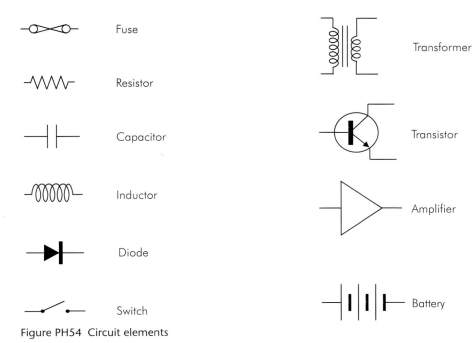

Figure PH54 Circuit elements

- **Resistance** is a measure of a device's ability to resist DC current. It is represented by R and measured in ohms.
- **Reactance** describes a device's ability to resist the flow of AC. The reactance of a device will be dependent on the frequency of AC applied. It is normally represented by X and is measured in ohms.
- **Impedance** for a device is obtained by mathematically combining its reactance and resistance. It is normally represented by Z and is measured in ohms.

$$Z = \sqrt{R^2 + X^2}$$

Note that impedance will also vary with frequency, because of the reactive component.

Circuit elements

Figure PH54 shows some symbols representing circuit elements that are commonly encountered. The properties of some of them are outlined below.

Resistance

Resistance opposes the flow of both AC and DC alike. A resistor in a circuit can be used to reduce currents or voltages. Often multiple resistors are used in a circuit. These can be combined in order to calculate the values of currents and voltages produced in different parts of the circuit.

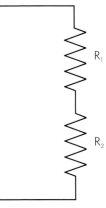

Figure PH55 Combination of series resistances

Series resistances

A series arrangement is 'end to end'. This is shown in Figure PH55. Combination of these values is by simple addition. Thus to calculate total resistance R_T, where $R_1 = 5\,\Omega$ and $R_2 = 3\,\Omega$

$$R_T = R_1 + R_2$$
$$= 8\,\Omega$$

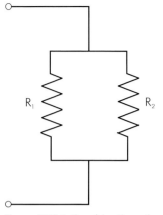

Figure PH56 Combination of parallel resistances

Parallel resistances

A parallel arrangement is 'side by side' and is shown in Figure PH56. For $R_1 = 5\ \Omega$ and $R_2 = 3\ \Omega$, the total resistance R_T is given by

$$1/R_T = 1/R_1 + 1/R_2$$
$$= 1/5 + 1/3$$
$$= 8/15$$

Thus $R_T = 1.9\ \Omega$.

Wheatstone bridge circuit

This circuit consists of a ring of four resistances supplied by a DC voltage across diagonally opposite corners of the ring A and C (Figure PH57). The values of the resistances are balanced using a variable resistor R_1, such that points B and C are at exactly the same potential. This occurs when

$$R_1/R_3 = R_2/R_4$$

When this condition is fulfilled, if a galvanometer, G, is connected between B and D no current will be detected and the bridge is *balanced* or *zeroed*. The bridge circuit is very sensitive to any variation in the value of the resistances, and if one of them changes a current will be detected on G.

The circuit is applied by using a strain gauge as one of the resistances (R_2), e.g. as in a piezoresistive pressure transducer. The pressure to be measured alters the resistance of the strain gauge such that the bridge circuit registers a current in G.

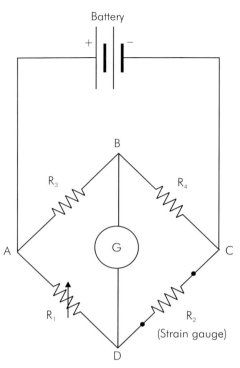

Figure PH57 Wheatstone bridge circuit

Capacitance

Capacitance describes the property of a device enabling it to store electric charge. A capacitor consists of two conducting plates separated by a thin layer of insulating material (or dielectric). When a voltage is applied across the plates, there is an initial surge of current as charge moves onto the plates, but when the plates have become charged no more current flows. Figure PH58 shows a capacitor charging circuit and the current and voltage changes occurring when the switch is closed. The amount of charge stored depends on the size of the capacitance, which is measured in farads (F). This in turn depends on the size of the capacitor plates, the separation of the plates and the dielectric material used. The physical size of a capacitor depends on the materials used and the working voltage, but a capacitance of 1 farad would be impractical in most circuits, being the size of a briefcase, and thus more practical units of microfarads (μF) and picofarads (pF) are used.

The charge (Q) stored can be calculated given the value of the capacitance (C) and the voltage (V) applied across the capacitor plates:

$$Q = CV \text{ coulombs}$$

(a)

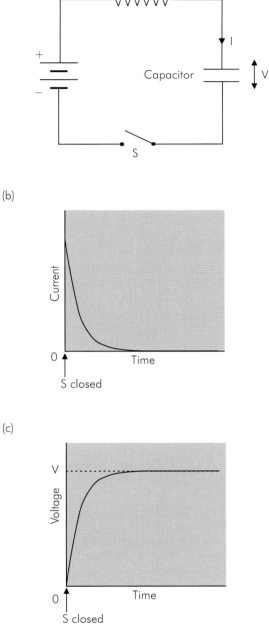

(b)

(c)

Figure PH58 Capacitance: (a) capacitor charging circuit; (b) current and (c) voltage changes that occur when the switch is closed

In a circuit a capacitor has the useful property of being able to *pass* AC signals, since electrostatic forces between the capacitor plates transmit AC current changes, but to *block* DC, since there is no direct contact between the plates. The resistance of a capacitor (to DC) is therefore very high since it is effectively an open circuit. However the reactance of a capacitor (to AC) is low and decreases with frequency. This enables it to be used to bypass unwanted AC signals to earth in cases of electrical interference. The frequency dependence of capacitors also means that they are useful components in filters.

Parallel capacitors

Parallel capacitors are shown in Figure PH59. Combination of these values is by simple addition. Thus to calculate total capacitance C_T, where $C_1 = 16\ \mu\text{F}$ and $C_2 = 32\ \mu\text{F}$:

$$C_T = C_1 + C_2$$
$$= 16 + 32$$
$$= 48\ \mu\text{F}$$

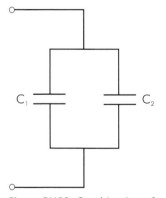

Figure PH59 Combination of parallel capacitors

Series capacitors

Figure PH60 shows series capacitors of value $C_1 = 16\ \mu\text{F}$ and $C_2 = 32\ \mu\text{F}$. To calculate the total resistance C_T:

$$1/C_T = 1/C_1 + 1/C_2$$
$$= 1/16 + 1/32$$
$$= 3/32$$

Thus, $C_T = 10.7\ \mu\text{F}$.

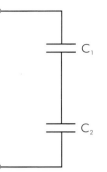

Figure PH60 Combination of series capacitors

Inductance

An inductor is made by forming a conductor into coils, which are often wound around a core (or *former*) of ferrous material. This construction has the effect of producing a concentrated magnetic field through the axis of the inductor and around it, whenever a current flows (Figure PH61).

When a voltage is applied across the terminals of an inductor, current does not flow immediately but increases slowly in step with the build up of the magnetic lines of force. Similarly, if the voltage is switched off, the current does not fall to zero immediately but dies down slowly, since as the magnetic field collapses it maintains the current flow for a while (Figure PH62).

The build-up and collapse of the magnetic field around an inductor tends to slow down changes in current flow, whenever the applied potential difference varies. The behaviour of inductances in an electrical circuit is thus analogous to the inertial effect of masses in a mechanical system. The unit of inductance is the henry (H).

An inductance has a relatively low resistance to DC, simply equal to that of the coils of wire. However, when AC is applied to an inductance, the continually varying current meets a comparatively high reactance. The reactance of an inductor increases with frequency. Inductors therefore tend to *block* AC but *pass* DC.

Inductances are used as components in filters and to 'smooth out' spikes and surges in power supplies.

Defibrillator circuit

A circuit using both capacitance and inductance is the defibrillator circuit. Its operation consists of two phases, *charging* and *discharging*. These phases are controlled by the switch S_1.

When charging (Figure PH63a) S_1 connects the capacitor to the DC power supply, which charges it to deliver

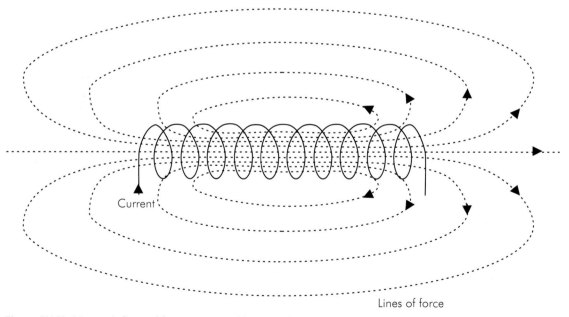

Current

Lines of force

Figure PH61 Magnetic lines of force generated by an inductance

(a)

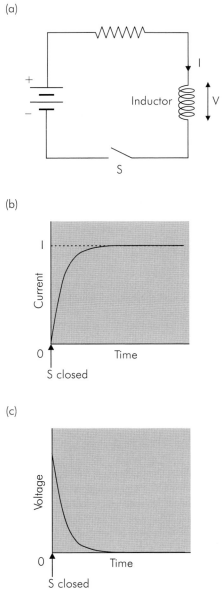

(b)

(c)

Figure PH62 Inductance: (a) circuit; (b) current and (c) voltage changes when the switch is closed

(a) Defibrillator charging

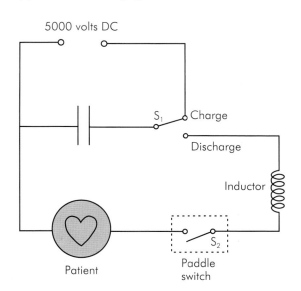

5000 volts DC

(b) Defibrillator discharging

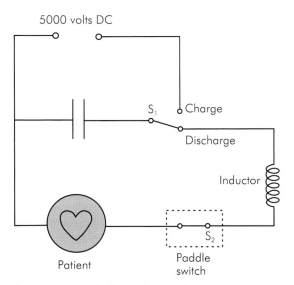

5000 volts DC

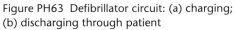

Figure PH63 Defibrillator circuit: (a) charging; (b) discharging through patient

the required amount of energy or number of joules set by the operator. The energy stored by a charged capacitor depends on its capacitance (C) and the applied voltage (V), since

Energy stored $= 1/2\,C V^2$ joules
For $C = 100\,\mu F$ and $V = 2000\,V$:
Energy stored $= 0.5\,(100 \times 10^{-6})(2000)^2$
$= 200\,J$

On discharge (Figure PH63b) S_1 connects the capacitor to the patient circuit, which enables the stored charge to be delivered to the patient via the switch (S_2) on the paddles. The inductor (L) in the discharge circuit has the effect of slowing down and spreading out the delivered pulse of energy to the myocardium, which makes it more effective than the shorter sharper spike waveform that would be delivered without the inductance.

Transformer

A transformer consists of two inductors wound around the same former. The close physical relationship between the two coils means that current changes in one circuit (the primary winding) will induce currents in the second coil (the secondary winding) via the coupling effect of the magnetic field (Figure PH64). The degree of coupling will depend on the number of turns in the primary winding (N_1) and the secondary winding (N_2), and the quality of the former. If an AC voltage V_1 is applied across the primary, the voltage produced across the secondary (V_2) will be given by

$$V_2 = V_1 \times N_2/N_1$$

A transformer can thus be used to *step up* or *step down* AC voltages in circuits. Transformers are commonly used in distributing the electrical power supply from the national grid to domestic users. An alternative use for transformers

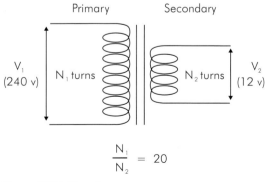

Figure PH64 Transformer

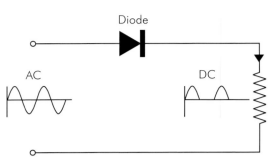

Figure PH65 Diode circuit converting AC to DC

is in transferring signals between circuits and in devices such as microphones or loudspeakers.

Diode

A diode is a semiconductor (silicon or germanium) device which only enables current to flow through it in one direction. It is often used to convert AC to DC (Figure PH65) in order to provide a DC power supply from the AC mains. This is commonly found in the mains adaptors used as a substitute for equipment batteries. Diodes are also used in protective circuits and to process signals in measurement systems.

Transistor

Transistors are also semiconductor devices. These are used to amplify small current signals, enabling small electrical signals of a few microamps to be converted to much greater signals of tens of milliamps. The basic transistor consists of a tiny slice of semiconductor material with connections to three regions: base, collector and emitter (Figure PH66). A common configuration allows a small signal fed into the base to produce an amplified signal in the collector circuit. In the early days of transistor electronics a circuit would be constructed using a few separate transistors. In modern electronics many thousands or even millions of transistors may be incorporated into a single semiconductor *chip*, which in turn is simply a single component in a more complex device such as a computer.

Electrical safety

The hazards associated with the use of electrical equipment are:

- Electric shock – macroshock
- Electric shock – microshock
- Diathermy hazards
- Burns
- Fire and explosion

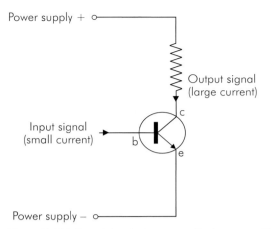

Figure PH66 Transistor: b, base; c, collector; e, emitter

Electric shock (macroshock)

Electric shock (macroshock) occurs with the external application of a voltage to the skin, causing an electric current to pass through the body tissues. Commonly electric shock occurs from the AC mains supply.

The mains supply in the UK consists of a *live* line carrying the generated voltage (240 V RMS) and a *neutral* line, which acts as a return for the current supplied. The neutral line is earthed at the generator. In an intact mains circuit the current supplied in the live line is equal to the return current in the neutral line.

Electric shock occurs from the mains supply, when the body forms a circuit between the live mains line and a local earth connection or the neutral mains line.

- Earthed circuit – The local earth connection may occur via the floor or ground (Figure PH67). Alternatively earthing may take place by inadvertent contact with earthed metalwork such as an anaesthetic machine or operating table (Figure PH68).
- Isolated circuit – In the absence of an earth connection, an individual or circuit is said to be electrically *isolated* or *floating*. However, current can still flow if contact with an alternative return path such as the neutral supply line is made (Figure PH69).

The effects of electric current flowing through body tissues depend on the following factors:
- Whether the current is AC or DC
- The magnitude of the current
- The tissues the current passes through
- The current density

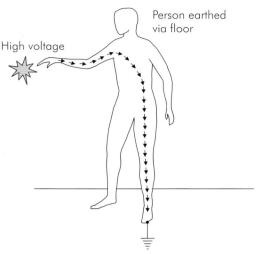

Figure PH67 Electric shock in person earthed via floor

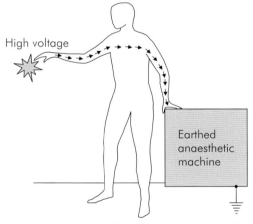

Figure PH68 Electric shock in person earthed by touching metalwork

- The duration of current passage
- Pre-existing disease

AC or DC current

DC produces a single muscle spasm on contact, which often throws the victim clear. Arrhythmias can be precipitated, but DC shock is also used to cardiovert arrhythmias. Prolonged exposure to low DC currents can produce chemical burns. AC will cause muscle spasm due to tetanic effects, which are maximal at mains frequency (50 Hz). When contact is made through the hand, muscle spasm may cause the individual to grip the contact uncontrollably,

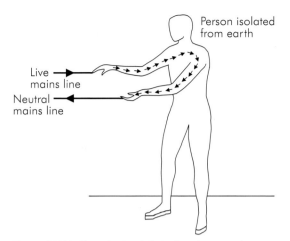

Figure PH69 Electric shock in isolated person by return through neutral line

prolonging duration of the shock. AC at mains frequency is also more likely to cause arrhythmias than higher frequencies. The risk of arrhythmias decreases significantly above 1 kHz, and at diathermy frequencies (>1 MHz) this risk is negligible. AC currents also cause localised sweat release, which lowers skin resistance and increases tissue current (see below). AC shock is about three times as dangerous as DC for the same magnitude of current.

Magnitude of the current
When an electric shock is received from the AC mains, different physiological effects are caused as the current increases in magnitude. These are summarised in Figure PH70.

Currents above 100 mA may not only disturb normal function in conducting tissues, but can disrupt epithelium and cell membranes. There may also be a direct heating

Current (mA)	Effects
0–5	Tingling sensation
5–10	Pain
10–50	Severe pain Muscle spasm
50–100	Respiratory muscle spasm Ventricular fibrillation Myocardial failure

Figure PH70 Physiological effects at different current levels in AC mains shock

effect on tissues, depending on current density (see below), duration of application and local cooling.

The main factors determining the magnitude of a current during an electric shock are:
- Voltage applied to the skin.
- Impedance (AC resistance) of the skin contact. Location of the skin, thickness and sweating can all affect skin contact resistance significantly. Skin contact resistance can vary between 1000 and 200 000 V.
- Impedance of the earth connection. When the earth connection occurs via the floor the impedance of footwear becomes important.
- Tissue impedance. This is usually low (<500 Ω).

Consider an electric shock received from the live mains wire (240 V) in an individual (Figure PH67) where the skin impedance is 2000 Ω, tissue impedance is 300 Ω and the earth contact resistance through shoes is 200 000 Ω.

If the current pathway lies through the right hand along the right arm, through the body and then via the feet to earth:

$$\text{Total resistance} = 1000 + 300 + 200000$$
$$= 201.3 \, k\Omega$$
$$\text{Current} = 240/201300$$
$$= 1.2 \, mA$$

Normally this current would not have any harmful effects in a person, although it may be discernable as a tingling sensation.

Tissues or organs through which the current passes
Currents passing through conducting tissues can disrupt normal physiological function. Consider an individual with one hand in contact with a live mains terminal and the other hand earthed through an anaesthetic machine (Figure PH68). The current pathway in this case is right hand and arm, chest, left arm and hand. The current flowing is given by:

$$\text{Total resistance} = 1000 + 300 + 1000$$
$$= 2.3 \, k\Omega$$
$$\text{Current} = 240/2300$$
$$= 104 \, mA$$

This current through the chest would not only deliver a painful shock but also carries a significant risk of inducing ventricular fibrillation or other arrhythmias, since it will pass through the heart.

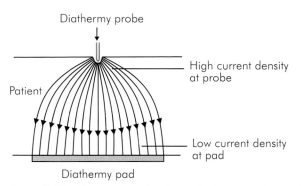

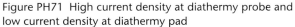

Figure PH71 High current density at diathermy probe and low current density at diathermy pad

Current density

This is obtained by dividing the total current flowing by the cross-sectional area that the current flows through. The effect of electric currents on tissues will be more dependent on current density in the tissue than on the total current passing through the tissue. If a current passes through a diathermy probe tip the current density will be much higher than in the case of the diathermy pad (Figure PH71). Thus tissue is burnt at the probe but not at the pad. If the pad is improperly applied, the contact surface area may be reduced and unwanted burns may occur. It is therefore important to ensure that diathermy electrode plates are properly and uniformly applied to the patient in order to avoid accidental burns.

Duration of current passage

The longer the duration of current flow, the more damage is caused to tissues in the current path, since the total amount of heat dissipated in the tissues depends on time.

$$\text{Power} = I^2R \text{ watts}$$
$$\text{Total heat} = I^2Rt \text{ joules}$$

where I = current (amps), R = resistance (ohms) and t = time (seconds).

A small DC current, which may not produce excessive heating of tissues locally, can still produce 'chemical' burns by an electrolytic effect.

Pre-existing disease

The presence of ischaemic heart disease in a patient increases the likelihood of problems such as arrhythmias.

Prevention of electric shock (macroshock)

Macroshock is prevented by a number of measures, including the design of equipment and circuits and the use of suitable footwear.

Equipment design

Equipment should be designed to suitable specifications. Different classes of equipment are specified for the medical working environment, and for use in different applications. The safety specifications may refer to the risk of electric shock, as follows:
- Class I – earthed
- Class II – double-insulated but not earthed
- Class III – low voltage (<24 V), battery-powered

Earth circuits

These are designed into equipment in order to reduce risk of electric shock and reduce interference. Earth connections reduce the risk of electric shock by maintaining exposed metalwork at zero potential. Such metalwork cannot then deliver an electric shock current if inadvertently contacted. However, such earth connections may also increase the risk of shock if an individual is already in contact with a high voltage, since contact with earthed metalwork can then complete the circuit (Figure PH68).

Earth connections can also provide a discharge pathway for static charges or leakage currents, which reduces the risk of **microshock**. Poor design of earth circuits, however, can actually generate leakage currents, which can act as a source of microshock. This occurs where multiple earth connections are used, each connection being at a slightly different potential, causing small currents to flow through earth circuits or patient.

The optimum earth circuit connects all earth circuits to earth at a single point via a good-quality contact. Earth casing or shielding around conductors carrying high-frequency AC reduces both the transmission and pick-up of interference signals, particularly in the case of high frequencies. Coaxial cables are often used, with an earthed outer conductor surrounding and screening an inner wire in sensitive circuits.

Isolated patient circuit

An option most commonly used is the isolated patient circuit, in which there is no earth connection to the patient. Faulty or obsolete apparatus may form an unwanted earth

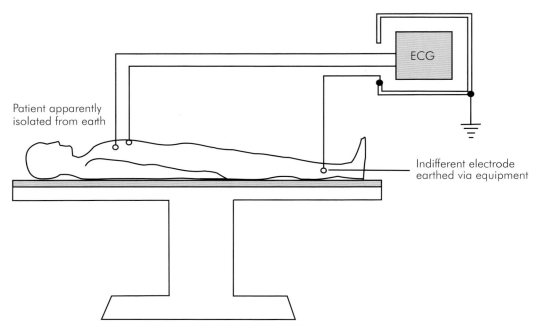

Patient apparently
isolated from earth

Indifferent electrode
earthed via equipment

Figure PH72 Unwanted earth connection via indifferent ECG electrode

connection via an indifferent ECG electrode, which can lead to macroshock and microshock risk (Figure PH72).

Leakage currents

This term refers to small electric currents ($<500 \ \mu A$) which arise unintentionally. These currents may originate through faulty equipment, faulty components, faulty earth connections or the accumulation of static charges. Such currents can either pass or 'leak' down to earth through a designed safety circuit (e.g. earth connection, antistatic shoes) or may flow through an unintentional pathway, creating a risk of microshock.

Isolating transformer

This system supplies all equipment attached to the patient via a transformer so that no equipment associated with the patient is directly connected to the mains.

Circuit breaker

This is a sensitive mains switch which operates to disconnect the mains whenever abnormal currents are detected due to dangerous equipment faults or the occurrence of an electric shock.

Suitable footwear

Footwear impedance should be designed to isolate the wearer from earth. The impedance should be high enough to prevent large current passing to earth (avoiding electric shock) in case of contact with a high-voltage source, but low enough to allow a leakage current to earth to prevent the wearer and clothing from accumulating a static charge. Such shoes normally have an impedance of between $100 \ k\Omega$ and $1 \ M\Omega$.

Ingress protection rating

Electrical equipment has safety information affixed to it to provide the user with information about which environments it is safe to use in. One such rating is the ingress protection (IP) rating. This is in the form 'IPxx', where x is a single-digit classification as shown in Figure PH73. The first digit indicates the resistance ingress by solid objects and the second digit the resistance to ingress by liquids. The higher the number, the better the protection. A third digit is occasionally used to indicate the resistance to impact. If ingress to solids has not been classified for a particular device then the first character will remain as x, for example in IPx3. This system is complementary to the electric insulation classification also denoted on the equipment ID plate.

	Solids protected against	Fluids protected against
0 (or x)	No protection	No protection
1	Solid objects up to 50 mm^2	Vertically falling drops of water
2	Solid objects up to 12 mm^2	Direct sprays of water up to 15 degrees from vertical
3	Solid objects up to 2.5 mm^2	Direct sprays of water up to 60 degrees from vertical
4	Solid objects up to 1 mm^2	Water sprayed from all directions – limited ingress permitted
5	Dust, limited ingress (no harmful deposits)	Low-pressure jets of water from all directions – limited ingress permitted
6	Dust total, no ingress	Strong jets of water – limited ingress permitted
7		The effect of immersion between 15 cm and 1 m
8		Long periods of immersion under pressure

Figure PH73 Ingress protection rating

Microshock

In microshock current is delivered internally to the myocardium, causing arrhythmias. The conducting pathway may be through an intravenous catheter or pulmonary artery catheter and its contained fluid. Figure PH74 shows a patient earthed via two circuits. One is via the pulmonary artery catheter monitor (E_2), and the other is via an indifferent ECG electrode (E_1). If the voltage at E_2 is greater than the voltage at E_1, even by 100 millivolts, then a leakage current may be generated, great enough to cause microshock. The magnitude of currents required to produce ventricular fibrillation in microshock is in the order of 100–150 μA. This is much smaller than in the case of macroshock. Figure PH75 shows the use of a single earth point to remove the leakage current in Figure PH74.

Some potential sources of microshock:

- Central venous catheter
- Pulmonary artery catheter
- Temporary external pacemaker
- Oesophageal temperature probe in lower third of oesophagus
- Statically charged staff touching any of the above

Prevention of microshock

- Appropriate equipment in good order. Equipment specifications may refer to leakage current generation and the risk of microshock. For example: CF (cardiac, floating) – leakage <50 μA through cardiac connection; BF (non-cardiac, floating) – leakage <500 μA through patient connection with single fault.
- Suitable footwear impedance.
- Antistatic flooring.
- Isolated patient circuit – with no earth connection to patient (e.g. Figure PH75).
- Isolating capacitor in diathermy (Figure PH76).
- Optimum design of earthing circuits for equipment.
- Correct humidity in theatre.

Diathermy hazards

Diathermy uses high-frequency (0.4–1.5 MHz) currents to generate heat in the tissues during surgery. This is applied via a probe to produce coagulation and cutting effects. The most common risks in the use of diathermy are of unwanted diathermy burns, as well as the usual risks of electric shock associated with the use of any electrical equipment. In addition, diathermy signals can cause interference in monitoring equipment and possibly indwelling pacemakers.

Prevention of diathermy hazards

- Use of isolated patient circuit.
- Use of isolating capacitor. In diathermy devices an isolating capacitor is used which effectively short-circuits high-frequency diathermy currents to earth, reducing the risk of unintentional diathermy burns. But at low frequencies (mains frequency and DC) the patient remains isolated, reducing the risk of macroshock and microshock (Figure PH76).
- Proper application of diathermy pad.

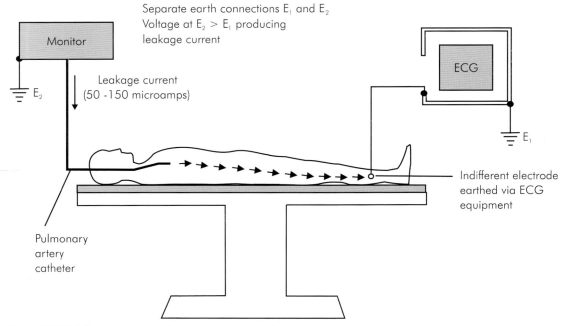

Figure PH74 Microshock via pulmonary artery catheter

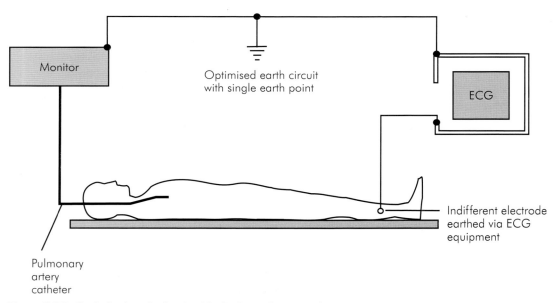

Figure PH75 Optimised earth circuit with single earth connection

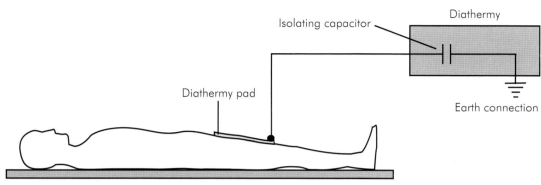

Figure PH76 Isolating capacitor in diathermy equipment

- Avoiding inadvertent patient contact with earthed metalwork.
- Use of bipolar diathermy. This form of diathermy uses a pair of probes, one to deliver the diathermy signal and the other to act as a return circuit. They are arranged as the arms of forceps, which restricts the current field to a small area surrounding the forceps tips. In this way no diathermy pad is required and no electric field exists in the peripheral parts of the patient's body. This reduces the risk of unwanted peripheral diathermy burns, and also decreases possible interference with monitoring equipment and pacemakers.

Electrical burns

There are several ways in which an electric shock can cause burns:

- Flash burns – This term describes the effect of arcing around the individual in high-voltage (>1000 V) shock, when electric arcing occurs to earth from the body or clothing.
- External burns – These may occur due to ignition of clothing or other inflammable materials around the individual, including gases or vapours.
- Tissue burns – These may occur at the point of contact with the high-voltage source or earthing point. They are localised and are due to the passage of high-density electric currents, sometimes with accompanying arcing.

Explosions and fire

In an operating theatre there is a risk of fire or explosion due to the ignition of gas mixtures. The mixture usually consists of a fuel with oxygen or another oxidising agent such as nitrous oxide.

Inflammable gas mixtures may simply burn, generating temperatures of several hundred degrees Celsius at atmospheric pressure.

Explosions are a much more violent reaction, generating a rapid rise in temperature to several thousand degrees Celsius, and a high-pressure shock wave which propagates outwards at speeds greater than the speed of sound.

For explosion or fire to occur the following are required:

- An inflammable agent. Examples include diethyl ether, cyclopropane, ethyl chloride and ethyl alcohol.
- An oxidising gas. These include oxygen, air and nitrous oxide.
- Inflammable or explosive concentrations. Inflammable agents will only burn between flammability limits in different oxidising gases, e.g. the concentration flammability limits for cyclopropane in air are 2.4% to 10%, while in oxygen the limits for cyclopropane are 2.5% to 60%. Explosions occur when the mixture reaches stoichiometric proportions. Stoichiometric concentrations occur when the proportions of inflammable agent and oxidising gas are the same as the ratios required by the chemical reaction. An excess concentration of inflammable agent or oxidising gas reduces the likelihood of explosion. The reaction for cyclopropane when it burns is:

$$2C_3H_6 + 9O_2 \rightarrow 6CO_2 + 6H_2O$$

Therefore a stoichiometric mixture consists of 2 parts cyclopropane to 9 parts oxygen, which is equivalent to an 18% concentration in oxygen or a 4.3% concentration in air.

- A source of ignition and activation energy. Examples are diathermy, electrostatic sparks and surgical lasers.

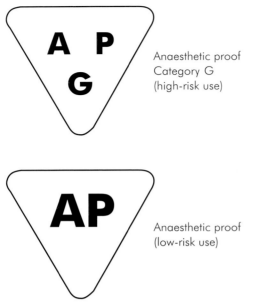

Anaesthetic proof
Category G
(high-risk use)

Anaesthetic proof
(low-risk use)

Figure PH77 APG and AP labels for equipment suitable for use with inflammable gas mixtures

Prevention of fire and explosion

- Use of non-flammable agents.
- Avoiding high-risk (5 cm radius) and low-risk (25 cm radius) zones with electrical equipment likely to generate sparks.
- Use of appropriate antistatic equipment, footwear and clothing.
- Awareness of equipment specifications (Figure PH77). The APG label refers to equipment which is safe to use within the high-risk zone, where oxygen and nitrous oxide may be the oxidising agents. The AP label is used for the low-risk zone, where anaesthetic gases and air mixtures provide the risk.
- Adequate air conditioning, with 5–10 air changes per hour.
- Appropriate scavenging system.
- Use of specialised equipment in the surgical field during laser surgery.

Ultrasound

Ultrasound scanning is becoming increasingly used in anaesthesia and critical care. It is applied in:

- Acquiring vascular access
- Performing nerve blocks
- Estimating cardiac output
- Detecting pleural effusions

Sound

Sound travels as waves composed of alternating regions of compression and rarefaction. The particles of the medium in which the sound wave is travelling move backwards and forwards about a mean position, in the direction of propagation of the wave (Figure PH78). A sound wave is therefore a longitudinal wave (compare this with the transverse nature of light waves, or surface waves) and requires a medium to propagate in (compare this with electromagnetic waves which can propagate through a vacuum).

The behaviour of sound waves is described by basic parameters and relationships that are common to all wave phenomena.

Frequency

The frequency (f) of a sound wave is the number of compression cycles which occur at any given point per second, and it is measured in hertz (Hz). The greater the frequency of a sound wave the higher its tone or pitch (e.g. in the musical scale middle C is 262 Hz, and top C on the piano is 4186 Hz). Some examples of frequency ranges for sound waves are shown in Figure PH79.

The audible frequency range varies according to age and species, and many examples of sound waves are generated outside the audible range for humans. The term *ultrasound* is used to describe sound waves at frequencies above the audible range. The ultrasound frequencies used in medical scanning are usually between 2 and 20 MHz.

Wavelength

Wavelength (λ) is the distance between two adjacent pressure peaks or troughs in a sound wave. It will vary with the medium that the wave is travelling in. The significance of the wavelength in ultrasound scanning is that detectable reflection of ultrasound waves will only occur from objects with dimensions much greater than the wavelength being used. Wavelength therefore becomes an important factor in determining the discriminative ability of an ultrasound scan. Detail in a scan will be greatest at shorter wavelengths (and higher frequencies – see below).

Velocity of propagation

Sound waves will travel through a given medium with a characteristic velocity of propagation (v). This will vary slightly with ambient conditions in the medium such as density, pressure and temperature. As with other wave phenomena, the velocity of propagation will be related

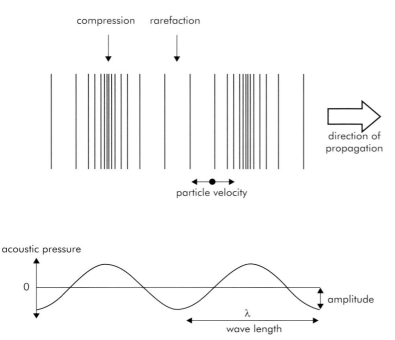

Figure PH78 Ultrasound wave, showing particle velocity and acoustic pressure

Quantity	Frequency range
Adult hearing	15 Hz to 20 kHz
Child hearing	15 Hz to 40 kHz
Bat hearing	up to 200 kHz
Medical ultrasound	2 MHz to 20 MHz

Figure PH79 Sound frequency ranges

to frequency (f) and wavelength (λ) by

$$v = f \times \lambda$$

The velocity of sound in air is 330 m s^{-1}, while in water it travels much faster at 1500 m s^{-1}. In clinical use, ultrasound passes through various tissues with different velocities of propagation. Some examples are shown in Figure PH80.

As noted above, the discrimination of detail in an ultrasound scan is dependent on wavelength, and will thus be greatest at high frequencies. Using frequencies of 10 MHz in soft tissues (assuming velocity of propagation, $v = 1540$ m s^{-1}) will give a wavelength of

$$\text{Wavelength, } \gamma = \frac{1540}{10\,000\,000}$$
$$= 1.5\,\text{mm}$$

Therefore objects with dimensions less than 1.5 mm will not be adequately visualised on the scan.

Acoustic impedance

As sound waves propagate through the particles (molecules) of a medium, the pressure peaks and troughs cause the particles to oscillate about their mean undisturbed position. These pressure changes and oscillations will gradually become attenuated as the wave progresses and its energy is dissipated. This process is analogous to the dissipation of electrical energy occurring when an electrical current passes through a resistance (or impedance) in a circuit. The local pressure increase produced in a sound wave is called the acoustic pressure (p), and it is equivalent to electrical potential in a circuit, while the particle velocity (v) produced by the wave is equivalent to electrical current. These parameters (p and v) are dependent on the medium, and their ratio represents a property of the medium known as its *acoustic impedance*.

$$\text{Acoustic impedance, } z = \frac{\text{acoustic pressure, } p}{\text{particle velocity, } v}$$

The acoustic impedance of a material describes how easily the substance attenuates sound waves passing through it.

Tissue	Velocity of sound (m s⁻¹)	Density (kg m⁻³)	Acoustic impedance (kg m⁻² s⁻¹) × 10⁻⁶
Gas	330	1.3	0.0004
Fat	1470	970	1.43
Blood	1570	1020	1.53
Muscle	1568	1040	1.63
Bone	4080	1700	6.12

Figure PH80 Velocities of propagation in different body tissues

It is related to the 'sponginess' of a substance, i.e. spongy materials will absorb sound energy more effectively. A measure of this property is the *modulus of elasticity* (E). A spongy material has a low modulus of elasticity.

A material's acoustic impedance is also related to its characteristic speed of sound (c) and its density (ρ), thus:

Acoustic impedance, $z = \rho \times c$

Some acoustic impedances for common tissues are shown in Figure PH80.

Reflection and acoustic impedance

Sound waves are reflected when they are incident on a smooth boundary between two media with different acoustic impedances (Figure PH81). This type of reflection is called *specular* or *mirror* reflection, since it is analogous to the reflection of light at a mirror. Specular reflection obeys the normal laws of reflection:

Angle of incidence = angle of reflection

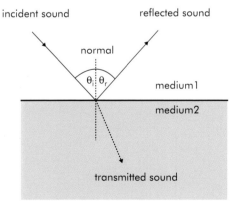

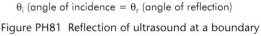

θ_i (angle of incidence = θ_r (angle of reflection)

Figure PH81 Reflection of ultrasound at a boundary

Some sound is transmitted across the boundary, while some is reflected. The amount of light transmitted depends on the acoustic impedances (Z_1 and Z_2). The percentage of sound reflected (R) at a boundary is given by

$R = I_R / I_i$

where I_i = incident intensity and I_R = reflected intensity.

$$R = \left[\frac{Z_1 - Z_2}{Z_1 + Z_2} \right]^2 \times 100\%$$

Consider the effect of differences in acoustic impedance on the reflected sound. If acoustic impedances differ by 10%, where $Z_1/Z_2 = 1.1$, then the amount of sound reflected will be $< 0.25\%$. However, when $Z_1/Z_2 = 10$, the amount of reflected sound is $> 80\%$. Acoustic impedances are therefore important in ultrasound scanning, for the following reasons:

- In order to obtain efficient transmission of sound from the ultrasound probe to the tissues, *matching* of acoustic impedances must be obtained by the use of appropriate gels, otherwise most of the sound energy is reflected from the boundary between probe and tissues.
- Since objects are only visualised by their reflected ultrasound, those objects with the greatest *mismatch* in acoustic impedance at their boundaries will show up brightly. Thus boundaries between different soft tissues will not be as bright as those between soft tissue and air, or soft tissue and bone.
- When there is a significant mismatch in acoustic impedance at a boundary between tissues most of the incident ultrasound is reflected, leaving a *shadow* behind the boundary or object. Common examples are bone surfaces or air spaces. Calculation of the reflected ultrasound shows that at a boundary between soft tissue and bone 30–40% of the incident ultrasound is

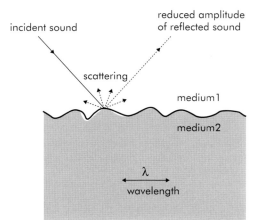

Figure PH82 Non-specular reflection of ultrasound at a boundary

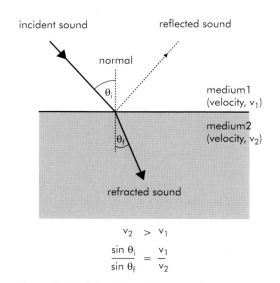

Figure PH83 Refraction of ultrasound

reflected, while at a boundary between soft tissue and air 99.99% reflection occurs. Thus the shadow created by an air-filled target is denser than that distal to a bony target.

Scatter

When sound waves are incident on objects or surface irregularities with dimensions comparable to or less than the wavelength, the sound waves are not reflected whole-sale as in specular reflection, but are scattered. This has the effect of reducing or attenuating the sound intensity without producing an image of a boundary or object. This is sometimes referred to as *non-specular* reflection (Figure PH82).

Refraction

When ultrasound is transmitted across a boundary between tissues the transmitted ultrasound is deviated from its original course. This is due to refraction. The devi-ation can be measured by the angle of refraction, which is dependent on the ratio of velocities of propagation in the two media. This phenomenon is analogous to the refrac-tion of light and obeys the same law, Snell's law:

$$\frac{\sin \theta_i}{\sin \theta_r} = \frac{\text{velocity of sound in medium 1}}{\text{velocity of sound in medium 2}}$$

Refraction effect in ultrasound scanning can lead to *focus-ing* effects behind fluid-filled objects (Figure PH83).

Power and acoustic intensity

The instantaneous energy content of a sound wave at any particular point in the wave is dependent on the kinetic energy and potential energy of the particles at that point. It is more meaningful to consider the power (P) generated by the sound wave, which is energy per second given to the medium particles (measured in joules per second = watts). By electrical analogy:

Acoustic power, P = acoustic pressure (p)
$$\times \text{particle velocity } (v)$$

A quantity used to compare effects of a sound wave on tissues is the acoustic intensity (I), where acoustic inten-sity is the power passing through unit cross-sectional area of tissue. In practice acoustic intensity is measured in milliwatts per square millimetre (mW mm^{-2}). Ultra-sound scanning is associated with acoustic intensitites of <1.0 mW mm^{-2}.

Acoustic intensities in an ultrasound field are compared using the logarithmic decibel (dB) scale:

$$\text{Change in acoustic intensity} = 10 \log_{10} \frac{I_1}{I_2} \text{dB}$$

Thus a reduction in acoustic intensity by 50% is referred to as a 3 dB loss in intensity.

Attenuation of sound-wave intensity

The intensity of sound waves in a scanned field varies throughout the field, and is generally reduced with increasing distance from the probe. The sound intensity is decreased by various mechanisms. These include:

- Absorption by tissues – which is dependent on frequency and accounts for most of the attenuation
- Reflection of the beam
- Scatter
- Divergence of the beam due to its not being perfectly parallel-sided

Averaged intensity units

When estimating the exposure of tissues to ultrasound energy it is useful to calculate an average value for acoustic intensity. Ultrasound fields produced when scanning patients are generated by pulses from the probe. The acoustic intensity in the tissues is therefore not constant in time, and neither is the acoustic pulse amplitude constant over the scanned field. Thus, in order to obtain a practical value, the peak acoustic intensity is averaged over both time and space (ISPTA: spatial-peak temporal-average intensity). The exposure of the tissues is then dependent on ISPTA and the duration of exposure.

Harmful effects of ultrasound on tissues

The clinical use of ultrasound is generally a safe procedure but ultrasound may damage tissues via its **heating effect**, **cavitation** and **mechanical effect**. The heating effect of ultrasound is the mechanism which has caused the most concern, and this is thought to be most significant in the dividing tissues of the fetus during its first 8 weeks. Prolonged temperature rises of >1.5 °C are considered to be hazardous to fetal tissues.

Heating effect

Absorption of ultrasound energy results in local increase in temperature. The factors which determine this temperature rise include:

- Total dose of ultrasound = mean intensity × duration
- Acoustic impedance
- Heat dissipation from the targeted area

These are important factors in determining the temperatures produced in tissues exposed to ultrasound. Thus bone is likely to suffer much higher temperature rises than soft tissues in an ultrasound field.

Safety levels

It has been estimated that temperature rises of more than 1 °C may be produced in tissues by B-mode scanning, and higher temperatures during Doppler mode because of the continuous-wave nature of the ultrasound in Doppler mode.

Significant thermal effects due to ultrasound are not recorded as occurring at intensities below $1 \, \mathrm{mW \, mm^{-2}}$ for unfocused ultrasound or below $10 \, \mathrm{mW \, mm^{-2}}$ for focused ultrasound. Duration of exposure for unfocused ultrasound is considered safe up to 500 seconds, and up to 50 seconds with focused ultrasound.

Cavitation

Cavitation refers to the production and excitation of gas bubbles in tissues exposed to ultrasound. Cavitation bubbles are mainly caused by the negative pressures produced by continuous-wave ultrasound (as in Doppler), but they are unlikely to occur during diagnostic scanning. Higher intensities, as used during therapeutic ultrasound by physiotherapists, may produce cavitation. Pre-existing gas bubbles or gas spaces in tissues (such as lung tissue) may also become excited by ultrasound waves and if violently excited may undergo collapse (collapse cavitation) with the generation of damaging effects and temperatures.

Mechanical effect

An object in a continuous-wave ultrasound field may experience a force due to incident sound waves on one surface, which is not balanced by an equal force on the opposite surface. It will therefore experience a net mechanical force moving it in the direction of travel of the ultrasound waves. Small objects such as red blood cells can be agglomerated in this way by Doppler-mode exposure.

Ultrasound scanners

Ultrasound imaging is achieved by the transmission of pulses of sound waves, each pulse containing 2–3 compression cycles. These pulses are emitted by a transducer (ultrasound probe) into the tissue field, and reflected from objects in the field back to the transducer, which also acts as a receiver.

Ultrasound transducers for generating and receiving ultrasound signals use the **piezoelectric effect**. This is a property of certain crystalline materials (commonly

(a)

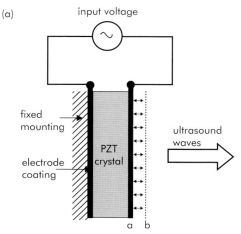

input voltage signal causes PZT crystal width
to oscillate between a and b, generating
ultrasound.

(b)

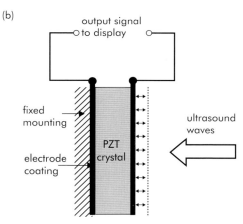

ultrasound waves cause PZT crystal width
to oscillate between a and b, generating
output signal.

Figure PH84 Piezoelectric effect: (a) transmitter,
(b) receiver

ceramic lead zirconate titanate, PZT) in which application of a voltage across opposite faces of a crystal causes
change in the width of the crystal. The crystal can thus
be used as an emitting transducer to produce ultrasound
from an electrical input signal (Figure PH84a).

The reciprocal effect can be applied to use the same
crystal as a receiving transducer, since sound waves incident
on the exposed surface of a crystal will cause a small change
in its dimensions, resulting in the production of a voltage
across its width (Figure PH84b).

Ultrasound scanning can be used in different modes.

A-mode

This scan mode is the most basic type, and simply detects
the range of a tissue boundary from the transducer. It
displays the reflected ultrasound pulses from a single
line scan on a time axis (Figure PH85). Its main advantage is that it can accurately give the time delay between
reflected pulses (hence distance between tissue boundaries/
thickness of fluid layer). In addition, reflected pulse amplitudes can give an idea of the acoustic attenuation of tissue
layers. This is not a particularly useful mode in clinical
practice.

B-mode

This scan mode extends the A-mode to two dimensions to
display the reflecting surfaces over a 'slice' of tissue. The
reflected pulse amplitudes are displayed using a brightness
scale. Surfaces producing high-amplitude reflections are
outlined as 'bright' or 'white'. This is the most widely used
mode in anaesthesia and can provide the most easily interpreted displays, which can be correlated with anatomical
cross sections (Figure PH86).

M-mode

This mode is used to detect the movement of reflecting
surfaces along a single scan line. It is the mode used in
cardiac work to monitor the movement of valves. M-mode
scanning is usually used in conjunction with B-mode scanning, the B-mode scan being used initially to select the best
single line for the M-mode scan.

The M-mode scan plots distance from transducer
on the vertical axis against time on the horizontal axis
(Figure PH87).

Doppler mode

When scanning in Doppler mode the velocity of moving
targets, such as the red cells in blood vessels, can be detected
and displayed using a colour scale on an M-mode scan. This
mode depends on a mechanism known as the Doppler
effect.

Typically blood flow moving towards the transducer
is displayed on a scale from red to yellow, with velocity
increasing towards yellow, while flow away from the transducer is displayed on a scale from dark blue to light blue.

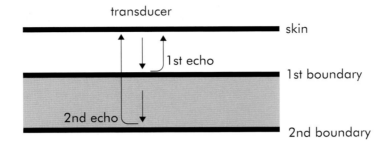

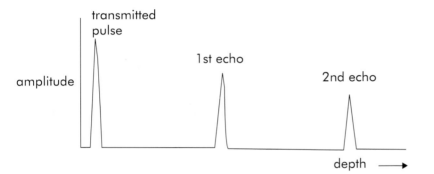

Figure PH85 A-mode ultrasound scan

It should be noted that these colours do not indicate the arterial or venous function of blood vessels. Usually venous flow velocities are too low to produce a display in Doppler mode.

Doppler effect

When ultrasound waves are reflected from a static target, the reflected wavelength equals the wavelength of the incident ultrasound wave (i.e. the reflected frequency equals the incident frequency, see Figure PH88a). If the target is moving towards the probe, the reflected sound wave peaks will be closer together than those in the incident wave. The wavelength of the reflected wavelength is thus shorter than the incident wavelength, and the reflected frequency is greater than the incident frequency (Figure PH88b). When the target is moving away from the probe, the opposite effect occurs, and the frequency of the reflected wave is lower than that of the incident wave (Figure PH88c). This alteration in frequency of the reflected ultrasound from

a moving target such as the blood in an artery gives rise to the characteristic sound signals during a Doppler scan. Should the direction of motion of the target be at right angles to the ultrasound beam, relative motion towards or away from the probe is minimised and a poor Doppler signal results. This change in frequency produced by motion of the target is known as the 'Doppler effect' and the difference in frequency between incident and reflected ultrasound waves is called the 'Doppler shift'. A classic example often quoted of the Doppler effect is the rise in tone of a train whistle as it approaches a listener, and its fall in tone as the train passes by and speeds away.

B-mode scanning for nerve blocks or vascular access

B-mode scanning irradiates a 'slice' of tissue with ultrasound using a probe. This probe consists of a linear array of crystal transducers, usually etched from a single block of PZT. The use of such an array enables the ultrasound beam to be swept electronically across the probe to

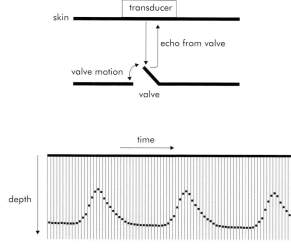

M-mode scan composed of serial time slots showing an ultrasound pulse echo from the valve as a black dot on the depth scale

Figure PH87 M-mode ultrasound scan

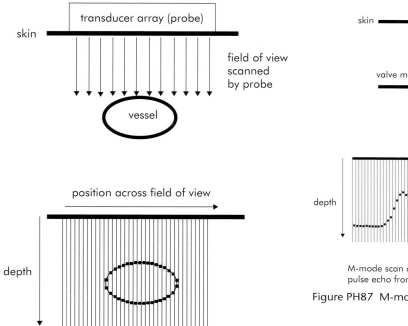

B-mode scan composed of serial pulse echoes as u/s beam is scanned electronically across transducer array (probe)

Figure PH86 B-mode ultrasound scan

produce the ultrasound field. Different types of probe can be used, varying in size, shape of field and frequency range. A common probe used in nerve blocks or vascular access is 28 mm wide, producing a parallel-sided field 1 mm thick. The depth of penetration can be adjusted depending on the machine and probe, but typically may range from 2 to 6 cm. This can be visualised as a field with the approximate dimensions of a credit card.

The usefulness of a B-mode scan will depend on its resolution of detail, the width of the field covered and the depth of penetration. The pulses of ultrasound produced will have a *mark–space ratio* which, together with the ultrasound frequency (and wavelength), the design of the probe and the power of the scanner, will determine the performance. The mark–space ratio is the ratio of the time spent at the high amplitude (mark) to the time spent at the low amplitude (space) of the signal. There is usually a trade-off between increasing frequency to obtain more detail in the scan and decreasing frequency to obtain more depth of penetration.

Interpretation of B-mode scans

When interpreting a B-mode scan a knowledge of the underlying anatomy is essential, and an awareness of limitations and artefacts is useful. A sample scan of the supraclavicular region is shown in Figure PH89, alongside a diagram of the corresponding anatomy.

Limitations and artefacts
- B-scan display – only represents a thin two-dimensional slice of tissue.
- Angle of incidence – maximal reflection occurs with reflection at angle of incidence = 0, i.e. when the ultrasound beam is at right angles to the target. Hence an injection needle will only be visualised if it lies within the 1 mm thickness of the ultrasound field and crosses the direction of the beam.
- Enhancement – occurs distal to fluid containing cysts or blood vessels, because of low attenuation within the target and refractive effects.
- Shadowing – occurs behind targets, either due to high reflection at the boundary (e.g. lung) or high attenuation (e.g. bone).

(a) Doppler effect – target stationary

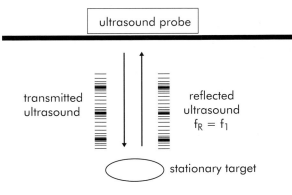

(b) Doppler effect – target moving towards ultrasound probe

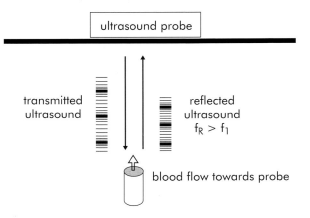

(c) Doppler effect – target moving away from ultrasound probe

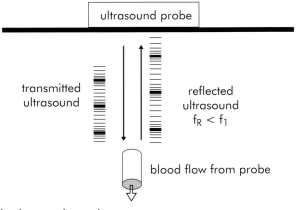

Figure PH88 Doppler-mode ultrasound scanning

(a)

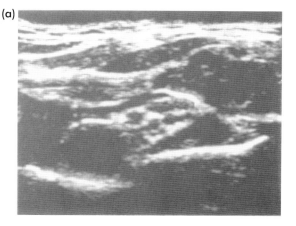

(b)

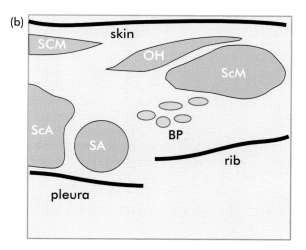

OH = omohyoid

ScM = scalenus medius

BP   = brachial plexus

SA   = subclavian artery

SCM = sternocleidomastoid

ScA = scalenus anterior

Figure PH89 Brachial plexus: (a) ultrasound scan;
(b) diagram of anatomy

Magnetic resonance imaging

Magnetic resonance imaging (MRI) was developed in the early 1970s and came into commercial use in the 1980s. It has the following advantages:

- Can display chemical differences between tissues
- Can display blood flow
- Can display 3D slices from axial, coronal, sagittal and oblique views

MRI scanning uses the interaction between the hydrogen molecules in body tissues and a superimposed magnetic field to image the tissues under examination. This does not involve the use of ionising radiation (x rays) or transmission of sound energy through the tissues.

Basic principles of MRI

The principle of MRI scanning uses the normal stable spinning state of nuclei in body tissues. The natural spin of the charged particles in a nucleus gives it magnetic properties causing it to behave as a microscopic bar magnet or magnetic dipole (Figure PH90). Application of a high-intensity external magnetic field causes all these microscopic magnetic dipoles to align with this external field. These nuclei are then disturbed by an electromagnetic radiofrequency (RF) pulse fired into the static magnetic field, which causes the tissue nuclei to acquire an added 'wobble' or *precession* to their original spin (Figure PH91a).

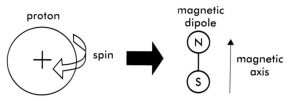

Figure PH90 Magnetic equivalence of a spinning proton

A gravitational analogy to this phenomenon is the spinning top, which can be disturbed from its stable vertical position, causing it to wobble or precess. Once the precession has been initiated, it will naturally die away or *decay*, as the spinning top realigns itself in a vertical position (Figure PH91b).

In MRI scanning, the precession of a nucleus has its own natural frequency, referred to as the *Larmor frequency*. This characteristic frequency depends on the structure of the nucleus and the magnitude of the magnetic field surrounding it. During precession the nucleus emits electromagnetic (radio) waves, which are received by the MRI scanner and can be processed to construct the MRI image. The RF pulse frequency can be set to the characteristic value for hydrogen nuclei (protons), enabling these nuclei

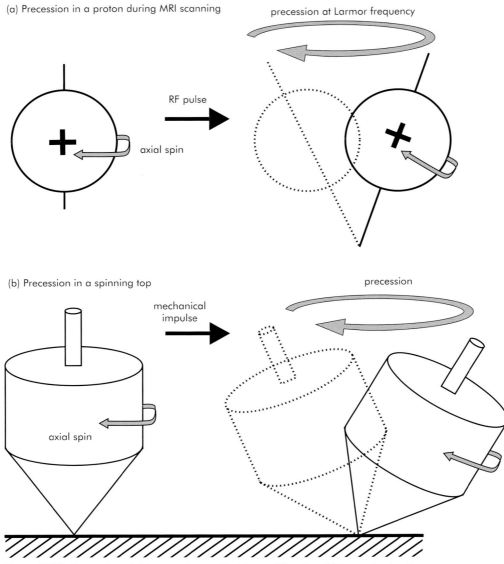

(a) Precession in a proton during MRI scanning

precession at Larmor frequency

RF pulse

axial spin

(b) Precession in a spinning top

precession

mechanical impulse

axial spin

Figure PH91 Precession: (a) in a proton excited by an RF pulse, (b) in a spinning top

to be selectively stimulated and visualised in the image. This is usually the case in MRI scanning, as hydrogen is the most abundant nucleus in tissues. This sequence of events is summarised in Figure PH92.

Changes in the magnetic field caused by the RF pulse

Some insight into how different tissues respond to the RF impulse can be obtained by considering the changes to

the magnetic field caused by the RF pulse. Reference axes are set by convention for the magnetic field in the MRI scanner (Figure PH93a). Initially all nuclei are aligned with the high-intensity magnetic field along the z axis (Figure PH93b). When disturbed by the RF impulse the axes of the hydrogen nuclei are all shifted by an angle α (Figure PH93c). This angle is the *flip angle* or angle of precession. The effect of the RF pulse is to add a transverse magnetic component to the magnetic field in plane xy at

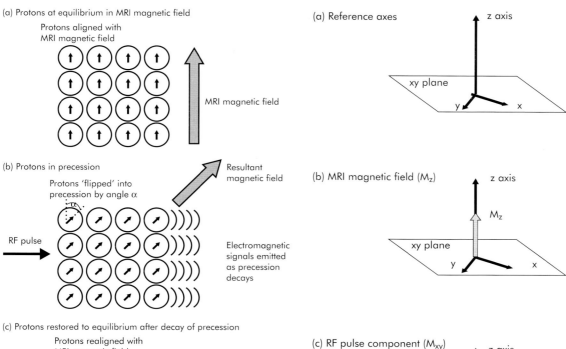

(a) Protons at equilibrium in MRI magnetic field

Protons aligned with
MRI magnetic field

MRI magnetic field

(b) Protons in precession

Protons 'flipped' into
precession by angle α

RF pulse

Resultant
magnetic field

Electromagnetic
signals emitted
as precession
decays

(c) Protons restored to equilibrium after decay of precession

Protons realigned with
MRI magnetic field

MRI magnetic field

Figure PH92 Alignment of protons in an MRI magnetic
field: (a) protons aligned at equilibrium; (b) precession of
protons and flip angle; (c) realignment of protons
following precession decay

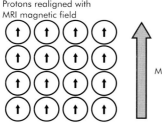

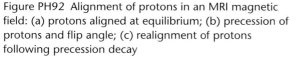

(a) Reference axes

z axis

xy plane

y   x

(b) MRI magnetic field (M_z)

z axis

M_z

xy plane

y   x

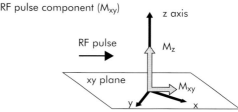

(c) RF pulse component (M_{xy})

z axis

RF pulse

M_z

xy plane

M_{xy}

y   x

(d) Resultant magnetic field (M_r)

z axis

M_r

xy plane

α

y   x

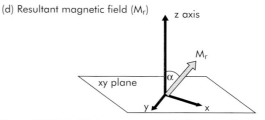

Figure PH93 (a) Reference axes in MRI magnetic field;
(b) MRI magnetic intensity vector (M_z); (c) RF pulse
transverse component vector (M_{xy}); (d) Resultant
magnetic field producing precession and 'flip' angle

right angles to the z axis (Figure PH93c). This produces a
resultant magnetic field, M_r (Figure PH93d) from vector
addition of the two components, a longitudinal component (M_z) and a transverse component (M_{xy}).

Relaxation time constants T1 and T2

After the RF pulse excites the hydrogen nuclei from their
equilibrium state into precession, the hydrogen nuclei
gradually *relax* back into their equilibrium state. As the
nuclei relax they lose the energy gained from the RF pulse
by transfer to the surrounding tissues and by emission of
Larmor-frequency electromagnetic waves. This relaxation
phase is important because it is during this phase that

Tissue	T1 (milliseconds)	T2 (milliseconds)
CSF	2160	160
Grey matter	810	100
White matter	680	90
Muscle	730	45
Fat	240	80

Figure PH94 Examples of T1 and T2 time constants for some different tissues in an equilibrium magnetic field of 1 T (tesla)

information leading to construction of the MRI image is collected. Individual tissues will produce different signals during the relaxation phase, and by varying the sequence of RF pulses applied differences between normal and abnormal tissues in the MRI image can be enhanced.

Relaxation is considered as consisting of two components:

- Relaxation of the transverse component, which is the decay of the precessional motion to zero. This process is an exponential process also contributed to by the loss of coherence or *dephasing* of the precessional spin of each nucleus. It is characterised by a time constant T2 (spin–spin time constant: the time taken to lose 37% of its maximum displacement value).
- Relaxation of the longitudinal component, or restoration of the longitudinal magnetic field. This is an inverse exponential process and characterised by a time constant T1 (spin–lattice time constant: the time taken to recover 63% of its original equilibrium value).

These T1 and T2 time constants vary for different tissues. Some sample times are shown in Figure PH94.

T1- and T2-weighted images

Different effects in the MR image can be achieved by weighting the image towards T1 or T2.

In a T1-weighted image, tissues with a long T1 time (e.g. CSF) will appear dark, while short-T1 tissues (e.g. fat) will appear bright.

In T2-weighted images tissues with long T2 (CSF) will appear bright, while short-T2 tissues (muscle) will appear dark. T1-weighted images usually show good contrast between tissues with clear boundaries. Fluids appear dark and fat appears bright, with other tissues intermediate greys. T1 weighting can enhance the contrast between grey and white matter compared to T2 weighting, because of the greater difference in T1 values as compared with

similar T2 times for the tissues. The *shorter* the T1 time the brighter the tissue on MRI image.

T2-weighted images show fluids as bright and other tissues as varying greys. Oedematous tissues appear brighter against normal tissues, and hence the appearance of pathological areas is often enhanced due to oedema. Abnormal collections of fluid can also be visualised more readily by using T2-weighted images. Note that, in contrast to T1 weighting, the *longer* the T2 time the brighter the tissue on MRI image.

Pulse sequences

The RF pulse used to excite the hydrogen nuclei or protons in the patient's tissues is actually a carefully selected and pre-adjusted sequence of pulses.

There are two main types of pulse sequence used, spin echo (SE) and gradient echo (GE). Both sequences can weight an MR image towards T1 or T2 to achieve the image quality required. SE sequence pulses produce the best-quality images, but use a longer-duration pulse sequence, which may take several minutes to obtain an image. GE sequencing is much more rapid because of a shorter pulse sequence, but image quality may be impaired by inhomogeneities in the main magnetic field.

The MRI scanner

An MRI image is obtained by placing the patient in the high-intensity magnetic field generated by a large-bore circular magnet. This magnetic field is generated within the magnet (in a tunnel) but an outer or *fringe* field exists which can cause interference with external apparatus or equipment. It is important that this magnetic field is free from inhomogeneities, which can impair the quality of the final image. Magnets used (Figure PH95) may be of the following types:

- Permanent – low field strength for their weight but non-uniform. No power consumption, but continual loss of field strength. Small fringe field.
- Resistive – good field strength and power to weight ratio. Power consumption heat generation (>30 kW).
- Superconducting – good power to weight ratio, with a high-quality field.

Magnetic field strength

Magnetic field strength is measured as the density of magnetic lines of force or magnetic flux density. The units of magnetic flux density are gauss (G) or tesla (T). The tesla is the SI unit.

$$1\,T = 10\,000\,G$$

	Permanent	Resistive	Superconducting
Strength (teslas)	0.06–0.2	0.1–0.3	0.5–2.0
Fringe field	small	small	large
Weight	up to 80 tonnes	2 tonnes	6 tonnes

Figure PH95 Magnet types and properties

The earth's magnetic field is approximately 50 µT (0.5 G). A simple bar magnet may produce a magnetic field of 5 mT (50 G). An MRI magnet produces a magnetic field intensity of 0.2–2 T, depending on clinical application.

MRI scanner coils

The tunnel inside an MRI scanner magnet is lined by systems of coils which perform the following functions.

- Gradient coils – superimpose magnetic gradients on the static magnetic field. These gradients provide a spatial reference framework which enables the scanner to pick out a 'slice' on the z axis and a point in the xy plane.
- Transmitter coils – transmit the RF pulse sequence.
- Receiver coils – receive the Larmor-frequency radio waves emitted during the relaxation phase. In some machines the same set of coils may be used for receiving and transmitting.

In addition there may be active shield coils around the outside of the scanner – these coils generate an opposing field to reduce the fringe magnetic field and radiation of RF signals from the scanner.

Biohazard effects of MRI exposure

Exposure to MRI scanning involves exposure to static and time-variant magnetic fields and radiofrequency (RF) electromagnetic waves. There are no known fatalities due to this type of radiation exposure. However, there are fatalities associated with MRI scanning due to hazards such as projectile injury from metallic objects in the MRI field, displacement of an aneurysm clip and pacemaker displacement or dysfunction. Some biological effects of exposure to RF or magnetic fields include:

- RF exposure may produce heating of tissues or heating of conductors (monitoring cables) in contact with the patient. Safety recommendations are designed to limit temperature rises to below 1 °C.

- Exposure to time-variant magnetic fields may produce peripheral nerve stimulation with associated discomfort, by inducing currents in the body.
- High-intensity static magnetic field exposure can produce mild sensory discomfort including vertigo, nausea and taste sensations. It is accepted that fields up to 2 T produce no harmful biological effects.
- There are no recorded effects on fetuses, pregnancies or fertility.

Although MRI scanning is considered to be a safe technique for patients and staff, the National Radiological Protection Board in the UK has issued guidelines for safety.

Light

The spectrum of electromagnetic radiation (Figure PH96) covers many different forms of radiation, ranging from low-frequency radio waves (as used in MRI) at the lower end of the spectrum to γ rays at the high-frequency end. Wavelengths of radio signals are hundreds of metres ($>10^2$ m), while those of γ radiation are in the order of 10^{-12} m or less. Light is a type of electromagnetic wave forming a narrow band of frequencies that are defined as those frequencies detectable by the human retina.

Light has a dualistic nature, and in some phenomena it is best considered as a stream of discrete particles or quanta of energy called photons. These phenomena include the action of light on photocells and photomultipliers, as applied in oximetry and spectrophotometry.

Transverse waves, light waves and light rays

A light wave can be visualised as being analogous to a surface wave on water occurring when a stone is dropped into a pond. The surface wave is formed by water particles moving up and down, and the shape of a wave as it moves across the surface is called a wavefront. The wave moves across the surface in a plane at right angles to the particle motion. This is called a *transverse wave*. The direction that waves travel in is often represented by a single straight line at right angles to the plane of particle motion giving rise to the wave. This is referred to as a *ray* (Figure PH97). Light waves are also transverse waves produced by the vibration of photons emitted from the light source (Figure PH98).

Wavelength of light

Wavelengths of light are normally quoted in nanometres (nm, 1 nm = 10^{-9} m), which have replaced the more

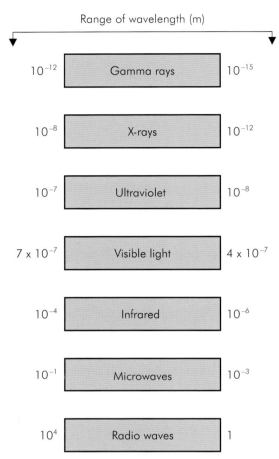

Figure PH96 Electromagnetic spectrum

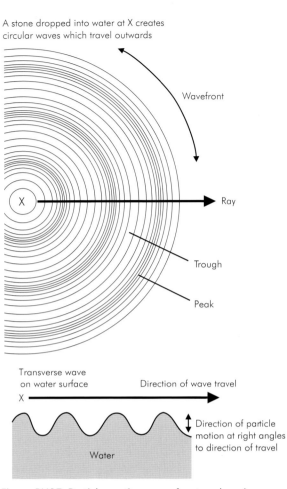

A stone dropped into water at X creates circular waves which travel outwards

Figure PH97 Particle motion, wavefront and ray in a transverse wave

traditional unit of the ångström (1 Å = 10^{-10} m). The lowest frequencies of visible light are dark red, with wavelengths of around 700 nm, while the highest frequencies visible are violet, with wavelengths of around 400 nm.

Speed of light

The speed of light in a vacuum is a fundamental constant in physics, which has a defined value of 299 792 458 metres per second. This value is now used to give the definition for the standard unit of length, the metre. The speed of light decreases with the density of the medium. Thus light travels more slowly in air and is even slower in glass.

Refraction of light

A consequence of the changes in the speed of light between different media is that the path of light is 'bent' when it travels across a boundary from one medium to another. Consider light travelling from air to glass, as shown in Figure PH99. The light path is represented by a 'ray' or line drawn at right angles to the wave front. As the ray crosses the boundary from air to glass it 'bends' towards the normal. When light passes from a dense medium to a less dense medium, its path is deviated away from the normal.

The refraction of the light can be quantified using two angles, the angle of incidence (i) and the angle of refraction (r). The deviation produced is dependent on the ratio of the speeds of light in air and glass (c_1 and c_2 respectively), which will be a constant.

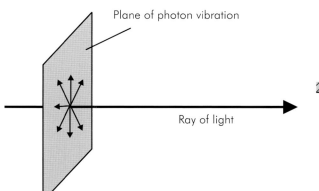

Figure PH98 Light ray, showing plane of photon vibration

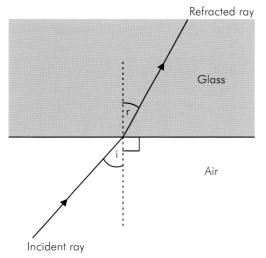

Figure PH99 Refraction of light

Snell's law states that for light travelling between two given media

$$\frac{\sin_i}{\sin_r} = \frac{c_1}{c_2}$$

The refractive properties of a medium are measured by its absolute refractive index (n), which is defined by

$$\text{refractive index} = \frac{\text{speed of light in a vacuum}}{\text{speed of light in medium}}$$

$$n = \frac{c}{c_1}$$

When considering light passing from air to a medium, the value of the refractive index relative to air is virtually the

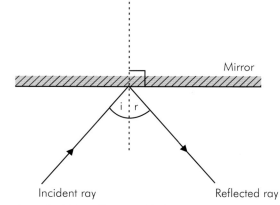

Figure PH100 Reflection of light

same as its absolute value, because the refractive index of air is 1.0003 (i.e. the speed of light in air is almost the same as in a vacuum). Snell's law then becomes

$$\frac{\sin i}{\sin r} = \frac{1}{n}$$

Refraction results in the apparent distortion of images and distances, when viewing objects in one medium from another. This is why a pool of water appears shallower than it actually is. Refraction is also responsible for the actions of lenses, including that in the eye. The refractive index for glass is typically 1.5, for water $n = 1.33$.

Reflection

When a light ray is reflected from a boundary between two media or from a surface (Figure PH100), the geometry is again defined by the angles made with the normal to the surface. In this case the angle of incidence (i) is always equal to the angle of reflection (r). Reflection is used in mirrors, and in the design of dish aerials or mirrors to focus light or other waves.

Total internal reflection

When light passes from a dense medium to a less dense medium (e.g. glass to air) Snell's law will only apply over a range of angles. This is because the angle of refraction is greater than the angle of incidence, the light being deviated away from the normal (Figure PH101a). As the angle of incidence increases, a value is reached when the angle of refraction becomes 90° (Figure PH101b). This value of the angle of incidence is called the critical angle (C). In this

(a) i < C

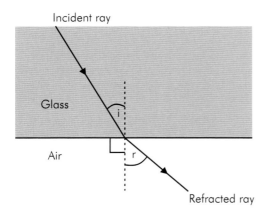

(b) i = C

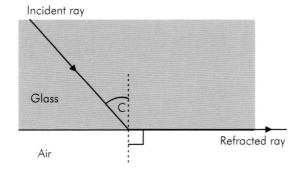

(c) i > C

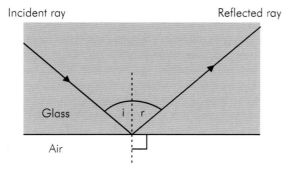

Figure PH101 Total internal reflection

case, applying Snell's law:

$$\frac{\sin C}{\sin 90°} = \frac{1}{n}$$

When the angle of incidence exceeds C, total internal reflection occurs (Figure PH101c). This is used in the construction of prisms to guide light in optical equipment, and also in the use of optical fibres to conduct light in fibreoptic equipment. The critical angle for glass is approximately 42°.

Polarised light

All electromagnetic waves, including light, are transverse waves. This means that the particle movement giving rise to the wave is in a plane at right angles to the direction in which the wave is travelling. Frequently the particle movement occurs in many different directions within the plane described. This is the case in light emitted by a high-temperature source such as a light filament or the sun, since it is emitted at random from the atoms in the source. This type of light is said to be *unpolarised*, and it can be considered to be a mixture of vertical and horizontal components.

Unpolarised light may be filtered so that only light with particle oscillation in a single direction (vertical or horizontal) is allowed to pass. The light is then said to be *polarised*. Light can be polarised by passage through different crystals (e.g. quinine iodosulphate, toumaline). Vertically polarised light can only pass through a crystal with its optical axis aligned vertically (Figure PH102). If such a crystal were then to be rotated through 90° (i.e. become horizontally aligned) it would only allow horizontally polarised light to pass.

Dextrorotatory (+) and levorotatory (−) substances

Many pharmacological compounds are optically active causing polarised light to rotate either clockwise to the right (+) or anticlockwise to the left (−). The optical activity of such substances can be investigated by using a combination of vertically aligned (polariser) and horizontally aligned (analyser) crystal filters (Figure PH103a). These in combination do not allow any light to pass. When an optically active substance is placed between the filters the vertically polarised light is rotated and some light passes through the analyser (Figure PH103b). The analyser is then rotated until the light passing through is once again extinguished (Figure PH103c). The rotation of the analyser must then

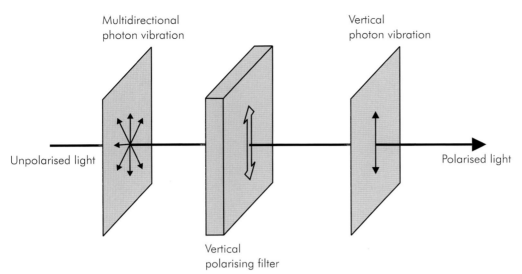

Figure PH102 Non-polarised light filtered to give polarised light

Multidirectional
photon vibration

Vertical
photon vibration

Unpolarised light

Polarised light

Vertical
polarising filter

match the rotation caused by the substance under test. For detail of optical isomerism see Section 3, Chapter 1.

Luminous intensity and the candela

It is required sometimes to quantify the luminous intensity or brightness of a source. This can be defined by the amount of light energy emitted per second (power) through unit solid angle (steradian) by the source, and is measured in candelas.

The candela is the luminous intensity of a source emitting light at 540×10^{12} Hz with an intensity of 1/630 watt per steradian.

Light transmission and absorbance (optical density)

When light passes through a substance some of the energy is absorbed. The absorption of light energy is dependent on the length of the path travelled and the absorptive properties of the substance. The absorption of monochromatic light (single wavelength) by a layer of solution or gas is used in absorption oximetry and spectrometry.

Consider the absorption of monochromatic radiation by a layer of substance. It is determined by a combination of two laws:

- **Lambert–Bouguer law** – When a layer of solution of known thickness (d), is transilluminated by monochromatic light, the transmitted light (I) is related to the incident light (I_O), by

$$I = I_O \, e^{-(ad)}$$

where (ad) is the *absorbance* or *optical density* of the layer of solution. This in turn is the product of its thickness (d) and the quantity (a) known as the extinction coefficient of the solution (Figure PH104). Thus, if the absorbance of the solution layer is 1.0, only 37% of the light is transmitted, but doubling the absorbance to 2.0 reduces the transmitted light to 13.5%.

- **Beer's law** – This states that for a solution, absorbance is a linear function of molar concentration.

Combining the above two laws gives:

- the **Lambert–Beer law**, which relates the transmitted light to both molar concentration and thickness of the solution layer by expressing the absorbance as:

$$\text{Absorbance} = \varepsilon c d$$

where

ε is molar extinction coefficient
c is molar concentration
d is thickness

To measure the concentration of a particular compound in a mixture, the mixture is transilluminated with monochromatic light at the wavelength where absorbance is maximal. The machine must be calibrated with a pure solution of the compound, and then the measured concentration can be calculated. Further details of this technique are given in Section 4, Chapter 2.

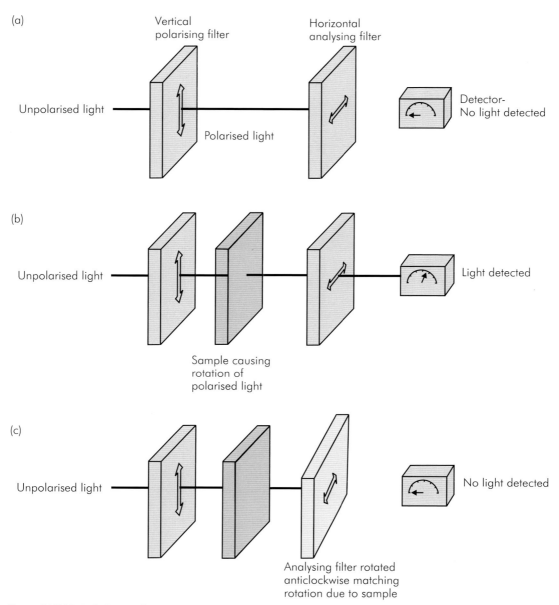

Figure PH103 Polariser and analyser filters set up to determine rotation by dextrorotatory (*d* or +) and levorotatory (*l* or −) compounds

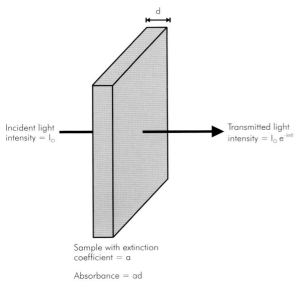

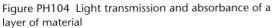

Figure PH104 Light transmission and absorbance of a layer of material

Lasers

Laser is an acronym derived from *light amplification by stimulated emission of radiation*, and is applied to devices which emit a special form of light radiation. Laser light has the following characteristics:

- It is monochromatic.
- All radiated waves are in phase.
- The light waves emitted do not diverge but remain in a narrow beam.
- High light energy intensities can be produced with a relatively low power source.

Stimulated emission

This describes the reaction when a high-energy atom is struck by an incoming photon. The high-energy-state atom is 'stimulated' to lose energy by giving out two light particles with the same phase and frequency. This process is called *stimulated emission* (Figure PH105a). These emitted photons can then each stimulate the further emission of photons by striking two further high-energy atoms. In this way, provided that a suitable population of high-energy atoms can be maintained, a cascade amplification process is set up, resulting in a high-energy light source emitting waves which are all in phase (Figure PH105b).

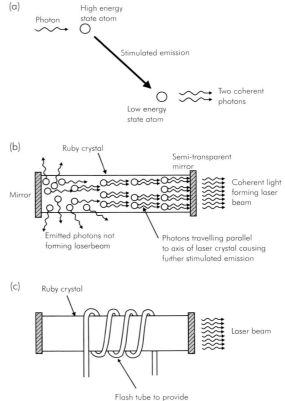

Figure PH105 Laser system, showing details of device

Laser construction

All lasers consist of three basic parts:

- A source of energy to raise the electrons from the ground state to an excited one (a process known as pumping).
- A suitable laser substance capable of stimulated emission.
- A system of mirrors to reflect light repeatedly backwards and forwards through the laser substance. This process amplifies the light many times over.

Figures PH105b and PH105c show simplified diagrams of a ruby laser. The pumping energy source is a flash tube, which feeds continuous or pulsed energy into the laser material to produce high-energy-state atoms. These undergo stimulated emission, producing photons which are then reflected backwards and forwards between the

Laser material	Application	Properties
Synthetic ruby	Early use in eye surgery	
Argon	Replacement for ruby laser in eye surgery. Used for retinal coagulation and repairing retinal detachment. Used for removal of birthmarks	Passes through vitreous and aqueous humour. Absorbed by haemoglobin. Also absorbed by pigmented skin. Can be transmitted by optical fibres for endoscopic application
Carbon dioxide	The most commonly used laser in surgery. Superficial surgery, removing thin layers of tissue at a time	Absorbed by water, therefore low penetration to <200 mm. Cannot be used endoscopically
Nd-YAG (neodymium yttrium aluminium garnet)	Coagulation and cutting	Not absorbed by water, therefore good penetration of tissues. Can be used endoscopically

Figure PH106 Properties of some surgical lasers

mirrored surfaces. The reflected photons in turn produce further stimulated emission, and an amplifying cascade is built up. At one end the mirror is partially transparent, allowing light to escape as a highly parallel coherent beam. This beam can then be focused to produce extremely high light power intensities.

Many substances can act as laser materials. The properties of some commonly used lasers in surgery are summarised in Figure PH106.

Laser safety

Lasers are classified according to their degree of hazard from class 1 (least dangerous) to class 4 (most dangerous). Domestic lasers (CD players, laser printers) are safe because of the wavelengths used and their low power. However, all surgical lasers are class 4, being inherently hazardous as they are specifically designed to damage tissue. Safety precautions when working with lasers include:

- Appropriate training for all staff.
- A designated suitably equipped area with all exposed surfaces matt-finished.
- All instruments with matt finish.
- No inflammable material in the vicinity of the patient or in the operating field.
- All theatre staff must wear protective eye glasses, and the patient's eyes and skin must be protected against stray laser light.
- The laser theatre must be well ventilated with a suitable smoke extraction system.

- Precautions against use of inflammable or explosive anaesthetic gases.

X rays

X rays are a form of electromagnetic radiation with wavelengths in the range 10^{-8} m to 10^{-12} m. The main properties of x rays in medical applications are their ability to penetrate tissue and their ionising effect. The latter represents a hazard in their use, but it is a property which is also used therapeutically in x-radiotherapy.

X rays are generated in an x ray tube, by bombarding a high-temperature anode with electrons generated by a cathode (Figure PH107). The electrons are accelerated in the tube using a high-voltage electric field. X ray machines are thus rated by the current and voltage that can be delivered: e.g. a portable x ray set may deliver 100 mA at 90 kV.

Radioactive isotopes and radiation

An element may exist in different forms due to variations in its nuclear structure. These different forms are called isotopes of the element. Each isotope will differ in atomic mass number but will possess the same atomic number. Some basic facts about the structure of an atom are:

- The nucleus consists of neutrons and protons and is orbited by electrons.
- The atomic mass number is equal to the number of neutrons plus the number of protons in the nucleus. It is the nearest integer to the atomic weight.

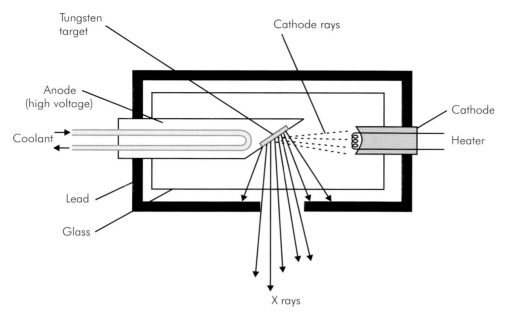

Figure PH107 X ray tube

Element		Atomic number	Neutrons	Atomic mass number	Stability
Hydrogen	^1_1H	1	0	1	stable
Deuterium	^2_1H	1	1	2	stable
Tritium	^3_1H	1	2	3	unstable
Carbon	$^{10}_6C$	6	4	10	unstable
Carbon	$^{12}_6C$	6	6	12	stable
Carbon	$^{14}_6C$	6	8	14	unstable

Figure PH108 Some of the stable and unstable isotopes of hydrogen and carbon

- The atomic number is equal to the number of protons in the nucleus, and determines which element is present.

Notation used to identify isotopes is as follows:

$$^{\text{atomic mass number}}_{\text{atomic number}} [\text{element symbol}]$$

Thus ^1_1H is the symbol for hydrogen.

Some isotopes are stable and retain their nuclear structure indefinitely, while other isotopes are unstable and decay spontaneously. Unstable isotopes are said to be radioactive, and they decay by emitting radiation. Some examples of stable and unstable isotopes are shown in Figure PH108.

Radioactive decay

Decay of a radioactive isotope involves the emission of nuclear particles from the substance, resulting in the formation of another isotope or another element. An example is the uranium series, which occurs when uranium decays. This series of reactions finally results in the formation of lead, but involves a chain of intermediate decay reactions. Some of these are illustrated in Figure PH109. Each of these reactions involves the emission of a specific type of particle with a characteristic mean

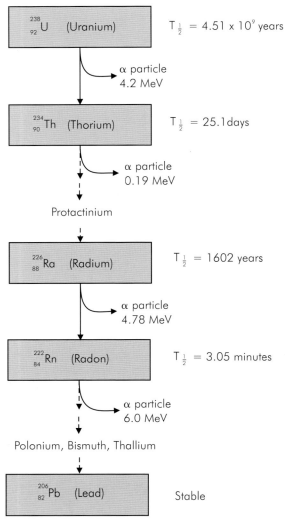

Figure PH109 Uranium series

energy level. Each reaction also has a particular half-life (see below).

The energy possessed by elementary particles (e.g. electrons or protons) is usually measured in electronvolts (eV). The electronvolt is defined as the change of kinetic energy occurring when a particle with a charge of e (the charge on an electron) moves through a potential difference of 1 volt.

$$1 \, eV = 1.602 \times 10^{-19} \text{ joules}$$
$$1 \, MeV = 1.602 \times 10^{-13} \text{ joules}$$

Radiation from radioactive isotopes

The types of radiation emitted from radioactive isotopes are:

- α **particles** – a combination of two protons and two neutrons (equivalent to a helium nucleus), e.g.

$$^{226}_{88}Ra \quad \rightarrow \quad ^{222}_{86}Rn \quad + \quad ^{4}_{2}He$$
$$\text{radium} \qquad \text{radon} \qquad \text{helium } (\alpha \text{ particle})$$

- β **particles** – an electron which is negatively charged, derived from a neutron splitting to give a proton and a high-energy electron. The creation of another proton in the nucleus will increase the atomic number of the atom and thus change the element present.

$$^{14}_{6}C \quad \rightarrow \quad ^{14}_{7}N \quad + \quad e^{-}$$
$$\text{carbon 14} \quad \text{nitrogen} \quad \text{electron } (\beta \text{ particle})$$

Sometimes an electron may be emitted from the nucleus with a positive charge, in which case it is called a positron.

- γ **radiation** – electromagnetic radiation with wavelengths $< 10^{-12}$ m, which is emitted during most nuclear reactions, usually following the emission of an α or β particle.

Decay half-life

The decay of a radioactive element from one isotopic form to the next form in its series follows an exponential decay curve, i.e.

$$N = N_0 \, e^{(-\lambda t)}$$

where N is the number of atoms of the element present at time $= t$, N_0 is the number of atoms present at time $= 0$, and λ is the decay constant for the element. λ is related to the decay time constant (K), for the element by

$$\lambda = 1/K$$

The half-life for the element ($T_{1/2}$) is the time for the mass of element to decay to a half of its initial mass, and is related to the time constant K by

$$T_{1/2} = 0.693 \, K$$

The half-life may have a value ranging from seconds to millions of years (Figure PH109).

Units of radioactivity

The activity of a radioactive sample is measured by the number of disintegrations occurring per second. The SI unit of measurement used is the becquerel (Bq), which is defined as

$$1 \text{ Bq} = 1 \text{ disintegration per second}$$

The curie is a traditional unit based on the activity of one gram of radium, where 1 curie $= 3.7 \times 10^{10}$ disintegrations per second $= 3.7 \times 10^{10}$ Bq.

Applications of radioactive isotopes

Radioactive isotopes are used in many applications clinically. These include:

- Measurements with labelled substances – chromium-51 in measurement of red cell volume
- Cancer therapy – use of yttrium-90 in pituitary tumours
- Diagnostic uses – imaging techniques with technetium-99 as in assessment of cardiac function

Measurement of exposure to ionising radiation

Exposure to ionising radiation can result in both short- and long-term sequelae.

The short-term effects of radiation exposure appear as the symptoms of acute radiation sickness. These are dose-dependent and include nausea, vomiting, anorexia, general lassitude and weakness, and can lead to death over a period of days or less. The long-term effects include an increased incidence of cancers and genetic defects in the population, which occur after a period of years. A dose of radiation can be measured by the effects it produces in different ways:

- Energy absorbed by irradiated air – The röntgen (R) is a unit used to measure x-radiation dosage. One röntgen is the dose of x-radiation giving 83.3 ergs of energy to 1 gram of air.
- Energy absorbed by body tissue – Radiation energy absorbed depends on the substance irradiated, and therefore the energy absorbed by body tissues will not be the same as that absorbed by air, even when exposed to the same dose of radiation. The SI unit of radiation dose absorbed by body tissues is the gray (Gy). One gray is the dose of radiation giving an absorbed energy of 1 joule per kilogram of soft tissue.

Description	Dose/time
Max permitted dose	5 mSv per year
Natural background dose	1.25 mSv per year
Dose causing nausea	1 Sv per few hours
Dose causing death within days	10 Sv per few hours

Figure PH110 Some estimated ionising radiation doses

Biological effect

Different types of ionising radiation provide different levels of biological hazard when absorbed. Thus even though the same amount of energy may be absorbed from different types of radiation, different sequelae may result. For instance, 200 kV x rays are less damaging than γ rays or β particles, and α particles are even more damaging in their ionising effect, by a factor of 10 or more. Therefore, to assess risk in exposure to ionising radiation, a unit of biological effectiveness is used. The SI unit of biological effectiveness is the sievert (Sv). One sievert is the radiation dose equivalent to 1 Gy of absorbed radiation from 200 kV x rays in terms of biological damage.

Thus if 1 Gy of radiation is absorbed from 200 kV x rays, the biological dose equivalent will be 1 Sv by definition. But an absorbed dose of 1 Gy from α particle radiation will have a dose equivalent to 10 Sv.

Biologically significant levels of ionising radiation have been estimated in terms of their acute effects and their effect on the incidence of cancer and genetic defects in the population. These are at best an estimate, since the rate of delivery of a given dose can vary as well as individual response. An average dose of 1 mSv per individual over a population is believed to increase the incidence of cancer by 13 and genetic defects by 8 per million of population during the following years. A whole-life exposure of 1 Sv is thought to reduce life span by 1 year.

Some estimated doses of ionising radiation are shown in Figure PH110.

Clinical measurement

M. Tidmarsh and E. S. Lin

Clinical measurement in anaesthesia is usually concerned with the direct measurement of a physical quantity such as the pressure, flow or concentration of a gas. Alternatively, assessment of a physiological parameter such as neuromuscular blockade, depth of anaesthesia or pain levels may be required. In these instances measurement is made indirectly, using a related physical variable such as a stimulated muscle twitch, the electroencephalogram or a visual analogue scale.

The process of measurement is performed using apparatus that can be referred to as the measurement system. This may be as simple as a ruler with pencil and paper or as sophisticated as the integrated electronic monitoring systems available in operating theatres and intensive care units.

In the final analysis data must be interpreted. The data obtained by making measurements can only be interpreted correctly if:

Fundamentals of Anaesthesia, 3rd edition, ed. Tim Smith, Colin Pinnock and Ted Lin. Published by Cambridge University Press. © Cambridge University Press 2008.

INPUT

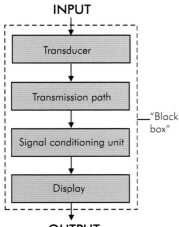

OUTPUT

Figure CM1 'Black box' analogy for a measurement system

- The relationship between the data and the physical quantity or parameter being measured is understood.
- The characteristics of the measurement system are known.

Measurement systems

Measurement of a physical quantity is a process in which the quantity being measured provides an input to a measurement system, which then processes this input to yield an output in the form of a reading or display. This concept is illustrated in Figure CM1, where a measurement system is represented as a 'black box' with an input and an output.

The measurement system consists of component 'black boxes' representing:

- A transducer – a detecting element to convert the quantity being measured (the input) into usable data or a signal, usually an electrical signal. Examples of common transducers are:
  - Microphone, which converts sound to an electrical signal
  - Thermistor, which converts temperature variations into an electrical signal
  - Piezoelectric crystal, which converts pressure variations into an electrical signal.
- A transmission path – the means by which the transducer signal is transferred to the signal-conditioning unit or the display unit. Examples include electrical or optic cables, a length of tubing or an infrared link.

Function	Analogue	Digital
Display	Oscilloscope	Digital voltmeter
	Moving coil meter	Light-emitting diodes
	Chart recorder	Liquid crystal display
Storage	Magnetic tape	Computer hard disk
	Chart	Floppy disc
		Magnetic tape
		CD-ROM
		USB flash drive

Figure CM2 Analogue and digital methods of signal display and storage

- A signal-conditioning unit – processes the transducer signal to make it suitable for display or storage. Signal processing includes functions such as amplification, filtering, and analogue-to-digital conversion. It may occur before or after the signal passes along the transmission path.
- A display or storage unit – provides the output of the system as a display and also stores the signals or data. It may employ analogue or digital methods, examples of which are shown in Figure CM2.

The performance of a measurement system can be characterised by its **static** and **dynamic** characteristics. These determine the relationship between the quantity being measured (input) and the reading (output).

Static characteristics

Static characteristics define the performance of a measurement system when it is dealing with an input which is not changing (or changing only slowly). Under these circumstances there is enough time for the system to reach a steady state before the measured quantity changes, so that the output follows changes in the input accurately. Static characteristics include:

- Accuracy – closeness between the measurement obtained and the true value of the quantity being measured. For example, if a pressure has a true value of 10 cmH$_2$O, an accurate system may read 10.01 cmH$_2$O and may be described as having an accuracy of 0.1%. In an inaccurate system reading 11 cmH$_2$O the accuracy may be quoted as 10% (Figure CM3a).
- Sensitivity – relationship between changes in the output reading of the system and changes in the

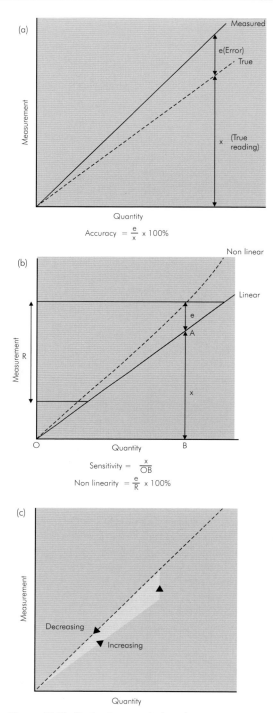

$$\text{Accuracy} = \frac{e}{x} \times 100\%$$

$$\text{Sensitivity} = \frac{x}{OB}$$

$$\text{Non linearity} = \frac{e}{R} \times 100\%$$

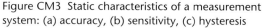

Figure CM3 Static characteristics of a measurement system: (a) accuracy, (b) sensitivity, (c) hysteresis

measured quantity. The sensitivity of a pressure measurement system may be described as the change in output signal voltage for a given change in pressure, e.g. 1 volt per cmH_2O for a sensitive system or 100 mV per cmH_2O for a system 10 times less sensitive. Less sensitive systems will cover a wider range of pressure measurement than sensitive systems (Figure CM3b).

- Linearity – in a linear measurement system the output reading varies in proportion to the measured quantity. Thus, in a linear pressure measurement system, if the pressure doubles the output voltage will double. When the output voltage is plotted against the input pressure, a straight line is obtained. The gradient of this line gives the sensitivity of the system. It is usually desirable for a system to be linear, and any non-linearity may be quoted as a percentage of the operating range of the instrument (Figure CM3b). Some instruments may be intrinsically non-linear, reflecting their underlying mechanism, e.g. hot wire ammeter, or rotameter.

- Hysteresis – a property of a measurement system that produces an error dependent on whether the measured value is decreasing or increasing. Hysteresis in a mechanical device is caused by elastic energy stored in the system, or frictional losses between moving parts. Figure CM3c shows how hysteresis in a measurement system produces errors in the measurement of increasing and decreasing pressures.

- Drift – variation in the reading from an instrument that is not caused by change in the measured quantity. It is usually caused by the effect of internal or external temperature changes on the measurement system, and unstable components in the system.

Dynamic characteristics

Every system requires a certain time to settle to a steady state when presented with a change in its input. This response time may affect the accuracy of the measurement, since if the input is changing rapidly the measuring system may not have adequate time to reach steady state, and thus will not give an accurate reading. The dynamic characteristics of a system reflect its ability to respond to rapidly changing inputs.

Step response of a system

An important dynamic characteristic of any measurement system is its response to a rapid increase in input or a *step function* (Figure CM4). This can be simulated by dipping a thermometer at room temperature into boiling water,

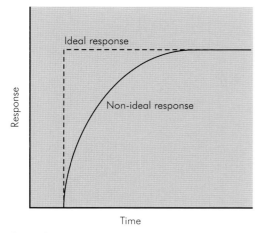

Figure CM4 Step input to a measurement system

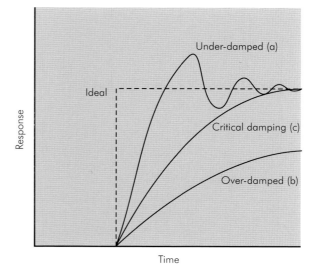

Figure CM5 Effects of damping on the step response of a system

or rapidly opening a tap connecting a pressure gauge to a pressurised container. In a perfect measuring instrument, the output or *step response* produced by a step input should also be a step function occurring instantaneously to give a reading of the measured quantity.

In practice, the step response differs from the ideal due to the properties of the system, and the output only reaches a true steady-state value after a finite time. The time lag for an instrument between a step input and the output reaching its final value is reflected by:
- Response time – time taken from occurrence of the step input to the instrument output reaching 90% of its final value
- Rise time – time taken for the output of the instrument to rise from 10% to 90% of its final value

Damping in a measurement system

The step response of an instrument may also fall short of the ideal in the shape of the output signal produced. Some examples are shown in Figure CM5, where in curve (a) the output overshoots and oscillates about the true value. In curve (b) the response does not reach the true value in the time plotted; in curve (c) the output reaches a steady reading of the true value within the shortest time compatible with no overshoot. The property that determines these effects in the step response is called the *damping* of the system.

All instruments will possess damping that affects their dynamic response. This includes mechanical, hydraulic, pneumatic and electrical devices. In an electromechanical

device such as a galvanometer there are mechanical moving parts such as the meter needle and bearings. Damping in these components arises from frictional effects on their movement. This may arise unintentionally or may be applied as part of the instrument design to control oscillation of the needle when it records a measurement. In a fluid- (gas or liquid) operated device, damping occurs due to viscous forces that oppose the motion of the fluid. In an electrical system, damping is provided electronically by electrical resistance that opposes the passage of electrical currents.

Damping is an important factor in the design of any system. In a measurement system it can lead to inaccuracy of the readings or display:
- **Under-damping** can result in oscillation and overestimation of the measurement.
- **Over-damping** can result in underestimation of the measurement.
- **Critical damping** is usually an optimum compromise resulting in the fastest steady-state reading for a particular system, with no overshoot or oscillation.

Frequency response of a measurement system

Any measurement system in practice will only respond to a restricted range of frequencies, either by design or due to the limitations of its components. Thus, if the system were to be tested with input signals of the same amplitude but different frequencies it would only produce an output

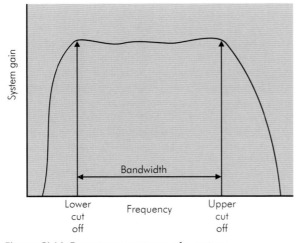

Figure CM6 Frequency response of a system

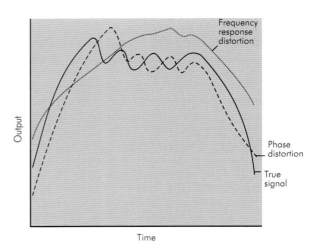

Figure CM7 Causes of signal distortion

over a limited range of frequencies. Within this frequency range the system may respond more sensitively to some frequencies than to others. The response of the system (system gain) plotted against signal frequency is called the *frequency response* of the system (Figure CM6).

Bandwidth

The highest frequency that a system responds to is the *high cutoff frequency*, above which input signals will produce no output. An example of such a cutoff is in the frequency response of the human auditory system, which at best may have a high cutoff frequency of 20 kHz. Similarly, a system may possess a *low cutoff frequency*, the lowest frequency audible by the human ear being 15 Hz. The frequency range between low and high cutoff frequencies is referred to as the *bandwidth*.

Distortion due to poor frequency response

Any input signal can be characterised by its frequency spectrum, which defines the different frequency components into which the signal can be resolved. The frequency response of a measurement system may not cover the spectrum of a signal, thus blocking part of the input signal. Alternatively, an instrument may be more sensitive or attenuate certain frequencies, causing it to give falsely high or low readings within its operating frequency range. This can occur at natural frequencies or resonances. Distortion of a signal is illustrated in Figure CM7.

It might initially be assumed that the ideal frequency response for a system would be one with equal sensitivity

at all frequencies from very low to very high (i.e. a flat response from 0 to ∞ Hz), but this would also enable *noise* to pass through the system with the measurement signal, thus causing error and distortion.

The frequency response of a mechanical system is determined by its inertial and compliance elements (equivalent to masses and springs), while in an electrical circuit it is determined by the inductances and capacitances. There is often a design compromise between providing accuracy and reducing noise levels.

Natural frequencies or resonances

A measurement system may possess natural frequencies or resonances determined by inertial and compliance elements in a mechanical system (or inductances and capacitances in an electrical circuit). These resonances appear as peaks in the system's frequency response and can produce distortion in a signal display and errors in the readings (Figure CM8). Good design practice can ensure that these resonances do not lie in the operating frequency range of the instrument, or ensure appropriate levels of damping to smooth out these unwanted peaks.

Phase shift response

Fourier analysis demonstrates how a signal is composed of a series of component frequencies. In a signal being measured each component wave will undergo a different delay in time or phase shift (a phase shift is a time delay expressed as an angle, i.e. the units are degrees or radians) introduced by its passage through the measurement system. If a measurement system significantly alters the

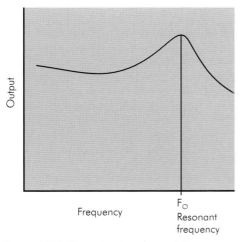

Figure CM8 Example of a resonant frequency

Signal	Voltage range	Frequency range (Hz)
Electroencephalogram (EEG)	1–500 µV	0–60
Electrocardiogram (ECG)	0.1–50 mV	0–100
Electromyogram (EMG)	0.01–100 mV	0–1000

Figure CM9 Common biological signals

relative phases between the components of a signal it can distort the signal. Any measurement system will have a *phase shift response*, consisting of the phase shift occurring at different frequencies, which can be plotted against the frequency axis. This phase shift response will be dependent on the components of the system, and can be responsible for distortion or errors in an instrument.

Electrical signals

In modern measuring instruments the transducer usually produces an electrical current or voltage, which varies according to the measured parameter. This voltage or current is a signal. Signals in clinical measurement are usually voltage signals or *biological potentials*. Most biological potentials vary in time, many in a repetitive or cyclical fashion (e.g. electrocardiogram, airway pressure during respiration). Some signals, such as the electroencephalogram and evoked potentials, are not cyclical but vary irregularly.

Biological potentials

The characteristics of some common biological potentials are outlined in Figure CM9.

Electrical signals can be described in the following ways:

- As a voltage (or current) varying in time. Any signal can be represented as a voltage (or current) plotted along the time axis, i.e. it is a *time-variant* signal. The height of the signal above the time axis is measured in volts, millivolts or microvolts (V, mV, µV) (Figure CM10). If a current, it will be in amps, milliamps or microamps (A, mA, µA). The amplitude of a signal is

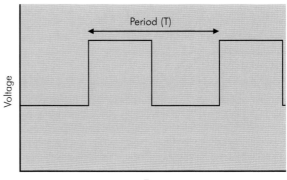

Figure CM10 Voltage signal that varies with time – square wave

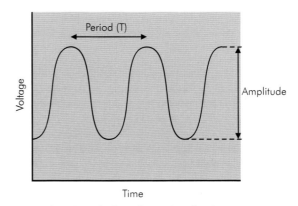

Figure CM11 Periodic voltage signal – sine wave

the range of variation (volts or amps) between maximum and minimum values (Figure CM11).

- As periodic or non-periodic. A signal that varies with a repeating pattern in time, at regular intervals, is said to be periodic (Figure CM11). Each cycle of the signal has the same shape or waveform, and possesses a *period* (T = duration of one cycle (s)), a *frequency* (Hz) and an *amplitude*, the maximum swing in voltage or

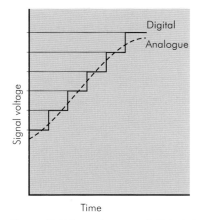

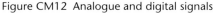

Figure CM12 Analogue and digital signals

current spanned by the signal. The simplest type of periodic signal is a sine wave.

- As analogue or digital. An *analogue* signal is continuous in time, and the magnitude of the signal varies smoothly without discernible increments. The signal is thus analogous to most natural varying processes. Signals produced by transducers are usually analogue signals. A *digital* signal is produced from an analogue signal by sampling the signal at regular intervals and recording the magnitude with changes in fixed increments rather than on a continuous varying scale. Such a signal can be represented completely by a set of numbers. This adapts the signal for processing by digital systems and manipulation by computer, which can have significant advantages (Figure CM12).
- As a series of frequency components. A mathematical method of analysis was invented by Jean Fourier (a French mathematician) in 1822. This has evolved both theoretically and practically to become one of the most powerful tools used in signal processing. Application of Fourier analysis to a signal enables it to be described by its *frequency spectrum*.

Frequency spectrum of a signal

Fourier analysis (Figure CM13) describes the conversion of a signal into its frequency components. Fourier analysis is most suitable for periodic signals, but can still be used for non-periodic waveforms using an approximation which treats the waveform as if it were a periodic signal with a very long period.

In describing a signal by its frequency spectrum consider that:

- Any signal varying continuously in time can be broken down into a collection of sine and cosine waves, which if added together yield the original signal.
- The component waves exist as sine–cosine pairs at the same frequency.
- Each pair of components has a combined amplitude and can be plotted as a point on the frequency axis giving the *frequency spectrum* for the signal.

Figure CM13 Fourier analysis

Electrical 'noise'

A signal may be modified by any of the components of the measurement system. If the changes introduced are intentional, they represent *signal processing* or *signal conditioning*. Unwanted alteration of the signal by the system is distortion and introduces error. The addition of unwanted components to the signal by the system or from outside electrical interference is called *noise*. These unwanted components can be added to a signal at any instant, changing its value and its appearance on display. This may occur due to noise being generated in the measurement system itself, or due to the *pick-up* of interference from external sources such as diathermy or fluorescent lighting.

Signal-to-noise (S/N) ratio

In some cases the noise signals may be so large as to obscure the measurement signal altogether. An awareness of the magnitude of noise components in the signal is necessary to assess the accuracy of the measurements. This can be expressed by the *S/N ratio*, which is the ratio of signal amplitude to noise amplitude expressed in decibels (Figure CM14).

Signal processing

Signal processing modifies a measurement signal by using various functions, for example:

- **Amplification** to make it suitable for display, storage or transmission. Many biological signals are very small in amplitude (e.g. electroencephalogram (EEG) signals may be microvolts, while ECG signals may be millivolts). Such signals are usually too small to drive display or storage units, and require amplification. Low-amplitude signals are also unsuitable for transmission since noise signals picked up may be of

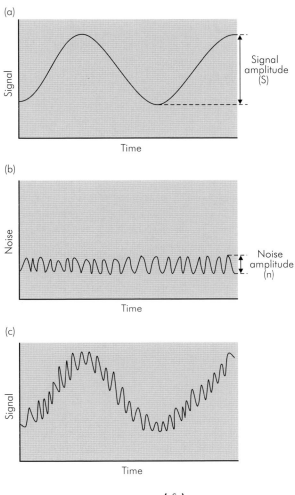

$$\text{Signal to noise ratio} = 10 \log \left(\frac{S}{n} \right) \text{ dB}$$

Figure CM14 Illustration of signal-to-noise ratio: (a) signal, (b) noise, (c) noisy signal

below a set threshold. A *notch* filter rejects a specific frequency, such as 50 Hz to avoid pick-up from mains cables.

- **Spectral analysis**. A signal is usually displayed as a time-varying voltage or current. In some cases (e.g. cerebral function monitoring) a display of the signal frequency spectrum is required, which can be achieved using electronic processing. A common method first converts the analogue signal to a digital signal, and then applies a mathematical algorithm called the Fast Fourier Transform (FFT). Transformation of a signal to its spectral components can make some processing functions such as filtering easier and more accurate. It also enables more complex analysis to be readily performed by computers.

- **Analogue-to-digital** (A-to-D) conversion. This is often required before applying other processing functions, and is always necessary in order for the signal to be stored and analysed in a computer. This is because most electronic manipulation of signals uses digital electronics as opposed to analogue methods.

- **Averaging** to remove noise. In some cases the amplitude of the measurement signal may only be a fraction of the noise amplitude (i.e. S/N ratio is very low), and when displayed the wanted signal may be completely obscured by noise. If the wanted signal is repetitive and the noise is random in time, multiple repetitions and summations of the combined signal lead to an increase of the S/N ratio as the random noise cancels itself out. This is called averaging, and is used in the extraction of evoked potentials, where the evoked signal is only a few millivolts in amplitude, hidden in background noise. Averaging >2000 repetitions may be required to obtain a clear signal.

similar or greater amplitude, giving a low S/N ratio and obscuring the signal.

- **Filtering** to remove noise. Often noise signals are in a different frequency range from the wanted measurement signal. In these cases the noise can be reduced by using filters to block out the unwanted frequencies. A *low-pass* filter rejects all frequencies above a given threshold. Such a filter would be used to avoid high-frequency interference from a source like diathermy. A *high-pass* filter rejects low frequencies

Amplifiers

As previously noted, the components of a measuring system can be considered as *black boxes* in the same way as the measurement system as a whole. Thus an amplifier is simply an electronic 'black box' which when presented with an electrical signal at its input produces an output which is of greater amplitude. The purpose of an amplifier in measuring systems is to increase the power of a low-amplitude signal in order that it can be used to drive a display or storage unit. An amplifier contains an electronic circuit that requires a power supply, and channels power from this power supply into the signal, increasing the voltage, the current, or both voltage and current.

Characteristics of an amplifier include:

- Gain, which is the ratio of the amplitude of the output signal (A_O) to the input signal (A_I). It is usually expressed as decibels (db). Such units may be used to express any ratio by taking 10 times the $\log_{10}$ of the ratio. Thus, if the output amplitude produced by an amplifier, A_O, is 100 times the input amplitude, A_I:

$$\begin{aligned} \text{Amplifier gain} &= 10 \log (A_O/A_I) \\ &= 10 \log 100 \\ &= 20 \text{ db} \end{aligned}$$

- Frequency response and phase response. An amplifier will be characterised by these responses as a result of its circuit design, just as the complete instrument will have these responses dependent on the combined effects of its component parts.
- Upper cutoff frequency, which is the upper frequency limit above which signals are blocked or cut off. Measured in hertz (Hz).
- Lower cutoff frequency, the lower frequency limit below which signals are blocked or cut off.
- Bandwidth, which is the extent of the frequency range passed by a system or amplifier, i.e. the amplifier only amplifies signals within this frequency range. It therefore lies between upper and lower cutoff frequencies and is also measured in frequency units (Hz).
- Input impedance, which is the electrical impedance 'seen' by the transducer signal at the input of the amplifier. Maximum power transfer takes place when the input impedance of the amplifier matches the output impedance of the transducer. Measured in ohms (Ω).
- Output impedance, the electrical impedance seen 'looking' back into the output terminals of the amplifier. Maximum transfer of signal power from the amplifier requires matching of the output impedance to the input impedance of the transmission path or the display unit.

Pressure measurement

Pressure is defined as force per unit area, and it may be measured in various units in the clinical setting. Some examples are shown in Figure CM15.

In anaesthesia, pressure measurements are usually applied to gases (cylinders, anaesthetic machines, breathing circuits) or liquids (intra-arterial pressure monitoring).

Quantity measured	Unit
Blood pressure	mmHg
Airway pressure	cmH_2O
Partial pressure of blood gas	kPa
Gas cylinder pressure	bar, psi

Figure CM15 Units in the clinical measurement of pressure

Pressures are not usually absolute measurements, but are generally measured relative to atmospheric pressure. When interpreting pressure measurements various factors should be considered, such as:

- Transmission path – Pressure transducers are often remote from the site at which pressure is sampled. The pressure is transmitted to the transducer by a length of tubing. The dynamic characteristics of this transmission path can significantly affect the final pressure measurements and signal displayed.
- Sampling site – Pressure may be sampled at a site remote from where the measurement is actually required, due to lack of access. Although static pressures may be equal throughout a closed system, pressures may differ significantly in a dynamic situation. A common example is the measurement of proximal airway pressures, which may not necessarily reflect distal airway pressures.
- Static or fluctuating conditions – If the pressure is not varying rapidly it can be considered as static, in which case the dynamic characteristics of the transmission path and measuring system may not affect the measurement significantly. This may not be the case when measuring a rapidly fluctuating pressure.

Common types of device used to measure pressure in gases or liquids include the aneroid gauge, the manometer and the piezoresistive strain gauge.

Aneroid gauge

This type of gauge is a mechanical device that uses the pressure being measured to operate a mechanism coupled to a pointer. It can be used to measure high or low pressures, and is usually employed when measuring pressures greater than one bar.

In the Bourdon gauge the measured pressure is applied to a spiral tube which uncoils as the pressure increases. This uncoiling movement is coupled to a pointer that indicates the pressure. Another form of aneroid mechanism relies

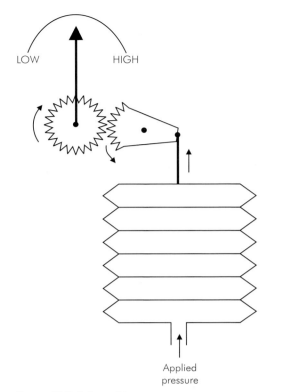

Figure CM16 Aneroid gauge

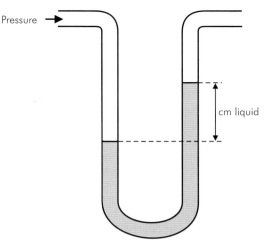

Figure CM17 Manometer

on the expansion of a capsule produced by connection to the sampled pressure. This expansion drives a pointer over a scale (Figure CM16).

- Advantages – simple technology, mechanically robust and convenient to use. Operate in any position and do not require power supply. Suitable for high or low pressures.
- Disadvantages – not suitable for very low pressures ($<5\ \mathrm{cmH_2O}$). Not easily recalibrated.

Manometer

The manometer is the most basic device for measuring pressure and, because of its simplicity, represents a standard method of calibrating other devices. The unknown pressure is measured by balancing it against the pressure due to a column of a liquid (Figure CM17). The liquids used most commonly are water for lower pressures and mercury for higher pressures. Common pressure units are thus $\mathrm{cmH_2O}$ and mmHg. Accuracy and sensitivity can be increased by angling the manometer tubing and using a liquid with a lower density than water (e.g. alcohol).

Surface tension between the liquid and the manometer tubing can cause an error, which causes the water manometer to read too high and the mercury manometer to under-read.

- Advantages – simplicity of mechanism and no need for calibration. A standard method used to calibrate other techniques of pressure measurement.
- Disadvantages – bulkiness of the device and lack of a direct reading.

Piezoresistive strain gauge

This device is based on a semiconductor material with piezoresistive properties that cause it to vary in electrical resistance when subjected to a mechanical strain. The semiconductor is deposited onto the surface of a thin diaphragm that flexes when a pressure difference is applied across it. The distortion of the diaphragm produces a strain in the piezoresistive material that forms one arm of a bridge circuit etched onto the diaphragm. This results in a small signal current from the transducer that can then be amplified and processed.

- Advantages – versatility, since it can be used for measurement of high or low pressures. The electronic signal and display make it suitable for online display, automated data logging and linking to a computer. It is also easily adaptable for measuring differential pressures, since the diaphragm can be mounted with each face of the diaphragm enclosed in its own chamber and isolated from the other. Differential pressures can be used to measure gas flows, with the use of a suitable pneumotachograph head.

- Disadvantages – requires power supply and signal-processing unit. Susceptible to electrical interference but has to be used in electronically hostile environments (operating theatres and intensive care units).

Blood pressure measurement

Blood pressure is a determinant of tissue perfusion, oxygen delivery and cardiac work. It varies between individuals and is subject to a diurnal rhythm (lowest when the subject sleeps).

Note that recorded blood pressures reflect not only cardiovascular performance but also artefact (Figure CM18). Failure to recognise this can result in errors of interpretation and inappropriate action. For example, changing the measurement site by 10 cm in height produces an error of 7.5 mmHg in the pressure measurement. For this reason, a standard reference point is taken, usually the level of the heart. Since blood flow is pulsatile, the blood pressure also varies according to the phase of the cardiac cycle.

- Cardiac output
- The pulsatile nature of blood flow
- Systemic vascular tone
- Hydrostatic pressure variation in the circulatory system
- The characteristics of the measurement system used

Figure CM18 Factors affecting blood pressure measurement

Methods of measuring blood pressure

The value of the displayed blood pressure is a function of the method used to measure it. The validity of any such measurements is strongly influenced by the observer's familiarity with the particular strengths and weaknesses of the technique employed. These can be divided into indirect and direct methods.

Indirect methods

These are most commonly based on an occlusive cuff, which is inflated to a pressure above that of the artery and then slowly deflated. Once the cuff pressure falls below that of the artery, pressure transients begin to pass beneath the cuff and can be measured. Blood pressure values are

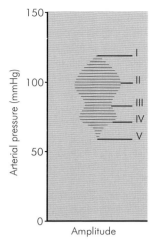

Figure CM19 Representation of Korotkov sounds:
Phase I – clear tapping synchronous with the pulse
Phase II – sounds become softer about 5–10 mmHg below phase I
Phase III – as the diastolic point approaches, sounds become more intense
Phase IV – sounds suddenly become muffled
Phase V – sounds disappear

derived from these pressure transients, and can be measured manually or automatically.

Manual occlusive cuff methods

Manual methods rely on auscultation and palpation and are historically the earliest, but have become superseded by automated non-invasive techniques that provide a continuous display of blood pressure.

Riva-Rocci (1896) described the use of an occlusive cuff to measure systolic pressure by palpation. Using an occlusive cuff, Korotkov (1905) first described the measurement of blood pressure by auscultation. *Korotkov sounds*, heard over the artery as the cuff pressure falls, are the result of turbulent blood flow, vibration in the arterial wall and pressure transients created as the extent of arterial occlusion decreases (Figure CM19).

Von Recklinghausen (1931) described a dual cuff (occlusive and sensing) technique, employing aneroid valves in series within a sealed metal block, the oscillotonometer. This provided a visual measure of systolic, diastolic, and mean arterial pressures displayed on a dial, connected by levers to an aneroid gauge.

- Advantages – simple and well established. Do not require sophisticated equipment or power supplies. Encourage patient contact.

- Disadvantages – dependent on operator technique and require manual intervention.

Automated occlusive cuff methods (oscillometry)

Oscillometry is the most common method of automatic blood pressure measurement in clinical practice. It is a development of von Recklinghausen's oscillotonometer. The accuracy of blood pressure measurement has been improved by coupling the rate of cuff deflation to heart rate. A single occlusive cuff is employed, using a dual sensing connection, which replaces the double cuff of the oscillotonometer. A pneumatic pump periodically inflates the cuff to a point 25–30 mmHg above the systolic pressure and allows air to escape through a bleed valve, producing controlled deflation (about 2–3 mmHg per second). Vibrations of the arterial wall produce pressure transients that are transmitted via a sensing channel to an electrical transducer in the apparatus. The data are then analysed by a microprocessor. Using algorithms that relate the rate of change of pressure transient amplitude to blood pressure, systolic, diastolic and mean arterial pressures are calculated. The effects of electrical noise are reduced by comparing successive arterial pulsations as the cuff pressure decreases. If these do not correlate the data are rejected.

Systolic pressure corresponds to the point where the amplitude of pulsations is increasing, and is about 25–50% of maximum. Diastolic pressure corresponds to the point where the amplitude of pulsations has declined to 80% of the maximal pulse amplitude. Mean arterial pressure is the maximum amplitude point.

- Advantages – the principal advantages of these instruments are that they free the operator's hands, allowing measurements to be obtained conveniently when access to the patient is difficult, allow calculation of the mean arterial pressure, have alarm capabilities, and provide the capacity for data transfer.
- Disadvantages – while correlating fairly well with invasive measurements, they are less accurate at extremes of blood pressure (will over-read at low pressures, and under-read at high pressures), and should not be regarded as any more accurate than manual techniques. All these instruments assume the presence of a regular cardiac cycle; when this is absent, e.g. in atrial fibrillation, blood pressure measurements become inconsistent. The automatic cuff increases the risk of underlying tissue damage (in the elderly, particularly when the frequency of measurement is high, and the instrument is used for prolonged periods). Incorrect cuff placement may be responsible for nerve entrapment injuries (the ulnar nerve at the elbow).

Penaz technique

In oscillometry blood pressure measurement relies on gradual deflation of a cuff, which limits the frequency of measurement. To overcome this limitation, Penaz first described a continuous non-invasive technique in 1973. This monitors the diameter of the digital artery using an infrared plethysmograph, which is mounted in a pneumatic cuff. The infrared signal responds to arterial dilatation and contraction during each cardiac cycle. By using a pump servo-controlled by the infrared signal, the infrared signal is maintained constant, at a value corresponding to mean arterial pressure, by inflating and deflating the cuff. Thus, as the artery dilates in systole cuff pressure is increased, and as arterial diameter reduces during diastole cuff pressure decreases. This duplicates the arterial pressure waveform in the cuff, which is then displayed on the machine.

- Advantages – provides a record of the changing trends in blood pressure, and in patients with normal, or vasodilated fingers, correlates well with invasive methods.
- Disadvantages – results are less reliable in patients with peripheral vascular disease. Small differences in cuff positioning or tightness result in significant changes in the measured pressure. These measurements display a downward drift because of relocation of tissue fluid, necessitating repeated calibration. When used for >20–30 minutes, the cuff causes discomfort. If peripheral blood flow is poor, there is the potential for vascular occlusive damage.

Doppler ultrasound

Employs an encapsulated array of transducer crystals that can transmit and receive ultrasound waves. These are coupled to the skin by a layer of silicone gel (preventing excessive reflection), and positioned directly over the artery. Movements in the arterial wall caused by pressure transients as they pass beneath the cuff cause Doppler shifts in the frequency of the transmitted ultrasound waves. The amplitude of the shift provides a measure of the systolic and diastolic pressures.

- Advantages – can be used for patients of all ages.
- Disadvantages – requires the accurate positioning of the transducers, and the use of the correct ultrasound

coupling medium. The signals are prone to movement artefact, and are distorted by diathermy and arrhythmias.

Sources of error in indirect methods

In comparison with direct methods of blood pressure measurement (the 'gold standard'), indirect methods tend slightly to under-read, with the diastolic pressure showing the greatest degree of variability. The sources of error include:

- Detection of Korotkov sounds, which are complex with a large proportion of the sound energy being below the audible range. This reduces sound transmission to the observer. In addition, observer detection of the sounds will be dependent on aural acuity. The generated sounds are flow-dependent, and factors affecting flow can thus introduce inaccuracy (e.g. in high-output states, and post exercise, Phase V may not occur).
- Cuff size. Width of the cuff effects the measured value of blood pressure: too narrow, and there is a tendency to overestimate; too wide, and there is a tendency to underestimate. As a consequence, there have been efforts to standardise the widths of blood pressure cuffs. The World Health Organization (WHO) recommends that adult cuffs should be 14 cm wide, and should cover two-thirds of the length of the upper arm, or its width should be 20% greater than the diameter of the arm. Suggested widths are shown in Figure CM20.
- Zero and calibration errors, particularly in aneroid devices.
- Pneumatic leaks.
- Speed of deflation. When too fast, there is insufficient time to detect audible change.

Age (years)	Cuff width (cm)
Adult	12–14
4–8	9
1–4	6
Neonate	2–5

Figure CM20 Recommended cuff widths for different ages

Direct method (intra-arterial pressure monitoring)

Intra-arterial pressure monitoring provides an invasive, continuous measure of blood pressure by beat-to-beat reproduction of the arterial pressure waveform. It is particularly useful in the following situations:

- Cardiovascular instability
- Where blood pressure manipulation is required (inotropes or vasodilators)
- Where non-invasive blood pressure measurement is likely to be difficult and/or inaccurate (obesity)

The method requires the insertion of a short parallel-sided cannula into an artery. A continuous flow of either saline or heparinised saline at rates between 1 and 4 ml per hour is used to reduce clot formation in the cannula. The cannula is connected by a short length of narrow-bore, non-compliant plastic tubing containing saline to a pressure transducer, which is usually of the piezoresistive strain gauge type. More recently, catheter-tip pressure transducers have been developed, but they remain comparatively expensive. The piezoresistive strain gauge produces a low-amplitude signal requiring signal processing before analysis and display.

The design of an intra-arterial pressure monitoring system must take into account the following considerations:

(1) The frequency and phase shift responses of the system have to be adequate to allow good reproduction of the arterial signal. An approximate guide is that acceptable accuracy requires a frequency response extending to 8–10 times the maximum heart rate expected. In humans, the most important information is contained within the frequency range 0–20 Hz. The system can thus be designed to have an upper cutoff frequency >20 Hz.

(2) The transducer and connecting tubing should be chosen to avoid natural frequencies or resonances occurring within the desired frequency response. Mechanical resonances due to the properties (compliance and inertial elements) of the transducer and column of saline in the connecting tubing can be shifted above the desired cutoff frequency by reducing the diameter of the connecting tubing.

(3) Components must also be chosen to provide the optimum degree of damping. Usually critical damping is aimed for, but since frequency response, phase shift response and damping requirements may conflict a compromise may have to be arrived at. It is important to be able to recognise abnormal levels of damping to interpret the arterial waveforms appropriately. Figure CM21 illustrates the effect of damping on arterial pressure waveforms.

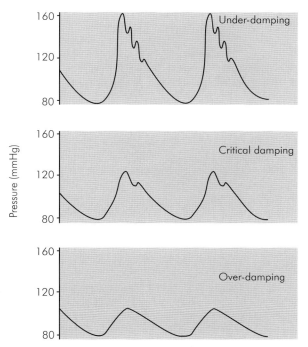

Figure CM21 Measurement system damping

Pressure (mmHg)

- Advantages – provides a continuous display of the pressure wave form, providing an immediate assessment of blood pressure that is regarded as the 'gold standard'.
- Disadvantages – cannulation can be difficult, particularly in low-output states, and may require consideration of multiple sites before success. Disconnection – if unrecognised this may result in serious blood loss and, in the extreme, exsanguination. Infection is particularly relevant in cases of prolonged use. Distal vascular insufficiency may result directly from cannulation, or arise from subsequent thrombosis of the cannulated artery. This risk is increased by insufficient collateral circulation, which should always be checked before cannulation. Emboli (air or thrombus) can cause distal vascular occlusion.

Sources of error in arterial pressure monitoring
- Air bubbles – a recording system with a high resonant frequency and critical damping is preferable. Standard pressure transducers have a natural frequency of about 100 Hz, but the addition of the connecting tubing, tap and cannula markedly reduces this. The presence of air

bubbles in the system also decreases the resonant frequency of the system and increases the damping.
- Catheter wall compliance – if compliant tubing is used to connect the cannula and transducer it will distend with the pulse wave, and like the presence of air will cause decreased resonant frequency and increased damping.
- Blood clots – if within the cannula will increase the flow resistance of the cannula and also the flow velocity of the saline. These factors also tend to increase system damping and decrease resonant frequency.
- Zero point – it is important to choose a zero reference point to minimise hydrostatic errors.

Measurement of gas flow
The measurement of gas flow and volumes is applied in clinical practice for the following uses:
- To test pulmonary function in patients
- To monitor gas flows in anaesthetic machines
- To monitor respiratory flows and tidal volumes in patient breathing circuits

Devices used in pulmonary function testing are outlined below.

Benedict–Roth spirometer
Consists of a light bell that traps a closed volume of air over water. The subject breathes in and out of this trapped gas, causing the bell to rise and fall following the inspired and expired volumes. A sensor or pen coupled to the bell traces its movement, giving a spirometric trace from which gas flow rates and lung volumes can be derived (Figure CM22). This device is relatively large and not portable.

Vitalograph
Records expiratory flow rates and volumes by collecting expired gas from the subject in a bellows. A recording pen is coupled to the bellows, tracing an expired-volume graph (Figure CM23). It is more portable than the Benedict–Roth spirometer but only measures forced expiratory volumes and flows. The results obtained are also very dependent on subject technique.

Wright respirometer
Another continuous volume recorder that has been designed specifically for clinical application. It operates by using the gas flow to drive a spinning vane (and is, thus, a type of anemometer), which is coupled by

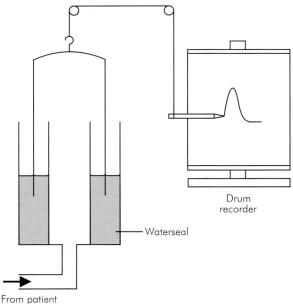

Figure CM22 Benedict–Roth spirometer

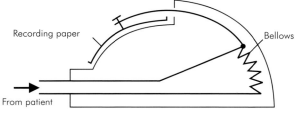

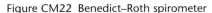

Figure CM23 Vitalograph

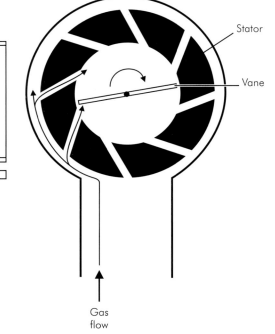

Figure CM24 Cross section of a Wright respirometer

clockwork gears to the display dials. The total volume that can be recorded is 1000 litres, and like the dry gas meter its accuracy and reliability is dependent on the mechanical quality of its clockwork mechanism. It can only measure unidirectional flow but has the advantage of being small and portable, and it requires no power supply. Flow rates can only be derived by averaging recorded volumes over time, and thus the device is labelled 'inferential' (Figure CM24).

Dry gas meter

Based on the gas meters used for measuring domestic gas consumption. It measures large volumes of gas by continually feeding the gas flow into a pair of reciprocating bellows. As each bellows fills alternately, its movement records an increase in volume by a clockwork counter and operates

inlet and exhaust valves to direct the gas flow through the machine. In this way the flow of very large volumes (10^6 litres) of gas can be measured, compared with the several litres capacity of the closed-volume spirometers. However, average flow rates can only be estimated over time, and cannot be measured directly.

Electronic volume meter

Here the spinning vane mechanism described in the Wright respirometer is adapted to give an electronic signal. One method uses a fixed-blade stator to create a spiral flow to drive the blades of the vane. The spinning blades interrupt a light signal from light-emitting diodes (LED), which is then picked up by photoelectric cells. These provide an electrical signal that can be processed and calibrated to give volume measurements. This device has the advantages of being free from the mechanical errors associated with clockwork mechanisms and of being able to measure volumes from bidirectional (inspiratory and expiratory) flow. It does, however, require a power supply, signal processing and display unit.

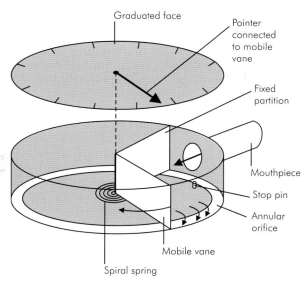

Figure CM25 Exploded diagram of a peak flow meter

Peak flow meter

This device records the maximum expiratory flow of a patient by using the expired gas to operate a shutter controlling a variable orifice through which the gas escapes to the atmosphere. The greater the expiratory flow the larger the orifice opened up by the shutter. The displacement of the shutter is non-returnable and is recorded by a pointer, which therefore records the maximum expiratory flow reached (Figure CM25).

Gas flow measurement in anaesthetic machines

Rotameter

Gas flows from an anaesthetic machine into a ventilator or patient circuit are most commonly measured using rotameters. The rotameter is a variable-orifice flowmeter in which the gas flow to be measured is passed upwards through a vertically mounted glass (or plastic) tube. This tube has a tapering internal diameter, wider at the top and narrower at the bottom. Gas flow through the rotameter is controlled by a needle valve at the bottom.

A bobbin with a smaller diameter than the internal diameter of the rotameter tube acts as a pointer, and is moved up or down the tube by the force of the gas flow as it increases or decreases. The bobbin may vary in design, but the most common type is shaped like a 'spinning top' with spiral grooves cut in the sides causing it to spin in the gas flow. The spin reduces friction and sticking of the

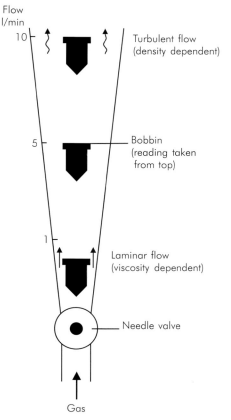

Figure CM26 Working principles of a rotameter

bobbin. Readings on this type of bobbin are taken from the top edge.

When the gas flow is steady the bobbin settles at a point where the force of the gas flow acting on it and passing round it equals the bobbin weight. At high flows the bobbin is near the top of the rotameter, and the cross section of the annular space around the bobbin is greater than at low flows, when the bobbin is near the bottom of the rotameter and the orifice cross section is small.

Gas flow pattern in a rotameter

The pattern of gas flow through a rotameter is a mixture of turbulent and laminar flow, due to the flow conditions as the gas passes the bobbin (Figure CM26). When the cross-sectional area open to flow is small, i.e. the bobbin is near the bottom of the rotameter, flow past the bobbin is like flow in a 'tube' (defined in this context by having diameter < length). This is because the cross-sectional area open to flow is small. In this case flow is laminar and gas viscosity is the main determinant of flow. When the bobbin is near the top of the rotameter at high flows, the annular cross-sectional area open to flow is large. Flow here is similar to that through an 'orifice', an orifice being defined by having diameter > length. In this case flow is turbulent and density becomes the most important gas property determining flow. The importance of the flow pattern is that because the viscosities and densities of gases can differ significantly (e.g. oxygen and helium have similar viscosities but their densities are 1.33 and 0.17 kgm^{-3}), a rotameter can only be calibrated accurately for a specific gas or mixture.

- Advantages – simple design and reliable; does not require power supply; no signal transmission path, conditioning unit or display to go wrong.
- Disadvantages – only calibrated for specific gas under standard pressure and temperature conditions. Actually part of the gas circuit: failure may therefore be hazardous, and the device is sensitive to circuit changes downstream.

Features of the rotameter block

Rotameters on an anaesthetic machine are arranged in an array, a different one for each gas. Different arrangements exist, but it is desirable for oxygen to enter the common flow last. In the design of the array, certain features need to be considered for increased safety:

- If the first gas to enter the flow line is oxygen (Figure CM27a), it can leak from the breakage of any subsequent rotameter, potentially giving rise to a hypoxic gas mixture. Thus the order of gases entering the flow line can increase the risk of hypoxia, and theoretically the safest position for oxygen would be last in order of entering the common flow (Figure CM27b). Changing the rotameter order would, however, bring its own risks, and therefore internal channelling is used to separate the individual gas flows. Thus, even when the oxygen control knob is **first** in order, channelling can ensure that oxygen is the **last** gas to enter the flow line (Figure CM27c).
- The oxygen control can be mechanically linked to other gases to prevent hypoxic mixtures being selected.
- Positioning vaporisers at the outlet of the rotameters can increase the pressure in the rotameters and thus affect their calibration, since the density of the gases becomes altered.

(a)
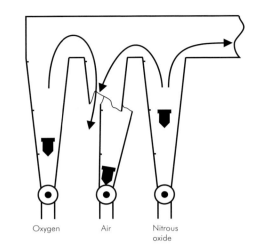

(b)
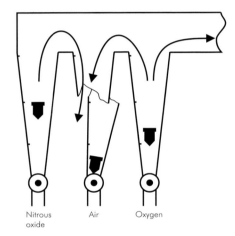

(c)
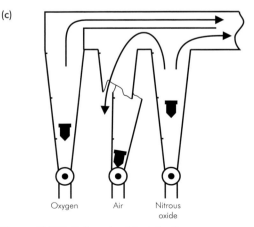

Figure CM27 Rotameter block faults

Gas flow measurement in breathing circuits

Pneumotachograph

The pneumotachograph obtains a signal (dependent on the gas flow) by the use of a pneumotachograph head, which is inserted into the breathing circuit, or through which a patient can breathe directly during pulmonary function testing. Common types of pneumotachograph heads are:

- Fixed resistance, where the signal is a differential pressure signal produced by gases flowing through a fixed flow resistance. These include the screen and Fleisch heads.
- Hot wire, in which a low signal is produced by the gas flow cooling a heated resistance wire.
- Pitot tube, in which the flow signal is dependent on the pressure difference between dynamic and static pressures in the centre of the pneumotachograph head.

The flow signal is passed to a signal-conditioning unit, from which it can be analysed and displayed. Tidal volumes are calculated by integrating the flow signal over the duration of inspiration or expiration. Linearity of a pneumotachograph head signal is important in making calibration and calculation of volumes easier. Flow should be corrected for changes in gas mixture. Correction will include gas **viscosity** if flow is laminar, but gas **density** for turbulent flow.

Screen pneumotachograph

The most commonly used design, consisting of a short connector with a gauze screen mounted across the middle, through which the gas flows (Figure CM28a). The diameter of the head must be large enough to ensure laminar flow through the screen. The screen acts as a flow resistance and produces a small pressure drop across it. This pressure drop is sampled by a pair of pressure ports, one on either side of the screen, which feed the differential pressure to a differential pressure transducer. The pressure transducer produces a small electrical signal for conditioning, analysis and display. This pneumotachograph head is linear over a wide range and of a convenient size, but turbulence may be produced at high flow rates.

Fleisch pneumotachograph

The pneumotachograph head passes the flow through an array of fine-bore ducts to ensure laminar flow over a wide range (Figure CM28b). It is larger and bulkier than the screen head.

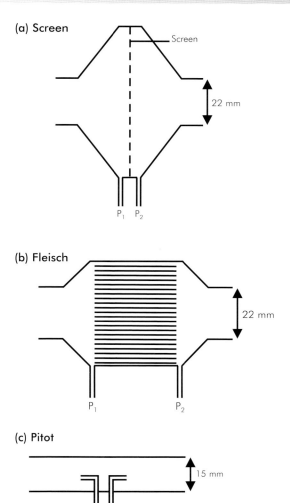

(a) Screen

Screen

22 mm

P_1 P_2

(b) Fleisch

22 mm

P_1 P_2

(c) Pitot

15 mm

P_1 P_2

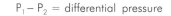

$P_1 - P_2 =$ differential pressure

Figure CM28 Pneumotachograph heads

Hot wire pneumotachograph

In this device two 'hot' wires are used mounted at right angles to each other, across the lumen of the pneumotachograph head. The hot wires are resistive wires heated by a controlled current passing through them. The gas flow produces cooling of the wires which is dependent on the flow rate, which in turn varies their resistance, giving a small electric signal. Disadvantages are limited frequency response and the requirement for a stabilised power supply.

Modified Pitot tube pneumotachograph

This device is based on the Pitot tube, which is used to measure local gas speed (as in an aircraft airspeed gauge). It consists of a connector with two small-diameter (1–2 mm) pressure-sampling tubes mounted axially in the centre of the gas flow path, the open ends of these tubes acting as pressure-sampling ports (Figure CM28c). One sampling port faces downstream and one upstream. The downstream port measures the *static* pressure. The upstream port gives a *total* pressure reading, which is greater than the static pressure, since gas impacts on the port creating an additional pressure (*dynamic* pressure) due to its kinetic energy. The difference between the total pressure and static pressure port is measured by a differential pressure transducer and is dependent on the square of the gas velocity. The pneumotachograph is calibrated for gas flow but is non-linear, requiring linearisation in the signal-processing unit. It has the advantage of being simple mechanically, small in size (and dead space) and cheap to produce. The flow through this head is turbulent.

Measurement of gas and vapour concentrations

In the past the analysis of gas concentrations, in gas mixtures and blood samples, relied on chemical methods. These were relatively slow, laborious and inaccurate compared with modern methods. They included:

- The Haldane apparatus – a volumetric technique based on gas absorption, which was used to measure component gases in a respiratory gas mixture. Oxygen was absorbed by passage through pyrogallol.
- The van Slyke apparatus – a method for the measurement of blood gases. Haemoglobin was released from red cells by inducing rapid haemolysis with saponin. CO_2 was displaced by lactic acid and oxygen displaced by potassium ferrocyanide, enabling volumetric measurements to be made.

Gas analysers based on physical principles have largely superseded these chemical methods. In addition to improving accuracy, they can provide continuous breath-to-breath measurement, and by generating a proportional electrical signal they facilitate data storage and processing.

Gas analysers

All modern gas analysers generate electrical signals that are proportional to the concentration of a measured component gas. The signals are small and require

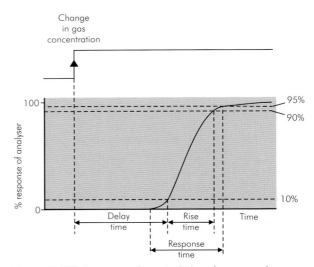

Figure CM29 Response characteristics of a gas analyser

signal conditioning to improve accuracy and compensate for non-linearity.

Step response of gas analysers

Gas analysers, like many other instruments, suffer a finite delay before registering a change in sample composition. This time lag may be measured as:

- Delay time – time from a stepped change in concentration/partial pressure at the sampling site to detection of a 10% increase at the sample chamber. Largely due to the time required for the sample to pass from sampling orifice to the measurement chamber.
- Rise time – time required for the display to rise from 10% to 90% of the stepped change in gas concentration/partial pressure at the sampling site.
- Response time – time from the gas reaching the sample chamber to the analyser displaying 95% of the final measurement (Figure CM29).

Types of gas analyser

Gas and vapour analysers can be usefully divided into discrete analysers (extremely accurate), or continuous analysers (less accurate).

(1) **Discrete analysers** are rarely used in clinical anaesthesia. An example of discrete analysis is provided by gas/liquid chromatography. In this method the unknown gas mixture is injected into a stream of carrier gas (e.g. nitrogen) flowing through a column of liquid-coated particles (e.g. polyethylene

glycol), the *stationary phase*. As the gas mixture passes through the column the various component gases are slowed down according to their solubility in the stationary-phase liquid, and thus appear separated out at the end of the column. On exit from the column the gases are assayed by a method such as infrared absorption or thermal conductivity detection, which yields a series of peaks corresponding to the component gases. The gases are identified by comparison of the time lags of the different peaks with those for known gas samples, and their concentrations are given by the height of their peaks. This method is very accurate and very sensitive, but expensive, and it is usually only used for research purposes.

(2) **Continuous analysers** include:
- Mass spectrometers
- Infrared absorption
- Ultraviolet absorption
- Paramagnetism
- Thermal conductivity
- Polarography
- Galvanic fuel cell

Mass spectrometers

These instruments can separate complex mixtures of gases. The sample is continuously drawn into the apparatus through a narrow sampling tube. Some of the sample passes into an evacuated steel ionising chamber, where it is ionised by a beam of electrons. The resulting mixture of ions then diffuses through a slit in the chamber, and a negatively charged plate accelerates them. These charged ions are then separated to give a spectrum (Figure CM30). There are two methods of separating the ions, based on magnetism and mass:

(1) **Magnetic sector method** – the ions, once accelerated, are deflected by a strong magnetic field, which separates out different particle streams according to mass and charge. Each of the deflected ion streams is then measured at a different detector plate. The number of detector plates (usually 4–6) determines the number of gases that can be measured. As most ions have the same charge, separation mainly depends on molecular mass.

(2) **Quadrupole method** – the spectrometer, despite possessing only one detector, can measure up to eight different species of particle. The ions reach the detector through a passage formed by four steel rods, the quadrupole. These rods are energised by a radio-frequency signal, which enables them selectively to allow ions with a specific mass to pass through to the detector. The quadrupole signal can be varied to scan for ions of different masses, thus producing a sequential assay for different gases. The mass range is less than that of a magnetic sector spectrometer, and the use of a single shared detector makes it less accurate.
- Advantages – versatile, allowing measurement of a variety of component gases in a mixture with a rapid response time ($<0.1\,$s).
- Disadvantages – needs complex equipment with high capital, installation and maintenance costs. The presence of water vapour can interfere with sample measurement and prolong the rise time, but many mass spectrometers incorporate a correction for the presence of water vapour.

Infrared (IR) absorption

A molecule composed of two or more dissimilar atoms will absorb IR light. Absorption of wavelengths between

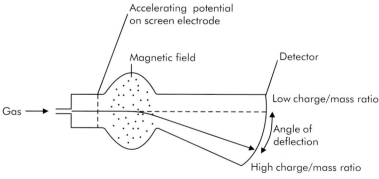

Figure CM30 Mass spectrometer

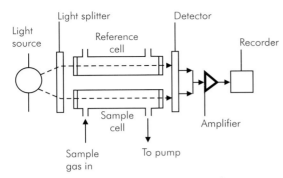

Figure CM31 Infrared absorption gas analyser

2.5 and 25 μm will cause covalent bonds to bend and vibrate, increasing the molecule's rotational speed. Different gas molecules absorb specific wavelengths of IR light. Thus, by detecting increased absorption at particular frequencies, gases can be identified and their concentrations determined. These instruments can be classified as:

(1) **Dispersive** – usually multiple gas analysers where the radiation from the IR source is split and delivered to the sample sequentially, e.g. IR spectrophotometer
(2) **Non-dispersive** – single gas analysers where only one wavelength is used, e.g. the capnograph specifically used for CO_2 (Figure CM31)

The most frequently used IR gas analyser is the IR spectrophotometer. Modern machines use specific LEDs to split the IR irradiation into different wavelengths. The sample chamber is trans-illuminated, and the absorption of IR radiation measured and compared with that of a reference chamber.

- Advantages – fast enough to follow breath-to-breath changes of CO_2, N_2O and volatile anaesthetics.
- Disadvantages – as the response time increases with molecular size (250 ms for CO_2, increasing to 750 ms for a volatile anaesthetic agent), rapid respiratory rates may decrease the accuracy of end-tidal and inspiratory volatile agent concentrations.

Ultraviolet (uv) absorption

Some gases composed of similar atoms will not absorb IR radiation (O_2, H_2, N_2), but will absorb UV light (as will halogenated vapours). These molecules all possess characteristic UV absorption spectra, absorbing light of very short wavelength. The only clinical analyser based on this method measures halothane, with a quoted accuracy of 0.2% over the range 0–5%.

- Advantages – acceptable accuracy.
- Disadvantages – absorbed quanta are of sufficient energy to disrupt the molecule, producing toxic breakdown products, which cannot be returned to the breathing circuit unless passed through soda lime. The response time is slow, >1 s.

Paramagnetism

Molecules can be either paramagnetic (attracted towards a magnetic field) or diamagnetic (repelled by a magnetic field). Paramagnetic molecules possess two unpaired electrons spinning in the same direction in the outer electron shell (e.g. oxygen). The Pauling analyser uses the ability of oxygen to distort a non-homogeneous magnetic field as the basis to detect the presence of oxygen in a gas mixture. The analyser consists of a cell with a sealed glass dumbbell (containing nitrogen, a weakly diamagnetic gas) and a mirror, suspended by wires (but free to rotate) between the poles of a magnet. The paramagnetic effect of oxygen displaces the dumbbell, causing it and the mirror to rotate. The degree of rotation of both dumbbell and mirror is proportional to the concentration of oxygen present in the mixture. By reflecting a beam of light off the suspended mirror, the degree of rotation can be detected using a photocell. The resulting electrical signal, after processing, provides a measure of oxygen concentration. No other gases of clinical interest have this property (Figure CM32).

Various modifications have been made to the basic design to compensate for external vibration, excessive gas flow rates, and pressurisation of the cell.

- Advantages – commercial versions of this type of analyser are compact, relatively cheap, and remain unaffected by other common gases.
- Disadvantages – slow response times (5–20 s), mainly the result of large sample chambers.

Thermal conductivity

A gas with a high thermal conductivity will conduct heat more readily than one with a low conductivity (e.g. in comparison with air, CO_2 has 35% conductivity, whereas helium has 600%). This is the basis of instruments known as katharometers. When a gas is passed over a heated wire, the wire is cooled to a temperature that depends on the temperature of the gas, its flow rate and the thermal conductivity of the gas.

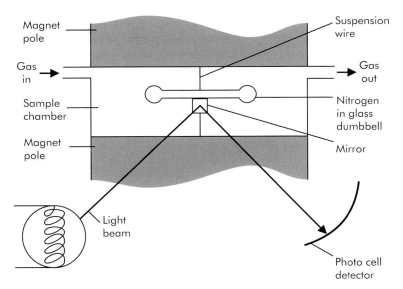

Figure CM32 Pauling type of paramagnetic analyser

The fall in wire temperature causes a decrease in electrical resistance. This fall in resistance is used to produce a small signal related to gas concentration, by connecting the wire as one arm of a Wheatstone bridge circuit. These analysers have been used mainly to measure CO_2 and helium concentrations, and have also found use in gas chromatography systems.
- Advantages – relatively simple and inexpensive technology.
- Disadvantages – slow response times (about 5 s) unless operated at low pressure (100 mmHg).

Electrochemical methods
These methods are based on an electrochemical reaction in buffer solution occurring between two electrodes and involving dissolved gas molecules. There are two main devices:
(1) **Polarographic electrode** – consists of a pair of electrodes of specific materials (depending on the gas being measured) in an electrolyte solution. When these electrodes are maintained at a potential difference, a current is produced between them through the electrolyte solution, which is dependent on the concentration of the gas in solution. In this device the reaction is driven by the voltage applied to the electrodes.
(2) **Fuel cell** – effectively a primary cell (as in a battery) consisting of two electrodes of specific materials in an electrolyte solution, which generates its own current through the solution due to the potential difference produced between the electrodes. Again the current in the solution is dependent on the dissolved gas concentration. This device drives the reaction itself, by the current it generates, but ultimately the reagents in the cell will be used up, and the reaction will cease. Hence, the name *fuel cell*.

Other methods of gas analysis
Several other physical properties have been used as the basis for analysers, notably:
- Solubility – the basis of the Dräger Narkotest®, which measures the effect of different concentrations of various volatile anaesthetic agents (cyclopropane, methoxyflurane, halothane, diethyl ether) on the length of four bands of silicon rubber. There is a linear relationship between the concentration of the volatile agent, and the measured length of the rubber bands. Measurements require correction for the presence of nitrous oxide.
- Density – the basis for the Waller chloroform balance. A sealed glass bulb filled with air is counterbalanced with a small weight in a gas-tight chamber. If a gas with a density greater than air is introduced into the chamber, there is an apparent decrease in the weight of the glass bulb. This reduction in weight is proportional to the difference in densities between air and

vapour/air mixture, and can be used as the basis to calculate the amount of volatile agent present.

- Refractive index – the difference in the velocity of light passing through a vacuum and through a transparent substance/gas determines the refractive index of that substance. The measured delay in the passage of light through a gas is dependent on the number of molecules present. The Rayleigh refractometer measures this transmission delay. If the refractive index of the gas is known, it is possible to calculate gas concentration.
- Velocity of sound – when a gas oscillates at a particular frequency, its structure will begin to resonate. The resonance depends on the velocity of sound in the gas mixture, which is in turn a function of gas composition.
- Raman light scattering – when a photon of light passes through a gas, it gives up a portion of its energy to the gas molecule. This is then re-emitted at a longer wavelength characteristic to that gas.

Sources of error in gas and vapour measurements
Gas sampling errors
Gas sampling errors can arise when sampling gases from a breathing circuit due to:

- Contamination – gas samples can become contaminated with secretions, debris, or water vapour.
- Poor gas mixing – significant concentration gradients may occur in a circuit and be sustained by laminar flow conditions, giving anomalous results.
- Altered vapour pressure – significant temperature gradients occur between inspired and expired gases, which can alter the vapour pressure in the sampled gas.
- Altered pattern of flow at the sampling point – excessive sampling rates can cause local flow and gas concentrations to change at the sampling point.
- Variation in absolute pressure – pressure may vary from point to point in a circuit, which can give rise to different results depending on the location of the sample site.

Instrument errors
A major source of instrument sampling error is the *ram-gas effect*. The flow velocity of gas as it enters the sampling port can alter sample composition. This effect can be reduced by using lower sampling rates, and ensuring that the sampling port is set at right angles to the main gas flow.

Patient errors
Chronic lung disease can lead to increased non-homogeneity of the alveolar time constants throughout the lung. This results in a corresponding variation of alveolar gas composition between different lung units. Thus, expiratory gas samples may not be representative of lung performance as a whole.

Oxygen measurement
Oxygen measurements in arterial blood can be made using various parameters including gas tension (PaO_2), blood oxygen content (CaO_2) and haemoglobin oxygen saturation (SaO_2).

These parameters are all related to each other in the oxygen dissociation curve. Current measurement techniques can be applied *in vitro*, i.e. remote from the patient using samples of gases or blood collected from the patient, or alternatively they can be applied directly to the patient, enabling *in vivo* measurements to be made. The in vivo measurements usually employ the same basic technology as the in vitro methods, but have been adapted to provide immediate bedside results.

In vitro oxygen measurement
Measurement in gas mixtures
Can be done using the following methods, which have been previously described:

- Paramagnetic analysers – have slow response times due to their large sample chambers, which limits their practical use.
- Mass spectrometers – although versatile, with a rapid response, these instruments are too complex and expensive for widespread use.

Measurement in blood samples
This is almost universally done using electrochemical methods and forms the basis for both in vitro and in vivo techniques. The two most common techniques already mentioned above are the polarographic (Clark) electrode and the galvanic fuel cell.

These devices are based on the electrochemical reduction of oxygen at a cathode, using electrons generated at the anode. For each molecule of O_2 reduced, four electrons move between the electrodes. This generates an electrical current that is proportional to the concentration of oxygen present in the sample. Application of Henry's law (the number of molecules in solution is proportional to the partial pressure) enables the partial pressure of oxygen to be calculated from the current measured.

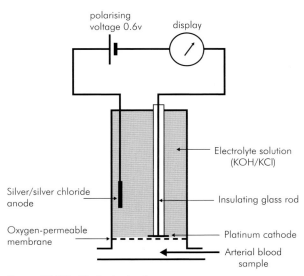

Figure CM33 Clark electrode

Clark electrode (polarographic electrode)

The Clark electrode is used to measure partial pressure of oxygen in arterial blood samples. This device is a system of two electrodes, a negative platinum cathode and a positive silver/silver chloride anode, which are immersed in electrolyte solution (KCl). It measures the concentration of oxygen in a sample (e.g. arterial blood) by allowing the oxygen in a sample to filter into the electrolyte solution via a permeable membrane. This membrane protects the electrode system from contamination by the sample (protein deposition on the electrodes) (Figure CM33).

Redox reactions occur at each electrode. The redox reaction which detects the oxygen from the sample occurs at the platinum cathode, which is sometimes referred to as the sensing electrode. This reaction reduces the oxygen in solution by combining it with H^+ and electrons, and is as follows:

$$O_2 + 4H^+ + 4e^- = 2H_2O^-$$

Effectively the platinum cathode behaves as a hydrogen electrode, the platinum acting as a catalyst for the dissociation of water which provides H^+ for the redox reaction. This dissociation also results in the production of hydroxyl ions in the electrolyte solution.

$$H_2O = 4H^+ + 4OH^-$$

Electrons are provided for O_2 reduction at the cathode by the reaction at the silver/silver chloride anode. This involves

the oxidation of silver in the anode by Cl^-. This occurs as follows:

$$4Ag + 4Cl^- = 4AgCl + 4e^-$$

The Cl^- is obtained from the electrolyte solution (KCl). As AgCl is formed at the anode, it is deposited on the silver, giving the dual composition (Ag/AgCl) of this electrode. The Cl^- removed from solution is replaced by the OH^- generated at the platinum electrode.

The electrode potentials of the anode and cathode produce a small voltage difference between them which opposes the flow of electrons from anode to cathode. This is because the silver anode is electropositive relative to the cathode (hydrogen). Therefore an external power source is required in order to maintain the electron flow between anode and cathode. A polarising voltage supply of 0.6 volts is used, which removes electrons from the anode and supplies them to the cathode.

The redox reactions are driven by the oxygen in solution at the platinum cathode. Hence the magnitude of the current generated at equilibrium is dependent on the concentration of oxygen in solution (which is equal to that in the sample).

- Advantages – robust and can be battery-powered, making it portable.
- Disadvantages – limited life span due to consumption of the silver in the anode. High maintenance in order to preserve accuracy. Need for replacement of the electrolyte solution and maintenance of the power supply.

Galvanic fuel cell

This device is similar to the Clark electrode in that it is composed of two electrodes in an electrolyte solution (KOH). The electrodes are a lead anode and a gold mesh cathode (Figure CM34).

The cathode is the sensing electrode at which the oxygen concentration is measured, the reduction of oxygen taking place as follows:

$$O_2 + 4H^+ + 4e^- = 2H_2O$$

This is similar to the case of the Clark electrode, and as before H^+ is obtained from the dissociation of water:

$$H_2O = 4H^+ + 4OH^-$$

Electrons are provided for this reaction by direct connection to the lead anode, at which the following reaction

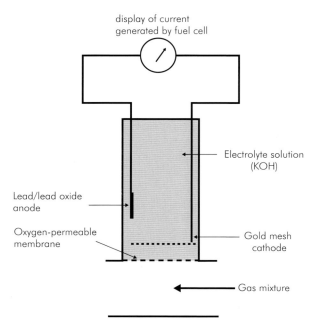

Figure CM34 Galvanic fuel cell

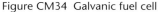

occurs:

$$2Pb + 4OH^- = PbO + H_2O + 2e^-$$

Although this reaction consumes OH^- from the electrolyte, the OH^- is replaced by the dissociation of water at the cathode.

In this case the electrons flow directly between anode and cathode due to the difference in their electrode potentials. Lead is electronegative compared to the cathode (hydrogen), and thus when the circuit is completed between the electrodes a small current flows under the influence of this small potential difference, with electrons passing from the anode to the cathode.

This device system is a primary cell which maintains itself by the consumption of externally supplied gas (i.e. the oxygen in the sample). Since the electrolyte solution is continually replenished by the redox reaction at the cathode, it has a longer working life than a simple galvanic cell in which the electrolyte solution is consumed by the redox reactions. Theoretically its working life is only determined chemically by consumption of the lead anode.

- Advantages – compact, does not require a power supply, inexpensive, low maintenance.
- Disadvantages – relatively slow response time (approximately 30 s), too slow to measure

breath-to-breath changes. Basic cells can be contaminated by N_2O, which reacts with the lead anode to produce nitrogen. Working life span 6–12 months.

Sources of error in electrochemical methods
- Blood gas factor – the measured oxygen values are lower for blood than for gas samples. This is thought to reflect the delay caused by oxygen diffusion in blood, and the localised depletion of oxygen that occurs at the cathode. It is a consistent effect requiring mathematical correction.
- Stability – as these systems utilise a two-point calibration (gas containing zero oxygen, and one containing a fixed concentration), calibration drift occurs when protein and lipid deposits build up on the membrane or bubbles form in the electrolyte solution. To prevent this, a combination of regular electrode cleaning and quality control is necessary.
- Interference – erroneous effects can result from substances other than oxygen being reduced at the cathode (including N_2O), which can be avoided by specific membrane selection.
- Temperature – modern blood gas analysers measure at 37 °C. If a patient has a temperature that differs by more than 2 °C mathematical correction is necessary.

In vivo oxygen measurement
Intravascular oxygen electrodes
This is a bipolar variant of the Clark electrode in which both the anode and the cathode are mounted within a fine tube covered by an oxygen-permeable membrane. The whole assembly is small enough to pass through an 18 G cannula. Response times vary between 5 and 60 seconds.
- Advantages – provide a continuous measurement of arterial oxygen tension.
- Disadvantages – as for the monopolar variant, the electrode is temperature-sensitive, and subject to calibration drift due to protein deposition. Access of oxygen to the cathode is flow-dependent, which can introduce error at low-blood-flow states (largely overcome by using a pulsed polarising current). Rapid response times are only achieved at the expense of poor accuracy at low flow rates.

Transcutaneous oxygen electrodes
These provide a measure of the oxygen that has diffused from capillaries in the dermis of the skin. The electrode

comprises a ring-shaped anode, a central cathode, and electrolyte solution enclosed by an oxygen-permeable membrane. The electrode housing contains a heating element and a thermistor to allow temperature compensation. The whole assembly is held in direct contact with the skin by adhesive tape. Locally heating the skin increases capillary blood flow, improving the correlation between transcutaneous and arterial PO_2. Transcutaneous PO_2 increases with local temperature up to the point where tissue damage occurs, about 44–46 °C.

- Advantages – useful in neonatal monitoring, particularly in detecting hyperoxia. Response times are a function of diffusion distance, and vary from 10–15 s in infants to 45–60 s in adults.
- Disadvantages – excessive heating can increase the oxygen diffusion distance (oedema) and eventually lead to burns. Heating also increases skin metabolism, and causes the ODC to shift to the right. Essentially, transcutaneous PO_2 is a better index of skin oxygen delivery than PaO_2 (correlation between cutaneous and arterial PO_2 is best in infants). Changes in cutaneous PO_2 lag behind changes in PaO_2.

Conjuctival oxygen tension electrode

The electrode consists of a ring cathode (gold or platinum), an anode (silver or silver/silver chloride), and a thermistor (for temperature compensation). These elements are covered by a membrane composed of either silicon oxide or polyethylene, and mounted on an ophthalmic former. This is placed under the eyelid in the conjuctival fornix (local anaesthesia is necessary for the awake patient), and held in place by the orbicularis occuli. Response times are similar to those obtained with transcutaneous electrodes.

Mass spectrometer

In addition to its in vitro application, the mass spectrometer can also be used as an in vivo analyser. In vivo the mass spectrometer is in direct continuity with the patient either via an intravascular perforated metal catheter covered with a gas-permeable membrane or by means of a transcutaneous oxygen electrode. The estimated response time varies between 3 and 50 seconds.

Optodes

This method is different from the others described, in that measurement does not depend on the consumption of oxygen. Oxygen will 'quench' the fluorescence of certain dyes. The magnitude of this quenching effect is a function of oxygen concentration. This provides the basis for the technique, which uses an intravascular probe, composed of an optical fibre with a dye-coated tip, covered by an oxygen-permeable membrane. Sequential illumination of the fibre causes the dye to fluoresce. The intensity of fluorescence is dependent on the concentration of oxygen present at the tip, and it is measured using a photomultiplier. The inclusion of a thermocouple allows for temperature compensation.

- Advantages – independent of blood flow. Initial results suggest favourable stability and response times.
- Disadvantages – probes are expensive and subject to fibrin deposition. In addition, prolonged use may result in the deterioration of the dye, making measurements invalid.

Carbon dioxide measurement

CO_2 is the metabolic end product of the aerobic oxidation of glucose. It is a soluble gas and is an important determinant of tissue pH. CO_2 is transported in the blood as carbamino-Hb compounds, as bicarbonate, or dissolved in solution.

The direct measurement of the partial pressure of CO_2 in arterial blood ($PaCO_2$) can provide information regarding pH, adequacy of ventilation and metabolic status.

The indirect measurement of end-tidal CO_2 reflects cardiac output, pulmonary blood flow, and can confirm correct endotracheal intubation.

The relationship between CO_2 and pH is described by the Henderson–Hasselbalch equation:

$$pH = pK_a + \log_{10} \frac{[HCO_3^-]}{[PaCO_2]}$$

An early method of measuring CO_2 levels indirectly was the Astrup technique, which used pH measurements to derive the PCO_2 level of a sample from a Siggard-Andersen diagram, by interpolation. This technique was time-consuming and inaccurate. Modern techniques measure either arterial or end-tidal CO_2 levels. These can be applied in vitro, where the measurements are made on blood or gas samples remote from the subject, or in vivo, where the oxygen measurement system is in direct continuity with the patient.

In vitro CO_2 measurement
The CO_2 electrode

This technique is used in modern blood gas analysers. It uses two electrodes, a glass pH electrode, and a silver/silver chloride reference electrode, both maintained at 37 °C.

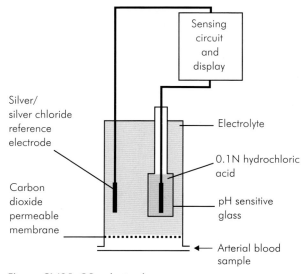

Figure CM35 CO_2 electrode

The glass electrode is covered by a layer of cellophane or nylon mesh with a thin layer of sodium bicarbonate between the electrode and the covering. Both electrodes are enclosed within a membrane (Teflon or silicon rubber) which is permeable to CO_2 but impermeable to blood cells, plasma and hydrogen ions (Figure CM35). Using a two-point calibration system, buffers of known CO_2 concentration are used to establish the relationship between pH and CO_2. The system relies on the carbonic acid equilibrium:

$$H_2O + CO_2 \rightleftharpoons H_2CO_3 \rightleftharpoons H^+ + HCO_3^-$$

The diffusion of CO_2 across the membrane causes the equilibrium to shift to the right in accordance with the law of mass action. This generates hydrogen ions and causes a fall in pH, which is proportional to the concentration of CO_2 (0.01 pH units for every 0.1 kP_a change in CO_2).
- Advantages – generally regarded as accurate and stable.
- Disadvantages – response times are governed by the permeability properties of the membrane, and the rate of conversion of CO_2 into bicarbonate (the rate of reaction can be accelerated by inclusion of the enzyme carbonic anhydrase). Accuracy depends on membrane integrity, since it is vital to ensure that the only change in pH at the electrode results from the shift in the carbonic acid equilibrium. This can be monitored by measurement of electrical resistance across the membrane.

In vivo CO_2 measurement
Transcutaneous electrodes
The measurement of transcutaneous CO_2 requires a modification of the basic CO_2 electrode. The electrode is part of a housing, which also contains a heating element and thermistor (for temperature compensation). This is held in direct contact with the skin by adhesive tape. The skin is heated to a temperature of 42–44 °C. This increases capillary blood flow, CO_2 production in the skin and CO_2 solubility. As described by Severinghaus, the measured transcutaneous CO_2 is usually greater than arterial CO_2 ($PaCO_2$):

$$\text{Transcutaneous } CO_2 = 1.33 \times PaCO_2 + 0.5 \text{ kP}_a$$

- Advantages – gives a continuous measurement of CO_2 concentration in capillary blood.
- Disadvantages – risk of skin burns. Response times are slow, and the correlation between transcutaneous and arterial CO_2 is variable.

Intravascular probes
Miniaturised versions of the CO_2 electrode have been commercially produced that are small enough to be inserted through an arterial cannula.

Optodes
Similar to the method used to measure oxygen, CO_2 is measured indirectly by recording the change in pH of a buffer, which in turn causes a change in the intensity of fluorescence of a pH-sensitive dye. The intravascular probe is composed of an optical fibre with a dye-coated tip covered by a thin layer of buffer. This is separated from the blood by a CO_2-permeable membrane. Any change in light intensity is proportional to the change in buffer pH, caused by the diffusion of CO_2 across the membrane. Changes in fluorescence are detected by a photomultiplier.

End-tidal CO_2 (ETCO$_2$)
ETCO$_2$ measurement is now an established clinical tool. In normal individuals, the ETCO$_2$ usually measures 0.5–0.8 kPa less than the arterial CO_2. The magnitude of this difference increases with respiratory disease, particularly where there is significant ventilation–perfusion mismatch. The capnograph provides a continuous display of repeated ETCO$_2$ estimations (Figure CM36).

The majority of the commercial capnographs are based on infrared spectrophotometry, and can be classified as

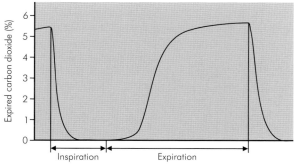

Figure CM36 Capnograph trace

either **sidestream** or **mainstream** monitors according to their sampling system.

Sidestream capnograph
The most common type of capnograph is the sidestream type, where the sample gas is drawn from the main respiratory flow through a side port via a narrow tube to the sample cuvette (flow rates between 50 and 500 ml min^{-1}). Following CO_2 measurement, the gas is either returned to the expiratory limb of the breathing circuit (of particular relevance to low-flow anaesthesia) or scavenged.
- Advantages – generally more convenient than mainstream monitors; the patient attachment is less bulky and more robust.
- Disadvantages – without elaborate water traps/filters to remove water vapour, the measured value of ETCO$_2$ would be invalid. A suction pump transfers the sample from the site of sampling to the measurement chamber; this sampling rate can in itself introduce error. The response time of these instruments tends to be longer than mainstream analysers.

Mainstream capnograph
In the mainstream capnograph the measuring head inserts into the breathing or ventilator circuit so that it carries the main gas flow. The capnograph head acts as the sampling chamber, and is trans-illuminated by IR light through side windows.
- Advantages – the position of the probe makes removal of a sample of gas from the breathing circuit unnecessary. The system is far less complicated (no suction pump required); the errors due to gas sampling are eliminated. Response times are significantly less than with the sidestream type.

- Disadvantages – probes are fragile, expensive, heavy, and require support, and direct contact with the skin may cause a burn. The sensor window must remain clean to prevent inaccuracy and calibration problems.

During anaesthesia the capnograph trace can provide immediate verification of successful tracheal intubation. However, in addition to this, both the shape of the capnogram and the value of the ETCO$_2$ measurement can reflect clinical changes (Figure CM37).

Measurement of pH
In 1909 Sorenson defined pH as the log to the base 10 of the reciprocal of the hydrogen ion concentration [H$^+$]:

$$pH = -\log_{10} [H^+]$$

Under normal conditions, buffer systems within the body (bicarbonate, phosphate, haemoglobin and protein) maintain the pH within a narrow range (7.38–7.42). The pH scale can be used as a clinical measure of acid–base status; this has both diagnostic and therapeutic value. The SI unit of pH is the hydrogen ion concentration expressed as nmol l^{-1}.

Indirect estimation of pH
Because of difficulty in measuring [H$^+$] directly, blood pH was estimated by derivation from the Henderson–Hasselbalch equation:

$$pH = pK_a + \log \frac{[HCO_3^-]}{H_2CO_3}$$

or

$$pH = pK_a + \log \frac{[HCO_3^-]}{\alpha PCO_2}$$

where pK$_a$ is the equilibrium constant for the dissociation of carbonic acid, and α is the solubility coefficient for CO_2. This method is inaccurate because the values of pK$_a$ and α vary with temperature.

pH electrode
To overcome the problems of indirect estimation of pH, a glass electrode was developed to enable measurement of blood pH directly. This method is employed in most modern blood gas analysers. First described in 1933, the glass electrode has been extensively modified to produce what is now a stable, sensitive instrument capable of pH measurement using increasingly smaller volumes of blood. The electrode itself is non-selective and will respond to more than one particular anion or cation. Specificity is

Change	Cause	Diagnosis
↓ ETCO$_2$	↑ alveolar ventilation	↑ respiratory rate, tidal volume
	↓ CO$_2$ production	Hypothermia
	↑ Dead space	Pulmonary embolus, shock, hypotension
	Technical error	Calibration error, air contamination
↑ ETCO$_2$	↓ alveolar ventilation	↓ respiratory rate, ↓ tidal volume
	↑ CO$_2$ production	Sepsis, hyperpyrexia, thyrotoxicosis
	↑ inspired CO$_2$	Rebreathing, CO$_2$ added to inspired gases, administration of NaHCO$_3$

Figure CM37 Causes of changes in end-tidal CO$_2$ concentrations

achieved by enclosing the electrode in a membrane with ion-selective permeability; in this way only H$^+$ ions have access to the electrode.

The actual pH electrode consists of two component electrodes:

- Silver/silver chloride electrode (Ag/AgCl)
- Mercury/mercury chloride electrode (Hg/Hg$_2$Cl$_2$), calomel

Each component electrode consists of a metal conductor and electrolyte solution, the metal conducts electrons, the electrolyte solution conducts ions. A potential difference or electromotive force (EMF) is generated at the interface of the two electrodes (electrode potential). If the temperature remains constant, the only remaining variable is the pH difference between the inner buffer solution of the electrode and the sample. A saturated solution of KCl provides a salt bridge that completes the circuit between the sample and the second calomel electrode. To minimise diffusion of KCl into the sample, a porous plug is placed at the end of the measurement pathway (Figure CM38).

As the pH electrode responds to the activity of H$^+$ rather than concentration, the electrodes must be calibrated using standard solutions of known pH. The pH scale of the electrode depends on the pH of the standard solutions rather than the absolute concentration of H$^+$. Modern blood gas analysers use two different buffers. The first (pH 6.841) has the same pH as the buffer inside the electrode and is taken as the arbitrary zero. The second buffer (pH 7.383) is used as a reference against which the blood pH is measured.

Pulse oximetry

Oximetry is a spectrophotometric technique (trans-illumination of a sample and measurement of absorbed

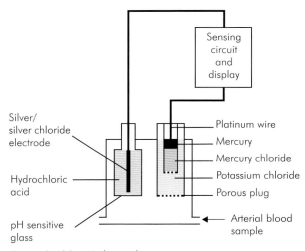

Figure CM38 pH electrode

radiation) that measures % haemoglobin saturation (SaO$_2$). In addition, it can also provide an indirect measure of oxygen tension and content, by use of the oxygen dissociation curve (ODC).

There are two forms of oximetry: **transmission** (or absorbance) and **reflectance** oximetry. Of the two techniques, transmission oximetry is the most commonly used for both in vitro and in vivo measurements.

Transmission oximetry
Basic principles

The absorption of radiation by a layer of solution is determined by the Lambert–Beer law, which relates the absorbance of transmitted light to the concentration, extinction coefficient and thickness of the solution. Details are in Section 4, Chapter 1, page 781. The Lambert–Beer

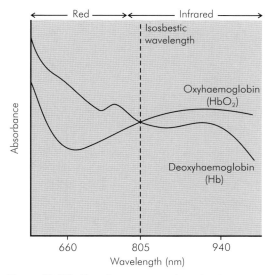

Figure CM39 Absorbance curves in oximetry

law does not describe the in vivo relationship exactly and still requires the use of corrective algorithms before haemoglobin saturation can be calculated. To measure the concentration of a particular compound in a mixture, the mixture is trans-illuminated with monochromatic light at the wavelength where absorbance is maximal. The machine must be calibrated with a pure solution of the compound, and then the measured concentration can be calculated.

Absorbance curves for HbO_2 and Hb

Absorbance can be plotted against wavelength to give curves for HbO_2 and Hb (Figure CM39). It can be seen that the absorbance of both compounds is high for shorter wavelengths (<600 nm) of light since they are both basically red in colour. However, at longer wavelengths in the red region of the electromagnetic spectrum, the absorbance of HbO_2 is less than that of Hb. This gives HbO_2 a brighter red appearance than Hb. At these longer wavelengths, the curves display secondary peaks in absorbance, one at 660 nm for deoxyhaemoglobin, and one at 940 nm for oxyhaemoglobin.

The isosbestic point is the point at which the absorbances for HbO_2 and Hb are equal, i.e. it is the point at which the absorbance curves cross. It is dependent only on haemoglobin concentration. Some earlier oximeters corrected for haemoglobin concentration using the wavelength at the isosbestic points.

Functional saturation

To determine haemoglobin saturation, monochromatic light at the two secondary peak wavelengths (660 and 940 nm) must be used to trans-illuminate the sample. Measurement of the absorbances at these wavelengths enables the concentrations of HbO_2 and Hb to be calculated, and hence the haemoglobin saturation. This saturation measurement is referred to as the *functional saturation*, since it is only based on the principal form of haemoglobin and ignores the presence of minor haemoglobin species such as carboxyhaemoglobin (HbCO), methaemoglobin (HbMet), sulphaemoglobin (HbSul) and fetal haemoglobin (HbF). It is calculated by:

$$\text{functional haemoglobin saturation} = \frac{100 \times [HbO_2]}{[HbO_2] + [Hb]}\%$$

Fractional saturation

Most co-oximeters measure light absorbance at a minimum of four different wavelengths. This enables measurement of the minor haemoglobin species in addition to the principal forms, oxyhaemoglobin and deoxyhaemoglobin. The more accurate *fractional saturation* may then be calculated by:

fractional haemoglobin saturation

$$= \frac{100 \times [HbO_2]}{[HbO_2] + [Hb] + [HbCO] + [HbMet]}\%$$

The two most commonly detected minor species of haemoglobin are HbMet and HbCO, which constitute <1% and <2% (in non-smokers) of the total of Hb concentration respectively. This means that under normal circumstances it is adequate to measure functional SaO_2.

Co-oximeter

This instrument requires haemolysis of the blood sample (either by chemical or by physical means) prior to measurement of haemoglobin saturation. It is often incorporated into a blood gas machine.

- Advantages – light absorbance is measured at several different wavelengths, enabling fractional saturation estimation.
- Disadvantages – unable to provide continuous saturation monitoring. Moderately high capital and maintenance costs to obtain fractional saturation, which is not normally significantly different from functional saturation.

Pulse oximeter

A pulse oximeter consists of a peripheral probe and a processing/display unit. The probe contains two LEDs that trans-illuminate the chosen tissue with monochromatic light at red (660 nm) and infrared (940 nm) wavelengths. A photodiode (PD) detects the transmitted light, converting it to an electrical signal. The functional haemoglobin saturation (SaO_2) is then calculated from the signal by the processing unit and displayed. One LED emits red and the other infrared light, but the PD is unable to differentiate between wavelengths. To overcome this problem only one LED trans-illuminates at a time, the LEDs switching on and off alternately. The pulses in the PD signal are then identified in time to give separate values for red and infrared absorbances. Multiple pulses are used in each measurement cycle to minimise any motion artefact, and a specific sequence is set up, including a period of no trans-illumination. This time period when both LEDs are switched off is used to provide a correction for ambient light conditions.

The trans-illumination signal of the pulse oximeter can be divided into two components:

- AC component – a rapidly changing signal that corresponds to the light absorbed during the pulsatile portion of arterial blood flow
- DC component – represents the light absorbed constantly by the resting volume of tissues and arterial blood

The AC component constitutes a small proportion of the total signal, but is the major determinant of accuracy. It ranges from 1% to 5% of the DC component in a normal pulse wave. These signals are processed by the internal algorithm of the device to calculate SaO_2.

Oximeters are calibrated using data previously obtained from human volunteer studies, in which saturations were recorded while the subjects breathed various inspired oxygen concentrations, including hypoxic levels. On ethical grounds, these studies were limited to minimum measured saturations of 80%. As a result, commercial oximeters are most accurate over the saturation range 80–100%. Any saturation values below this level are obtained by extrapolation, and suffer from increasing errors. Even within the normal range, the intrinsic error of some oximeters has been estimated to vary between 0% and 13%.

The response time of the device is particularly important. Prolonged response time can be attributed to:

- Instrumental delay – relating to the averaging time used to reduce movement artefact. Increasing the averaging time prolongs the response time.
- Circulatory delay – response time is the time taken for changes in central saturation to reach the peripheral circulation. It varies according to probe site (about 10–15 s for an ear probe, >60 s for a finger probe). Both cold-induced vasoconstriction and venous engorgement can increase response times two- to threefold.

Reflectance oximetry

Used for continuous invasive measurement, i.e. monitoring mixed venous saturation with an oximetric pulmonary artery catheter (OPAC). Light of specific wavelength passes along a fibreoptic channel to the tip of the catheter, where it is reflected back up a second channel in the OPAC by the passing blood. The intensity of the reflected light is measured by a photodiode.

Sources of error in oximetry

- LEDs – each emits light over a narrow spectral range either side of the central or principal wavelength, i.e. 660 or 940 nm. This can vary up to ± 15 nm between LEDs of the same type, introducing an error in the measurement of absorbance and the calculation of SaO_2. Oximeters compensate for this by using internal software.
- Ambient light – can be minimised by using shielded probes, and sequential LED cycling.
- Low perfusion states – amplitude of the probe signal amplitude depends on tissue perfusion (decreased perfusion reduces signal amplitude). The oximeter attempts to compensate by amplifying the total signal (AC and DC components). This has the effect of making the S/N ratio worse. Under poor conditions the noise may become the predominant signal. When this occurs, the ratio of scaled signals for both 660 and 940 nm approaches unity, corresponding to a falsely displayed saturation of 85%. To prevent this happening, modern machines have S/N ratio limits, which will interrupt the display if exceeded.
- Motion artefact – can be reduced by increasing the signal averaging time, but only at the expense of response time. Alternatively, some oximeters employ sophisticated internal algorithms that help identify obviously spurious readings.
- External dyes. Methylene blue has the most dramatic effect – as concentration increases, SaO_2 values

decrease. This reduces oximeter readings by up to 65% at a concentration of 2–5 mg kg^{-1} for between 10 and 60 minutes. Some dark nail polishes can also interfere with oximetry.

- Effect of additional haemoglobin species on absorbance:
  - HbMet – light absorption is greater than both principal species at 940 nm, and simulates reduced Hb at 660 nm. At high saturations (>85%) the true value is underestimated; at low values (<85%) it is overestimated.
  - HbCO – has minimal absorbance at 940 nm, but has a similar absorbance to HbO$_2$ at 660 nm; this results in overestimation of SaO$_2$.
  - HbF – essentially the same absorption spectra as adult haemoglobin and has no effect on oximetry.
  - HbS – no reported effect on oximetry. It should be noted that in patients with sickle disease there is a shift in the ODC to the right. Thus, for any given PaO$_2$, the corresponding saturation is less than expected.
- Anaemia – there is a linear trend to underestimate SaO$_2$ as the concentration falls; at haemoglobin levels of 8 g 100 ml^{-1} this can be 10–15%. Polycythaemia has no effect. Accuracy is less at low saturation levels in anaemic patients.
- Diathermy – interference effect largely depends on the particular oximeter. This can be reduced by using suppression filters.

Neuromuscular measurement

Neuromuscular measurement is used in the following applications:
- Assessment of neuromuscular blockade during surgical anaesthesia, to guide the use of muscle relaxants
- Identification of the type of neuromuscular blockade present (depolarising, non-depolarising or type II block)
- Localisation of peripheral nerves for regional techniques

Methods of neuromuscular measurement

The basic technique involves two stages: first the pulsed electrical stimulation of a peripheral motor nerve, and second the assessment of the muscular response.

Electrical stimulation of a peripheral nerve

Needle or surface electrodes are located over or close to a peripheral motor nerve.

A standard electrical pulse stimulates the nerve, producing a measurable muscle twitch. It should be noted that muscle response is related to delivered current and not applied voltage. The electrical characteristics of the stimulator pulse should include:
- A square-wave pulse with a uniform amplitude.
- A pulse current amplitude appropriate for the particular application, i.e. low amplitude (0.5–5.0 mA) for needle electrodes and higher amplitude for skin electrodes (10–40 mA).
- An optimal pulse length of 0.2 ms. This is a result of the compromise between current pulse amplitude and duration of current flow, since excessive values of either increase the risk of neural damage.
- Various patterns of pulses, including single or trains of pulses at 1–2 Hz and tetanic bursts at between 50 and 100 Hz.

All currently used nerve stimulators are battery-powered and are isolated electrically from all other objects. Skin electrodes are used for intraoperative neuromuscular monitoring and require relatively high current pulse amplitudes. This provides *supramaximal* stimulation that ensures maximum recruitment of muscle fibres, thus providing a baseline for a control twitch when using relaxants. Peripheral nerve location for local anaesthetic blocks is performed using needle electrodes, insulated except for the needle tips. These stimulate with much lower currents. Dual-function stimulators with controls for both neuromuscular monitoring (external mode) and nerve location (internal mode) are now commercially available.

Assessment of neuromuscular blockade

The assessment of muscular response to electrical stimulation provides the basis for neuromuscular monitoring. A variety of methods providing an indirect measure of contractile force have been employed. These include:
- Vision and touch
- Mechanomyography
- Acceleromyography
- Electromyography

For effective clinical application of neuromuscular blockade monitoring, the method of assessment needs to combine accuracy with practical convenience. When monitoring neuromuscular blockade, it is important to realise that different muscle groups demonstrate different sensitivities to muscle relaxants.

Vision and touch

The muscle twitch that results from the electrical stimulation is assessed either by observation (i.e. either degree of contraction or a simple count of pulse when using *train of four*), or by palpation.

- Advantages – simple and convenient.
- Disadvantages – inaccurate, and provides only a gross assessment of muscle response.

Mechanomyography

In this method the muscle becomes a force-displacement transducer. A small preload is attached to the muscle to maintain isometric conditions. Electrical stimulation causes the muscle to contract against the preload, generating a tension that is proportional to the force of contraction. This *generated tension* is converted to an electrical signal, which can then be measured. For access and convenience, adductor pollicis is the muscle normally used.

- Advantages – more accurate than 'vision and touch'.
- Disadvantages – correct positioning of the transducer, selection of the preload, and immobilisation of the hand, makes this method inconvenient and difficult to maintain.

Acceleromyography

This method requires careful positioning of a joint, usually a digit, such that the distal end remains free-hanging. Electrical stimulation of the appropriate motor nerve causes muscle contraction and movement of the digit. The measured acceleration of the distal part is directly proportional to the force of muscle contraction. By fixing a piezoelectric wafer to the distal part of the digit, it is possible to covert the measured acceleration into an electrical signal, which can then be measured.

- Advantages – more objective than 'vision and touch'.
- Disadvantages – as with mechanomyography there are problems with joint positioning, which make this technique inconvenient and inconsistent.

Electromyography

This measures muscle activity by recording the magnitude of the evoked compound action potentials from either skin or needle electrodes overlying a particular muscle (adductor pollicis or the hypothenar eminence is the most commonly used site). The active electrode is placed over the motor nerve, and the indifferent electrode is placed over the tendon insertion.

- Advantages – avoids the mechanical problems of using and calibrating transducers attached to joints.

- Disadvantages – simple alteration in hand position can alter electrode geometry sufficiently to change the measured response.

Stimulation patterns in neuromuscular monitoring

Several patterns of current pulses for neuromuscular stimulation have been developed to improve sensitivity in the monitoring. These are designed to exaggerate specific characteristics of non-depolarising muscle blockade, e.g. *fade*, which describes decreased muscle twitch amplitude with repeat stimulation, and *post-tetanic facilitation*, an increase in the response following tetanic stimulation due to increased mobilisation of acetylcholine. The various stimulation patterns include:

- Single twitch
- Train of four
- Tetanic stimulation
- Post-tetanic count
- Double burst

Single twitch

A supramaximal electrical stimulus is delivered at 1 Hz. At this frequency there is sufficient time for complete muscle fibre recovery between stimuli, avoiding any misinterpretation of twitch height arising from fade. The ratio of the measured twitch height after relaxant administration (T1) to the control twitch height before relaxant (Tc) provides a measure of muscle relaxation. Normal muscle function corresponds to a T1/Tc ratio of 1.0. This falls steadily to zero as receptor occupancy increases from 75% to 100%, reflecting acetylcholine receptor occupancy at the neuromuscular junction.

- Advantages – useful for assessment of neuromuscular blockade with depolarising relaxants (suxamethonium chloride), where there is neither fade nor post-tetanic facilitation.
- Disadvantages – limited application due to the narrow range of receptor occupancy detected (i.e. 25%) and the requirement for a means of measuring twitch height, e.g. mechanomyography.

Train of four (TOF)

This pattern consists of four identical stimuli delivered at 2 Hz. Non-depolarising muscle relaxants cause a reduction in height of the first twitch compared with a pre-relaxant supramaximal stimulus, and also a serial reduction in height of the four response twitches. There is a

Detectable twitches	% Receptor blockade
4	>75
3	75
2	80
1	90
0	100

Figure CM40 Acetylcholine receptor occupancy corresponding to number of TOF twitches detectable

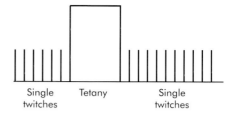

Normal neuromuscular junction

Single twitches   Tetany   Single twitches

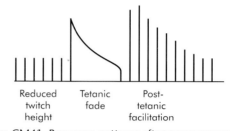

Non-depolarising agent present

Reduced twitch height   Tetanic fade   Post-tetanic facilitation

Figure CM41 Response patterns after neuromuscular stimulation

relationship between receptor occupancy and the number of visually detectable twitches (Figure CM40).

The degree of neuromuscular blockade can be more objectively assessed by calculating the ratio of the fourth (T4) and first (T1) measured twitch heights (T4/T1). The consensus of opinion is that for adequate respiratory function, the T4/T1 ratio must be >70%.

- Advantages – more sensitive than the single twitch. Gives a quantitative result with simple visual assessment.
- Disadvantages – although more sensitive than the single twitch, TOF remains a basically inaccurate method. The fade of TOF pulses on administration of relaxant does not correlate with the reappearance of TOF pulses during recovery.

Tetanic stimulation

The extent of detectable fade following a tetanic stimulation depends on the degree of muscle blockade and the amplitude and duration of the tetanic burst.

By increasing the amplitude of the tetanic burst, it is possible to detect fade at much lower levels of receptor occupancy. A tetanic burst of 50 Hz for 5 seconds produces a muscle response comparable with a maximal voluntary effort. The absence of fade following this stimulus can be interpreted as the return to full muscle power (Figure CM41).

- Advantages – can be used to assess neuromuscular blockade at relatively low levels of receptor occupancy.
- Disadvantages – cannot quantify receptor occupancy from post-tetanic fade. It is an unpleasant sensation in the conscious patient, and leaves an unpleasant sensory aftermath when applied to the unconscious patient.

Post-tetanic count (PTC)

This pattern is sometimes known as post-tetanic potentiation or facilitation. Intense muscle blockade can completely abolish the response to a train of four. Tetanic stimulation increases the mobilisation of acetylcholine (ACh) in the presynaptic membrane. Subsequent electrical stimulation using twitches at 1-second intervals releases supranormal concentrations of ACh, sufficient to overcome the effect of non-depolarising relaxants. The number of resultant twitches (PTC) depends on the frequency of the tetanic burst, the amplitude and duration of the burst, and the degree of neuromuscular blockade present.

This method can produce a response at relatively high levels of receptor occupancy, and a PTC < 5 indicates profound neuromuscular blockade. A PTC > 15 is at least equivalent to two twitches of a TOF, and at this level successful pharmacological reversal of the remaining muscle blockade is possible.

Double burst

This variant pattern was introduced to improve the manual assessment of fade. This consists of two tetanic bursts of 50 Hz. Each burst is composed of three tetanic twitches (at 20 ms intervals), the bursts being separated by 750 ms. Muscle response is clinically detected as just two separate twitches (T1 and T2). The T2/T1 ratio is closely related to the TOF ratio (Figure CM42).

Normal neuromuscular junction

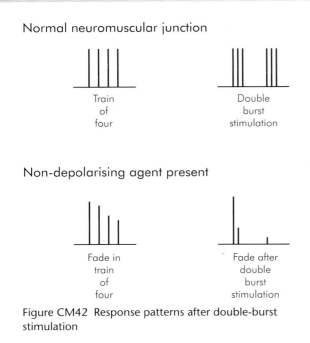

Figure CM42 Response patterns after double-burst stimulation

Parameter	Measurement	Score
P	< Control + 15	0
	< Control + 30	1
	> Control + 30	2
R	< Control + 15	0
	< Control + 30	1
	> Control + 30	2
S	Nil	0
	Skin moist to touch	1
	Visible beads of sweat	2
T	No excess tears, eye open	0
	Excess tears, eye open	1
	Tear overflow, eye closed	2

Figure CM43 Evans scoring system for depth of anaesthesia

Measurement of depth of anaesthesia

In 1845, Snow made the first documented attempt to assess anaesthetic depth, describing five levels of ether anaesthesia. This was refined by Guedel during the First World War, who developed the chart classification of ether anaesthesia based on lacrimation, pupil size and position, respiratory pattern and peripheral movements. Advances in anaesthesia (in particular the introduction of curare soon after the Second World War) made previous classifications obsolete. As a consequence a new system was developed based on the graded assessment of autonomic activity, which includes lacrimation, a parameter surviving from Guedel's chart classification.

The ideal measuring system for assessing anaesthetic depth would:

- Identify a universally acceptable indicator of conscious awareness
- Translate this measurement into a convenient clinical scale
- Eliminate the risk of conscious awareness

To date no system fulfils any of these criteria.

Clinically applied methods for assessment of anaesthetic depth include the following:

- Tunstall's isolated arm technique – provides a gross visual indicator of inadequate anaesthesia by detecting movement in forearm muscles isolated from the effect of muscle relaxants by a tourniquet
- Integrated clinical scores (e.g. Evans score)
- Lower oesophageal contractility
- Frontalis electromyogram
- Electroencephalogram
- Evoked responses – include auditory evoked responses (AER), brain-stem evoked responses (BSER) and visual evoked responses (VER)

Integrated clinical scores

The most commonly quoted score is the Evans or PRST score. This scoring system was designed to assess the elements of autonomic activity: P (systolic blood pressure), R (heart rate), S (sweating) and T (tears). The scoring system is outlined in Figure CM43.

In practice scores range from 0 to 8: the midpoint of the range is rarely exceeded, reflecting the redundancy within this scoring system.

- Advantages – simple, requiring no specialised equipment.
- Disadvantages – parameters are not specific for the effects of anaesthesia. Values vary widely among individuals and can be significantly affected by various drugs and pre-existing disease states.

Lower oesophageal contractility

There are two types of smooth muscle contraction detectable in the lower oesophagus:

- Provoked lower oesophageal contractions (PLOC) – result from sudden distension of the oesophagus, as if due to the arrival of a food bolus. PLOC are induced by the rapid inflation of a balloon catheter in the lower oesophagus. This causes smooth muscle contraction and is detected by a more distally placed pressure transducer. The dose–response curve for PLOC is more shallow than that for spontaneous lower oesophageal contractions.
- Spontaneous lower oesophageal contractions (SLOC) – arise spontaneously and can be induced by emotion and stress in the awake individual. It is believed that SLOC are under the control of a central oesophageal motility centre, the activity of which is influenced by higher centres. SLOC arise spontaneously, and can be detected by the same pressure transducer.

An attempt to improve the available information by combining the measurement of SLOC frequency and PLOC amplitude led to derivation of the oesophageal contractility index (OCI):

$$OCI = 70 \times (SLOC\ rate + PLOC\ amplitude)$$

- Advantages – easy to interpret, can be used in the presence of muscle relaxants.
- Disadvantages – consensus opinion is against this method being a reliable measure of anaesthetic depth.

Frontalis electromyogram (FEMG)

The frontalis muscle was chosen for this purpose because it receives both visceral and somatic fibres from the facial nerve, and it is less sensitive than other muscles to the effects of muscle relaxants. The dual nerve supply means that this muscle can be influenced by autonomic activity. Using two surface electrodes, compound action potentials from this muscle are recorded.

- Advantages – non-invasive, convenient and easy to apply electrodes.
- Disadvantages – recording EMG signals poses technical problems due to low amplitude and interference. There is a wide inter-individual variability in measured FEMG.

Electroencephalogram (EEG)

This method provides a continuous non-invasive assessment of cerebral activity. The generated electrical signal is the summated product of excitatory and inhibitory post-synaptic activity controlled and paced by subthalamic

Band	Frequency range (Hz)
α	8–13
β	>13
δ	<4
θ	4–7

Figure CM44 Frequency bands in the EEG signal

nuclei. To have any clinical use, these signals require extensive processing. The EEG is a varying voltage signal, with amplitudes between 1 and 500 μV. For the purposes of interpretation, the frequency spectrum is divided into four bands (Figure CM44).

If the EEG frequency spectrum for a patient undergoing deepening anaesthesia is plotted, sequential changes are noted. The EEG of an awake patient has a low amplitude and high frequency. Deepening anaesthesia causes a progressive increase in signal amplitude and reduces frequency. All volatile anaesthetics induce these sequential changes in the EEG signal.

- Advantages – EEG monitoring reflects cerebral electrical activity rather than peripheral muscular or autonomic function.
- Disadvantages – unreliable predictors of depth of anaesthesia. At best they provide a trend of information that needs to be combined with clinical observation.

Note that the EEG represents a general indicator of cerebral perfusion and metabolic activity. Hypoxia, hypotension, cerebral oedema and metabolic encephalopathy can significantly depress signal output. Any change in the character of the EEG signal needs to be interpreted with this in mind, and cannot be entirely attributed to anaesthesia. Interpretation is further complicated in that different anaesthetic agents have different effects on the EEG signal.

Cerebral function analysing monitor (CFAM)

This device produces a continuous display of an analysed EEG signal from two symmetrical pairs of scalp electrodes. The top trace displayed shows the mean amplitude of the signals plotted in time (within 90% confidence limits), while the bottom traces show the power amplitude in each frequency band. Thus, at any instant the CFAM display shows the overall mean amplitude and relative power in each frequency band (α, β, θ and δ).

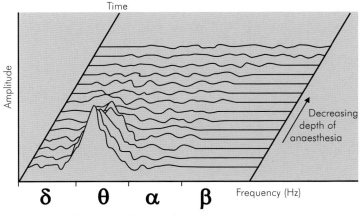

Figure CM45 Compressed spectral array

Compressed spectral array

This system plots sequential segments of the EEG power spectrum, to give a three-dimensional picture of power amplitude vertically (y axis), frequency horizontally (x axis) and time (z axis). This creates a three-dimensional plot of 'peaks' and 'valleys' showing how the power spectrum of the EEG changes with the course of time (Figure CM45).

Evoked responses

These signals are of very low amplitude (1–2 µV) compared with the EEG background trace (10–300 µV) and electrical noise due to neuromuscular activity. They are extracted from the background EEG and noise signal by computer averaging. The signals consist of a series of identifiable peaks and troughs, each with a time delay relative to the stimulus, which is referred to as the *latency*. The early signal (from 0 to 10 ms) is the *brainstem response*, based on its presumed origin. Signals between 10 and 100 ms are middle latency and contain the *early cortical response.* Signals beyond this (100–1000 ms) represent the *late cortical response* arising mainly from the frontal cortex and association areas.

The signal latencies are increased and the peaks and troughs are attenuated, or even abolished, by anaesthesia, sedation and sleep. There is an increasing volume of data that suggests that the early cortical waves of the AER can detect dose-related changes in a range of general anaesthetic agents, respond to surgical stimulation, and correlate with the explicit and implicit memory of events during anaesthesia.

- Brain-stem evoked responses (BSER) are generated using an auditory stimulus and are sometimes referred to as auditory evoked responses (AER). The signal has six distinguishable peaks (I–VI), the anatomical origin of which has caused much debate. It is suggested that the first is derived from the cochlear nerve, the second from the cochlear nucleus, the third from the superior olivary complex, and the fourth and fifth from the inferior colliculus. BSER are not affected significantly by IV anaesthetic agents, thus limiting their usefulness in total IV anaesthesia.
- Visual evoked response (VER) arises from stimulation of the visual pathway by a pulsed flash of light. This modified flash test produces variable results, and as such is more suited to a qualitative rather than a quantitative assessment. The signals represent a mainly cortical response.

Temperature measurement

Temperature scales

- Fahrenheit (1714) developed this temperature scale using the first mercury thermometer. The zero point was set using a mixture of sodium chloride and ice. According to this scale, ice melted at 32 °F, water boiled at 212 °F and body temperature was assumed to be 100 °F.
- Celsius (1742) developed a scale (also known as centigrade) with two fixed points, 0 °C for the melting point of ice and 100 °C for the boiling point of water.
- Kelvin (absolute temperature scale) – uses absolute zero and the triple point of water, 273.16 K. The

boiling point of water according to this scale is approximately 373 K.

Conversion between temperature scales
Simple conversion between temperature scales can be made as follows:

Celsius to Fahrenheit ($^\circ$F) = ($^\circ$C × 9/5) + 32
Fahrenheit to Celsius ($^\circ$C) = ($^\circ$F − 32) × 5/9
Celsius to Kelvin (K) = ($^\circ$C + 273.15)

Temperature measurement site
Small temperature gradients exist between different parts of the body in normal subjects. The ability of a measured value to reflect core temperature depends on the site chosen. This will also determine the response time, i.e. the speed with which a change in body temperature is registered. The following sites may be used:

- Oesophagus – correct probe position is in the lower 25% of the oesophagus. When correctly placed, the measured values provide a good estimate of cerebral blood temperature. If placed above this level, however, the probe may under-read due to the cooling effect of the inspired gases.
- Nasopharynx – probe should be positioned just behind the soft palate. This provides a less accurate measure of core temperature than the oesophageal probe.
- Tympanic membrane – aural canal temperature provides an accurate measure of hypothalamic temperature. It has a short response time and correlates well with the results obtained from an oesophageal probe.
- Blood – blood temperature can be measured using the thermistor of a pulmonary flotation catheter. This method provides the best continuous measure of core temperature.
- Rectum – rectal temperature is influenced by the heat generated by gut flora, the cooling effect of blood returning from the lower limbs and the insulation of the temperature probe by faeces. The rectal temperature is normally 0.5–1.0% higher than core temperature, and compared with other sites the response time is slow.

Thermometers
These can be classified as:
(1) **Direct-reading** thermometers – where the display and site of measurement are in direct contact

(2) **Remote-reading** thermometers – where the display is distant from the site of measurement

The choice of thermometer is determined by the application, the clinical environment, the required accuracy, and whether a continuous display is needed.
Clinical measurement of temperature uses the following devices:
- Liquid expansion thermometer
- Chemical thermometer
- Resistance thermometer
- Thermistor
- Thermocouple

Note that dial thermometers usually measure the environmental temperature.

Direct-reading thermometers
Liquid expansion thermometers
These consist of a glass bulb filled with either alcohol or mercury, which is connected to a narrow evacuated glass capillary tube. When warmed, the liquid expands, causing a column of liquid to rise up the capillary tube. The temperature corresponds to a point on a calibrated temperature scale measured by the height of the fluid column. If the cross-sectional area of the capillary tube is constant, then the relationship between expansion of the liquid and the column height will remain linear.
- Advantages – simple, no power supply required.
- Disadvantages – poor visual display of temperature, slow response time, limited temperature range (requiring a low-reading thermometer for hypothermia), cannot be read remotely, easily broken, unsuitable for insertion into cavities.

Chemical thermometers
Chemical thermometers consist of a series of cells, each containing a mixture of chemicals, the colour of which is temperature-dependent. The particular chemical mixture is chosen to suit the required temperature range, and the colour change usually occurs within 30 seconds. The older single-use thermometers relied on a series of dye-containing crystals. The newer reusable thermometers use liquid crystal technology. In these, the solid crystals are colourless, and as they melt the realignment of the composite molecules produces the change in colour.
- Advantages – fast response time, no breakage problem, disposable.
- Disadvantages – usually only possible to differentiate temperature intervals of about 0.5 $^\circ$C.

Dial thermometers

Two types:

(1) **Bimetallic** – a typical example consists of a flattened spiral spring composed of two dissimilar metals each with a different coefficient of expansion. One end of the spring is fixed, the other attached to a pointer. As the temperature increases the spring either winds or unwinds, causing the pointer to move across a temperature scale.

(2) **Pressure gauge** type – based on the Bourdon pressure gauge and consists of a hollow spiral metal tube. This tube forms a spring and terminates at one end in a temperature-sensing bulb. The bulb contains either volatile liquid or vapour that expands as the temperature increases, causing an increase in pressure within the tube. This results in an unwinding movement which is coupled to a pointer on a temperature scale.

- Advantages – relatively cheap and robust, providing a continuous easily readable measurement.
- Disadvantages – accuracy of these thermometers is poor and they are prone to calibration errors.

Remote-reading thermometers
Resistance thermometers

Resistance thermometers utilise the change in electrical resistance of a coil of wire with temperature. This occurs according to the relationship

$$R_t = R_0(1 + at + bt^2)$$

where R_t is the resistance at temperature $t\,°C$, R_0 is the resistance at $0\,°C$, and a and b are constants.

The change in resistance is detected using a Wheatstone bridge circuit and galvanometer. Platinum is most commonly used for this purpose because it resists corrosion, and has a large temperature coefficient of resistance. This type of thermometer has the ability to measure very small changes in temperature, i.e. $\pm 0.0001\,°C$. Over the range 0–$100\,°C$, the relationship between temperature and resistance is largely linear.

- Advantages – accuracy.
- Disadvantages – physical size of the coil, making it difficult to produce a small probe; fragile, slow response time.

Thermistors

Composed of the fused oxides of heavy metals (including of manganese, nickel, zinc, cobalt and iron), a thermistor is a semiconductor that possesses a negative temperature coefficient of resistance. The components are compressed into minute beads (ranging in diameter from 0.012 to 0.25 cm) which have very small thermal capacities and rapid response times (as little as 0.2 s). A greater temperature coefficient makes thermistors more sensitive than wire resistance thermometers.

- Advantages – small size, rapid response time.
- Disadvantages – relationship between resistance and temperature is non-linear and subject to wide variation. This requires signal conditioning and calibration. Thermistors from the same batch show wide variation in their electrical resistance, and as they age their electrical resistance changes. Thermistors exhibit hysteresis, and the relationship between resistance and temperature is different when heating up from that when cooling. To minimise these effects, commercial thermistors are batched and pre-aged.

Thermocouples

A thermocouple is an electric circuit composed of two different metals, joined to form two separate identical junctions. If these junctions are maintained at different temperatures, an electromotive force (EMF) is generated that is proportional to the temperature difference between the two junctions and can be measured using a galvanometer. This is the *Seebeck effect*.

The metals commonly used include copper–constantin (copper/nickel alloy), and platinum–rhodium.

- Advantages – junctions may be very small and versatile. Low thermal capacity means rapid response times. Acceptable accuracy ($\pm 0.1\,°C$). All junctions made with the same metals behave identically. Relatively cheap.
- Disadvantages – voltage output per degree Celsius is small (about 50 mV) and requires signal amplification. The non-linear relationship between EMF and temperature requires signal processing to correct.

Humidity measurement

Historically the measurement of humidity was an important contribution to the safe practice of anaesthesia. The combination of static electric sparks, and the use of flammable anaesthetic gases (e.g. ether) constituted a significant risk to both patient and anaesthetist. One of the measures used to reduce static electricity, and hence the incidence of fires and explosions, was to maintain the relative humidity in the operating theatre above 50%. While this is no longer a major consideration in current practice, an understanding of humidity, with its influence on thermal balance and respiratory function, is important. Failure to adequately humidify respiratory gases by using a heat and moisture exchanger (HME) or circle circuit can result in:

- Failure to maintain patient temperature
- Mucosal drying and decreased ciliary activity
- Increased viscosity of secretions

Definition of humidity

Humidity can be defined in two ways:

(1) **Absolute humidity** – mass of water vapour present in a given volume of gas at defined temperature and pressure (expressed as g H_2O m^{-3} gas)

(2) **Relative humidity** – mass of water vapour present in a given volume of gas, expressed as a percentage of the mass of water vapour required to saturate the same volume of gas at identical temperature and pressure

Note particularly that the amount of water vapour required to saturate a known volume of gas increases with temperature, so a gas saturated at room temperature ($20\,°C$) contains less water than the same volume saturated at body temperature ($37\,°C$).

From its definition, relative humidity (RH) can be calculated from the ratio of the mass of water vapour present (m_P) to the mass required for saturation (m_S):

$$RH = \frac{m_P}{m_S}$$

However, from the gas laws, mass of a gas in a mixture is proportional to the partial pressure it exerts, thus:

$$RH = \frac{\text{water vapour pressure}}{\text{saturated water vapour pressure}}$$

Hygrometers

A hygrometer is a device that measures humidity. Examples include:

- Regnault's hygrometer (Figure CM46) – based on the cooling effect of evaporating ether on the temperature of a silver tube. When the temperature of the tube decreases to the *dew point*, small droplets of water condense on the outside. The temperature of the ether at the dew point corresponds to the absolute humidity of the surrounding air, and can be determined from tables.
- Hair hygrometer – hair protein is organised into β-pleated sheets. This biochemical structure elongates in the presence of moist heat. The increase in hair length is proportional to the humidity of the

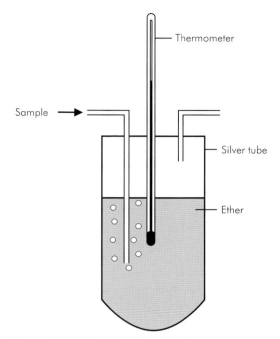

Figure CM46 Regnault's hygrometer

surrounding air. If one end of the hair is fixed to a light lever, the change in length can be amplified and measured. Once calibrated, the instrument can be used to measure relative humidity. The accuracy is poor, and the measured range is limited to between 15% and 85% relative humidity (though this is still adequate to measure humidity in the operating theatre).

- Wet and dry bulb thermometers (Figure CM47) – uses two mercury bulb thermometers, a *dry* thermometer that is exposed to air and a *wet* thermometer that is surrounded by a wick that draws water from a small reservoir. The temperature of the wet thermometer depends on the rate of evaporation of water from the wick, and hence the humidity of the surrounding air. This temperature will always be lower than that recorded on the dry thermometer. The difference between the two recorded temperatures decreases as the humidity increases. Using specific tables, the relative humidity can be obtained from the measured temperature difference.
- Humidity transducers – measure a change in electrical current in response to a change in humidity. The electrical conductivity of certain substances varies depending on the amount of absorbed water. When such a substance is incorporated into a simple

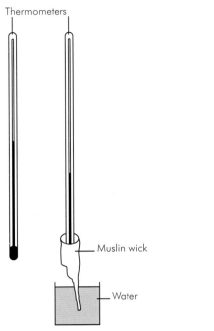

Thermometers

— Muslin wick

— Water

Figure CM47 Wet and dry bulb thermometer

Dimension	Parameter measured or described
Physical	Location
	Intensity and character
	Frequency and duration
Functional	Aggravating and relieving factors
	Disability, e.g. walking distance, self care
	Productivity, e.g. employment, recreation
Behavioural	Rubbing, grimacing, guarding, vocalisation
	Gait and posture
	Medication frequency and dosage
Affect	Degree of depression
Cognition	Degree of understanding

Figure CM48 Dimensions characterising pain

electrical circuit as either a resistor or a capacitor, any increase in the humidity results as a detectable change in either resistance or capacitance. This method provides a rapid, sensitive measure of humidity and is often used in control systems for air-conditioning systems. These transducers display hysteresis.

Measurement of pain

Pain is one of the most difficult physiological phenomena to quantify, but its impact on the individual patient, and on health care in general, make assessment an essential part of clinical practice. Pain has been defined by the International Association for the Study of Pain as 'an unpleasant sensory and emotional experience associated with actual or potential tissue damage'. For details of the physiology of pain, see Section 2, Chapter 10.

Pain is multidimensional (Figure CM48), and has to be assessed using both objective and subjective methods of measurement:

- An observer performs **objective** measurement. In addition to assessment of the pain dimensions outlined in Figure CM48, objective measurements also include measurements associated with the physical changes accompanying pain.

- **Subjective** measurement consists of data that are self-reported by the patient.

Most of the methods of assessing pain dimensions are common to both patient and observer.

A further dimension defining the nature of a pain condition is the classification into acute and chronic pain (see Section 2, Chapter 10, page 429). Physiological changes are associated with both acute and chronic pain conditions. In acute pain, these signs are reflected by autonomic changes, which can be recorded and scored. They are particularly useful when assessing pain in unconscious or obtunded patients, but are not specifically associated with pain and are open to misinterpretation (Figure CM49).

Single-dimension pain measurement

Single-dimension measurements can be applied to both acute and chronic pain situations, and include:

- Use of body chart for pain location – a simple diagram on which the patient or observer marks the areas corresponding to the pain.
- Visual analogue scale – a straight line drawn between two extremes, e.g. 'no pain' and 'worst pain imaginable'. The patient marks a point on this line to represent their current status. It can be used for various parameters such as pain, mood, pain relief and disability. The value is taken as the distance of the mark along the scale from the origin. The validity of

Pain	Signs
Acute pain	Heart rate
	Blood pressure
	Respiratory rate
	Lacrimation
	Sweating
Chronic pain	Changes in limb size and muscle bulk
	Changes in skin temperature and sweating
	Localised swelling
	Muscle spasm

Figure CM49 Physical signs associated with pain

these scales is questioned concerning their reproducibility and reliability. Current opinion is that visual analogue scales are reliable when used with the appropriate group of patients and under controlled circumstances. These scales are not suitable for very young children, in the immediate postoperative period, or with the visually impaired.

- Numerical ranking or pictorial ranking – an alternative to using visual analogue scales, and may be more suitable for some groups of patients (e.g. children). These scales are marked by numbers, or pictures of faces, to represent increasing or decreasing pain. The gradation is thus not continuous, but is limited to a finite number of choices. This may make the results more reproducible in some cases and the method may be easier to use for patients, but a loss of sensitivity can result.
- Word descriptor ranking – here assessment is dependent on a choice of a word descriptor from a list. The assessment is obtained by scoring for each word to give a pain rating index (PRI). Alternatively, using free choice from non-scored word lists, the total number of words chosen (NWC) can be recorded. Multiple word descriptor lists can be used to produce multidimensional pain assessment. This method can be adapted for visually impaired patients.

Multidimensional pain measurement

These methods can be applied to produce a more complete assessment of a pain condition by combining assessment of multiple pain dimensions. They include:

- McGill questionnaire – first described by Melzack in 1975. It consists of a body map and word descriptor sections for evaluating the intensity and other characteristics of pain. It is a relatively involved questionnaire taking around 20 minutes or more to complete, depending on patient skills. This limits its application since it is not suitable for children, highly anxious patients or patients in the immediate postoperative period. It is commonly used in research.
- Memorial pain assessment card – a collection of linear analogue scales for different pain dimensions such as intensity, pain relief or mood. It can also include a limited set of word descriptor lists.
- Pain observation chart – can be designed for patients to record a number of pain dimensions on a diary basis, e.g. pain intensity, pain relief and drug side effects to optimise drug regimes. Alternatively pain charts can be designed for observers or carers to record objective assessment data on a diary/timetable basis, to optimise postoperative analgesia.
- Beck depression inventory – provides a self-reported index of depression that can be used to quantify changes in depression levels due to treatment of chronic pain conditions.

Assessment of pain in children

Pain assessment in children is dependent on the age and skills of the child, and is affected significantly by their interaction with their parents. Some of the methods used are summarised in Figure CM50.

Age (years)	Method
Infant	Observation – crying, motor withdrawal
1–3	Observation – crying, withdrawal, facial expression, lip smacking, aggressive behaviour
3–5	Pictorial-ranking scales
	Colour-matching scales
5–12	Visual analogue scales
	Number-ranking scales
>12	Multidimensional scales

Figure CM50 Methods of pain assessment in children

CHAPTER 3

Anaesthetic equipment

E. S. Lin

Medical gas pipeline services

The medical gas pipeline system (MGPS) provides wall gas and vacuum supplies at working areas such as operating theatres, resuscitation and recovery areas. The MGPS consists of the following:

- Oxygen (at 420 kPa)
- Nitrous oxide
- Medical air (at 700 and 420 kPa)
- Medical vacuum
- Scavenging vacuum

The gases and services are distributed by a medical pipeline network to specialised terminal outlets. Equipment can then be connected to these outlets by non-interchangeable flexible hosing.

The MGPS distribution network consists of especially cleaned and degreased medical-quality copper pipes. These

Fundamentals of Anaesthesia, 3rd edition, ed. Tim Smith, Colin Pinnock and Ted Lin. Published by Cambridge University Press. © Cambridge University Press 2008.

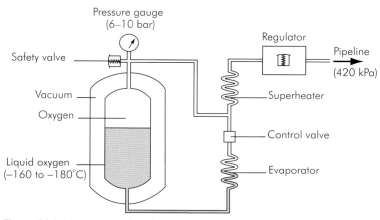

Figure EQ1 Vacuum-insulated evaporator

are colour-coded and installed to government-specified standards. Different areas of the network are isolated by special valves connected into the network by non-interchangeable threaded (NIST) unions.

The pipeline terminal outlets consist of Schrader sockets that are clearly labelled and colour-coded for the service or gas. They are matched for a specific connecting flexible pipeline by a collar indexing system. Each flexible pipeline is colour-coded with unique terminal and equipment ends. The terminal end consists of an indexed Schrader probe that fits into its specific terminal socket. The other end of the hose is a non-interchangeable (NIST) union, which connects on to a piece of equipment. These design features of the hoses and terminal sockets ensure that the gases or services cannot be cross-connected to equipment.

Oxygen supply

Oxygen is stored centrally in a vacuum-insulated evaporator (VIE). This consists of an inner stainless-steel tank with an outer steel jacket. A vacuum is maintained between the tank and jacket for insulation. The VIE has the following features:

- It contains liquid and gaseous oxygen with an inner temperature between -160 and $-180\ ^{\circ}\mathrm{C}$ (lower than the critical temperature of oxygen, which is $-118\ ^{\circ}\mathrm{C}$, but higher than the boiling point at 1 atm, $-183\ ^{\circ}\mathrm{C}$).
- The pressure within the VIE is approximately 1100–1300 kPa, varying with oxygen demand.
- There is a main outlet at the top of the VIE, for oxygen withdrawal to supply the distribution pipeline.
- Liquid oxygen may also be withdrawn via a separate outlet and fed through a superheater, in order to 'top

up' the supply line and maintain pressure during periods of high demand.
- A reserve supply, provided by a cylinder bank, is available in case of VIE failure.
- The VIE normally contains enough oxygen for 10 days' supply, while the reserves are adequate for 24 hours' use.

A schematic diagram of a VIE is shown in Figure EQ1.

Nitrous oxide supply

Nitrous oxide is supplied from a central bank of gas cylinders, which contain a mixture of liquid and gas (critical temperature of nitrous oxide is 36.5 °C). These are connected to the distribution pipeline network by a control panel, which regulates the gas pressure. The control may also provide local heating in order to avoid condensation and freezing due to the cooling caused by the evaporation of the liquid nitrous oxide. A reserve bank of cylinders is also provided.

Medical compressed air

Compressed air for medical use must be much purer than its industrial equivalent. It is generated by compressors and will contain oil mist as well as water vapour. In a hospital two types of supply are required, a low-pressure supply (420 kPa) for anaesthetic machines and ventilators, and a higher-pressure supply (700 kPa) to provide power for surgical equipment. The pipeline network may be supplied either by a bank of air cylinders or by a local compressor system. If a local compressor is used care must be taken to ensure the purity of the compressed air produced.

Content	Gas/vapour	Cylinder pressure kPa (psi)	Boiling point at 1 atm (°C)	Critical temperature (°C)
Oxygen	gas	13 700 (1980)	−183	−118
Nitrous oxide	vapour	4400 (640)	−89	36.5
Entonox	gas and vapour	13 700 (1980)	gas separation at −6°C	
Air	gas	13 700 (1980)		
Carbon dioxide	vapour	5000 (723)	−78.5	31
Helium	gas	13 700 (1980)	−269	−268

Figure EQ2 Gases and vapours supplied in cylinders

Substance	Gas/vapour	Symbol	Colour coding	
			Cylinder	Shoulder
Oxygen	gas	O_2	black	white
Nitrous oxide	vapour	N_2O	blue	blue
Entonox	gas and vapour	N_2O/O_2	blue	white/blue
Air	gas	AIR	black	white/black
Carbon dioxide	vapour	CO_2	grey	grey
Helium	gas	He	brown	brown

Figure EQ3 Colour coding of gas cylinders (for UK and ISO)

Medical vacuum

Medical vacuum is required for suction, and BS4957 specifications suggest a vacuum level of 53 kPa (400 mmHg). Medical vacuum is also required for scavenging of anaesthetic gases, but it is not recommended that the same vacuum supply is used for both purposes because:

- Suction requires relatively low flow rates but high levels of vacuum, which if applied inadvertently to a patient's airway would be harmful.
- Scavenging requires low vacuum levels with high flow rates. The high flow rates used to remove waste anaesthetic gases could reduce suction levels during surgery.
- Waste anaesthetic gases contain volatile vapours which may be absorbed by lubricants and ultimately cause system failure.

Suction vacuum systems incorporate bacterial filtration and drainage to dispose of aspirated body fluids.

Gas cylinders

Gases and vapours are supplied from cylinders in the absence or failure of piped gas supplies. The cylinders are made of molybdenum steel, which is stronger than carbon steel. This enables cylinders to be made lighter in weight and with thinner walls. They are used to supply the gases and vapours shown in Figure EQ2.

Cylinder identification

Cylinders possess various markings on the cylinder or its label which include:

- Tare weight of cylinder
- Hydraulic test pressure of cylinder
- Identity of gas (symbol)
- Density of gas
- Serial number of cylinder
- Owner of cylinder and manufacturer of gases

The cylinders are also identified visually by a symbol and colour coding, as listed in Figure EQ3.

Pin index system (PIS)

Gas cylinders are also identified mechanically by a pin indexing system, which conforms to both British Standard (BS) and equivalent International Standards Organisation

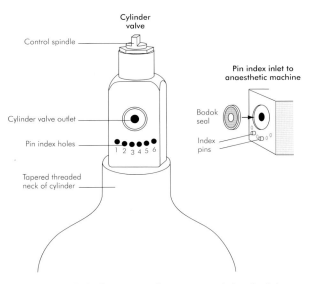

Figure EQ4 Pin index system for gases, and detail of the cylinder head

Pin index positions:

Nitrous oxide	·	·	3	·	5	·	
Oxygen	·	2	·	·	5	·	
Air	1	·	·	·	5	·	
Carbon dioxide	1	·	·	·	·	6	
Entonox							7

(ISO) specifications. This system prevents the wrong cylinder from being connected to an anaesthetic machine.

The pin index system is designed into the outlet valve block of the cylinder, and is illustrated in Figure EQ4. The cylinder valve block face matches up to the inlet port of the anaesthetic machine. This face contains the gas outlet from the cylinder, which is made gas-tight by a metal and rubber ring seal, the Bodok seal. Beneath the outlet are six possible positions for indexing holes. Pins on the anaesthetic machine inlet fit into these holes. If the positions of these pins do not match the index holes on the valve block outlet, the cylinder cannot be fitted to that particular inlet on the anaesthetic machine. Figure EQ4 shows PIS positions for some of the gases commonly used, and details of the cylinder head arrangement.

Cylinder testing

Cylinders are hydraulically tested every 5 years using water under high pressure. Water or water vapour remaining in a cylinder may represent a hazard because it may condense and freeze (affecting the operation of the outlet valve) if the cylinder empties rapidly. Random cylinders from a batch may be destructively tested by the manufacturers using water under pressure.

Cylinders may be inspected endoscopically for cracks and defects on their inner surfaces, and they can also be tested ultrasonically.

Estimation of cylinder contents

The contents of a cylinder, for both gases and vapours, are estimated by weighing the cylinder and subtracting the weight of the empty cylinder or *tare weight*. The tare weight is recorded on the cylinder itself. Cylinder contents can thus be estimated by weighing a cylinder and subtracting the tare weight of the cylinder.

Gases

In the case of gases, such as oxygen and air, cylinders are initially filled to a given pressure (13 700 kPa). Since gases are not liquefied in the cylinder (temperature < critical temperature), the cylinder contents can also be estimated by the cylinder pressure. This gradually decreases as the cylinder empties. The mass of gas present is directly proportional to the pressure according to the universal gas law, and the volume of the contents available at atmospheric pressure can be estimated using Boyle's law.

Vapours

In the case of vapours (such as nitrous oxide or carbon dioxide) the contents of the cylinders are a mixture of gas and liquid. The cylinders are initially filled to a given *filling ratio*. The filling ratio is defined as the weight of the substance contained divided by the weight of a volume of water equal to the internal volume of the cylinder. This ratio is set at 0.75, since if the cylinders are overfilled there is a risk of rupture with increases in ambient temperature.

The cylinder pressure cannot be used to estimate cylinder contents in the case of a vapour, because it does not vary as the cylinder empties. This is because the cylinder pressure is maintained at saturated vapour pressure (SVP) while liquid is present. The cylinder pressure only falls when the cylinder is nearly empty and all of the liquid contents have evaporated. Cylinder pressure, in the case of vapour content only, varies if the temperature changes. This can occur when the cylinder is emptied rapidly, due to absorption of latent heat of vaporisation causing cooling of the contents. Under these circumstances the cylinder pressure will decrease with cooling but will be restored as the cylinder warms up again (Figure EQ5).

(a) Slow emptying of cylinder

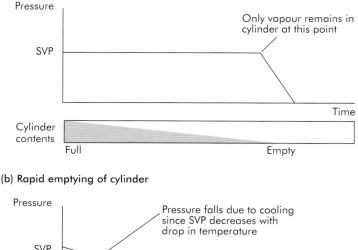

(b) Rapid emptying of cylinder

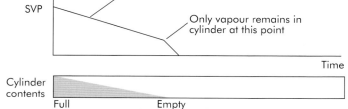

Figure EQ5 Pressure and temperature changes in a cylinder containing vapour

Pressure regulators

The high pressure inside gas cylinders is reduced by a pressure regulator before connection to equipment such as an anaesthetic machine. An example of a single-stage regulator which might be used to reduce oxygen cylinder pressure from 13 700 kPa to 420 kPa is shown in Figure EQ6. Cylinder pressure (P) is reduced to the supply pressure (p) as oxygen passes through the small inlet valve (area $=$ a) into the control chamber. The pressure in the control chamber (p) is controlled by a compression spring acting on a diaphragm (area $=$ A) which is coupled mechanically to the inlet valve. The supply pressure is thus controlled by the force (F) in the spring. This can be expressed by the following equation:

$F =$ Force acting on conical valve
   $+$ Force acting on diaphragm

$= Pa + pA$

It is assumed that the force in the spring remains constant, i.e. the range of movement in the spring is small compared to its total length. Then any change in the supply or cylinder pressures will cause a compensating change as the diaphragm moves and varies the effective area of the inlet valve. In the above equation, if F is constant, a decrease in pA (drop in supply pressure due to increased demand) causes an increase in Pa (increased flow from cylinder). Alternatively if Pa decreases (due to cylinder pressure falling as it empties), pA will increase (increased flow from cylinder).

Thus the pressure regulator not only reduces the cylinder pressure to a suitable supply pressure but also compensates for changes in demand or cylinder pressure. The sensitivity of this control depends on the ratio of the area of the diaphragm to the area of the valve, which is usually 200 to 1.

Anaesthetic machines

Surgical anaesthesia is usually provided through a continuous-flow anaesthetic machine which consists of the following components:

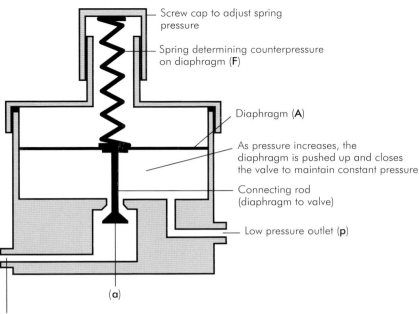

Screw cap to adjust spring pressure

Spring determining counterpressure on diaphragm (**F**)

Diaphragm (**A**)

As pressure increases, the diaphragm is pushed up and closes the valve to maintain constant pressure

Connecting rod (diaphragm to valve)

Low pressure outlet (**p**)

(**a**)

High pressure inlet (**P**)

Figure EQ6 Single-stage pressure regulator

- Metal framework and pipeline circuitry
- Medical gas pipeline service connections
- Connections for gas cylinders and pressure gauges for cylinder contents
- Safety mechanisms
- Back bar including vaporiser connections
- Common gas outlet and auxiliary gas outlets
- Vaporisers
- Rotameters (see Section 4, Chapter 2, pages 804–5)
- Scavenging circuitry
- Suction circuitry

The basic arrangement of these components is illustrated in Figure EQ7. Modern machines often incorporate electronic monitoring, safety features and a mechanical ventilator.

Metal framework and pipeline circuitry

The metal framework of the anaesthetic machine is usually made of stainless steel and is electrically earthed via anti-static wheels, which reduce risks of electric shock, interference with rotameters, and fire or explosion of inflammable agents. The frame incorporates pipeline circuitry with both fixed and detachable joints. The pipes are usually brass or copper with brazed fixed joints. More recently nylon pipes have been introduced. Detachable joints are screw-threaded and sealed with a compressible washer, O-ring seal or polytetrafluoroethylene (PTFE) tape. Different diameter pipes are used for each gas to prevent cross connection.

Medical gas pipeline service (MGPS) connections

Non-interchangeable screw-threaded (NIST) connections are used for MGPS supplies. Flexible colour-coded hoses are used to connect to gas-specific wall terminals. The machine end of these hoses is a male NIST connector which is made gas-specific by:
- A non-interchangeable threaded nut
- A specific diameter shoulder with O-ring seal
- A specific diameter forward shaft

The machine MGPS connections are the female counterparts of the above hose connectors. They also incorporate metal gauze filters and one-way non-return valves to prevent retrograde leakage.

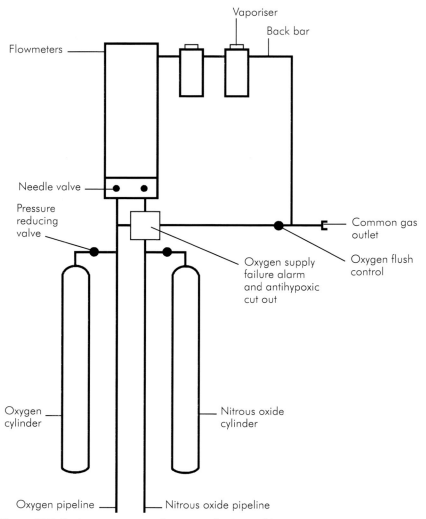

Figure EQ7 Basic components of an anaesthetic machine

Pin index system (PIS) connections for gas cylinders

The PIS connections for the cylinder gas supplies consist of a gas inlet with the male counterpart of the PIS, i.e. pins corresponding to the indexing holes on the cylinder valve block. A yoke with an arrangement secured by a screw fitting holds the cylinder valve block in place. The cylinder inlets also incorporate metal gauze filters and one-way non-return valves to prevent retrograde leakage. Retrograde leakage through gas inlets, if great enough, has been known to alter the gas mixture delivered to the patient, and can lead to the delivery of a hypoxic mixture. The PIS connection is made gas-tight by a metal and rubber ring seal in the cylinder valve block (Bodok seal). Pin index positions have been described in Figure EQ4.

Safety mechanisms

Several safety mechanisms are incorporated into the design of an anaesthetic machine. These include:

- **Secondary pressure regulators** – Smooth out gas pressure fluctuations within the anaesthetic machine, which occur due to changes in pipeline pressure or variations in demand from the machine. Such fluctuations in machine pressure can cause inaccuracies in the fresh gas mixture, or disturb the performance of rotameters and oxygen monitors. Secondary pressure regulators are set to pressures below the anticipated pressure fluctuations and are designed to maintain working pressures within 10% over a wide range of flow rates, from hundreds of millilitres to tens of litres.

- **Oxygen failure warning device** – Monitoring of the delivered fresh gas oxygen concentration is mandatory, but the anaesthetic machine also has a built-in oxygen failure device. This is mounted upstream of the rotameter block and is designed according to BS4272 specifications, which include:

  ○ Audible alarm > 60 db at a distance of 1 metre from the machine, for 7 seconds or more
  ○ Activation when the oxygen supply falls to 200 kPa
  ○ Power supply derived from the oxygen supply pressure
  ○ Alarm that cannot be switched off or reset until the oxygen supply is restored
  ○ Alarm coupled to a gas cutoff valve that cuts off anaesthetic gases and opens the machine pipeline circuitry to air

An early oxygen failure warning device was the Ritchie whistle (1960), and many modern devices are similar in principle. Figure EQ8 shows how such a device works.

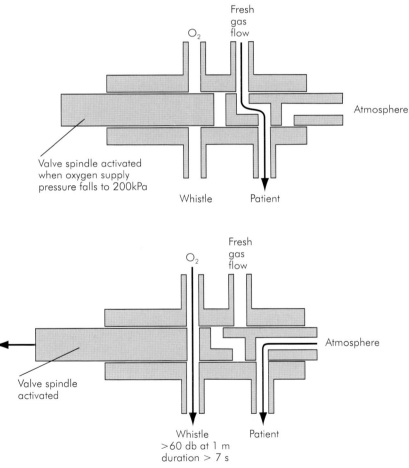

Figure EQ8 Oxygen failure warning device (Ritchie whistle)

- **Oxygen bypass circuit** – Bypasses the rotameter block and back bar to provide an emergency oxygen flow of at least 30 litres per minute to the common gas outlet. The control is usually a push-button situated near the common gas outlet, which is recessed to prevent accidental operation, and which cannot be locked, to prevent barotrauma to the patient.

Back bar

The back bar is the horizontal part of the anaesthetic machine circuit between the rotameter block and the common gas outlet. It is downstream of the rotameter block and feeds fresh gas mixture to the common gas outlet. Vaporisers are mounted on the back bar, enabling volatile agents to be added to the fresh gases. The pressure in the back bar is approximately 1 kPa at the outlet end, and may be 7–10 kPa at the rotameter end, depending on:

- Total gas flow
- Circuit connection to common gas outlet
- Vaporisers used and their settings

Total occlusion of the common gas outlet produces pressures of approximately 30 kPa in the back bar. The maximum pressure that can be produced in the back bar is limited by a 'blow off', or pressure relief valve at the outlet end (threshold set to 30–40 kPa). This protects the rotameter block and vaporisers from overpressure damage, and to a very limited degree protects the patient from barotrauma.

Vaporiser connections

The connection system for vaporisers (and the vaporisers themselves), are designed with the following features:

- Prevention of gas leakage from the back bar with or without a vaporiser in place
- Prevention of volatile agent leakage into the back-bar circuit
- Convenient installation and removal of vaporisers
- Safety interlock mechanism to prevent use of more than one volatile agent simultaneously

Figure EQ9 illustrates some of these design features. The potential hazards caused by poor design or usage of the vaporiser connection system include:

- Leakage of gas causing inadequate fresh gas mixtures or pressures to be delivered to the patient
- Leakage of volatile agent into the fresh gas flow
- Damage or injury caused by difficulty in attaching or detaching vaporisers

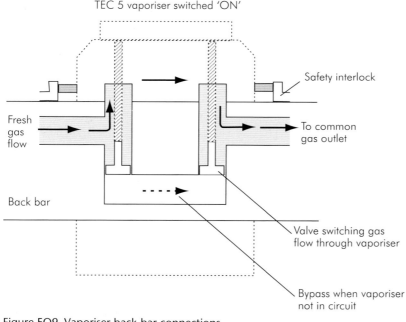

Figure EQ9 Vaporiser back-bar connections

- Contamination of downstream vaporisers by upstream volatile agent, when no safety interlock mechanism is present
- Contamination of soda lime in the breathing circuit by trichloroethylene (no longer used in the UK), which produces a neurotoxin

In early machines, where more than one vaporiser could be switched on at a time, a more volatile agent (e.g. halothane), if placed upstream, could be absorbed by a less volatile agent (e.g. trichloroethylene). This could lead to the release of a maximal concentration (determined by the saturated vapour pressure) of the absorbed agent on subsequent use of the downstream vaporiser. In modern machines with a good safety interlock mechanism, the sequence of vaporisers on the back bar presents no significant hazard.

Gas outlets

The common gas outlet is a 22 mm male (external) and 15 mm female (internal) tapered outlet which supplies fresh gas mixture to the patient breathing circuit or a mechanical ventilator. It may be mounted on a swivel (Cardiff swivel) for increased convenience. It can withstand bending moments of up to 10 Nm (equivalent approximately to 40–50 kg weight hanging from the outlet). It may be threaded to prevent accidental disconnection.

The auxiliary gas outlets are Schrader oxygen or air sockets, which can be used to power devices such as a ventilator or a Venturi injector.

Anaesthetic machine maintenance

Servicing of machines should follow manufacturer's guidelines. Typically servicing is performed at 3- to 6-month intervals. Each machine should have an attached logbook to record commissioning date, servicing dates, faults, repairs and modifications.

Anaesthetic machine checklist

The anaesthetic machine should be checked by the anaesthetist before each operating session. A checklist is published by the Association of Anaesthetists of Great Britain and Ireland (2004) as a card, which is usually attached to each machine. This is reproduced at the end of the chapter in Figure EQ41.

Vaporisers

The functions of a vaporiser are:
- To produce vaporisation of the volatile anaesthetic agent.

Volatile agent	SVP (kPa) at 20 °C	BP (°C) at 100 kPa	MAC
Halothane	31.9	51	0.76
Enflurane	23.1	56	1.68
Isoflurane	31.5	48	1.15
Sevoflurane	21.3	58	2
Desflurane	88.5	23	6

Figure EQ10 Properties of some commonly used volatile agents

- To mix the vapour with the fresh gas flow to the patient.
- To control the mixture so that a given concentration of volatile agent is delivered to the patient, in spite of varying gas flow rates and ambient temperature conditions.

The design of a vaporiser is determined by the clinical application and the volatile agent being used. Choice of a vaporiser for use in the absence of compressed gas supplies will differ from that where piped supplies are available, while a vaporiser suitable for use with desflurane will be very different from one for use with isoflurane. The important properties of volatile agents when considering vaporiser design are saturated vapour pressure (SVP), boiling point (BP) and minimum alveolar concentration (MAC). These are shown for some commonly used agents in Figure EQ10.

Two different types of vaporiser are considered here, **variable bypass** and **measured flow**.

Variable bypass vaporiser

In this vaporiser the fresh gas flow to the patient circuit is split into two streams by a flow-splitting valve. One stream bypasses the vaporising chamber and is free from volatile agent. The other stream passes through the vaporiser chamber and becomes saturated with vapour. This second stream then rejoins the bypass flow to give the required concentration of vapour in the fresh gas flow to the patient (Figure EQ11). The final vapour concentration is controlled by using the flow-splitting valve to vary the fraction of the gas flow passing through the vaporiser chamber. Accuracy is therefore dependent on the flow-splitting valve maintaining a constant *flow-splitting ratio* over the range of flow rates used. There are two main types of variable bypass vaporiser, described below: **plenum vaporisers** and **draw-over vaporisers**.

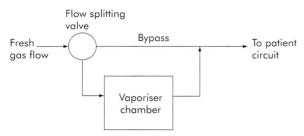

Figure EQ11   Principles of a variable bypass vaporiser

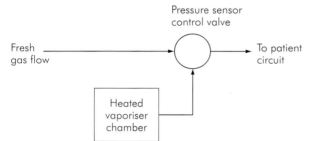

Figure EQ12   Principles of measured flow vaporiser

Measured flow vaporiser

This vaporiser has a chamber in which the volatile agent is heated by an electrical element to produce pure vapour under pressure. The pressure produced in the chamber is equal to the saturated vapour pressure (SVP) of the volatile agent at the preset temperature. The vaporiser then controls the addition of the pressurised vapour to the fresh gas flow using a pressure sensor-controlled valve, to maintain a given volatile percentage in the patient's inspired gases. This type of device is used for desflurane (Figure EQ12).

Plenum variable bypass vaporisers

Examples – Ohmeda TEC 5, Blease Datum, Drager Vapor

In the plenum vaporiser (Latin *plenum*, full) the inspired gases are at higher than atmospheric pressure (back-bar pressure 1–8 kPa) and pressurise the vaporiser chamber. Pressurisation increases the density of the carrier gas in the chamber, thus ensuring better mixing with the vapour at low flows. When the vaporiser chamber is at atmospheric pressure, carrier gas density is less than vapour density, and at low flow rates gas will tend to pass across the top of the chamber without mixing.

The plenum vaporiser is the most commonly used type in hospital practice. Plenum vaporisers have a relatively

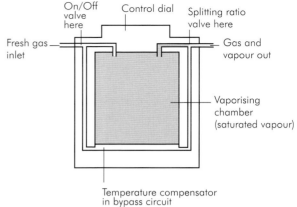

Figure EQ13   Basic design of a plenum vaporiser

high flow resistance (approximately 0.4 kPa per litre per minute of flow) and are therefore unsuitable for placing 'in line' in a spontaneously breathing circuit.

To illustrate: in order to develop a peak inspiratory flow rate of 30 litres per minute through this vaporiser, a patient would need to develop a peak inspiratory pressure of $30 \times 0.4 = 12$ kPa (>120 cmH$_2$O), compared with a normal inspiratory pressure of <2 kPa. Effectively the plenum vaporiser acts as a flow restrictor, and for a spontaneously breathing patient a circuit with a reservoir bag is usually needed to supply the peak inspiratory flow rates. Figure EQ13 illustrates the design of a simple plenum vaporiser.

Flow-splitting ratio

The performance of variable bypass vaporisers depends on the flow-splitting ratio, which is the ratio of the bypass flow to the gas flow through the chamber.

For example, if total gas flow through the anaesthetic machine back bar is 5 litres per minute, and flow through the vaporiser is 0.2 litres per minute, what is the flow splitting ratio?

$$\text{Vaporiser chamber flow} = 0.2$$
$$\text{Bypass flow} = 5.0 - 0.2 = 4.8$$
$$\text{Flow splitting ratio} = 4.8/0.2 = 24$$

So consider the concentration of vapour in an isoflurane vaporiser chamber at 20 °C (SVP for isoflurane at 20 °C = 31.5 kPa; assume ambient pressure in the vaporiser chamber to be 105 kPa).

Saturated vapour concentration in the vaporiser chamber is given by the ratio

$$\frac{SVP}{\text{pressure in vaporiser chamber}} \times 100\% = \frac{31.5}{105} \times 100\%$$
$$= 30\%$$

To find the flow-splitting ratio required to produce a final concentration of 1% isoflurane:

Final concentration
$$= \frac{\text{concentration in vaporiser chamber}}{(\text{flow splitting ratio} + 1)}$$

To obtain 1% isoflurane the vapour must be diluted by a factor of 30. Therefore a flow-splitting ratio of 29 is required, i.e. 1/30 (3.3%) of the total flow must pass through the chamber.

It can be seen that the more potent the volatile agent the greater the dilution of the vapour required, and the greater the flow-splitting ratio.

Draw-over variable bypass vaporisers

Examples – Epstein, Macintosh, Oxford (EMO), Goldman, Oxford Miniature

In the draw-over vaporiser the inspiratory gases are at atmospheric pressure and are drawn through the vaporiser chamber by the inspiratory efforts of the patient. The vaporiser and flow-splitting valve must therefore have low resistance. This type of vaporiser has the advantage that atmospheric air can be used as the carrier gas (supplemented by cylinder oxygen if required).

However, accuracy is poor in this type of vaporiser since flow rates vary considerably through the vaporiser with the respiratory cycle. The ability of the flow-splitting valve to maintain a constant splitting ratio becomes poor over the wide range of flows. At low flow rates the resistance of the flow-splitting valve will become relatively more significant and gases will tend to bypass the vaporiser, causing a fall in volatile concentrations. At high flow rates there will be increased dilution of the vapour in the vaporiser chamber and again concentrations will tend to be reduced. Figure EQ14 shows a simple draw-over vaporiser.

Measured flow vaporisers

Example – Ohmeda TEC 6 Desflurane vaporiser

The measured flow vaporisers produce a separate independent flow of vapour or saturated carrier gas. This flow is then metered into the patient's fresh gas flow to produce

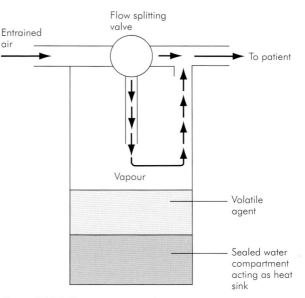

Figure EQ14 Draw-over vaporiser

the required concentration of volatile agent (Figure EQ15). Thus no splitting of the fresh gas flow occurs. This method is used in the desflurane vaporiser (TEC 6) because the boiling point of desflurane at sea level is 23.6 °C, which is approximately room temperature. In such a case, use of a plenum vaporiser with an intermittently boiling volatile agent would make its performance unpredictable. The desflurane vaporiser therefore heats the volatile agent to 39 °C to produce a chamber pressure of approximately 194 kPa. A continuous flow of desflurane vapour from the chamber is then added to the fresh gas flow via the concentration control valve.

The desflurane vaporiser has features which include:
- Mains supply, with back-up battery
- Three built-in heaters to boil the desflurane and to prevent condensation in different parts of the vaporiser
- A warm-up time of 10 minutes, during which the control dial is locked
- Electronic circuitry to indicate 'ready for use', to warn of low levels of desflurane or disconnection, and to switch off when tilted
- Supplies concentrations up to 18% (3 MAC)

Vaporiser performance

Vaporiser performance is dependent on the range of flow rates, the ambient conditions, the carrier gas mixture used, together with the design and maintenance of the vaporiser.

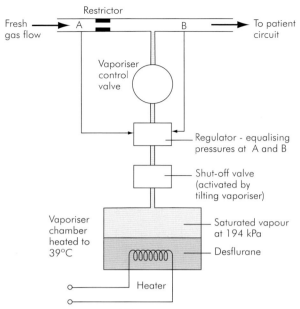

Figure EQ15 Measured flow vaporiser

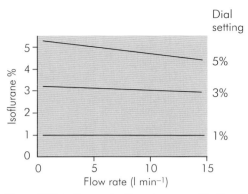

Figure EQ16 Concentration changes with flow in a plenum vaporiser

Flow rate

Flow rate of carrier gas passing through the vaporiser is important because as flow rate increases, an increasing amount of vapour is required to saturate the carrier gas. At higher flow rates the carrier gas in the vaporiser chamber may not become fully saturated, and thus the concentration of the volatile agent delivered to the patient tends to fall. Figure EQ16 shows how volatile agent concentration might vary with increasing flow rate in a plenum vaporiser. In addition, high flow rates will accentuate the temperature effects in the chamber (see below). Performance of a vaporiser will therefore be more consistent if variations in flow rates are minimised. A large surface area for vaporisation in the vaporiser chamber will be able to maintain saturation of the carrier gas over a wider range of flow rates.

Temperature

The concentration of vapour in the vaporiser chamber is dependent on the SVP of the volatile agent and the ambient pressure in the chamber. Temperature affects the performance of a vaporiser due to the variation of SVP with temperature. A main cause of temperature falling in the chamber is the absorption of latent heat as vaporisation occurs. This will become more marked at higher flow rates when the rate of vaporisation is increased.

Compensation to correct for such fluctuations is achieved by adjusting the gas flow through the vaporiser chamber. Temperature compensation was performed manually in early vaporisers by altering the flow-splitting valve according to the temperature in the vaporiser. However, this has been superseded by automatic devices, such as a bimetallic-strip-controlled flow valve, built into the chamber outlet of modern models. This valve automatically increases the flow through the vaporiser chamber should temperature in the chamber start to fall.

Further compensation is obtained by increasing the thermal capacity of the vaporiser in order to smooth out temperature fluctuations. This was achieved in the EMO draw-over vaporiser by filling a compartment in the base of the vaporiser with water. Alternatively, in the later plenum vaporisers, a large heavy mass of copper is incorporated into the vaporiser body. This enhanced thermal capacity acts as a heat source in case of temperature falls, and a heat sink should ambient temperature rise, thus smoothing out the effects of temperature fluctuations. Figure EQ17 shows how vaporiser performance might vary with temperature in a typical modern vaporiser.

Atmospheric pressure

From the calculation example for plenum vaporisers given above (see *Flow-splitting ratio*), the concentration of volatile agent in the vaporiser chamber is dependent on the ratio

$$\frac{SVP}{\text{Pressure in the vaporiser chamber}}$$

The pressure in the vaporiser chamber is essentially atmospheric pressure, so if atmospheric pressure is increased the final volatile concentration delivered will be reduced. On the other hand, at altitude, where atmospheric pressure is reduced, the volatile concentration delivered is increased.

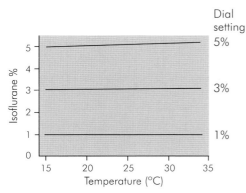

Figure EQ17 Concentration changes with temperature in a plenum vaporiser (TEC 4) at 5 litres per minute oxygen flow

It should be noted that although the delivered concentration may increase at altitude, the partial pressure exerted by the volatile agent in the tissues will remain unchanged.

'Pumping effect'

This effect is produced by repetitive changes in circuit resistance at the common gas outlet. It can be produced when the outlet is periodically obstructed by assisting ventilation or attaching a minute volume divider ventilator (e.g. Manley) to the outlet. This results in alternating compression and release of the saturated gas in the vaporiser chamber, which in turn produces surges of volatile agent concentration in the patient circuit. Mechanisms to reduce this pumping effect include increasing the flow resistance of the vaporiser and insertion of a non-return valve at the outlet of the vaporiser.

Carrier gas composition

Increasing the nitrous oxide content of the carrier gas can produce a small reduction in the volatile concentration delivered. This is because the nitrous oxide reduces the viscosity and increases the density of the gas mixture, which decreases the gas flow through the vaporiser chamber due to the flow-splitting valve characteristics. Nitrous oxide also has increased solubility in volatile agents, which can cause a further transient fall in volatile agent concentration when the nitrous oxide fraction is increased. This effect is not significant clinically.

Mechanical stability

Poor fitting of the vaporiser to the back bar can result in gas leaks, loss of back-bar pressure or tilting, which can allow leakage of volatile agent into the bypass circuit.

Regular checking of vaporiser seating and improvements in vaporiser and back-bar design can minimise the risk of these problems.

Overfilling

Direct leakage of volatile agent into the patient circuit can also be caused by overfilling of the vaporiser, and it is potentially fatal. Care should be taken in filling and checking vaporisers.

Vaporiser maintenance

Vaporisers should be serviced annually, and calibration should also be checked regularly. Drainage and cleaning of vaporiser chambers (2-weekly intervals) can prevent the build-up of unwanted substances (such as thymol, a waxy stabilising agent used in halothane), which can reduce evaporation rates in the vaporiser chamber and cause moving parts to stick if they accumulate.

Design features of a vaporiser

The desirable features of a vaporiser depend to some extent on the specific application (portable or fixed, compressed gas supplies available or not), but some general specifications include:

- Large surface area for vaporisation in the vaporiser chamber
- Large heat sink
- Temperature compensation valve to control flow through the vaporiser
- Accurate flow-splitting valve
- Low flow resistance for draw-over vaporiser
- Stable mechanical mounting
- Safeguard against leakage into patient circuit
- Safety interlock device
- Clear liquid-level gauge
- Agent-specific filling port
- Easy emptying and cleaning

Breathing systems

Breathing system describes the equipment used to deliver fresh gases and volatile agents to a patient. The following general terms are used to describe breathing systems:

(1) **Open system** – In its simplest form a breathing system may just be a method of augmenting room air, an open hose and a cupped hand, nasal cannulae delivering oxygen or a clear plastic oxygen mask. These are referred to as *open* breathing systems.

(2) **Closed system** – This controls the gas mixture delivered to the patient, using a sealed mask and

circuit. Closed systems can be classified into *rebreathing* and *non-rebreathing* systems.

 - *Rebreathing* – is the inhalation of previously expired gases including carbon dioxide and water vapour. Many of the breathing systems used in practice allow rebreathing, but are normally used with high enough fresh gas flow rates to prevent rebreathing. These types of system include the Bain and Magill circuits, and are described below in the Mapleson classification.
 - *Non-rebreathing* – describes breathing systems in which rebreathing is prevented. This can be achieved by a non-rebreathing valve, a carbon dioxide absorber or high fresh gas flow rates in a rebreathing system.

Most practical breathing systems function as semi-closed and partially rebreathing systems. They are often capable of operating as non-rebreathing systems, depending on the magnitude of fresh gas flow (FGF) used.

Breathing system performance
Breathing systems may have to work in different environments, each of which may influence the design of the circuit. The optimum circuit for a given application will be a compromise between various features, which include:

- Low dead space. **Apparatus dead space** is the volume between the patient and the expiratory valve. **Functional dead space** extends to all of the volume contaminated with expired gases during each ventilatory cycle. It may be greater than apparatus dead space in an inefficient circuit, or less in other cases, where FGF flushes out expired gases before inspiration (Figure EQ18).
- Efficient operation in both spontaneously breathing (SV) patients and those requiring controlled/assisted ventilation (CV). Efficiency in this context is measured by minimum fresh gas flow (FGF) required to prevent rebreathing, expressed as a multiple of the patient's minute volume (MV). The Magill attachment requires an FGF of greater than 0.7 MV to prevent rebreathing in a spontaneously breathing patient.
- Economical use of fresh gas supply and volatile agent. Economy of usage of anaesthetic gases is needed where supplies are restricted, or to minimise costs. In the operating theatre piped gas supplies are usually available. In other areas gas supplies may be limited, and occasionally pressurised supplies may not even be available. Environmental considerations and pollution are also a concern in the work environment.

(a) Apparatus dead space

(b) Functional dead space during spontaneous breathing

(c) Functional dead space during assisted ventilation

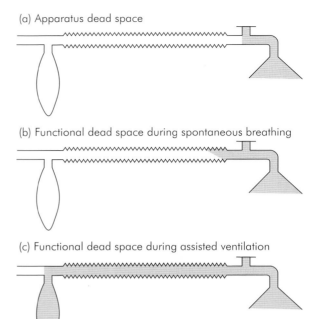

Figure EQ18 Functional dead space within Magill circuit

- Physical size or weight. The weight and bulk of a circuit's components may be a factor discouraging its use, as the circuit may drag on endotracheal tubes or laryngeal masks, and displace them from a patient's airway. Factors such as apparatus dead space are likely to be in proportion to the size of the circuit's components. It is not always convenient to use breathing systems via an anaesthetic machine in resuscitation areas, and a simpler system such as the Waters circuit may be more practical.

Breathing system components
A breathing system may consist of all or some of the following components:
- Face mask
- Gas hoses and connectors
- Adjustable pressure-limiting (APL) expiratory valve (Figure EQ19)
- Reservoir bag (inflating or self-inflating)
- Carbon dioxide absorber
- A valve to switch between controlled (CV) and spontaneous (SV) ventilation modes
- One-way valves to prevent rebreathing

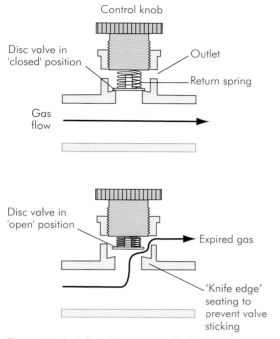

Figure EQ19 Adjustable pressure-limiting expiratory valve

Masks and hoses

Used to be made of black rubber, which was antistatic and autoclavable. Modern equivalents are lightweight, disposable and transparent or semi-transparent. These features make the components easier to handle, cheaper and safer. Hoses come in three standard sizes: 22 mm diameter for adult breathing circuits, 15 mm diameter for paediatric breathing circuits and 30 mm diameter for scavenging circuits.

Hose connectors

Standard male and female sizes to fit the hose diameters. They are also designed with standardised tapers to allow convenient but secure push-fitting between circuit components. 22 mm (15 mm for paediatric circuits) connections fit the breathing circuit hoses together and to valves, reservoir bags and masks. 15 mm connectors join the circuit to endotracheal tubes and laryngeal masks. Tapers are designed according to ISO and BS standards. Some connectors possess 22 mm external and 15 mm internal tapers to facilitate connection between the circuit hoses and an endotracheal tube or laryngeal mask.

Reservoir bags

Come in 0.5 litre, 2 litre and 4 litre sizes and are made of black rubber or distensible synthetic. The compliance of the bag is designed to be low enough to prevent development of harmful pressures if the system valves are accidentally closed.

Mapleson classification for breathing systems

This system classifies breathing systems according to the configuration of the following components:
- Reservoir bag
- Flexible hosing
- Adustable pressure-limiting expiratory valve
- Face mask

The different configurations are described and illustrated in Figure EQ20.

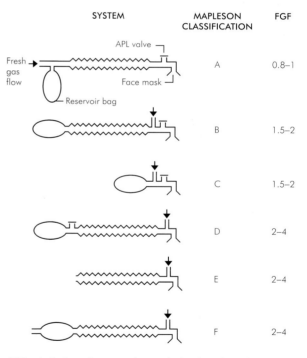

FGF is the fresh gas flow required to avoid rebreathing during spontaneous ventilation quoted as multiples of minute volume

Figure EQ20 Mapleson classification system for breathing systems

Circuit	Mapleson	Comments
Magill	A	Good for SV. May be used for CV but requires twice MV. APL valve convenient near patient, but drags on endotracheal tube or mask.
Lack	A	Coaxial circuit delivering FGF via outer hose. Expiratory limb through inner with APL valve at anaesthetic machine. Disadvantages are high inspiratory resistance and large apparatus dead space. Also parallel twin-hose Lack circuit offers low flow resistances but more bulky.
Bain	D	Coaxial circuit. FGF delivered through inner hose. Suitable for SV or CV; less efficient for SV than Magill but more efficient for CV. Disadvantages of coaxial system are that cracks or disconnection in inner hose may go unnoticed.
Waters circuit	C	Practical circuit for resuscitation. Requires low-pressure oxygen supply. Low dead space. Suitable for SV or CV.
Ayre's T-piece	E	Suitable for paediatrics. The expiratory limb forms apparatus dead space but also acts as an inspiratory reservoir. This limb should be equal to the tidal volume to prevent dilution of inspired gases by entrained air. Requires 2–4 times MV to avoid rebreathing.
Jackson–Rees modification of Ayre's T-piece	F	Paediatric circuit. Open-ended reservoir modification of bag in expiratory limb.
Humphrey	ADE	Twin-hose system which switches between Mapleson A for SV and D/E for CV.

Figure EQ21 Examples of commonly used circuits

Practical breathing systems

Various breathing systems have been developed empirically for different applications.

Some systems consist of the basic components described in the Mapleson classification (above) and therefore fit into the system described. Some examples are described in Figure EQ21.

Circle system

A typical circle system is shown in Figure EQ22. The system consists of a carbon dioxide absorber, a reservoir bag, one-way valves to ensure unidirectional gas flow and hoses with a Y-piece to connect the patient into the circuit. The circle system can be used with a spontaneously breathing patient, or control/assist can be given manually using the reservoir bag.

The optimum configuration for the components has the FGF and reservoir bag located in between the carbon dioxide absorber and the one-way inspiratory valve. This arrangement minimises the inspiratory resistance of the circuit.

The circle system has the following advantages:
- Low FGF rates can be used without causing rebreathing of expired carbon dioxide, resulting in economy of anaesthetic gas usage.
- Recirculation of volatile agent gives economy and low pollution rates.
- Low functional dead space, equal to the volume of the patient Y-piece, due to removal of carbon dioxide by the absorber.

The disadvantages of the circle system are:
- More components than simpler systems (such as Magill or Bain) create a bulky system requiring a separate mounting on the anaesthetic machine.
- One-way valves to ensure unidirectional flow increase flow resistances and are a potential source of problems such as sticking.
- Inspiratory and expiratory flow resistances are higher than in the case of the Magill or Bain systems. These higher flow resistances are dependent on FGF rates in the circle. Low FGF rates increase inspiratory resistance but decrease expiratory resistance. High FGF rates

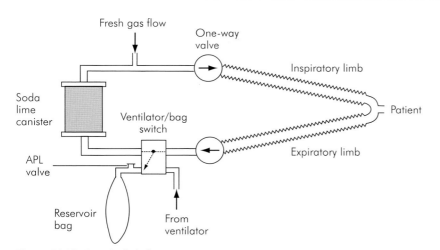

Figure EQ22 A typical circle system

produce the opposite effect, decreasing inspiratory resistance and increasing expiratory resistance. Work of breathing is therefore lowest with high FGF rates. This effect is not significant in a fit adult, but can become important in frail patients or children.

Controlled ventilation (CV) with the circle system

CV can be applied using the circle system, by using a 'bag in the bottle' type of ventilator. This effectively acts as a 'bag squeezer', and the ventilator is connected into the circle system in place of the reservoir bag. In such a case the tidal volume delivered may depend on both the ventilator setting and the FGF. Modern circle systems incorporate ventilators which monitor the delivered tidal volume and compensate for changes in FGF.

An alternative arrangement is the use of a servo-type ventilator which delivers 'driving' gas (oxygen) via the reservoir bag limb and allows expiration through the same limb. In such a configuration the driving gas must not 'contaminate' the patient circuit. This means FGF must be greater than MV, and the length of the reservoir limb tubing must have a volume greater than 1.5 times the tidal volume.

Use of volatile agents with the circle

When volatile agents are used with the circle the commonest configuration is with a plenum vaporiser located out of the circle (vaporiser outside circle, VOC). The FGF thus passes through the vaporiser first, and then into the circle system. In the past draw-over vaporisers were used positioned in the circle system (vaporiser inside circle, VIC).

Both methods have disadvantages at low FGF. In summary:

- **VOC** – Expired gas dilutes the inspired gases and reduces inspired volatile concentrations, until equilibrium is reached, when end-tidal volatile concentrations equal inspired concentrations. Also the performance of many plenum vaporisers may be inaccurate at low flow rates.
- **VIC** – Inspired gases are recirculated through the vaporiser, resulting in continually increasing volatile concentrations, which may reach saturation levels.

Carbon dioxide absorption

Carbon dioxide absorption is used to prevent rebreathing, and is most commonly used in the circle system in combination with low FGF rates. A combination of chemical reactions is used to absorb carbon dioxide. First carbon dioxide is dissolved in water to form carbonic acid, and the carbonic acid then reacts with calcium hydroxide to form calcium carbonate and water:

$$CO_2 + H_2O = H_2CO_3 = H^+ + HCO_3^-$$
$$Ca(OH)_2 + H^+ + HCO_3^- = CaCO_3^- + 2H_2O$$

This reaction is exothermic and produces water, providing a warm moist environment in the carbon dioxide absorber for the FGF to pass through. The pH of the reagents increases as the reaction proceeds, enabling an indicator to be used to show when the calcium hydroxide is exhausted.

Some practical points concerning the use of carbon dioxide absorbers are as follows:

- **FGF rates** – Use of carbon dioxide absorption with the circle system can reduce FGF rate to a few hundred millilitres per minute, once equilibrium has been reached. This FGF is required to replace absorbed oxygen ($100-300$ ml min^{-1}) and gases lost through leakage and the APL valve.
- **Calcium hydroxide preparation** – The most commonly used preparation is soda lime, which is a mixture of 80% $Ca(OH)_2$, 4% $NaOH$ and 16% H_2O. The soda lime is in the form of granules, which are designed to be small enough to give low spaces between granules and thus high efficiency absorption, but not so small as to provide excessive resistance to gas flow.
- **Soda lime** – The absorption capacity of soda lime is in the order of 25 litres of carbon dioxide per 100 g of soda lime. The colour change indicating exhaustion of the granules (commonly pink to white) may occur before full-capacity absorption due to surface reaction on the granules. This can lead to apparent regeneration of granules as the surface and core of the

granule equilibrate when used soda lime is left standing. Soda lime dust is caustic and can cause morbidity if a soda lime canister is located too close to the patient's airway in the breathing system. This can occur in the to-and-fro configuration used with a Waters canister (Mapleson C) system. 'Channelling' may occur in soda lime canisters which are poorly packed. This is the formation of channels through the soda lime granules through which gases pass without adequate exposure to the soda lime, and it results in incomplete carbon dioxide absorption

Oxygen delivery systems

Various systems exist to provide enhanced fraction of inspired oxygen (FiO_2) for the spontaneously breathing patient. These can be required in locations such as recovery areas, resuscitation areas, labour suites and ambulances. The types of device used include nasal cannulae, face masks and attachments for enhancing the FiO_2 through laryngeal masks or endotracheal tubes (see also Section 1, Chapter 4: pages 68–9).

Oxygen delivery systems may be described in terms of **variable** or **fixed performance**, and **low, medium** or **high dependency**. Figure EQ23 summarises some characteristics of commonly used devices.

Device	Type	FIO$_2$	Comments
Nasal cannulae	Variable, no capacity	0.21–0.3	Alternative for patients who cannot tolerate masks. Performance unpredictable, affected by nasal obstruction and mouth breathing.
Face mask	Variable, low capacity	0.21–0.5	Performance depends on entrainment through holes in mask and around mask. Enhanced by flap valves. Increases functional dead space.
Face mask with reservoir and non-rebreathing valve	Variable, large capacity	0.21–0.80	Provides high F$_I$O$_2$. Suitable for head-injury patient. Recommended by ATLS.
Venturi face mask	Fixed	0.24–0.60	Performance depends on colour-coded Venturi jets. F$_I$O$_2$ determined by jet size and entrainment ratio. Requires reservoir tubing between jet and face mask. Dependent on tidal volume.
Venturi T-piece	Fixed	0.24–0.60	Used for laryngeal masks or endotracheal tubes. F$_I$O$_2$ determined by jet size and entrainment ratio. Requires high flow rates and reservoir tubing in expiratory limb.

Figure EQ23 Oxygen delivery systems for spontaneously breathing patients

No capacity device

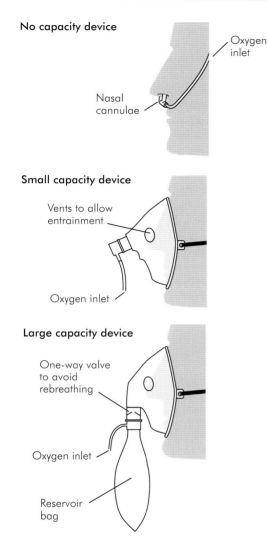

Oxygen inlet

Nasal cannulae

Small capacity device

Vents to allow entrainment

Oxygen inlet

Large capacity device

One-way valve to avoid rebreathing

Oxygen inlet

Reservoir bag

Figure EQ24 Variable-performance oxygen delivery systems

Variable performance

This term refers to the F_IO_2 delivered by a particular system. In a variable-performance system (Figure EQ24) the F_IO_2 delivered is dependent on the oxygen flow rate. The range of flow rates used is usually between 2 and 15 litres per minute, and such devices are capable of producing F_IO_2 up to 0.8–0.9. Variable-performance systems require an inspiratory oxygen reservoir in order to achieve the higher F_IO_2 levels, and may be classified as being of 'no capacity' if they have no reservoir capacity (nasal cannulae), 'small capacity' in the case of face masks, and 'large capacity' when a reservoir bag is included. Non-return valves are also incorporated in order to restrict entrainment in face masks and to prevent rebreathing from reservoir bags. The F_IO_2 delivered in the variable performance systems depends on:

- Oxygen flow rate
- Tidal volume
- Respiratory rate
- Capacity of the system
- Use of non-return valves

Fixed performance

A fixed-performance device (Figure EQ25) delivers an F_IO_2 which is independent of the oxygen flow rate used. These systems are usually based on a Venturi jet that is fed by the oxygen supply and entrains room air. They are often applied in patients with chronic respiratory disease in whom oxygen-dependent respiratory drive is suspected.

Low dependency

Describes systems used to increase F_IO_2 in patients breathing spontaneously at atmospheric pressure.

Medium dependency

Describes a system which supplies a degree of positive airway pressure to a spontaneously breathing patient (e.g. a continuous positive airway pressure (CPAP) system). These systems are used in high dependency areas or intensive care units.

High dependency

Describes systems used to control the F_IO_2 in patients requiring mechanical ventilation.

Resuscitation breathing systems

Such systems are used during resuscitation, to apply artificial ventilation to patients who are not breathing spontaneously. They also allow the patient to breathe spontaneously through them. There are two commonly used systems: the Ambu system and the Laerdal system.

The basic components of these systems are:
- **Self-inflating bag** – This has a volume of approximately 1500 ml for an adult (500 ml for a child, 250 ml for an infant). The walls are reinforced to make the bag self-inflating. One end of the bag is the inlet

Venturi mask

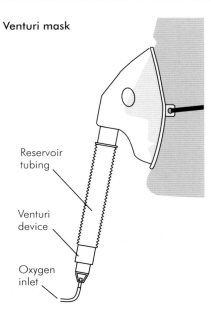

Reservoir
tubing

Venturi
device

Oxygen
inlet

Venturi T-piece

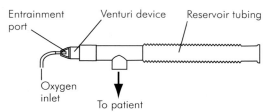

Entrainment
port

Venturi device

Reservoir tubing

Oxygen
inlet

To patient

Figure EQ25 Fixed performance oxygen delivery systems

inflation). During expiration the spring closes the airway to the bag and opens it to the atmosphere. High pressures in the bag can hold the bobbin in the inspiratory position. The Ambu valve (type E) uses a double leaf valve to produce the same reciprocal

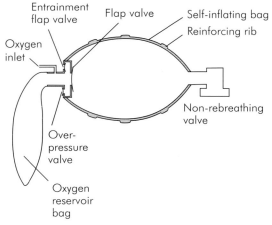

Entrainment
flap valve

Flap valve

Self-inflating bag

Reinforcing rib

Oxygen
inlet

Non-rebreathing
valve

Over-
pressure
valve

Oxygen
reservoir
bag

Figure EQ26 Self-inflating bag

INSPIRATION

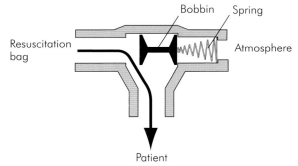

Bobbin

Spring

Resuscitation
bag

Atmosphere

Patient

for fresh gas, and this is sealed by a flap valve. This also possesses an inlet for oxygen supplementation. The other end of the bag is connected to the patient via a non-rebreathing valve (Figure EQ26).

• **Non-rebreathing valve** – There are several designs for this valve in common use. These include the Rubens valve, the Laerdal valve and different types of Ambu valve. These valves open the patient's airway to the bag during inspiration, and then during expiration close the connection to the bag and allow the patient's gases to expire to the atmosphere. Figure EQ27 and EQ28 show examples of some non-rebreathing valves used in resuscitation systems. The Rubens valve possesses a spring-loaded bobbin which slides to open the patient's airway to the bag during inspiration (or

EXPIRATION

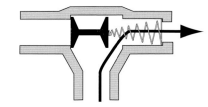

Figure EQ27 Rubens non-rebreathing valve

INSPIRATION

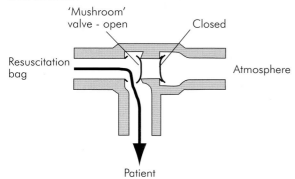

EXPIRATION

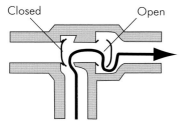

Figure EQ28 Ambu non-rebreathing valve

inspiratory and expiratory functions of the valve.

- **Oxygen reservoir bag** – This is fitted over the fresh gas inlet to the self-inflating bag and is inflated by the supplementary oxygen supply. It also possesses an inlet flap valve to allow entrainment from the atmosphere should the demand of the patient exceed its capacity. Without the reservoir bag the delivered FIO_2 is limited to less than 0.5. Using a reservoir bag can increase the FIO_2 to 1.
- **Oxygen supply** – This enters the bag or reservoir via narrow-bore tubing and a nipple connector. The flow rate used is between 2 and 15 litres per minute. The final inspired oxygen concentration delivered to the patient will depend on the oxygen flow rate, respiratory rate, tidal volume and whether a reservoir is used.

Endotracheal tubes

The endotracheal tube (ETT) is a plastic or rubber tube inserted into the trachea. It provides the definitive airway, allowing positive-pressure ventilation while preventing contamination of the lungs from the contents of the pharynx. The original tubes were made by Rowbotham and Magill in 1920 from rubber tubing of varying diameter and cut to the correct length by hand. Both oral and nasal tubes were designed, and these were connected to the breathing circuit by a metal adapter. Later developments included the cuff with pilot balloon, double lumen tubes for thoracic surgery, and anatomically shaped tubes such as the Oxford or RAE (Ring, Adair, Elwyn) tubes.

Red rubber produced inflammatory reactions at the site of contact and has been superseded by non-irritant transparent plastic. The tubes are often marked with the initials IT (implant tested) or Z79 (which refers to a room number related to the toxicity subcommittee of ANSI) to indicate compliance with the standards defined by the American National Standards Institute. The tube is marked with the internal and external diameters in millimetres, the length in centimetres, and usually also a radio-opaque line to aid visualisation on chest x ray. High-volume cuffs when inflated are associated with a lower pressure on the tracheal mucosa and are appropriate for long operations or intensive care use. The pressure in the cuff can also increase as nitrous oxide diffuses through the thin plastic wall. While this can be prevented by filling the balloon with saline, some tubes have been designed with an oversize pilot balloon (Brandt pattern) or with a cuff filled with self-expanding foam and the connecting tube left open to the atmosphere. The requirements of ENT surgery have led to designs which minimise the obstruction to the surgeon's vision (microlaryngoscopy tubes), or which cannot be kinked (wire-reinforced tubes), and tubes resistant to ignition by the operating laser.

To describe a tube, identify the following features:
- Single or double lumen
- Material
- Cuff and pilot balloon with self-sealing valve
- Bevel with or without eyes
- Special features

Laryngeal mask airway

First produced commercially in 1986 to the design of Dr Archie Brain, the LMA offered an airway intermediate between the face mask and the tracheal tube, and represents one of the most significant advances of the past quarter-century. It consists of a wide tube terminating at one end in a 15 mm connection and at the other in an inflatable cuff that is placed over the laryngeal opening. When inflated, the cuff provides an airtight seal sufficient to permit gentle positive-pressure ventilation if the chest compliance is normal, although it does not protect the trachea from soiling by stomach contents and should not therefore be used if aspiration is a possibility. The LMA is produced in a range of sizes from #1 (neonate) to #5 for large adults. There is a standard pattern and a reinforced pattern for use in ENT surgery. The construction materials withstand repeated cleaning and autoclaving for up to 40 times and this should be noted on the record card that is supplied by the manufacturer. The intubating LMA allows for the passage of an ETT through the lumen, blindly into the trachea. The LMA is latex-free in all its variants.

Scavenging systems

An appropriate scavenging system is mandatory in each anaesthetic room and operating theatre in order to avoid pollution by anaesthetic gases and agents. Although there are no studies proving side effects caused by chronic exposure to low levels of anaesthetic gases or vapours, the alleged side effects include:

- Increased incidence of spontaneous abortion
- Vitamin B_{12} inactivation by nitrous oxide with neurological sequelae
- Increased incidence of female births
- Reduced fertility in females exposed to nitrous oxide
- Increased incidence of minor congenital abnormalities
- Increased incidence of leukaemia and lymphoma in exposed females

Recommended levels of pollutants

There is legal requirement under a code of practice drawn up by the Health and Safety Commission to control exposure levels of many pollutants including anaesthetic agents. Some of the recommended maximum levels of exposure (averaged over any 8-hour time period) (COSHH) are listed in Figure EQ29.

Types of scavenging system

Scavenging systems are designed to collect the waste gases and vapours from the anaesthetic machine and dispose of them, without affecting the breathing or ventilation of the patient, and without affecting the safe operation of the

Pollutant	Maximum level (ppm)
Nitrous oxide	100
Halothane	10
Enflurane	50
Isoflurane	50

Figure EQ29 Maximum anaesthetic pollutant levels recommended by the HSC

anaesthetic machine. The different types of scavenging system include **passive** systems, **active** systems and **absorber** systems.

All scavenging systems require a device for collecting the waste gas from the breathing system, ventilator or patient. To cope with wide fluctuations in gas flow (from 0 to 130 litres per minute) there needs to be a reservoir to collect waste gases. The patient may either be protected by positive and negative pressure relief valves or, in an active system, by an open-ended reservoir. The standard size of connections is 30 mm to avoid wrong connections, and the risk of obstruction of the patient's expiratory pathway must be minimised. Figure EQ30 shows the design of scavenging systems.

Passive systems

Early scavenging systems were passive in that the patient's expiratory effort was required to propel waste gas down an additional length of tubing to the outside atmosphere. While the flow of gas could be assisted either by placing the end near the air-conditioning outlet or by terminating the roof vent with an extractor cowl, these systems were notably inefficient. Despite a maximal tubing resistance of 0.5 cmH$_2$O the increased resistance to expiration and the potential for complete obstruction represented a distinct hazard to the patient without measurably protecting the theatre staff.

Active systems

Modern active scavenging is usually driven by a fan unit remote to the theatre unit which produces a sub-atmospheric pressure capable of large gas flows ($75 \, l \, min^{-1}$, peak flow $130 \, l \, min^{-1}$ per patient) in a piped distribution system. Distribution is terminated in each theatre, where it is connected to the reservoir collection system. The

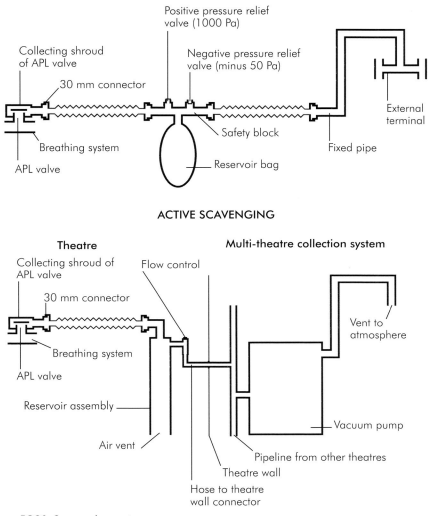

PASSIVE SCAVENGING

Positive pressure relief valve (1000 Pa)

Collecting shroud of APL valve

Negative pressure relief valve (minus 50 Pa)

30 mm connector

External terminal

Safety block

Breathing system

Fixed pipe

APL valve

Reservoir bag

ACTIVE SCAVENGING

Theatre

Multi-theatre collection system

Collecting shroud of APL valve

Flow control

30 mm connector

Vent to atmosphere

Breathing system

APL valve

Reservoir assembly

Vacuum pump

Air vent

Pipeline from other theatres

Theatre wall

Hose to theatre wall connector

Figure EQ30 Scavenging systems

reservoir usually houses a visual flow indicator, which should be periodically checked to ensure the system is working. The system should operate within the pressures of $-0.5\ cmH_2O$ and $+5\ cmH_2O$ at $30\ l\ min^{-1}$ flow.

Absorbers

Absorbers are usually based on activated charcoal and can, to a limited extent, absorb volatile agents (which may be released again by the use of heat).

Mechanical ventilators

A mechanical ventilator is designed to automatically inflate the lungs when a patient is unable to breathe spontaneously. This is most commonly achieved by applying positive pressure to the patient's airway, as in CV. Alternative techniques also include high-frequency methods such as high-frequency jet ventilation (HFJV), and the use of negative pressure applied to the patient's chest wall (cuirass).

A ventilator can be described by different characteristics, which can be divided into:

- **Ventilation cycle parameters** – This term refers to the parameters (pressure, flow rate) which are defined during the inspiratory and expiratory phases of each ventilation cycle. It also defines how the ventilator switches between inspiratory and expiratory phases. Detailed discussion is presented below under *Mapleson classification for ventilators.*
- **Mechanics** – The mechanism and power supply used to generate the ventilation cycle, e.g. minute volume divider, 'bag in the bottle'. These characteristics will often determine its physical size and power requirements.
- **Clinical features** – The features which determine its clinical field of application (operating theatre, ICU, neonatal unit). These include its ability to provide ancillary modes such as positive end-expiratory pressure (PEEP), continuous positive airway pressure (CPAP) and synchronised intermittent mandatory ventilation (SIMV).

Ideal characteristics of a ventilator

The ideal specifications for a ventilator will vary according to its clinical application. Clearly the requirements of a ventilator for the intensive care unit will be very different from those for a ventilator to be used in an ambulance. Usually clinical application will dictate the physical parameters of the ventilation cycle and the mechanics of the ventilator.

Within the limitations of its clinical application a ventilator should:

- Provide appropriate ventilation modes for its particular application
- Have easy switching between automatic and manual functions
- Be simple and practical to use
- Be mechanically well designed and reliable
- Have appropriate, reliable and readily visible monitoring and alarms
- Be easy to clean and sterilise

Mapleson classification for ventilators

This scheme classifies positive-pressure ventilators according to the different phases of the ventilation cycle:

- Inspiratory phase
- Cycling between inspiration and expiration (inspiratory cycling)

- Expiratory phase
- Cycling between expiration and inspiration (expiratory cycling, inspiratory triggering)

Inspiratory phase

During inspiration either pressure or flow rate can be determined by the ventilator mechanism. Thus a ventilator can be described either as a **pressure generator** or as a **flow generator**.

Flow generators and pressure generators are basically different in mechanical design. A pressure generator must be capable of providing high flow rates at the preset inspiratory pressure, which means it must have a low internal impedance to flow. In the case of the flow generator, in order for it to deliver the preset flow rate irrespective of variations in lung compliance, its internal impedance must be very high to attenuate the effect of variations in lung compliance on ventilator performance.

Some properties of pressure and flow generators are listed in Figure EQ31.

Ventilator performance and reduced lung compliance

As can be seen from Figure EQ31, inspiratory pressures and flow rates are affected by both lung compliance and the type of ventilator used. The differences between pressure and flow generators when ventilating patients with normal or reduced lung compliances can be illustrated by the pressure and flow curves during a ventilation cycle. The flow curve also gives information about the tidal volume, since volume is obtained from the area under the flow curve. The inspired tidal volume delivered is thus equal to the area under the flow curve during inspiration. Expired tidal volume is given by the area under the flow curve during expiration.

Figure EQ32 shows a **pressure generator** delivering constant inspiratory pressure. Flow rate increases to a peak during inspiration and then decreases exponentially during expiration, which is passive. The areas (tidal volumes) under the inspiratory and expiratory parts of the flow curve are approximately equal. When lung compliance is reduced the peak inspiratory flow rate reached is lower and the inspiratory and expiratory tidal volumes are reduced.

Figure EQ33 shows a **flow generator** delivering constant flow during inspiration with a **preset tidal volume**. Inspiratory pressure will rise rapidly initially and

Property	Pressure generators	Flow generators
Inspiratory pressure	Inspiratory pressure and pattern (e.g. constant, sinusoidal, triangular) preset on ventilator	Inspiratory pressure will vary according to respiratory mechanics of patient. High inspiratory pressures may be produced with low lung compliance (e.g. acute respiratory distress syndrome)
Inspiratory flow rate	Inspiratory flow rate (and hence tidal volume) will vary according to respiratory mechanics of patient. High flow rates may be produced with high lung compliance (e.g. neonates)	Inspiratory flow rate and pattern (e.g. constant, ramp) preset on ventilator
Tidal volume	Tidal volume will vary according to lung compliance. Decreased lung compliance will reduce tidal volume	Preset tidal volume will be delivered at the expense of airway pressure, unless an inspiratory pressure limit is preset
Risk of barotrauma	Low risk	High risk unless pressure limit preset on ventilator
Risk of volutrauma (excessive tidal volumes)	High risk unless limit on tidal volume preset on ventilator	Low risk
Compensation for leakage	Some limited ability to compensate for small leaks in circuitry between ventilator and patient, since ventilator always acts to deliver preset inspiratory pressure	Any leakage from connecting circuit will be lost as it is counted by ventilator as delivered flow (tidal volume)
Clinical application	Suitable for paediatrics or neonates because of low risk of barotrauma and ability to compensate for small leaks. Requires tidal volume limit. Safer for emphysematous lungs	Appropriate for ICU because of ability to deliver flow (tidal volume) with low lung compliance. Requires inspiratory pressure limitation to reduce risk of barotrauma

Figure EQ31 Comparison between pressure and flow generator ventilators

reach a peak, which then decreases exponentially during expiration. When lung compliance is reduced the ventilator still delivers the same constant inspired flow with the same duration (preset tidal volume), but peak inspiratory pressure is increased. The lower the compliance (i.e. the stiffer the lungs), the greater the inspiratory pressures required to deliver the preset flow and tidal volume.

Figure EQ34 shows a **flow generator** delivering constant flow with **pressure limitation** and a **preset tidal volume**. With normal lung compliance the pressure limit is not exceeded and an inspiratory pressure curve as in Figure EQ33 is produced. When reduced lung compliance is present the inspiratory pressures are increased. If the pressure exceeds the preset limit, inspiration is cut short and the tidal volume delivered is reduced below the preset value.

Cycling between inspiration and expiration (inspiratory cycling)

The change between inspiration and expiration can be triggered by various parameters. This function is referred to as cycling, and it may be described as follows:

- Volume cycling – Inspiration stops and expiration begins when the preset tidal volume is delivered. An inspiratory pause may be used, which prolongs the inspiratory phase.
- Pressure cycling – Inspiration occurs up to a preset inspiratory pressure, at which expiration is then triggered.

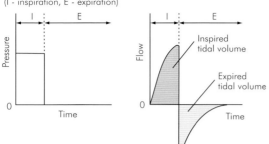

(a) Pressure generator with constant inspiratory pressure
(I - inspiration, E - expiration)

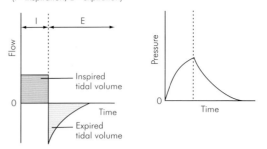

(a) Flow generator with preset tidal volume
(I - inspiration, E - expiration)

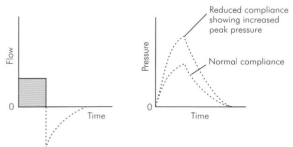

(b) Effect of reduced compliance on flow generator with preset tidal volume

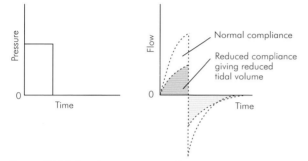

(b) Effect of reduced compliance in pressure generator

Figure EQ32 Inspiratory patterns from a pressure generator

- Time cycling – The inspiratory phase occurs for a fixed duration, which is preset, and at the end of this time expiration is triggered. This type of cycling will effectively preset tidal volume in a flow generator.

Expiratory phase

Expiration is normally passive, but during the expiratory phase positive pressure can be applied to give positive end-expiratory pressure (PEEP). This technique is usually applied in the intensive care unit to improve oxygenation and recruit lung volume in patients with certain lung pathologies such as acute respiratory distress syndrome. Surgical anaesthesia in the operating theatre does not usually involve the use of PEEP.

Cycling between expiration and inspiration (expiratory cycling)

The change from expiration to inspiration usually occurs on a timed basis (i.e. expiratory time cycling) as determined by the preset ventilation frequency. For example,

Figure EQ33 Inspiratory patterns from a flow generator with preset tidal volume

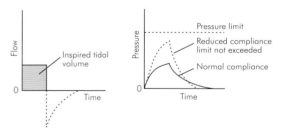

(a) Flow generator with preset tidal volume and pressure limitation

(b) Effect of reduced compliance on flow generator with pressure limitation causing reduction of tidal volume

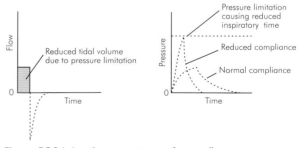

Figure EQ34 Inspiratory patterns from a flow generator with pressure limitation and preset tidal volume

Ventilator	Mechanism	Comments
Minute volume divider	Driven by the fresh gas supply. The fresh gas flow passes into bellows, which divide it up into tidal volumes by filling repeatedly. The first bellows empty into second bellows, which deliver the tidal volume to the patient.	Simple reliable mechanism. No additional power supply required. Limited capability for patients with abnormal lungs. Workhorse ventilator for theatres and anaesthetic rooms.
'Bag in bottle' or 'bag squeezer'	Fresh gas flow for the patient enters bellows (bag) mounted in a container (bottle). The ventilator compresses the bellows downwards, by pressurising the bottle during inspiration. The bag is then opened to an expiratory port during expiration. Different sizes of bellows used for adults and children. Modern versions microprocessor-controlled.	The patient circuit is isolated from the ventilator circuit. This means the ventilator is used as a servoventilator, to ventilate the patient through a separate breathing system such as a circle or Bain. Often incorporated into anaesthetic machines.
Microprocessor-controlled electronic ventilator	Usually employs a bellows mechanism driven mechanically (e.g. spring-loaded). Sophisticated electronics and monitoring to provide accurate control and triggered modes of ventilation.	Used for intensive care. Complex and software-driven. Provides ancillary modes for difficult lung pathologies (ARDS, bullous lung disease) and weaning.
High-frequency jet ventilator	Uses high MGPS supply (400 kPa) to inject into an endotracheal tube, tracheostomy tube or other interface circuit, which connects to the patient's airway. The ventilator–patient interface is an important factor in determining performance.	Used for intensive care and thoracic surgery. Does not require a sealed airway to ventilate patient. Increased risk of barotrauma and problems with humidification when applied for prolonged periods.

Figure EQ35 Ventilator mechanics

if a frequency of 12 breaths per minute is preset, then expiratory cycling will occur (i.e. inspiration will be triggered) every 5 seconds.

Alternatively, inspiration may be triggered by negative pressure changes or flow rates generated by the patient's own spontaneous inspiratory efforts. This approach is adopted in supported or assisted ventilation modes (e.g. SIMV) used to give ventilatory support to patients with some degree of spontaneous respiratory effort or who are being weaned from mechanical ventilation.

Ventilator mechanics

The mechanical design of ventilators centres around the driving mechanism which delivers fresh gas to the patient. Secondary aspects such as the power supply, control mechanisms, monitoring and reliability are often equally important in determining the ventilator's clinical performance. Some examples of the different mechanical designs used for ventilators are summarised in Figure EQ35. A ventilator may have the advantages of simplicity and reliability, or may be very complex in design, in order to cope with more specialised clinical applications.

Clinical features of ventilators

Most ventilators can be used to ventilate normal lungs. For the more specialised clinical applications, for patients with respiratory pathology, or for weaning from mechanical ventilation, additional clinical features or ancillary modes may be required in a ventilator. Some examples of these modes are outlined in Figure EQ36.

Humidifiers

Humidity refers to the amount of water vapour present in a gas or the atmosphere. It is defined in two ways:
(1) **Absolute humidity (AH)** is the mass of water vapour present in a given volume of air or gas (g m^{-3} or

Mode	Description	Comments
Positive end-expiratory pressure (PEEP)	0–15 cmH$_2$O of positive airway pressure maintained during expiration.	Applied to improve oxygenation, recruit lung volume and prevent micro-atelectasis.
Continuous positive airway pressure (CPAP)	0–15 cmH$_2$O of positive airway pressure maintained during inspiration and expiration.	Applied to assist patients' spontaneous breathing by improving oxygenation and reducing the work of breathing.
Intermittent mandatory ventilation (IMV)	This mode supports patients who are breathing spontaneously, but inadequately. It supplies a minimum minute volume, as a preset number of mandatory breaths per minute. The patient breathes spontaneously between mandatory breaths.	Applied to patients who are being weaned from mechanical ventilation. A disadvantage is that mandatory breaths may 'stack' on top of spontaneous breaths, giving high airway pressures.
Synchronised intermittent mandatory ventilation (SIMV)	This form of IMV synchronises the mandatory breaths with the patient's spontaneous breathing.	Avoids 'stacking' of mandatory breaths and spontaneous breaths.
Pressure support (PS)	An 'assisted' mode in which the ventilator provides a mechanical breath when triggered by the patient's spontaneous effort. The ventilator is set to act as a pressure generator in this mode.	Used as a supporting mode in spontaneously breathing patients being weaned from mechanical ventilation or with respiratory failure.

Figure EQ36 Ancillary modes in ventilators

kg m^{-3}). This value will not vary with the temperature of the air.

(2) **Relative humidity (RH)** is the ratio of the mass of water present in a given volume of air at a given temperature, to the mass of water required to saturate that given volume at the same temperature. RH is usually expressed as a percentage, and will decrease as temperature increases. Fully saturated air at 20 °C contains 17 g m^{-3} while at 37 °C it contains 43 g m^{-3}.

It is important for us to control the humidity of medical gases and the atmosphere in order to decrease the risk of the following problems:

- Heat and moisture loss from the patient's respiratory tract
- Damage to the mucosa of the respiratory tract
- Corrosion or frost damage to gas pipes, cylinders and valves
- Discomfort and fatigue of operating theatre staff
- Accumulation of static electrical charges (risk of microshock) in operating theatre

Humidifiers for medical gases

Ideally inspired fresh gases should be supplied at body temperature with an RH of 100% (i.e. saturated). Inspiration of cool unhumidified gases by a patient can potentially lead to a loss of more than 10% (>10 W) of basal metabolic energy requirements. In addition the prolonged use of under-humidified gases in a ventilated patient can cause severe damage to the mucosa (inflammation, ulceration) and lungs (inspissation of secretions, micro-atelectasis).

Various mechanisms have been used to humidify inspired gases. The most commonly used types of humidifier are listed below.

Bottle humidifier

This method, often seen on wards, relies on passing or bubbling oxygen through a bottle containing water at room temperature. From the values for water content at room temperature and body temperature, it can be seen that this is at best only likely to achieve an RH of approximately 40% at body temperature. In practice, complete saturation of the gas is not even achieved at room temperature.

Soda lime absorber in the circle breathing system

This device is primarily used to prevent rebreathing at low flow rates, by absorbing carbon dioxide. The reaction of the carbon dioxide with the soda lime results in the production of calcium carbonate, heat and water. As a result an RH of 60–70% can be produced in the inspired gases at body temperature.

Heat and moisture exchanger (HME)

These passive devices consist of a capsule containing a condensing filter (stainless-steel mesh), hygroscopic material (paper coated with calcium chloride), or hydrophobic material (ceramic fibres). The capsule is fitted with 22 mm and 15 mm ports so that it can be fitted in-line between the breathing circuit and the patient's airway (endotracheal tube or laryngeal mask). Expired gases, saturated with water vapour, pass through the capsule, causing water to be deposited and heat to be retained by the contained element. Condensation causes a further temperature rise (latent heat of evaporation), producing a warm, moist environment for the incoming cool dry inspired fresh gas flow to pass through. Effective operation of the HME relies on the humidity and temperature gradient between the capsule and the fresh gas flow, and can result in an RH of 60–70% at body temperature. The HME is made of low thermal conductivity plastic to preserve the temperature inside the capsule. It may also be combined with a port for end-tidal CO_2 monitoring and a bacterial/viral filter.

Disadvantages with the use of this device include increased dead space, increased flow resistance, water accumulation in the filter and decreased efficiency with large tidal volumes.

Hot water bath

This consists of a thermostatically controlled water tank through which the inspired fresh gas flow is passed (Figure EQ37). Temperature is monitored at the airway by a thermistor which feeds back to control the water temperature. The water tank has a large surface area to ensure full saturation of the inspired gases. Performance depends on fresh gas flow rate passing through the humidifier. 100%

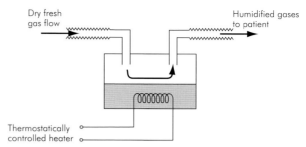

Figure EQ37 Water bath humidifier

RH (full saturation) can be achieved by setting the water tank temperature higher than body temperature to allow for cooling in the patient circuit.

Disadvantages with this method include risk of scalding and electric shock, risk of water and condensation passing into the patient's respiratory tract (so humidifier and water traps must be kept below level of patient), risk of infection due to colonisation of humidifier, and the need for a power supply.

Nebulisers

These devices produce a fine mist of water droplets in the inspired gases, and can be used to deliver drugs as well as humidification. The diameter of these droplets may range from less than 1 μm up to 20 μm, depending on the mechanism used to produce the droplets. Droplets of less than 1 μm in diameter can reach the lower airways and alveoli, while larger particles of 5–10 μm tend to deposit in the trachea and pharynx. Since the water is in the form of droplets, there is no saturation limit to the amount of water contained by the inspiratory gases, and excessive quantities of water can be readily deposited in the trachea and larger airways, particularly with the smaller particles. Different mechanisms are used to nebulise solutions, including:

- **Gas jet nebuliser** – This device is driven by a high-pressure gas jet passing across the top of a small tube fed by water from a reservoir (Figure EQ38). The negative pressure produced at the jet orifice entrains water from the tube, creating a spray, which is broken into finer droplets by impact on an anvil. This method produces a majority of droplets in the range of 2–5 μm diameter.
- **Ultrasonic nebuliser** – This method uses an ultrasonic (1–3 MHz) transducer to break up a water feed dripping on to it. The resultant droplets are finer than

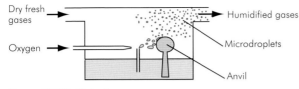

Figure EQ38 Nebuliser

those produced by the gas jet nebuliser, and are in the range 0.5–2 μm. This is the more effective technique for delivering nebulised drugs. Disadvantages of nebulisers are that they are more complex devices than other techniques, can easily result in excessive delivery of water to the respiratory system, and have variable performance according to the droplet sizes produced.

Intravenous equipment

Historically, vascular pressures, especially the central venous pressure, were measured using a water column manometer and three-way tap. More information is obtained if the pressure changes can be converted to an electronic signal and processed by a monitor. The waveform can be displayed and stored as a trend, calculations are performed automatically and staff alerted when preset limits are exceeded. Transducers are incorporated into a modified giving set incorporating a sampling port and a flushing device that delivers 3 millilitres of fluid per hour to keep the catheter patent. A coloured stripe aids identification – red for arterial line, blue for central venous, yellow for pulmonary artery catheter. Disposable, one-piece transducer sets are designed so that the compliance of the tubing and transducer are matched to transmit the pressure wave with minimal distortion. Earlier arrangements made with separate components were prone to either over- or under-damping of the waveform and hence inaccurate systolic or diastolic readings. The value for mean arterial pressure can usually be relied upon, since it is least distorted, and arguably should be charted instead of the more familiar systolic and diastolic values. Coincidentally, it is also the more accurate when measured by automated cuff methods.

Intravenous cannulae

These vary from the simple winged steel needle of the 'butterfly' pattern to the multi-lumen central venous catheter. The winged steel needle is now rarely used in the UK except for subcutaneous infusions. It has been superseded by the plastic cannula over needle pattern, which is associated with a much lower incidence of extravasation. Those made of translucent plastic are somewhat easier to place, but the smoothness and mechanical strength of the material are important considerations. Some needle types are made ultra-sharp with a double-angled bevel, and all include a flashback chamber to indicate successful venepuncture. Cannulae are colour-coded by the manufacturer to indicate the gauge. Some terminate with a Luer lock fitting whereas others also have an injection port. Other designs have resulted from attempts to reduce needle-stick injuries.

Although central venous catheters can be placed by an over-the-needle approach this limits the length of the combination to about 15 cm. A 'through-the-needle' method enables longer catheters to be placed, but then larger diameter catheters require even larger needles. A safer approach was pioneered by Seldinger, who used a fine-gauge needle to seek the central vein into which he inserted a thin guide wire. The track was then enlarged with a vein dilator passed over the wire, allowing the larger-diameter catheter to be similarly placed. Those intended for short-term monitoring or drug administration are sutured to the skin by the hub. This method of fixation is not appropriate for lines intended to be used over a period of weeks or months for chemotherapy or long-term parenteral nutrition. Instead, such lines are retained by having a cuff of fibrous material bonded to the line that becomes firmly anchored by the ingrowth of scar tissue after 2–3 weeks.

Intravenous giving sets

Giving sets consist of a clear plastic tube terminating at one end in a Luer lock adapter for the IV cannula and the other end in a spike for insertion into the bag of fluid. Manually controlled adult sets produce a drop size of 20 per millilitre, whereas paediatric sets are more easily regulated since the drop size is 60 per millilitre. While some automated drip controllers use standard giving sets, the majority require the use of the manufacturer's own disposables. Simple giving sets intended just for low-viscocity crystalloid administration deliver an acceptable flow rate through cheaper, narrow-gauge tubing. Blood is more viscous and is best given through wider tubing and a drip chamber that incorporates a 150 μm mesh filter. Most designs either terminate in a rubber end or have a dedicated injection port so that bolus doses of drugs can be given. Additional filters can be placed in-line to remove undesirable leucocytes and platelet aggregates from fresh blood. Crystalloid filters with an even finer mesh can retain microscopic particles of undissolved drugs, plastic, glass, rubber and bacteria as well as preventing air embolism. In theory, drugs too can be adsorbed onto these filters and the plastic of the giving sets, but this is only a problem with very potent drugs given in microgram doses.

Blood warmers

The earliest method of warming refrigerated blood was the use of an extended giving set that was dipped into an electrically heated water bath. Later versions consisted of a modified giving set sandwiched between electrically heated dry plates. At slow flow rates, though the blood leaves the warmer at 37 °C it cools significantly before reaching the patient. The maximum flow rate of the dry plate type is limited even when using a pneumatic pressure bag. If the blood loss can be measured in litres per minute there are designs ('level 1' blood warmer) which will permit resuscitation at this rate. The conducting tubing is all large-bore, and obviously the intravenous cannula should be as large as possible too.

Regional anaesthesia equipment

Although standard intravenous needles can be used for regional anaesthesia, success rates can be improved by using needles specifically designed for the purpose. These have a shorter bevel, which, although more difficult to insert through the skin, affords a greater 'feel' as it penetrates the tissues, and this results in less trauma to the nerve. The needles come in a range of sizes and some incorporate a short length of flexible plastic tubing so that movement of the tip is minimised during the injection of local anaesthetic. Other needles are electrically insulated for connection to a nerve stimulator. These are battery-powered devices that produce a small current at the tip of the advancing needle, which produces parasthesiae or motor stimulation when correctly placed.

Spinal needles

These are needles modified to access the subarachnoid space. Adult needles are 10 cm long and are produced in a range of sizes and tip types. Needles of size 22 G to 29 G are used in anaesthesia, whereas the larger 18 G needle is only needed to obtain CSF if it is expected to be purulent in suspected meningitis. The needles incorporate an inner stylet that helps to stiffen the needle during its insertion and prevents the lumen from being occluded by a core of tissue. The hubs are made of translucent plastic so that the emerging CSF can be easily seen. Usually the plastic component of the needle is colour-coded to identify the needle gauge. While an incidence of headache is inevitable after dural puncture, it is related to the size of the hole or tear in the dura. This can be minimised by using a needle with an *atraumatic* tip such as the pencil-tipped Whitacre or Sprotte type, and by using the smallest possible gauge.

Epidural needles and catheters

A modified needle is used to place a catheter into the epidural space. The most widely used needle in the UK is the Tuohy (1945) needle. Adult needles are 10 cm long and marked at 1 cm intervals. They are either 16 or 18 G and come with a metal or plastic stylet. The hub has a Luer lock fitting to accept the *loss of resistance syringe* (glass or plastic) and is supplied with or without wings. The bevel has been rounded to a blunt Huber tip designed to give the maximum 'feel' when inserted through the ligaments and not be so sharp as to penetrate the more delicate dura. The angled tip helps direct the epidural catheter in the desired direction. While there are epidural catheters that are open-ended, the most widely used pattern in the UK has a blind end, with the local anaesthetic exiting by three small holes near the tip. This style is said to be less likely to enter a dural vein and should reduce the chances of intravascular injection of local anaesthetic. The catheter is marked in centimetres at the distal end to aid placement of the intended length in the epidural space. The proximal end is fitted to a Luer lock connector, and all injections should be given through a filter to remove particles of glass or bacteria.

The increasing popularity of the combined spinal and epidural (CSE) technique for obstetric analgesia has resulted in the introduction of kits containing modified epidural needles, catheters and matching spinal needles.

Infusions of drugs into the epidural space are best delivered from one of the purpose-designed pumps now available. Potential confusion with drip controllers is prevented, and the additional security features are an important safeguard so that patients or their relatives or unauthorised staff are prevented from altering the infusion rates.

Methods of sterilisation

There is a range of methods for cleaning equipment, from decontamination through disinfection to sterilisation:

- Decontamination – the physical removal of infected material by washing or scrubbing
- Disinfection – the killing of non-sporing organisms
- Sterilisation – the killing of all micro-organisms including viruses, fungi and spores

Methods of disinfection and sterilisation are listed in Figure EQ39.

Increasingly filtration is used as a method of controlling transfer of infected material, for example the protection of ventilators. The various labels which are used in medical products after sterilisation are shown in Figure EQ40.

References and further reading

Al-Shaikh B, Stacey S. *Essentials of Anaesthetic Equipment*, 2nd edn. Edinburgh: Churchill Livingstone, 2002.

Association of Anaesthetists of Great Britain and Ireland. *Checking Anaesthetic Equipment 3*. London: AAGBI, 2004.

Mapleson WW. The elimination of rebreathing in various semi closed anaesthetic systems. *Br J Anaesth* 1954; **26**: 323–32.

Disinfection

(1) Pasteurisation
  ○ 20 minutes at 70 °C or
  ○ 10 minutes at 80 °C or
  ○ 5 minutes at 100 °C

(2) Chemical
  ○ formaldehyde or
  ○ 70% alcohol or
  ○ 0.1–0.5% chlorhexidine or
  ○ 2% gluteraldehyde or
  ○ 10% hypochlorite solution or
  ○ hydrogen peroxide or
  ○ phenol

Sterilisation

(1) Dry heat
  ○ 150 °C for 30 minutes

(2) Moist heat (steam under pressure: autoclaving)
  ○ 30 minutes at 1 atmosphere 122 °C or
  ○ 10 minutes at 1.5 atmospheres 126 °C or
  ○ 3 minutes at 2 atmospheres 134 °C

(3) Ethylene oxide

(4) Gamma irradiation

Figure EQ39 Methods of sterilisation and disinfection

Symbols used on medical devices and their packaging

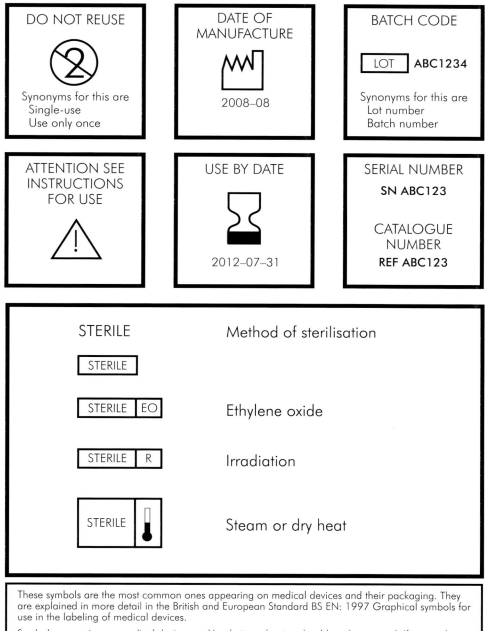

These symbols are the most common ones appearing on medical devices and their packaging. They are explained in more detail in the British and European Standard BS EN: 1997 Graphical symbols for use in the labeling of medical devices.

Symbols appearing on medical devices and/or their packaging should not be ignored. If a user does not understand a symbol, they should first look in the instructions for use or user manual for an explanation.

Figure EQ40 Symbols used on medical devices and their packaging

The following checks should be made prior to each operating session.

In addition, checks 2, 6 and 9 (Monitoring, Breathing System and Ancillary Equipment) should be made prior to each new patient during a session.

1. **Check that the anaesthetic machine is connected to the electricity supply (if appropriate) and switched on.**
   Note: Some anaesthetic workstations may enter an integral self-test programme when switched on; those functions tested by such a programme need not be retested.
   - Take note of any information or labelling on the anaesthetic machine referring to the current status of the machine. Particular attention should be paid to recent servicing. Servicing labels should be fixed in the service logbook.

2. **Check that all monitoring devices, in particular the oxygen analyser, pulse oximeter and capnograph, are functioning and have appropriate alarm limits.**
   - Check that gas sampling lines are properly attached and free of obstructions.
   - Check that an appropriate frequency of recording non-invasive blood pressure is selected.
   (Some monitors need to be in stand-by mode to avoid unnecessary alarms before being connected to the patient.)

3. **Check with a 'tug test' that each pipeline is correctly inserted into the appropriate gas supply terminal.**
   Note: Carbon dioxide cylinders should not be present on the anaesthetic machine unless requested by the anaesthetist. A blanking plug should be fitted to any empty cylinder yoke.
   - Check that the anaesthetic machine is connected to a supply of oxygen and that an adequate supply of oxygen is available from a reserve oxygen cylinder.
   - Check that adequate supplies of other gases (nitrous oxide, air) are available and connected as appropriate.
   - Check that all pipeline pressure gauges in use on the anaesthetic machine indicate 400–500 kPa.

4. **Check the operation of flowmeters (where fitted).**
   - Check that each flow valve operates smoothly and that the bobbin moves freely throughout its range.
   - Check the anti-hypoxia device is working correctly.
   - Check the operation of the emergency oxygen bypass control.

5. **Check the vaporiser(s).**
   - Check that each vaporiser is adequately, but not over, filled.
   - Check that each vaporiser is correctly seated on the back bar and not tilted.
   - Check the vaporiser for leaks (with vaporiser on and off) by temporarily occluding the common gas outlet.
   - Turn the vaporiser(s) off when checks are completed.
   - Repeat the leak test immediately after changing any vaporiser.

6. **Check the breathing system to be employed.**
   Note: A new single-use bacterial/viral filter and angle-piece/catheter mount must be used for each patient. Packaging should not be removed until point of use.
   - Inspect the system for correct configuration. All connections should be secured by 'push and twist'.
   - Perform a pressure leak test on the breathing system by occluding the patient-end and compressing the reservoir bag. Bain-type coaxial systems should have the inner tube compressed for the leak test.
   - Check the correct operation of all valves, including unidirectional valves within a circle, and all exhaust valves.
   - Check for patency and flow of gas through the whole breathing system including the filter and anglepiece/catheter mount.

Figure EQ41 Association of Anaesthetists of Great Britain and Ireland: checklist for anaesthetic equipment 2004

7. **Check that the ventilator is configured appropriately for its intended use.**
   - Check that the ventilator tubing is correctly configured and securely attached.
   - Set the controls for use and ensure that an adequate pressure is generated during the inspiratory phase.
   - Check the pressure relief valve functions.
   - Check that the disconnect alarms function correctly.
   - Ensure that an alternative means to ventilate the patient's lungs is available (see 10, below).

8. **Check that the anaesthetic gas scavenging system is switched on and is functioning correctly.**
   - Check that the tubing is attached to the appropriate exhaust port of the breathing system, ventilator or workstation.

9. **Check that all ancillary equipment which may be needed is present and working.**
   - This includes laryngoscopes, intubation aids, intubation forceps, bougies etc. and appropriately sized facemasks, airways, tracheal tubes and connectors, which must be checked for patency.
   - Check that the suction apparatus is functioning and that all connectors are secure.
   - Check that the patient trolley, bed or operating table can be rapidly tilted head down.

10. **Check that an alternative means to ventilate the patient is immediately available (e.g. self-inflating bag and oxygen cylinder).**
    - Check that the self-inflating bag and cylinder of oxygen are functioning correctly and the cylinder contains an adequate supply of oxygen.

11. **Recording**
    - Sign and date the logbook kept with the anaesthetic machine to confirm the machine has been checked.
    - Record on each patient's anaesthetic chart that the anaesthetic machine, breathing system and monitoring has been checked.

Figure EQ41 (*Cont.*)

CHAPTER 4

Basic statistics

E. S. Lin

Introduction

A knowledge of statistics is required in designing studies for research, analysing the data collected in studies, and writing for publication – as well as for the critical assessment of published research work. Statistical techniques are also a key component of evidence-based medicine, used in systematic reviews and meta-analysis. This chapter reviews the application of statistical methods in:
- Describing data
- Collecting data
- Testing and interpreting data

Data description

Types of data

Data are obtained by recording measurements or observations, and can be classified into different types. The data may consist of numbers (**numerical data**) or group names/labels (**categorical data**). It is important to choose the appropriate statistical test to suit the type of data.

Numerical data

Obtained from measurements (e.g. height, weight) or counts (e.g. number of operations, number of children). Numerical data can be divided into continuous and discrete data:
- *Continuous data* – can take any value over the range measured, depending only on the accuracy of the measurement device.
- *Discrete data* – can only take whole-number or integer values.

Categorical data

Consists of group names or labels. Categorical data can be further divided into unordered and ordered data.
- *Unordered* – the data comes from groups which are mutually exclusive and not ordered in any way, e.g. blood group (A, B, O), gender (M, F).
- *Ordered* – the data groups are mutually exclusive and also ordered or ranked, e.g. socioeconomic class, staging of a disease.

Displaying data

Raw data usually consist of a collection of numbers and labels (Figures ST1 and ST2).

Noradrenaline infusion rate (ml hr^{-1})	1.1	2.3	3.0	4.5	5.2	6.7
Mean BP (mmHg)	56	78	80	88	87	90

Figure ST1 Numerical data for noradrenaline infusion in a patient

Postoperative pain at 4 hours	none	mild	moderate	severe
Group 1	23	11	9	2
Group 2	31	6	6	0

Figure ST2 Categorical data for two postoperative analgesics

Fundamentals of Anaesthesia, 3rd edition, ed. Tim Smith, Colin Pinnock and Ted Lin. Published by Cambridge University Press. © Cambridge University Press 2008.

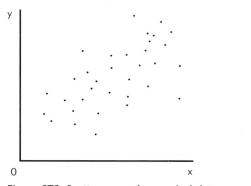

Figure ST3 Scattergram of numerical data

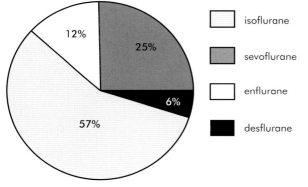

Use of volatile agents 2001–2003 St Elsewhere Hospital

12%

25%

57%

6%

☐ isoflurane

▨ sevoflurane

☐ enflurane

■ desflurane

Figure ST4 Pie chart of categorical data

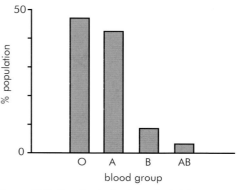

Occurrence of ABO blood groups in the UK

Figure ST5 Bar chart of categorical data

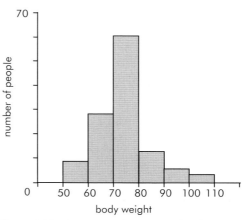

Figure ST6 Histogram – frequency distribution of continuous numerical data

Graphical display gives a visual summary of the data. Graphs and charts are useful in characterising data because:

- With a small number of points a relationship can be sought between the independent (x) and dependent (y) variable.
- With a large number of data points, grouping the data points into categories or ranges enables the distribution to be visualised.

Figures ST3 to ST6 illustrate some common types of graph. Small numbers of numerical data, plotting y against x, can be displayed as a *scattergram* (Figure ST3). Larger numbers of categorical data can be plotted as a *pie chart* (Figure ST4). A *bar chart* can also be used to represent categorical data. Figure ST5 illustrates the occurrence of blood groups in the UK, by plotting the percentage of population for each blood group. Sometimes continuous numerical data can be plotted as a *histogram* (a form of bar chart in which the area

of each bar is proportional to the number of observations) in order to produce a frequency distribution.

Frequency distributions

Plotting numbers of data points in each category for categorical data produces a histogram showing the *frequency distribution*. Continuous numerical data may also be represented in this way by dividing the variable into ranges and plotting the frequency of data points occurring in each range. Figure ST6 shows body weights for a sample of people. In this sample the number of people in each range (vertical axis) is plotted against body weight (horizontal axis). The following points can be made about frequency distributions:

- The area under a frequency distribution is proportional to the total number of data points (total number of people) in a sample.
- For large samples or whole populations the frequency distribution tends towards a smooth curve.
- A frequency distribution can be normalised by converting frequencies to relative frequencies, dividing each frequency by the total number of points in the sample. This makes comparisons between samples easier. When sample sizes are large the normalised frequency distribution approximates to the *probability density* function for the population.

Probability

Statistical methods are required because of biological variation between individuals. We cannot obtain black and white answers from our interpretation of data, we can only obtain a probability of a value being representative for a population, or for a hypothesis being true or false.

Probability is usually expressed as a number from 0 to 1. If the probability of an event occurring is 0 it will not occur, and if the probability is 1 the event is certain to occur. For example:

- In any individual, the probability of death occurring in their lifetime is 1 ($P = 1$).
- The probability of 'heads' occurring when a coin is tossed is 0.5 ($P = 0.5$).
- The probability of being blood group B in the UK is 0.08 ($P = 0.08$).

It is often useful to plot the probabilities for a variable having a specific value or falling into a particular category, as this gives an overall view of how the variable is distributed throughout the population. This curve is called a *probability density curve.*

Probability density curves

A probability density curve plots the probability of occurrence (probability density) against value of variable for a population. Frequency distribution curves for samples from a whole population approximate to the probability density curve if the frequencies are converted to relative frequencies and the sample numbers are large.

Probability density curves are useful in describing the distribution of data values in populations. Naturally

occurring data tend to follow recognised probability density curves, which can be defined by characteristic equations. These equations represent families of curves which depend on the values of parameters in the equations.

Probability density curves can also be derived for statistical parameters such as t and χ^2. These parameters are sometimes simply referred to as statistics, and are calculated from the data obtained in research studies. Such curves enable probabilities to be derived for specific values of the parameters. These probabilities (or p numbers) are the end product, when data are statistically tested for the null hypothesis (see below).

A probability density curve has the following properties:

- The height of the curve at any point equals the probability of that value of x occurring.
- The maximum height of the curve cannot be greater than 1.
- The area under the curve between any two values of x equals the probability of x occurring in that range of values.
- The total area under the curve equals 1, since the curve covers all probabilities for the variable x.

Recognised probability density curves

Commonly occurring curves describing data include:

- *Normal distribution* – This is the most common probability density curve in biological data. It is based on the idea of a representative or average value for a population, and is a symmetrical bell-shaped curve. The normal distribution describes many numerical variables – e.g. blood pressure, body temperature, body weight, haemoglobin level – and it is central to many statistical methods. The curve is defined by its mean value (μ) and its standard deviation (σ). Figure ST7 shows two normal distributions with different mean values μ_1 and μ_2 ($\mu_2 > \mu_1$), and different standard deviations σ_1 and σ_2 ($\sigma_2 < \sigma_1$).

For example, consider plotting a probability density curve for systolic BP, over the whole population in the UK (this can only be approximated to by taking a very large sample). If the probability density is plotted against systolic BP, a normal distribution curve is obtained (Figure ST8). The mean, mode and median are 120 mmHg. There are much lower probabilities for pressures 180 mmHg or 60 mmHg occurring. These occur in the outermost portions of the curve, called the *tails*. The shaded area equals the probability of systolic blood pressures >180 mmHg occurring. The

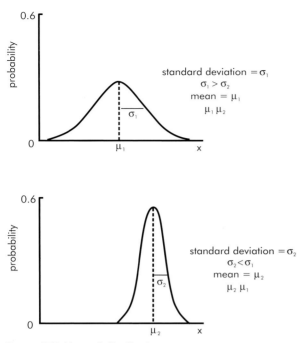

Figure ST7 Normal distribution

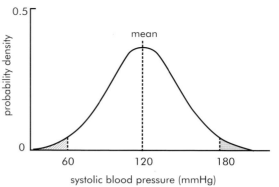

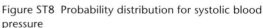

Figure ST8 Probability distribution for systolic blood pressure

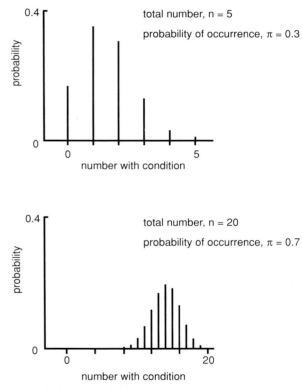

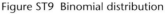

Figure ST9 Binomial distribution

hatched area equals the probability of systolic blood pressures <60 mmHg occurring.

- *Binomial distribution* – These curves describe the probability distribution of proportions. Proportions occur in a sample in which a binary variable is recorded. Binary variables only have two possible values or states, e.g. 0 or 1, dead or alive, diseased or disease-free, ventilated or spontaneously breathing. Consider recording deaths in a sample (n) of ICU admissions. A number (r) will have died and a number ($n-r$) survive. These curves plot probability against the number of individuals (r) with the chosen outcome. The binomial distribution curves alter shape according to the total number (n) of individuals in the sample, and the probability (π) of the chosen outcome occurring. Figure ST9 shows a binomial distribution plotting probability against r. It is skewed for $\pi < 0.5$ or $\pi > 0.5$ and becomes symmetrical at $\pi = 0.5$. The shape of the distribution curve also varies with n and tends towards a normal distribution as n increases (>40).
- *Poisson distribution* – This is used to describe the probability distribution of rates of occurrence, e.g. the respiratory rate of a patient (breaths per minute), the

number of ICU admissions per week, the incidence of prostatic cancer per year. The Poisson distribution plots probability against the rate of events occurring. These probability density curves only depend on the average rate of events recorded over a period of time

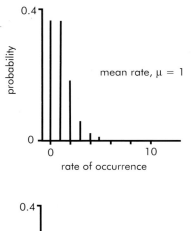

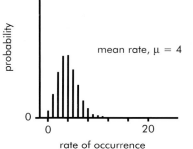

Figure ST10 Poisson distribution

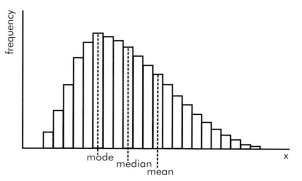

Figure ST11 Mean, mode, median – skewed distribution

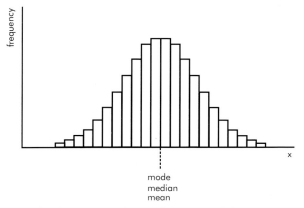

Figure ST12 Mean, mode, median – normal distribution

(μ). The distribution is skewed for low values of μ (<10), but tends towards a normal distribution when μ is high (>20) (Figure ST10).

Describing numerical data
Consider a set of values for a variable x. The values are $x_1 + x_2 + x_3 \ldots x_n$ and have been divided into ranges and plotted as a frequency distribution in Figure ST11. These data can then be described by two main characteristics:
- An **average** or representative value
- A measure of the **spread** of values

The average value
There are three choices for a representative value.
- The mode – This is the most commonly occurring value in the set of data values.
- The median – This is the value in the data set which has an equal number of data points above it and below it. It is sometimes called the geometrical mean, as the area above the median equals the area below.

- The mean – This is short for the arithmetical mean value, and is the most useful of these choices. It is calculated first by summing all the values:

$$\text{Sum of values} = x_1 + x_2 + x_3 \ldots x_0$$

Using mathematical notation $= \Sigma_{i=0}^{i=n} x_i$ (abbreviated to Σx_i)

Then the mean, $m = \Sigma_{x_i} / n$

In Figure ST11 it can be seen that the frequency distribution is not symmetrical but is *skewed*. The mode, median and mean are all given by different values of x. Medical variables usually have a normal shaped frequency distribution, which is symmetrical and has mean, mode and median values all coinciding (Figure ST12).

The spread of values
The spread of a set of data can be calculated numerically in the case of a normal distribution, and is given by the

standard deviation (s) which is derived from the variance (s²).

Calculation of variance (s²)

Consider the above set of data, consisting of *n* values for a variable *x*. Then, using the above calculation, the mean, *m*, can be calculated. The variance is calculated from the deviations of each value from the mean and the number of degrees of freedom (DF), where $DF = n - 1$.

The deviation of each value from the mean is given by

$$\text{Deviation} = x_i - m$$

$$\text{Squared deviation} = (x_i - m)^2$$

$$\text{Sum of squared deviations} = \Sigma(x_i - m)^2$$

$$\text{Variance } (s^2) = \frac{\Sigma(x_i - m)^2}{DF} = \frac{\Sigma(x_i - m)^2}{n - 1}$$

$$\text{Standard deviation}(s) = \text{square root of variance}$$

$$= \sqrt{\frac{\Sigma(x_i - m)^2}{n - 1}}$$

In a normal distribution the standard deviation gives a measure of the spread of values. Figure ST13 shows the frequency distribution for a normally distributed variable *x*, in which the mean value is *m* and the standard deviation is *s*. Then 68% of the values lie within the area $m \pm s$ (light shaded area), and 96% lie within $m \pm 2s$ (light and dark shaded areas). The smaller the standard deviation the more the data points cluster around the mean value, and the narrower the frequency distribution.

Sampling

Recording a number of numerical values from a whole population is known as sampling. The larger the number of data points recorded the closer the information obtained from the sample is to the true situation for the whole population. In a population of a million people, taking a sample from 10 individuals is not likely to be as accurate in representing the whole population as sampling 1000 individuals.

In descriptive statistics a convention exists of representing sample parameters with Roman (normal) letters, but using Greek letters to represent true parameters for the whole population.

Figure ST14 shows how a sample with mean, *m*, and standard deviation, *s*, is related to a normally distributed population with mean, μ, and standard deviation, σ. The population frequency distribution is represented by the broken line, while the sample is represented by the smaller histogram. Note the following:

- The population distribution is shown as a smooth curve because it usually covers a very large number of individuals.
- The area of the sample histogram is small compared to the area of the population distribution curve, because the number of individuals in the sample is small compared to the population.
- The sample mean, *m*, is only an estimate of the true population mean, μ. It is unlikely that the sample mean will coincide with the population mean. Therefore there will be an error (error = μ − m) in the estimated mean. A *standard error of the mean* (SEM) can be calculated for samples.

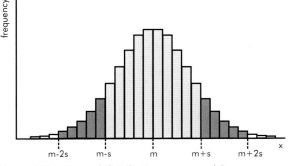

Figure ST13 Normal distribution – *m, s* and 2*s*

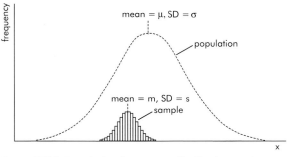

Figure ST14 Population frequency distribution and sample frequency distribution

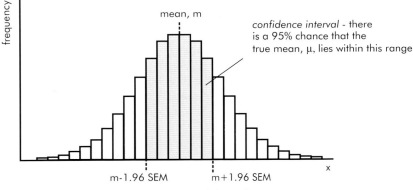

Figure ST15 Confidence interval and confidence limits

Standard error of the mean (SEM)

When a mean value is calculated from a sample set of data, the value obtained (m) is only an estimate of the true mean (μ). The true mean can only be calculated by measuring every value in the population. However a standard error of the mean can be calculated using the standard deviation (s) of the sample, and the number of data points in the sample (n):

$$\text{SEM} = \frac{s}{\sqrt{n}}$$

If a number of samples were to be taken from a population, each sample would provide its own estimate ($m_1, m_2, \ldots$) of the true mean (μ). These estimates ($m_1, m_2, \ldots$) would form a normal distribution centred about μ. The SEM is the standard deviation of this distribution, and gives an idea of how close the estimated mean value is likely to be to the true mean value. In order to quantify this 'closeness', the *confidence limits* have to be calculated.

Confidence limits

When reporting a calculated mean value, it is sometimes quoted as $m \pm \text{SEM}$. This only gives an idea of the ratio between mean value and SEM. Consider a calculated mean value

$$= m \pm \text{SEM}$$
$$= 10 \pm 2$$

It is not immediately apparent where the real mean (μ) lies in relation to the estimate (m). In order to clarify this, a *confidence interval* (CI) is determined around m, within which a reader can be confident the true mean (μ) lies. The wider the CI is the poorer the estimate. The CI is defined by two values, the *confidence limits* (CL). There is a 95% probability of the CI containing the true mean (μ). In a normally distributed sample, the confidence limits are calculated from the SEM by

$$\text{Confidence limits (CL)} = \pm 1.96\,(\text{SEM})$$

Thus in the above example the mean value can now be quoted as

$$m = 10(6.08,\ 13.92)$$

A reader then knows that the estimated mean is 10 and there is a 95% chance of the true mean lying within the range 6.08 to 13.92 (Figure ST15).

Describing categorical data

As discussed above, categorical data takes the form of variables which are labelled rather than measured. A common situation, referred to previously, is to sample a group of individuals in whom there are only two possible outcomes (categories) of interest. In such cases the data are described as binary, and the sample is considered in terms of proportions.

Proportions

Consider a group of n individuals, in whom there exist two possible categories. Let the number of individuals in one category be r, out of the total number n. This can be expressed as a proportion r/n.

For example, 10 (r) deaths occurred out of a sample of 100 (n) admissions to ICU. The proportion of deaths (p) is given by

$$p = r/n$$

$$\text{Proportion of deaths} = 0.1$$

Proportions obtained by sampling follow a binomial distribution curve (see above).

Confidence limits for a proportion (p) can be obtained from

$$CL = p \pm 1.96\sqrt{p(1-p)n}$$

Thus in the above example the confidence limits can be quoted as

$$CL = 0.1 \pm 0.0588$$

Proportion of deaths $= 0.1(0.041, 0.16)$

Contingency tables

Studies are often designed to look for differences in outcome between two or more groups of patients who have been exposed to different treatments or risk factors. The results can be conveniently displayed in a contingency table. In a contingency table the *column variable* labels each column with an outcome, while the *row variable* assigns each group to a row. In its simplest form it appears as a 2×2 table.

Consider a study examining the incidence of influenza in two groups of patients, one treated with a vaccine and the other not vaccinated. There are only two outcomes for the patients, either they catch influenza or they do not. The contingency table thus appears as in Figure ST16.

Larger contingency tables occur in studies examining multiple outcomes (increased number of columns) or more than two groups (increased number of rows. Contingency tables are important in the analysis of categorical data because of the use of the chi-squared test when testing non-parametric data. It should be noted, however, that many studies comparing proportions in two groups result in a 2×2 contingency table, which can be tested

more effectively using parametric tests as described below (see *Parametric and non-parametric tests*, pages 877–8).

Data collection

Several different types of study can be designed. These can be broadly divided into:

*   *Observational studies* – In these the investigator simply observes events occurring. Observational studies may be either cross-sectional (observations at one instant of time) or longitudinal (observations following the time course of events, e.g. plasma concentrations of a drug to determine pharmacokinetic parameters).
*   *Experimental studies* – In these an investigator influences the outcome, e.g. administering a drug to observe its effect on blood pressure.

Experimental studies

Many experimental studies in medicine seek an answer by comparison, as in the comparison of the effects of two drugs, or the comparison of a drug against placebo. Experimental studies may fall into one or more of the following categories:

*   *Parallel* – Here data are collected from two groups of different patients that have been treated differently. Data groups are independent and data comparison is *between individuals*.
*   *Cross-over* – In these studies each group of patients passes through different phases of treatment and non-treatment sequentially. Therefore each patient is used as his or her own control. Thus data groups are related or paired and *within-individual* comparisons are made. This has the theoretical advantage of reducing the effects of individual variation.
*   *Cohort* – This a single group of patients whose progress is followed to provide data.
*   *Case–control* – This type of study collects data from a treated group and an untreated group who are the controls.
*   *Clinical trial* – This is a study designed to assess the efficacy of a new treatment or medication. The design of clinical trials is discussed in detail in Section 3, Chapter 19.

The design of an experimental study must take account of a number of issues, including:

*   *Randomisation* – This refers to the method of selecting individuals for each of the groups in a study, and it is one of the important ways of reducing bias.

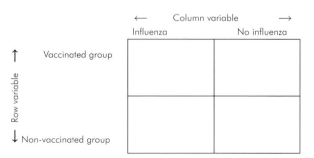
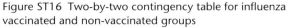

Figure ST16 Two-by-two contingency table for influenza vaccinated and non-vaccinated groups

Randomisation is usually performed by tossing a coin, using a random number generator program in a computer, or by using random number tables.

- *Bias* – This is any systematic departure of results from the real situation, and may arise for different reasons. *Observer bias* occurs when an observer consistently under-records or over-records specific data values. *Selection bias* occurs when patients are not randomised into their study groups, or they are not representative of the population the results are to be applied to. *Publication bias* occurs when either favourable or unfavourable results are preferentially selected for publication. *Patient bias* may be introduced by patients who are trying to 'help' the investigators by only reporting positive results.

- *Sample numbers* – This is an important feature when designing a study because the size of sample groups will affect the SEMs obtained on statistical testing and can therefore determine the significance of the results. Appropriate selection of sample numbers is aided by power calculation (see below).

- *Blinding* – In a study comparing treatments and controls, observer and patient biases can be reduced by 'blinding' both patients and observers to the status of the individual patient under study. *Double blinding* means that neither the patient nor the observer knows whether the patient is a control or is receiving treatment; where only the patient can be blinded this is called *single blinding*.

- *Replication* – Measurements can be made more precise if they are repeated when made and an average taken.

Types of hypothesis

Studies often compare data collected from two groups. The question asked by such studies can be reduced to proving or rejecting a simple hypothesis. There are two types of hypothesis:

- *Null hypothesis* (H_0) – there is no difference between the two groups studied.

- *Alternative hypothesis* (H_1) – there is a difference between the groups studied.

Consider a study of two groups of subjects, one treated with a new medication and the other treated with placebo. The question to be answered is, 'Is the new medication effective?'

By convention the hypothesis to be proved or rejected is taken to be the null hypothesis. The null hypothesis states there is no difference between the groups. Thus if the null hypothesis is proved no significant difference exists between groups and the treatment is therefore ineffective. However if the null hypothesis is rejected, then a difference exists between groups, and the treatment is effective. This leads to the definition of two types of error.

Types of error

Testing the null hypothesis leads to the definition of two types of error (Figure ST17):

- *Type I error* – rejecting the null hypothesis when it is true (i.e. finding a false difference between groups). This is equivalent to finding a positive effect of treatment when there is none. The probability of making a type I error is also equal to α, which is used as a label for the level of significance (see below).

- *Type II error* – accepting the null hypothesis when it is untrue (i.e. missing a true difference between groups). This is equivalent to overlooking a therapeutic effect of treatment. It can also be regarded as a lack ability of the study to detect a difference between groups. This ability is referred to as the *power* of the study. The probability of making a type II error is called β.

Power of a study

The power of a study is described above as its ability to detect a difference between groups or an effect of treatment. Power can be defined mathematically as the probability of not obtaining a type II error (i.e. missing a true difference):

Power of a study $= 1 - \beta$

Error	Definition	Probability	Comment
Type I	False rejection of H_0	α – also significance level	Detects false difference/effect
Type II	False acceptance of H_0	β – related to power	Misses true difference/effect
		Power $= 1 - \beta$	

Figure ST17 Type I and Type II errors (H_0 = null hypothesis)

Since β is the probability of making a type II error, power increases as β decreases. A good level of power for a study is 0.8 (i.e. β = 0.2).

The power of a study depends on various factors:
- *Sample size* – larger sample sizes increase study power.
- *Treatment effect* – the more effective the treatment the greater will be the difference (d) between groups, and study power will increase.
- *Variability of measurements* – less variability in measurements increases study power. Variability is represented by the variance of the measurements (s^2).
- *Level of significance* – a greater value for the significance level (α) increases the power of a study. Thus setting $\alpha = 0.05$ produces a more powerful study than setting $\alpha = 0.001$. (See *Level of significance*, below).

Calculating numbers of patients required in a study

Consider the common example of comparing the efficacy of two analgesics in two groups of patients using visual analogue scores (VAS). The number of patients (n) in each group required can be estimated as follows:
- Select power required, usually β = 0.9 (90%). Find percentage point (b) in normal distribution corresponding to $100 - \beta$ (e.g. for β = 90%, $b = 1.29$),
- Select level of significance, usually $\alpha = 0.05$. Find percentage point (a) in normal distribution corresponding to α (e.g. for $\alpha = 0.05$, $a = 1.96$)
- Estimate variances of measurements by pilot study or from previous work (s_1^2 and s_2^2), e.g. let variance of VAS measurements in pilot study be 14, thus assume $s_1^2 = s_2^2 = 14$
- Select outcome measure (VAS) and anticipated difference in effect (d). In this case the difference in mean VAS values, e.g. let $d = 3$

Then the number of patients in each group to be studied is given by

$$n = \frac{(a+b)^2(s_1^2 + s_2^2)}{d^2}$$
$$= \frac{(1.96 + 1.28)^2(14 + 14)}{9}$$
$$= \frac{10.5 \times 28}{9}$$
$$= 32.6$$

Therefore a minimum of 33 patients in each group is required to produce a study power of 90% with the estimated parameters and treatment effect difference suggested above. This calculation will be varied according to the study design, e.g. if a proportion is the outcome measure selected, as in determining the efficacy of a vaccine.

Data interpretation

P-number

However convincing data obtained by research studies may appear to be in demonstrating differences between sample groups, there is always a possibility that apparent differences are not meaningful, having arisen simply by chance. By convention, statistical testing is performed to determine the probability of the null hypothesis (H_0) being true. This probability is referred to as the *P*-number or simply *P*.

If the *P*-number is less than a chosen value, called the level of significance (α), then H_0 is rejected and the differences found are accepted as being statistically significant. If the *P*-number is greater than the level of significance (α), then H_0 is accepted and there are no significant differences between groups.

In clinical research α is usually chosen as $\alpha = 0.05$, i.e. H_0 is only rejected when the probability for it being true is $\leq 5\%$.

Obtaining P-numbers

The choice of an appropriate statistical test depends on the type and form of data recorded. Statistical tests usually involve complex or repetitive arithmetic, readily performed by computers, and result in a value for a specific parameter or *statistic* depending on the test applied (e.g. a *t*-test will give a value for *t*, a χ^2 test will give a value for χ^2).

These statistics have known probability density curves. Figure ST18 shows probability density curves for *t*. Different curves are produced by differing *degrees of freedom* (DF). The DF relate to the numbers of data points in each group and the number of groups tested. In the case of a *t*-test, using the value of *t* obtained by testing the data, a corresponding *P*-number (probability for H_0 being true) can be looked up in numerical tables representing the probability density curves for *t*.

For example, consider a comparison between two groups, drug and placebo, involving 501 patients (DF = 500). If H_0 is true there is no difference between groups and the drug is ineffective. If H_0 is rejected, there is a difference between groups and the drug is effective. Applying a

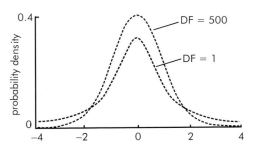

Figure ST18 Probability distribution for t, DF $= 1$ and DF $= 500$

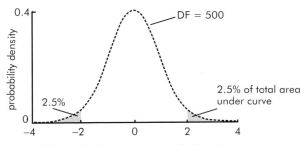

Figure ST19 t distribution – two-tailed testing

t-test to the data gives a value of $t = 2$, and the appropriate section in the t table may show:

t	P
1	0.03
2	0.04
3	0.05

Looking at the distribution curve in Figure ST18, it can be seen that $t = 2$ is at the upper end (tail) of the distribution curve, where probabilities for the null hypothesis being true are low. From the t table, $P = 0.04$, so the null hypothesis can be rejected and the drug can be considered to be effective.

Level of significance (α)

Consider the probability density curve for t in the above example (Figure ST19). The shaded area in the upper tail equals the probability of H_0 being true for all values of $t \geq 2$. Similarly $t = -2$ defines a small area at the lower tail of the curve which equals the probability of H_0 being true for $t \leq -2$. Because the probability levels are very low for values of t in these tail areas, it is unlikely that H_0 is true, and H_0 can be safely rejected. These areas therefore represent rejection areas for H_0.

In clinical research 95% probability ($P = 0.95$) is usually accepted as 'proving the case', so if $P \geq 0.95$ H_0 is accepted.

P	The probability that H_0 is true
α	The level of significance. Usually $\alpha = 0.05$
$P \leq \alpha$	H_0 is rejected – differences between groups are statistically significant
$P \geq \alpha$	H_0 is accepted – differences between groups are not statistically significant

Figure ST20 Summary for P-number (P) and level of significance (α)

Another way of expressing this is to say that if $P < 0.05$, H_0 is rejected. Therefore the total area for rejection of H_0 is the sum of the two shaded tail areas, which is equal to 5%. This is called the level of significance (α). Usually

$$\alpha = 0.05$$

Note that if H_0 is rejected falsely due to poor-quality or inaccurate data, a type I error has occurred. Thus the probability of making a type I error must also be equal to α (see *Types of error*, page 875).

Consider data demonstrating a difference in mean blood pressure between two groups of patients, one group treated with an antihypertensive and the other group treated with placebo. Statistical testing of the data may give $P = 0.03$ for the difference between the groups. This result means that there is only a 3% probability of H_0 being true. For $\alpha = 0.05$, H_0 is rejected, the difference is significant, and the antihypertensive is effective.

The relationship between P and α is summarised in Figure ST20.

Single-tailed and two-tailed testing

This refers to the setting of the significance level (α). In the above discussion α is shown to be equal to the area of rejection of H_0 in the probability density curve for t. This area consists of the 2 'tails' in the distribution. This is the usual situation, and is referred to as **two-tailed testing** or two-sided testing.

Under some circumstances it may be valid to assume that t can not assume negative values, in which case the upper tail rejection area can be increased from 2.5% to 5%, still maintaining the level of significance at $\alpha = 0.05$. This is **single-tailed testing**, and it can only be used under certain circumstances.

In a study investigating the difference between a treatment group and a control group, the results may demonstrate one of three outcomes:

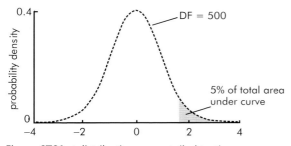

Figure ST21 *t* distribution – one-tailed testing

- Treatment is the same as control and H_0 accepted. This means the treatment is ineffective.
- Treatment produces better outcomes. The treatment is effective and H_0 is rejected (upper tail).
- Treatment produces worse outcomes. The treatment is harmful and H_0 is rejected (lower tail).

Usually clinical studies are subjected to two-tailed testing, allowing for better or worse outcomes. Occasionally, however, a single-tailed test is used, because it can be assumed that the treatment can only affect the patient one way, i.e. make them better.

For example, consider testing a placebo treatment against no treatment. This assumes that the placebo can only make a patient feel better or the same, but not worse. This comparison can only reject the null hypothesis on the basis of the 'treatment' being better, and only one tail of the statistic probability distribution is used.

Single-tailed testing increases the rejection area at the single tail, compared to two-tailed testing (Figure ST21). This can sometimes bring borderline *P*-numbers, which fail to demonstrate a significant difference, into significance. However, the assumptions made to justify single-tailed testing have to be valid.

Parametric and non-parametric tests

When tests are applied to data that fit a known probability density curve (i.e. one represented by a characteristic equation with defined parameters) these tests are referred to as **parametric tests**. Several defined probability density curves are well known. The most familiar is the *normal distribution* (bell-shaped curve, assumed in many biological and physiological data sets). Others include the *binomial distribution* and the *Poisson distribution* (see Figures ST8 and ST9).

In medical studies the data often follow a normal distribution, and parametric testing is often associated with normally distributed data. Parametric tests include the Student's *t*-test. However, binomially distributed data occur in a significant number of clinical studies and appropriate parametric tests can be applied to these data.

When testing data in which the probability density curve can not be assumed, **non-parametric tests** are used. These include ranking tests and the chi-squared test.

The chi-squared test is applied to data in the form of contingency tables. It is therefore usually used for non-parametric data presented in this form. Chi-squared testing may also be used for parametric data fitted to a contingency table, but it is less specific than the appropriate parametric tests and is therefore not usually used in this context.

Statistical tests

The type of testing used depends on the data collected. As noted above, the first consideration is whether data are parametric or non-parametric. Next the number of groups from which the data are collected must be considered. In practice comparisons between two groups form a large portion of medical studies. In this section the main emphasis will be on these types of data.

Comparing numerical data from two groups

When normally distributed numerical data are collected from two groups of patients, the mean values for each group are usually compared, and this is commonly done with the *Student's t-test*. For data that do not fit a known probability density curve the most commonly used non-parametric test is the *Wilcoxon rank sum test*.

Student's t-test

This test compares the means of two small samples of numerical data, and determines whether the difference between the means is significant. The test obtains a value for the statistic *t*, which can be used to obtain a *P*-number from tables. The null hypothesis states that there is no difference between the groups, and the *P*-number represents the probability that this hypothesis is true. Thus if $P > 0.05$, the difference between the means is not significant.

The *t* statistic is calculated from the difference between the means and the standard error for this difference as

$$t = \frac{\text{difference in means}}{\text{standard error of difference in means}}$$

Given two independent sample groups of n_1 individuals and n_2 individuals, with means m_1 and m_2 and standard deviations s_1 and s_2:

$$\text{Difference in means} = m_1 - m_2$$

$$\text{SEM of difference in means} = SEM_1 + SEM_2$$

$$t = \frac{m_1 - m_2}{\sqrt{s_1^2/n_1 + s_2^2/n_2}}$$

If the two samples of data come from the same individuals, such as in a cross-over study, then the samples are said to be *paired* and the SEM is reduced. There is therefore an advantage in using paired data.

Consider comparing blood pressure measurements to find the effect of a new antihypertensive in one group of ($n_1 = 12$) patients against placebo in another group ($n_2 = 10$). If analysis of the results produced a statistic $t = 2.2$, looking up this value in the t tables for degrees of freedom (DF) $= n_1 + n_2 - 2 = 20$ gives the following:

t	P
1.7	0.1
2.1	0.05
2.8	0.01

This gives a probability $P < 0.05$ for the null hypothesis, and therefore makes the difference between groups significant and the antihypertensive effective.

Ranking tests

When non-parametric numerical data are recorded, the data can not be assumed to fit a known probability density curve. Comparison between two groups then requires a non-parametric test such as the *Wilcoxon rank sum test*. Ranking combines the two groups to be compared into one single large group, and assigns each individual a rank according to the magnitude of the data measurement. The ranks are then summed for each group, and the rank sums are compared.

For example, consider recording the average weekly alcohol consumption (units) of 12 individuals, 5 females (n_1) and 7 males (n_2) (Figure ST22). Is there a significant difference in alcohol consumption between males and females?

Rank sum for females $= 3 + 4.5 + 7 + 9.5 + 11.5 = 35.5$
  Rank sum for males $= 1 + 2 + 4.5 + 6 + 8 + 9.5 + 11.5$
    $= 42.5$

For samples of $n \leq 15$, the statistic for the test (z) is taken as the rank sum of the smaller group (n_1). Thus here $z = 35.5$.

Referring to the Wilcoxon two-sample rank sum table, the relevant line (for $n_1 = 5$ and $n_2 = 7$) shows the ranges

Sex	Consumption	Rank
F	0	11.5
M	10	8
M	15	6
F	16	4.5
F	18	3
M	22	1
M	0	11.5
M	16	4.5
M	20	2
F	8	9.5
M	8	9.5
F	14	7

Figure ST22 Average weekly alcohol consumption of 5 women and 7 men

for z:

		Two-tailed P value		
n_1	n_2	0.05	0.01	0.001
5	7	17,38	15,40	

At $P = 0.05$, this table shows a range of values for z between 17 and 38. Here $z = 35.5$, and the null hypothesis is accepted. There is no difference in alcohol consumption between males and females.

If the results were different and $z < 17$, then $P < 0.05$ and the null hypothesis would be rejected – i.e. female alcohol consumption is less than that of males. Similarly, for $z > 38$, the results would have demonstrated that females consume more alcohol than males.

Testing categorical data from two groups

Categorical data are usually presented in the form of a contingency table (see page 874). The *chi-squared test* is a non-specific test for the differences between group data as they appear in the contingency table. This is described first below. No assumptions need to be made about the probability distributions of the recorded data.

Chi-squared test

This test is used to test the relationship between the row and column variables in a contingency table. It does not provide a specific answer to a question such as 'what are the odds of catching a particular disease if vaccinated or not vaccinated' as in the proportion testing below. It provides

	Outcome 1	Outcome 2
Group A ($n = 10$)	2 (5)	8 (5)
Group B ($n = 20$)	13 (10)	7 (10)
Totals	15	15

Figure ST23 Example contingency table for χ^2 test

an estimate of how significant the differences observed between column and row variables in the contingency table are. As with other tests, the null hypothesis (H_0) is tested for. In this case H_0 is that there is no difference between groups, and therefore both rows are samples from the same population.

A χ^2 value is determined by comparing the observed values in the table with expected values. The expected values are calculated as if there was no difference between the groups (rows).

Consider a simple 2×2 contingency table for two groups of patients (Figure ST23). The *observed* numbers in each category for each group are shown outside the brackets.

If there were no difference between groups, all of the patients could be considered as one big group of 30 patients. In such a case equal numbers would be expected in each of the outcome columns for each group. The *expected* values would then be those bracketed in the contingency table, and using these the χ^2 value can be calculated. Using the χ^2 value, a P-number can be obtained by looking it up in the appropriate table for χ^2. The value for χ^2 is calculated by

$$\chi^2 = \Sigma \frac{(\text{observed} - \text{expected})^2}{\text{expected}}$$

In the example shown in Figure ST23:

$$\chi^2 = \frac{(2-5)^2}{5} + \frac{(8-5)^2}{5} + \frac{(13-10)^2}{10} + \frac{(7-10)^2}{10}$$

$$\chi^2 = 5.4$$

In order to obtain a value for the P-number the degrees of freedom (DF) for the contingency table must be identified. For a 2×2 table DF $= 1$. The P-number is then obtained by looking up its value in the section of the χ^2 table for DF $= 1$, which is shown below:

χ^2	P
3.84	0.5
5.02	0.025
6.63	0.01

Thus for $\chi^2 = 5.4$, $P < 0.025$. This means that the differences between the groups shown in the contingency table are significant.

Comparison of two proportions

A proportion is obtained from a group of patients who can be divided into either of two outcomes (outcome X or outcome Y), e.g. dead or alive, disease-positive or disease-free. Such outcomes are referred to as *binary* outcomes, since there are only two possibilities.

In simple studies, proportions are compared between two groups, one of which (Group A) has been treated, tested, or exposed to a risk factor, while the other group (Group B) is a control. The results of such a comparison may be expressed in three different ways, as a *risk difference*, a *relative risk* or an *odds ratio*.

Some examples of such studies (with the basic question to be asked of the results in brackets) might be:

- Incidence of prostatic cancer in two groups: smokers and non-smokers (is smoking a risk factor for prostatic cancer?)
- Incidence of influenza in two groups: vaccinated and non-vaccinated (is vaccination effective against influenza?)
- Incidence of primary hepatoma in two groups: Hep B Ag positive and Hep B Ag negative (is Hep B Ag a risk factor for primary hepatoma?)

Such data will present as a 2×2 contingency table. Consider the example in Figure ST24, showing influenza rates in two groups, one vaccinated and the other not vaccinated. The basic question to be answered with these data is 'How effective is the vaccine?' This table can be interpreted in different ways, by calculating:

- The difference in risk (probability of contracting influenza) between vaccinated and non-vaccinated groups. This is the **risk difference**.
- The ratio of the risk in the vaccinated group to that in the non-vaccinated group. This is the **relative risk**.
- The odds of contracting influenza in the vaccinated group, compared with the odds in the non-vaccinated group. This is the **odds ratio**.

	Influenza	No influenza	Total
Vaccinated	30	300	330
Not vaccinated	80	270	350

Figure ST24 Example 2×2 table for comparison of proportions – influenza vaccination

Risk

Risk can be defined as the probability of a condition occurring in a sample group. If 30 patients out of the vaccinated sample of 330 shown in Figure ST24 contracted influenza, the risk (probability) of contracting influenza in that group is calculated as $30/330 = 0.09$.

Risk difference (absolute risk reduction, ARR)

Risk difference is the difference in risk of contracting a condition between treated and untreated groups. Normally treatment would be expected to reduce the risk of a disease occurring, and this difference is sometimes referred to as the *absolute risk reduction* (ARR), which is usually expressed as a percentage.

$$\text{Risk in the vaccinated group, } r_1 = 30/330$$
$$= 0.09$$
$$\text{Risk in the non-vaccinated group, } r_2 = 80/350$$
$$= 0.23$$
$$\text{Risk difference, } r_1 - r_2 = 0.09 - 0.23$$
$$= -0.14$$
$$ARR = 14\%$$

This means that vaccination decreases the risk of contracting influenza by 0.14 (14%).

Number needed to treat (NNT)

This is defined as the number of patients that need to be treated in order to save one disease event. If ARR is expressed as a percentage (i.e. the number of disease events saved per 100 patients), then

$$NNT = 100/ARR$$

In the example from Figure ST24:

$$NNT = 100/14$$
$$= 7.14$$

Number needed to harm (NNH)

A treatment may cause an increase in a disease condition as an unwanted side effect, e.g. increased incidence of peptic ulceration with the use of NSAIDs. In such a case there may be a positive risk difference between the control group ($r_2 = 0.1$) and the treated group ($r_1 = 0.2$).

$$\text{Risk difference, } r_1 - r_2 = 0.2 - 0.1$$
$$= 0.1$$
$$ARR = 10\%$$
$$NNH = 100/10$$
$$= 10$$

Relative risk

Relative risk is the ratio of the risk in the treated group to the risk in the untreated group. Sometimes this ratio is presented in terms of the *relative risk reduction* (RRR), often quoted as a percentage.

$$\text{Risk in the vaccinated group, } r_1 = 0.09$$
$$\text{Risk in the non-vaccinated group, } r_1 = 0.23$$
$$\text{Relative risk, } r_1/r_2 = 0.09/0.23$$
$$= 0.39$$

This means that the risk of contracting influenza in the vaccinated group is only 39% of the risk in the unvaccinated group. Alternatively, this can be stated by saying that vaccination reduces the number of influenza cases by $100\% - 39\%$: a relative risk *reduction* (RRR) of 61%. RRR can also be obtained by ARR divided by control event rate (or control-group risk, r_2). In this case ARR/CER $= 0.14/0.23 = 0.61$.

Odds ratio

Rather than calculating risk (probability) proportions can be expressed as *odds*. The odds of an event occurring are defined as the ratio

$$\text{Odds} = \frac{\text{Probability of event occurring}}{\text{Probability of event not occurring}}$$

The odds of contracting influenza in the vaccinated group are given by

$$\text{Odds}_1 = 30/300$$
$$= 0.1$$

The odds of contracting influenza in the non-vaccinated group are given by

$$\text{Odds}_2 = 80/270$$
$$= 0.29$$

The *odds ratio* (OR) is then calculated as $\text{Odds}_1/\text{Odds}_2$:

$$OR = 0.1/0.29$$
$$= 0.34$$

This means that the odds of contracting influenza in the vaccinated group are only 34% of those in the non-vaccinated group.

Odds ratio is the most commonly used method of comparing two proportions. It has the following properties:

- Odds ratio (OR) approximates to relative risk (RR) when the outcome is rare.

	Diabetes present	Diabetes absent
Test positive	12	38
Test negative	4	46

Figure ST25 Example 2 × 2 table for a diabetes screening test

- When the outcome is common, the relative risk does not discriminate well because with common outcomes relative risk tends to a value of 1. This is not so with OR.
- OR is the measure of choice in case–control studies, where a group of case studies are compared with a sample of control cases.

Diagnostic or screening tests

A study may be performed to assess the value of a diagnostic or screening test, e.g. PSA for prostatic cancer, BIS score >35 for awareness, Mallampati score for difficult airway. Such tests do not perform perfectly, and in some cases the condition may be missed (*false negatives*) while in others the test may give a *false positive* result.

Testing a group of patients will result in a 2×2 contingency table.

Consider the example shown in Figure ST25, in which 100 people are screened for diabetes with a single fasting blood sugar. Subsequent glucose tolerance testing reveals the true diabetics. Out of the 100 subjects, 50 test positive and 50 test negative, but only 16 are true diabetics.

Sensitivity

How good is the test at picking up the condition in patients who have diabetes?

$$\text{Sensitivity} = \frac{\text{true positives}}{\text{total with condition}}$$
$$= 12/16$$
$$= 0.75$$

A high blood sugar result will pick up 75% of diabetics.

Specificity

How good is the test at confirming the absence of the condition?

$$\text{Specificity} = \frac{\text{true negatives}}{\text{total without condition}}$$
$$= 46/84$$
$$= 0.55$$

A low blood sugar result will only pick out 55% of people without diabetes. 45% of patients who do not have diabetes will have a false-positive blood sugar.

Positive predictive value (PPV)

How good is the test at predicting the condition when the result is positive?

$$\text{PPV} = \frac{\text{true positives}}{\text{total positives}}$$
$$= 12/50$$
$$= 0.24$$

A positive blood sugar result gives a 24% chance of diabetes being present.

Negative predictive value (NPV)

How good is the test at predicting absence of the condition when the result is negative?

$$\text{NPV} = \frac{\text{true negatives}}{\text{total negatives}}$$
$$= 46/50$$
$$= 0.92$$

A negative blood sugar result gives a 92% chance of diabetes being absent.

Likelihood ratio (LR)

Given a positive result in the test, what is the likelihood that a person has the condition compared to the likelihood of obtaining a positive result in somebody free from the condition?

$$\text{LR} = \frac{\text{sensitivity}}{1 - \text{specificity}}$$
$$= 0.75/(1 - 0.55)$$
$$= 1.67$$

Given a positive result, a person is 1.67 times as likely to have diabetes as to be free from the condition.

Multiple groups
Parametric data

When more than two groups are studied, data may be analysed by **analysis of variance** (ANOVA). Consider investigating the postoperative analgesic requirements for patients from k different cities, with n patients in each group. The data obtained would give k different mean values ($m_1 \ldots m_k$).

Is there a true difference between the means? Or is the variation in the mean values simply due to individual variation rather than geographical variation? The null hypothesis is that no difference exists and the groups are all from the same population.

ANOVA compares the variance across the mean values ($m_1 \ldots m_k$) to the variance within each group of n patients. This statistic is called F, and it has a known F distribution that can be used to give P-numbers for values obtained from ANOVA testing. The number of degrees of freedom (DF) in this test is specified for the number of groups ($k - 1$) and the number of patients in each group ($n - 1$).

This test is known as *one-way analysis of variance* because a single factor is being tested for. It is equivalent to repeated t-testing between pairs of groups. The calculation is complex, but it is commonly available on computer software.

Non-parametric data

The Kruskal–Wallis test can be used to analyse non-parametric data from more than two groups. This test is an extension of the Wilcoxon rank sum test, and is not described further here.

Testing relationships

Data may be collected in order to try and define a relationship between two variables. If a relationship is found this is used as a model, and predictions can be made using this model. The simplest relationship mathematically is a linear one, and plotting a graph of one variable against the other will produce a straight-line graph.

Correlation

Correlation describes the strength of relationship between two numerical variables, e.g. height and body weight, age and systolic blood pressure. This is quantified by measuring these variables in a sample of the population and calculating their correlation coefficient, r. (The full name for r is the Pearson product moment correlation coefficient.)

If two variables x and y are measured in a group of individuals they can be plotted against each other to produce a scatter plot. The shape of this scatter plot will be determined by their degree of association (Figure ST26):
- If all of the points lie perfectly on a straight line the variables are said to be linearly correlated, and $r = +1$ or -1, depending on whether the gradient of the straight line is positive or negative.

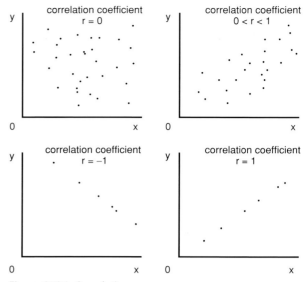

Figure ST26   Correlation

- If the points form a shapeless cloud with no apparent axis or direction the variables are uncorrelated and $r = 0$.
- For intermediate degrees of correlation a best-fit straight line can be drawn through the data points, and r will assume values between 0 and ± 1.

Correlation describes a purely mathematical relationship and does not imply any causal relationship. For example, random fasting blood sugar levels may show some degree of correlation with shoe size. This does not mean that wearing big shoes causes high blood sugars, but simply implies an associative relationship rather than a causal one.

Testing for correlation between two variables

As in other statistical tests, when testing for correlation between two variables the null hypothesis ($r = 0$) is tested for and a P-number is determined from statistical tables. If $P < 0.05$ for the value of r and the given sample, then the null hypothesis is rejected and the variables are considered to be linearly correlated.

Calculation of the value of r is laborious and is commonly available in commercial software packages. Manually, r is calculated by first determining the mean values for x and y. Let these mean values be x_m and y_m.

Then find the differences between the coordinates of each data point (x, y) and the mean point (x_m, y_m). The arithmetic is given in the following formula:

$$r = \frac{\Sigma(x - x_m)(y - y_m)}{\Sigma(x - x_m)^2(y - y_m)^2}$$

A value for r on its own is not enough to assess the degree of correlation in the data. This is because r is dependent on the size of the sample. If there are only two points in the sample $r = 1$ by definition. The greater the number of points the lower the value of r that is significant. With normally distributed data, five points in a sample might give $r = 0.8$, which is not significant. However, a sample of 150 points may yield a value of $r = 0.2$ which is significant.

Points to note about correlation:
- The Pearson correlation coefficient is calculated for normally distributed variables. For non-parametric data use Spearman's rank correlation coefficient.
- A value for r^2 is sometimes calculated, and this is useful as a measure of the fraction of the variability in one variable that is due to the linear relationship with the other variable.
- The correlation found in a sample of data only exists within the boundaries of the range of data points examined.

Linear regression

Linear regression takes the process of investigating the relationship between two variables a step further than correlation analysis. **Linear correlation** enables an observer to assess the degree of linear association between two variables but provides no further information upon which predictions can be made. **Linear regression** is used to mathematically model the relationship between two continuous variables by identifying the gradient and intercept of the best-fit line. Consider the measurement of two continuous variables x and y from a sample of a population (Figure ST27). These data can be plotted as a scatter diagram. Linear regression is used to define the best straight line fitting the points of the scatter diagram. Here it is assumed that one variable, x, is independent, and that the other variable, y, is dependent on x. In this case the equation for the best-fit straight line (or regression line) is given by

$$y = bx + a$$

where b is the gradient of the regression line and a is the intercept. The coefficients b and a are also called the *regression coefficients*. The regression line is thus a mathematical

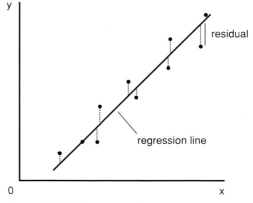

Figure ST27 Linear regression

model for the relationship between y and x, and is sometimes referred to as the regression of y on x. By knowing the coefficients a and b, any value of y can be calculated for a given value of x using the regression line.

Performing linear regression analysis

In order to calculate the regression coefficients a and b, a method of *least squares* is used. This method selects the best straight line, which minimises the sum of the vertical distance of each point from the regression line (the sum of the residuals). Figure ST27 shows a regression line for a set of data points. The residuals are shown as dotted lines. The regression line is chosen so as to minimise the sum of these residuals. Certain assumptions are made when using this method:

- There is a linear relationship between x and y.
- The observations in the sample are independent.
- The variables y and x are normally distributed.
- The variance of the y values at all values of x is the same.

Calculation of the gradient (b) and the intercept (a) are usually performed on readily available software. Manual calculation is reasonably straightforward but laborious. Initially mean values x_m ($= \Sigma\, x/n$) and y_m ($= \Sigma\, y/n$) are calculated:

$$\text{gradient, } b = \frac{\Sigma(x - x_m)(y - y_m)}{\Sigma(x - x_m)^2}$$

intercept, $a = y_m - bx_m$

The null hypothesis in linear regression is that the gradient is zero, in which case there is no linear relationship between x and y. A probability can thus be calculated, which if $P <$

0.05 will reject the null hypothesis and indicate significance for the regression coefficients.

Goodness of fit for the regression line to the data is assessed by calculating a value for correlation coefficient squared (r^2). This is the proportion of the variability in y due to the linear relationship with x. If this is high (>0.7) the line is a 'good' fit.

Systematic reviews

Many research studies may be performed over a period of decades before a particular treatment becomes employed routinely in clinical practice. Part of this process is reviewing the results from the different studies in order to reach a conclusion as to the efficacy of the treatment.

A conventional review is a 'narrative' or 'expert' review by an author, who gives a subjective opinion based on selected literature. Such a review can be misleading due to bias introduced by the selection of literature and differing methods of assessing results across studies.

A **systematic review** attempts to reduce this bias by using systematically assembled collections of literature and a standardised method of analysing the collected results.

Systematic reviews of appropriate collections of medical literature are provided by the Cochrane Collaboration. This is an independent international organisation, which originated in 1993 and provides continually updated literature reviews (via the internet or CD-ROM) covering a wide range of medical interventions and other topics.

Meta-analysis

The collective analysis of results from different studies is known as **meta-analysis**. In order to combine the results from different studies there must be criteria for selecting the studies to be included in the meta-analysis:

- The studies must be of the same type, producing the same format of results. The most common type of study included is a randomised controlled trial comparing two groups.
- The studies should have the same type of outcome. This can be a *fixed effect* or *binary outcome*, e.g. dead or alive. Such studies produce a 2 × 2 contingency table, which is usually analysed to give an odds ratio (OR) or absolute risk reduction (ARR). This is the most common type of study in meta-analyses.
- Alternatively the studies can have variable outcome, or *random effect*. These studies require a more complex analysis to combine their results.
- The studies must be statistically *homogeneous*. This means there should not be considerable variation

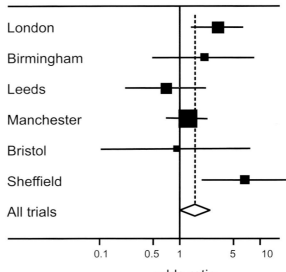

Figure ST28 Forest plot for meta-analysis

between the outcome measures. Statistical homogeneity can be tested for, and may be quoted as a Q number.

Although systematic reviews and meta-analyses can be more powerful than individual studies they are still subject to their own sources of bias. These include:

- *Publication bias* – Trials that demonstrate a positive effect are more likely to be published than those that show a negative or non-significant effect.
- *Variable trial quality* – Differences in methodology can exaggerate outcome results, e.g. inadequate randomisation of allocation, small samples, poor blinding.
- *Heterogeneity* – Statistical heterogeneity can be tested for, but clinical heterogeneity may cause incompatibility due to population differences or differences in definition of variables.

Meta-analysis for a fixed effect most commonly results in a *forest plot*, which combines the results from a number of studies. For example, consider a systematic review and meta-analysis for a new thromboprophylactic drug. This has been tested on hip-replacement patients, and six studies from different centres have met the inclusion criteria and been selected for review. The results are presented as odds ratios (OR) for positive venograms with confidence intervals (CI). The results of the meta-analysis are shown in Figure ST28. This shows the study labels (trial centres) with the corresponding OR and CI on the axes. The horizontal axis is the OR and CI, while the vertical axis is the line for no effect (OR = 1). At the bottom of the diagram is the summary result for the meta-analysis, showing the resultant OR (open diamond), with the width of the diamond representing the resultant CI. The results from the individual trials are weighted before combination to allow for differences in quality of data. Different methods of weighting are used. One method is inverse variance weighting, while another is Mantel–Haenszel weighting. Degree of weighting is indicated by the width of the solid square representing the OR for each trial.

Appendix: Primary FRCA syllabus

This appendix uses the FRCA syllabus to guide the exploration of FoA$_3$ as an alternative to the index. Whilst closely following the syllabus, FoA$_3$ does not rigidly follow its organisation.

The most relevant section and chapter for each heading are indicated (e.g., S2C14). Each topic is given a *single* page reference to indicate a starting point. Under a particular heading, references to pages in other chapters point the reader to areas of FoA$_3$ that might not otherwise be viewed. This helps to integrate and cross-reference the material in the four sections of the book and exam. A few topics are outside the book's scope, and some are dealt with too diffusely to merit a single page number.

Reproduced with permission from Royal College of Anaesthetists, *The CCT in Anaesthesia II: Competency Based Basic Level (ST years 1 and 2) Training and Assessmente.* January 2007.

8   Regional anaesthesia   Section 1, Chapter 7

Vertebral column

Surface anatomy

18   Physiology and biochemistry

Biochemistry

Body fluids and their functions and constituents   Section 2, Chapter 2

21   Statistical methods

Index